Table A — The Genetic Code

Second Position

First Position (5' end)	U	C	A	G	Third Position (3' end)
U	UUU, UUC — Phe (F); UUA, UUG — Leu (L)	UCU, UCC, UCA, UCG — Ser (S)	UAU, UAC — Tyr (Y); UAA — stop; UAG — stop	UGU, UGC — Cys (C); UGA — stop; UGG — Trp (W)	U C A G
C	CUU, CUC, CUA, CUG — Leu (L)	CCU, CCC, CCA, CCG — Pro (P)	CAU, CAC — His (H); CAA, CAG — Gln (Q)	CGU, CGC, CGA, CGG — Arg (R)	U C A G
A	AUU, AUC, AUA — Ile (I); AUG — Met (M)	ACU, ACC, ACA, ACG — Thr (T)	AAU, AAC — Asn (N); AAA, AAG — Lys (K)	AGU, AGC — Ser (S); AGA, AGG — Arg (R)	U C A G
G	GUU, GUC, GUA, GUG — Val (V)	GCU, GCC, GCA, GCG — Ala (A)	GAU, GAC — Asp (D); GAA, GAG — Glu (E)	GGU, GGC, GGA, GGG — Gly (G)	U C A G

Table B — Redundancy of the Genetic Code

Amino Acid	Abbreviation 3-letter	Abbreviation 1-letter	Codons
Alanine	Ala	A	GCA, GCC, GCG, GCU
Arginine	Arg	R	AGA, AGG, CGA, CGC, CGG, CGU
Asparagine	Asn	N	AAC, AAU
Aspartic acid	Asp	D	GAC, GAU
Cysteine	Cys	C	UGC, UGU
Glutamic acid	Glu	E	GAA, GAG
Glutamine	Gln	Q	CAA, CAG
Glycine	Gly	G	GGA, GGC, GGG, GGU
Histidine	His	H	CAC, CAU
Isoleucine	Ile	I	AUA, AUC, AUU
Leucine	Leu	L	UUA, UUG, CUA, CUC, CUG, CUU
Lysine	Lys	K	AAA, AAG
Methionine	Met	M	AUG
Phenylalanine	Phe	F	UUC, UUU
Proline	Pro	P	CCA, CCC, CCG, CCU
Serine	Ser	S	AGC, AGU, UCA, UCC, UCG, UCU
Threonine	Thr	T	ACA, ACC, ACG, ACU
Tryptophan	Trp	W	UGG
Tyrosine	Tyr	Y	UAC, UAU
Valine	Val	V	GUA, GUC, GUG, GUU

Unparalleled Problem-Solving Support

Genetic Analysis expertly guides students through the core ideas of genetics while introducing them to real-world applications and supporting them with unparalleled problem-solving guidance.

A consistent approach to problem solving is used in every **Genetic Analysis** worked example to help students understand the logic and purpose of each step in the problem-solving process.

Each example guides students with a unique, consistent, three-step approach that trains them to **Evaluate, Deduce,** and then **Solve** problems.

Every example is presented in a clear, **two-column format** that helps students see the Solution Strategy in one column and its corresponding execution in a separate Solution Step column.

"Break It Down" prompts help students get started with formulating an approach to solving a problem.

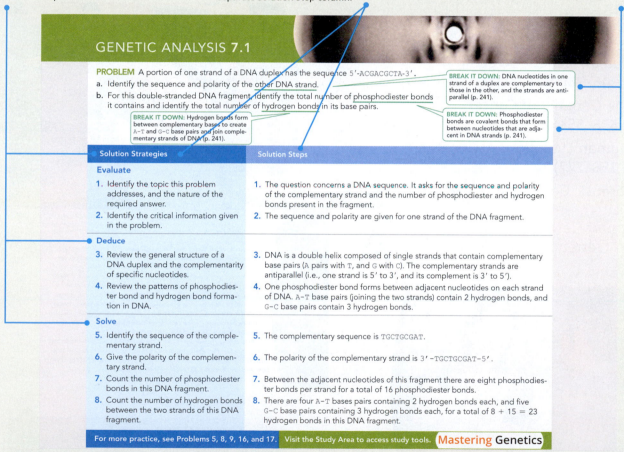

GENETIC ANALYSIS 7.1

PROBLEM A portion of one strand of a DNA duplex has the sequence 5'-ACGACGCTA-3'.
a. Identify the sequence and polarity of the other DNA strand.
b. For this double-stranded DNA fragment, identify the total number of phosphodiester bonds it contains and identify the total number of hydrogen bonds in its base pairs.

BREAK IT DOWN: DNA nucleotides in one strand of a duplex are complementary to those in the other, and the strands are antiparallel (p. 241).

BREAK IT DOWN: Phosphodiester bonds are covalent bonds that form between nucleotides that are adjacent in DNA strands (p. 241).

BREAK IT DOWN: Hydrogen bonds form between complementary bases to create A–T and G–C base pairs and join complementary strands of DNA (p. 241).

Solution Strategies	Solution Steps
Evaluate	
1. Identify the topic this problem addresses, and the nature of the required answer.	1. The question concerns a DNA sequence. It asks for the sequence and polarity of the complementary strand and the number of phosphodiester and hydrogen bonds present in the fragment.
2. Identify the critical information given in the problem.	2. The sequence and polarity are given for one strand of the DNA fragment.
Deduce	
3. Review the general structure of a DNA duplex and the complementarity of specific nucleotides.	3. DNA is a double helix composed of single strands that contain complementary base pairs (A pairs with T, and G with C). The complementary strands are antiparallel (i.e., one strand is 5' to 3', and its complement is 3' to 5').
4. Review the patterns of phosphodiester bond and hydrogen bond formation in DNA.	4. One phosphodiester bond forms between adjacent nucleotides on each strand of DNA. A–T base pairs (joining the two strands) contain 2 hydrogen bonds, and G–C base pairs contain 3 hydrogen bonds.
Solve	
5. Identify the sequence of the complementary strand.	5. The complementary sequence is TGCTGCGAT.
6. Give the polarity of the complementary strand.	6. The polarity of the complementary strand is 3'–TGCTGCGAT–5'.
7. Count the number of phosphodiester bonds in this DNA fragment.	7. Between the adjacent nucleotides of this fragment there are eight phosphodiester bonds per strand for a total of 16 phosphodiester bonds.
8. Count the number of hydrogen bonds between the two strands of this DNA fragment.	8. There are four A–T bases pairs containing 2 hydrogen bonds each, and five G–C base pairs containing 3 hydrogen bonds each, for a total of 8 + 15 = 23 hydrogen bonds in this DNA fragment.

For more practice, see Problems 5, 8, 9, 16, and 17. Visit the Study Area to access study tools. **Mastering** Genetics

PREPARING FOR PROBLEM SOLVING

In addition to the list of problem-solving tips and suggestions given here, you can go to the Study Guide and Solutions Manual that accompanies this book for help at solving problems.

1. Be familiar with and able to describe the structure of DNA.

2. Know the four DNA nucleotide bases and be able to describe complementary base pairing and the antiparallel alignment of strands. If required by your instructor, know the structure of the DNA bases.

3. Be able to describe the evidence that identified DNA as the hereditary material.

4. Understand the overall process of DNA replication and be able to diagram the general structure of a replication bubble.

5. Be able to identify the major enzymatic activities during DNA replication.

6. Be prepared to use an understanding of DNA replication processes and biochemical activities to analyze and predict the results of experiments involving DNA replication.

7. Understand the polymerase chain reaction (PCR) process and results.

8. Be able to describe dideoxy DNA sequencing and to analyze DNA sequencing results.

NEW! Preparing for Problem Solving feature in every chapter identifies specific knowledge and skills students need to answer end of chapter problems.

Applications of Genetics

This edition introduces five Application Chapters—brief chapters focused on specific applied topics in human genetics. Each topic is highly relevant and engaging, and the Application Chapters illustrate some of the practical uses of genetics and genetic analysis.

The Application Chapters are integrated into the book, each following relevant prerequisite material (see table of contents). The five Application Chapters are:

- A: Human Hereditary Disease and Genetic Counseling (pp. 223–234)
- B: Human Genetic Screening (pp. 346–360)
- C: The Genetics of Cancer (pp. 538–551)
- D: Human Evolutionary Genetics (pp. 758–777)
- E: Forensic Genetics (pp. 778–791)

APPLICATION B

Human Genetic Screening

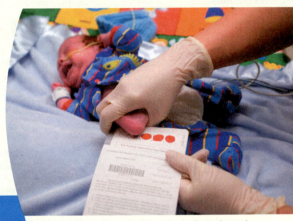

A heel stick is a minimally invasive procedure, being used here to collect a small amount of blood from a newborn infant. The blood is used to screen for disorders on the Recommended Uniform Screening Panel (RUSP) list of human hereditary diseases, as discussed in this chapter.

Kristen Powers is not the most famous graduate of Stanford University, but she is one of the bravest. In 2003, when Kristen was 9 years old, her mother Nicola was diagnosed with the autosomal dominant neurological disorder Huntington disease (HD). HD is a devastating and fatal disease. It usually strikes people in their thirties or forties, with initial symptoms that include a loss of balance and coordination. Over the next few years the symptoms progress. People with the disease move with increasing jerkiness, lose the ability to walk and perform daily tasks, experience behavioral changes, and ultimately develop dementia and require full-time care. Nicola Powers was 37 years of age when she was diagnosed, and she died in 2011 at the age of 45.

Nicola had not known that HD ran in her family. She had lost touch with her biological father after her parents' divorce and did not find out he had HD until after her own diagnosis. By then, Kristen and her younger brother Nate had been born, and they each had a 50% chance of having the disease.

APPLICATION A

Human Hereditary Disease and Genetic Counseling

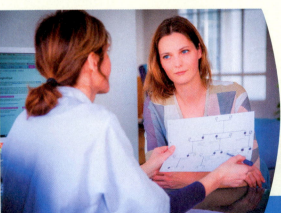

Genetic counseling, a central activity in medical genetics, seeks to provide individuals, couples, and families with medical and genetic information they can use to make informed decisions about genetic testing and medical treatment, in person-to-person meetings involving physicians, genetic counselors, and consultands.

When B.K. was born in San Francisco, California, in July 2015, he appeared to be a healthy baby boy. Among the myriad forms B.K.'s parents signed at the hospital was one informing them that B.K. would undergo mandated newborn genetic testing for almost four dozen different hereditary conditions within 24 hours of his birth. All the conditions tested are rare, but each can be treated to eliminate or substantially reduce the symptoms and complications of the disease. California, like all U.S. states and many other countries, mandates tests for several dozen rare genetic diseases of all newborns. We discuss this testing again later in the chapter and more fully in Application Chapter B: Human Genetic Screening.

Parents almost never hear about the results of these newborn genetic tests because a positive result is rare. But B.K.'s parents were told of a result indicating that B.K. had argininemia, commonly abbreviated ARG. B.K.'s parents had

NEW! Each Application Chapter includes problems, many of which are assignable in Mastering Genetics.

New Questions Support Active Learning

New types of questions help engage students while they read the book and when they are in the classroom. Questions related to key figures and problems for group work help support instructor efforts to build students' critical thinking and problem solving skills.

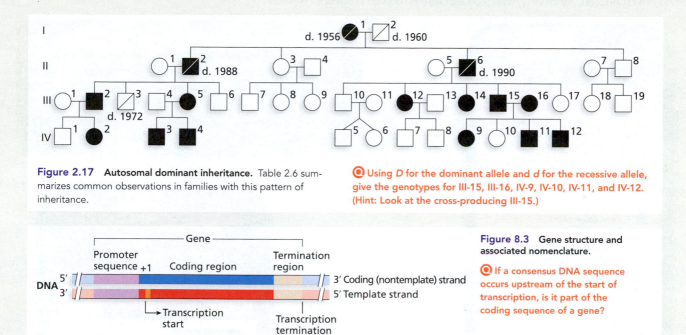

Figure 2.17 Autosomal dominant inheritance. Table 2.6 summarizes common observations in families with this pattern of inheritance.

❓ Using *D* for the dominant allele and *d* for the recessive allele, give the genotypes for III-15, III-16, IV-9, IV-10, IV-11, and IV-12. (Hint: Look at the cross-producing III-15.)

Figure 8.3 Gene structure and associated nomenclature.

❓ If a consensus DNA sequence occurs upstream of the start of transcription, is it part of the coding sequence of a gene?

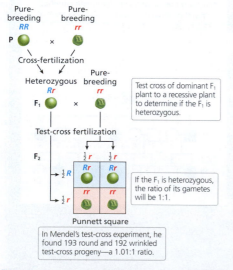

Figure 2.6 Test-cross analysis of F₁ plants. A test cross between an F₁ plant and one that is homozygous recessive produces progeny with a 1:1 ratio of the dominant to the recessive phenotype if the F₁ plant is heterozygous.

❓ If a test-cross experiment identical to the one shown here produces 826 progeny plants, how many plants are expected in each phenotype category?

NEW! Caption Queries accompany many figures in the book, helping students focus on the illustrations and more fully understand the content. Some questions ask students to solve a problem using information from the figure, some require an explanation, and others ask students to expand on the information or idea in the figure. As an instructor resource, we provide Caption Queries for all book figures as clicker questions for in-class use.

Collaboration and Discussion

NEW! Collaboration and Discussion Problems have been added to every end of chapter question set to facilitate group work and hands-on problem solving in class.

Learn Genetics Concepts and Problem Solving

Mastering™ Genetics is an online homework, tutorial, and assessment platform designed to improve results by helping students quickly master concepts. Students benefit from self-paced tutorials that feature personalized wrong-answer feedback and hints that emulate the office-hour experience and help keep students on track. Learn more at www.pearson.com/mastering/genetics

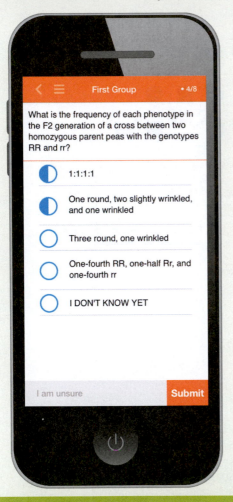

NEW! Dynamic Study Modules personalize each student's learning experience. Available for assignments or for self-study, these chapter-based modules help prepare students for class so they'll be ready for discussions or problem solving. These modules are accessible on smartphones, tablets, and computers.

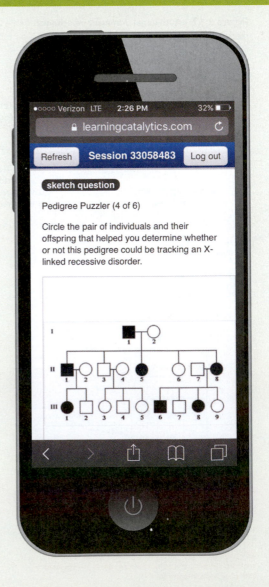

Learning Catalytics™ helps generate class discussion, customize lectures, and promote peer-to-peer learning with real-time analytics. Learning Catalytics is a student response tool that uses students' smartphones, tablets, or laptops to engage them in more interactive tasks and thinking.

- Help your students develop critical thinking skills
- Monitor responses to find out where your students are struggling
- Rely on real-time data to adjust your teaching strategy

With Mastering Genetics

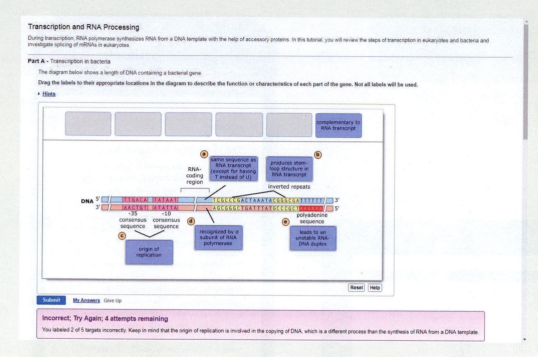

Transcription and RNA Processing

During transcription, RNA polymerase synthesizes RNA from a DNA template with the help of accessory proteins. In this tutorial, you will review the steps of transcription in eukaryotes and bacteria and investigate splicing of mRNAs in eukaryotes.

Part A - Transcription in bacteria

The diagram below shows a length of DNA containing a bacterial gene.

Drag the labels to their appropriate locations in the diagram to describe the function or characteristics of each part of the gene. Not all labels will be used.

▸ Hints

Submit   My Answers   Give Up

Incorrect; Try Again; 4 attempts remaining

You labeled 2 of 5 targets incorrectly. Keep in mind that the origin of replication is involved in the copying of DNA, which is a different process than the synthesis of RNA from a DNA template.

Activities feature personalized wrong-answer feedback and hints that emulate the office-hour experience to guide student learning. New tutorials include coverage of topics like CRISPR-Cas.

140 Practice Problems offer more opportunities to develop problem-solving skills. These questions appear only in Mastering Genetics and include targeted wrong answer feedback to guide students to the correct answer.

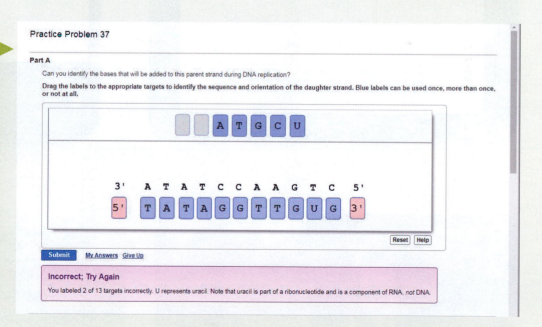

Practice Problem 37

Part A

Can you identify the bases that will be added to this parent strand during DNA replication?

Drag the labels to the appropriate targets to identify the sequence and orientation of the daughter strand. Blue labels can be used once, more than once, or not at all.

Submit   My Answers   Give Up

Incorrect; Try Again

You labeled 2 of 13 targets incorrectly. U represents uracil. Note that uracil is part of a ribonucleotide and is a component of RNA, *not* DNA.

Access the text anytime, anywhere with Pearson eText

NEW! Pearson eText is built to adapt to the device readers are using—smartphone, tablet, or computer.

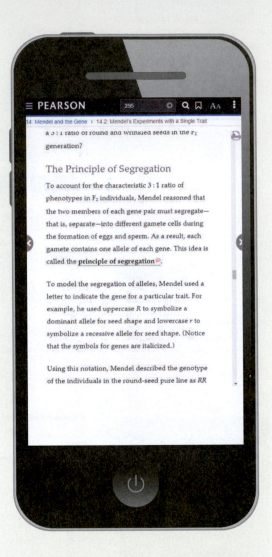

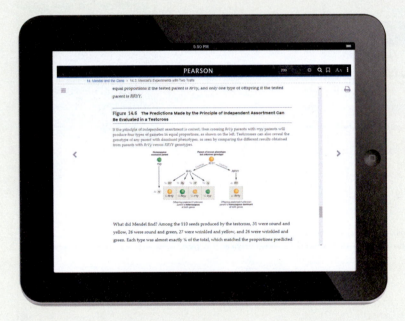

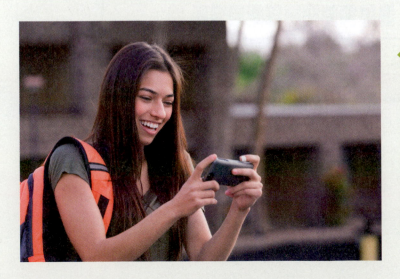

Pearson eText Mobile App offers offline access and can be downloaded for most iOS and Android phones/tablets from the Apple App Store or Google Play.

- Seamlessly integrated videos
- Accessible (screen-reader ready)
- Configurable reading settings, including resizable type and night reading mode
- Instructor and student note-taking, highlighting, bookmarking, and search

Genetic Analysis

AN INTEGRATED APPROACH

Third Edition

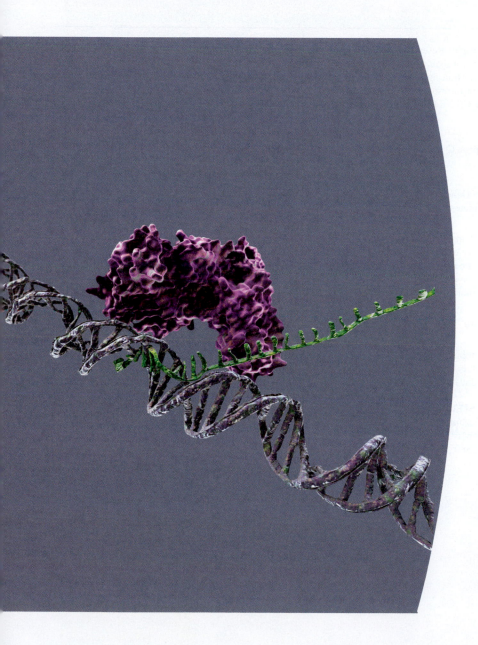

Mark F. Sanders
University of California at Davis

John L. Bowman
Monash University,
Melbourne, Australia
University of California at Davis

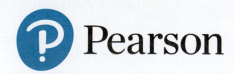

330 Hudson Street, NY NY 10013

Director, Courseware Portfolio Manager: *Beth Wilbur*
Courseware Portfolio Manager: *Michael Gillespie*
Content Producer: *Melanie Field*
Development Editor: *Moira Lerner*
Courseware Sr. Analysts, Content Development: *Margot Otway, Barbara Price*
Courseware Editorial Assistant: *Summer Giles*
Courseware Director, Content Development: *Ginnie Simione Jutson*
Managing Producer: *Michael Early*
Full Service Project Manager: *Thomas Russell*
Full Service Vendor: *SPi Global*

Design Manager: *Mark Ong*
Interior and Cover Design: *Cadence*
Rights and Permissions Project Manager: *Linda DeMasi*
Photo Researcher: *Maureen Spuhler*
Rich Media Content Producer: *Chloé Veylit*
Manufacturing Buyer: *Stacey Weinberger*
Product Marketing Manager: *Christa Pelaez*
Field Marketing Manager: *Kelly Galli*
Cover Photo Credit: *Gunilla Elam/Science Photo Library*
Illustrator: *Lachina*

Library of Congress Cataloging-in-Publication Data

Names: Sanders, Mark Frederick, author. | Bowman, John L., author.
Title: Genetic analysis : an integrated approach / Mark F. Sanders, John L. Bowman.
  Description: Third edition. | New York : Pearson Education, Inc., [2019] |
    Includes bibliographical references and index.
  Identifiers: LCCN 2017052380 | ISBN 9780134605173 | ISBN 0134605179
  Subjects: | MESH: Genetic Phenomena | Genetic Techniques
  Classification: LCC QH430 | NLM QU 500 | DDC 616/.042--dc23
  LC record available at https://lccn.loc.gov/2017052380

1 17

ISBN-10: 0134605179
ISBN-13: 9780134605173

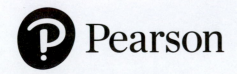

Table of Contents

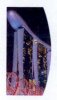

1
The Molecular Basis of Heredity, Variation, and Evolution 1

1.1 Modern Genetics Is in Its Second Century 2
The Development of Modern Genetics 2
The Four Phases of Modern Genetics 3
Genetics—Central to Modern Biology 5

1.2 The Structure of DNA Suggests a Mechanism for Replication 6
The Discovery of DNA Structure 6
DNA Nucleotides 7
DNA Replication 9
Genetic Analysis 1.1 10
Experimental Insight 1.1 10

1.3 DNA Transcription and Messenger RNA Translation Express Genes 11
Transcription 12
Translation 13
Genetic Analysis 1.2 14

1.4 Genetic Variation Can Be Detected by Examining DNA, RNA, and Proteins 15
Gel Electrophoresis 15
Stains, Blots, and Probes 16
DNA Sequencing and Genomics 18
Proteomics and Other "-omic" Analyses 18

1.5 Evolution Has a Genetic Basis 19
Darwin's Theory of Evolution 19
Four Evolutionary Processes 20
Tracing Evolutionary Relationships 21
Genetic Analysis 1.3 24
Case Study Ancient DNA: Genetics Looks into the Past 24
Summary 26 • *Preparing for Problem Solving* 27 • *Problems* 27

2
Transmission Genetics 30

2.1 Gregor Mendel Discovered the Basic Principles of Genetic Transmission 31
Mendel's Modern Experimental Approach 31
Five Critical Experimental Innovations 33

2.2 Monohybrid Crosses Reveal the Segregation of Alleles 34
Identifying Dominant and Recessive Traits 34
Evidence of Particulate Inheritance and Rejection of the Blending Theory 36
Segregation of Alleles 36
Hypothesis Testing by Test-Cross Analysis 37
Hypothesis Testing by F_2 Self-Fertilization 38
Genetic Analysis 2.1 39

2.3 Dihybrid and Trihybrid Crosses Reveal the Independent Assortment of Alleles 40
Dihybrid-Cross Analysis of Two Genes 40
Experimental Insight 2.1 41
Testing Independent Assortment by Test-Cross Analysis 43
Genetic Analysis 2.2 44
Testing Independent Assortment by Trihybrid-Cross Analysis 45
The Rediscovery of Mendel's Work 46
Experimental Insight 2.2 46

2.4 Probability Theory Predicts Mendelian Ratios 47
The Product Rule 47
The Sum Rule 47
Conditional Probability 47
Binomial Probability 48

2.5 Chi-Square Analysis Tests the Fit between Observed Values and Expected Outcomes 49
Chi-Square Analysis 50
Chi-Square Analysis of Mendel's Data 50

2.6   Autosomal Inheritance and Molecular Genetics Parallel the Predictions of Mendel's Hereditary Principles   51

Autosomal Dominant Inheritance   52

Autosomal Recessive Inheritance   53

Prospective and Retrospective Predictions in Human Genetics   53

Molecular Genetics of Mendel's Traits   54

Genetic Analysis   2.3   55

Case Study   OMIM, Gene Mutations, and Human Hereditary Disease   57
Summary   59 • *Preparing for Problem Solving   60* • *Problems   60*

3
Cell Division and Chromosome Heredity   67

3.1   Mitosis Divides Somatic Cells   68

The Cell Cycle   68

Substages of M Phase   69

Chromosome Movement and Distribution   72

Completion of Cell Division   73

Cell Cycle Checkpoints   74

3.2   Meiosis Produces Cells for Sexual Reproduction   75

Meiosis Features Two Cell Divisions   75

Meiosis I   76

Meiosis II   79

Meiosis Generates Mendelian Ratios   80

3.3   The Chromosome Theory of Heredity Proposes That Genes Are Carried on Chromosomes   82

Genetic Analysis   3.1   84

X-Linked Inheritance   85

Testing the Chromosome Theory of Heredity   86

3.4   Sex Determination Is Chromosomal and Genetic   87

Sex Determination in *Drosophila*   87

Genetic Analysis   3.2   88

Mammalian Sex Determination   89

Diversity of Sex Determination   89

Experimental Insight   3.1   90

3.5   Human Sex-Linked Transmission Follows Distinct Patterns   91

Expression of X-Linked Recessive Traits   92

X-Linked Dominant Trait Transmission   93

Y-Linked Inheritance   93

Genetic Analysis   3.3   95

3.6   Dosage Compensation Equalizes the Expression of Sex-Linked Genes   96

Case Study   The (Degenerative) Evolution of the Mammalian Y Chromosome   97
Summary   99 • *Preparing for Problem Solving   99* • *Problems   100*

4
Gene Interaction   105

4.1   Interactions between Alleles Produce Dominance Relationships   106

The Molecular Basis of Dominance   106

Functional Effects of Mutation   107

Notational Systems for Genes and Allele Relationships   109

Incomplete Dominance   110

Codominance   110

Dominance Relationships of ABO Alleles   110

Genetic Analysis   4.1   113

Allelic Series   113

Lethal Alleles   116

Delayed Age of Onset   118

4.2   Some Genes Produce Variable Phenotypes   118

Sex-Limited Traits   119

Sex-Influenced Traits   119

Incomplete Penetrance   120

Variable Expressivity   120

Gene–Environment Interactions   121

Pleiotropic Genes   122

4.3   Gene Interaction Modifies Mendelian Ratios   122

Gene Interaction in Pathways   122

The One Gene–One Enzyme Hypothesis   124

Experimental Insight   4.1   125

Genetic Dissection to Investigate Gene Action   127

Genetic Analysis   4.2   128

Epistasis and Its Results   129

4.4 Complementation Analysis Distinguishes Mutations in the Same Gene from Mutations in Different Genes 133

Genetic Analysis **4.3** 134

Case Study *Complementation Groups in a Human Cancer-Prone Disorder* 136
Summary 137 • *Preparing for Problem Solving* 138 • *Problems* 138

5

Genetic Linkage and Mapping in Eukaryotes 145

5.1 Linked Genes Do Not Assort Independently 146

Detecting Genetic Linkage 147

The Discovery of Genetic Linkage 149

Detecting Autosomal Genetic Linkage through Test-Cross Analysis 150

Cytological Evidence of Recombination 153

Genetic Analysis **5.1** 154

5.2 Genetic Linkage Mapping Is Based on Recombination Frequency between Genes 155

The First Genetic Linkage Map 155

Map Units 156

Chi-Square Analysis of Genetic Linkage Data 156

5.3 Three-Point Test-Cross Analysis Maps Genes 156

Identifying Parental, Single-Crossover, and Double-Crossover Gametes in Three-Point Mapping 157

Constructing a Three-Point Recombination Map 158

Determining Gamete Frequencies from Genetic Maps 161

Correction of Genetic Map Distances 162

Genetic Analysis **5.2** 163

5.4 Multiple Factors Cause Recombination to Vary 164

Sex Affects Recombination 164

Recombination Is Dominated by Hotspots 165

Genome Sequence Analysis Reveals Recombination Hotspot Distribution 166

5.5 Human Genes Are Mapped Using Specialized Methods 166

Mapping with Genetic Markers 166

The Inheritance of Disease-Causing Genes Linked to Genetic Markers 167

Allelic Phase 168

Lod Score Analysis 169

Experimental Insight **5.1** 171

Genetic Analysis **5.3** 172

Genome-Wide Association Studies 172

Linkage Disequilibrium and Evolutionary Analysis 174

Case Study *Mapping the Gene for Cystic Fibrosis* 175
Summary 176 • *Preparing for Problem Solving* 177 • *Problems* 177

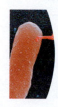

6

Genetic Analysis and Mapping in Bacteria and Bacteriophages 185

6.1 Specialized Methods Are Used for Genetic Analysis of Bacteria 186

Bacterial Culture and Growth Analysis 186

Characteristics of Bacterial Genomes 188

Plasmids in Bacterial Cells 189

Research Technique **6.1** 189

6.2 Bacteria Transfer Genes by Conjugation 191

Conjugation Identified 193

Transfer of the F Factor 194

Formation of an Hfr Chromosome 196

Hfr Gene Transfer 196

Interrupted Mating and Time-of-Entry Mapping 198

Time-of-Entry Mapping Experiments 198

Genetic Analysis **6.1** 199

Consolidation of Hfr Maps 200

Conjugation with F′ Strains Produces Partial Diploids 201

Plasmids and Conjugation in Archaea 203

6.3 Bacterial Transformation Produces Genetic Recombination 203

Genetic Analysis **6.2** 204

Steps in Transformation 205

Mapping by Transformation 205

6.4 Bacterial Transduction Is Mediated by Bacteriophages 205

Bacteriophage Life Cycles 205

Generalized Transduction 208

Cotransduction 209

Cotransduction Mapping 209

Specialized Transduction 211

6.5   Bacteriophage Chromosomes Are Mapped by Fine-Structure Analysis 211

Genetic Analysis 6.3   212

Genetic Complementation Analysis   213

Intragenic Recombination Analysis   213

Deletion-Mapping Analysis   214

6.6   Lateral Gene Transfer Alters Genomes 214

Lateral Gene Transfer and Genome Evolution   215

Identifying Lateral Gene Transfer in Genomes   216

Case Study The Evolution of Antibiotic Resistance and Its Impact on Medical Practice 217
Summary 218 • *Preparing for Problem Solving* 219 • *Problems* 219

APPLICATION A
Human Hereditary Disease and Genetic Counseling

A.1   Hereditary Disease and Disease Genes 225

Types of Hereditary Disease   225

Genetic Testing and Diagnosis   226

A.2   Genetic Counseling 227

Indicators and Goals of Genetic Counseling   227

Assessing and Communicating Risks and Options   228

Ethical Issues in Genetic Medicine   231

Genetic Counseling and Ethical Issues   232

In Closing   233
Problems 234

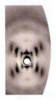

7
DNA Structure and Replication 235

7.1   DNA Is the Hereditary Molecule of Life 236

Chromosomes Contain DNA   236

A Transformation Factor Responsible for Heredity   236

DNA Is the Transformation Factor   238

DNA Is the Hereditary Molecule   238

7.2   The DNA Double Helix Consists of Two Complementary and Antiparallel Strands 240

DNA Nucleotides   240

The DNA Duplex   241

Genetic Analysis 7.1   244

7.3   DNA Replication Is Semiconservative and Bidirectional 244

Three Competing Models of Replication   245

The Meselson–Stahl Experiment   245

Origin and Directionality of Replication in Bacterial DNA   247

Multiple Replication Origins in Eukaryotes   248

7.4   DNA Replication Precisely Duplicates the Genetic Material 249

DNA Sequences at Replication Origins   249

Molecular Biology of Replication Initiation   253

Continuous and Discontinuous Strand Replication   253

RNA Primer Removal and Okazaki Fragment Ligation   254

Synthesis of Leading and Lagging Strands at the Replication Fork   255

DNA Proofreading   256

Supercoiling and Topoisomerases   257

Replication at the Ends of Linear Chromosomes   257

Genetic Analysis 7.2   258

7.5   Methods of Molecular Genetic Analysis Make Use of DNA Replication Processes 260

The Polymerase Chain Reaction   261

Separation of PCR Products   262

Dideoxynucleotide DNA Sequencing   263

New Generations of DNA Sequencing Technology   266

Genetic Analysis 7.3   267

Case Study DNA Helicase Gene Mutations and Human Progeroid Syndrome 269
Summary 270 • *Preparing for Problem Solving* 271 • *Problems* 271

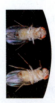

8
Molecular Biology of Transcription and RNA Processing 275

8.1   RNA Transcripts Carry the Messages of Genes 276

RNA Nucleotides and Structure   276

Experimental Discovery of Messenger RNA   277

Categories of RNA   278

8.2   Bacterial Transcription Is a Four-Stage Process 279

Bacterial RNA Polymerase   280

Bacterial Promoters   280

Transcription Initiation   281

Genetic Analysis **8.1**   283

Transcription Elongation and Termination   284

Transcription Termination Mechanisms   284

8.3 Eukaryotic Transcription Is More Diversified and Complex than Bacterial Transcription   286

Polymerase II Transcription of mRNA in Eukaryotes   287

Research Technique **8.1**   288

Pol II Promoter Recognition   289

Detecting Promoter Consensus Elements   290

Other Regulatory Sequences and Chromatin-Based Regulation of RNA Pol II Transcription   291

RNA Polymerase I Promoters   292

RNA Polymerase III Promoters   292

Archaeal Promoters and Transcription   292

The Evolutionary Implications of Comparative Transcription   293

8.4 Posttranscriptional Processing Modifies RNA Molecules   294

Capping 5′ Pre-mRNA   294

Polyadenylation of 3′ Pre-mRNA   295

The Torpedo Model of Transcription Termination   296

Introns   296

Pre-mRNA Splicing   297

Splicing Signal Sequences   298

A Gene Expression Machine Couples Transcription and Pre-mRNA Processing   298

Alternative Patterns of RNA Transcription and Alternative RNA Splicing   301

Self-Splicing Introns   302

Genetic Analysis **8.2**   303

Ribosomal RNA Processing   304

Transfer RNA Processing   304

RNA Editing   307

Case Study *Sexy Splicing: Alternative mRNA Splicing and Sex Determination in Drosophila*   307
Summary   308 • *Preparing for Problem Solving   309* • *Problems   309*

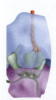

9

The Molecular Biology of Translation   314

9.1 Polypeptides Are Amino Acid Chains That Are Assembled at Ribosomes   315

Amino Acid Structure   315

Polypeptide and Transcript Structure   315

Ribosome Structures   317

A Three-Dimensional View of the Ribosome   319

Research Technique **9.1**   319

9.2 Translation Occurs in Three Phases   320

Translation Initiation   320

Polypeptide Elongation   324

Genetic Analysis **9.1**   326

Translation Termination   327

9.3 Translation Is Fast and Efficient   327

The Translational Complex   327

Translation of Polycistronic mRNA   329

9.4 The Genetic Code Translates Messenger RNA into Polypeptide   329

The Genetic Code Displays Third-Base Wobble   330

The (Almost) Universal Genetic Code   331

Genetic Analysis **9.2**   332

Charging tRNA Molecules   333

Protein Folding and Posttranslational Polypeptide Processing   333

The Signal Hypothesis   334

9.5 Experiments Deciphered the Genetic Code   334

No Overlap in the Genetic Code   335

A Triplet Genetic Code   336

No Gaps in the Genetic Code   336

Deciphering the Genetic Code   337

Genetic Analysis **9.3**   339

Case Study *Antibiotics and Translation Interference   340*
Summary   340 • *Preparing for Problem Solving   341* • *Problems   342*

APPLICATION **B**
Human Genetic Screening

B.1 Presymptomatic Diagnosis of Huntington's Disease   348

Trinucleotide Repeat Expansion   348

Detecting the Number of Repeats   348

B.2 Newborn Genetic Screening   349

Phenylketonuria and the First Newborn Genetic Test   349

Living with PKU   350

The Recommended Uniform Screening Panel   351

B.3   Genetic Testing to Identify Carriers   353

Testing Blood Proteins   353

DNA-Based Carrier Screening and Diagnostic Verification   353

Carrier Screening Criteria   353

Pharmacogenetic Screening   354

B.4   Prenatal Genetic Testing   354

Invasive Screening Using Amniocentesis or Chorionic Villus Sampling   354

Noninvasive Prenatal Testing   356

Maternal Serum Screening   356

Preimplantation Genetic Screening   356

B.5   Direct-to-Consumer Genetic Testing   357

B.6   Opportunities and Choices   359

Problems   359

10
Eukaryotic Chromosome Abnormalities and Molecular Organization   361

10.1   Chromosome Number and Shape Vary among Organisms   362

Chromosomes in Nuclei   362

Chromosome Visualization   363

Chromosome Banding   364

Heterochromatin and Euchromatin   365

10.2   Nondisjunction Leads to Changes in Chromosome Number   366

Chromosome Nondisjunction   366

Gene Dosage Alteration   366

Genetic Analysis 10.1   368

Aneuploidy in Humans   368

Mosaicism   370

Uniparental Disomy   371

10.3   Changes in Euploid Content Lead to Polyploidy   371

Causes of Autopolyploidy and Allopolyploidy   371

Genetic Analysis 10.2   372

Consequences of Polyploidy   373

Polyploidy and Evolution   374

10.4   Chromosome Breakage Causes Mutation by Loss, Gain, and Rearrangement of Chromosomes   375

Partial Chromosome Deletion   375

Unequal Crossover   376

Detecting Duplication and Deletion   377

Deletion Mapping   377

10.5   Chromosome Breakage Leads to Inversion and Translocation of Chromosomes   378

Chromosome Inversion   378

Genetic Analysis 10.3   379

Experimental Insight 10.1   382

Chromosome Translocation   383

10.6   Eukaryotic Chromosomes Are Organized into Chromatin   385

Chromatin Compaction   386

Histone Proteins and Nucleosomes   386

Higher Order Chromatin Organization and Chromosome Structure   389

Nucleosome Disassembly, Synthesis, and Reassembly during Replication   389

Position Effect Variegation: Effect of Chromatin State on Transcription   390

Case Study Human Chromosome Evolution   392
Summary   393 • *Preparing for Problem Solving   394* • *Problems   394*

11
Gene Mutation, DNA Repair, and Homologous Recombination   399

11.1   Mutations Are Rare and Random and Alter DNA Sequence   400

Proof of the Random Mutation Hypothesis   400

Germ-Line and Somatic Mutations   401

Point Mutations   401

Base-Pair Substitution Mutations   401

Frameshift Mutations   402

Regulatory Mutations   402

Experimental Insight 11.1   404

Forward Mutation and Reversion   405

11.2 Gene Mutations May Arise from Spontaneous Events 405
Spontaneous DNA Replication Errors 405
Genetic Analysis 11.1 407
Spontaneous Nucleotide Base Changes 409

11.3 Mutations May Be Caused by Chemicals or Ionizing Radiation 410
Chemical Mutagens 410
Radiation-Induced DNA Damage 412
The Ames Test 413

11.4 Repair Systems Correct Some DNA Damage 415
Direct Repair of DNA Damage 415
Genetic Analysis 11.2 416
DNA Damage-Signaling Systems 419

11.5 Proteins Control Translesion DNA Synthesis and the Repair of Double-Strand Breaks 420
Translesion DNA Synthesis 420
Double-Strand Break Repair 420

11.6 DNA Double-Strand Breaks Initiate Homologous Recombination 422
The Holliday Model 422
The Bacterial RecBCD Pathway 422
The Double-Stranded Break Model of Homologous Recombination 422

11.7 Transposable Genetic Elements Move throughout the Genome 425
The Characteristics and Classification of Transposable Elements 425
The Mutagenic Effect of Transposition 426
Transposable Elements in Bacterial Genomes 426
Transposable Elements in Eukaryotic Genomes 427
The Discovery of *Ds* and *Ac* Elements in Maize 427
Genetic Analysis 11.3 428
Drosophila P Elements 429
Retrotransposons 430

Case Study Mendel's Peas Are Shaped by Transposition 431
Summary 432 • *Preparing for Problem Solving* 434 • Problems 434

12 Regulation of Gene Expression in Bacteria and Bacteriophage 439

12.1 Transcriptional Control of Gene Expression Requires DNA–Protein Interaction 440
Negative and Positive Control of Transcription 441
Regulatory DNA-Binding Proteins 441

12.2 The *lac* Operon Is an Inducible Operon System under Negative and Positive Control 443
Lactose Metabolism 443
lac Operon Structure 444
lac Operon Function 444

12.3 Mutational Analysis Deciphers Genetic Regulation of the *lac* Operon 447
Analysis of Structural Gene Mutations 447
lac Operon Regulatory Mutations 448
Molecular Analysis of the *lac* Operon 451
Genetic Analysis 12.1 452
Experimental Insight 12.1 453

12.4 Transcription from the Tryptophan Operon Is Repressible and Attenuated 454
Feedback Inhibition of Tryptophan Synthesis 455
Attenuation of the *trp* Operon 456
Attenuation Mutations 459
Attenuation in Other Amino Acid Operon Systems 459

12.5 Bacteria Regulate the Transcription of Stress Response Genes and Also Translation 459
Alternative Sigma Factors and Stress Response 459
Genetic Analysis 12.2 460
Translational Regulation in Bacteria 461

12.6 Riboswitches Regulate Bacterial Transcription, Translation, and mRNA Stability 462
Riboswitch Regulation of Transcription 462
Riboswitch Regulation of Translation 463
Riboswitch Control of mRNA Stability 464

12.7 Antiterminators and Repressors Control Lambda Phage Infection of *E. coli* 464

The Lambda Phage Genome   465

Early Gene Transcription   465

Cro Protein and the Lytic Cycle   466

The λ Repressor Protein and Lysogeny   468

Resumption of the Lytic Cycle following Lysogeny Induction   468

Case Study Vibrio cholerae—*Stress Response Leads to Serious Infection Through Positive Control of Transcription* 469
Summary 470 • *Preparing for Problem Solving* 471 • *Problems* 471

13
Regulation of Gene Expression in Eukaryotes 476

13.1 Cis-Acting Regulatory Sequences Bind Trans-Acting Regulatory Proteins to Control Eukaryotic Transcription 478

Overview of Transcriptional Regulatory Interactions in Eukaryotes   479

Integration and Modularity of Eukaryotic Regulatory Sequences   480

Locus Control Regions   481

Enhancer-Sequence Conservation   482

Yeast as a Simple Model for Eukaryotic Transcription   482

Insulator Sequences   484

13.2 Chromatin Remodeling and Modification Regulates Eukaryotic Transcription 484

PEV Mutations   485

Overview of Chromatin Remodeling and Chromatin Modification   486

Open and Covered Promoters   486

Mechanisms of Chromatin Remodeling   487

Chemical Modifications of Chromatin   488

Genetic Analysis **13.1**   490

An Example of Inducible Transcriptional Regulation in *S. cerevisiae*   493

Facultative Heterochromatin and Developmental Genes   494

Epigenetic Heritability   494

lncRNAs and Inactivation of Eutherian Mammalian Female X Chromosomes   496

Genomic Imprinting   497

Nucleotide Methylation   498

13.3 RNA-Mediated Mechanisms Control Gene Expression 498

Gene Silencing by Double-Stranded RNA   499

Constitutive Heterochromatin Maintenance   501

The Evolution and Applications of RNAi   502

Case Study Environmental Epigenetics   502
Summary 503 • *Preparing for Problem Solving* 504 • *Problems* 504

14
Analysis of Gene Function by Forward Genetics and Reverse Genetics 507

14.1 Forward Genetic Screens Identify Genes by Their Mutant Phenotypes 509

General Design of Forward Genetic Screens   509

Specific Strategies of Forward Genetic Screens   509

Analysis of Mutageneses   513

Identifying Interacting and Redundant Genes Using Modifier Screens   514

Genetic Analysis **14.1**   515

14.2 Genes Identified by Mutant Phenotype Are Cloned Using Recombinant DNA Technology 516

Cloning Genes by Complementation   516

Genome Sequencing to Determine Gene Identification   517

14.3 Reverse Genetics Investigates Gene Action by Progressing from Gene Identification to Phenotype 519

Genome Editing   519

Use of Homologous Recombination in Reverse Genetics   522

Use of Insertion Mutants in Reverse Genetics   524

RNA Interference in Gene Activity   525

Reverse Genetics by TILLING   525

Genetic Analysis **14.2**   527

14.4 Transgenes Provide a Means of Dissecting Gene Function 527

Monitoring Gene Expression with Reporter Genes   528

Enhancer Trapping   531

Investigating Gene Function with Chimeric Genes   532

Case Study Reverse Genetics and Genetic Redundancy in Flower Development   533
Summary 535 • *Preparing for Problem Solving* 535 • *Problems* 535

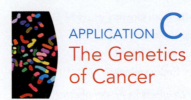

APPLICATION **C**
The Genetics of Cancer

C.1 Cancer Is a Somatic Genetic Disease that Is Only Occasionally Inherited 540

C.2 What Is Cancer and What Are the Characteristics of Cancer? 540
Progression of Abnormalities 540
The Hallmarks of Cancer Cells and Malignant Tumors 541

C.3 The Genetic Basis of Cancer 543
Single Gene Mutations and Cancer Development 543
The Genetic Progression of Cancer Development and Cancer Predisposition 546
Breast and Ovarian Cancer and the Inheritance of Cancer Susceptibility 548

C.4 Cancer Cell Genome Sequencing and Improvements in Therapy 549
The Cancer Genome Atlas 549
Epigenetic Irregularities 549
Targeted Cancer Therapy 550
Problems 550

15
Recombinant DNA Technology and Its Applications 552

15.1 Specific DNA Sequences Are Identified and Manipulated Using Recombinant DNA Technology 553
Restriction Enzymes 553
Experimental Insight **15.1** 554
Genetic Analysis **15.1** 556
Molecular Cloning 557
DNA Libraries 562
Advances in Altering and Synthesizing DNA Molecules 564

15.2 Introducing Foreign Genes into Genomes Creates Transgenic Organisms 565
Expression of Heterologous Genes in Bacterial and Fungal Hosts 565
Experimental Insight **15.2** 569
Transformation of Plant Genomes by *Agrobacterium* 570
Transgenic Animals 574
Manipulation of DNA Sequences in Vivo 578

15.3 Gene Therapy Uses Recombinant DNA Technology 579
Two Forms of Gene Therapy 579
Somatic Gene Therapy Using ES Cells 579
Genetic Analysis **15.2** 580

15.4 Cloning of Plants and Animals Produces Genetically Identical Individuals 583
Case Study Gene Drive Alleles Can Rapidly Spread Through Populations 585
Summary 587 • Preparing for Problem Solving 588 • Problems 588

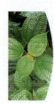

16
Genomics: Genetics from a Whole-Genome Perspective 593

16.1 Structural Genomics Provides a Catalog of Genes in a Genome 594
Whole-Genome Shotgun Sequencing 596
Reference Genomes and Resequencing 599
Metagenomics 600
Experimental Insight **16.1** 601

16.2 Annotation Ascribes Biological Function to DNA Sequences 602
Experimental Approaches to Structural Annotation 602
Computational Approaches to Structural Annotation 602
Functional Gene Annotation 603
Research Technique **16.1** 604
Related Genes and Protein Motifs 605
Variation in Genome Organization among Species 605
Three Insights from Genome Sequences 606

16.3 Evolutionary Genomics Traces the History of Genomes 607
The Tree of Life 608
Interspecific Genome Comparisons: Gene Content 608
Research Technique **16.2** 610
Genetic Analysis **16.1** 614
Interspecific Genome Comparisons: Genome Annotation 615
Interspecific Genome Comparisons: Gene Order 616

16.4 Functional Genomics Aims to Elucidate Gene Function 618
Transcriptomics 619

Other "-omes" and "-omics"   621

Use of Yeast Mutants to Categorize Genes   624

Genetic Networks   625

Case Study *Genomic Analysis of Insect Guts May Fuel the World*   627
Summary   628 • *Preparing for Problem Solving*   628 • *Problems*   629

17
Organellar Inheritance and the Evolution of Organellar Genomes   632

17.1 Organellar Inheritance Transmits Genes Carried on Organellar Chromosomes   633
The Discovery of Organellar Inheritance   633

Homoplasmy and Heteroplasmy   634

Genome Replication in Organelles   635

Replicative Segregation of Organelle Genomes   635

17.2 Modes of Organellar Inheritance Depend on the Organism   636
Mitochondrial Inheritance in Mammals   637

Genetic Analysis 17.1   639

Mating Type and Chloroplast Segregation in *Chlamydomonas*   640

Biparental Inheritance in *Saccharomyces cerevisiae*   641

Genetic Analysis 17.2   643

Summary of Organellar Inheritance   644

17.3 Mitochondria Are the Energy Factories of Eukaryotic Cells   644
Mitochondrial Genome Structure and Gene Content   645

Mitochondrial Transcription and Translation   646

17.4 Chloroplasts Are the Sites of Photosynthesis   648
Chloroplast Genome Structure and Gene Content   648

Chloroplast Transcription and Translation   649

Editing of Chloroplast mRNA   650

17.5 The Endosymbiosis Theory Explains Mitochondrial and Chloroplast Evolution   651
Separate Evolution of Mitochondria and Chloroplasts   651

Experimental Insight 17.1   652

Continual DNA Transfer from Organelles   654

Encoding of Organellar Proteins   655

The Origin of the Eukaryotic Lineage   656

Secondary and Tertiary Endosymbioses   656

Case Study *Ototoxic Deafness: A Mitochondrial Gene–Environment Interaction*   658
Summary   659 • *Preparing for Problem Solving*   660 • *Problems*   660

18
Developmental Genetics   663

18.1 Development Is the Building of a Multicellular Organism   664
Cell Differentiation   665

Pattern Formation   665

18.2 *Drosophila* Development Is a Paradigm for Animal Development   666
The Developmental Toolkit of *Drosophila*   667

Maternal Effects on Pattern Formation   669

Coordinate Gene Patterning of the Anterior–Posterior Axis   669

Domains of Gap Gene Expression   670

Regulation of Pair-Rule Genes   671

Specification of Parasegments by *Hox* Genes   673

Downstream Targets of *Hox* Genes   675

Hox Genes throughout Metazoans   676

Genetic Analysis 18.1   677

Stabilization of Cellular Memory by Chromatin Architecture   678

18.3 Cellular Interactions Specify Cell Fate   679
Inductive Signaling between Cells   679

Lateral Inhibition   682

Cell Death During Development   682

18.4 "Evolution Behaves Like a Tinkerer"   683
Evolution through Co-option   683

Constraints on Co-option   685

18.5 Plants Represent an Independent Experiment in Multicellular Evolution   685
Development at Meristems   685

Combinatorial Homeotic Activity in Floral-Organ Identity   686

Genetic Analysis **18.2**   689

Case Study *Cyclopia and Polydactyly—
Different* Shh *Mutations with Distinctive
Phenotypes* 690
Summary   691 • *Preparing for Problem
Solving*   692 • Problems   692

19
Genetic Analysis of Quantitative Traits   696

19.1 Quantitative Traits Display Continuous Phenotype Variation   697
Genetic Potential   697
Major Gene Effects   698
Additive Gene Effects   698
Continuous Phenotypic Variation from Multiple Additive Genes   699
Allele Segregation in Quantitative Trait Production   701
Effects of Environmental Factors on Phenotypic Variation   702
Genetic Analysis **19.1**   703
Threshold Traits   704

19.2 Quantitative Trait Analysis Is Statistical   706
Statistical Description of Phenotypic Variation   706
Partitioning Phenotypic Variance   707
Partitioning Genetic Variance   708

19.3 Heritability Measures the Genetic Component of Phenotypic Variation   708
Genetic Analysis **19.2**   709
Broad Sense Heritability   710
Twin Studies   710
Narrow Sense Heritability and Artificial Selection   712

19.4 Quantitative Trait Loci Are the Genes That Contribute to Quantitative Traits   713
QTL Mapping Strategies   714
Identification of QTL Genes   716
Genome-Wide Association Studies   717

Case Study *The Genetics of Autism Spectrum Disorders*   718
Summary   719 • *Preparing for Problem Solving*   720 • Problems   720

20
Population Genetics and Evolution at the Population, Species, and Molecular Levels   725

20.1 The Hardy–Weinberg Equilibrium Describes the Relationship of Allele and Genotype Frequencies in Populations   726
Populations and Gene Pools   727
The Hardy–Weinberg Equilibrium   727
Determining Autosomal Allele Frequencies in Populations   729
The Hardy–Weinberg Equilibrium for More than Two Alleles   731
The Chi-Square Test of Hardy–Weinberg Predictions   731
Genetic Analysis **20.1**   732

20.2 Natural Selection Operates through Differential Reproductive Fitness within a Population   732
Differential Reproductive Fitness and Relative Fitness   733
Directional Natural Selection   733
Natural Selection Favoring Heterozygotes   735
Genetic Analysis **20.2**   736

20.3 Mutation Diversifies Gene Pools   736
Quantifying the Effects of Mutation on Allele Frequencies   737
Mutation–Selection Balance   737

20.4 Gene Flow Occurs by the Movement of Organisms and Genes between Populations   737
Effects of Gene Flow   738
Allele Frequency Equilibrium and Equalization   739

20.5 Genetic Drift Causes Allele Frequency Change by Sampling Error   739
The Founder Effect   740
Genetic Bottlenecks   740

20.6 Inbreeding Alters Genotype Frequencies but Not Allele Frequencies   741
The Coefficient of Inbreeding   741
Inbreeding Depression   743

20.7   New Species Evolve by Reproductive Isolation   743

   Genetic Analysis   **20.3**   744

   Processes of Speciation   744

   Reproductive Isolation and Speciation   746

   The Molecular Genetics of Evolution in Darwin's Finches   748

20.8   Molecular Evolution Changes Genes and Genomes through Time   748

   Vertebrate Steroid Receptor Evolution   749

   Case Study   Sickle Cell Disease Evolution and Natural Selection in Humans   750
   Summary   751 • *Preparing for Problem Solving*   752 • *Problems*   753

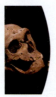

APPLICATION D
Human Evolutionary Genetics

D.1   Genome Sequences Reveal Extent of Human Genetic Diversity   759

   SNP Variation in Humans   760

   Variation in CNVs   761

D.2   Diversity of Extant Humans Suggests an African Origin   761

   Mitochondrial Eve   762

   Y Chromosome Phylogeny   762

   Autosomal Loci   763

D.3   Comparisons between Great Apes Identify Human-Specific Traits   763

   Revelations of Great Ape Genomes   763

   Comparing the Human and Chimpanzee Genomes   765

D.4   Ancient DNA Reveals the Recent History of Our Species   766

   Neandertals   768

   Denisovans   769

   Finding Genes that Make Us Human   770

D.5   Human Migrations around the Globe   770

   Europe   770

   Australia   771

D.6   Genetic Evidence for Adaptation to New Environments   772

   Lactose Tolerance   772

   Skin Pigmentation   774

   High Altitude   774

D.7   Domestication of Plants and Animals: Maize   775

D.8   The Future   776

   Problems   777

APPLICATION E
Forensic Genetics

E.1   CODIS and Forensic Genetic Analysis   780

   CODIS History and Markers   780

   Electrophoretic Analysis   781

   Forensic Analysis Using CODIS   782

   Paternity Testing   784

   Individual Identification   785

   Remains Identified following the 9-11 Attack   785

   Identification of the Disappeared in Argentina   786

E.2   DNA Analysis for Genealogy, Genetic Ancestry, and Genetic Health Risk Assessment   786

   Assessing Genealogical Relationships   786

   Assessing Genetic Ancestry   787

   Genetic Health Risk Assessment   788

   Late-Onset Alzheimer Disease   788

   Celiac Disease   789

   One Side of the Equation   789

   Problems   789

References and Additional Reading   R-1

Appendix: Answers   A-1

Glossary   G-1

Credits   C-1

Index   I-1

About the Authors

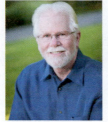

Mark F. Sanders has been a faculty member in the Department of Molecular and Cellular Biology at the University of California, Davis, since 1985. In that time, he has taught more than 150 genetics courses to nearly 35,000 undergraduate students. Although he specializes in teaching the genetics course for which this book is written, his genetics teaching experience also includes a genetics laboratory course, an advanced human genetics course for biology majors, and a human heredity course for nonscience majors, as well as introductory biology and courses in population genetics and evolution. He has also served as an advisor to undergraduate students and in undergraduate education administration, and he has directed several undergraduate education programs.

Dr. Sanders received his B.A. degree in Anthropology from San Francisco State University, his M.A. and Ph.D. degrees in Biological Anthropology from the University of California, Los Angeles, and 4 years of training as a postdoctoral researcher studying inherited susceptibility to human breast and ovarian cancer at the University of California, Berkeley.

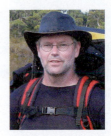

John L. Bowman is a professor in the School of Biological Sciences at Monash University in Melbourne, Australia, and an adjunct professor in the Department of Plant Biology at the University of California, Davis, in the United States. He received a B.S. in Biochemistry at the University of Illinois at Urbana-Champaign in 1986 and a Ph.D. in Biology from the California Institute of Technology in Pasadena, California. His Ph.D. research focused on how the identities of floral organs are specified in *Arabidopsis* (described in Chapter 18), and he conducted postdoctoral research at Monash University on the regulation of floral development. From 1996 to 2006, his laboratory at UC Davis investigated developmental genetics of plants, focusing on how leaves are patterned. From 2006 to 2011, he was a Federation Fellow at Monash University, where his laboratory is studying land plant evolution using a developmental genetics approach. He was elected a Fellow of the Australian Academy of Science in 2014. At UC Davis he taught genetics, "from Mendel to cancer," to undergraduate students, and he continues to teach genetics courses at Monash University.

Dedication

To my extraordinary wife and partner Ita. She is a treasure whose support, patience, and encouragement throughout this ongoing project make me very fortunate. To my wonderful children Jana and Nick, to their spouses John and Molly, to my grandson Lincoln, and to all my students, from whom I have learned as much as I have taught.

Mark F. Sanders

For my parents, Lois and Noel, who taught me to love and revere nature, and Tizita, my partner in our personal genetics experiments. And to all my genetics students who have inspired me over the years, I hope that the inspiration was mutual.

John L. Bowman

We dedicate this third edition of *Genetic Analysis: An Integrated Approach* to our friend and colleague Mel Green, who passed away in October 2017 at the age of 101. Mel was a stellar geneticist and was engaged in genetics until the end. Over his long career, he made numerous important contributions to genetics, inspiring scores of geneticists including the authors of this textbook.

Preface

We are now almost two decades into the second century of modern genetics, and the expansion of knowledge in this rapidly progressing field continues at a dizzying pace. Topics that seemed impenetrable just a few years ago are coming into focus. Novel approaches to old problems are providing profound insights into the genomics, development, and evolution of organisms in all three domains of life. CRISPR–Cas9, which was discovered in basic research on bacterial immunity, has been developed into a genome-editing system that has revolutionized the manipulation of genomic sequences in living cells. Advancements in genomics, proteomics, transcriptomics, and other enterprises of the "omic" world have opened avenues for research that were unimaginable in years past. And the resulting advancements in knowledge are quickly being turned into new applications. These are great times to be a geneticist or a student studying genetics!

In keeping with these exciting times of revolutionary change in our field, our textbooks too must undergo change. This third edition of *Genetic Analysis: An Integrated Approach* contains some significant changes that have been made with students foremost in our minds. As authors and instructors of genetics, we have had front row seats in the discipline and in the classroom. Between the two of us, we have more than 50 years' experience and experimentation in teaching genetics. We have used that experience to produce this new edition. We hope that it conveys the excitement we feel about genetics and the dynamism at work in the field, and that it offers students new and interesting examples of and insights into our favorite scientific discipline. As teachers and student mentors, our highest goal is to see students succeed. To accomplish this we seek to motivate students to pursue and explore genetics more fully and to incorporate what they learn into their thinking and plans for their future. We hope teachers and students alike will find motivation and encouragement in the subject matter and examples in this book.

Our Integrated Approach

This third edition, like its predecessors, carries the unique subtitle *An Integrated Approach*. The phrase embodies our pedagogical approach, consisting of three principles: (1) to integrate problem solving throughout the text—not relegating it to the ends of chapters—and consistently to model a powerful, three-step problem-solving approach (Evaluate, Deduce, and Solve) in every worked example; (2) to integrate an evolutionary perspective throughout the book; and (3) to integrate descriptions of Mendelian genetics with molecular genetics and genomics so as to demonstrate the value of each of these different approaches for investigating the same

basic sets of observations. In this edition, we adhere to and strengthen the integration that has resonated strongly with instructors and students.

New to This Edition

As was the case in our previous editions, our aim above all is to assist the student by making the learning of genetics easier, more interesting, and more effective. Thus, three specific goals have driven this revision, and each is supported by new features that help accomplish it. Goal 1 is to provide more interesting, real-world applications of genetics. We have addressed this goal by writing five "Application Chapters" that each highlight a particular applied topic in human genetics. Goal 2 is to make the job of learning the details of genetics easier. We have addressed this goal by writing "Caption Queries" to accompany chapter figures and by providing a new feature, titled "Preparing for Problem Solving," at the end of each chapter. Goal 3 is to facilitate group work and discussion of genetics problems and concepts among classmates. We have addressed this goal in part through the Caption Queries and in part by providing a new category of chapter problems, called "Collaboration and Discussion," that are specifically designed to be tackled in groups. Along with these important pedagogical changes, this revision is also important for incorporating new genetic information that is defining the future of the field. The following descriptions highlight key new features and information designed to accomplish our revision goals.

Application Chapters

Many students come to genetics curious about human heredity and about how genetic principles are applied in real-world activities. This edition, like the previous ones, features numerous human examples to help illustrate the operation of genetic principles, and it features five new Application Chapters—short chapters focused on specific applied topics in human genetics and evolutionary genetics. The Application Chapters are written to give students information on topics of particular interest and to illustrate some of the practical uses of genetics and genetic analysis. Each of these special chapters is about half the length of a typical textbook chapter, and each has a specific applied focus. They are spaced periodically throughout the book in such a way that each of them comes just after the key prerequisite material has been presented. Importantly, these new Application Chapters do not add to the length of the book. We have made reorganization and revision decisions that have maintained the depth of coverage while allowing for the addition of the Application Chapters in a space-neutral way.

Every Application Chapter opens with a story that exemplifies why the topic of the chapter is important, and each contains several end-of-chapter problems to guide student learning and discussion. The five Application Chapters are:

- **Application Chapter A – Human Hereditary Disease and Genetic Counseling** This chapter describes the role of genetic counselors and the genetic information and analysis they employ in medical decision-making. Students interested in human hereditary transmission, as well as those potentially interested in careers in medical genetics or genetic counseling, will find satisfying discussions of these topics in this chapter.

- **Application Chapter B – Human Genetic Screening** Numerous invasive and non-invasive methods of screening for inherited conditions are described in this chapter, and their results are discussed. Topics include carrier screening; pre-natal, newborn, and pre-symptomatic genetic testing; and amniocentesis and chorionic villus sampling.

- **Application Chapter C – The Genetics of Cancer** This chapter discusses cancer from two perspectives. The first is an overview of the major hallmarks of cancer that have been articulated over the last decade or so. The second is a discussion of cancers that have a simpler genetic basis and cancers for which inherited susceptibility has been identified. New, immune system–based approaches to cancer treatment are also discussed.

- **Application Chapter D – Human Evolutionary Genetics** This chapter presents the current interpretation of human evolution from a genomic perspective and describes the relationship of modern humans to their archaic predecessors. The discussion includes up-to-date information on Neandertal and Denisovan genome sequencing, along with recent evidence on interbreeding among archaic human populations.

- **Application Chapter E – Forensic Genetics** This chapter focuses on the uses and analysis of DNA in the contexts of crime scene analysis, paternity testing, and direct-to-consumer genealogy, genetic ancestry testing, and genetic health risk assessment. Examples of genetic analysis using the Combined DNA Index System (CODIS) and of genetic analysis to determine the paternity index and combined paternity index are given. Descriptions of the direct-to-consumer genetic analyses provided by AncestryDNA and 23andMe are part of the chapter as well.

Caption Queries

Textbook figures are an integral part of the pedagogical apparatus of a textbook, but they are only effective if the reader takes the time to look at and understand them. How does one help students examine a figure attentively enough to derive the critical content and meaning? One way is by asking questions about the figure. In this revision, we have written Caption Queries for virtually every figure in the book to help students dissect the illustrated content and more fully understand its meaning and importance. Several Caption Queries have been printed below their corresponding figure in the chapter itself, and all Caption Queries are available as clicker questions for classroom use and in Mastering Genetics as assignable homework. Some Caption Queries require the student to solve a problem using information from the figure, some require an explanation be provided, and others ask students to expand on the information or idea in the figure. All Caption Queries, whatever their form, will help students focus on the figures and derive a better understanding of their content.

Caption Queries serve a second purpose as well. Genetics instructors are becoming increasingly interested in the pedagogical approach known as "flipping the classroom." This approach has students do their textbook reading and review of lecture, PowerPoint®, and other course materials outside of class, leaving class time open for discussion, problem solving, and inquiry-based learning. In our own classrooms, we have found that asking questions about chapter figures is an effective way to stimulate discussion and jump-start problem solving and inquiry-based learning. The clicker versions of Caption Queries can be the first line of interactive questions in this approach.

Preparing for Problem Solving

Building on the strong problem-solving guidance of our Genetic Analysis worked examples (the three-step problem-solving approach described momentarily), we have added a new chapter feature titled Preparing for Problem Solving, located between the Chapter Summary and the end-of-chapter problems. This feature is a list identifying the specific knowledge and skills required to answer chapter problems. The listed items draw students' attention back to the major ideas described in the chapter and to the practical skills that were modeled there, before the students begin working on end-of-chapter problems.

Collaboration and Discussion Problems

Having students work in groups to solve problems is an increasingly popular and productive way to encourage participation in, and to enhance, active learning. In this revision, each end-of-chapter problem set has been expanded to include several new problems in a section titled Collaboration and Discussion. As the name implies, these problems are designed to be evaluated and solved by small groups of students working together. Whether assigned as homework or as part of flipped classroom activities, these exercises offer an array of opportunities for comprehensive and hands-on problem solving.

Redesigned Chapter Content

The content and coverage of all chapters has been reworked in this revision to keep up with changes in the field and keep all discussions timely. Several chapter revisions reflect changes in approaches to genetic analysis. In Chapter 5 ("Genetic Linkage and Mapping in Eukaryotes"), for example, the discussion of mapping of molecular genetic markers has been substantially expanded. To make way for this expansion, discussion of tetrad analysis in yeast has been dropped. Chapter 13 ("Regulation of Gene Expression in Eukaryotes") has undergone revision to feature more discussion of epigenetic regulation and the roles of epigenetic readers, writers, and erasers. Chapters 14 ("Analysis of Gene Function by Forward Genetics and Reverse Genetics") and 15 ("Recombinant DNA Technology and Its Application") have a greatly expanded descriptions of the CRISPR–Cas9 system and its applications in gene editing and gene drive systems. Chapter 16 ("Genomics: Genetics from a Whole-Genome Perspective") has undergone substantial revision to feature new genomic approaches.

Several chapters include important new information that became available just as writing was being completed. Among numerous examples are the discussion in Chapter 7 ("DNA Structure and Replication") of the apparently stochastic pattern of DNA replication initiation in *E. coli* that was described in mid-2017; and the description in Application Chapter C (Genetics of Cancer) of the CAR-T cell method for treating certain cancers that was recommended for approval by a panel of the U.S. Food and Drug Administration in mid-2017.

A chapter from the first two editions, "The Integration of Genetic Approaches: Understanding Sickle Cell Disease," has been removed in this edition to help make room for the inclusion of the Application Chapters. We know many professors are fond of this chapter, and they can access it in Mastering Genetics or in custom versions of this text.

Maintaining What Works

While making numerous pedagogical and content changes in this third edition of *Genetic Analysis: An Integrated Approach*, we have maintained all of the features that made previous editions of the book so popular and effective. These include the systematic problem-solving approach, the pervasive evolutionary perspective, and the consistent cross connections drawn throughout between transmission and molecular genetics.

A Problem-Solving Approach

To help train students to become more effective problem solvers, we employ a unique problem-solving feature called Genetic Analysis that gives students a consistent, repeatable method to help them learn and practice problem solving.

Genetic Analysis teaches how to start thinking about a problem, what the end goal is, and what kind of analysis is required to get there. The three steps of this problem-solving framework are *Evaluate*, *Deduce*, and *Solve*.

Evaluate: Students learn to identify the topic of the problem, specify the nature or format of the requested answer, and identify critical information given in the problem.

Deduce: Students learn how to use conceptual knowledge to analyze data, make connections, and infer additional information or next steps.

Solve: Students learn how to accurately apply analytical tools and to execute their plan to solve a given problem.

Irrespective of the type of problem presented to them, this framework guides students through the stages of solving it and gives them the confidence to undertake new problems.

Each Genetic Analysis worked example is laid out in a two-column format to help students easily follow the steps of the Solution Strategy that are enumerated in the left-hand column and executed in the right-hand column. "Break It Down" comments point to key elements in the problem statement of each example, as an aid to students, who often struggle to identify the concepts and information that are critical to starting the problem-solving process. We also include problem-solving Tips to help with critical steps, as well as warnings of common Pitfalls to avoid; these suggestions and admonitions are gathered from our teaching experience. It is also important to note that the Genetic Analysis examples are integrated into the chapters, right after discussions of important content, to help students immediately apply the concepts they are learning. Each chapter includes two or three Genetic Analysis problems, and the book contains nearly 50 in all.

Complementing the Genetic Analysis problems are strong end-of-chapter problems that are divided into three groups. Chapter Concept problems come first and review the critical information, principles, and analytical tools discussed in the chapter. These are followed by Application and Integration problems that are more challenging and broader in scope. Last come the chapter's Collaboration and Discussion questions, a new addition described above. All solutions to the end-of-chapter problems in the *Study Guide and Solutions Manual* use the evaluate–deduce–solve model to reinforce the book's problem-solving approach.

An Evolutionary Perspective

Geneticists are acutely aware of evolutionary relationships between genes, genomes, and organisms. Evolutionary processes at the organismal level, discovered through comparative biology, can shed light on the function of genes and organization of genomes at the molecular level.

Likewise, the function of genes and organization of genomes informs the evolutionary model. The integration of evolution and of the evolutionary perspective remains a central organizing theme of this third edition, greatly strengthened through enhanced coverage of molecular genetic evolution. For example, Chapter 20 includes updated discussion of the molecular genetic evolution of Darwin's finches, and Application Chapter D includes extensive discussion of the role of interbreeding between Neandertals and archaic humans in forming the modern human genome.

Connecting Transmission and Molecular Genetics

Experiments that shed light on principles of transmission genetics preceded by several decades the discovery of the structure and function of DNA and its role in inherited molecular variation. Yet biologists already recognized that DNA variation is the basis of inherited morphological variation observed in transmission genetics. Understanding how these two approaches to genetics are connected is vital to thinking like a geneticist. We have retained the integration of transmission genetics and molecular genetics in the text and have enhanced this feature in two ways: first, through additional discussion of the molecular basis of hereditary variation, including the mutations that underlie the four identified genes examined by Mendel, and second, with a much more robust genomic approach.

Pathways through the Book

This book is written with a Mendel-first approach that many instructors find to be the most effective pedagogical approach for teaching genetics. We are cognizant, however, that the scope of information covered in genetics courses varies and that instructor preferences differ. We have kept such differences and alternative approaches in mind while writing the book. Thus, we provide *four pathways* through the book that instructors can use to meet their varying course goals and objectives. Each pathway features integration of problem solving through the inclusion of Genetic Analysis worked examples in each chapter.

1. Mendel-First Approach

Ch 1–20

This pathway provides a traditional approach that begins with Mendelian genetics but integrates that material with evolutionary concepts and connects it solidly to molecular genetics. This approach is exemplified by the discussion in Chapter 2 of genes responsible for four of Mendel's traits, followed in Chapters 10 and 11 by a description of the molecular basis of mutations of those genes.

2. Molecular-First Approach

Ch 1 → Ch 7–9 → Ch 2–6 → Ch 10–20

This pathway provides a molecular-first approach, to develop a clear understanding of the molecular basis of heredity and variation before delving into the analysis of hereditary transmission.

3. Quantitative Genetics Focus

Ch 1, 2, 4 → Ch 19 → Ch 3, 4–18 → Ch 20

This pathway incorporates quantitative genetics early in the course by introducing polygenic inheritance (Chapter 4) and following it up with a comprehensive discussion of quantitative genetics (Chapter 19).

4. Population Genetics Focus

Ch 1–2 → Ch 20 → Ch 3–19

This pathway incorporates population genetics early in the course. Instructors can use the introduction to evolutionary principles and processes (Chapter 1) and the role of genes and alleles in transmission (Chapter 2) and then address evolution at the population level and at higher levels (Chapter 20).

Chapter Features

A principal goal of our writing style, chapter format, and design and illustration program is to engage the reader intellectually and to invite continuous reading, all the while explaining complex and difficult ideas with maximum clarity. Our conversational tone encourages student reading and comprehension, and our attractive design and realistic art program visually engage students and put them at ease. Experienced instructors of genetics know that students are more engaged when they can relate concepts to the real world. To that end, we use real experimental data to illustrate genetic principles and analyses as well as to familiarize students with exciting research and creative researchers in the field. We also discuss a broad array of organisms—such as humans, bacteria, yeast, plants, fruit flies, nematodes, vertebrates, and viruses—to exemplify genetic principles.

Careful thought has been given to our chapter features; each of them serves to improve student learning. The following list illustrates how we highlight central ideas, problems, and methods that are important for understanding genetics.

- **Essential Ideas:** Each chapter begins with a short list of concepts that embody the principal ideas of the chapter.
- **Genetic Analysis:** Our key problem-solving feature that guides students through the problem-solving process by using the *evaluate–deduce–solve* framework.
- **Foundation Figures:** Highly detailed illustrations of pivotal concepts in genetics.

- **Caption Queries:** Questions that help students dissect the illustrated content of book figures and more fully understand their meaning and importance.

- **Experimental Insights:** Discussions of critical or illustrative experiments, including the observed results of the experiments and the conclusions drawn from their analysis.

- **Research Techniques:** Explorations of important research methods, illustrating the results and interpretations.

- **Case Studies:** Short, real-world examples, at the end of every chapter, that highlight central ideas or concepts of the chapter while reminding students of some practical applications of genetics.

- **Preparing for Problem Solving:** Immediately preceding the end-of-chapter problems, this list of approaches and suggestions briefly highlights the tools and concepts students will use most often in answering chapter problems.

Mastering Genetics

http://www.masteringgenetics.com

A key reviewing and testing tool offered with this textbook is Mastering Genetics, the most powerful online homework and assessment system available. Tutorials follow the Socratic method, coaching students to the correct answer by providing feedback specific to a student's misconceptions as well as proffering hints students can access if they get stuck. The interactive approach of the tutorials provides a unique way for students to learn genetics concepts while developing and honing their problem-solving skills. In addition to tutorials, Mastering Genetics includes animations, quizzes, and end-of-chapter problems from the textbook. This exclusive product of Pearson greatly enhances the learning of genetics. Its features include:

- New tutorials on topics like CRISPR–Cas, to help students master important and challenging concepts.

- New Dynamic Study Modules. These interactive flashcards present multiple sets of questions and provide extensive feedback so students can test, learn, and retest until they achieve mastery of the textbook material. Whether assigned for credit or used for self-study, they are powerful pre-class activities that help prepare students for more involved content coverage or problem solving in class.

- eText 2.0, a dynamic digital version of the textbook, adapts to the size of the screen being used, includes embedded videos and hotlinked glossary, and allows student and instructor note-taking, highlighting, bookmarking, and searches.

- Practice Problems, similar to end-of-chapter questions in scope and level of difficulty, are found only in Mastering Genetics. Solutions are not available in the *Study Guide and Solutions Manual*, and the bank of questions

extends your options for assigning challenging problems. Each problem includes specific wrong-answer feedback to help students learn from their mistakes and to guide them toward the correct answer.

- Inclusion of nearly 90% of the end-of-chapter questions among the assignment possibilities in the item library. The broad range of answer types the questions require, in addition to multiple choice, includes sorting, labeling, numerical, and ranking.

- Learning Catalytics is a "bring your own device" (smartphone, tablet, or laptop) assessment and active classroom system that expands the possibilities for student engagement. Instructors can create their own questions, draw from community content shared by colleagues, or access Pearson's library of question clusters that explore challenging topics through two- to five-question series that focus on a single scenario or data set, build in difficulty, and require higher-level thinking.

Student Supplements

Mastering Genetics

http://www.masteringgenetics.com

Used by over one million science students, the Mastering platform is the most effective and widely employed online tutorial, homework, and assessment system for the sciences; it helps students perform better on homework and exams. As an instructor-assigned homework system, Mastering Genetics is designed to provide students with a variety of assessment tools to help them understand key topics and concepts and to build problem-solving skills. Mastering Genetics tutorials guide students through the toughest topics in genetics with self-paced tutorials that provide individualized coaching offering hints and feedback specific to a student's individual misconceptions. Students can also explore the Mastering Genetics Study Area, which includes animations, chapter quizzes, the eText, and other study aids. The interactive eText 2.0 allows students to highlight text, add study notes, and watch embedded videos.

Study Guide and Solutions Manual

ISBN: 0134832256 / 9780134832258

Heavily updated and accuracy-checked by Peter Mirabito from the University of Kentucky, the *Study Guide and Solutions Manual* is divided into four sections: Genetics Problem-Solving Toolkit, Types of Genetics Problems, Solutions to End-of-Chapter Problems, and Test Yourself. In the "toolkit" section, students are reminded of key terms and concepts and key relationships they need to know to solve the problems in each chapter. This material is followed, in the second section of the manual, by a breakdown of the types of problems students will encounter in the end-of-chapter problems, the key strategies for solving each problem type, variations on the problem type that may also be encountered, and a worked example modeled after the Genetic Analysis feature of the main textbook. The solutions provided in the third section of the manual also reflect the *evaluate–deduce–solve* strategy of the Genetic Analysis feature. Finally, for more practice, we've included five to ten Test Yourself problems and accompanying solutions for each chapter in the textbook.

Instructor Supplements

Mastering Genetics

Mastering Genetics engages and motivates students to learn and allows you to easily assign automatically graded activities. Tutorials provide students with personalized coaching and feedback. Using the gradebook, you can quickly monitor and display student results. Mastering Genetics easily captures data to demonstrate assessment outcomes. Resources include:

- In-depth tutorials that coach students with hints and feedback specific to their misconceptions.

- An item library of thousands of assignable questions, including reading quizzes and end-of-chapter problems. You can use publisher-created prebuilt assignments to get started quickly. Each question can be easily edited to precisely match the language you use.

- A gradebook that provides you with quick results and easy-to-interpret insights into student performance.

TestGen Test Bank

ISBN: 0134872762 / 9780134872766

Test questions are available as part of the TestGen EQ Testing Software, a text-specific testing program that is networkable for administering tests. It also allows instructors to view and edit questions, export the questions as tests, and print them out in a variety of formats.

Instructor Resources

A robust suite of instructor resources offers adopters of the text a comprehensive and innovative selection of lecture presentation and teaching tools. Developed to meet the needs of veteran and newer instructors alike, these resources include:

- The JPEG files of all tables and line drawings from the text. Drawings have labels individually enhanced for optimal projection results and also are provided in unlabeled versions.

- Most of the text photos, including all photos with pedagogical significance, as JPEG files.

- A set of PowerPoint® presentations consisting of a thorough lecture outline for each chapter augmented by key text illustrations and animations.

- PowerPoint® presentations containing a comprehensive set of in-class Classroom Response System (CRS) questions for each chapter.

- PowerPoint® presentations containing clicker-based Caption Query questions for all figures in the text.

- In Word and PDF files, a complete set of the assessment materials and study questions and answers from the test bank. Files are also available in TestGen format.

We Welcome Your Comments and Suggestions

Genetics is continuously changing, and textbooks must also change continuously to keep pace with the field and to meet the needs of instructors and students. Communication with our talented and dedicated users is a critical driver of change. We welcome all suggestions and comments and invite you to contact us directly. Please send comments or questions about the book to us at **mfsanders@ucdavis.edu** or **john.bowman@monash.edu**.

Acknowledgments

In our first edition, we described the adage that begins with the words "It takes a village . . . " as aptly applying to the development and assembly of our textbook. This new edition too has been a true team effort, and we are grateful to all of our teammates. We particularly wish to thank our editorial team led by our senior editor Michael Gillespie, our developmental editor Moira Lerner Nelson, and our content producer Melanie Field for their guidance and assistance in bringing this new edition to life. Margot Otway and Barbara Price also brought their developmental editing expertise to improving the art and page layouts. Our thanks to proofreader Pete Shanks for his keen attention to detail. We also thank our compatriot Peter Mirabito, author of the *Study Guide and Solutions Manual*, for his work assembling an exceptionally useful supplement. Beth Wilbur, Adam Jaworski, and Ginnie Simione Jutson have also been essential supporters who have made this new edition a reality.

On the production side, we thank the fine artists at Lachina who have managed to turn our rudimentary cartoons into instructive pieces of art. We thank the production team at SPi Global led by Thomas Russell.

The Pearson Education marketing team led by Kelly Galli and Christa Pelaez have provided expert guidance in bringing our textbook to the attention of genetics instructors throughout North America and indeed around the world.

Finally, and perhaps most importantly, we thank the scores of gifted genetics instructors and the thousands of genetics students who used the previous editions of our book and the many reviewers and accuracy checkers whose contributions have been invaluable. Many of our users and all of our reviewers have provided comments and feedback that have immeasurably improved this third edition. We particularly want to thank Ben Harrison at the University of Alaska, Anchorage; Pamela Sandstrom at the University of

Nevada, Reno; Christopher Halweg at North Carolina State University; and Nancy Staub at Gonzaga University for their more than generous expert advice.

Reviewers

Jade Atallah, *University of Toronto*
Michelle Boissiere, *Xavier University of Louisiana*
Sarah Chavez, *Washington University*
Claire Cronmiller, *University of Virginia*
Robert Dotson, *Tulane University*
Steven Finkel, *University of Southern California*
Benjamin Harrison, *University of Alaska Anchorage*
Laura Hill, *University of Vermont*
Adam Hrincevich, *Louisiana State University*
Steven Karpowicz, *University of Central Oklahoma*
Kirkwood Land, *University of the Pacific*
Craig Miller, *University of California at Berkeley*
Jessica Muhlin, *Maine Maritime Academy*
Anna Newman, *University of Houston*
Joanne Odden, *Pacific University Oregon*
Matthew Skerritt, *Corning Community College*
Nancy Staub, *Gonzaga University*
David Waddell, *University of North Florida*
Cynthia Wagner, *University of Maryland Baltimore County*
Rahul Warrior, *University of California at Irvine*

Supplements and Media Contributors

Laura Hill Bermingham, *University of Vermont*
Pat Calie, *Eastern Kentucky University*
Christy Fillman, *University of Colorado–Boulder*
Kathleen Fitzpatrick, *Simon Fraser University*
Michelle Gaudette, *Tufts University*
Christopher Halweg, *North Carolina State University*
Jutta Heller, *Loyola University*
Steven Karpowicz, *University of Central Oklahoma*
David Kass, *Eastern Michigan University*
Fordyce Lux III, *Metropolitan State College*
Peter Mirabito, *University of Kentucky*
Pam Osenkowski, *Loyola University*
Jennifer Osterhage, *University of Kentucky*
Louise Paquin, *McDaniel College*
Fiona Rawle, *University of Toronto Mississauga*
Pamela Sandstrom, *University of Nevada, Reno*
Tara Stoulig, *Southeastern Louisiana State*
Kevin Thornton, *University of California at Irvine*
Douglas Thrower, *University of California, Santa Barbara*
Sarah Van Vickle-Chavez, *Washington University in St. Louis*
Dennis Venema, *Trinity Western University*
Andrew J. Wood, *Southern Illinois University*

The Molecular Basis of Heredity, Variation, and Evolution

CHAPTER OUTLINE

1.1 Modern Genetics Is in Its Second Century

1.2 The Structure of DNA Suggests a Mechanism for Replication

1.3 DNA Transcription and Messenger RNA Translation Express Genes

1.4 Genetic Variation Can Be Detected by Examining DNA, RNA, and Proteins

1.5 Evolution Has a Genetic Basis

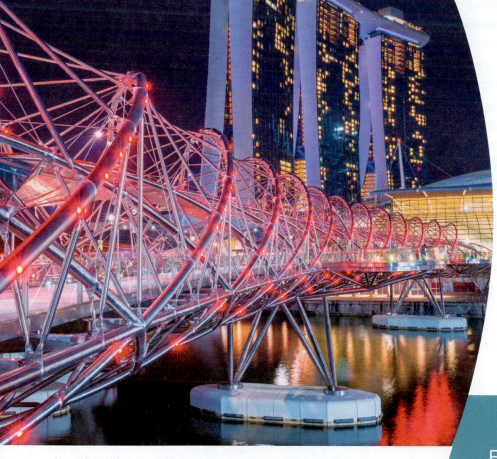

The Helix Bridge is a 280-meter pedestrian bridge spanning the marina in downtown Singapore. The bridge design is inspired by the structure of DNA and features two twisting helices with colored lights representing the A–T and G–C base pairs.

ESSENTIAL IDEAS

- Modern genetics developed during the 20th century and is a prominent discipline of the biological sciences.

- DNA replication produces exact copies of the original molecule.

- The "central dogma of biology" describing the relationship between DNA, RNA, and protein is a foundation of molecular biology.

- Gene expression is a two-step process that first produces an RNA transcript of a gene and then synthesizes an amino acid string by translation of RNA.

- Inherited variation can be detected by laboratory methods that examine DNA, RNA, and proteins.

- Evolution is a foundation of modern genetics that occurs through four processes.

L ife is astounding, both in the richness of its history and in its diversity. From the single-celled organisms that evolved billions of years ago have descended millions of species of microorganisms, plants, and animals. These species are connected by a shared evolutionary past that is revealed by the study of genetics, the science that explores genome composition and organization and the transmission, expression, variation, and evolution of hereditary characteristics of organisms.

Genetics is a dynamic discipline that finds applications everywhere humans interact with one another and with other organisms. In research laboratories, on farms, in grocery stores, in medical offices, in courtrooms, and in other settings, genetics plays a prominent and expanding role in our lives. Modern genetics is an increasingly genome- and gene-based discipline—that is, it is increasingly focused on the entirety of the hereditary information carried by organisms and on the molecular processes that control and regulate the expression of genes. Despite its increasingly gene-focused emphasis, however, genetics retains a strong interest in traditional areas of inquiry and investigation—heredity, variation, and evolution. The fascinating discipline of genetics explores the basis of life—past and present—and its study will provide you with an exciting and rewarding journey.

In this chapter, we survey the scope of modern genetics and reacquaint you with some basic information about deoxyribonucleic acid—DNA, the carrier of genetic information. We begin with a brief overview of the origins and contemporary range of genetic science. Next we retrace some of the fundamentals of *DNA replication,* and of *transcription* and *translation* (the two main components of gene expression), by reviewing what you learned about these processes in previous biology courses. We also look at some research techniques that are indispensable for studying genetic variation in the laboratory; and we meet the most prominent of the modern-day "-omic" avenues of research and investigation in genetics. The chapter's final section describes the central position of evolution in genetics and discusses the roles of heredity and variation in evolution.

1.1 Modern Genetics Is in Its Second Century

Humans have been implicitly aware of genetics for more than 10,000 years (**Figure 1.1**). From the time of the domestication of rice in Asia, maize in Central America, and wheat in the Middle East, humans have recognized that desirable traits found in plants and animals can be reproduced and enhanced in succeeding generations through selective mating. On the other hand, explicit exploration and understanding of the hereditary principles of genetics—what we might think of as the science of modern genetics—is a much more recent development.

The Development of Modern Genetics

In a sense, modern genetics can trace its early roots back to the invention of the compound microscope in the 1590s by a father and son team of Dutch eyeglass makers, Hans and Zacharias Jansen. The genesis of ideas about cells—their origins, structure, contents—was made possible by the Jansen's invention, and by numerous improvements in microscope technology over the centuries. Collectively, these developments paved the way for theories like the cell theory and the germ plasm theory that are foundational to modern genetics.

In 1665, Robert Hooke first described cells he observed in thin sections of cork. In the 1670s and 1680s, Anton van Leeuwenhoek, often called the father of microbiology, described the abundance of tiny single-celled organisms in pond water and made numerous observations of bacteria. In the 1830s, Matthias Schleiden and Theodor Schwann described cells in plants and in animals, respectively, and are credited with proposing the cell theory that states all life is composed of cells and that cells are the basic building blocks of organisms. Rudolph Virchow expanded and extended the ideas of the cell theory in 1855, declaring that "every cell stems from another cell." Virchow's contribution was important for giving the cell theory an evolutionary basis. In 1831, Robert Brown provided the first description of the nucleus of a cell; and after descriptions by others of the contents of the nucleus—including chromosomes—Walter Fleming, Theodor Boveri, and Walter Sutton in the 1880s described chromosome separation during cell division, cementing the importance of the cell theory and giving rise to the germ plasm theory.

It was August Weismann who proposed the germ plasm theory, in 1889, bringing together multiple threads of evidence linking chromosomes and heredity. The germ plasm theory posits that reproductive organs (ovaries and testes, for example) carry full sets of genetic information and that the sperm and egg cells they produce carry the genetic information brought together in fertilization. This was followed by the proposal of Edmund Beecher Wilson in 1895 that DNA, known at the time as "nuclein," was the hereditary molecule and a component of chromosomes (whose separation during cell division was observed, as noted above, by Fleming, Boveri, and Sutton). Just a few years later, a British physician-scientist named Archibald Garrod identified the first human hereditary condition, an autosomal recessive disorder called alkaptonuria, by examining several generations of British families with the condition.

The ideas embodied in the cell theory, the germ plasm theory, and Wilson's proposal that DNA was the hereditary molecule took shape against a backdrop of other developments in 19th century biology. The most important of these was Charles Darwin's theory of evolution by natural selection in 1859. Darwin recognized the importance of heredity in his theory of evolution, but despite his attempts to decipher a mechanism, he was never able to describe how organisms transmitted their hereditary traits. Little did Darwin know that the explanation for hereditary transmission was already available. In 1866, Gregor Mendel published the descriptions and analysis of his experiments of the inheritance of seven traits in pea plants. Although Mendel's work would lie in obscurity for nearly 35 years—until more than a decade after his death—his experiments and analysis form the foundation of modern genetics.

(a)

(b)

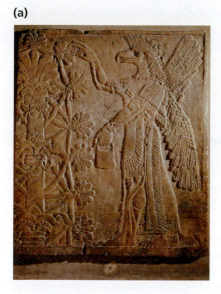

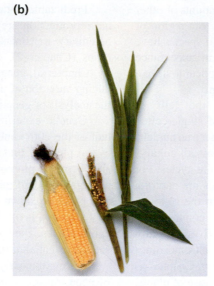

Figure 1.1 **Ancient applications of genetics.** (a) An early record of human genetic manipulation is this Assyrian relief (882–859 BCE) showing priests in bird masks artificially pollinating date palms. (b) Modern maize (left) developed through human domestication of its wild ancestor teosinte (right).

The Four Phases of Modern Genetics

In 1900, three botanists working independently of one another—Carl Correns in Germany, Hugo de Vries in Holland, and Erich von Tschermak in Austria—reached strikingly similar conclusions about the pattern of transmission of hereditary traits in plants. Each reported that his results mirrored those published in 1866 by an obscure amateur botanist and Augustinian monk named Gregor Mendel. (Mendel's work is discussed in Chapter 2.) Although Correns, de Vries, and Tschermak had actually *rediscovered* an explanation of hereditary transmission that Mendel had published 34 years earlier, their announcement of the identification of principles of hereditary transmission gave modern genetics its start.

Biologists immediately began testing, verifying, and expanding on the newly appreciated explanation of heredity. In 1901, during a train ride from Cambridge to London, William Bateson read the publication by Archibald Garrod describing the pattern of occurrence of alkaptonuria and immediately realized that Garrod's description depicted "exactly the conditions most likely to enable a rare, usually recessive character to show itself." According to his own retelling, Bateson was converted into a firm believer in Mendelism during that train ride. Garrod—with Bateson's interpretive assistance—having produced the first documented example of a human hereditary disorder, continued to study alkaptonuria for decades, eventually devising the designation "inborn error of metabolism," a phrase still used today to describe many recessive genetic conditions.

From that starting point in the first years of the 20th century, modern genetics has moved through four phases that we discuss below and then explore in greater detail as we advance through the book. The first phase was the identification of the cellular and chromosomal basis of heredity. The second phase was the identification of DNA as the hereditary material. Phase three was the description of the

informational and regulatory processes of heredity, that is, the encoding of information in genes and the processes of transcription and translation. The current and fourth phase of modern genetics can be described as the genomic era. This phase began in the 1980s with the completion of the first genome sequences, but it reached popular recognition in 2001 when the complete human genome was produced.

Location of the Genetic Material Fleming, Sutton, and Boveri independently used microscopy to observe chromosome movement during cell division in reproductive cells. They each noted that the patterns of chromosome movement mirrored the transmission of the newly rediscovered Mendelian hereditary units. This finding implied that the hereditary units, or *genes,* posited by Mendel are located on *chromosomes.* We now know that **genes**—the physical units of heredity—are composed of defined DNA sequences that collectively control gene *transcription* (described later in the chapter) and contain the information to produce RNA molecules, one category of which is called messenger RNA, or mRNA, and is used to produce proteins by *translation* (described later in the chapter). **Chromosomes** consist of single long molecules of double-stranded DNA that in plants and animals are bound by many different kinds of protein that give chromosomes their structure and can affect the transcription of genes the chromosomes carry. The chromosomes of sexually reproducing organisms typically occur in pairs known as **homologous pairs,** or, more simply, as **homologs.** Each chromosome carries many genes, and homologs carry genes for the same traits in the same order on each member of the pair.

Bacteria and archaea are single-celled organisms that do not have a true nucleus. In almost all cases, species of bacteria and archaea have a single, usually circular chromosome. As a consequence, in the genome of these organisms, there is just one copy of each gene, a condition described as **haploid.** Bacterial and archaeal chromosomes are bound by a relatively small amount of protein. Limited amounts of other proteins help localize bacterial chromosomes to a region of the cell known as the **nucleoid**. Some archaeal species have chromosomes and associated proteins that in appearance resemble those in bacteria, but other species appear to have a more eukaryote-like chromosome organization.

In contrast to bacteria and archaea, the cells of eukaryotes—a classification that includes all single-celled and multicellular plants and animals—contain a true nucleus holding multiple sets of chromosomes. Almost all eukaryotes have haploid and **diploid** stages in their life cycles. For example, sperm and eggs produced in animals are haploid, having one copy of each chromosome pair in the genome. In the diploid state, the eukaryotic genome contains two copies—a homologous pair—of each gene. (Even in a diploid cell, genes located on eukaryotic sex chromosomes might not be present in two copies, as we see in Chapter 4.) Numerous eukaryotic genomes, particularly those of plants, contain more than two copies of each chromosome—a genome composition known as **polyploidy**.

In addition to the chromosomes carried in their nuclei—the so-called nuclear chromosomes—plant and animal cells also contain genetic material in specialized organelles called **mitochondria** (singular: *mitochondrion*), and plant cells contain a third type of gene-containing organelle called **chloroplasts.** Many of these organelles are present by the dozens in each cell, and each mitochondrion or chloroplast carries one or more copies of its own chromosome. Mitochondrial and chloroplast genes produce proteins that work with proteins produced by nuclear genes to perform essential functions in cells—mitochondria are essential for the production of adenosine triphosphate (ATP) that is the principal source of cellular energy, and chloroplasts are necessary for photosynthesis. Mitochondria and chloroplasts are transmitted in the cytoplasm during cell division, and the term **cytoplasmic inheritance** is used to refer to the random distribution of mitochondria and chloroplasts among daughter cells.

Mitochondria and chloroplasts have an evolutionary history, having descended from ancient parasitic bacterial invasion of eukaryotic cells. Since the time of their acquisition by eukaryotes, mitochondria and chloroplasts have evolved an endosymbiotic relationship with their eukaryotic hosts, and the precise genetic content of mitochondria and chloroplasts varies by eukaryotic host species (see Chapter 17).

A complete set of nuclear chromosomes are transmitted during the cell-division process called **mitosis**, to produce genetically identical daughter cells. In contrast, sexual reproduction to produce offspring occurs by the cell-division process called **meiosis**, that produces reproductive or sex cells, often identified as **gametes**—sperm and egg in animals and pollen and egg in plants. The gametes of a diploid species are haploid and contain one chromosome from each of the homologous pairs of chromosomes in the genome. The union of haploid gametes at fertilization produces a diploid fertilized egg that begins mitotic division to produce the zygote.

Predictable patterns of gene transmission during sexual reproduction are a focus of later chapters that discuss hereditary transmission and the analysis of transmission ratios (Chapter 2), cell division and chromosome heredity (Chapter 3), gene action and interaction of genes in producing variation of physical characteristics (Chapter 4), and the analysis of genetic linkage between genes (Chapter 5).

Genetic experiments taking place in roughly the first half of the 20th century developed the concept of the gene as the physical unit of heredity and revealed the relationship between **phenotype**, meaning the observable traits of an organism, and **genotype**, meaning the genetic constitution of an organism. Biologists also described how hereditary variation is attributable to alternative forms of a gene, called **alleles.** The alleles of a gene have differences in DNA sequence that alter the product of the gene.

During the early decades of the 20th century, the study of gene transmission was established as a central focus of genetics. The concepts of gene action and gene interaction in producing phenotype variation were described, as was the concept of mapping genes along chromosomes. It was also during this period that evolutionary biologists developed gene-based models of evolution. These, too, are integral to genetic analysis, and their use continues to the present day.

Identifying the Genetic Material An experiment conducted in 1944 by Oswald Avery, Colin MacLeod, and Maclyn McCarty identified *deoxyribonucleic acid (DNA)* as the hereditary material and is commonly credited with inaugurating the "molecular era" in genetics (see Chapter 7). This new era, which spanned the second half of the 20th century and continues to the present day, began an effort to discover the molecular structure of DNA. Molecular genetic research reached a milestone in 1953, when the experimental work of many biologists, including, most famously, James Watson, Francis Crick, Maurice Wilkins, and Rosalind Franklin, led to the identification of the double-helical structure of DNA. A few years later, in 1958, the general mechanism of DNA replication was ascertained. We examine details of this work in Chapter 7.

Describing the Nature and Processing of Genetic Information By the mid-1960s, the basic mechanisms of DNA transcription and messenger RNA (mRNA) translation were laid out, and the genetic code by which mRNA is translated into proteins was deciphered. This period also saw the first descriptions of mechanisms that regulate transcription in cells of different types or in response to a wide variety of stimuli from outside and inside cells. Chapters 8 and 9 are devoted to discussions of transcription and translation, and Chapters 12 and 13 describe processes that regulate gene expression in bacteria and in eukaryotes.

The Genomics Era Gene cloning and the development of recombinant DNA technologies developed and progressed rapidly during the 1970s. By the early 1980s, biologists realized that to properly understand the unity and complexity of life, they would have to study and compare the **genomes** of species—the complete sets of DNA sequences, including all genes and regions controlling genes. This realization launched the "genomics era" in genetics, which continues to expand rapidly today.

Since the inception of genome sequencing, biologists have deciphered thousands of genomes that range in size from a few tens of thousands of DNA base pairs in the simplest viral genomes to tens of billions of base pairs in the largest plant and animal genomes. Fittingly, in 2001, a century after Garrod and Bateson's historic identification of alkaptonuria as a human hereditary disease, collaborative scientific groups from around the world published the completed "first draft" of the human genome. Collective efforts like the Human Genome Project and the other genome sequencing projects that have been and will be undertaken promise to provide databases that will make the second century of genetics every bit as remarkable as its first century. Chapters 14, 15, and 16 are primarily devoted to descriptions of the analysis and functions of genomes.

Genetics—Central to Modern Biology

One of the foundations of modern biology is the demonstration that all life on Earth shares a common origin in the form of the "*last universal common ancestor*," or **LUCA** (**Figure 1.2**). All life is descended from this common ancestor and is most commonly divided into three major domains. These three domains of life are **Eukarya**, **Bacteria**, and **Archaea**.

The three-domain model of life is originally derived from the research of Carl Woese and colleagues in the mid-1970s. In contrast to earlier models, which were based on morphology alone, Woese used molecular sequences to determine phylogenetic relationships between existing organisms and thus to trace the evolution of life. Woese used the sequence of ribosomal RNA (rRNA), a small molecule produced directly from DNA in all organisms, as his basis for comparison. His premise was simple—evolutionary theory predicts that closely related species will have more similarity in their rRNA sequences than will species that are less closely related. Furthermore, species that are members of the same evolutionary lineage will share certain rRNA sequence changes that are not shared with species outside the lineage. Since Woese's work, many researchers have used other molecules to refine and propose additional details to the three-domain model. The tree of life remains a work in progress, but the three-domain model is well established. We use this model in subsequent chapters to compare and contrast molecular features, activities, and processes that shed additional light on the evolutionary relationships between the three domains.

A second foundation of biology is the recognition that the hereditary material—the molecular substance that

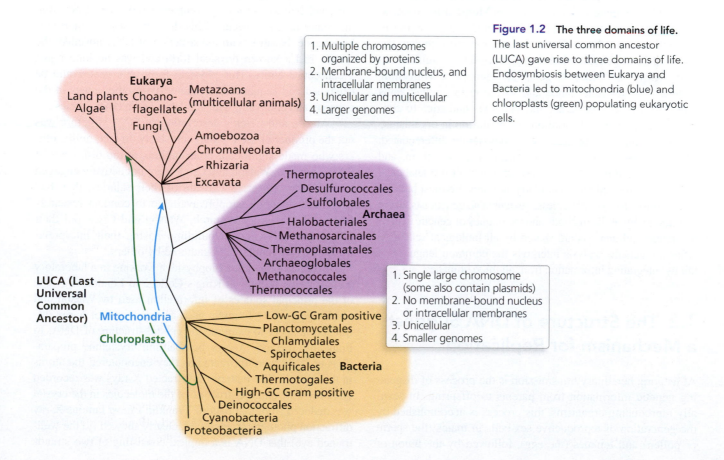

Figure 1.2 The three domains of life. The last universal common ancestor (LUCA) gave rise to three domains of life. Endosymbiosis between Eukarya and Bacteria led to mitochondria (blue) and chloroplasts (green) populating eukaryotic cells.

conveys and stores genetic information—is **deoxyribonucleic acid (DNA)** in all organisms. Certain viruses use **ribonucleic acid (RNA)** as their hereditary material. Most biologists argue that viruses are not alive. Rather, they are obligate intracellular parasites that are noncellular and must invade host cells to reproduce, at the expense of the host cell. In living organisms, DNA has a double-stranded structure described as a **DNA double helix**, or as a **DNA duplex**, consisting of two strands joined together in accordance with specific biochemical rules. Certain viral genomes consist of a small single-stranded DNA molecule that replicates to form a DNA duplex in a host cell.

Eukarya, Bacteria, and Archaea share general mechanisms of **DNA replication**, the process that precisely duplicates the DNA duplex prior to cell division, and they also share general mechanisms of gene expression, the processes through which the genetic information guides development and functioning of an organism. All organisms express their genetic information by a two-step process that begins with **transcription**, a process in which one strand of DNA is used to direct the synthesis of a single strand of RNA. Transcription produces various forms of RNA, including **messenger RNA (mRNA),** which in all organisms undergoes **translation** to produce proteins at structures called **ribosomes**.

As the biological discipline devoted to the examination of all aspects of heredity and variation, between generations and through evolutionary time, genetics is central to modern biology. Modern genetics has three major branches. **Transmission genetics,** also known as **Mendelian genetics**, is the study of the transmission of traits and characteristics in successive generations. **Evolutionary genetics** studies the origins of and genetic relationships between organisms and examines the evolution of genes and genomes. **Molecular genetics** studies inheritance and variation in nucleic acids (DNA and RNA), proteins, and genomes and tries to connect them to inherited variation and evolution in organisms.

These branches of genetics are not rigidly differentiated. There is substantial cross-communication among them, and it is rare to find a geneticist today who doesn't use analytical approaches from all three. Similarly, not only are most biological scientists, to a greater or lesser extent, also geneticists, but in addition many of the methods and techniques of genetic experimentation and analysis are shared by all biological scientists. After all, genetic analysis interprets the common language of life by integrating information from all three branches.

1.2 The Structure of DNA Suggests a Mechanism for Replication

At its core, hereditary transmission is the process of dispersing genetic information from parents to offspring. In sexually reproducing organisms, this process is accomplished by the generation of reproductive sex cells in males (the sperm or pollen) and females (the egg), followed by the union of egg and sperm (animals) or pollen (plants) or spores (yeast) at fertilization, with the subsequent development of an organism. DNA is the hereditary molecule in reproductive cells. Similarly, in somatic (body) cells of plants and animals and in organisms that reproduce by asexual processes, DNA is the hereditary molecule that ensures that successive generations of cells are identical. Clearly, then, discovering the molecular structure of DNA would be the key that opened the door to two fundamental areas of inquiry: (1) how DNA could carry the diverse array of genetic information present in the various genomes of animals and plants; and (2) how the molecule replicated. In this section, we review basic concepts of DNA structure and DNA replication. The molecular details of DNA structure and replication are provided in Chapter 7.

The Discovery of DNA Structure

In the early 1950s, James Watson, an American in his mid-20s who had recently completed a doctoral degree, and Francis Crick, a British biochemist in his mid-30s, began working together at the University of Cambridge, England, to solve the puzzle of DNA structure. Their now-legendary collaboration culminated in a 1953 publication that ignited the molecular era in genetics.

Watson and Crick's paper accurately described the molecular structure of DNA as a double helix composed of two strands of DNA, with an invariant sugar-phosphate backbone on the outside and nucleotide bases—adenine, thymine, guanine, and cytosine—forming complementary base pairs within the center of the molecule. This discovery was of enormous importance, because with the structure of DNA unveiled, the "gene" had a known physical form and was no longer just a conceptual entity. This physical form of a gene could be examined and sequenced, compared with other genes in the genome, and compared with similar genes in other species.

Watson and Crick's description of DNA structure was not the product of their work exclusively. In fact, unlike others who made significant contributions to the discovery of DNA structure, Watson and Crick were not actively engaged in laboratory research. Outside of their salaries, they had very little financial support available to conduct research. In lieu of laboratory research, Watson and Crick put their efforts into DNA-model building, basing their interpretations on experimental data gathered by others.

Rosalind Franklin, a biophysicist working in a laboratory with Maurice Wilkins at King's College in London, was one of the principal sources of information used by Watson and Crick (**Figure 1.3**). Franklin used an early form of X-ray diffraction imagery to examine the crystal structure of DNA. In Franklin's method, X-rays bombarding crystalline preparations of DNA were diffracted as they encountered the atoms in the crystals. The pattern of diffracted X-rays was recorded on X-ray film, and the structure of the molecules in the crystal was deduced from that pattern. Franklin's most famous X-ray diffraction photograph, Photo 51, clearly showed (to the well-trained eye) that DNA is a duplex, consisting of two strands

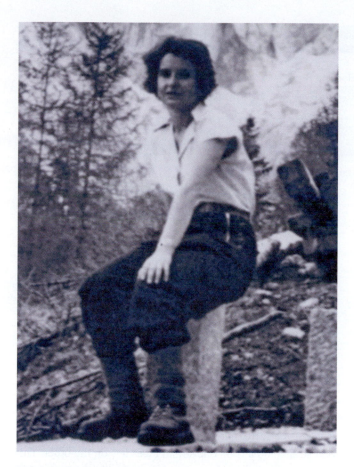

Figure 1.3 **Rosalind Franklin, shown here on holiday, used X-ray diffraction to investigate the structure of DNA.**

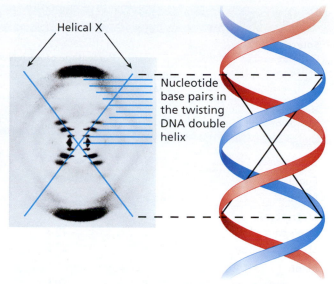

Figure 1.4 **Rosalind Franklin's Photo 51, revealing DNA to be a double helix.** The photo is an image of DNA viewed down the center of the helix from the top. The "rungs" of the twisting helix are base pairs, and the "X" superimposed on the photo identifies the helical shape of the molecule.

twisted around one another in a double helix. **Figure 1.4** shows Photo 51 and provides a schematic interpretation of its distinctive image. The photo captures a DNA double helix from the top. The "X" superimposed on the photo traces the spiral of nucleotide base pairs as it recedes from the focal plane.

There is considerable controversy surrounding the use of Franklin's Photo 51 by Watson and Crick. The essential story is that Wilkins, who did not get along with Franklin, took Photo 51 from a drawer in Franklin's laboratory space and showed it to Watson without Franklin's consent or knowledge. Watson and Wilkins have both admitted in later years that the story is true and that Watson's knowledge of the photo's contents violated scientific ethics. When Watson and Crick published their paper describing DNA structure in the British science periodical *Nature* in 1953, the article following theirs in the same volume was authored by Franklin and Wilkins and provided supporting evidence, including Photo 51. Watson, Crick, and Wilkins were awarded the Nobel Prize in Physiology or Medicine in 1962 for their work on DNA structure. Franklin did not share in the award since she died in 1958, at the age of 38, of ovarian cancer. The Nobel Prize is not awarded posthumously.

In devising their DNA model, Watson and Crick combined Franklin's X-ray diffraction data with information published a few years earlier by Erwin Chargaff. Chargaff had determined the percentages of the four DNA nucleotide bases in the genomes of a wide array of organisms and had concluded that (allowing for experimental error) the percentages of adenine and thymine are approximately equal to one another and that the percentages of cytosine and guanine are equal to one another as well (**Table 1.1**). Known as **Chargaff's rule**, this information helped Watson and Crick formulate the hypothesis that DNA nucleotides are arranged in **complementary base pairs**. Adenine, on one strand of the double helix, pairs only with thymine on the other DNA strand, and cytosine pairs only with guanine to form the other base pair. With these data, their own knowledge of biochemistry, and their analysis of incorrect models of DNA structure, Watson and Crick built a table-top model of DNA out of implements and materials scattered around their largely inactive research laboratory space—wire, tin, tape, and paper, supported by ring stands and clamps (**Figure 1.5**).

DNA Nucleotides

Each strand of the double helix is composed of **DNA nucleotides** that have three principal components: a five-carbon deoxyribose sugar, a phosphate group, and one of four nitrogen-containing nucleotide bases, designated **adenine** (A), **guanine** (G), **thymine** (T), and **cytosine** (C) (**Figure 1.6**). The nucleotides forming a strand are linked together by a covalent **phosphodiester bond** between the 5′ phosphate group of one nucleotide and the 3′ hydroxyl (OH) group of the adjacent nucleotide. Phosphodiester bonding leads to alternation of deoxyribose sugars and phosphate groups along the strand and gives the molecule a sugar-phosphate backbone.

Table 1.1	Nucleotide-Base Composition of Various Genomes					
Source Genome	Percentage of Each Nucleotide Base				Ratios	
	Adenine (A)	Guanine (G)	Cytosine (C)	Thymine (T)	G+C	G/C
Bacteria						
E. coli (B)	23.8	26.8	26.3	23.1	53.1	1.02
Yeast						
S. cerevisiae	31.3	18.7	17.1	32.9	35.8	1.09
Fungi						
N. crassa	23.0	27.1	26.6	23.3	53.7	1.02
Invertebrate						
C. elegans	31.2	19.3	20.5	29.1	39.8	0.94
D. melanogaster	27.3	22.5	22.5	27.6	45.0	1.00
Plant						
A. thaliana	29.1	20.5	20.7	29.7	41.2	0.99
Vertebrate						
M. musculus	29.2	21.7	19.7	29.4	41.4	1.10
H. sapiens	30.6	19.7	19.8	30.3	39.5	0.99

The nucleotide bases are hydrophobic (water-avoiding) and naturally orient toward the water-free interior of the duplex. The bases can occur in any order along one strand of the molecule, but DNA is most stable as a duplex of two strands that have complementary base sequences, so that an A on one strand faces a T on the second strand and a G on one strand faces a C on the other. This complementary base pairing is the basis of Chargaff's rule and produces equal percentages of A and T and of C and G in double-stranded DNA molecules. **Hydrogen bonds**, noncovalent bonds consisting of weak electrostatic attractions, form between complementary base pairs to join the two DNA strands into a double helix. Two hydrogen bonds form between each A–T base pair and three hydrogen bonds are formed between each G–C base pair. Each strand of DNA has a 5′ end and a 3′ end. These designations refer to the phosphate group (5′) and hydroxyl group (3′) at the opposite ends of each strand of DNA and establish **strand polarity**, that is, the 5′-to-3′ orientation of each strand. The differences at each end of a strand allow the ends to be readily distinguished from one another. (Complementary strands of DNA are **antiparallel**, meaning that the polarities of the complementary strands run in opposite directions—one strand is oriented 5′ to 3′ and the complementary strand is oriented 3′ to 5′. Genetic Analysis 1.1 guides you through a problem that tests your understanding of base-pair complementation and complementary strand polarity.

If you are like many biology students, you have probably wondered from time to time what DNA actually looks like, both on the macroscopic and microscopic level. Even today's best microscopes have difficulty capturing high-resolution images of DNA, although computer-aided techniques for analyzing molecular structure can produce an interpretation of its microscopic appearance, as you'll see, for example, in Chapters 7, 8, and 9. However, you do not need sophisticated instrumentation to produce a sample of DNA that you can hold in your hand. Experimental Insight 1.1 presents a

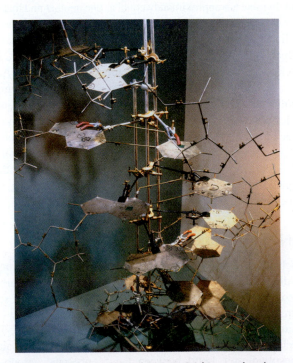

Figure 1.5 James Watson and Francis Crick's metal-and-wire model of DNA constructed in 1953.

Ⓠ Notice that the A-T base pairs and the G-C base pairs in this model are each connected by two wires. If the wires represent hydrogen bonds, what is wrong with the model? (See also Figure 1.6)

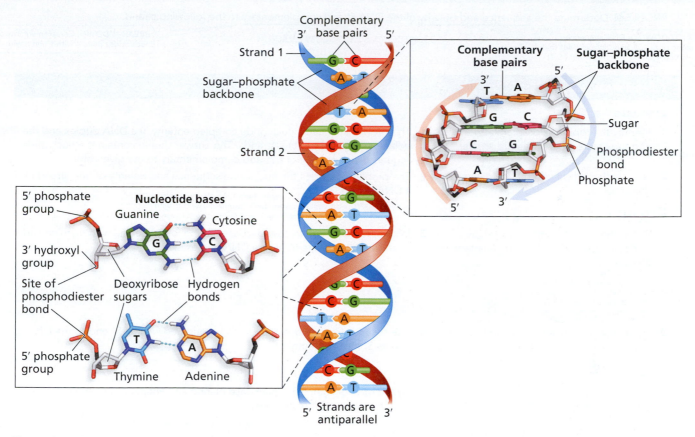

Figure 1.6 DNA composition and structure. DNA nucleotides contain a deoxyribose sugar, a phosphate group, and a nucleotide base (A, T, G, or C). Phosphodiester bonds join adjacent nucleotides in each strand, and hydrogen bonds join complementary nucleotides of strands that have antiparallel orientation.

simple recipe for DNA isolation you can do at home with common and safe household compounds.

DNA Replication

The identification of the double-helical structure of DNA established a starting point for a new set of questions about heredity. The first of these questions concerned how DNA replicates. After correctly describing DNA structure in their 1953 paper, Watson and Crick closed with a directive for future research on the question of DNA replication: "It has not escaped our notice that the specific base-pairing we have proposed immediately suggests a possible copying mechanism for the genetic material."

Indeed, as a consequence of the A-T and G-C complementary base-pairing rules, it was evident that each single strand of DNA contains the information necessary to generate the second strand of DNA and that DNA replication generates two identical DNA duplexes from the original parental duplex during each replication cycle. At the time Watson and Crick described the structure of DNA, however, the mechanism of replication was not known. It would take another 5 years for Matthew Meselson and Franklin Stahl, in an ingenious experiment of simple design, to prove that DNA replicates by a *semiconservative* mechanism (see Chapter 7).

In **semiconservative replication,** the mechanism by which DNA usually replicates, the two complementary strands of original DNA separate from one another, and each strand acts as a template to direct the synthesis of a new, complementary strand of DNA with antiparallel polarity. The mechanism is termed "semiconservative" because after the completion of DNA replication, each new duplex is composed of one **parental strand** (conserved from the original DNA) and one newly synthesized **daughter strand** (**Figure 1.7**).

DNA replication begins at an origin of replication, with the breaking of hydrogen bonds that hold the strands together. (This process is much like what happens when a zipper comes undone.) DNA polymerases are the enzymes active in DNA replication. Using each parental DNA strand as a template, these enzymes identify the nucleotide that is complementary to the first unpaired nucleotide on the parental strand and then catalyze formation of a phosphodiester bond to join the new nucleotide to the previous nucleotide in the nascent (growing) daughter strand.

The biochemistry of nucleic acids and DNA polymerases dictates that DNA strands elongate only in the 5′-to-3′ direction. In other words, nucleotides are added exclusively to the 3′ end of the nascent strand, leading to 5′-to-3′ growth. Like the parental duplex, each new DNA duplex contains antiparallel strands. Each parental strand–daughter strand combination forms a new double helix of DNA that is an exact replica of the original parental duplex.

PROBLEM Determine the sequence and polarity of the DNA strand complementary to the following strand:

3′-...ACGGATCCTCCCTAGTGCGTAATACG...-5′

BREAK IT DOWN: A DNA sequence is a string of A, G, T, and C nucleotides that is 5′ on one end and 3′ on the other (p. 7).

BREAK IT DOWN: Complementarity of DNA nucleotides pairs A with T and G with C (p. 8).

Solution Strategies	Solution Steps
Evaluate	
1. Identify the topic this problem addresses and the nature of the required answer.	1. This problem concerns nucleotide complementarity in a DNA duplex and the polarity of complementary strands. The answer should contain the nucleotide sequence and polarity of a strand complementary to the given one.
2. Identify the critical information given in the problem.	2. The problem provides the nucleotide sequence and polarity of one strand of a DNA duplex.
	PITFALL: Always check the polarity of a strand you are given; don't assume it's written with either the 5′ or 3′ end facing a certain way.
Deduce	
3. Recall the base-pairing relationships of DNA nucleotides in complementary strands.	3. In complementary DNA strands, base pairing joins adenine with thymine and guanine with cytosine to form a DNA duplex.
TIP: Complementary DNA strands are antiparallel, with one strand 3′ → 5′ and the other 5′ → 3′.	
4. Recall the polarity relationship of complementary DNA strands.	4. The second strand of this duplex will be oriented with its 5′ end to the left and its 3′ end to the right.
Solve	
5. Give the sequence and polarity of the complementary DNA strand.	5. By the rules of complementary base pairing and antiparallel strand orientation, the second DNA strand is
	5′-TGCCTAGGAGGGATCACGCATTATGC-3′

For more practice, see Problems 12, 15, and 16.   Visit the Study Area to access study tools.   **Mastering Genetics**

EXPERIMENTAL INSIGHT 1.1

DNA Isolation on Your Kitchen Countertop—Try This at Home!

For all the abundance of DNA in cells, its molecular structure is too small to see without the aid of the most powerful electron microscopes. However, that doesn't mean DNA must remain invisible to the naked eye. The key to seeing it is simply a question of volume. If enough DNA is collected together, it can be seen—although not, of course, in its molecular detail. Using a rich source of DNA (such as onions, which are available year-round, or strawberries, whose nuclei contain eight copies of each chromosome) and a few familiar household items, you can collect a visible sample of DNA in about 30 minutes.

INGREDIENTS

1 small peeled onion (about 1 cup) or about 1 cup strawberries with leaves removed

1 to 2 cups water with 1 teaspoon of dissolved salt per cup

2 tablespoons dishwashing liquid

1 tablespoon meat tenderizer (containing "papain" from papaya)

4 to 6 ounces isopropyl ("rubbing") alcohol (95% is best, but 70% is sufficient)

EQUIPMENT

Food processor (for onion) or a potato masher or ricer (for strawberries)

Small bowl

Clear glass jar or container with vertical sides

Cheesecloth to layer over the top of the glass container with a few inches to spare all around

1 rubber band to go around the glass container

1 chopstick or a similar wooden implement

DIRECTIONS

1. Peel onion and finely chop in food processor or thoroughly mash strawberries in bowl.

2. Add 1 to 2 cups water to onion and process into a fine slurry. Pour slurry into small bowl. If using strawberries, add about 1 cup water and mash into a fine slurry.

3. Add 2 tablespoons liquid dishwashing soap to slurry and stir gently. Be careful not to let the soap get foamy. Let mixture stand at least 10 to 15 minutes (longer is fine) while the soap breaks down the cell and nuclear membranes.

4. Add 1 tablespoon meat tenderizer to mixture, stir gently, and let stand at least 10 to 15 minutes (longer is fine). The papain will digest much of the protein released by the ruptured cells and also the proteins attached to DNA.

5. Place 2 to 3 layers cheesecloth loosely over the opening of the glass container, allowing the cloth to form a small "bowl" inside the opening. Use the rubber band to hold the cheesecloth in place. Pour the slurry mixture through the cheesecloth, scooping out the onion or strawberry debris as it fills the cheesecloth bowl. Approximately

8 to 12 ounces of "juice" will collect at the bottom of the container. Discard the cheesecloth and its contents.

6. Pour the alcohol into the juice and stir very briefly. Let the juice mixture stand for at least 5 to 10 minutes. As the juice settles, the alcohol rises to the top, and the large mass of floating cottony material in it is DNA.

7. When the alcohol has completely separated from the juice, you can "spool" the DNA onto a chopstick by slowly twirling the stick in the cottony DNA.

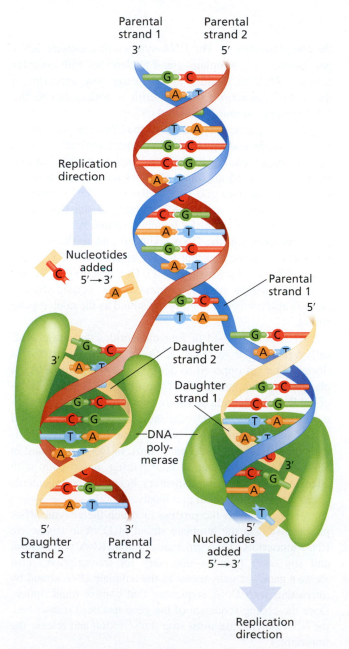

Figure 1.7 Semiconservative DNA replication. Each parental DNA strand serves as the template for synthesis of its daughter strand. DNA polymerase synthesizes daughter strands one nucleotide at a time.

1.3 DNA Transcription and Messenger RNA Translation Express Genes

The **central dogma of biology** is a statement describing the flow of hereditary information. It summarizes the critical relationships between DNA, RNA, and protein; the functional role that DNA plays in maintaining, directing, and regulating the expression of genetic information; and the roles played by RNA and proteins in gene function. Francis Crick proposed the original version of the central dogma, shown in **Figure 1.8a**, in 1956 to encapsulate the role DNA plays in directing transcription of RNA and, in turn, the role messenger RNA plays in translation of proteins. As Crick told the story years later, he wrote this concept as "DNA → RNA → protein" (spoken as "DNA to RNA to protein") on a slip of paper and taped it to the wall above his desk to remind himself of the direction of information transfer during the expression of genetic information. The most important idea it conveys is that DNA does not code directly for protein. Rather, DNA makes up the genome of an organism and is a permanent repository of genetic information in each cell, directing gene expression by the transcription of DNA to RNA and, ultimately, the production of proteins.

Over the decades since Crick first introduced the central dogma, biologists have developed a clear understanding of the role of DNA in maintaining and expressing genetic information. Most of the details of the two-stage process by which genetic information in sequences of DNA is transcribed to RNA and then translated to protein are known, as described in later chapters (transcription in Chapter 8 and translation in Chapter 9). For example, biologists now know that several forms of RNA are found in cells, and all these RNA molecules are transcribed from DNA and play a variety of roles in cells, but only mRNA is translated.

Two important categories of RNA that are not translated but nonetheless play critical roles in translation are ribosomal RNA and transfer RNA. **Ribosomal RNA (rRNA)** forms part of the ribosomes, the plentiful cellular structures where protein assembly takes place. **Transfer RNA (tRNA)**

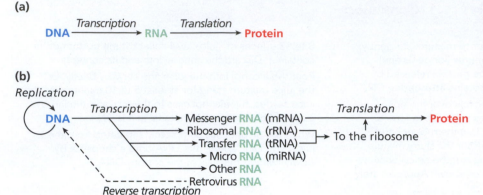

Figure 1.8 The central dogma of biology. (a) Francis Crick's original central dogma of biology. **(b)** The updated central dogma of biology.

In one sentence each, write your own definition of transcription and of translation.

carries **amino acids**, the building blocks of proteins, to ribosomes. An updated central dogma of biology is shown in **Figure 1.8b**. In addition to mRNA, rRNA, and tRNA, the figure identifies **reverse transcription**, a form of information flow in which an enzyme called reverse transcriptase synthesizes DNA from an RNA template that comes from RNA-containing viruses (retroviruses). The figure also identifies micro-RNA (miRNA), the focus of a rapidly emerging new area of RNA investigation that studies the role of these small RNA molecules in the regulation of gene expression in plants and animals (see Chapter 13).

Transcription

Transcription is the process by which information in a DNA sequence is converted into an RNA sequence. Transcription uses one strand of the DNA making up a gene to direct synthesis of a single-stranded RNA transcript. The DNA strand from which the transcript is synthesized is called

the **template strand**. The RNA-synthesizing enzyme RNA polymerase pairs template-strand nucleotides with complementary RNA nucleotides to synthesize new transcript in the 5′-to-3′ direction; the transcript is antiparallel to the DNA template strand (**Figure 1.9**).

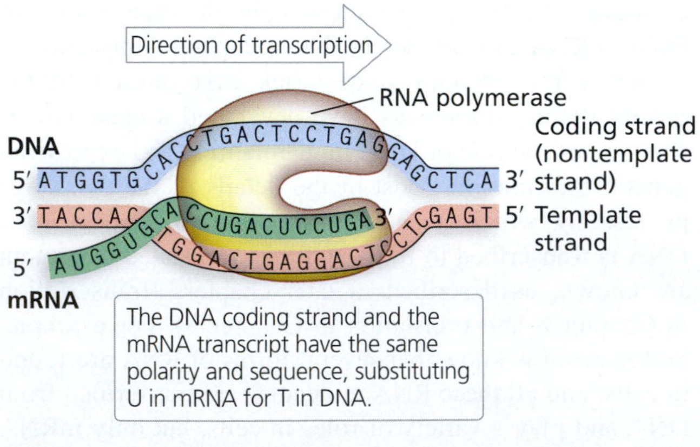

The complementary partner of the DNA template strand is known as the **coding strand**. In the past, the coding strand has also been identified as the "nontemplate strand," but that term is rarely used anymore. Because the coding strand is both complementary and antiparallel to the DNA template strand, it has the same 5′ → 3′ polarity as the RNA transcript synthesized from the template strand; moreover, the RNA transcript and the DNA coding strand are identical in nucleotide sequence, except for the appearance of U in the place of T (see discussion below). Our descriptions in this book will refer to this DNA strand as the "coding strand," but it is also correct to identify the strand as the nontemplate strand.

RNA is composed of four nucleotides that are chemically very similar to DNA. RNA nucleotides consist of a ribose sugar (as opposed to deoxyribose found in DNA), a phosphate group, and one of four nitrogenous bases. Three of the RNA nucleotide bases are adenine, cytosine, and guanine. They are identical to the same nucleotide bases found in DNA. The fourth RNA base is **uracil (U)**. It is chemically closely related to thymine; thus, in DNA–RNA and in RNA–RNA complementary base pairing, uracil pairs with adenine. All other complementary base-pair arrangements are as we described them previously.

Transcription is the process in which the enzyme RNA polymerase uses the template strand of DNA to synthesize RNA transcripts. To begin transcription, RNA polymerase, and any other proteins necessary for transcription, must locate a gene and gain access to the template DNA strand by interacting with DNA sequences that control transcription. Once the coding sequence of the gene has been transcribed, the RNA polymerase must stop transcription and release the transcript.

Promoters are the most common type of DNA sequences controlling transcription. Promoters are recognized by RNA polymerase, and they direct RNA

Figure 1.9 The correspondence of mRNA to DNA template and coding strands. RNA and DNA share the nucleotide bases adenine (A), guanine (G), and cytosine (C), but RNA contains uracil (U), whereas DNA contains thymine (T).

Write out the complementary base-pair relationship of DNA nucleotides to RNA nucleotides.

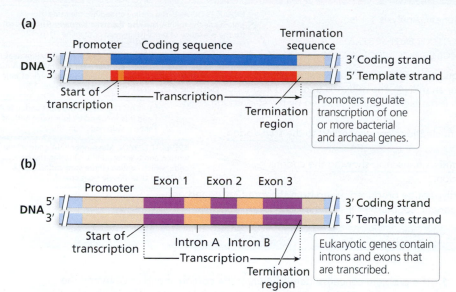

Figure 1.10 **Gene structure.** Coding sequences contain information to be transcribed into RNA. Promoter sequences regulate the initiation of transcription, and termination sequences control the cessation of transcription. **(a)** Bacterial and most, but not all, archaeal genes contain a single coding sequence per gene, although a promoter may regulate the transcription of more than one gene. **(b)** In eukaryotic genes, the coding sequence is split up into exons, which are separated by introns.

polymerase to a nearby gene. Promoters themselves are regulatory sequences and are not transcribed. Instead, the transcription of a gene begins near the promoter at the **start of transcription**, the DNA location where transcription of a sequence begins. Transcription ends at the **termination sequence**, where another DNA sequence facilitates the cessation of transcription (**Figure 1.10a**). In bacteria and archaea, protein-producing genes are transcribed into mRNA that is quickly translated to produce the protein. Eukaryotic genes have a different structure than do bacterial and most archaeal genes. Nearly all eukaryotic genes are subdivided into **exons**, which contain the coding information that will be used during translation, and **introns**, which intervene between exons and are removed from the transcript before translation (**Figure 1.10b**). Bacterial genes do not contain introns, and only a tiny number of archaeal genes are suspected to contain introns. The removal of introns from eukaryotic mRNA and other modifications before translation occur in the nucleus (see Chapter 8).

Translation

Translation converts the genetic message of mRNA into sequences of amino acids using the *genetic code*. The amino acids are joined to one another by a covalent bond called a **peptide bond**. The resulting string of amino acids is a **polypeptide**, which upon folding makes up all or part of a **protein**.

Translation of mRNA occurs at ribosomes, where sets of three consecutive nucleotides in the mRNA, each set called a **codon,** specify the amino acid at each position of a polypeptide. Each mRNA codon is a triplet of RNA nucleotides coded by three complementary DNA nucleotides on the template strand. The DNA nucleotides complementary to codon nucleotides are known as the DNA triplet (**Figure 1.11a**). Translation begins with mRNA attaching to a ribosome in a manner that places the **start codon,** the

codon specifying the first amino acid of a polypeptide, in the necessary location (**Figure 1.11b**). The start codon is most commonly 5'-AUG-3', and is the codon at which translation begins. The ribosome reads the start codon and then each subsequent codon, as the ribosome moves $5' \rightarrow 3'$ along the mRNA to assemble the amino acid string.

Amino acids are transported to ribosomes by transfer RNAs (tRNAs). At each codon, complementary base pairing occurs between codon nucleotides and a three-nucleotide sequence of tRNA called an **anticodon**. This interaction assembles amino acids in the order dictated by the mRNA sequence. Ribosomal proteins power the continuous progression of the ribosome along mRNA and catalyze peptide bond formation in the growing polypeptide chain. Translation continues until the ribosome encounters a **stop codon** thus bringing translation to a halt.

The **genetic code**, through which mRNA codons specify amino acids, was deciphered by a series of experiments that took place during the early 1960s. The experiments revealed that the genetic code contains 64 codons; every codon consists of three positions that are each filled by one of the four RNA nucleotides. An mRNA codon is read in the 5'-to-3' direction: The first base of the codon is at its 5' end, the third base is at its 3' end, and the second base is in the middle.

A total of 61 of the 64 codons specify amino acids, and the other 3 are the stop codons. The 64 codons and their amino acids are displayed in **Table A** (inside the book front cover) using the three-letter and one-letter abbreviations for the amino acids. **Table B** (also inside the book front cover) lists the names and abbreviations of each amino acid, along with their codons. The genetic code is redundant, with individual amino acids encoded by as many as six codons and as few as one codon.

Genetic Analysis 1.2 allows you to work through the transcription and translation of the DNA sequence assessed in Genetic Analysis 1.1.

PROBLEM The DNA duplex identified in Genetic Analysis 1.1 is

```
3'-...ACGGATCCTCCCTAGTGCGTAATACG...-5'
5'-...TGCCTAGGAGGGATCACGCATTATGC...-3'
```

One strand of the double-stranded DNA sequence serves as the coding strand and the other as the template strand that is transcribed to produce an mRNA. The mRNA is translated into a polypeptide containing five amino acids, the first of which is methionine (Met), encoded by the start codon AUG. The mRNA also contains a stop codon.

a. Identify the DNA coding strand and the nucleotides corresponding to the start codon, amino acid codons, and the stop codon.

b. Write the sequence and polarity of the mRNA transcript, showing the codons for the five amino acids and the stop codon.

c. Write the amino acid sequence of the polypeptide produced, using both the three-letter and one-letter codes for the sequence. (See the genetic code tables inside the front cover).

BREAK IT DOWN: The coding strand has the same 5' → 3' polarity as the mRNA and also the same base sequence except for the presence of uracil (U) instead of thymine (T) (p. 12).

BREAK IT DOWN: Translation uses mRNA codons (three consecutive mRNA nucleotides) to direct the assembly of polypeptides (strings of amino acids) (p. 13).

BREAK IT DOWN: The start codon is AUG, and it is followed by four more codons and then a stop codon (p. 13).

BREAK IT DOWN: Messenger RNA codons are written and translated 5' to 3' using the genetic code, which contains three stop codons, UAA, UAG, and UGA (inside front cover).

Solution Strategies	Solution Steps
Evaluate	
1. Identify the topic this problem addresses and the nature of the required answer.	1. The problem concerns identification of the coding strand of DNA and the sequence of mRNA encoding five amino acids in a polypeptide and the stop codon. The amino acid sequence is also required.
2. Identify the critical information given in the problem.	2. The double-stranded DNA sequence is given. It contains a sequence corresponding to the start codon (AUG), encodes five amino acids, and contains a stop codon.
Deduce	
3. Scan the double-stranded DNA sequence to identify possible DNA coding-strand triplets and triplets that might be a start codon.	3. The double-stranded DNA sequence contains two possible triplets corresponding to start codons (5'-ATG-3'), one on each strand. Each is highlighted here in bold:

```
3'-ACGGATCCTCCCTAGTGC**GTA**ATACG-5'
5'-TGCCTAGGAGGGATCACGCATT**ATG**C-3'
```

PITFALL: Don't simply read left to right. Instead, identify strand polarity and read 5' → 3'.

TIP: The start codon in mRNA is 5'-AUG-3' (methionine), coded by the template-DNA strand triplet 5'- ATG -3'.

4. Scan the double-stranded DNA to identify possible DNA coding-strand triplets corresponding to possible stop codons.	4. Four DNA triplets potentially correspond to a stop codon. Each corresponding stop codon is shown in bold type here:

```
3'-ACG**GAT**CCTCCCT**AGT**GCGTA**AAT**CG-5'
5'-...TGCC**TAG**GAGGGATCACGCATTATGC...-3'
```

TIP: There are three stop codons, UAA, UAG, and UGA, corresponding to DNA coding-strand triplets TAA, TAG, and TGA, respectively.

Solve	**Answer a**
5. Determine which 5'-ATG-3' DNA triplet is followed by four additional codons (12 nucleotides) encoding amino acids and then by a stop codon and therefore corresponds to the authentic start codon.	5. The potential start codon in the upper strand (5'-ATG-3') corresponds to the authentic start codon (AUG). The following 12 nucleotides correspond to the amino acid codons and the stop codon (5'-TAG-3', which corresponds to the UAG stop codon of mRNA).

TIP: The total length of this region would be 18 nucleotides.

Answer b

| 6. Determine the mRNA sequence and polarity, showing the codons. | 6. The mRNA sequence is |

```
5'-AUG CGU GAU CCC UCC UAG-3'
   Start                 Stop
```

Answer c

| 7. Determine the amino acid sequence of the polypeptide encoded by this mRNA. | 7. The polypeptide encoded by this mRNA is Met-Arg-Asp-Pro-Ser, or M-R-D-P-S. |

For more practice, see Problems 19, 20, and 29. Visit the Study Area to access study tools. **Mastering Genetics**

(a)

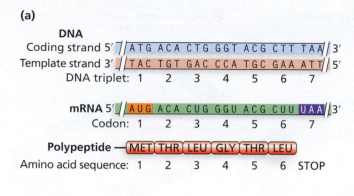

(b)

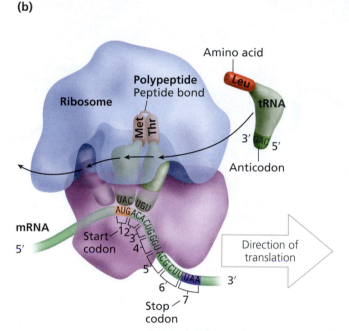

Figure 1.11 **Overview of transcription and translation.** **(a)** Messenger RNA codons are complementary and antiparallel to DNA triplets of the template strand. **(b)** Ribosomes initiate translation of mRNA at the start codon and move along the mRNA in the 3′ direction, adding each new amino acid to the nascent polypeptide by reading each codon. Transfer RNA molecules carry amino acids to ribosomes, where the tRNA anticodon sequences interact with codon sequences of mRNA. Translation terminates when the ribosome encounters a stop codon.

1.4 Genetic Variation Can Be Detected by Examining DNA, RNA, and Proteins

Many experimental techniques are used to identify variation in DNA, RNA, and proteins. A few of these are described in later chapters when knowing the details of a technique is necessary for understanding the analysis of experimental results. But one technical approach to the assessment of nucleic acid and protein variation—*gel electrophoresis*—forms the basis for several other techniques and is worth presenting in advance.

Gel Electrophoresis

Gel electrophoresis is a method for separating different protein or nucleic acid molecules or fragments from one another using an electrical field. The electrical field is created in a semisolid medium called a "gel," and it separates different proteins or nucleic acid molecules from one another on the basis of each molecule's charge, shape, and size characteristics. The gel material used in gel electrophoresis is most commonly either **agarose**, a noninteracting form of cellulose, or **polyacrylamide**, a synthetic material. Both types of gels create a matrix that interferes with the movement of biological molecules in the electrical field but doesn't react with them chemically. The gel matrix–based retardation of molecular movement causes the molecules to separate from one another.

Figure 1.12 shows the preparation of an agarose gel. Agarose is a dry powder that is melted in a hot, liquid buffer and poured into a plastic mold. A "comb" is placed near one end to create indentations known as "wells" as the gel cools into a semisolid form. The final consistency of an agarose gel is that of a dense jello. The wells (after the comb is removed) are the spots where experimental samples containing DNA, RNA, or protein will be loaded for electrophoretic separation. Each well is the **origin of migration** for a sample, and it serves as the starting point for molecular migration in one of the "lanes" of the gel. After biological samples are loaded into the wells, an electrical current is applied, and the samples migrate through the gel.

Most proteins, as well as DNA and RNA, are negatively charged at physiological pH (about 7.0). As a result, during an electrophoresis run, the molecules in a lane move toward the positively charged end of the gel at a rate determined by one or more distinguishing characteristics of the molecules. These molecular characteristics are (1) the molecular weight, related to the number of nucleotides or amino acids that make up the molecule; (2) the molecular charge, meaning the degree of negative charge the molecule carries; and (3) the molecular shape, or molecular conformation. The movement of protein in electrophoresis is usually influenced by all three of these molecular parameters. The movement of DNA or RNA is often a matter of molecular weight alone (i.e., how many nucleotides the molecules contain), particularly if all the nucleic acid molecules in the samples are linear.

After a sufficient period is allowed for migration, the electrical current is turned off and the results of molecular separation can be observed. The final position of a particular molecule of protein, DNA, or RNA is identified as the **electrophoretic mobility** of the molecule. The electrophoretic mobilities of the experimental molecules in a gel can be compared with one another, compared between gels, and compared with molecular weight or size marker standards (molecules with known electrophoretic mobilities) to ascertain information about variation.

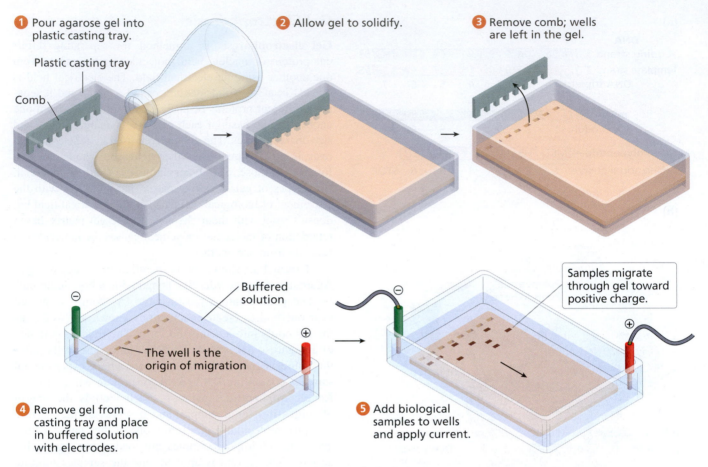

❶ Pour agarose gel into plastic casting tray.

❷ Allow gel to solidify.

❸ Remove comb; wells are left in the gel.

Plastic casting tray

Comb

Buffered solution

The well is the origin of migration

❹ Remove gel from casting tray and place in buffered solution with electrodes.

❺ Add biological samples to wells and apply current.

Samples migrate through gel toward positive charge.

Figure 1.12   Gel electrophoresis, an essential laboratory technique in biological science research.

The first use of gel electrophoresis was in 1949, when Linus Pauling used it to determine that inherited variation of the red blood cell protein hemoglobin was responsible for the hereditary anemia known as sickle cell disease (SCD). The hemoglobin protein is composed of two different globin molecules, and one of these globins, called β-globin, is inherited in a variant form to produce SCD. The wild-type β-globin protein is designated β^A and the mutant β-globin protein is designated β^S. People in Pauling's study had one of three genotypes. Those that were $\beta^S\beta^S$ had SCD, and those that were either $\beta^A\beta^A$ or $\beta^A\beta^S$ did not have the disease. Pauling sought to distinguish these three hemoglobin genotypes from one another by detecting the different type or types of β-globin protein each contained. Pauling's electrophoretic analysis revealed that the protein band seen in the $\beta^S\beta^S$ lane of **Figure 1.13** had lower electrophoretic mobility (smaller distance migrated from the origin) than the protein band detected in the $\beta^A\beta^A$ lane. A single band is detected in each of these lanes, suggesting that all the protein in the lane is identical. In contrast, when an electrophoresis lane contained protein from a $\beta^A\beta^S$ individual, the protein in that lane separated into two bands, each corresponding to the electrophoretic mobility of a different one of the protein bands in the other lanes.

Stains, Blots, and Probes

In Pauling's electrophoretic analysis of hemoglobin, the protein under study had already been isolated from other substances in his samples, so the staining revealed either one or two "bands" in the gel, each consisting of a protein with a distinct electrophoretic mobility—and nothing else. Typically, however, gel electrophoresis of proteins, DNA, or RNA contains many different molecules that can be stained to make their positions known for analysis. The bands can be stained in such a way that *all* separated substances are visualized, or they can be stained in such a way that only a specific protein or a specific sequence of DNA or RNA will show up. General stains or dyes are those that label all of the different proteins or all the nucleic acid bands in a gel. Specific labels, on the other hand, bind to just a single kind of protein or a particular nucleic acid sequence.

When an investigator wants to see all of the molecules present in a DNA or RNA electrophoretic gel, a general labeling compound called **ethidium bromide (EtBr)** can be used as a chemical tag. EtBr attaches to all DNA or RNA in a gel by binding to the sugar-phosphate backbone. The exposure of gels containing EtBr-stained nucleic acids to ultraviolet light excites the EtBr and causes it to emit

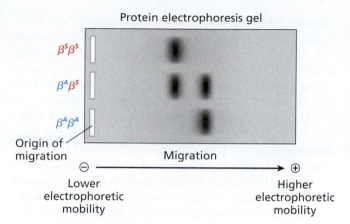

Figure 1.13 Gel electrophoresis of hemoglobin protein, first performed by Linus Pauling.

Q Why does the gel lane containing the hemoglobin from the $\beta^A\beta^S$ individual have two protein bands?

fluorescent light, allowing bands in EtBr-stained DNA or RNA gels to be visualized and photographed (**Figure 1.14a**). Molecular weight size markers consisting of DNA fragments of known length serve as control samples for this gel and are in lanes 1 and 8 of Figure 1.14a. Experimental samples are in lanes 2 through 7. For protein electrophoresis gels, general protein stains—stains that bind to any protein—can be used to discover the location of each protein run through the gel (**Figure 1.14b**). Protein standards, that is, proteins with known electrophoretic mobilities, serve as controls for the protein electrophoresis gel and are in lane 1. Experimental samples in lanes 2 through 5 can be compared with the standards in lane 1 to aid assessment.

Two innovations in gel electrophoresis methods have made the identification of specific proteins and the detection of specific sequences in mRNAs and DNA fragments possible. The first is the development of methods for "blotting," a general name for the transfer of nucleic acids or proteins from an electrophoresis gel to a membrane that can withstand rigorous treatment and analysis. The membrane is most often a durable synthetic material that can serve as a permanent record of gel results. **Southern blotting** (named after its inventor, Edwin Southern) is the term applied to DNA transfer; **northern blotting** (named by tongue-in-cheek analogy with Southern blotting) identifies the transfer of mRNA from a gel to a membrane; and **western blotting** is the term identifying the gel-to-membrane transfer of proteins.

The second innovation is the development of **molecular probes**, traceable molecules that bind to specific target proteins or nucleic acid sequences. In the identification of specific proteins, antibodies are used as molecular probes. Antibodies are produced by the immune system, and they bind to specific target proteins. If the material in a gel is DNA or RNA and an investigator wants to locate a particular molecule or fragment in the sample, the molecular probe will be a single-stranded nucleic acid containing a sequence capable of binding through complementary base pairing to its target nucleic acid. This process is known as **hybridization**.

Molecular probes are essential for identifying a particular nucleic acid molecule or a specific protein in an electrophoresis experiment because there can be thousands of molecules in a gel sample. In a way, the process of searching for a protein, DNA, or RNA target molecule in an electrophoresis gel is analogous to trying to find a specific word or phrase in a text document. Just as word processing programs locate a desired word or phrase by searching for a

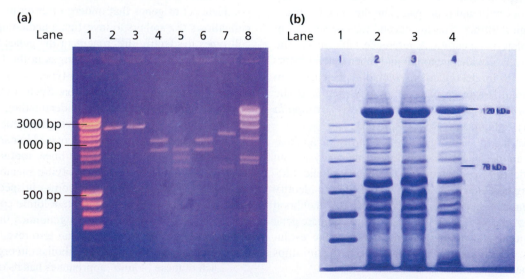

Figure 1.14 Visualization of nucleic acids and proteins in electrophoresis gels. **(a)** The nucleic acids DNA and RNA are visualized using the compound ethidium bromide (EtBr) that binds to nucleic acid molecules and emits fluorescent light when excited by ultraviolet light. Molecular weight size markers in lanes 1 and 8 (bp = base pairs) aid in determining the size of molecules in the different bands in the experimental lanes 2 through 7. **(b)** General protein stains bind to proteins in electrophoresis gels to reveal bands. Protein standards in lane 1 (kDa = kilodaltons) aid in determining the sizes of proteins in experimental lanes 2 through 4.

specific string of letters in response to a "find" command, biologists use molecular probes to locate target nucleic acid sequences or target proteins dispersed by electrophoresis.

DNA Sequencing and Genomics

Genomics is the field that focuses on the sequencing, interpretation, and comparison of genomes of different organisms. Genomic data collection and analysis involve an array of molecular techniques and analytical strategies that aid in identification and examination of the totality of the DNA in a cell, nucleus, or organelle (mitochondria and chloroplasts) carried by a species. Indeed, genomics has made critical contributions to many areas of biological investigation. From medicine to the study of hereditary variation to the study of evolution, genomic data are proving critically important.

Much has changed in DNA sequencing since it began in the 1980s. Genome sequencing is accomplished today by automated high-throughput methods, so-called next-generation sequencing that is thousands of times faster, and far cheaper, than the original genome sequencing methods (see Chapters 7 and 18 for details and applications).

To date, thousands of genome sequences have been compiled. Among the smallest genomes are those of viruses, mitochondria, and chloroplasts, which generally contain tens of thousands to a few hundred thousand base pairs. In contrast, the largest sequenced genomes are those of some plant species that carry multiple sets of chromosomes from their progenitors and have billions of base pairs. Genome sizes are usually reported in **megabases (Mb)**, with 1 Mb equal to 1 million base pairs.

Certain selected species known as "model organisms" are commonly used in genetics and genomics experiments. They are selected because their biology is well known, they are easy to work with and propagate, and they can be investigated through multiple experiments and thus be seen from a more complete perspective. A reference table inside the book back cover provides genomic and other critical information about nine model organisms, including the bacterium *E. coli*, the small flowering plant *Arabidopsis thaliana,* the yeast *Saccharomyces cerevisiae*, the fruit fly *Drosophila melanogaster*, and humans (*Homo sapiens*).

Genomics has a seemingly limitless array of applications. For example, genomic techniques and analyses can be used to identify specific genes, to identify allelic variants producing hereditary diseases, to map genes, to identify regions of genomes that increase or decrease the likelihood of an organism expressing a particular trait, to compare gene sequences within and among species, to trace the evolution of genes, and to identify the evolutionary relationships between related organisms.

The Human Genome Project, completed in 2000, was a landmark achievement that, by producing the nucleotide sequence of an entire representative human genome, set a new course for the genetic investigation of humans. In so doing, it made some striking discoveries. For example, 45% of the human genome consists of transposable genetic elements. These are mobile DNA sequences that can move throughout the genome (see Section 11.7). It also showed that almost 26% of the genome consists of noncoding introns, and only 1.5% of the genome consists of protein-coding exons. Section 16.1 provides additional details of the content and genetic annotation of the human genome.

Genome sequencing and analysis are not limited to living species. Several extinct species have recently had their genomes sequenced for comparison with those of living relatives. These species include the mastodon (for comparison to the elephant), the quagga (for comparison to the zebra), and two extinct lineages of early humans, Neandertal and Denisovans (for comparison to the modern human genome). We look at the interesting results of the Neandertal–Denisovan–*Homo sapiens* genome comparisons in the Case Study that concludes the chapter.

Proteomics and Other "-omic" Analyses

On the heels of genomic sequencing, additional arenas of "-omic" investigations and analyses have developed.

Proteomics, the study of the **proteome,** the complete set of proteins encoded in a genome, examines the functions of proteins, their localization, their regulation, and their interactions in a comprehensive way. In other words, rather than analyzing the structure and function of individual proteins and looking one by one for interacting partners, proteomics is a methodology for examining large numbers of proteins at once. Multiple techniques are used to collect and analyze the proteomes of organisms. Among the numerous applications for proteomics is the use of proteomic analyses to decipher complex networks of protein–protein interaction in cells to find the number and types of such interactions there (see Section 11.1).

Transcriptomics, the study of the **transcriptome**, the complete set of genes that undergo transcription in a given cell, allows researchers to investigate and compare different cell types to identify differences in the genes that are transcribed there, to characterize changes in the levels of gene transcription within a single cell type, or to see how biological changes affect transcription. Such studies can make important contributions to the understanding of biological abnormalities in cancer by identifying the genes whose transcription is either increased or decreased in cancer cells versus normal cells. Along the same lines, **metabolomics**, the study of chemical processes involving metabolites, examines metabolic processes and outcomes in specific cells, tissues, organs, and organisms. Metabolomic comparisons of related organisms ties directly to genomics through shared genetic ancestry. Metabolomics can also reveal new genetic adaptations that have altered metabolism in organisms.

Each of these "-omic" approaches has its own goals, but collectively they also share a common goal—to contribute to the comprehensive understanding of complex biological systems. **Systems biology,** a comprehensive, systems-oriented approach to understanding biological complexity, has become possible through the development and integration of genomics, proteomics, transcriptomics, and metabolomics.

One overarching goal of the biological sciences—to which genetics is a principal contributing discipline—is to achieve an all-inclusive understanding of the normal and abnormal biology of organisms through systems biology.

Applied to humans, for example, systems biology aims to understand how cells work in health and disease, to explain the details of how a single cell develops into a complete organism, and even to explain phenomena as complex as learning, memory, personality, and the development of personality disorders. These enormously complex attributes of organisms result in part from networks of interactions between genes, proteins, metabolites, and environmental influences. They are the most challenging objects of study in modern biology, requiring both the understanding of genetic principles and analysis and the use and application of new tools and technologies for data collection and assessment. This is the exciting and dynamic world in which modern genetics operates.

1.5 Evolution Has a Genetic Basis

As biologists survey varieties of life, assess the genetic similarities and differences between species, and explore the relationships of modern organisms to one another and to their extinct ancestors, it becomes apparent that all life is connected through DNA. Richard Dawkins, a biologist and author of several books on evolution, made note of this molecular connection, observing that life "is a river of DNA, flowing and branching through geologic time." This shared DNA connecting all organisms throughout time is a basis for identifying and studying relationships between organisms and tracing their evolutionary histories.

Life is not static or uniform, of course; it evolves as DNA diverges into separate "branches" whose metaphorical forking leads to new species. The Dawkins quote suggests that for heredity to maintain genetic continuity across generations and for variation to develop between organisms and evolve new species, the biochemical processes that replicate DNA and express the genetic information must also be universal. From this perspective the universality of DNA as the hereditary molecule of life, the shared processes of DNA replication and transcription, and the use of the same genetic code by all life are consistent with the idea of a single origin of life that has evolved into the millions of species inhabiting Earth today as well as other millions that preceded them but are now extinct.

Life on Earth originated from a single source during the Archaean Eon that lasted from 4 billion to 2.5 billion years ago. In 2011, an international group of scientists led by David Wacey discovered fossils of a sulphur-metabolizing single-celled organism in 3.49-billion-year-old rocks from Western Australia (**Figure 1.15**). At that time in Earth's history there was very little oxygen present, and the first living organisms, likely not much different from those identified in fossil form, metabolized sulphur-containing compounds for growth. Organisms with similar metabolism exist today around hot springs and thermal vents.

These early life-forms have given rise to a dazzling array of species, most now extinct. Some of those extinct ancestors, however, gave rise to the modern species that inhabit every conceivable ecological niche on Earth, from the most temperate to the most extreme.

Darwin's Theory of Evolution

Over the millennia since life originated, untold millions of species have come and gone, through the operation of shared processes that faithfully replicated their DNA and passed it on to the next generation while also allowing for the accumulation of variation that drives diversification. This variation, the changes life has undergone, is explained by the theory of **evolution**, which says that all organisms are related by common ancestry and have diversified over time. The four widely recognized evolutionary processes are described below, but first some general comments on Charles Darwin's theory of *evolution by natural selection*.

This view of evolution was proposed separately and independently by both Darwin and Alfred Wallace in the late 1850s. Both authors based their proposals on firsthand observations of the distribution and diversity of life across the globe. Each author described higher rates of survival and reproduction of certain forms of a species over alternative forms through the process of natural selection that favors the survival and reproduction of the most fit individuals in each generation. Unlike the other processes we describe in this overview of evolution, natural selection works at the phenotypic level, but like all evolutionary processes, its effectiveness is based on underlying genetic variation. Natural selection operating to favor one morphological form over others increases the frequency of the favored form in the population and, by doing so, increases the frequencies of the alleles controlling the favored form. Over many generations, forms that produce more offspring also leave more copies of the alleles that control the

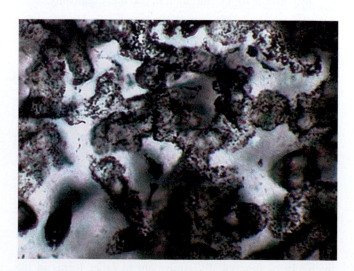

Figure 1.15 Ancient fossilized single-celled organisms. These single-celled sulphur-metabolizing organisms are fossilized in 3.49-billion-year-old rocks collected in Western Australia.

phenotype, creating the hallmark of evolutionary change—change in the genetic makeup of the population.

Darwin's theory of evolution by natural selection is now a firmly established scientific fact incorporating three principles of population genetics that were obvious to many naturalists in Darwin's day but were not assembled into a coherent model until Darwin articulated their connection in his 1859 publication *The Origin of Species by Means of Natural Selection.* Darwin's union of observation and principles into an evolutionary theory had a revolutionary effect on biology and laid the foundation of the modern biological sciences. Darwin's principles of populations are

1. Variation exists among the individual members of populations with regard to the expression of traits.

2. Hereditary transmission allows the variation in traits to be passed from one generation to the next.

3. Certain variant forms of traits give the individuals that carry them a higher rate of survival and reproduction in particular environmental conditions. These organisms leave more offspring and increase the frequency of the variant form in the population.

Yet although Darwin laid out the general process by which species evolved, he never understood the underlying hereditary mechanisms that allowed the process to occur. Today, however, nearly 160 years after Darwin introduced his revolutionary proposal, biologists fully understand the role of genetics in evolution. With regard to Darwin's evolutionary principles, biology has established that

1. Phenotypic variation of expressed traits reflects inherited genetic variation. DNA-sequence differences (allelic variation) must be the cause of phenotypic variation if evolution is to occur.

2. Hereditary transmission of phenotypic variation requires that offspring inherit and express the alleles that were responsible for the variation in parental organisms.

3. Organisms carrying alleles that are favored by natural selection have a reproductive advantage over organisms that do not carry favored alleles. The former group therefore leave more copies of their alleles in the next generation, causing the population to evolve through a change in allele frequency.

In other words, progressive phenotypic change in a population is paralleled by genetic changes.

In this particular process of evolution—evolution by natural selection—one form reproduces in greater numbers than others in a population because of being better adapted to the conditions driving natural selection. This process, also known as adaptive evolution, is common; but many examples of so-called nonadaptive evolution (or neutral evolution), the evolution of characteristics that are reproductively or functionally equivalent to other forms in the population, are also observed. Nonadaptive traits are neutral with respect to natural selection, conferring neither a selective advantage nor a selective disadvantage to their bearer, yet their evolutionary basis is fundamentally the same as that of adaptive evolution, as the following paragraphs attest.

Four Evolutionary Processes

The foundations of evolutionary genetics (which, you will recall, studies and compares genetic changes in populations and species over time) were established in the first four decades of the 20th century by several notable evolutionary biologists and innumerable lesser-known individuals. Interestingly, this work took place before DNA was identified as the hereditary material and before the chemical structure of genes was defined and understood. Ronald Fisher, Sewall Wright, J. B. S. Haldane, and many others devised mathematical and statistical models of gene frequency distribution and evolution in populations and species, leading to evolutionary hypotheses that have been tested and verified countless times in laboratory and natural populations.

Through this massive body of work, evolutionary biology has confirmed Darwin's model of the evolution of species by natural selection and expanded the description of evolution to include three additional processes. Thus, biologists identify four processes of evolution, each leading to *changes in the frequencies of alleles in a population over time,* a hallmark characteristic of evolutionary change. The four evolutionary processes are

1. **Natural selection**—the differential survival and reproduction of members of a population owing to possession of favored traits. Population members with the best-adapted morphological form are best able to survive and reproduce, and they leave more offspring than those possessing less-adaptive forms. Over time, the frequency of the best-adapted form and the alleles that produce it increase in the population.

2. **Migration**—the movement of individual organisms from one population to another. This migratory movement transfers alleles from one population to another, and if the allele frequencies between the populations are different and if the number of migrating individuals is large enough, migration can rapidly alter allele frequencies.

3. **Mutation**—the slow acquisition of inherited variation that increases the diversity of populations and serves as the "raw material" of evolutionary change. Mutation, occurring in many different ways in genomes, provides the genetic diversity that is essential for evolution.

4. **Genetic drift**—the random change of allele frequencies due to chance in randomly mating populations. Genetic drift occurs in all populations, but it is most pronounced in very small populations, where statistically significant fluctuations in allele frequencies can occur from one generation to the next.

By the middle of the 20th century, the **modern synthesis of evolution**—the name given to the merging of evolutionary theory with the results of experimental, mathematical, and molecular population biology—emerged as a unified view of evolution. The modern synthesis tells the story of morphological and molecular evolution of plant and animal species using experimentally verified processes and mechanisms.

Among the best-known principal architects of the modern synthesis are Theodosius Dobzhansky and Ernst Mayr, who drew together ideas from Darwin, Fisher, Wright, Haldane, and others to demonstrate how evolution operates in real populations. Dobzhansky and Mayr profoundly influenced the thinking and research of generations of biologists by demonstrating that evolutionary events revealed by laboratory investigations and in natural populations are consistent with the predictions made by Fisher, Wright, and Haldane. In simple terms, Dobzhansky and Mayr showed that evolution in populations and evolution in species occur as predicted by evolutionary theory. Today, having been fleshed out by the work of countless researchers, the modern synthesis gives a clear and virtually complete picture of the factors that produce the evolutionary changes in populations and of the mechanisms that produce the evolution of species. Evolutionary examples are incorporated into many of the chapters of this book, and Chapter 20 is devoted specifically to evolution in species and in populations.

Tracing Evolutionary Relationships

Evolutionary biologists investigate evolution by looking for evidence of morphological (physical) and molecular (DNA, RNA, and protein) changes in populations and organisms over time. Both morphological and molecular comparisons can be used to identify relationships between living species and to reveal ancestor–descendant relationships. These similarities and differences can be depicted in a diagram called a **phylogenetic tree**, a branching diagram that describes the ancestor–descendant relationships among species or other taxa. The tree of life shown in Figure 1.3 is one type of phylogenetic tree. These trees summarize the evolutionary histories of species by using branching points in the tree to represent the common ancestors of descendant organisms.

The most commonly used approach to phylogenetic tree construction is the **cladistic** approach, which depicts species' evolutionary relationships by sorting the species into groups called **clades,** or **monophyletic groups**, based on **shared derived characteristics**, or **synaptomorphies**, either morphological or molecular. Synaptomorphies are shared by organisms that are members of a clade. Such sharing of traits is interpreted to indicate that the common ancestor shared by clade members also possessed the trait. Synaptomorphies, whether they are of body morphology, proteins, or nucleic acid sequence, occur through **homology**, the presence of the trait or sequence in a common ancestor. An example of morphological homology is limb structure in vertebrates. The limbs of humans, horses, bats, and seals have different functions, but they share the same underlying structure in terms of the number and arrangement of bones in the limbs. These similarities are due to the common ancestry of vertebrates.

In some apparent cases of synaptomorphy, the similarities are not a result of sharing a close common ancestor. Instead, convergent evolution has led unrelated organisms to display similar-looking traits. Such instances are known as **homoplasmy**. One example of homoplasmy is the presence of wings in birds and bats. These wings—despite the similarities brought about by convergent evolution—have independent origins.

Figure 1.16 shows a phylogenetic tree for 14 finch species that inhabit the Galápagos Islands. These finch

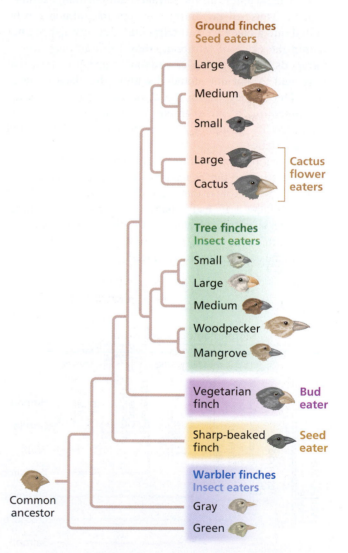

Figure 1.16 Morphological evolution. A phylogenetic tree based on morphological and other characteristics shows the apparent evolutionary relationships between 14 species of finches inhabiting the Galápagos Islands.

Q What role did geographic isolation play in the evolution of Darwin's finches?

species were one of the groups studied by Darwin as he formulated his evolutionary theory. The tree shown here is based on a number of morphological and behavioral characteristics, including the beak shape, beak size, feeding habits, and habitat of each species, as well as its degree of isolation or separation from other species in the Galápagos Islands.

Constructing Phylogenetic Trees Using Morphology and Anatomy Consider the features shared by various animals listed in **Figure 1.17**. One morphological feature common to all these animals is the presence of a backbone. This feature unites these animals into a clade we know as vertebrates that all share a common vertebrate ancestor. A second morphological feature, the presence of four legs, unites all the tetrapod animals and excludes salmon. Thus, all the animals except the salmon can be united into a clade we call tetrapods. Because fish are not within the clade of tetrapods, they form an *outgroup* to tetrapods. An **outgroup** is a taxon or group of taxa that is related to, but not included within, the clade in question. The species within the clade of interest are called the **ingroup.** In our example, each successive clade is identified by grouping species based on other shared characteristics.

After a phylogenetic tree has been constructed, it may be used to infer the characters of ancestral species. For example, we can infer that the common ancestor of all the taxa in Figure 1.17 had a backbone, which would therefore be an ancestral character; but it did not have four legs, which in this case would be a derived character that evolved later, in the common ancestry of tetrapods.

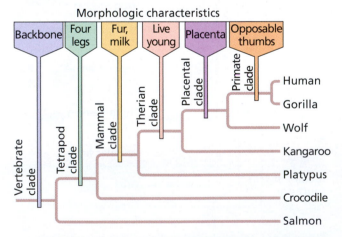

Figure 1.17   The identification of clades based on morphological characters. Organisms are assessed for the presence or absence of a series of morphological characters, and those that share derived characteristics form clades. The origins of specific traits can be traced on the phylogenetic tree.

Constructing Phylogenetic Trees Using Proteins or Nucleic Acids Phylogenetic trees based on molecular characteristics are constructed in the same manner as those based on morphological characteristics, except the shared features are DNA sequences or the amino acid sequences of proteins. Descendant groups have nucleic acid or amino acid sequences that are derived from ancient sequences possessed by their common ancestors (i.e., homology). As a consequence of DNA sequence homology, the most closely related molecular sequences are those that have the smallest number of differences between them, and they are carried by the most closely related species.

Figure 1.18 examines the first 15 nucleotides of the β-globin gene from seven species (**a** to **g**). In the figure, the sequences have been aligned vertically, and the number of differences between the top sequence and each of the other sequences is noted in the first step of the figure.

A common method of constructing a phylogenetic tree begins with pairwise comparisons of genes or nucleotide sequences, grouping the most similar sequences or genes closest together (on the assumption that they are the most closely related) and subsequently bringing in the more distantly related sequences to add to the tree. Analysis in this example begins with sequences **a** and **b,** since they are identical, and then successively attaches more distantly related sequences to the tree. Sequence information from **c,** which differs from **a** and **b** at one nucleotide, is appended next, followed by the other sequences. A completed phylogenetic tree constructed by following these steps recapitulates the known phylogeny of vertebrates.

Genetic Analysis 1.3 guides you in constructing a simple phylogenetic tree.

The availability of DNA sequence data and genomic data has revolutionized how we construct and view phylogenies. Some groups that were traditionally grouped together, such as mammals, birds, and amphibians, do prove, from DNA sequence and genomic data, to be monophyletic groups. However, analyses have indicated that reptiles and fish are not monophyletic groups. For example, crocodiles are now known to be more closely related to birds than to other reptiles. Similarly, morphological and molecular analyses of dinosaurs (recall it is sometimes possible to obtain some molecular information from extinct species) suggest they are the sister group of birds, implying that extant birds are a kind of modern-day descendant of dinosaurs.

In addition to evolution of the coding sequences of genes, molecular evolution also occurs in regulatory sequences. These sequences are essential for gene transcription and operate either through the activity of proteins that bind to specific regulatory DNA sequences and activate or repress transcription or through protein binding to DNA that blocks transcription. Numerous evolutionary analyses and genome sequence comparisons have identified the important role of this type of evolutionary change in the diversification of organisms.

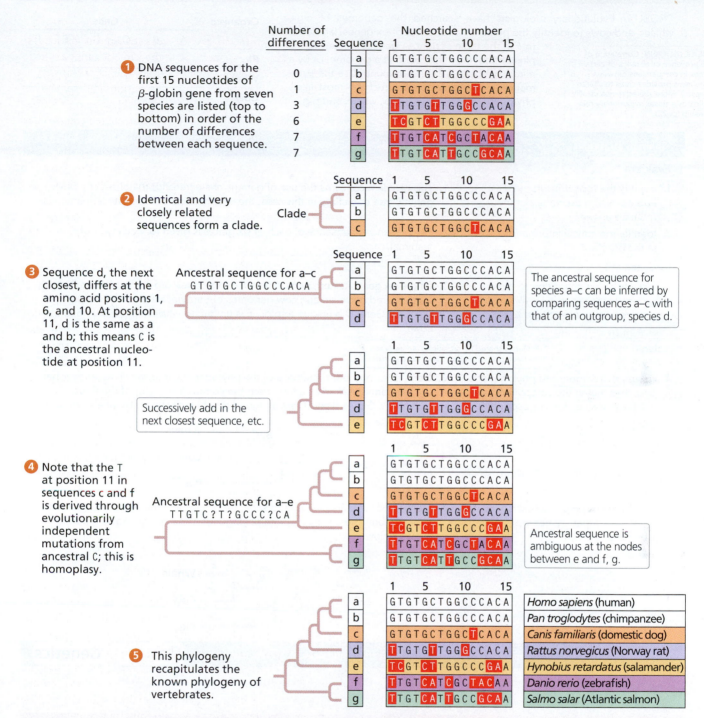

Figure 1.18 Construction of a phylogenetic tree based on molecular characters, using the principle of homology.

Q **How is change in DNA sequence through mutation related to the concept of gene homology?**

PROBLEM Evolutionary biologists have searched the genomes of pigs, whales, and cows to identify the presence or absence of six genes, labeled A to F in the table at right. A gene is marked with a plus symbol (+) if it is found in a genome, or by a minus symbol (−) if it is not found. Use the information in the table to construct the most likely phylogenetic tree relating cow, whale, and pig.

> **BREAK IT DOWN:** Correlation of the presence or absence of certain genes in comparisons between organisms provides clues to shared ancestry. More shared genes usually indicates a closer evolutionary relationship (p. 22).

Organism	Gene					
	A	B	C	D	E	F
Pig	+	−	−	+	−	−
Whale	+	+	+	−	+	−
Cow	+	+	+	−	−	+

Solution Strategies	Solution Steps
Evaluate	
1. Identify the topic this problem addresses and the nature of the required answer.	1. This problem concerns the use of genetic characteristics to construct a phylogenetic tree depicting, in this case, the relationships between three mammals.
2. Identify the critical information given in the problem.	2. The presence or absence of each of six genes is given for each type of mammal.
Deduce	
3. Identify genes shared by all three groups, genes shared by two of the groups, and genes unique to one group.	3. Of the six genes tested, gene A is found in all three organisms. Genes B and C are shared by whale and cow genomes but are not detected in the pig genome. Gene D is unique to pigs, E is unique to whales, and F is unique to cows.
Solve	

> **TIP:** Genes shared by organisms are likely to have been present in their common ancestor.

4. Assign shared genes to phylogenetic branches that in the completed tree will be shared by the corresponding organisms.	4. Gene A is assigned to the base of the phylogenetic tree, which ascends (when the diagram is viewed as a tree) from the common ancestor of the three organisms. Genes B and C are assigned to a branch shared by whale and cow.

5. Assign genes unique to each genome to branches that are not shared by other organisms.	5. Genes D, E, and F are unique to separate groups and therefore are placed on separate branches. The complete phylogenetic tree containing all genes is shown below.

For more practice, see Problems 22, 25, and 21.   Visit the Study Area to access study tools.   **Mastering Genetics**

CASE STUDY

Ancient DNA: Genetics Looks into the Past

In 1878 the last member of a now extinct relative of the zebra died in the wild in South Africa. The animal, known as the quagga ("kwa-ga") was once numerous in South Africa, but hunting wiped the species out. A few quaggas were captured for exhibition in zoos, including the Amsterdam Zoo, where the last living quagga died in 1883, and the Regent's Park Zoo in London, where the only known photographs of a quagga was taken in 1870 (**Figure 1.19**).

One hundred years after the death of the last quagga, a group of molecular biologists working with the American biochemist Allan Wilson visited a dusty warehouse in South Africa and scraped some 125-year-old dried muscle tissue off the back of several quagga hides that had languished there for decades. The researchers were hoping to find DNA derived from the intracellular organelles called mitochondria that might have been preserved in the desiccated tissue. The samples they brought back to the laboratory for analysis yielded a tiny amount of highly fragmented mitochondrial DNA (mtDNA), but it was sufficient for making a comparison between quagga mtDNA and mtDNA from living mountain zebras. The results,

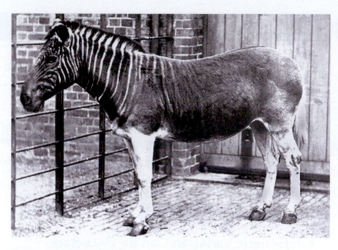

Figure 1.19 The last captive quagga. This animal was photographed at the Regents Park Zoo in London is 1870.

published in 1984, were consistent with the 3 to 4 million years of evolution estimated to have taken place since mountain zebras and quaggas shared a common ancestor. The research by Wilson and his colleagues was the first to demonstrate that old tissue samples could yield DNA that could be sequenced and analyzed. In the period that followed, several additional ancient samples yielded mtDNA, and within a few years the first samples of ancient nuclear DNA were also obtained. These efforts inaugurated more than 35 years of research seeking to sequence ancient genomes. The genomes of hominins, a group made up of modern humans and very closely related ancestral species, are a principal focus of this research.

Thanks primarily to pioneering work by Svante Pääbo and his many colleagues and collaborators, ancient nuclear DNA from numerous animals and many archaic hominins, some of it tens of thousands of years old, has been collected and sequenced. Bones, teeth, and hair are the sources of ancient DNA. Bone or tooth samples are collected, pulverized, and processed through a series of highly exacting steps to yield archaic DNA. Hair, which can carry a root bulb or associated skin cells, is a good source of DNA when it is available, have also been shown to yield archaic DNA.

The improvements in collection of ancient DNA suitable for genome sequence analysis are a major scientific achievement. In practice, however, it is the gathering of fragmentary DNA of hominin origin along with dramatic improvements in methods of cloning and sequencing that has advanced the field of ancient DNA sequencing. Until very recently it was thought necessary to use recognizable human remains, in the form of bones, hair, or teeth, as the source of DNA. However, research published in 2017 by Matthias Meyers and colleagues revealed that sediments from caves inhabited by archaic hominins and more modern humans contain DNA. Much of this DNA is from animals, plants, fungi, and bacteria and other microorganisms, but DNA from the human lineage can be identified in the mixture and isolated for analysis. This new DNA source promises to provide genetic information on archaic hominins even when no bones are found.

There are several complications to working with ancient hominin DNA, whatever the source. The yield of high-quality ancient DNA is very low—the DNA yield from ancient bones, for example, is several hundredfold less than from fresh bones—and ancient hominin DNA is heavily contaminated

with DNA of various plants, animals, and microbes. The DNA that is collected is generally highly fragmented, with most fragments measuring 50 base pairs or less. But novel DNA cloning methods developed in 2010 by Matthias Meyer and others for use on ancient DNA have increased the amount of DNA that is usable for sequencing by about 500-fold, making archaic hominin genome sequencing much easier.

Ancient DNA samples provide two principal avenues for exploration of the genetic origins of modern humans. One is through genomic sequencing of nuclear DNA and mtDNA, allowing researchers to compare modern human genomes with those of archaic hominins such as Neandertals to search for similarities, differences, and signs of interbreeding. The second avenue is the examination of nuclear genomic sequences from modern humans who lived between 50,000 and 5,000 years ago to reconstruct the evolutionary history of the modern human genome.

DNA sequence analyses support the fossil and archaeological evidence that the genus *Homo* originated and diversified in Africa and that archaic hominins moved out of Africa in numerous waves over a span of 400,000 years or more. Only the most recent wave, beginning about 60,000 years ago, is responsible for modern-day human populations outside of Africa. In addition to the DNA of these migrating humans, genomic DNA from two archaic hominins—Neandertals in Europe, Eurasia, and parts of the near east, and Denisovans, in central Europe and Asia—is available for examination. The genomic evidence clearly indicates interbreeding between Neandertals and Denisovans, and also between both of these archaic forms and more modern humans whose descendants populate Europe, Eurasia, Australia, and the Pacific Islands. The proportions of Neandertal DNA and of Denisovan DNA in modern human genomes are small—about 2% to 5% in populations outside of Africa. The evidence also indicates that while a few Neandertal and Denisovan genes remain in the modern human genome, the proportion of Neandertal and Denisovan DNA has decreased steadily over the last 40,000 to 50,000 years. This suggests that, for the most part, Neandertal and Denisovan genes were not evolutionarily advantageous to modern humans.

Studies of the evolution of the human genome over the last 40,000 to 50,000 years have been greatly aided by advances in DNA cloning that have led to completion of the genome sequences of thousands of ancient humans. The most comprehensive research, led by David Reich and colleagues, has sequenced the genomes of ancient humans who lived between 5000 and 50,000 years ago in Europe and Eurasia. With these data, Reich and colleagues have shown that an initial migratory wave of humans who moved out of Africa beginning about 60,000 years ago established resident populations in Europe and Eurasia that can be dated to 40,000 to 50,000 years ago. Additional waves founded several population centers over the next 25,000 years or so. Immediately following the retreat of glaciation in Europe and Eurasia about 14,000 years ago, extensive contact took place between populations, resulting in a high degree of genetic mixing. These events formed the foundations of the human genome of today. Interestingly, this genomic sequence information matches up quite well with the archaeological and linguistic evidence, suggesting that modern humans have been moving and sharing both their ideas and their genes for millennia. Application Chapter D: Human Evolutionary Genetics contains further, more detailed discussion of archaic human DNA and the evolutionary hypotheses generated by its analyses.

1.1 Modern Genetics Is in Its Second Century

- Genetic principles first outlined by Gregor Mendel in 1865 were "rediscovered" in 1900 and so made modern genetics a 20th-century scientific discipline.

- Study of the transmission of morphological variation during the first half of the 20th century established transmission genetics as a central focus of genetic analysis.

- The analysis of DNA, RNA, and protein beginning in the second half of the 20th century established genetics as a molecular discipline.

- Life on Earth has three domains—Bacteria, Archaea, and Eukarya—that share a common evolutionary history.

1.2 The Structure of DNA Suggests a Mechanism for Replication

- Deoxyribonucleic acid (DNA) is the genetic material. DNA is a double helix containing two strands of nucleotides that are composed of a five-carbon deoxyribose sugar, a phosphate group, and one of four nucleotide bases: adenine (A), thymine (T), cytosine (C), or guanine (G).

- Nucleotides in a DNA strand are joined by covalent phosphodiester bonds between the 5′ phosphate of one nucleotide and the 3′ OH of the adjoining nucleotide.

- DNA strands are joined by hydrogen bonds that form between complementary base pairs. A pairs with T and C pairs with G.

- Strands of the DNA duplex are antiparallel; one strand is oriented 5′ → 3′, and the complementary strand is oriented 3′ → 5′.

- DNA replicates by a semiconservative process that produces exact copies of the original DNA double helix.

- DNA polymerase uses one strand of DNA as a template to synthesize a complementary daughter strand one nucleotide at a time in the 5′-to-3′ direction.

1.3 DNA Transcription and Messenger RNA Translation Express Genes

- The central dogma of biology (DNA → RNA → protein) identifies DNA as an information repository and describes how DNA dictates protein structure through a messenger RNA intermediary that in turn directs polypeptide synthesis.

- Transcription is the process that synthesizes single-stranded RNA from a template DNA strand.

- RNA transcripts have the same 5′ → 3′ polarity and sequence as the coding strand of DNA; they differ only in the presence of U rather than T.

- Certain DNA sequences, most commonly promoters, bind RNA polymerase and other transcriptional proteins.

- Translation is the process that uses messenger RNA (mRNA) sequences to synthesize proteins.

- Messenger RNA codons base-pair with tRNA anticodons at the ribosome.

- Each tRNA carries a specific amino acid that is added to the growing polypeptide chain.

- The genetic code contains 61 codons that specify amino acids and 3 that are stop codons.

1.4 Genetic Variation Can Be Detected by Examining DNA, RNA, and Proteins

- Gel electrophoresis efficiently separates different proteins, DNA fragments, or RNA based on their electrophoretic mobility.

- Following gel electrophoresis of DNA fragments, Southern blotting uses labeled single-stranded nucleic acid molecular probes to bind to a specific target DNA sequence on a fragment by complementary base pairing (hybridization).

- Northern blotting is performed by hybridizing a labeled single-stranded nucleic acid probe to mRNA.

- Western blotting uses labeled antibodies as molecular probes to bind to target proteins.

- Genomics, proteomics, transcriptomics, and metabolomics are new investigative strategies that can help decipher complex problems of systems biology.

1.5 Evolution Has a Genetic Basis

- Four processes—natural selection, migration, mutation, and genetic drift—drive the evolution of populations and species.

- The evolution of adaptive morphological characters occurs through natural selection pressures exerted on species by their environments. Nonadaptive characters that are neutral with respect to natural selection evolve by other evolutionary processes.

- The modern synthesis of evolution is the name applied to the union of transmission genetics, molecular genetics, Darwinian evolution, and modern evolutionary genetics.

- Phylogenetic trees describe the evolutionary relationships among modern species and trace their descent from common ancestors to identify the most likely pattern of evolution.

- Shared derived characteristics are molecular or morphological attributes that evolve in descendant species from ancient characters found in a common ancestor.

- Molecular phylogenies trace the evolution of nucleic acid or protein sequences from common ancestors to modern species.

PREPARING FOR PROBLEM SOLVING

In addition to the list of problem-solving tips and suggestions given here, you can go to the Study Guide and Solutions Manual that accompanies this book for help at solving problems.

1. Understand the basic terminology of genetics. Key terms are in **bold** when they are first defined and used in descriptions. Key terms are also defined in the Glossary at the back of the textbook.

2. Recognize the levels at which genetic information and expression are described and analyzed: the molecular level (DNA, RNA, protein, etc.), the sequence level (gene, allele, wild type, mutant, etc.), the microscopic

level (chromosome, nucleus, ribosome, etc.), and the phenotypic level (wild type, mutant, etc.).

3. Be prepared to describe and analyze the relationships between DNA, RNA, and protein.

4. Reacquaint yourself with the fundamentals of DNA replication, transcription, and translation before studying the chapters where these processes are described in detail.

5. Understand the four processes that drive evolutionary change.

6. Be prepared to construct and analyze phylogenetic trees.

PROBLEMS

Mastering Genetics Visit for instructor-assigned tutorials and problems.

Chapter Concepts

For answers to selected even-numbered problems, see Appendix: Answers.

1. Genetics affects many aspects of our lives. Identify three ways genetics affects your life or the life of a family member or friend. The effects can be regularly encountered or can be one time only or occasional.

2. How do you think the determination that DNA is the hereditary material affected the direction of biological research?

3. A commentator once described genetics as "the queen of the biological sciences." The statement was meant to imply that genetics is of overarching importance in the biological sciences. Do you agree with this statement? In what ways do you think the statement is accurate?

4. All life shares DNA as the hereditary material. From an evolutionary perspective, why do you think this is the case?

5. Define the terms *allele, chromosome,* and *gene* and explain how they relate to one another. Develop an analogy between these terms and the process of using a street map to locate a new apartment to live in next year (i.e., consider which term is analogous to a street, which to a type of building, and which to an apartment floor plan).

6. Define the terms *genotype* and *phenotype,* and relate them to one another.

7. Define *natural selection,* and describe how natural selection operates as a mechanism of evolutionary change.

8. Describe the modern synthesis of evolution, and explain how it connects Darwinian evolution to molecular evolution.

9. What are the four processes of evolution? Briefly describe each process.

10. Define each of the following terms:
    a. transcription
    b. allele
    c. central dogma of biology
    d. translation
    e. DNA replication
    f. gene
    g. chromosome
    h. antiparallel
    i. phenotype
    j. complementary base pair
    k. nucleic acid strand polarity
    l. genotype
    m. natural selection
    n. mutation
    o. modern synthesis of evolution

11. Compare and contrast the genome, the proteome, and the transcriptome of an organism.

12. With respect to transcription describe the relationship and sequence correspondence of the RNA transcript and the DNA template strand. Describe the relationship and sequence correspondence of the mRNA transcript to the DNA coding strand.

13. Plant agriculture and animal domestication developed independently several times and in different locations in human history. Do a brief Internet search and then list the approximate locations, time periods, and crops developed in three of these agricultural events. What role do you think ideas about heredity may have played in these events?

14. Briefly describe the contribution each of the following people made to the development of genetics or genetic analysis.
    a. Archibald Garrod
    b. Rosalind Franklin
    c. Robert Hooke
    d. William Bateson
    e. Rudolph Virchow
    f. Edmund B. Wilson

Application and Integration

For answers to selected even-numbered problems, see Appendix: Answers.

15. If thymine makes up 21% of the DNA nucleotides in the genome of a plant species, what are the percentages of the other nucleotides in the genome?

16. What reactive chemical groups are found at the 5′ and 3′ carbons of nucleotides? What is the name of the bond formed when nucleotides are joined in a single strand? Is this bond covalent or noncovalent?

17. Identify two differences in chemical composition that distinguish DNA from RNA.

18. What is the central dogma of biology? Identify and describe the molecular processes that accomplish the flow of genetic information described in the central dogma.

19. A portion of a polypeptide contains the amino acids Trp-Lys-Met-Ala-Val. Write the possible mRNA and template-strand DNA sequences. (Hint: Use A/G and T/C to indicate that either adenine/guanine or thymine/cytosine could occur in a particular position, and use N to indicate that any DNA nucleotide could appear.)

20. The following segment of DNA is the template strand transcribed into mRNA:

    5′-...GACATGGAA...-3′

    a. What is the sequence of mRNA created from this sequence?
    b. What is the amino acid sequence produced by translation?

21. Using the following amino acid sequences obtained from different species of apes, construct a phylogenetic tree of the apes.

Pongo pygmaeus	G G P H Y R L I A V E D
Pongo abelii	G G P H Y R L I A V E D
Pan paniscus	G A P H F R L L A V E E
Pan troglodytes	G A P H F R L L A V E E
Gorilla gorilla	G A P H F R L I A V E E
Gorilla beringei	G A P H F R L I A V E E
Homo sapiens	G A P H F N L L A V E E
Hylobates lar	G G P H Y R L I S V E D
Hoolock hoolock	G G P H Y R L I S V D D
Common ancestor	G G P H Y R L I S V D D

22. Examine Figure 1.17 and answer the following questions.
    a. How many clades are shown in the figure?
    b. What characteristic is shared by all clades in the figure?
    c. What characteristics are shared by the mammalian clade and the primate clade? What characteristic distinguishes the primates from other members of the mammalian clade?

23. Fill in the missing nucleotides (so there are three per block) and the missing amino acid abbreviations in the graphic shown here.

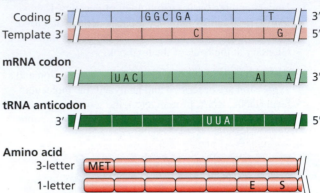

24. Suppose a genotype for a protein-producing gene can have any combination of three alleles, A_1, A_2, and A_3.
    a. List all the possible genotypes involving these three alleles.
    b. Each allele produces a protein with a distinct electrophoretic mobility. Allele A_1 has the highest electrophoretic mobility, A_3 has the lowest electrophoretic mobility, and the electrophoretic mobility of A_2 is intermediate between them. Draw the appearance of gel electrophoresis protein bands for each of the possible genotypes. Be sure to label each lane of the gel with the corresponding genotype.

25. Shorter fragments of DNA (those with fewer base pairs) have a higher electrophoretic mobility then larger fragments. Thinking about electrophoresis gels as creating a matrix through which fragments must migrate, briefly explain why the size of a DNA fragment affects its electrophoretic mobility.

26. Four nucleic-acid samples are analyzed to determine the percentages of the nucleotides they contain. Survey the data in the table to determine which samples are DNA and which are RNA, and specify whether each sample is double-stranded or single-stranded. Justify each answer.

	A	G	T	U	C
Sample 1	22%	28%	22%	0	28%
Sample 2	30%	30%	0	20%	20%
Sample 3	18%	32%	0	18%	32%
Sample 4	29%	29%	21%	0	21%

27. What is meant by the term *homology*? How is that different from the meaning of *homoplasmy*?

28. If one is constructing a phylogeny of reptiles using DNA sequence data, which taxon (birds, mammals, amphibians, or fish) might be suitable to use as an outgroup?

29. Consider the following segment of DNA:

```
5'-...ATGCCAGTCACTGACTTG...-3'
3'-...TACGGTCAGTGACTGAAC...-5'
```

a. How many phosphodiester bonds are required to form this segment of double-stranded DNA?
b. How many hydrogen bonds are present in this DNA segment?
c. If the lower strand of DNA serves as the template transcribed into mRNA, how many peptide bonds are present in the polypeptide fragment into which the mRNA is translated?

Collaboration and Discussion

For answers to selected even-numbered problems, see Appendix: Answers.

30. Ethical and social issues have become a large part of the public discussion of genetics and genetic testing. Choose two of the propositions presented here and prepare a list of arguments for and against them.
    a. The results of genetic testing for susceptibility to cancer, heart disease, and diabetes should be available to insurance companies and current or prospective employers to provide more information for decision making.
    b. Prenatal genetic testing and genetic testing of newborn infants should be available for hereditary conditions that can be treated or managed.
    c. Prenatal genetic testing and genetic testing later in life should be available for hereditary conditions that cannot currently be treated or effectively managed.
    d. Gene therapy should be used on humans when it can correct a hereditary condition such as sickle cell disease.

31. In certain cases, genetic testing can identify mutant alleles that greatly increase a person's chance of developing a disease such as breast cancer or colon cancer. Between 50 and 70% of people with these particular mutations will develop cancer, but the rest will not. Imagine you are either a 30-year-old woman with a family history of breast cancer or a 30-year-old man with a family history of colon cancer (choose one). Each person can undergo genetic testing to identify a mutation that greatly increases susceptibility to the disease. Putting yourself in the place of the person you have chosen, provide answers to the following questions.
    a. If you have a spouse or partner, are you obligated to tell that person the result of the genetic test? Why or why not?
    b. If you have children, are you obligated to tell the children the result of the genetic test? Why or why not?
    c. If you were the spouse or partner of the person you have selected, would you encourage or would you discourage the person from having the genetic test? Why?
    d. If this person that you have selected were you, do you think you would have the genetic test or not? Can you explain the reasons for your answer?

32. What information presented in this chapter and what information familiar to you from previous general biology courses is consistent with all life having a common origin?

33. It is common to study the biology and genetics of bacteria, yeast, fruit flies, and mice to understand biological and genetic processes in humans. Why do you think this is the case?

2

Transmission Genetics

CHAPTER OUTLINE

2.1 Gregor Mendel Discovered the Basic Principles of Genetic Transmission

2.2 Monohybrid Crosses Reveal the Segregation of Alleles

2.3 Dihybrid and Trihybrid Crosses Reveal the Independent Assortment of Alleles

2.4 Probability Theory Predicts Mendelian Ratios

2.5 Chi-Square Analysis Tests the Fit between Observed Values and Expected Outcomes

2.6 Autosomal Inheritance and Molecular Genetics Parallel the Predictions of Mendel's Hereditary Principles

ESSENTIAL IDEAS

- Mendel's hereditary experiments with pea plants identified two laws of heredity known as segregation and independent assortment.

- Consistent and predictable phenotype ratios in generations descending from two parents differing for a single trait support the law of segregation.

- The inheritance of two or more traits is predicted by the law of independent assortment.

- The rules of probability predict genetic inheritance.

- The statistical method known as chi-square analysis is used to evaluate how closely the predicted outcomes of genetic crosses match experimental observations.

- The inheritance of certain traits in human families follows the hereditary laws of segregation and independent assortment.

- Genes controlling four traits described by Mendel have been identified and the activity of their alleles characterized.

This statue of Gregor Mendel stands in the garden outside the entrance to the Mendel Science Center on the Philadelphia, Pennsylvania campus of Villanova University. It was sculpted in 1998 by James Peniston and was inspired by the statue of Mendel at the St. Thomas monastery in Brno, Czech Republic. You can take a virtual tour of the Brno's Mendel museum at www.mendel-museum.com.

When Gregor Mendel identified and described two fundamental laws of hereditary transmission, he ushered in a new era of understanding in biology. The terms *Mendelian genetics* and *Mendelism* were coined to recognize this contribution, and they are used as synonyms for **transmission genetics**, the field that describes and investigates the patterns of transmission of genes and traits from parents to offspring. Like his contemporary Charles Darwin, who elegantly described the process of evolution by natural selection, Mendel articulated a new way to view the world.

Mendel was one of a long list of amateur botanists of the 18th and early 19th centuries who conducted what were then called studies of plant hybridization in many species, including the edible pea plant (*Pisum sativum*) that was the subject of Mendel's experiments. Unlike those who preceded him, however, Mendel was able to describe the *mechanism* of hereditary transmission, thanks in large part to his unique and superior experimental design. Mendel's experimental approach allowed him to formulate and test genetic hypotheses with a level of rigor that no one had achieved before him or would achieve for another 35 years.

In this chapter, we discuss the design and results of Mendel's experiments and the two laws of heredity they revealed. We will see (1) how Mendel's unprecedented experimental designs enabled him to detect genetic phenomena that escaped identification by his predecessors and (2) how the transmission of traits can be predicted using random probability theory. The chapter concludes with a description of the molecular genetics of the four genes known to control traits described by Mendel. We begin, however, with a short biography of Mendel that explains how his educational experiences shaped his approach to scientific exploration.

2.1 Gregor Mendel Discovered the Basic Principles of Genetic Transmission

Born in 1822 to a farming family of modest means in the village of Hynčice that is now part of the Czech Republic, Johann (later known by his clerical name, Gregor) Mendel completed the equivalent of high school at age 18 with a certificate attesting to exceptional academic abilities. He began his higher education at the Olomouc Philosophical Institute in 1840, but these studies took a severe toll on his mental and physical health, and he gave them up after the first year. In 1843, after attempting unsuccessfully to restart his education at Olomouc, he decided to pursue higher learning by entering the priesthood instead. Based on its strong reputation in teacher training and a recommendation from a former teacher at Olomouc, he selected St. Thomas monastery in the Czech city of Brno. Mendel's duties at St. Thomas included temporary teaching of natural science at a middle school in Brno. His keen interest in teaching science and his desire to become a permanent teacher led monastery administrators to send Mendel to the University of Vienna in 1851 to study natural science as preparation for a teaching examination.

In Vienna, Mendel studied plant physiology and plant biology with Professor Franz Unger and physics with Professor Christian Doppler as well as Doppler's successor,

Professor Andreas von Ettinghausen. From Professor Unger, Mendel learned to think critically about prevailing theories of plant reproduction and hybridization. Doppler, an experimental physicist famous for describing the Doppler effect, espoused a "particulate" view of physics and taught Mendel how to study individual characteristics separately in experiments. Professor Ettinghausen taught Mendel the principles of combinatorial mathematics, the analysis of finite, or countable, sets of numbers. This branch of mathematics is central to probability theory. Mendel would apply all these lessons to his later research. In 1853, Mendel returned to Brno, where he took and passed the written portion of the permanent teachers' examination but apparently never completed the oral portion, remaining a "temporary" teacher at the school in Brno until he became abbot of the monastery in 1868.

In the summer of 1856, after a 3-year period during which he pondered how he might pursue his interest in natural science, Mendel began his work on the heredity of traits in the edible pea plant *Pisum sativum*. This species was widely used in experimentation at the time, and Mendel had no trouble gathering seeds that produced plants with distinguishing traits. Mendel began his studies by gathering 34 different varieties of peas. Over the next 2 years, he tested each variety for its ability to uniformly reproduce identical characteristics from one generation to the next. Ultimately, he settled on 14 strains of *Pisum* representing seven individual traits, each of which had two easily distinguished forms of expression in a seed or plant (**Figure 2.1**). Such traits are called *dichotomous*. Mendel worked with these 14 strains for the next 5 years, concluding his experiments in 1863.

On February 8 and March 8, 1865, Mendel discussed his work on peas at two meetings of the Natural History Society of Brunn (Brno). The society published his report in its *Proceedings* the following year, 1866. After publication of his work, Mendel corresponded with several prominent botanists in Europe, most notably Karl Naegeli. Mendel's letters to Naegeli have scientific significance because they clearly lay out his experiments, his results, and his conclusions. Unfortunately, neither Naegeli nor any of his contemporaries seemed to grasp the importance of Mendel's work.

After becoming abbot of the monastery in 1868, Mendel gave up his work in genetics but continued to pursue his interests in bee keeping and meteorology. As abbot, he became involved in business activities in and around Brno, including holding a seat on the board of directors of a local bank and running a brewery that generated income for St. Thomas. He faithfully served the monastery until his death in 1884. Mendel died in scientific obscurity, never having had the importance of his experiments understood or appreciated. Sixteen years after his death, in 1900, biologists would rediscover and replicate his experiments and launch a revolution in biology.

Mendel's Modern Experimental Approach

Mendel successfully identified principles of hereditary transmission that eluded investigators who preceded him and continued to elude investigators for many years after

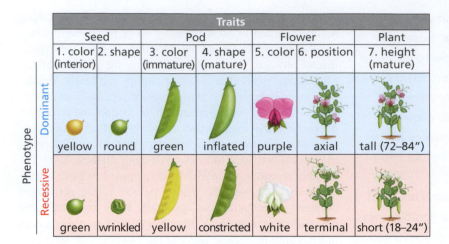

Traits						
Seed		Pod		Flower		Plant
1. color (interior)	2. shape	3. color (immature)	4. shape (mature)	5. color	6. position	7. height (mature)
Dominant						
yellow	round	green	inflated	purple	axial	tall (72–84")
Recessive						
green	wrinkled	yellow	constricted	white	terminal	short (18–24")

Figure 2.1 **The seven dichotomous traits of** *Pisum sativum* **studied by Mendel.** Each trait has a dominant phenotype and a recessive phenotype that are easily distinguished. (These terms are defined in Section 2.2.)

his death. Was Mendel more insightful? Did he make fortuitous choices by selecting *Pisum sativum* as his experimental organism and in selecting his seven characteristics? Did he have a superior approach to genetic experimentation and analysis? The answer to each of these questions is yes.

Mendel's superior insight came principally from his familiarity with quantitative thinking and his understanding of the particulate nature of matter, learned through the study of physics with Doppler. Central to Mendel's experimental success was counting the number of progeny with specific phenotypes. This logical and now routine component of data gathering was the key to Mendel's ability to formulate the hypotheses that explained his results.

Mendel made a fortuitous choice in selecting the pea plant as his experimental organism. Pea plant flowers have both male (anther) and female (ovule) reproductive structures, and they naturally reproduce by **self-fertilization** (**Figure 2.2**). Pea plant fertilization can also be manipulated by experimenters: they cut away the anthers to prevent the flower from producing pollen, and then they use a small paintbrush to manually fertilize the emasculated flower with pollen from a different plant. This **artificial cross-fertilization** allows experimenters (like Mendel) to perform controlled genetic crosses, as explained below (**Figure 2.3**).

Mendel's experiments were designed to identify the mechanism of hereditary transmission in pea plants and, specifically, to test the **blending theory of heredity** that was the predominant hereditary theory at the time. The blending theory viewed the traits of progeny as a mixture of the characteristics possessed by the two parental forms. Under this theory, progeny were believed to display characteristics that were approximately intermediate between those of the parents. For example, the blending theory would predict that crossing a black cat and a white cat would produce gray kittens, and that the original black or white colors would never reappear if the gray kittens were bred to one another. Mendel reasoned that if the blending theory were true, he would see evidence of it in each trait. If no blending were seen in individual traits, the blending theory would be disproved.

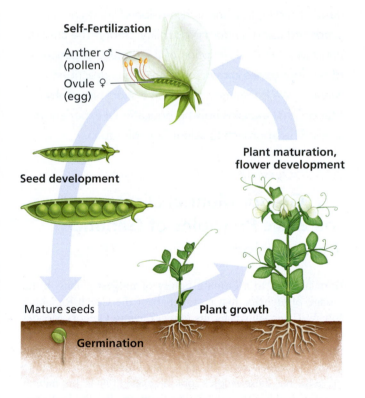

Figure 2.2 **Life cycle of** *Pisum sativum***.** Seeds (peas) are planted and germinate, growing into mature flowering plants. Plants self-fertilize when eggs in the flower ovule are fertilized by pollen produced from anthers in the same plant. Immature seeds arise from individual fertilized eggs in the pod that forms as seeds develop. After seeds mature, they are dispersed to renew the cycle.

What ultimately paved the way for Mendel's success at correctly describing two fundamental laws of heredity was his radically new experimental design. Most importantly, the design of Mendel's experiments was hypothesis driven. In other words, following an initial observation, he devised a hypothesis to explain the observation and then carried out an independent experiment to test the hypothesis. In fact,

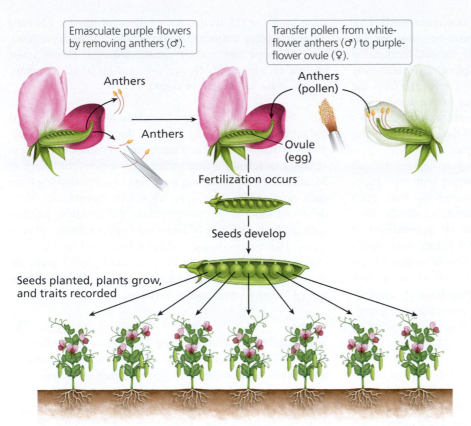

Emasculate purple flowers by removing anthers (♂).

Transfer pollen from white-flower anthers (♂) to purple-flower ovule (♀).

Anthers

Anthers

Anthers (pollen)

Ovule (egg)

Fertilization occurs

Seeds develop

Seeds planted, plants grow, and traits recorded

Figure 2.3 Artificial cross-fertilization of pea plants. Removing anthers emasculates the flower and prevents self-fertilization. Applying pollen from another flower fertilizes eggs in the emasculated flower.

Q Why did Mendel remove the anthers of the plants he used in controlled genetic-cross experiments?

the experimental design Mendel constructed is an example of the hypothesis-driven experimental approach scientists use today, known as the *scientific method*. This method of experimentation has six steps:

1. Make initial observations about a phenomenon or process.
2. Formulate a testable hypothesis to explain the observations.
3. Design a controlled experiment to test the hypothesis.
4. Collect data from the controlled experiment.
5. Interpret the experimental results, comparing the observed results with those expected under the assumptions of the hypothesis.
6. Draw reasonable conclusions, reformulating or retesting the hypothesis if necessary.

Mendel followed these steps to collect data on individual traits of the pea plant, formulate hypotheses to explain his phenotypic observations, and conduct independent experiments to test his predictions.

Five Critical Experimental Innovations

In addition to his use of the scientific method, five specific features of Mendel's breeding experiments distinguish them from those of his contemporaries and were critical to his success: (1) controlled crosses between plants; (2) use of pure-breeding strains to begin the experimental controlled

crosses; (3) selection of dichotomous traits; (4) quantification of results; and (5) use of replicate, reciprocal, and test crosses. These innovations are introduced briefly here and explored in greater detail as the chapter proceeds.

Controlled Crosses between Plants   In nature, pea plants self-fertilize (see Figure 2.2). Self-fertilization occurs when sperm-containing pollen from the anther fertilizes an egg within the ovule. Fertilized ovules develop in the ovary and then mature in the seed pod. A mature seed pod usually contains five to seven peas, each of which results from a different fertilization event. In genetic experiments, peas can be collected and counted by their phenotypes or can be planted to produce pea plants that are counted by their traits.

Pea plants are also capable of cross-pollination. In nature, plants are cross-pollinated by insects, birds, mammals, and wind. Mendel used his familiarity with plants to carry out artificial cross-fertilization, employing carefully selected plants as pollen and egg donors to ensure that the progeny could be used to test a hereditary hypothesis. By restricting reproduction to those plants he identified beforehand as likely to yield informative results, Mendel performed what are now known as **controlled genetic crosses** between selected organisms.

Pure-Breeding Strains to Begin Experimental Crosses
During the 2 years before beginning his hereditary experiments, Mendel performed dozens of controlled genetic crosses to obtain strains that consistently produced a single

phenotype without variation. Strains that consistently produce the same phenotype are called **pure-breeding strains** or **true-breeding strains**. For example, the self-fertilization of a pure-breeding purple-flowered plant will yield only purple flowers among progeny plants. Two plants from the same pure-breeding line can be crossed to one another and will produce progeny with the same phenotype. Mendel's work ultimately led to the production of the 14 pure-breeding strains for the seven traits shown in Figure 2.1.

Mendel structured the experimental crosses for all seven traits in the same way. He began with two pure-breeding parental plants for a dichotomous trait, each having a different one of the two phenotypes for the trait. These were the **parental generation (P generation)** of the cross. The pure-breeding parental plants were artificially cross-fertilized to produce the **first filial generation (F_1 generation**; **Figure 2.4**). The F_1 plants were then crossed to produce the **second filial generation (F_2 generation)**. The **third filial generation (F_3 generation)** was produced by crossing plants from the F_2 generation, and so on for as many generations as needed.

Selection of Single Traits with Two Phenotypes

Each of the seven traits Mendel studied had two forms. The two phenotypes are readily distinguished from one another, so there can be no ambiguity of assignment. For example, one trait was seed color: every seed was either yellow or green.

The alternative forms of the seven traits Mendel studied are illustrated in Figure 2.1. The 14 pure-breeding strains

were bred for (1) seed color (yellow or green), (2) seed shape (round or wrinkled), (3) pod color (green or yellow), (4) pod shape (inflated or constricted), (5) flower color (purple or white), (6) flower position (axial or terminal), and (7) plant height (tall or short).

Quantification of Results

Each time Mendel made a controlled cross, he carefully counted the number of progeny plants of each phenotype. This seemingly simple act—now standard in scientific data gathering—was revolutionary in Mendel's day. By obtaining large numbers of offspring from each cross and by expressing his results numerically, Mendel could more easily analyze them for revealing patterns such as the occurrence of consistent ratios between phenotypes. These ratios were critically important to Mendel's discovery of the rules by which he could predict transmission of alleles during reproduction, and they are the foundation of Mendel's two laws of heredity.

Replicate-, Reciprocal-, and Test-Cross Analysis

The final features that distinguished Mendel's experiments are his use of three genetic-cross strategies that have become tried-and-true approaches to genetic analysis. Rather than simply counting the results of a single cross, for example, Mendel made many **replicate crosses**, producing hundreds of F_1 plants and several thousand F_2 plants by repeating the same cross several times.

Mendel also performed **reciprocal crosses**, in which plants with the same phenotypes are crossed but the sexes of the donating parents are switched. The plant providing the egg in the first cross is used as a source of pollen in the reciprocal cross. Reciprocal crosses are always performed in pairs,

Finally, Mendel performed **test crosses**. These are crosses designed to identify the alleles carried by an organism whose genetic makeup is not certain. We discuss the structure of test crosses and their value as tools of genetic analysis in the following sections.

2.2 Monohybrid Crosses Reveal the Segregation of Alleles

In this section we explore the results and interpretation of Mendel's experiments on the seven traits by focusing on Mendel's examination of two traits, pea color (yellow or green) and pea shape (round or wrinkled). The results and interpretations for those traits apply equally well to the five other traits Mendel examined. The uniformity of Mendel's experimental results and interpretations are due to his decision to conduct experiments on each trait in the same way.

Identifying Dominant and Recessive Traits

Beginning each experiment with different pure-breeding parental plants to produce an F_1 generation, Mendel consistently found that all of the F_1 plants had the same phenotype

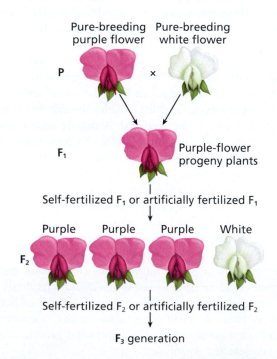

Figure 2.4 Controlled genetic crosses of pea plants. Plants of the P generation are artificially cross-fertilized to produce the F_1 generation. Self-fertilization or crossing of F_1-generation plants to one another produces the F_2 generation. F_2 plants either self-fertilize or are crossed to one another to produce the F_3 generation.

as one of the pure-breeding parents. For example, when Mendel crossed pure-breeding yellow-pea–producing plants and pure-breeding green-pea producers, he found that all the F_1 plants produced yellow peas and none produced green peas (**Figure 2.5**). Mendel identified yellow as the **dominant phenotype** on the basis of its presence in the F_1, and he identified green as the **recessive phenotype** since it is not seen among F_1 progeny.

Employing letters as symbols to represent each trait, Mendel proposed a pattern of transmission from parents to offspring that explained his phenotypic observations in the F_1 and later generations. Today, numerous notational systems for identifying genes and alleles are used, often differing in their particulars along species lines, but the use of letters remains a universal feature. A table describing gene naming (gene nomenclature) and other information about the genes and genomes of model genetic organisms is located inside the book back cover. Most commonly, a dominant trait is shown with an uppercase letter, and a recessive trait is shown in lowercase.

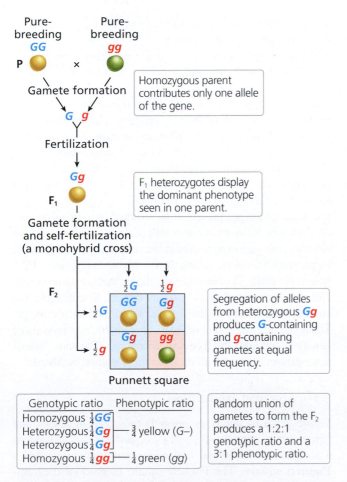

Figure 2.5 Segregation of alleles for seed color. In the cross between yellow-seeded and green-seeded pure-breeding parental plants, F_1 progeny display the dominant yellow phenotype. A 3:1 phenotypic ratio and a 1:2:1 genotypic ratio are observed in the F_2 generation.

Using this scheme, Mendel signified a pure-breeding organism as having a genotype consisting of two identical symbols representing two copies of an allele. This gives us a second way of thinking about pure-breeding organisms, namely that they have a **homozygous genotype**, GG or gg in the example shown in Figure 2.5. If a homozygous plant is self-fertilized, or if two pure-breeding plants expressing the same trait are crossed, the progeny have the same phenotype for the trait and the same homozygous genotype as the parents. In contrast, in a genetic cross between pure-breeding parents with *different* traits, the progeny all have a **heterozygous genotype**, consisting of one genotype symbol from each of the pure-breeding parents, or Gg in this example. Looking more closely at the example in Figure 2.5, note that while the phenotype of the F_1 is the same as that of the yellow parental plant, the genotype is not. This observation is explained momentarily.

Mendel next crossed F_1 yellow plants to produce the F_2 and observed reemergence of the recessive green phenotype. Among the F_2, Mendel found that approximately three-fourths (75%) of the peas were yellow and the remaining one-fourth (25%) were green. To repeat, the yellow : green ratio in the F_2 is $\frac{3}{4} : \frac{1}{4}$, or roughly 3:1. Mendel correctly interpreted these results to indicate that F_2 offspring with the dominant trait were a mixture of two genotypes—GG and Gg—and that plants with the recessive trait were homozygous recessive—gg. More generally, the dominant phenotype F_2 can be classified as having the genotype G–("G blank"), indicating that the genotype is either GG or Gg.

Mendel made similar observations for his experiments testing inheritance of pea shape. Replicate and reciprocal crosses of pure-breeding round-pea–producing plants with pure-breeding wrinkled-pea–producing plants produced F_1 plants bearing exclusively round peas. This result identifies round as the dominant phenotype and wrinkled as the recessive phenotype. His F_1 cross produced F_2 peas in the ratio 75% round to 25% wrinkled—once again a roughly 3:1 ratio.

Tabulating results over several growing seasons for all seven traits, Mendel counted more than 20,000 F_2 peas or plants. **Table 2.1** displays Mendel's results, revealing three consistent features: (1) dominance of one phenotype over the other in the F_1 generation, (2) reemergence of the recessive phenotype in the F_2 generation, and (3) a ratio of approximately 3:1 (dominant : recessive) among F_2 phenotypes. Mendel determined that yellow is dominant to green and round is dominant to wrinkled based on F_1 results. Green pea color and wrinkled pea shape reemerge in the F_2, which displays a consistent 3:1 ratio between the dominant and recessive phenotypes. For example, Mendel classified 8023 F_2 peas by their color and 7324 F_2 peas by their shape. Among the F_2 peas classified by color, he found 6022 yellow seeds and 2001 green seeds, a ratio of almost exactly three to one. Of the F_2 seeds classified for pea shape, 5474 were round and 1850 were wrinkled, again a ratio of very nearly three to one. Data for each of the other five characteristics revealed the same 3:1 ratio of dominant to recessive in the F_2.

Table 2.1   Mendel's Observations for Seven Monohybrid Traits in the F_1 and F_2 Generations

Crosses between Pure-Breeding Parental Phenotypes	F_1 Phenotype	F_2 Phenotypes		F_2 Phenotype Ratio
		Dominant	Recessive	
Round × wrinkled seeds[a]	All round seeds	5474 round	1850 wrinkled	2.96:1
Yellow × green seeds (interior seed color)	All yellow seeds	6022 yellow	2001 green	3.01:1
Purple × white flowers[b] (gray × white seed coat, or exterior seed color)	All purple flowers (gray seed coat)	705 purple	224 white	3.15:1
Axial × terminal flowers	All axial flowers	651 axial	207 terminal	3.14:1
Green × yellow pods	All green pods	428 green	152 yellow	2.82:1
Inflated × constricted pods	All inflated pods	882 inflated	299 constricted	2.95:1
Tall × short plants	All tall plants	787 tall	277 short	2.84:1
TOTAL		14,949	5010	2.98:1

[a] The dominant phenotype is written first and always appears as the F_1 phenotype.
[b] A single gene controls both flower color and seed-coat color. Mendel discussed both traits but recognized they were controlled by the same gene.

Evidence of Particulate Inheritance and Rejection of the Blending Theory

Mendel's F_1 experimental results reject the blending theory of heredity. Specifically, the observation that all F_1 progeny have the same phenotype as one of the pure-breeding parents (i.e., the dominant phenotype) contradicts the blending theory prediction that the F_1 would display a phenotype that is a blend of the two parental phenotypes. The persistence of the dominant phenotype and the reemergence of the recessive phenotype in the F_2 also run counter to the predictions of the blending theory.

Having rejected the blending theory, Mendel examined his experimental results and proposed a new hereditary hypothesis—that each trait is determined by two "particles of heredity"—what today we call "alleles." Mendel used the German word *elemente*, a term meaning "unit or element," to describe the two discrete units of hereditary information for each trait. This idea is the basis of Mendel's theory of **particulate inheritance**, which proposes that each plant carries two particles of heredity (i.e., two alleles) for each trait. A plant receives one unit of heredity (allele) in the egg and a second one in pollen. Each parental plant passes just one of its two alleles to offspring during reproduction. This means that inheritance of one G allele from the homozygous yellow parental plant is sufficient to produce the yellow phenotype, defining the G allele as the **dominant allele**. In contrast, the g allele that produces the green phenotype in the homozygous parental plant is the **recessive allele**. The recessive allele only produces the recessive phenotype when it is in a homozygous genotype.

After establishing that crosses of pure-breeding parental plants produce F_1 plants that always have the dominant phenotype, Mendel crossed F_1 plants ($Gg \times Gg$) to produce the F_2 generation (see Figure 2.5). This is a **monohybrid cross**, a term referring to a cross between two organisms that have the same heterozygous genotype for one gene. A monohybrid cross in pea plants can be made by either crossing heterozygous F_1 with one another or by allowing F_1 plants to self-fertilize. With a dominant and a recessive allele in their heterozygous genotype, these F_1 plants donate one or the other of the alleles to each of their F_2 progeny. The result of these monohybrid crosses is a 3:1 **phenotypic ratio** among the F_2. In other words, Mendel observed that approximately 75% of the F_2 had the dominant phenotype and 25% had the recessive phenotype. He also correctly predicted that the F_2 generation would have three genotypes: The two homozygous genotypes (the same genotypes present in the original pure-breeding parents) each occur in about one-fourth of the F_2 progeny, and the heterozygous genotype occurs in the remaining one-half of the F_2 progeny. Therefore, among the F_2, Mendel predicted a 1:2:1 **genotypic ratio**. The one-fourth of the F_2 that are homozygous GG plus the one-half of F_2 progeny that are heterozygous Gg are the three-fourths of the F_2 with the dominant phenotype. The remaining one-fourth of the F_2 contain the homozygous gg genotype and have the recessive phenotype. The same inheritance pattern occurs for all the other traits studied by Mendel.

Segregation of Alleles

Figure 2.5 uses letters as symbols to represent alleles and genotypes in parental, F_1, and F_2 organisms and introduces a simple and functional tool of genetic analysis called a **Punnett square**. The Punnett square method of diagramming the genetic content of gametes and their union to form offspring is named in honor of Sir Reginald Punnett, a famous geneticist of the early 20th century. The Punnett square separates the two alleles carried by each reproducing organism, placing the reproductive cells, or gametes, from one parent along the vertical margin of the diagram, and those from the other parent along the horizontal margin. The squares within the body of the Punnett diagram show the results expected from the random union of the male and female gametes, each square identifying a possible genotype of offspring produced by gamete union.

Having formed the concept of particulate inheritance and having carefully counted the number of plants in each phenotype category, Mendel was able to frame a hypothesis to explain his results. This first hypothesis of Mendel's is known as the **law of segregation**, sometimes also known as **Mendel's first law**. It describes the particulate nature of inheritance, identifies the segregation (separation) of alleles during gamete formation (we discuss this process more fully in Chapter 3), and proposes the random union of gametes to produce progeny in predictable proportions:

> **The law of segregation** *The two alleles for each trait will separate (segregate) from one another during gamete formation, and each allele will have an equal probability* $\left(\frac{1}{2}\right)$ *of inclusion in a gamete. Random union of gametes at fertilization will unite one gamete from each parent to produce progeny in ratios that are determined by chance.*

The law of segregation means that when pure-breeding parents with different homozygous genotypes are crossed, all their F_1 progeny have the dominant phenotype and have a heterozygous genotype. In the case of reproduction of heterozygous F_1 plants, the law of segregation means that one-half of the reproductive cells of each F_1 parent are expected to contain the dominant allele and one-half are expected to contain the recessive allele. The random union of reproductive cells from the heterozygous F_1 plants leads to the 3:1 phenotypic ratio and the 1:2:1 genotypic ratio of the F_2.

Hypothesis Testing by Test-Cross Analysis

Mendel proposed the law of segregation to explain the phenotype proportions he observed in the F_1 and F_2 generations of his breeding experiments, but two critical parts of his hypothesis could not be seen by observation of F_1 and F_2 phenotypes, and Mendel needed to demonstrate they were true to validate his hypothesis. Specifically, Mendel predicted that all the F_1 progeny in his experiment were heterozygous and that among the F_2 progeny with the dominant phenotype were plants with the homozygous genotype and plants with the heterozygous genotype.

To test the hypothesis that the F_1 were heterozygous, Mendel devised what is known in genetics as a test cross. This is the cross of an organism that has the dominant phenotype to one that has the recessive phenotype to determine whether the dominant organism has the homozygous genotype or the heterozygous genotype. If the plant with the dominant phenotype is homozygous, then all the progeny of the test cross will have the dominant phenotype. In contrast, if the dominant organism is

heterozygous, then there will be a roughly 1:1 ratio of progeny with the dominant phenotype to progeny with the recessive phenotype.

One of Mendel's test crosses of F_1 plants to recessive plants is shown in **Figure 2.6**. Based on his segregation hypothesis, Mendel predicted that test-cross progeny phenotypes would be 50% dominant and 50% recessive. Figure 2.6 illustrates Mendel's test cross between an F_1 plant producing round seeds (and suspected to have a heterozygous genotype) and a pure-breeding wrinkled-seed plant, known to be homozygous *rr*. In the test cross, the wrinkled-seed plant, being homozygous *rr*, produces only *r*-containing gametes. If the F_1 plant is indeed heterozygous, it should produce reproductive cells with *R* and *r* genotypes at a frequency of $\frac{1}{2}$ each. Consequently, the progeny of the cross should be $\frac{1}{2}$ *Rr* and $\frac{1}{2}$ *rr*, resulting in a 1:1 ratio of round : wrinkled. As the figure indicates, Mendel performed this cross and observed 193 round peas and 192 wrinkled peas, or a 1:1 ratio, in test-cross progeny. Mendel reported test-cross results for five of his traits and observed a 1:1 ratio in each case (**Table 2.2**). These results verify the prediction that the F_1 progeny of pure-breeding crosses are heterozygous. If the F_1 were homozygous dominant instead of heterozygous, the test-cross progeny would all have the dominant phenotype instead of the observed 1:1 ratio.

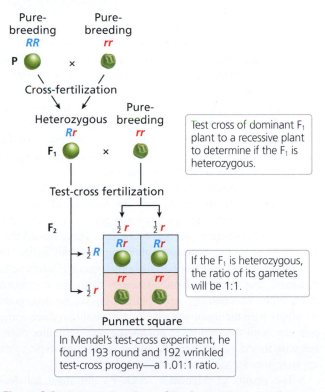

Figure 2.6   Test-cross analysis of F_1 plants. A test cross between an F_1 plant and one that is homozygous recessive produces progeny with a 1:1 ratio of the dominant to the recessive phenotype if the F_1 plant is heterozygous.

🔴 **If a test-cross experiment identical to the one shown here produces 826 progeny plants, how many plants are expected in each phenotype category?**

Table 2.2	Test-Cross Results from Mendel's Experiments		
Test Cross	**Test-Cross Progeny**		**Ratio**
	Dominant	**Recessive**	
Round seed (*Rr*) × wrinkled seed (*rr*)	193 round (*Rr*)	192 wrinkled (*rr*)	1.01:1
Yellow seed (*Gg*) × green seed (*gg*)	196 yellow (*Gg*)	189 green (*gg*)	1.04:1
Purple flower (*Pp*) × white flower (*pp*)	85 purple (*Pp*)	81 white (*pp*)	1.05:1
Tall plants (*Tt*) × short plants (*tt*)	87 tall (*Tt*)	79 short (*tt*)	1.10:1
TOTAL	561	541	1.04:1

Genetic Analysis 2.1 guides you in predicting the genotypes resulting from three crosses by examining phenotype ratios among progeny.

Hypothesis Testing by F₂ Self-Fertilization

The second pivotal component of Mendel's segregation hypothesis concerns the genotypes of F_2 progeny. Specifically, Mendel's hypothesis predicts that F_2 plants with the dominant phenotype can be either homozygous or heterozygous. His hypothesis further predicts that F_2 plants with the dominant phenotype are twice as likely to be heterozygous as homozygous. Figure 2.5 illustrates this prediction. Notice that among the three-fourths of the F_2 progeny that have the dominant (yellow) phenotype, two-thirds are heterozygous (*Gg*) and one-third are homozygous (*GG*).

Mendel allowed self-fertilization of the F_2 plants with the dominant phenotype, to test the validity of his proposal that heterozygotes and homozygotes occur at a 2:1 ratio among dominant plants (**Figure 2.7**). He reasoned that F_2 plants with the dominant phenotype (round seeds, in this figure) could be identified as homozygous if when self-fertilized they produced only progeny with the dominant phenotype. In contrast, self-fertilization of heterozygous F_2 plants with the dominant phenotype would produce some progeny with the dominant phenotype and a smaller number with the recessive (here, wrinkled seed) phenotype, in an approximate 3:1 ratio.

The results of Mendel's seven F_2 dominant self-fertilization experiments are shown in **Table 2.3**. His largest sample was for seed shape: he self-fertilized 565 round-seeded F_2 plants and found that 193 of the plants (34.2%) produced only round peas in progeny, demonstrating that these plants were homozygous for the dominant allele (*RR*). Self-fertilization of the other 372 round-pea–producing F_2 plants (65.8%) produced both round peas and wrinkled

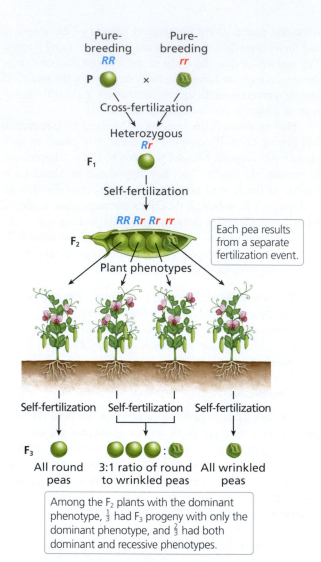

Figure 2.7   Determination of the genotype of F₂ plants by the production of F₃ progeny. F_2 plants are self-fertilized and their F_3 progeny are examined. Among the dominant (round) F_2, approximately one-third are expected to be homozygous for the dominant allele (*RR*). These plants produce progeny that have only round peas. The remaining two-thirds of the dominant F_2 are expected to be heterozygous, and produce both round and wrinkled peas in progeny. All F_2 wrinkled peas are homozygous recessive (*rr*) and produce only wrinkled peas as progeny.

peas in progeny plants. The ratio 372:193 is very close to the 2:1 ratio of heterozygous to homozygous genotypes that Mendel predicted would constitute the dominant, round-pea–producing F_2 plants.

Mendel's self-fertilization results consistently show a 2:1 ratio among dominant F_2 plants for each of the seven traits examined. These results validate the proposal that gametes unite at random to produce progeny. Taken together, the test-cross experiments and the dominant F_2 self-fertilization experiments represent successfully designed and executed independent experiments for testing components of Mendel's segregation hypothesis. In these tests, Mendel made predictions about the experimental

PROBLEM The presence of short hairs on the leaves of tomato plants is a dominant trait controlled by the allele *H*. The corresponding recessive trait, smooth leaf, is found in plants with the genotype *hh*. The table at right shows the progeny of three independent crosses of parental plants with genotypes and phenotypes that are unknown.

> **BREAK IT DOWN:** Dominant and recessive alleles dictate that hairy-leaf plants are *HH* or *Hh*; smooth-leaf plants are *hh* (p. 36).

Examine the relative numbers of the phenotypes in the progeny of each cross, and use that information to determine the parental genotypes for each cross. Use a Punnett square to diagram Cross 1.

> **BREAK IT DOWN:** Use a Punnett square to accurately organize gamete production and gamete union (p. 36).

> **BREAK IT DOWN:** Phenotype ratios among progeny identify the genotypes of parents in a cross (p. 35).

	Number of Progeny	
Cross	Hairy Leaf	Smooth Leaf
1	32	11
2	42	45
3	0	24

Solution Strategies	Solution Steps

Evaluate

1. Identify the topic of this problem and the kind of information the answer should contain.

2. Identify the critical information given in the problem.

> **TIP:** The numbers of progeny with each phenotype can be expressed as a ratio.

1. The problem presents the leaf-form phenotypes of progeny produced by three separate crosses of parental plants with unknown genotypes and phenotypes. The answer must identify parental genotypes and phenotypes for each cross and use a Punnett square to diagram Cross 1.

2. The information given for each cross is the number of progeny with hairy (dominant) and smooth (recessive) leaves. Interpretation of the phenotype ratio of progeny is required to determine parental genotypes and phenotypes.

Deduce

3. Examine the progeny of Cross 1, and determine the approximate ratio of progeny phenotypes.

> **PITFALL:** Genetics experiments produce finite numbers of progeny, so phenotypes may vary from expected ratios. Don't expect to see precise ratios in real data.

4. Examine the progeny of Cross 2, and determine the approximate ratio of progeny phenotypes.

5. Examine the progeny of Cross 3, and determine the approximate ratio of progeny phenotypes.

3. Ratio of phenotypes in Cross 1 progeny:

$$\frac{32}{11} = 2.91 : 1$$

This is an approximate 3:1 ratio. The recessive phenotype appears in about $\frac{1}{4}$ of the progeny $\left(\frac{11}{43}\right)$, and the remaining $\frac{3}{4}$ $\left(\frac{32}{43}\right)$ have the dominant phenotype.

4. Ratio of phenotypes for Cross 2:

$$\frac{42}{45} = 0.93 : 1$$

This is an approximate 1:1 ratio in which the dominant phenotype is seen in about one-half of the progeny $\left(\frac{42}{97}\right)$ and the recessive phenotype is seen in the other half of the progeny $\left(\frac{45}{97}\right)$.

5. Cross 3 produced only the recessive phenotype, so the ratio is 0:1.

Solve

6. Based on the results of Cross 1, identify the genotypes and phenotypes of the parental plants in the cross. Construct a Punnett square to illustrate this cross.

> **TIP:** There are two alleles for this gene, and three genotypes are possible. The recessive phenotype is found in plants with the *hh* genotype, whereas the dominant phenotype will be found in plants that are *Hh* and *HH*.

7. Based on the results of Cross 2, identify the genotypes and phenotypes of the parents.

8. Based on the results of Cross 3, identify the parental genotypes and phenotypes.

6. The recessive progeny in this cross have the genotype *hh*, so each parent in Cross 1 must carry a copy of *h*. The dominant progeny are either *HH* or *Hh*. The 3:1 progeny phenotype ratio is consistent with a parental cross *Hh* × *Hh*. The Punnett square for this cross is consistent with the observed 3:1 ratio:

7. Both parental plants in Cross 2 carry at least one copy of *h*. The 1:1 progeny ratio is consistent with the ratio expected for a test cross of a heterozygous organism to one that is homozygous recessive. This cross is *Hh* × *hh*.

8. Cross 3 produces only *hh* progeny. This is expected for a pure-breeding cross between two homozygous organisms. This cross is *hh* × *hh*.

For more practice, see Problems 10, 14, and 29.   Visit the Study Area to access study tools.   **Mastering Genetics**

Table 2.3	Results of Mendel's Experiments to Identify F$_2$-Plant Genotypes by Their F$_3$ Progeny		
Trait[a]	Heterozygous F$_2$ Plants[b]	Homozygous F$_2$ Plants[c]	Ratio[d]
Seed shape	372	193	1.93:1
Seed color	353	166	2.13:1
Flower color	64	36	1.78:1
Pod shape	71	29	2.45:1
Pod color	125	75	1.67:1
Flower position	67	33	2.03:1
Plant height	72	28	2.57:1
TOTAL	1124	560	2.01:1

[a] Mendel self-fertilized only F$_2$ plants with the dominant phenotype in this experiment.
[b] F$_2$ plants were heterozygous if the F$_3$ progeny they produced by self-fertilization had both dominant and recessive phenotypes.
[c] F$_2$ plants were homozygous if the F$_3$ progeny they produced by self-fertilization had only the dominant phenotype.
[d] The expected ratio of heterozygous to homozygous F$_2$ plants was 2.00:1.

outcomes and then verified the results by counting the progeny produced. The resulting data supported his segregation hypothesis and illustrate how Mendel anticipated modern scientific methods, using approaches that would not be consistently applied to genetic experiments for several decades.

Mendelian genetics is all around us. You'll even find it in the produce aisle of your local grocery store! **Experimental Insight 2.1** describes an experiment in Mendelian genetics using ears of corn that have a mixture of yellow and white kernels.

2.3 Dihybrid and Trihybrid Crosses Reveal the Independent Assortment of Alleles

Each of the seven traits investigated by Mendel showed the same pattern of hereditary transmission that is explained by the law of segregation. The predictability of phenotype proportions in F$_1$ and F$_2$ test-cross and self-fertilization progeny suggests that the same mechanism is responsible for allelic segregation in each one of the selected traits. But what about the inheritance of two or more traits simultaneously? Is there a pattern or ratio of phenotypes that allowed Mendel to propose a transmission mechanism when two or more genes are examined at the same time? Mendel believed that the law of segregation applied to all genes simultaneously, and he devised experiments to test this theory that led to his identification of a second law of heredity.

Dihybrid-Cross Analysis of Two Genes

To test the simultaneous transmission of two traits in the pea plant, Mendel performed a series of **dihybrid crosses**, crosses between organisms that differ in two traits. These tests followed an experimental strategy that paralleled his investigation of allelic segregation of single traits.

As **Figure 2.8** illustrates, Mendel began each dihybrid cross with pure-breeding lines. Any combination of two pure-breeding traits in parental plants can be used, but here we see Mendel's experimental cross in which one parent is pure-breeding for the two dominant pea traits of round and yellow (*RRGG*) and the other parent is pure-breeding for the recessive pea traits wrinkled and green (*rrgg*). The gametes, whether pollen or egg, produced by the round, yellow plant contain one allele for each type of gene and are *RG*. In contrast, gametes from the wrinkled, green plant are *rg*. Mendel's model predicts that all of the F$_1$ progeny will therefore have the genotype *RrGg*. These F$_1$ are described as *dihybrid*, meaning heterozygous for two traits, and display the dominant parental phenotypes round and yellow.

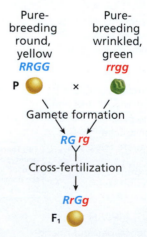

Figure 2.8 Dihybrid-cross analysis. Pure-breeding parental plants *RRGG* (round, yellow) and *rrgg* (wrinkled, green) are cross-fertilized to produce F$_1$ progeny that are dihybrid (*RrGg*) and display the two dominant phenotypes round and yellow.

Q **For this cross why doesn't it matter whether the round, yellow plant provides pollen and the wrinkled, green plant provides eggs or vice versa?**

EXPERIMENTAL INSIGHT 2.1

Mendelism in the Produce Aisle

Many of the appealing characteristics of fruits and vegetables available in grocery stores and at farmer's markets are the result of intensive selective breeding, a form of natural selection generated by breeders, who select which organisms are to reproduce and determine the crosses that will occur. For example, in recent years many new vegetable varieties have been introduced into the marketplace. Among these is a variety of corn that goes by several names, including "bicolor," "peaches and cream," and "yellow and white." Most of the kernels on a cob of bicolored corn are yellow, but a sizable number are white. With close inspection and a little quantitative analysis, you should be able to identify the genetic mechanism that produces this variation in color.

An ear of corn is a mini–genetic experiment: Each kernel on the ear, like each pea in a pod, is a separate seed,

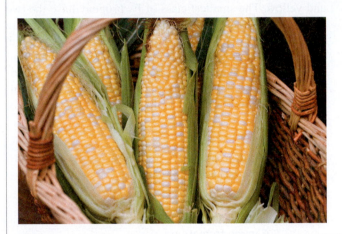

produced by a fertilization event independent of the events that produced adjacent kernels. This means that each mature ear of corn carries hundreds of progeny for analysis.

Bicolor corn originates with the cross of two pure-breeding corn lines, one producing yellow kernels and the other producing white kernels. The yellow plant is *WW*, and the white plant is *ww*. When seed company geneticists cross these parental stocks, the kernels on the F$_1$ plants are yellow and have the heterozygous *Ww* genotype. This F$_1$ seed is allowed to mature and is packaged for sale to farmers and home gardeners, who plant it to produce a crop. The seed is commonly labeled "hybrid," meaning "monohybrid," to reflect the heterozygosity at the kernel-color gene. Owing to segregation of alleles at the kernel-color gene, the plants that grow from this F$_1$ seed produce both yellow (*W–*) and white (*ww*) kernels on each ear.

If you saw some of this corn in your grocery store, how would you verify that the genetic basis of its yellow and white kernels is the segregation of two alleles at a single gene? The answer is that you would count the number of yellow kernels and the number of white kernels on ears of bicolor corn with the expectation of a ratio of approximately 3:1 between the yellow and white kernels.

Recent genetics classes of one of the authors examined several dozen ears of bicolor corn and counted 9304 yellow kernels and 3052 white kernels. Among the total of 12,356 kernels, this meant 75.3% were yellow and 24.7% were white, a ratio of 3.05:1. You will use these data in Problem 20 at the end of the chapter to do a statistical test to see if the observed data fit the hypothesis that this trait is the product of the segregation of alleles of a single gene. The next time you shop for fruits and vegetables, keep in mind that you are looking at Mendelian genetics in action!

If the assortment of alleles for each gene is independent of the assortment for other genes, gametes produced by these F$_1$ plants are equally likely to contain *any* combination of one allele for seed shape and one allele for seed color. Probabilities of each combination of alleles for each gene are predicted by recognizing that four combinations of alleles will be found in the gametes—*RG*, *Rg*, *rG*, and *rg*—and that each combination is expected to occur with a frequency of $\frac{1}{4}$.

Figure 2.9 shows a diagrammatic aid called the **forked-line diagram** that is used in this instance to help determine gamete genotypes and frequencies. The forked-line diagram illustrates that one-half of all gametes produced by an *RrGg* plant will contain *R* and one-half will contain *r*. If the segregation of *G* and *g* is independent of the *R* and *r* alleles, then one-half of the gametes containing *R* will also carry *G* and the other half will carry *g*. The same is true for *r*-bearing gametes; one-half will carry *G* and the remaining half will carry *g*. The frequency of each of the four gamete genotypes is $\left(\frac{1}{2}\right)\left(\frac{1}{2}\right) = \frac{1}{4}$.

A Punnett square can be used to illustrate the random union of these four different gametes to produce F$_2$ progeny

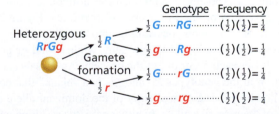

Figure 2.9   The forked-line method for determining gamete genotype frequency. The $\frac{1}{2}$ probabilities of the alleles are multiplied to determine the probability of each gamete genotype.

🔘 Reproduce this forked-line diagram switching the traits to flower color (purple versus white) and plant height (tall versus short), using allele symbols *W* and *w* for flower color and *T* and *t* for plant height.

(**Figure 2.10**). Each gamete has a predicted frequency of $\frac{1}{4}$, and each cell of the Punnett square has a predicted frequency of $\left(\frac{1}{4}\right)\left(\frac{1}{4}\right) = \frac{1}{16}$. Among F$_2$ progeny, four phenotypes are observed, displaying (1) both dominant phenotypes, (2) the dominant phenotype for one trait and the recessive phenotype for the other (there are two versions of this), or

Punnett square				Summary	
	$\frac{1}{4}RG$	$\frac{1}{4}Rg$	$\frac{1}{4}rG$	$\frac{1}{4}rg$	Genotypes / Phenotypes
$\frac{1}{4}RG$	$\frac{1}{16}RRGG$	$\frac{1}{16}RRGg$	$\frac{1}{16}RrGG$	$\frac{1}{16}RrGg$	$RRGG=\frac{1}{16}$ $RrGG=\frac{2}{16}$ $RRGg=\frac{2}{16}$ $RrGg=\frac{4}{16}$ — $\frac{9}{16}$ R–G–
$\frac{1}{4}Rg$	$\frac{1}{16}RRGg$	$\frac{1}{16}RRgg$	$\frac{1}{16}RrGg$	$\frac{1}{16}Rrgg$	$RRgg=\frac{1}{16}$ $Rrgg=\frac{2}{16}$ — $\frac{3}{16}$ R–gg
$\frac{1}{4}rG$	$\frac{1}{16}RrGG$	$\frac{1}{16}RrGg$	$\frac{1}{16}rrGG$	$\frac{1}{16}rrGg$	$rrGG=\frac{1}{16}$ $rrGg=\frac{2}{16}$ — $\frac{3}{16}$ rrG–
$\frac{1}{4}rg$	$\frac{1}{16}RrGg$	$\frac{1}{16}Rrgg$	$\frac{1}{16}rrGg$	$\frac{1}{16}rrgg$	$rrgg=\frac{1}{16}$ — $\frac{1}{16}$ rrgg

Figure 2.10   Independent assortment of alleles of two genes. Crossing dihybrid F_1 ($RrGg$) organisms to one another produces nine genotypes distributed in a 9:3:3:1 phenotypic ratio among F_2 progeny.

(3) both recessive phenotypes. The F_2 phenotypes appear in the ratio $\frac{9}{16}:\frac{3}{16}:\frac{3}{16}:\frac{1}{16}$.

By examining the F_2 phenotype proportions, we can see the relationship between the 3:1 ratio for each trait and the 9:3:3:1 ratio when the two traits are considered simultaneously. When pea shape and pea color are considered individually, monohybrid crosses produce F_2 that are $\frac{3}{4}$ dominant and $\frac{1}{4}$ recessive. The cross of two dihybrids also yields proportions of $\frac{3}{4}$ dominant to $\frac{1}{4}$ recessive for each trait, making the prediction of phenotypic ratios among the F_2 for both traits combined a problem of combinatorial arithmetic involving the segregation of alleles for each of two traits. Figure 2.10 reminds us that genotypes falling into the $R–$ and the $G–$ classes each occur in $\frac{3}{4}$ of the progeny, while rr and gg genotype classes each occur in $\frac{1}{4}$ of the progeny. As we saw earlier, the dash in the genotypes $R–$ and $G–$ is a "blank" that could be filled by either a second copy of the dominant allele or a copy of the recessive allele. In either case, the resulting genotype—for example, RR or Rr—produces the dominant phenotype. The co-occurrence of the two dominant phenotypes (round, yellow) is therefore expected to have a frequency of $\left(\frac{3}{4}\right)\left(\frac{3}{4}\right)=\frac{9}{16}$, the two recessive phenotypes (wrinkled, green) will occur with a frequency of $\left(\frac{1}{4}\right)\left(\frac{1}{4}\right)=\frac{1}{16}$, and the two phenotypic classes that display one dominant and one recessive trait (round, green and wrinkled, yellow) will each be found in a frequency of $\left(\frac{3}{4}\right)\left(\frac{1}{4}\right)=\frac{3}{16}$.

This outcome illustrates Mendel's **law of independent assortment**, also known as **Mendel's second law.**

The law of independent assortment During gamete formation, the segregation of alleles of one gene is independent of the segregation of alleles of another gene.

Mendel's conclusions regarding independent assortment were based on results he obtained from several dihybrid cross experiments, such as the one involving pea color and pea shape shown in **Figure 2.11**. After crossing the pure-breeding parents and allowing self-fertilization of the F_1, Mendel counted the phenotypes among the F_2 and found that both of the original parental phenotypes (round, yellow and wrinkled, green) were present along with two *nonparental* phenotypes: round, green and wrinkled, yellow. Among the F_2 produced in his experiment, Mendel found 315 round, yellow plants; 108 round, green plants; 101 wrinkled, yellow plants; and 32 wrinkled, green plants (Figure 2.11a).

This F_2 observation contains two features of pivotal importance to Mendel's hypothesis. First, parental and nonparental phenotypes are seen at frequencies that differ from one another. The most numerous class of F_2 progeny display the dominant parental phenotypes for each trait, round and yellow. The smallest class of F_2 progeny have the two recessive parental phenotypes, wrinkled and green; and the two nonparental F_2 classes (round, green and wrinkled, yellow) are intermediate and approximately equal in number. From these numbers, Mendel recognized that the ratios between the dominant and recessive forms of each trait followed the familiar 3:1 pattern. In looking at pea shape, for

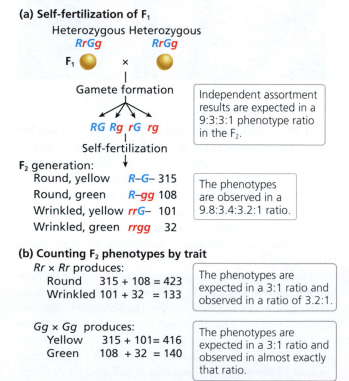

(a) Self-fertilization of F_1

Heterozygous   Heterozygous
RrGg   *RrGg*

F_1 ⊙   ×   ⊙

Gamete formation

RG Rg rG rg

> Independent assortment results are expected in a 9:3:3:1 phenotype ratio in the F_2.

Self-fertilization

F_2 generation:
Round, yellow   *R–G–* 315
Round, green   *R–gg* 108
Wrinkled, yellow *rrG–* 101
Wrinkled, green *rrgg* 32

> The phenotypes are observed in a 9.8:3.4:3.2:1 ratio.

(b) Counting F_2 phenotypes by trait

Rr × Rr produces:
Round   315 + 108 = 423
Wrinkled 101 + 32 = 133

> The phenotypes are expected in a 3:1 ratio and observed in a ratio of 3.2:1.

Gg × Gg produces:
Yellow   315 + 101 = 416
Green   108 + 32 = 140

> The phenotypes are expected in a 3:1 ratio and observed in almost exactly that ratio.

Figure 2.11   Phenotype proportions in the progeny of a dihybrid cross performed by Mendel. (a) The phenotypic ratio Mendel observed was close to the expected ratio of 9:3:3:1. (b) For each trait considered individually, the phenotype ratio in the progeny from the same cross is approximately 3:1.

example, Mendel found that 423 (315 + 108) plants were round and that 133 (101 + 32) plants were wrinkled. The ratio 423:133 reduces to approximately 3:1. Similarly, for pea color he found a ratio of 416 (315 + 101) yellow to 140 (108 + 32) green—a ratio of approximately 3:1 (Figure 2.11b). Considering each trait individually, the cross of heterozygous F_1 plants has produced an F_2 generation in which $\frac{3}{4}$ of the progeny have the dominant phenotype and $\frac{1}{4}$ have the recessive phenotype.

Second, Mendel predicted that if alleles of each gene unite at random to produce the F_2, then the expected F_2-progeny phenotypes will occur in predictable frequencies. He hypothesized that F_2 progeny displaying the two dominant traits (round and yellow) will occur at a frequency of $\left(\frac{3}{4}\right)\left(\frac{3}{4}\right) = \frac{9}{16}$. Similarly, progeny carrying the two recessive traits (wrinkled and green) are expected at a frequency of $\left(\frac{1}{4}\right)\left(\frac{1}{4}\right) = \frac{1}{16}$, and each of the nonparental phenotypes is expected at a frequency of $\left(\frac{3}{4}\right)\left(\frac{1}{4}\right) = \frac{3}{16}$. Independent assortment of alleles at the two genes therefore leads to an expected distribution among the F_2 of

round, yellow	R–G–	$\frac{9}{16}$
round, green	R–gg	$\frac{3}{16}$
wrinkled, yellow	rrG–	$\frac{3}{16}$
wrinkled, green	rrgg	$\frac{1}{16}$

Mendel's count of 315 round, yellow; 108 round, green; 101 wrinkled, yellow; and 32 wrinkled, green (see Figure 2.11) can be converted to a ratio by dividing each number by 32, the value of the smallest class. The division by 32 reduces Mendel's observed ratio to approximately 9:3:3:1 as predicted by his model. From this result, Mendel hypothesized that independent assortment in a dihybrid organism produces four different gamete genotypes at equal frequencies. Random union of the gametes then produces four phenotypic classes as a result of dominance relationships at each gene, and the ratio of these F_2 phenotypic classes is expected to be 9:3:3:1. **Genetic Analysis 2.2** guides you through a problem involving prediction of the ratios of phenotypes in offspring from three different dihybrid crosses involving the same traits.

Testing Independent Assortment by Test-Cross Analysis

Mendel's hypothesis of independent assortment rested on the assumption that when two of his pure-breeding lines differing in two traits were crossed, the F_1 were dihybrid, $RrGg$ in the case we have been discussing. To prove this assumption was correct, Mendel once again turned to test-cross analysis. Having proposed that the F_1 plants with round, yellow seeds were dihybrid and had the genotype $RrGg$, he predicted that the test cross of a dihybrid ($RrGg$) to a pure-breeding wrinkled, green plant ($rrgg$) would

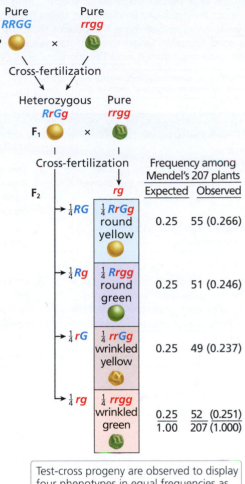

Figure 2.12 **Mendel's test cross to verify independent assortment.** Mendel predicted and observed an approximate 1:1:1:1 ratio among progeny, supporting his hypothesis of independent assortment.

produce four offspring phenotypes at a frequency of $\frac{1}{4}$ each. **Figure 2.12** shows that the dihybrid F_1 plant was expected to produce four different gamete genotypes. Recalling the logic of the forked-line diagram, remember that one-half of the gametes are expected to contain R and one-half to contain r. Gametes carry G and g independently of R or r, meaning that four different combinations of these alleles are possible in gametes: RG, rG, Rg, and rg, each occurring at an expected frequency of $\left(\frac{1}{2}\right)\left(\frac{1}{2}\right) = \frac{1}{4}$. In contrast, the homozygous recessive green, wrinkled ($rrgg$) plant can produce only an rg gamete. In the figure, we see that the test-cross progeny are expected to have four genotypes, each corresponding to a different phenotype. The predicted progeny are expected to be $\frac{1}{4}$ $RrGg$ (round, yellow) and $\frac{1}{4}$ $Rrgg$ (round, green), $\frac{1}{4}$ $rrGg$ (wrinkled, yellow) and $\frac{1}{4}$ $rrgg$ (wrinkled, green).

PROBLEM In a certain mammalian species, long fur and the appearance of white spots are produced by dominant alleles *F* and *S*, respectively, which assort independently. The genotype *ff* produces short fur, and the genotype *ss* produces solid fur color. Given the parental genotypes for each of the following crosses, determine the expected proportions of all progeny phenotypes.

	Male		Female
Cross 1:	*FF Ss*	×	*Ff ss*
Cross 2:	*ff Ss*	×	*Ff Ss*
Cross 3:	*Ff Ss*	×	*Ff Ss*

BREAK IT DOWN: If genes assort independently, fur length will be independent of the presence or absence of spots (p. 42).

BREAK IT DOWN: Use a Punnett square or a forked-line diagram to accurately predict cross outcomes (p. 41).

Solution Strategies	Solution Steps

Evaluate

1. Identify the topic of this problem and the kind of information the answer should contain.

2. Identify the critical information given in the problem.

1. This is a transmission genetic problem in which parental genotypes are given. Answers must predict the phenotypes of progeny and their expected proportions. These are predicted by determining the parental gametes and their proportions.

2. Genotypes of parents are given for each cross. The genotypes are used to predict the genotypes of parental gametes and the gamete proportions.

Deduce

3. For Cross 1, identify the genetically different gametes that can be produced by each parent and calculate the predicted proportion of each gamete.

TIP: A forked-line diagram is a useful tool for predicting the alleles in gametes and gamete frequencies.

3. Each of the parents can produce two genetically different gametes at predicted frequencies of $\frac{1}{2}$ each.

Cross 1

Male

$1F \left\langle \begin{array}{l} \frac{1}{2}S \cdots FS \cdots (1)(\frac{1}{2}) = \frac{1}{2} \\ \frac{1}{2}s \cdots Fs \cdots (1)(\frac{1}{2}) = \frac{1}{2} \end{array} \right.$

Female

$\frac{1}{2}F \longrightarrow 1s \cdots Fs \cdots (\frac{1}{2})(1) = \frac{1}{2}$
$\frac{1}{2}f \longrightarrow 1s \cdots fs \cdots (\frac{1}{2})(1) = \frac{1}{2}$

4. Identify the content and frequency of the genetically different gametes produced by the parents in Cross 2.

PITFALL: Carefully identify the genotype of each parent to avoid errors.

4. The male produces two types of gametes at a predicted frequency of $\frac{1}{2}$ each. The female produces four genetically different gametes at frequencies of $\frac{1}{4}$ each.

Cross 2

Male

$1f \left\langle \begin{array}{l} \frac{1}{2}S \cdots fS \cdots (1)(\frac{1}{2}) = \frac{1}{2} \\ \frac{1}{2}s \cdots fs \cdots (1)(\frac{1}{2}) = \frac{1}{2} \end{array} \right.$

Female

$\frac{1}{2}F \left\langle \begin{array}{l} \frac{1}{2}S \cdots FS \cdots (\frac{1}{2})(\frac{1}{2}) = \frac{1}{4} \\ \frac{1}{2}s \cdots Fs \cdots (\frac{1}{2})(\frac{1}{2}) = \frac{1}{4} \end{array} \right.$
$\frac{1}{2}f \left\langle \begin{array}{l} \frac{1}{2}S \cdots fS \cdots (\frac{1}{2})(\frac{1}{2}) = \frac{1}{4} \\ \frac{1}{2}s \cdots fs \cdots (\frac{1}{2})(\frac{1}{2}) = \frac{1}{4} \end{array} \right.$

5. Predict the gamete content and frequencies for the parents in Cross 3.

5. Both parents are dihybrids that produce four genetically different gametes at frequencies of $\frac{1}{4}$ each.

Cross 3

Male

$\frac{1}{2}F \left\langle \begin{array}{l} \frac{1}{2}S \cdots FS \cdots (\frac{1}{2})(\frac{1}{2}) = \frac{1}{4} \\ \frac{1}{2}s \cdots Fs \cdots (\frac{1}{2})(\frac{1}{2}) = \frac{1}{4} \end{array} \right.$
$\frac{1}{2}f \left\langle \begin{array}{l} \frac{1}{2}S \cdots fS \cdots (\frac{1}{2})(\frac{1}{2}) = \frac{1}{4} \\ \frac{1}{2}s \cdots fs \cdots (\frac{1}{2})(\frac{1}{2}) = \frac{1}{4} \end{array} \right.$

Female

$\frac{1}{2}F \left\langle \begin{array}{l} \frac{1}{2}S \cdots FS \cdots (\frac{1}{2})(\frac{1}{2}) = \frac{1}{4} \\ \frac{1}{2}s \cdots Fs \cdots (\frac{1}{2})(\frac{1}{2}) = \frac{1}{4} \end{array} \right.$
$\frac{1}{2}f \left\langle \begin{array}{l} \frac{1}{2}S \cdots fS \cdots (\frac{1}{2})(\frac{1}{2}) = \frac{1}{4} \\ \frac{1}{2}s \cdots fs \cdots (\frac{1}{2})(\frac{1}{2}) = \frac{1}{4} \end{array} \right.$

Solve

6. Construct a Punnett square for Cross 1 and predict the progeny phenotypes and proportions.

6. The predicted Cross 1 progeny are $\frac{1}{2}$ long, spotted and $\frac{1}{2}$ long, solid.

♂ / ♀	FS	Fs
Fs	FFSs	FFss
fs	FfSs	Ffss

7. Construct a Punnett square for Cross 2 and predict the progeny phenotypes and proportions.

7. The progeny predicted from Cross 2 are $\frac{3}{8}$ long, spotted; $\frac{1}{8}$ long, solid; $\frac{3}{8}$ short, spotted; and $\frac{1}{8}$ short, solid.

♂ / ♀	fS	fs
FS	FfSS	FfSs
Fs	FfSs	Ffss
fS	ffSS	ffSs
fs	ffSs	ffss

8. Construct a Punnett square for Cross 3 and predict the progeny phenotypes and proportions.

8. The progeny produced by Cross 3 are predicted to be $\frac{9}{16}$ long, spotted; $\frac{3}{16}$ long, solid; $\frac{3}{16}$ short, spotted; and $\frac{1}{16}$ short, solid.

♂ / ♀	FS	Fs	fS	fs
FS	FFSS	FFSs	FfSS	FfSs
Fs	FFSs	FFss	FfSs	Ffss
fS	FfSS	FfSs	ffSS	ffSs
fs	FfSs	Ffss	ffSs	ffss

For more practice, see Problems 6, 12, and 27.

Visit the Study Area to access study tools. **Mastering Genetics**

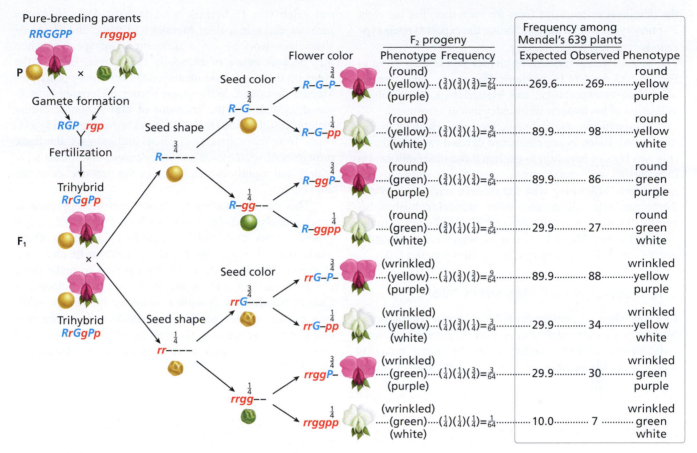

Figure 2.13 Trihybrid cross to verify independent assortment. The forked-line method can be used to determine the expected phenotype frequencies produced by a trihybrid cross. Expected and observed results for the F$_2$ generation of Mendel's trihybrid-cross experiment supported his hypothesis of independent assortment.

Q Thinking about the relationships of the alleles involved, (a) explain why the expected frequency of round, yellow, purple F$_2$ plants is greater than the expected frequency of wrinkled, green, white ones and (b) explain the reason for the difference between the expected frequencies of round, green, purple plants and wrinkled, yellow, white plants.

Mendel performed this cross, and his results almost exactly matched expectation. He found that the 207 test-cross progeny were composed of 55 round, yellow; 51 round, green; 49 wrinkled, yellow; and 52 wrinkled, green plants. This result confirmed the dihybrid genotype of the F$_1$ plant and supported the hypothesis that alleles for pea shape assort independently of those for pea color during gamete formation and that gametes unite at random to form offspring.

Testing Independent Assortment by Trihybrid-Cross Analysis

Mendel further tested the hypothesis of independent assortment by examining the results of a **trihybrid cross**, a cross involving three traits—in this case, seed shape, seed color, and flower color. He began this experiment by crossing a pure-breeding round, yellow, purple-flowered parental plant (*RRGGPP*) to a pure-breeding wrinkled, green, white-flowered plant (*rrggpp*) (**Figure 2.13**). The F$_1$ are presumed to be trihybrid (*RrGgPp*), and these plants are crossed with one another (or they can be self-fertilized) to produce the F$_2$.

The forked-line diagram in Figure 2.13 shows the number and expected frequency of gamete genotypes generated by the trihybrid F$_1$, and it predicts the phenotype distribution of the F$_2$. In the general case, assuming there are two alleles for each gene, the number of different gamete genotypes is expressed as 2^n, where $n =$ the number of genes involved. In this example, there are three genes ($n = 3$), and $2^3 = 8$ different combinations of alleles possible for the three traits in gametes from the trihybrid plant. The frequency of each gamete genotype is determined as $\left(\frac{1}{2}\right)^n$, or $\left(\frac{1}{2}\right)^3 = \frac{1}{8}$.

The diagram also predicts the expected frequency of the eight phenotypic classes in the F$_2$. For the general case where there are two phenotypes (dominant and recessive) for each trait, there are 2^n phenotypes in the F$_2$. Once again, $n =$ the number of genes. In this example, there are $2^3 = 8$ phenotypes in the F$_2$ progeny. Computation of each expected phenotype frequency is based on the expected frequencies of $\frac{3}{4}$ dominant and $\frac{1}{4}$ recessive for each trait. The expected frequency of each trihybrid class is the product of three fractions representing the predicted probabilities of the dominant or recessive form for each trait. For the eight F_2 phenotypes from a trihybrid cross, the expected phenotype ratio is $\frac{27}{64} : \frac{9}{64} : \frac{9}{64} : \frac{3}{64} : \frac{9}{64} : \frac{3}{64} : \frac{3}{64} : \frac{1}{64}$.

Mendel's experimental results for this test are given in Figure 2.13 for 639 F_2 progeny. The results were remarkably close to expectation, and Mendel took this result as validation of his hypothesis of independent assortment.

In conclusion, Mendel made observations about hereditary transmission in pea plants and devised two hypotheses (his two laws of heredity) to explain those observations. He then carried out separate experiments to test and verify his hypotheses, in keeping with the modern scientific method. Three and one-half decades after Mendel published his results, his work was rediscovered. That led quickly to the confirmation of Mendel's two laws, which are the foundation of our understanding of transmission genetics today.

The Rediscovery of Mendel's Work

In 1900, after remaining virtually unknown for 34 years, Mendel's experimental results and interpretations were rediscovered almost simultaneously by three botanists working independently of one another. Carl Correns and Erich von Tschermak were both working on *Pisum sativum*, the same plant Mendel had used, and Hugo de Vries was working on a different plant species, when they became aware of Mendel's 1866 paper. Each of the three, on their own, had identified the hereditary principles Mendel described. With support from the contemporaneous discoveries of the behavior of chromosomes during meiotic cell division, followed quickly by confirming evidence from other species of plants and animals, the basic principles of segregation and independent assortment were widely and rapidly disseminated in the first decade of the 20th century.

This chapter started by saying that the approach to genetic analysis it describes is often dubbed Mendelian genetics. After all, Mendel was the first scientist to offer a mechanism to explain the hereditary patterns he observed. However, Mendel was not the first person to make these observations. As **Experimental Insight 2.2** shows, if Charles Naudin had thought to quantify the results of his own crosses of pea plants, he could have been the first scientist to succeed at explaining heredity. Just think, this whole discussion might have been known as "Naudinian genetics"!

EXPERIMENTAL INSIGHT 2.2

Naudinian Genetics, Anyone?

Before Mendel, many "plant hybridists" experimented with pea plants and other plants, attempting to discern the mechanisms of plant reproduction and the process of hereditary transmission of traits. Mendel cited the work of several early hybridists in his 1866 paper.

Several of these plant hybridists came close to discovering the hereditary principles that today bear Mendel's name; none succeeded fully. For example, in 1823, Thomas Andrew Knight determined that gray seed coat is dominant to white and that self-fertilization of certain gray-seeded plants produces both gray and white seed in progeny plants. In 1822, John Goss, working with a pea variety that had blue and white seeds, reported that crossing a pure-breeding white-seeded plant with a pure-breeding blue-seeded plant produced only blue seeds in first-generation plants, and that self-fertilization then produced a second generation with a mixture of white and blue seeds in plants. Carl Friedrich Gaertner came tantalizingly close to explaining segregation in 1827 when he reported results of a cross between pure-breeding gold-kernel maize and pure-breeding red-striped maize. All the F_1 had gold kernels, and among the F_2, 328 plants had only gold kernels and 103 had red-striped kernels. If Gaertner had been able to correctly interpret his data, he would have identified a 3.18:1 ratio in the F_2. Alas, he never did and missed his "golden" opportunity to explain simple heredity.

Similar fates befell other plant hybridists, but arguably the one who came closest to explaining heredity prior to Mendel was Charles Naudin, who in 1863 seemed poised to beat Mendel to the punch by 2 years. In that year, Naudin reported the following:

▌ The results of reciprocal crosses are identical. (*Similar observations by Mendel were important in his identification of the particulate nature of hereditary factors.*)

▌ F_1 progeny display a single phenotype (*as Mendel reported 2 years later*).

▌ F_2 progeny display two phenotypes. (*These observations are the result of the segregation of alleles.*)

▌ The hereditary units for traits are separated in pollen and egg formation. (*This concept was fundamental to the segregation observation of Mendel.*)

▌ Nonparental combinations of phenotypes appear in the F_2 generation. (*This is identical to Mendel's independent assortment observation.*)

After making these observations, why wasn't Naudin able to propose a hereditary mechanism to explain them? The answer is that Naudin, like his predecessors and others who would follow, failed to quantify his results. Naudin did not report the number of plants falling into different phenotypic categories, and he was therefore unable to recognize the ratios between phenotypic classes that are the key to interpreting hereditary transmission. Without quantitative data, Naudin was unable to formulate a testable hypothesis.

Alas, poor Naudin! Were it not for his failure to see the necessity of quantifying experimental results, we might well be discussing Naudinian genetics in this chapter instead of Mendelian genetics!

2.4 Probability Theory Predicts Mendelian Ratios

Mendel recognized that chance, or random probability, the same process that determines the outcome of coin flips and rolls of the dice, is the arithmetic principle underlying the operation of the law of segregation and the law of independent assortment. Our discussion of Mendel's experiments has demonstrated that the basic rules of Mendelian inheritance are based on chance. The Mendelian probabilities we have described are formally expressed by four rules of probability theory—the *product rule*, the *sum rule*, *conditional probability*, and *binomial probability*. In this section, we look more closely at these rules as they relate to the prediction of the outcomes of genetic crosses.

The Product Rule

If two or more events are *independent* of one another, their joint probability, the likelihood of their simultaneous or consecutive occurrence, is the product of the probabilities of each one individually. The **product rule**, also called the **multiplication rule**, describes these circumstances.

You have already used the product rule several times in determining the outcomes of genetic crosses, and you were probably familiar with it (though perhaps not by name) even before you started this chapter. As an example of your familiarity with this rule, consider two consecutive flips of a coin and ask, "What is the chance that both flips are heads?" The answer is $\frac{1}{4}$, or one in four, which is obtained by multiplying the $\frac{1}{2}$ chance of heads on the first coin flip times the $\frac{1}{2}$ chance of heads on the second coin flip. Figure 2.5 shows how the product rule is used to determine the chance of producing an F_2 plant with the recessive phenotype by crossing heterozygous F_1 plants that are Gg. The probability of producing the recessive phenotype is $\left(\frac{1}{2}\right)\left(\frac{1}{2}\right) = \frac{1}{4}$. Similarly, in Figure 2.9, the probability of any gamete from a dihybrid organism having a specific one of the four possible genotypes is predicted by applying the product rule in the forked-line diagram. Likewise, in Figure 2.10, the probability that F_2 offspring will be homozygous recessive for both traits from a cross of F_1 dihybrid plants with the genotype $RrGg$ is predicted by applying the product rule.

The Sum Rule

The **sum rule**, also called the **addition rule**, calculates the joint probability of occurrence of any set of two or more outcomes when the possible outcomes for the individual events are *mutually exclusive* by summing the probabilities of each outcome. This rule is applied when more than one outcome satisfies the conditions of the probability question. Mutually exclusive events in this context are alternative outcomes, only one of which can occur to the exclusion of the other outcomes.

Again, you are probably already familiar with the use of this rule. Think once more about two consecutive flips of a coin, and this time ask, "What is the chance the result

will be one head and one tail in either order?" The answer is $\frac{1}{2}$, which is obtained by adding the $\frac{1}{4}$ chance (i.e., $\frac{1}{2} \times \frac{1}{2}$) of getting a head first followed by a tail plus the $\frac{1}{4}$ chance (i.e., $\frac{1}{2} \times \frac{1}{2}$) of getting a tail first followed by a head. You also applied the sum rule to several genetic calculations in the preceding section. For example, in Figure 2.5 the probability that F_2 progeny of the cross $Gg \times Gg$ will be heterozygous is determined by adding the probabilities of the two ways of obtaining the genotype: $\frac{1}{4} + \frac{1}{4} = \frac{1}{2}$. Similarly, in Figure 2.10, the probability that an F_2 progeny of the cross of dihybrid heterozygotes ($RrGg$) will have the two dominant phenotypes is obtained by applying the sum rule. This probability is $\frac{1}{16} + \frac{2}{16} + \frac{2}{16} + \frac{4}{16} = \frac{9}{16}$.

Conditional Probability

Certain questions of genetic probability can be asked *before* a cross is made. An example is a question of Mendelian probability such as, "What is the chance two heterozygotes have a child with the heterozygous genotype?" In this case, the product rule and the sum rule are used to predict a $\frac{1}{2}$ probability that the heterozygous genotype will be produced by the cross. This is known in probability terms as a **prior probability**. Certain other genetic probability questions are asked *after* a cross has been made, such as questions about the probability that an organism produced by a cross has a particular genotype given that the organism has a particular phenotype. This kind of probability is called **conditional probability**, and it is applied when specific information about the outcome of the cross modifies, or "conditions," the probability calculation.

An example of such a conditional probability might ask about the F_2 progeny of an F_1 cross $Gg \times Gg$, "What is the probability that yellow-seeded progeny plants are heterozygous Gg like the parents?" Yellow seed is present in $\frac{3}{4}$ of the progeny, but this phenotypic class contains two genotypes, GG and Gg, that are not equally frequent: the genotype Gg is found in $\frac{2}{3}$ of the yellow F_2 progeny, and the other yellow F_2 are GG (see Figure 2.5). Under the conditional criterion that the only progeny phenotype considered is yellow seeds, any nonyellow seeds are eliminated from the analysis. Looking only at the yellow-seeded progeny, we find that they have a $\frac{2}{3}$ probability of being Gg.

Mendel dealt with a version of this conditional probability question, asking "If the yellow-seeded F_2 are allowed to self-fertilize, what proportion of them are expected to breed true?" He asked this question as he devised an independent test of his segregation hypothesis (see Table 2.3 and the accompanying discussion). In Mendel's test of his segregation hypothesis, he predicted that $\frac{1}{3}$ of the F_2 with the dominant phenotype would be homozygous and that $\frac{2}{3}$ would be heterozygous. He found that $\frac{1}{3}$ of the dominant F_2 bred true and that the other $\frac{2}{3}$ produced progeny of both phenotypes and were heterozygous.

Genetic Analysis 2.3 in Section 2.6 will guide you in using conditional probability to predict the likelihood of a particular outcome of a mating between two prospective parents.

Binomial Probability

In determining the probabilities of certain kinds of outcomes, just one event need be predicted. The chance of obtaining a head or a tail on a coin flip or the chance of making the genetic-cross $Gg \times Gg$ and getting gg are examples. In contrast, questions concerning a combination or sequence of such events require a different approach. For example, determining the probability of getting four yellow and two green peas in a six-seeded pod produced by a $Gg \times Gg$ cross or the risk of a recessive phenotype occurring in one or more of the children of a couple who are each heterozygous carriers of a recessive disease-producing allele requires computation of all the different outcome patterns possible for the cross in question. To make these determinations, we use **binomial probability** calculations, expanding the binomial expression to reflect the number of outcome combinations and the probability of each combination.

Construction of a Binomial Expansion Formula A binomial expression contains two variables, each representing the frequency of one of the two alternative outcomes. We can express the likelihood of one outcome as having a frequency p and the alternative outcome as having a frequency q. Since the events p and q are the only outcomes possible, the sum of the two frequencies is $(p + q) = 1$. If we are examining the probabilities of the outcomes for a series of two alternative events, such as multiple flips of a coin or the sex of several successive children born to a couple, we can expand the binomial to the power of the number of successive events (n) to calculate the probabilities. The binomial expansion formula is written as $(p + q)^n$.

In some kinds of probability problems, the values of the binomial variables p and q will be equal; that is, $p = q = \frac{1}{2}$, as in the probability of producing a head or a tail from a coin flip. In other cases, the two binomial values will not be equal, as in the probability that heterozygous parents will mate and produce a child with a recessive trait $\left(\frac{1}{4}\right)$ versus a child with the dominant trait $\left(\frac{3}{4}\right)$.

Let's use combinatorial probability to predict the likelihood of different numbers of heads and tails produced from three consecutive flips of a coin. A combinatorial approach allows us to list all the different orders of heads and tails and to group the like combinations of outcomes into sets, or classes. The following table shows that there are 2^3, or eight, different orders of heads and tails in three coin flips. This value is determined based on two possible outcomes (which is the integer) for three successive events (which is the exponent). The outcomes can be grouped into four sets according to number of heads and number of tails in each set.

	0 heads 3 tails	1 head 2 tails	2 heads 1 tail	3 heads 0 tails
	TTT	TTH THT HTT	THH HTH HHT	HHH
Probability:	$\frac{1}{8}$	$\frac{3}{8}$	$\frac{3}{8}$	$\frac{1}{8}$

We can see that there is only one order in which to get either three heads (HHH) or three tails (TTT). Each of these two outcome classes (HHH or TTT) has a probability of $\left(\frac{1}{2}\right)^3$ or $\frac{1}{8}$. (Notice that we use the product rule to obtain each probability.) But what about an outcome class of two tails and one head, with three possible orders, or two heads and one tail, with three possible orders? Here we must recognize that each one of the possible orders has a probability of $\left(\frac{1}{2}\right)^3 = \frac{1}{8}$, and we use the sum rule to add together the chances of the similar results. For both of these outcome classes (one head and two tails; two heads and one tail), using the sum rule, the probability is $\frac{1}{8} + \frac{1}{8} + \frac{1}{8} = \frac{3}{8}$.

To arrive at this conclusion arithmetically, we use the binomial expansion to the third power $\left[(p + q)^3\right]$ to represent the three successive coin flips. The general equation for this binomial expands as follows:

$$(p + q)^3 = p^3 + 3p^2q + 3pq^2 + q^3$$

Inserting the coin flip probability values of $^1/_2$ for both p and q, the result is

$$\left(\frac{1}{2} + \frac{1}{2}\right)^3 = \frac{1}{8} + \frac{3}{8} + \frac{3}{8} + \frac{1}{8}$$

Application of Binomial Probability to Progeny Phenotypes Binomial probability and the binomial expansion can be used whenever a probability question addresses a repeating series of events that have two alternative outcomes. Let's look at the production of yellow and green peas in pods with six peas each. In this example, the dominant allele G determines yellow color, the recessive allele g determines green color, and the cross-producing progeny peas is a self-fertilization of a yellow-seeded heterozygous (Gg) plant. The probability that a seed is yellow is $\frac{3}{4}$, since the genotype would be either GG or Gg, and the probability that the seed is green, and therefore has the gg genotype, is $\frac{1}{4}$. We will use the variable p to represent the probability of yellow seeds and the variable q to represent the probability of green seeds.

To repeat, there are two possible color outcomes for each pea in our example and six peas per pod ($n = 6$), for a total of 2^n (2^6), or 64, different orders of peas in their pods. The combinations of yellow and green peas in each pod fall into seven outcome classes. For example, five yellow and one green seed is one class, another is three yellow and three green, and so on. In most binomial genetic cases, the number of classes is $n + 1$, as it is in this case.

Our goal in this example is to determine the expected frequency of each outcome class. To do so, we must first ask how many of the 64 different orders of peas occur in each of the seven classes. The answer to this question can be found using the formula $P = n!/(x! \, y!)$, where n is the number of events, x is the number of occurrences of one of the outcomes, and y is the number of occurrences of the other outcome. The ! symbol indicates the factorial operation. Using this equation for the case of four yellow and two green peas in a six-seeded pod, there are $6!/(4! \, 2!) = 720/48 = 15$ different orders. To avoid having to make this calculation for

n (number of events)	Binomial coefficients	Total number of combinations
0	1	1
1	1 1	2
2	1 2 1	4
3	1 3 3 1	8
4	1 4 6 4 1	16
5	1 5 10 10 5 1	32
6	1 6 15 20 15 6 1	64
7	1 7 21 35 35 21 7 1	128
8	1 8 28 56 70 56 28 8 1	256
9	1 9 36 84 126 126 84 36 9 1	512
10	1 10 45 120 210 252 210 120 45 10 1	1024
11	1 11 55 165 330 462 462 330 165 55 11 1	2048
12	1 12 66 220 495 792 924 792 495 220 66 12 1	4096

Figure 2.14 Pascal's triangle of binomial coefficients $(p + q)$ raised to the nth power. Each line of the table shows the distribution of the total number of outcome combinations for a given value of n (number of events). For example, for $(p + q)^2$, use the $n = 2$ line, which predicts a total of four outcome combinations distributed in a 1:2:1 or $\frac{1}{4}:\frac{1}{2}:\frac{1}{4}$ ratio. An application using the highlighted line $n = 6$ is discussed in the text.

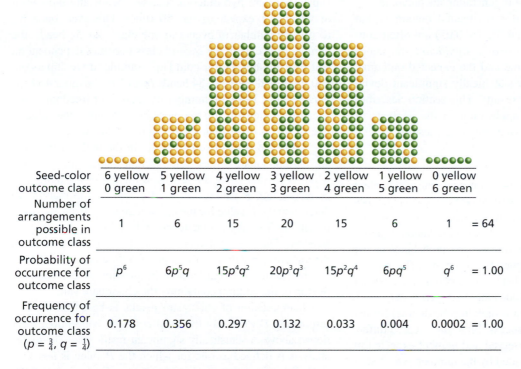

Seed-color outcome class	6 yellow 0 green	5 yellow 1 green	4 yellow 2 green	3 yellow 3 green	2 yellow 4 green	1 yellow 5 green	0 yellow 6 green	
Number of arrangements possible in outcome class	1	6	15	20	15	6	1	= 64
Probability of occurrence for outcome class	p^6	$6p^5q$	$15p^4q^2$	$20p^3q^3$	$15p^2q^4$	$6pq^5$	q^6	= 1.00
Frequency of occurrence for outcome class ($p = \frac{3}{4}$, $q = \frac{1}{4}$)	0.178	0.356	0.297	0.132	0.033	0.004	0.0002	= 1.00

Figure 2.15 Binomial-probability calculation of seed-color phenotype in six-seeded pods. Pascal's triangle has been used to find the coefficients for the binomial equation expanded to $n = 6$. The 64 different outcomes are displayed in seven classes, and the equation is used to compute the expected frequency of each class.

every binomial expansion problem, a convenient shortcut called **Pascal's triangle** can be used (**Figure 2.14**).

Figure 2.15 makes use of the values taken from the $n = 6$ line of Pascal's triangle (highlighted in Figure 2.14). These coefficients of the binomial expansion for $n = 6$ give the proportions of each of the seven outcome classes for this example. The coefficients are 1, 6, 15, 20, 15, 6, and 1, and they add up to a total of 64 different combinations. The coefficients are used to multiply the binomial probability of each outcome class. For this case where $p = \frac{3}{4}$ and $q = \frac{1}{4}$ the expected frequency of obtaining six yellow peas in a pod, for example, is calculated as $1(p^6) = \left(\frac{3}{4}\right)^6 = 0.178$; for pods containing three yellow and three green peas, the frequency is $20\left[\left(\frac{3}{4}\right)^3\left(\frac{1}{4}\right)^3\right] = 0.132$; the proportion of pods containing two yellow and four green peas is $15\left[\left(\frac{3}{4}\right)^2\left(\frac{1}{4}\right)^4\right] = 0.033$; and so on. The complete set of expected frequencies for different combinations of seed color is shown at the bottom of Figure 2.15. Notice that the

sum of category probabilities and the sum of category frequencies are each 1.00. This correspondence verifies that all possible outcomes have been taken into account.

2.5 Chi-Square Analysis Tests the Fit between Observed Values and Expected Outcomes

Sections 2.1 through 2.4 contain numerous examples of how the principles of probability can be used to predict the likelihood of different outcomes of genetic crosses. These genetic calculations make predictions of expected outcomes based on Mendel's two hereditary laws. But how do experimenters assess the general applicability of the experimental outcomes? Genetic experiments almost never produce the exact outcome expected. How can we decide, for example, that

Mendel's F_2 results in Table 2.1 (none of them an exact 3:1 ratio) are compatible with his segregation hypothesis predicting a 3:1 phenotype ratio? Similarly, are the observed results of Mendel's experiment shown in Figure 2.13 compatible with the predicted outcome?

Qualitative statements such as "the observed results support the hypothesis because they are close to the expected results" are unacceptable for scientific work. Instead, a quantitative approach, or in this case a statistical approach, is needed to objectively compare the results of an experimental cross with the results predicted by probability. Mendel did not have appropriate statistical tools available to him. But in the early 1900s, the *chi-square test* was derived as a statistical test for comparing observed experimental results with the results that are expected when chance is generating the outcome.

By convention, observed experimental outcomes that have a probability of less than 5% (< 0.05) are often considered to represent a *statistically significant* difference between the observed outcome and the expected outcome. Chi-square analysis tests for statistically significant deviation in genetic experimental results. This section describes the chi-square test and its application to the analysis of genetic data, including some of Mendel's F_2 results.

Chi-Square Analysis

The **chi-square (χ^2) test** is the most common statistical method used in genetics for comparing observed experimental outcomes with the results predicted by the hypothesis. Chi-square testing quantifies how closely an experimental observation matches the expected outcome by determining the probability of the observed outcome. The chi-square test has proven flexible and accurate in measuring the fit between observed and expected experimental results across a wide range of experiments.

Determining the chi-square value for the data set from a genetic cross is a two-step process. First, the squared difference between the number observed and number expected in each outcome category is divided by the number expected in the category; and second, the values obtained are summed for all outcome classes. The χ^2 formula is

$$\chi^2 = \sum \frac{(O - E)^2}{E}$$

where O is the observed number of offspring in each outcome class, E is the number expected for each class, and the summation (Σ) is taken over all outcome classes.

Chi-square values are not directly comparable from one experiment to the next. Instead, each experimental chi-square value is interpreted in terms of the results expected for an experiment *of that size*. The interpretation is done by means of a **probability value (*P* value)**, which is a quantitative expression of the probability that the results of another experiment of the same size and structure will *deviate as much or more from expected results by chance*. *P* values in chi-square analysis are directly related to how closely the observed and expected results match one another. High values for *P* (values close to 1) are associated with low χ^2 values. These occur when the observed

and expected results are very similar to one another—in other words, when the experimental outcome closely matches the expected results. On the other hand, low *P* values correspond to high chi-square values. They indicate substantial difference between observed and expected outcomes. The greater the difference between observed and expected results of an experiment, the greater the χ^2 value and the lower the *P* value.

The *P* value for each experiment is dependent on the number of **degrees of freedom (*df*)** in the experiment being examined. For each experiment, the *df* value is most often equal to the number of outcome classes (n) minus 1, or ($n - 1$). In a statistical sense, this *df* is equal to the number of independent variables in an experiment. For example, suppose we were conducting a chi-square test of 100 coin flips. There are two outcome classes, heads and tails, each of which we expect to see 50 times. However, once we record the number of events in one class, say 54 heads, the number of events in the second class becomes dependent on that first number. In our coin flip example, if we flip a coin 100 times and there are 54 heads recorded, the other 46 flips must be tails. Here the number of degrees of freedom is one because, while there are two possible outcomes, the value of one is always dependent on the value of the other.

Table 2.4 is a chi-square table. In the body of the table are the chi-square values for different degrees of freedom, which are listed along the left-hand margin of the table. The corresponding *P* values are listed along the top margin. To determine the *P* value for the chi-square value from an experiment, the first step is to determine the number of degrees of freedom. The second step is to locate the chi-square value on the line corresponding to the degrees of freedom. The *P* value for the result of the experiment in question is then found at the top of the column containing the chi-square value.

Interpretation of chi-square results is based on the corresponding *P* value. By the most common convention, mentioned above, a statistically significant result from chi-square analysis is defined as one for which the *P* value is *less than 0.05*. This means that there is less than a 5% chance (< 0.05) of obtaining the experimental observation by chance. Using this criterion, when the results of a genetic experiment produce a *P* value of less than 0.05, the hypothesis of chance is *rejected*. In other words, if the *P* value is less than 0.05, the difference between the observed and expected results is considered statistically significant, and the experimental hypothesis is rejected. Conversely, *P* values greater than 0.05 indicate a nonsignificant deviation between observed and expected values. These values result in *failure to reject* the chance hypothesis.

Chi-Square Analysis of Mendel's Data

Modern statistical methods allow us to do something Mendel could not do—test his experimental data for its compatibility with the predictions of the laws of segregation and independent assortment. Table 2.1 contains data from Mendel for F_2 segregation of the seven traits he tested. In the first row of the table, we see that Mendel examined 7324 F_2 seeds for round or wrinkled phenotypes. Among these, he counted

Table 2.4	The Chi-Square Table									
	Probability (P) Value									
df	0.95	0.90	0.70	0.50	0.30	0.20	0.10	0.05	0.01	0.001
1	0.004	0.016	0.15	0.46	1.07	1.64	2.17	3.84	6.64	10.83
2	0.10	0.21	0.71	1.39	2.41	3.22	4.61	5.99	9.21	13.82
3	0.35	0.58	1.42	2.37	3.67	4.64	6.25	7.82	11.35	16.27
4	0.71	1.06	2.20	3.36	4.88	5.99	7.78	9.49	13.28	18.47
5	1.15	1.61	3.00	4.35	6.06	7.29	9.24	11.07	15.09	20.52
6	1.64	2.20	3.83	5.35	7.23	8.56	10.65	12.59	16.81	22.46
7	2.17	2.83	4.67	6.35	8.38	9.80	12.02	14.07	18.48	24.32
8	2.73	3.49	5.53	7.34	9.52	11.03	13.36	15.51	20.09	26.13
9	3.33	4.17	6.39	8.34	10.66	12.24	14.68	16.92	21.67	27.88
10	3.94	4.87	7.27	9.34	11.78	13.44	15.99	18.31	23.21	29.59
11	4.58	5.58	8.15	10.34	12.90	14.63	17.28	19.68	24.73	31.26
12	5.23	6.30	9.03	11.34	14.01	15.81	18.55	21.03	26.22	32.91
13	5.89	7.04	9.93	12.34	15.12	16.99	19.81	22.36	27.69	34.53
14	6.57	7.79	10.82	13.34	16.22	18.15	21.06	23.69	29.14	36.12
15	7.26	8.55	11.72	14.34	17.32	19.31	22.31	25.00	30.58	37.70
	Fail to reject chance hypothesis							Reject chance hypothesis		

Note: Chi-square values are in the body of the table, degrees of freedom are at the far left side, and probability values are at the top of each column of chi-square values.

5474 round and 1850 wrinkled. Based on the predictions of his segregation hypothesis, Mendel expected that 75% of the F_2 would be round and the remaining 25% wrinkled. That means he expected $(7324)(0.75) = 5493$ round seeds and $(7324)(0.25) = 1831$ wrinkled seeds. There is 1 degree of freedom in the experiment, and the chi-square is calculated as

$$\chi^2 = (5474 - 5493)^2/5493 + (1850 - 1831)^2/1831$$
$$= 0.066 + 0.197 = 0.263$$

For $df = 1$, the P value falls between 0.50 and 0.70 (see Table 2.4). This is well above the cutoff value of 0.05 and consequently represents a nonsignificant deviation between the observed outcome and the values expected for an experiment of this size. We fail to reject the hypothesis that chance is responsible for the observed outcome, and we can say, therefore, that Mendel's F_2 data for seed shape are consistent with the predictions of the law of segregation.

Figure 2.11 provides data Mendel collected on seed shape and seed color that we can use to test whether his results were consistent with his predictions of independent assortment. Based on the predicted $\frac{9}{16} : \frac{3}{16} : \frac{3}{16} : \frac{1}{16}$, or 9:3:3:1, ratio (and converting the fractions to decimal numbers: $\frac{9}{16} = 0.5625$, $\frac{3}{16} = 0.1875$, and $\frac{1}{16} = 0.0625$), the 556 F_2 produced by Mendel would be expected to have the following distribution:

Round, yellow	$(556)(0.5625) = 312.75$
Round, green	$(556)(0.1875) = 104.25$
Wrinkled, yellow	$(556)(0.1875) = 104.25$
Wrinkled, green	$(556)(0.0625) = \underline{34.75}$
	556.00

The chi-square value is calculated as

$$\chi^2 = (315 - 312.75)^2/312.75 + (108 - 104.25)^2/104.25$$
$$+ (101 - 104.25)^2/104.25 + (32 - 34.75)^2/34.75$$
$$= 0.016 + 0.135 + 0.101 + 0.218 = 0.470$$

In this case, $df = 3$, and the P value falls between 0.90 and 0.95. This indicates a nonsignificant deviation, because the P value is above the 0.05 cutoff value. Mendel's F_2 data for seed color and seed shape are therefore also consistent with the predictions of independent assortment. A third example of chi-square analysis, using trihybrid-cross results from one of Mendel's experiments, is shown in Table 2.5. From statistical analysis of these data we conclude that Mendel's results are consistent with the predictions of segregation and independent assortment.

2.6 Autosomal Inheritance and Molecular Genetics Parallel the Predictions of Mendel's Hereditary Principles

Immediately after the rediscovery of Mendel's rules of hereditary transmission in 1900, biologists began testing Mendel's findings in species other than pea plants. These studies were undertaken in an effort to verify the principles of heredity and to expand their application. One of the species in which hereditary transmission was studied was our own. This section discusses some of the elements of hereditary transmission in humans.

Table 2.5	Chi-Square Analysis of Mendel's Trihybrid-Cross Data	
Mendel's Observation[a]		
Phenotype	Number	Number Expected
Round, yellow, purple	269	269.58
Round, yellow, white	98	89.86
Round, green, purple	86	89.86
Round, green, white	27	29.95
Wrinkled, yellow, purple	88	89.86
Wrinkled, yellow, white	34	29.95
Wrinkled, green, purple	30	29.95
Wrinkled, green, white	7	9.98
Total	639	638.99

Chi-square calculation $\Sigma[(O - E)^2/E]$

$$\chi^2 = (269 - 269.58)^2/269.58 + (98 - 89.86)^2/89.86$$
$$+ (86 - 89.86)^2/89.86 + (27 - 29.95)^2/29.95$$
$$+ (88 - 89.86)^2/89.86 + (34 - 29.95)^2/29.95$$
$$+ (30 - 29.95)^2/29.95 + (7 - 9.98)^2/9.98$$
$$= 2.67$$

$df = 7$

$P\ value > 0.90$

[a] Data are taken from Figure 2.13.

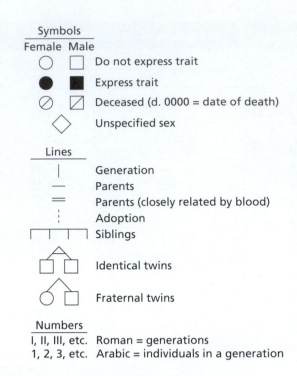

Figure 2.16 Common pedigree symbols.

In addition to the examination of Mendelian transmission in other species, the latter part of the 20th century saw the development of the field of molecular genetics. The rapid progress of molecular genetics has led, full circle, to identification of the genes responsible for four of the seven traits Mendel studied. The last part of this section explores the connections between molecular genetic variation and the phenotypic variation of traits that Mendel described.

With the benefit of well over a century of research, geneticists now understand that the patterns of hereditary transmission Mendel described are those of **autosomal inheritance**. This term refers to the transmission of genes that are carried on the paired chromosomes known as autosomes (examples of *homologous pairs*, as described in Chapter 1). In diploid organisms, like humans, one chromosome of each autosomal pair of chromosomes is inherited from the father and the other copy from the mother. Humans have 22 pairs of autosomal chromosomes (a total of 44 autosomes) and these are commonly identified by the numbers 1 through 22. The other two human chromosomes are the **sex chromosomes**, designated X and Y. Thus, humans have 46 chromosomes: 44 are autosomes and two are sex chromosomes, with two X chromosomes found in females and an X and a Y chromosome found in males. We discuss these chromosomes and their inheritance more fully in Chapter 3.

The study of hereditary transmission in humans and numerous other species is assisted graphically by the construction of **pedigrees**, or family trees. A pedigree is drawn using a kind of symbolic shorthand designed to trace the inheritance of traits. In standard pedigree notation, males are represented by squares and females by circles (**Figure 2.16**). A filled circle or square indicates that the phenotype of interest is present. A line through a symbol indicates the person is deceased. Parents are connected to each other by a horizontal line from which a vertical line descends to their progeny. Individuals in a pedigree are numbered by a Roman numeral (I, II, III, etc.) to indicate their generation combined with an Arabic numeral (1, 2, 3, etc.) that identifies each organism in a generation. Identifying an individual by a Roman numeral followed by an Arabic numeral, as in I-2 or III-6, is an efficient way to ensure clarity in referring to particular organisms and, in the case of humans, allows protection of privacy by not requiring the use of names.

Often, the reason for studying an inherited variation in a single gene carried on a human autosomal chromosome or sex chromosome is that the variant produces a condition or disorder. Frequently, although there are numerous exceptions, the condition or disorder is "rare"—meaning that the variant trait occurs in about 1% or less of the population. At present, almost 20,000 human hereditary conditions are known to be caused by inherited variation of single genes. Some of these conditions are so rare they occur in just a few individuals in the world, while others are relatively common in certain populations. The Online Mendelian Index of Man (OMIM) that we briefly describe in the Case Study at the end of this chapter is a continuously updated catalog of human hereditary conditions and variants.

Autosomal Dominant Inheritance

The pedigree in **Figure 2.17** shows characteristics commonly observed for **autosomal dominant inheritance** of a disease. To be classified as autosomal dominant, a trait must appear both in individuals who have a heterozygous genotype

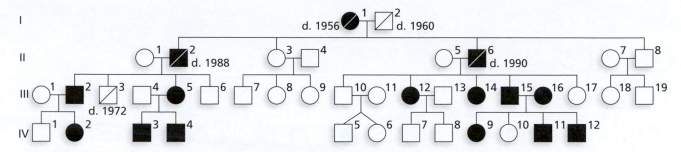

Figure 2.17 **Autosomal dominant inheritance.** Table 2.6 summarizes common observations in families with this pattern of inheritance.

Using *D* for the dominant allele and *d* for the recessive allele, give the genotypes for III-15, III-16, IV-9, IV-10, IV-11, and IV-12. (Hint: Look at the cross-producing III-15.)

Table 2.6	Common Characteristics of the Inheritance of Autosomal Dominant Traits Seen in Pedigrees (see Figure 2.17)

1. Males and females have the trait in about equal frequency. (There are seven females and eight males with the dominant trait in Figure 2.17.)
2. Each person with the trait has at least one parent with the trait. (Note this feature in each generation.)
3. Parents of either sex can transmit the trait to a child of either sex. (See generations I and II, for example.)
4. If neither parent has the trait, none of their children will have it. (See progeny of II-3 and II-4, and of II-7 and II-8, for example.)

If the trait is rare (less than about 1%), . . .

5. . . . a person with the trait is very likely heterozygous. In cases where one parent has the trait and the other does not, the chance a child will inherit the trait is 50%. (See generations I and II, for example.)
6. . . . and both parents have it (i.e., both parents are very likely to be heterozygous), they can produce children who do not have the trait. (See progeny of III-15 and III-16.)

(e.g., *Aa*) and in those with a certain homozygous genotype (e.g., *AA*). There are several common characteristics of autosomal dominant traits that can be evident in pedigrees. Table 2.6 lists some major ones, all of which can be seen in the pedigree in Figure 2.17. For example, the first common feature of autosomal dominant traits is that males and females will show the trait in approximately equal numbers. In Figure 2.17, the 15 individuals having the dominant trait (darkened circles and squares) are 7 females and 8 males.

Autosomal Recessive Inheritance

Figure 2.18 shows a human pedigree displaying the characteristics commonly observed for **autosomal recessive inheritance**. In this pattern of heredity, the recessive phenotype appears only in those individuals who have the genotype that is homozygous for the recessive allele (e.g., *aa*). The major common characteristics of autosomal recessive inheritance in pedigrees differ in several ways from those seen for autosomal dominant traits. Table 2.7 lists common characteristics of autosomal recessive traits that can be observed in the Figure 2.18 pedigree.

Prospective and Retrospective Predictions in Human Genetics

In the context of testing his hereditary laws, Mendel made prospective predictions about the outcomes of certain crosses. In other words, when setting up specific crosses between pea plants, he would make a prediction beforehand about the percentages of dominant and recessive phenotypes he expected to see among the cross progeny. That kind of prospective prediction occurs in the field of human genetics. If, for example, a man and a woman know that each is heterozygous for an autosomal recessive disease, they can ask the question, "What is the chance a child of ours will have the recessive condition?" In this case, the genetic cross is $Aa \times Aa$, and there is a $\frac{1}{4}$ chance that any offspring will have the homozygous genotype *aa*.

The study of heredity can also be retrospective. One feature making the study of inheritance in humans different from that in other organisms is that human heredity is *often* examined *after reproduction has taken place*, when questions may arise about the genotypes of individuals even though their phenotypes are known. For example, it is usually only after an adverse hereditary outcome has been detected in a family that the inheritance of the unusual trait becomes a subject of attention by medical genetic professionals. Construction of a pedigree may show the family to have a history of the hereditary condition; alternatively, it may show the hereditary condition to have previously been unknown in the family. In either case, an adverse reproductive outcome is the trigger for medical genetic investigation of the family.

Figure 2.19a shows a pedigree in which both parents (I-1 and I-2) have the dominant phenotype. The parental genotypes for this trait are initially unknown. They have had four children: three of the children also have the dominant phenotype (II-1, II-3, and II-4), but one child (II-2)

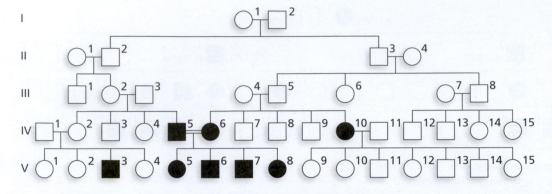

Figure 2.18 **Autosomal recessive inheritance.** Table 2.7 summarizes common observations for families with this pattern of inheritance.

Table 2.7	Common Characteristics of the Inheritance of Autosomal Recessive Traits Seen in Pedigrees (see Figure 2.18)

1. Males and females with the trait are approximately equally frequent. (Four males and four females in the pedigree in Figure 2.18 have the recessive trait.)
2. Often, a child with the recessive trait has parents who both have the dominant trait and are heterozygous carriers. (See progeny of III-4 and III-5, for example.)
3. If both parents have the trait (i.e., both are homozygous recessive), all their children will have the trait. (See progeny of IV-5 and IV-6.)
4. The trait is not seen in every generation. Instead, it is usually seen among siblings. (See generation V.)

If the trait is rare (less than about 1%), . . .

5. . . . and just one of the parents has the trait (i.e., this parent is homozygous recessive), a child can only have the trait if the other parent is heterozygous. This is a very low probability event. (See progeny of IV-10 and IV-11.)

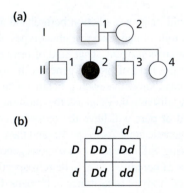

Figure 2.19 **Reconstructing genotypes and determining genotype probabilities.** **(a)** Parents who have a dominant phenotype and produce a child with a recessive phenotype (*dd*) must be heterozygous (*Dd*). The siblings with the dominant phenotype are *D–*. **(b)** Punnett square for the cross of heterozygous parents.

has an autosomal recessive condition. Through retrospective genetic analysis based on the family pedigree, we can obtain some of the missing genotypic information. Using allele symbols *D* and *d* for the dominant and recessive alleles of the gene, and knowing that II-2 has the recessive trait, we can assign her the genotype *dd*. This means that she must have received a recessive allele from each of her parents, who must each be heterozygous carriers of the condition. Therefore, both I-1 and I-2 have the genotype *Dd*. The three other children have the dominant phenotype but their genotypes are unknown. **Figure 2.19b**

shows a Punnett square with the possible outcomes for the *Dd* × *Dd* parental cross.

In the pedigree, the three children with the dominant phenotype can be assigned the *D–* genotype to indicate that they have at least one copy of the dominant allele. Their second allele is unknown without additional information. To make estimates of the two possibilities, recall the earlier discussion of conditional probability in Section 2.4. It tells us to focus only on the children with the dominant phenotype as the group of interest. Within this group, as the Punnett square shows, each child has a $\frac{1}{3}$ chance of being *DD* and a $\frac{2}{3}$ chance of being *Dd*.

Genetic Analysis 2.3 uses a pedigree to ask prospective questions about reproduction involving a man and a woman who each might be heterozygous carriers of this recessive condition.

Molecular Genetics of Mendel's Traits

Interest in Mendel's traits continues. Today, molecular genetics approaches are used to identify the genes responsible for the phenotypic variations he observed. The goal of these molecular analyses is to describe the variations in nucleic acid (DNA and RNA) and the variations in polypeptides (enzymes and other proteins) that are responsible for the dichotomous phenotypes. The success of these molecular genetic methods at uncovering the causes of Mendel's traits highlights a cornerstone of modern genetics: that the principles of Mendelian transmission genetics integrate seamlessly with those of molecular genetic analysis. Another way to say this is that the molecular genetic and the transmission

GENETIC ANALYSIS 2.3

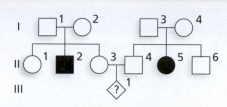

PROBLEM The pedigree provided here shows a woman (II-3) and a man (II-4) who each have a sibling with an autosomal recessive condition (II-2 and II-5). They seek to determine the chance that their first child (III-1) will have the condition. The child has not yet been conceived. Neither the man nor the woman has the condition, nor do the parents of either of them (see generation I). Using only the genetic information given, perform the following tasks:

> **BREAK IT DOWN:** Review the transmission pattern and genotypes associated with the inheritance of autosomal recessive traits (pp. 53–54).

> **TIP:** If both alleles of a genotype are not known with certainty, the genotype of a person with the dominant phenotype can be given as *D–*.

a. Using *D* to represent the dominant allele and *d* to represent the recessive allele, assign genotypes to all members of the pedigree. If a complete genotype (showing both alleles) cannot be given, provide the genotype information that is known. Explain your reasoning.

b. Calculate the chance that child III-1 will have the recessive condition. Show your work.

> **TIP:** Even if a genotype is not known with certainty it may be possible to estimate the likelihood of each possible genotype.

Solution Strategies	Solution Steps
Evaluate	
1. Identify the topic of this problem and the kind of information the answer should contain.	1. The problem concerns the transmission of an autosomal recessive trait in a family. The problem requires deducing either complete or partial genotypes of family members based on the transmission pattern. The genotypes of II-3 and II-4 can be evaluated as conditional probabilities.
2. Identify the critical information given in the problem.	2. The autosomal recessive condition is present in one sibling each of II-3 and II-4. The phenotypes of the pedigree members in generations I and II are known, allowing genotype deductions to be made and genotype probabilities inferred for II-3 and II-4.
Deduce	
3. Deduce the genotypes of the members of generation I based on the emergence of the recessive condition in generation II.	3. The recessive condition occurs when an individual has the genotype *dd*. Since the parental pairs in generation I have each produced a child with the recessive condition, and since none of those four parents has the recessive condition (i.e., they all have the dominant phenotype), the members of each parental pair must have the heterozygous *Dd* genotype.
4. State what is known about the genotypes of members of generation II. > **TIP:** Use a Punnett square to accurately determine the possible genotypes.	4. All members of generation II are produced from crosses that are *Dd* × *Dd*. II-2 and II-5 have the recessive phenotype and must have the genotype *dd*. All other family members in generation II are either *DD* or *Dd*. Because their genotypes are only partly known, the genotypes of II-1, II-3, II-4, and II-6 can be written as *D–*.
5. Assign the probabilities of each possible genotype for II-3 and II-4. > **PITFALL:** To avoid errors, first consider which genotype or genotypes are *not possible* for these two individuals and then assess the likelihood of the remaining possibilities.	5. Both II-3 and II-4 have the dominant phenotype, so neither can have the *dd* genotype. The Punnett square shows that for their possible *D–* genotypes, each of them has a two in three ($\frac{2}{3}$) chance of having the *Dd* genotype and a one in three ($\frac{1}{3}$) chance of having the *DD* genotype. 		*D*	*d*	 |---|---|---| 	**D**	*DD*	*Dd*	 	**d**	*Dd*	*dd*	
Solve	
6. Assign genotypes to members of generation I and generation II, except II-3 and II-4.	**Answer a** 6. The pedigree shown here includes the complete and partial genotypes assigned to members of generations I and II. 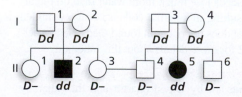

(continued)

Solution Strategies	Solution Steps
7. Determine the genotypes of II-3 and II-4 that would have to be present if they were to produce a child with the recessive condition.	7. To have the recessive phenotype, the child of II-3 and II-4 must have the *dd* genotype. Each of its parents must be *Dd* for this to occur. If we look at the Punnett square and consider only the genotypes that meet the condition of producing a dominant phenotype, we see that each parent has a $\frac{2}{3}$ chance of being heterozygous. The probability that both are heterozygous is $\left(\frac{2}{3}\right)\left(\frac{2}{3}\right) = \frac{4}{9}$.
8. Calculate the chance that III-1 would have the recessive condition. TIP: Use the product rule to determine the probabilities of mating outcomes.	**Answer b** 8. The chance that both II-3 and II-4 are heterozygous is $\frac{4}{9}$. The cross of these heterozygotes (*Dd* × *Dd*) would have a $\frac{1}{4}$ chance of producing a child that is *d*. This probability is $\left(\frac{4}{9}\right)\left(\frac{1}{4}\right) = \frac{1}{9}$. In other words, given the available information, there is a one in nine chance that this couple will have a child with the recessive phenotype.

For more practice, see Problems 3, 16, and 40.   Visit the Study Area to access study tools.   **Mastering** Genetics

genetic modes of analysis are two sides of the same coin. The Mendelian patterns of transmission of phenotype variation are traceable through examination of variation in the hereditary molecules DNA and RNA, and in protein.

Mendel did not leave any neatly labeled packets of seeds for later researchers to analyze, so the process of pinpointing the exact traits he examined and the genes and proteins responsible for them has been complicated. The first successful identification of one of Mendel's genes was in 1990, and since then, three other of his genes have been identified. Discussion in this section and in **Table 2.8** identifies these four genes, describes the differences in function of the protein products of the dominant and recessive alleles, and summarizes the processes that lead to the different phenotypes. In each case, the mutations generating the recessive allele significantly reduce or entirely eliminate the normal production or function of the protein product of the dominant allele.

Seed Shape (Round and Wrinkled, Gene *Sbe1*) In 1990, research published by Madan Bhattacharyya and colleagues described the identification and molecular analysis of a gene responsible for round and wrinkled seed shape. The *Sbe1* gene produces the starch-branching enzyme that helps convert a linear form of starch called amylose into a complex branched form of starch called amylopectin. As a consequence of the action of fully functional starch-branching enzyme, round seeds have a much higher percentage of amylopectin and a much lower percentage of amylose than do wrinkled seeds, which do not have functional starch-branching enzyme. Amylose readily loses sugar molecules, leading to high concentrations of free sugar in the developing seeds and, consequently, excessive water uptake that swells them. As seeds mature they naturally dehydrate. The maturing wrinkled seeds lose much more water than do maturing round seeds, resulting in a partial collapse of the wrinkled seed membranes that does not occur in round seeds. See Experimental Insight 11.2 for more details about this mutation.

Stem Length (Tall and Short, Gene *Le*) In 1997, two research groups, one led by David Martin and the other by Diane Lester, determined that a gene called *Le* controls the variation in stem length that Mendel saw as tall and short

plants. The *Le* gene produces an enzyme called gibberellin 3β-hydroxylase. This enzyme catalyzes one step of the biochemical pathway synthesizing the plant growth hormone gibberellin. Tall plants produce sufficient gibberellin to grow tall. However, a mutation in the recessive allele results in a very low level of gibberellin production and leads to short stems. See Experimental Insight 10.1 for more details about this mutation.

Seed Color (Yellow and Green, Gene *Sgr*) Two studies published in 2007, one by Ian Armstead and colleagues and the other by Sylvain Aubry and colleagues, identified a gene known as "stay-green," or *Sgr*. The protein produced by *Sgr* in plants with the dominant yellow seed phenotype is an enzyme that catalyzes a step in the breakdown of chlorophyll, a green-colored compound, as the seed matures. A mutation producing the recessive allele prevents production of the chlorophyll-breakdown enzyme. The absence of chlorophyll breakdown results in the retention of green color in mutant seeds. See Experimental Insight 10.1 for more details about this mutation.

Flower Color (Purple and White, Gene *bHLH*) In 2010, the gene responsible for the white-flower mutation in Mendel's pea plants was identified. A research group led by Roger Hellens determined that mutation of the *bHLH* gene in pea plants produces the recessive mutant white flowers rather than purple flowers, the dominant phenotype. The protein product of *bHLH* is a transcription factor protein that interacts with other proteins to activate the transcription of certain genes. Some of the genes whose transcription is activated are in the pathway that produces the purple-colored plant pigment called anthocyanin. Purple-flowered plants produce enough of the *bHLH* gene product to activate transcription of anthocyanin-producing genes. White-flowered plants, however, have a defect of the *bHLH* gene product and are unable to activate transcription of the anthocyanin-producing genes. See Experimental Insight 10.1 for more details about this mutation.

A common feature of each of the genes controlling Mendel's traits is that, coincidentally, the more frequent of the two alleles of the pair is dominant to a mutant allele that is recessive. This is a consequence of the loss of function on

Table 2.8	Molecular Identification and Characterization of Four of Mendel's Traits			
Trait	Gene and Gene Product	Dominant Allele and Function	Mutant Allele and Function	Reference
Seed shape (round and wrinkled seeds)	The gene is *Sbe1*, producing starch-branching enzyme.	The dominant allele (*R*) produces starch-branching enzyme that converts amylase, a linear starch, into amylopectin, a complex branched starch.	The recessive mutant allele (*r*) contains an inserted segment about 800 base pairs in length. The transcript of the mutant allele does not produce an enzyme product, resulting in a loss of function.	Bhattacharyya, M. K., et al. 1990. *Cell* 60: 115–122.
Stem length (tall and short plants)	The gene is *Le*, producing gibberellin 3β-hydroxylase (G3βH).	G3βH produced by the dominant allele *Le* converts a precursor in the synthesis of the plant growth hormone gibberellin that causes plants to grow tall.	The recessive mutant *le* allele contains a base substitution that results in an amino acid change. The mutant G3βH has less than 5% the activity of the dominant-allele product and produces little gibberellin, leading to short plants.	Lester, D. R., et al. 1997. *Plant Cell* 9: 1435–1443. Martin, D. N., et al. 1997. *Proc. Natl. Acad. Sci., USA* 94: 8907–8911.
Seed color (yellow seed and green seed)	The gene was originally named *I* gene and was later renamed *Sgr* (called "stay green"). The gene produces an enzyme that helps break down chlorophyll.	The dominant allele (*I*) produces an enzyme that catalyzes one step in the chlorophyll breakdown pathway, which turns seeds yellow as they mature.	The recessive mutant allele (*i*) contains two base substitutions and a base pair insertion. The resulting mutant polypeptide has no function, leading to a blockage of the chlorophyll breakdown pathway and causing mutant seeds to retain their immature green color.	Armstead, I., et al. 2007. *Science* 315: 73. Aubry, S., et al. 2008. *Plant Mol. Biol.* 67: 243–256.
Flower color (purple flower and white flower)	Originally named gene *A* and renamed *bHLH*, the gene produces a protein that activates transcription of target genes.	The dominant allele (*A*) produces a protein that activates transcription of genes required to synthesize the purple-colored plant pigment called anthocyanin.	The recessive mutant allele (*a*) contains a base substitution that results in production of abnormal mRNA. The mutant mRNA does not produce the transcription-activating protein, thus blocking anthocyanin production and resulting in the development of white flowers.	Hellens, R. P., et al. 2010. *PLoS One* 5: 1–8.

Note: For a comprehensive review, see Reid, J. B., and J. J. Ross. 2011. *Genetics* 189: 3–10.

the part of the mutant alleles. For each of these genes, the presence of one or two copies of the dominant allele results in the dominant phenotype, whereas the mutant phenotype is produced in plants that are homozygous for the mutant allele. We discuss this and other kinds of dominance relationships between alleles in Section 4.1.

In broader terms, the conclusions from molecular studies identifying genes Mendel examined in his crosses are that (1) the inheritance of allelic variants precisely parallels the pattern of transmission of phenotypic variation and (2) phenotypic variation in pea plants results from differences in the structure and function of the proteins produced by the alleles. Molecular genetic analysis has led to (3) identification of the DNA-sequence differences between alleles, determination of the impact of those differences on mRNA, and description of the alteration of protein structures resulting from each mRNA; and also to (4) functional analysis of the protein product of each allele to describe the role it plays in producing the phenotype.

CASE STUDY

OMIM, Gene Mutations, and Human Hereditary Disease

The human genome consists of the DNA making up the 22 pairs of autosomal chromosome pairs and the one pair of sex chromosomes (two X chromosomes in females and an X and a Y chromosome in males) that are located in the nucleus of each cell. The human genome also includes the small amount of DNA that makes up the single chromosome of mitochondria that inhabit the cytoplasm of cells. We discuss mitochondria and their genes in Chapter 17. In all, there are a little more than 3 billion DNA bases in the human genome, and the genome encodes approximately 22,500 genes, although the exact number remains the subject of active research.

Many human genes are involved in determining elements of the human phenotype, which includes both the outward appearance of the body and its many biochemical and metabolic processes. As we will describe in later chapters, no gene really works alone to determine a phenotypic characteristic. Instead, genes work together in pathways that involve the action of different genes at different steps of the process to produce a trait or to execute a biological function. Despite this cooperation among genes, or perhaps because of it, mutations of single genes can disrupt or block a pathway. Gene mutations that prevent production of the normal protein or produce an abnormal amount of the normal protein can lead to phenotypic abnormalities that are often identified as hereditary diseases in humans. How many genes have mutations that are implicated in the production of such hereditary diseases?

CATALOGING HEREDITARY DISEASES AND DISEASE GENES

One way to answer this question is to determine how many single-gene mutations are described as the source of a hereditary disease or condition. The Online Mendelian Index in Man (OMIM) is a continuously updated, public database containing a list of human genes and phenotypes associated with gene mutations. The official home page of OMIM is at http://www.omim.org. A searchable research page is located at https://www.ncbi.nlm.nih.gov/omim. From this page you can also search numerous other database websites maintained by the U.S. National Institutes of Health (NIH), the National Laboratory of Medicine (NLM), or the National Center for Biological Information (NCBI).

In 2016, OMIM celebrated its 50th anniversary. It began in 1966 as the brainchild of Victor McKusick, a physician who took a great interest in human genetics and in the roles genes play in human disease. OMIM started out as a comprehensive catalog then called the Mendelian Index in Man (MIM), with 1486 entries, most of them genetic disease phenotypes. McKusick and his staff assembled this first list, and they maintained and periodically updated the list for many years. Twelve editions of a thick book containing the complete MIM list were published annually from 1966 to 1988. In 1987, the published information was first made available on the Internet, and in 1995 the content was made available to the public on the worldwide web. Since that time the catalog has been known as OMIM.

Today, OMIM contains more than 24,000 entries. More than 8000 of these are hereditary diseases and 16,000 are human genes, from all 22 autosomes, the X chromosome, and the Y chromosome. **Table 2.9** gives the number of genes on each type of chromosome that are currently found on OMIM. Of the hereditary diseases listed on OMIM, almost 5900 have a known molecular basis. This means that the abnormality that causes the disease is known. The genes causing about 3650 of these diseases have been identified.

If you were interested in searching OMIM for information on a genetic disease, you could go to either the official home-page or the searchable website and enter the name of the disease or condition. For example, if you enter "cystic fibrosis" in the search bar at either site you will be given a number of clickable pages. If you select the page "*602421 cystic fibrosis transmembrane conductance regulator; CFTR" you will be taken to a synopsis of the autosomal recessive condition cystic fibrosis that is caused by mutations of the CFTR gene. The asterisk (*) preceding the six-digit number indicates that a gene is known for this condition. Any other genetic condition of interest can be searched in a similar manner. Often you will see a hash character (#) before a six-digit number. This indicates that the information is for a phenotypic description. Often a "cytogenetic location" is given. This indicates the chromosome location of a gene causing or contributing to a disease. We discuss deciphering these chromosome location designations in Chapter 10.

Each OMIM entry is accompanied by a six-digit number according to the following scheme:

1----- and 2----- (100,000 and up and 200,000 and up) are autosomal genes or phenotypes listed before May 15, 1995.

3----- (300,000 and up) are X-linked genes and phenotypes.

4----- (400,000 and up) are Y-linked genes and phenotypes.

5----- (500,000 and up) are mitochondrial genes and phenotypes (see Chapter 17).

6----- (600,000 and up) are autosomal genes and phenotypes listed after May 15, 1995.

THE FREQUENCY OF GENE MUTATIONS

How frequently do mutations of OMIM-listed genes cause a hereditary condition to appear in a newborn infant? This question is a little more difficult to answer for three reasons. First, most abnormalities present at the birth of a newborn infant *are not* the result of gene mutation. Instead, most abnormalities at birth result from an error in fetal development that can be caused by disease agents, malnutrition, exposure to drugs or chemicals, or a number of other factors. Second, some of the hereditary diseases listed in OMIM are not present at birth. Instead, the symptoms of these conditions take several months to several decades to develop. Finally, hereditary abnormalities resulting from errors in the number or structure of chromosomes are their own category of birth defects, not listed in OMIM. We discuss chromosome changes and their consequences in Chapter 10.

To apply some numbers to the question, however, we can take statistics on births and birth defects from the U.S. Centers for Disease Control (CDC). For 2014, the most recent full year for which the data have been published, the CDC reports that 3,988,076 babies were born in the United States. Nearly 97% of these babies were born healthy, but about 3%, or 1 in 33, have some kind of abnormality detected at birth. Between 20% and 30% of these birth defects are caused either by gene mutations or by abnormalities of chromosome number or structure;

Table 2.9	Hereditary Conditions and Gene Mutations in OMIM[a]				
	Autosomal	**X-Linked**	**Y-Linked**	**Mitochondrial**	**Total**
Genes described	14,562	714	49	35	15,360
Total entries[b]	22,274	1258	60	66	23,658

[a] OMIM statistics as of September 2016 (http://www.omim.org/statistics/entry).
[b] Genes plus hereditary conditions not yet associated with a gene.

the remainder are developmental abnormalities. The CDC estimates that in 2014 about 1 in 110 to 1 in 150 babies had defects caused by an inherited gene mutation, and an additional 1 in 150 to 1 in 200 babies were born with chromosome defects.

As we move on in this book we will pay special attention to a number of topics relating to human genome sequence variation, including inherited human diseases, testing for human genetic diseases, and the management and applications of information concerning human genetic variation and inherited diseases. Much of this discussion takes place in the application chapters distributed throughout the book. For example, Application Chapter B titled "Human Genetic Testing" discusses genetic tests performed on newborn infants and genetic testing done later in life to identify the presence of genetic disease or a mutation that can cause genetic disease. Application Chapter A titled "Human Hereditary Disease and Genetic Counseling" discusses how genetic information is managed and presented to families in a medical context. The other application chapters, on cancer genetics, human evolutionary genetics, and on DNA analysis in forensic genetics applications, describe additional uses of human genetic information.

SUMMARY

Mastering Genetics For activities, animations, and review quizzes, go to the Study Area.

2.1 Gregor Mendel Discovered the Basic Principles of Genetic Transmission

- A broad education in science and mathematics prepared Mendel to design hybridization experiments that could reveal the principles of hereditary transmission.

2.2 Monohybrid Crosses Reveal the Segregation of Alleles

- Mendel's experimental design had five important features: controlled crosses, use of pure-breeding parental strains, examination of discreet traits, quantification of results, and the use of replicate and reciprocal crosses.
- Crosses between pure-breeding parental plants with different phenotypes produce monohybrid F_1 progeny with the dominant phenotype.
- Monohybrid crosses produce a 3:1 ratio of the dominant to the recessive phenotype among F_2 progeny and demonstrate the operation of the law of segregation.
- The law of segregation states that two alleles of a gene will separate from one another during gamete formation, each allele has an equal probability of inclusion in a gamete, and gametes unite at random during reproduction.
- Mendel used test-cross analysis to demonstrate that F_1 plants are monohybrid, and he used the self-fertilization of F_2 plants with the dominant phenotype to demonstrate that the latter have a 2:1 ratio of heterozygotes to homozygotes.

2.3 Dihybrid and Trihybrid Crosses Reveal the Independent Assortment of Alleles

- The F_2 progeny of dihybrid F_1 plants display a 9:3:3:1 phenotype ratio that demonstrates the operation of the law of independent assortment.
- Mendel used trihybrid-cross analysis to demonstrate that alleles of multiple genes are transmitted in accordance with the predictions of the law of independent assortment.

2.4 Probability Theory Predicts Mendelian Ratios

- The product rule of probability is used to determine the likelihood of two or more independent events occurring simultaneously or consecutively. The joint probability in this case is determined by multiplying the probabilities of the independent events.
- The sum rule of probability is applied when two or more outcomes are possible. In this case, the individual probabilities of the outcomes are added together to determine the joint probability.
- Conditional probability is the probability of outcomes that are contingent on particular conditions.
- Binomial probability theory describes the outcomes of an experiment in terms of the number of outcome classes and the frequency of each class.

2.5 Chi-Square Analysis Tests the Fit between Observed Values and Expected Outcomes

- The chi-square test (χ^2) is used to compare observed results with the results predicted by a genetic hypothesis that is based on chance. It shows how closely predictions match results.
- The significance of a chi-square value is determined by the P (probability) value corresponding to the number of degrees of freedom in the experiment.

2.6 Autosomal Inheritance and Molecular Genetics Parallel the Predicitions of Mendel's Hereditary Principles

- Traits transmitted by autosomal inheritance are equally likely in males and females.
- Autosomal dominant inheritance produces a vertical pattern of transmission in which each organism with the dominant trait has at least one parent with the trait.
- Traits transmitted in an autosomal recessive pattern are usually distributed in a horizontal pattern in which offspring with the recessive trait frequently descend from parents that are heterozygous and have the dominant phenotype.
- Molecular analysis of four of Mendel's traits illustrates how transmission genetics and molecular genetics characterize the same hereditary processes at different levels.

PREPARING FOR PROBLEM SOLVING

In addition to the list of problem-solving tips and suggestions given here, you can go to the Study Guide and Solutions Manual that accompanies this book for help at solving problems.

1. Be familiar with Mendel's laws of segregation and independent assortment and the ways in which probability determines the outcomes of genetic crosses involving these two laws.

2. Familiarize yourself with monohybrid and dihybrid crosses and the ratios they generate in offspring.

3. Review test crosses and the phenotype ratios produced from test crosses.

4. Use the Punnett square and the forked-line method to predict the expected genotypic or phenotypic proportions from genetic crosses.

5. Work backward from offspring genotypes or phenotypes to predict the genotypes or phenotypes of parents in a cross.

6. Recognize the use of the product rule and the sum rule in predicting offspring genotype and phenotype proportions.

7. Recognize the circumstances that dictate the use of conditional probability, and understand the uses of binomial probability.

8. Be familiar with the use of chi-square analysis to test the fit between the observed results of a cross and the results that are expected.

PROBLEMS

Mastering Genetics   Visit for instructor-assigned tutorials and problems.

Chapter Concepts

For answers to selected even-numbered problems, see Appendix: Answers.

1. Compare and contrast the following terms:
   a. dominant and recessive
   b. genotype and phenotype
   c. homozygous and heterozygous
   d. monohybrid cross and test cross
   e. dihybrid cross and trihybrid cross

2. For the cross $BB \times Bb$, what is the expected genotype ratio? What is the expected phenotype ratio?

3. For the cross $Aabb \times aaBb$, what is the expected genotype ratio? What is the expected phenotype ratio?

4. In mice, black coat color is dominant to white coat color. In the pedigree shown here, mice with a black coat are represented by darkened symbols, and those with white coats are shown as open symbols. Using allele symbols B and b, determine the genotypes for each mouse .

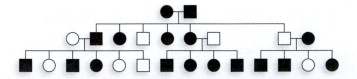

5. Two parents plan to have three children. What is the probability that the children will be two girls and one boy?

6. Consider the cross $AaBbCC \times AABbCc$.
   a. How many different gamete genotypes can each organism produce?
   b. Use a Punnett square to predict the expected ratio of offspring phenotypes.

   c. Use the forked-line method to predict the expected ratio of offspring phenotypes.

7. If a chi-square test produces a chi-square value of 7.83 with 4 degrees of freedom,
   a. In what interval range does the P value fall?
   b. Is the result sufficient to reject the chance hypothesis?
   c. Above what chi-square value would you reject the chance hypothesis for an experiment with 7 degrees of freedom?

8. Determine whether the statements below are true or false. If a statement is false, provide the correct information or revise the statement to make it correct.
   a. If a dihybrid cross is performed, the expected genotypic ratio is 9:3:3:1.
   b. A student uses the product rule to predict that the probability of flipping a coin twice and getting a head and then a tail is $\frac{1}{4}$.
   c. A test cross between a heterozygous parent and a homozygous recessive parent is expected to produce a 1:1 genotypic and phenotypic ratio.
   d. The outcome of a trihybrid cross is predicted by the law of segregation.
   e. Reciprocal crosses that produce identical results demonstrate that a strain is pure-breeding.
   f. If a woman is heterozygous for albinism, an autosomal recessive condition that results in the absence of skin pigment, the proportion of her gametes carrying the allele that allows pigment expression is expected to be 75%.
   g. The progeny of a trihybrid cross are expected to have one of 27 different genotypes.

h. If a dihybrid F_1 plant is self-fertilized,
   (1) $\frac{9}{16}$ of the progeny will have the same phenotype as the F_1 parent.
   (2) $\frac{1}{16}$ of the progeny will be true-breeding.
   (3) $\frac{1}{2}$ of the progeny will be heterozygous at one or both loci.

9. In the datura plant, purple flower color is controlled by a dominant allele P. White flowers are found in plants homozygous for the recessive allele p. Suppose that a purple-flowered datura plant with an unknown genotype is self-fertilized and that its progeny are 28 purple-flowered plants and 10 white-flowered plants.
   a. Use the results of the self-fertilization to determine the genotype of the original purple-flowered plant.
   b. If one of the purple-flowered progeny plants is selected at random and self-fertilized, what is the probability it will breed true?

10. The dorsal pigment pattern of frogs can be either "leopard" (white pigment between dark spots) or "mottled" (pigment between spots appears mottled). The trait is controlled by an autosomal gene. Males and females are selected from pure-breeding populations, and a pair of reciprocal crosses is performed. The cross results are shown below.

    Cross 1:   P: Male leopard × female mottled
                F_1: All mottled
                F_2: 70 mottled, 22 leopard
    Cross 2:   P: Male mottled × female leopard
                F_1: All mottled
                F_2: 50 mottled, 18 leopard

   a. Which of the phenotypes is dominant? Explain your answer.
   b. Compare and contrast the results of the reciprocal crosses in the context of autosomal gene inheritance.
   c. In the F_2 progeny from both crosses, what proportion is expected to be homozygous? What proportion is expected to be heterozygous?
   d. Propose two different genetic crosses that would allow you to determine the genotype of one mottled frog from the F_2 generation.

11. Black skin color is dominant to pink skin color in pigs. Two heterozygous black pigs are crossed.
   a. What is the probability that their offspring will have pink skin?
   b. What is the probability that the first and second offspring will have black skin?
   c. If these pigs produce a total of three piglets, what is the probability that two will be pink and one will be black?

12. A male mouse with brown fur color is mated to two different female mice with black fur. Black female 1 produces a litter of 9 black and 7 brown pups. Black female 2 produces 14 black pups.
   a. What is the mode of inheritance of black and brown fur color in mice?

   b. Choose symbols for each allele, and identify the genotypes of the brown male and the two black females.

13. Figure 2.12 shows the results of Mendel's test-cross analysis of independent assortment. In this experiment, he first crossed pure-breeding round, yellow plants to pure-breeding wrinkled, green plants. The round yellow F_1 are crossed to pure-breeding wrinkled, green plants. Use chi-square analysis to show that Mendel's results do not differ significantly from those expected.

14. An experienced goldfish breeder receives two unusual male goldfish. One is black rather than gold, and the other has a single tail fin rather than a split tail fin. The breeder crosses the black male to a female that is gold. All the F_1 are gold. She also crosses the single-finned male to a female with a split tail fin. All the F_1 have a split tail fin. She then crosses the black male to F_1 gold females and, separately, crosses the single-finned male to F_1 split-finned females. The results of the crosses are shown below.

    Black male × F_1 gold female:
        Gold   32
        Black   34
    Single-finned male × F_1 split-finned female:
        Split fin   41
        Single fin   39

   a. What do the results of these crosses suggest about the inheritance of color and tail fin shape in goldfish?
   b. Is black color dominant or recessive? Explain. Is single tail dominant or recessive? Explain.
   c. Use chi-square analysis to test your hereditary hypothesis for each trait.

15. The accompanying pedigree shows the transmission of albinism (absence of skin pigment) in a human family.

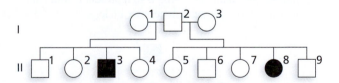

   a. What is the most likely mode of transmission of albinism in this family?
   b. Using allelic symbols of your choice, identify the genotypes of the male and his two mates in generation I.
   c. The female I-1 and her mate, male I-2, had four children, one of whom has albinism. What is the probability that they could have had a total of four children with *any other outcome* except one child with albinism and three with normal pigmentation?
   d. What is the probability that female I-3 is a heterozygous carrier of the allele for albinism?
   e. One child of female I-3 has albinism. What is the probability that any of the other four children are carriers of the allele for albinism?

16. A geneticist crosses a pure-breeding strain of peas producing yellow, wrinkled seeds with one that is pure-breeding for green, round seeds.
    a. Use a Punnett square to predict the F_2 progeny that would be expected if the F_1 are allowed to self-fertilize.
    b. What proportion of the F_2 progeny are expected to have yellow seeds? Wrinkled seeds? Green seeds? Round seeds?
    c. What is the expected phenotype distribution among the F_2 progeny?

17. Suppose an F_1 plant from Problem 16 is crossed to the pure-breeding green, round parental strain. Use a forked-line diagram to predict the phenotypic distribution of the resulting progeny.

18. In pea plants, the appearance of flowers along the main stem is a dominant phenotype called "axial" and is controlled by an allele T. The recessive phenotype, produced by an allele t, has flowers only at the end of the stem and is called "terminal." Pod form displays a dominant phenotype, "inflated," controlled by an allele C, and a recessive "constricted" form, produced by the c allele. A cross is made between a pure-breeding axial, constricted plant and a plant that is pure-breeding terminal, inflated.

a. The F_1 progeny of this cross are allowed to self-fertilize. What is the expected phenotypic distribution among the F_2 progeny?
b. Suppose that all of the F_2 progeny with terminal flowers, i.e., plants with terminal flowers and inflated pods and plants with terminal flowers and constricted pods, are saved and allowed to self-fertilize to produce a partial F_3 generation. What is the expected phenotypic distribution among these F_3 plants?
c. If an F_1 plant from the initial cross described above is crossed with a plant that is terminal, constricted, what is the expected distribution among the resulting progeny?
d. If the plants with terminal flowers produced by the cross in part (c) are saved and allowed to self-fertilize, what is the expected phenotypic distribution among the progeny?

19. If two six-sided dice are rolled, what is the probability that the total number of spots showing is
    a. 4?
    b. 7?
    c. greater than 5?
    d. an odd number?

Application and Integration
For answers to selected even-numbered problems, see Appendix: Answers.

20. Experimental Insight 2.1 describes data, collected by a genetics class like yours, on the numbers of kernels of different colors in bicolor corn. To test the hypothesis that the presence of kernels of different colors in each ear is the result of the segregation of two alleles of a single gene, the class counted 12,356 kernels and found that 9304 were yellow and 3052 were white. Use chi-square analysis to evaluate the fit between the segregation hypothesis and the class results.

21. The accompanying pedigree shows the transmission of a phenotypic character. Using B to represent a dominant allele and b to represent a recessive allele,

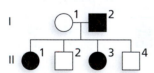

    a. Give the genotype(s) possible for each member of the family, assuming the trait is autosomal dominant.
    b. Give the genotype(s) possible for each member of the family, assuming the trait is autosomal recessive.

22. The seeds in bush bean pods are each the product of an independent fertilization event. Green seed color is dominant to white seed color in bush beans. If a heterozygous plant with green seeds self-fertilizes, what is the probability that 6 seeds in a single pod of the progeny plant will consist of
    a. 3 green and 3 white seeds?
    b. all green seeds?
    c. at least 1 white seed?

23. List all the different gametes that are possible from the following genotypes.
    a. *AABbCcDd*
    b. *AabbCcDD*
    c. *AaBbCcDd*
    d. *AabbCCdd*

24. Organisms with the genotypes *AABbCcDd* and *AaBbCcDd* are crossed. What are the expected proportions of the following progeny?
    a. *A–B–C–D–*
    b. *AabbCcDd*
    c. a phenotype identical to either parent
    d. *A–B–ccdd*

25. Blue moon beans produce beans that are either the dominant color blue or the recessive color white. The bean pods for this species always contain four seeds each. If two heterozygous plants that each have the *Bb* genotype are crossed, what are the predicted frequencies of each of the five outcome classes for combinations of blue and white seeds in pods?

26. In the fruit fly *Drosophila*, a rudimentary wing called "vestigial" and dark body color called "ebony" are inherited as independently assorting genes and are recessive to their dominant counterparts full wing and gray body color. Dihybrid dominant-phenotype males and females are crossed, and 3200 progeny are produced. How many progeny flies are expected to be found in each phenotypic class?

27. In pea plants, plant height, seed shape, and seed color are governed by three independently assorting genes. The three genes have dominant and recessive alleles, with tall

(T) dominant to short (t), round (R) dominant to wrinkled (r), and yellow (G) dominant to green (g).

a. If a true-breeding tall, wrinkled, yellow plant is crossed to a true-breeding short, round, green plant, what phenotypic ratios are expected in the F_1 and F_2?

b. What proportion of the F_2 are expected to be tall, wrinkled, yellow? $ttRRGg$?

c. What proportion of the F_2 that produce round, green seeds (regardless of the height of the plant) are expected to breed true?

28. A variety of pea plant called Blue Persian produces a tall plant with blue seeds. A second variety of pea plant called Spanish Dwarf produces a short plant with white seed. The two varieties are crossed, and the resulting seeds are collected. All of the seeds are white; and when planted, they produce all tall plants. These tall F_1 plants are allowed to self-fertilize. The results for seed color and plant stature in the F_2 generation are as follows:

F_2 Plant Phenotype	Number
Blue seed, tall plant	97
White seed, tall plant	270
Blue seed, short plant	33
White seed, short plant	100
TOTAL	500

a. Which phenotypes are dominant, and which are recessive? Why?

b. What is the expected distribution of phenotypes in the F_2 generation?

c. State the hypothesis being tested in this experiment.

d. Examine the data in the table by the chi-square test and determine whether they conform to expectations of the hypothesis.

29. In tomato plants, the production of red fruit color is under the control of an allele R. Yellow tomatoes are rr. The dominant phenotype for fruit shape is under the control of an allele T, which produces two lobes. Multilobed fruit, the recessive phenotype, have the genotype tt. Two different crosses are made between parental plants of unknown genotype and phenotype. Use the progeny phenotype ratios to determine the genotypes and phenotypes of each parent.

Cross 1 progeny:	$\frac{3}{8}$ two-lobed, red
	$\frac{3}{8}$ two-lobed, yellow
	$\frac{1}{8}$ multilobed, red
	$\frac{1}{8}$ multilobed, yellow
Cross 2 progeny:	$\frac{1}{4}$ two-lobed, red
	$\frac{1}{4}$ two-lobed, yellow
	$\frac{1}{4}$ multilobed, red
	$\frac{1}{4}$ multilobed, yellow

30. A male and a female are each heterozygous for both cystic fibrosis (CF) and phenylketonuria (PKU). Both conditions are autosomal recessive, and they assort independently.

a. What proportion of the children of this couple will have neither condition?

b. What proportion of the children will have either PKU or CF but not both?

c. What proportion of the children will be carriers of one or both conditions?

31. A woman expressing a dominant phenotype is heterozygous (Dd) for the gene.

a. What is the probability that the dominant allele carried by the woman will be inherited by a grandchild?

b. What is the probability that two grandchildren of the woman who are first cousins to one another will each inherit the dominant allele?

c. Draw a pedigree that illustrates the transmission of the dominant trait from the grandmother to two of her grandchildren who are first cousins.

32. Two parents who are each known to be carriers of an autosomal recessive allele have four children. None of the children has the recessive condition. What is the probability that one or more of the children is a carrier of the recessive allele?

33. An organism having the genotype $AaBbCcDdEe$ is self-fertilized. Assuming the five genes assort independently, determine the following proportions:

a. gametes that are expected to carry only dominant alleles

b. progeny that are expected to have a genotype identical to that of the parent

c. progeny that are expected to have a phenotype identical to that of the parent

d. gametes that are expected to be $ABcde$

e. progeny that are expected to have the genotype $AabbCcDdE–$

34. A man and a woman are each heterozygous carriers of an autosomal recessive mutation of a disorder that is fatal in infancy. They both want to have multiple children, but they are concerned about the risk of the disorder appearing in one or more of their children. In separate calculations, determine the probabilities of the couple having five children with 0, 1, 2, 3, 4, and all 5 children being affected by the disorder.

35. For a single dice roll, there is a $\frac{1}{6}$ chance that any particular number will appear. For a pair of dice, each specific combination of numbers has a probability of $\frac{1}{36}$ occurring. Most total values of two dice can occur more than one way. As a test of random probability theory, a student decides to roll a pair of six-sided dice 300 times and tabulate the results. She tabulates the number of times each different total value of the two dice occurs. Her results are the following:

Total Value of Two Dice	Number of Times Rolled
2	7
3	11
4	23
5	36
6	42
7	53
8	40
9	38
10	30
11	12
12	8
TOTAL	300

The student tells you that her results fail to prove that random chance is the explanation for the outcome of this experiment. Is she correct or incorrect? Support your answer.

36. You have four guinea pigs for a genetic study. One male and one female are from a strain that is pure-breeding for short brown fur. A second male and female are from a strain that is pure-breeding for long white fur. You are asked to perform two *different* experiments to test the proposal that short fur is dominant to long fur and that brown is dominant to white. You may use any of the four original pure-breeding guinea pigs or any of their offspring in experimental matings. Design two different experiments (crossing different animals and using different combinations of phenotypes) to test the dominance relationships of alleles for fur length and color, and make predictions for each cross based on the proposed relationships. Anticipate that the litter size will be 12 for each mating and that female guinea pigs can produce three litters in their lifetime.

37. Galactosemia is an autosomal recessive disorder caused by the inability to metabolize galactose, a component of the lactose found in mammalian milk. Galactosemia can be partially managed by eliminating dietary intake of lactose and galactose. Amanda is healthy, as are her parents, but her brother Alonzo has galactosemia. Brice has a similar family history. He and his parents are healthy, but his sister Brianna has galactosemia. Amanda and Brice are planning a family and seek genetic counseling. Based on the information provided, complete the following activities and answer the questions.
    a. Draw a pedigree that includes Amanda, Brice, and their siblings and parents. Identify the genotype of each person, using G and g to represent the dominant and recessive alleles, respectively.
    b. What is the probability that Amanda is a carrier of the allele for galactosemia? What is the probability that Brice is a carrier? Explain your reasoning for each answer.
    c. What is the probability that the first child of Amanda and Brice will have galactosemia? Show your work.

d. If the first child has galactosemia, what is the probability that the second child will have galactosemia? Explain the reasoning for your answer.

38. Sweet yellow tomatoes with a pear shape bring a high price per basket to growers. Pear shape, yellow color, and terminal flower position are recessive traits produced by alleles f, r, and t, respectively. The dominant phenotypes for each trait—full shape, red color, and axial flower position—are the product of dominant alleles F, R, and T. A farmer has two pure-breeding tomato lines. One is full, yellow, terminal and the other is pear, red, axial. Design a breeding experiment that will produce a line of tomato that is pure-breeding for pear shape, yellow color, and axial flower position.

39. A cross between a spicy variety of *Capsicum annum* pepper and a sweet (nonspicy) variety produces F_1 progeny plants that all have spicy peppers. The F_1 are crossed, and among the F_2 plants are 56 that produce spicy peppers and 20 that produce sweet peppers. Dr. Ara B. Dopsis, an expert on pepper plants, discovers a gene he designates *Pun1* that he believes is responsible for spicy versus sweet flavor of peppers. Dr. Dopsis proposes that a dominant allele P produces spicy peppers and that a recessive mutant allele p results in sweet peppers.
    a. Are the data on the parental cross and the F_1 and F_2 consistent with the proposal made by Dr. Dopsis? Explain why or why not, using P and p to indicate probable genotypes of pepper plants.
    b. Assuming the proposal is correct, what proportion of the spicy F_2 pepper plants do you expect will be pure-breeding? Explain your answer.

40. Alkaptonuria is an infrequent autosomal recessive condition. It is first noticed in newborns when the urine in their diapers turns black upon exposure to air. The condition is caused by the defective transport of the amino acid phenylalanine through the intestinal walls during digestion. About 4 people per 1000 are carriers of alkaptonuria.

    Sara and James had never heard of alkaptonuria and were shocked to discover that their first child had the condition. Sara's sister Mary and her husband Frank are planning to have a family and are concerned about the possibility of alkaptonuria in one of their children.

    The four adults (Sara, James, Mary, and Frank) seek information from a neighbor who is a retired physician. After discussing their family histories, the neighbor says, "I never took genetics, but I know from my many years in practice that Sara and James are both carriers of this recessive condition. Since their first child had the condition, there is a very low chance that the next child will also have it, because the odds of having two children with a recessive condition are very low. Mary and Frank have no chance of having a child with alkaptonuria because Frank has no family history of the condition." The two couples each have babies and *both* babies have alkaptonuria.
    a. What are the genotypes of the four adults?
    b. What was incorrect about the information given to Sara and James? What is incorrect about the information given to Mary and Frank?

c. What is the probability that the second child of Mary and Frank will have alkaptonuria?

d. What is the chance that the third child of Sara and James will be free of the condition?

e. The couples are worried that one of their grandchildren will inherit alkaptonuria. How would you assess the risk that one of the offspring of a child with alkaptonuria will inherit the condition?

41. Humans vary in many ways from one another. Among many minor phenotypic differences are the following five independently assorting traits that (sort of) have a dominant and a recessive phenotype: (1) forearm hair (alleles F and f)—the presence of hair on the forearm is dominant to the absence of hair on the forearm; (2) earlobe form (alleles E and e)—unattached earlobes are dominant to attached earlobes; (3) widow's peak (alleles W and w)—a distinct "V" shape to the hairline at the top of the forehead is dominant to a straight hairline; (4) hitchhiker's thumb (alleles H and h)—the ability to bend the thumb back beyond vertical is dominant and the inability to do so is recessive; and (5) freckling (alleles D and d)—the appearance of freckles is dominant to the absence of freckles. In reality, the genetics of these traits are more complicated than single gene variation, but assume for the purposes of this problem that the patterns in families match those of other single-gene variants.

If a couple with the genotypes $Ff\ Ee\ Ww\ Hh\ Dd$ and $Ff\ Ee\ Ww\ Hh\ Dd$ have children, what is the chance the children will inherit the following characteristics?

a. the same phenotype as the parents

b. four dominant traits and one recessive trait

c. all recessive traits

d. the genotype $Ff\ EE\ Ww\ hh\ dd$

42. In chickens, the presence of feathers on the legs is due to a dominant allele (F), and the absence of leg feathers is due to a recessive allele (f). The comb on the top of the head can be either pea-shaped, a phenotype that is controlled by a dominant allele (P), or a single comb controlled by a recessive allele (p). The two genes assort independently. Assume that a pure-breeding rooster that has feathered legs and a single comb is crossed with a pure-breeding hen that has no leg feathers and a pea-shaped comb. The F_1 are crossed to produce the F_2. Among the resulting F_2, however, only birds with a single comb and feathered legs are allowed to mate. These chickens mate at random to produce F_3 progeny. What are the expected genotypic and phenotypic ratios among the resulting F_3 progeny?

43. A pure-breeding fruit fly with the recessive mutation cut wing, caused by the homozygous cc genotype, is crossed to a pure-breeding fly with normal wings, genotype CC. Their F_1 progeny all have normal wings. F_1 flies are crossed, and the F_2 progeny have a 3:1 ratio of normal wing to cut wing. One male F_2 fly with normal wings is selected at random and mated to an F_2 female with normal wings. Using all possible genotypes of the F_2 flies selected for this cross, list all possible crosses between the two flies involved in this mating, and determine the probability of each possible outcome.

44. Situs inversus is a congenital condition in which the major visceral organs are reversed from their normal positions. Investigations into the genetics of this abnormality revealed that individuals with at least one dominant allele (SI) of an autosomal gene are normal but, surprisingly, of individuals that are homozygous for a recessive allele (si), $\frac{1}{2}$ are situs inversus and $\frac{1}{2}$ are normal.

a. What genotypes and phenotypes are expected in progeny from a cross of two $si\ si$ individuals?

b. What genotypes and phenotypes are expected in progeny from a cross of two $SI\ si$ individuals?

45. Domestic dogs evolved from ancestral grey wolves. Wolves have coats of short, straight hair and lack "furnishings," a growth pattern marked by eyebrows and a mustache found in some domestic dogs. In domestic dogs, coat variation is controlled by allelic variation in three genes. Recessive mutant alleles in the *FGF5* gene result in long hair, while dogs carrying the dominant ancestral allele have short hair. Likewise, recessive mutant alleles in the *KRT71* gene result in curly hair, whereas dogs with an ancestral dominant allele have straight hair. Dominant mutant alleles in the *RSPO2* gene cause the presence of furnishings, while dogs homozygous for the ancestral recessive allele have no furnishings.

A pure-breeding curly- and long-haired poodle with furnishings was crossed to a pure-breeding short- and straight-haired border collie lacking furnishings.

a. What are the genotypes and phenotypes of the puppies?

b. If dogs of the F_1 generation are interbred, what proportions of genotypes and phenotypes are expected in the F_2?

46. Alleles of the *IGF-1* gene in dogs, encoding insulin-like growth factor, largely determine whether a domestic dog will be large or small. Dogs with an ancestral dominant allele are large, whereas dogs homozygous for the mutant recessive allele are small. Chondrodysplasia, a short-legged phenotype (as in dachshunds and basset hounds), is caused by a dominant gain-of-function allele of the *FGF4* gene. The *MSTN* gene encodes myostatin, a regulator of muscle development. Dogs with a dominant ancestral allele of the *MTSN* gene have normal muscle development, while dogs homozygous for recessive mutants in the *MTSN* gene are "double muscled" and have trouble running quickly. However, dogs heterozygous for the mutant allele run faster than either of the homozygotes.

You breed a pure-breeding small basset hound of normal musculature with a pure-breeding "bully" whippet, a double-muscled large dog with normal legs.

a. What are the genotypes and phenotypes of the F_1 puppies?

b. If the F_1 of this cross is interbred, what proportion of the F_2 are expected to be fast runners and what proportion normal-speed runners?

47. The accompanying pedigree shows a family in which one child (II-1) has an autosomal recessive condition. On the basis of this fact alone, provide the following information.

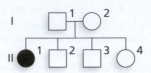

   a. Using *A* for the dominant allele and *a* for the recessive allele, give the genotypes for I-1, I-2, and II-1.
   b. Using the same alleles, give the possible genotypes for II-2, II-3, and II-4.

   c. What are the probabilities for each of the possible genotypes for II-2, II-3, and II-4?
   d. What is the probability that all three of the children in generation II who have the dominant phenotype are *Aa*?
   e. What is the chance that among the three children in generation II who have the dominant phenotype, one of them is *AA* and two of them are *Aa*? (Hint: Consider all possible orders of genotypes.)

Collaboration and Discussion

For answers to selected even-numbered problems, see Appendix: Answers.

48. A pea plant that has the genotype *RrGgwwdd* is crossed to a plant that has the *rrGgWwDd* genotype. The *R* gene controls round versus wrinkled seed, the *G* gene controls yellow versus green seed, the *W* gene controls purple versus white flower, and the *D* gene controls tall versus short plants. Determine the following;
   a. What are the phenotypes of each plant?
   b. What proportion of the progeny are expected to have the genotype *RrGGwwDd*?
   c. What proportion of the progeny are expected to have the genotype *rrggwwdd*?
   d. What proportion of the progeny are expected to be round, yellow, purple, and tall?

49. Go to the OMIM website (http://www.ncbi.nlm.nih.gov/omim) and locate the Search button at the top of the page. Use the Search function to look up, one by one, the following three human hereditary diseases that are relatively common in certain populations: "Tay–Sachs disease" (select OMIM number 272800 from the search results list); "cystic fibrosis" (select OMIM number 602421 from the search results list); and "sickle cell anemia" (select OMIM 603903 from the search results list). For each of these diseases, look through the information and provide the following details:
   a. On which chromosome is the gene for the disease located?
   b. What gene is mutated in the disease?
   c. Briefly describe the disease.
   d. In which population(s) does the disease most commonly occur?

50. Select a human hereditary disease or condition you would like to know more about. Using the OMIM website (http://www.ncbi.nlm.nih.gov/omim) search for the disease and prepare a short synopsis of your findings. Include the following information:
   a. The gene mutated in the disease and its chromosome location.
   b. A description of the disease or condition.
   c. Any available information about the population(s) in which the disease is most common.

51. For a number of human hereditary conditions, genetic testing is available to identify heterozygous carriers. Some heterozygous carrier testing programs are community-based, often as part of an organized effort targeting specific populations in which a disease and carriers of a disease are relatively frequent. For example, carrier genetic testing programs for Tay–Sachs disease target Ashkenazi Jewish populations; and sickle cell disease carrier testing programs target African American populations. The testing is usually free or available at minimal cost, the wait time for results is short, and the results are confidential and unavailable to third parties such as insurance companies. Neither the Tay–Sachs nor sickle cell allele produces serious consequences for heterozygous carriers.
   a. From a genetic perspective, what is the value of the information obtained by genetic testing of the type described?
   b. In a broader sense, what is the value of a community-based effort targeting specific populations for selected diseases?
   c. Do you personally think you would participate in the kind of carrier genetic testing described if you were a member of a population targeted for such testing?

52. In humans, the ability to bend the thumb back beyond vertical is called hitchhiker's thumb and is dominant to the inability to do so (OMIM 274200; see Problem 41). Also, the presence of attached earlobes is recessive to unattached earlobes (OMIM 128900).
   a. Check your own phenotype and those of several friends or classmates.
   b. Using all available and willing members of your family, or members of another family if yours is not easily accessible, trace the transmission of both traits in a pedigree. Use allelic symbols *H* and *h* for the thumb and *E* and *e* for earlobes, and identify the genotypes for each family member as completely as possible. Bring the pedigree back to share with your group.

Cell Division and Chromosome Heredity

3

CHAPTER OUTLINE

3.1 Mitosis Divides Somatic Cells

3.2 Meiosis Produces Cells for Sexual Reproduction

3.3 The Chromosome Theory of Heredity Proposes That Genes Are Carried on Chromosomes

3.4 Sex Determination Is Chromosomal and Genetic

3.5 Human Sex-Linked Transmission Follows Distinct Patterns

3.6 Dosage Compensation Equalizes the Expression of Sex-Linked Genes

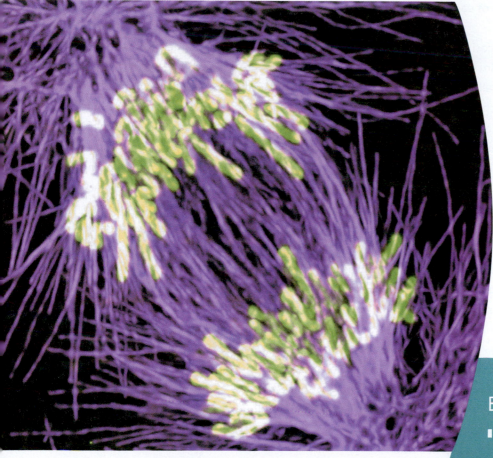

Cell division is a complex but precisely controlled process. In this cell in the anaphase segment of cell division, chromosomes are stained green and micro-tubules are stained blue. The chromosomes are in the process of migrating to opposite poles of the cell.

ESSENTIAL IDEAS

- The cell cycle consists of interphase, during which cells carry out regular functions and replicate their DNA, and M phase, the cell-division segment of the cycle.

- Mitosis divides somatic cells and produces two genetically identical daughter cells.

- Meiosis occurs in germ-line cells and produces four genetically different haploid cells that form gametes for reproduction.

- The separation of chromosomes and sister chromatids during meiosis is the mechanical basis of Mendel's law of segregation and law of independent assortment.

- The chromosome theory of heredity identified chromosomes as the cell structures containing genes.

- Sex determination is controlled by chromosomal and genetic factors that vary among species.

- Dosage compensation equalizes the expression of sex-linked genes of males and females of animal species.

A number of years ago, at the moment of conception that culminated in your birth, two gametes united to form the single fertilized cell—the zygote—from which you developed. Your chromosomal sex was determined in that instant. Your mother's egg carried an X chromosome, and your sex was determined by whether your father's sperm carried an X chromosome, making you female (XX), or a Y chromosome, making you male (XY). Shortly after fertilization, cell division began that over the next few hours increased the tiny zygote to two cells, then four cells, then eight cells, and so on. Over several days, these cell divisions continued while the mass of cells, called a trophoblast, moved down the fallopian tube toward the uterus. About 1 week after fertilization, the cluster of hundreds of cells, now called a blastocyst, implanted into the uterine wall; and within 2 weeks of conception, genetically controlled processes of cell differentiation and cell specialization began to form the first embryonic organs and structures. These processes eventually determined the structure and function of each cell in your body.

Since then, your body has produced thousands of generations of cells. The mechanism of cell division that produced most of them is called **mitosis**. It is an ongoing process that with each division creates two identical **daughter cells**. These two cells are exact genetic replicas of one another and of the parental cell from which they are derived. Mitosis produces somatic cells, the structural cells of the body. It is responsible for the growth and maintenance of your body, its organs, and its various structures; it repairs the damage and injury your body sustains, and it produces new cells to replace those that undergo programmed cell death (apoptosis). While you have been reading this passage, approximately 200 cells in your body have undergone mitotic division.

There are trillions of somatic cells in your body, and nearly all of them contain a nucleus in which the chromosomes are located. Human somatic cells are like those of most other animals in that their nuclei contain two sets of chromosomes: Each chromosome belongs to a homologous pair, and the total number of chromosomes is called the **diploid number**. Your somatic cell nuclei contain 46 chromosomes each, in 23 homologous pairs, so your diploid number is 46. The diploid number varies among species (each species having its characteristic number of pairs), so the characteristic diploid number for animal species in general is described as $2n$. Some plant cell nuclei, such as those of pea plants, also have two sets of chromosomes and are diploid. Commonly, however, plant cells carry more than two chromosome sets. They may be triploid ($3n$), tetraploid ($4n$), hexaploid ($6n$), octoploid ($8n$), or some other multiple of n. The value n represents the **haploid number** of chromosomes, and it is one-half the diploid number. Humans have a diploid number of $2n = 46$, so the human haploid number is $n = 23$.

Gametes, produced from **germ-line cells**, are the germinal, or reproductive, cells: sperm and egg in animals or pollen and egg in plants. Germ-line cells divide by **meiosis**. Meiotic cell division reduces the number of chromosomes in the nucleus of each daughter cell by one-half to the haploid number. In humans, the number of chromosomes in each egg and sperm nucleus is 23. Each of the 23 human chromosome pairs has one representative in each sperm or egg. The union of the sperm and egg nuclei at fertilization produces the fertilized egg with 46 chromosomes in its nucleus. Thus human reproduction, like that of other sexually reproducing organisms ensures that exactly one-half of the genetic information in an offspring comes from each parent.

In this chapter, we examine both mitosis and meiosis, and we look closely at the connection between meiotic cell division and Mendel's laws of heredity. We also explore patterns of sex determination in eukaryotes and look at processes that equalize the expression of genes carried on **sex chromosomes**, the chromosomes that determine sex. In addition, we study the special patterns of inheritance of genes on the X chromosome, and we see how the discovery of genes on the X chromosome supported the **chromosome theory of heredity**, the theory that chromosomes are the cell structures that carry genes.

3.1 Mitosis Divides Somatic Cells

Mitosis is among the most fundamental and important processes occurring in cells. It is a genetically controlled process that follows a precise script to enable organisms to grow and develop normally and to maintain the structures and functions of their organs, tissues, and other bodily components. Life depends on the orderly progression and proper regulation of mitosis. If too little cell division takes place or cell division occurs too slowly, an organism may fail to develop at all, or it may have morphologic abnormalities. On the other hand, too much cell division can lead to growth of structures beyond their normal boundaries, likewise producing morphologic abnormality and possible death.

The Cell Cycle

Cell division is regulated by genetic control of the **cell cycle**, the life cycle cells must pass through to replicate their DNA and divide. Since well-regulated cell division is such an integral part of life, it will not surprise you to learn that

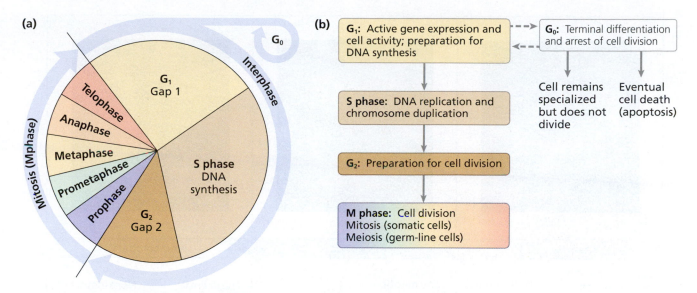

Figure 3.1   The cell cycle. (a) The cell cycle is divided into interphase and M phase, which are each further subdivided. The cycles are not drawn to scale. **(b)** An overview of cell cycle activities.

the cell cycles of all eukaryotes are similar and that much of the molecular machinery that controls the cell cycle is evolutionarily conserved in plants and animals. Furthermore, in powerful testament to the single origin of life, plants and animals share a number of cell cycle genes with the Bacteria and Archaea domains of life.

The eukaryotic cell cycle is divided into two principal phases—**M phase**, a short segment of the cell cycle during which cells divide, and **interphase**, the longer period between one M phase and the next (**Figure 3.1a**). Interphase consists of three successive stages, G_1, S, and G_2. During interphase the cell expresses genetic information, it replicates its chromosomes, and it prepares for entry into M phase. M phase is divided into multiple substages that correspond to the progress of the cell during its division.

When viewed under a light microscope, somatic cells in interphase may appear rather placid, but their outward appearance gives little indication of the complex activity taking place inside. Gene expression occurs continuously throughout the cell cycle, but during the G_1 **(or Gap 1) phase** of interphase, it is particularly high (**Figure 3.1b**). Cells of different types vary in how many genes they express, in how they function in the body, and in how they interact with other cells. Consequently, the duration of G_1 varies among different types of cells in the body. Some types of cells are rapidly dividing and spend only a short time, perhaps as little as a few hours, in G_1. Other cells linger in G_1 for periods of days, weeks, or more.

As they approach the end of G_1, cells follow one of two alternative paths. Most cells enter the **S phase**, or **synthesis phase**, during which DNA replication (DNA synthesis) takes place. On the other hand, a small subset of specialized cells transition from G_1 into a nondividing state called G_0 ("G zero"), a kind of semiperpetual G_1-like state in which

cells express their genetic information and carry out normal functions but do not progress through the cell cycle (see Figure 3.1b). Several kinds of cells in your body, including certain cells in your eyes and bones, reach a mature state of differentiation, enter G_0, and rarely if ever divide again. Most G_0 cells maintain their specialized functions until they enter programmed cell death (apoptosis) and die. Cells only rarely leave G_0 and resume the cell cycle.

DNA replication takes place during S phase and results in a doubling of the amount of DNA in the nucleus—by creating two identical **sister chromatids** that are joined to form each chromosome. Prior to S phase, each chromosome is composed of a long DNA double helix. During S phase, the DNA strands separate, and each acts as a template to direct the synthesis of a new daughter strand of DNA. This DNA synthesis forms the sister chromatids that are genetically identical to one another. The completion of S phase brings about the transition to the G_2, or **Gap 2**, phase of the cell cycle, during which cells prepare for division. Interphase ends when cells enter M phase, from which two identical daughter cells emerge.

The successive generations of cells produced through mitosis as one cell cycle follows the next are known as cell lines or cell lineages. Each cell line or cell lineage contains identical cells (i.e., clones) that are all descended from a single founder cell. Mitosis ensures that the genetic information in cells is faithfully passed to successive generations of cell lineages.

Substages of M Phase

M phase follows interphase and is divided into five substages— **prophase**, **prometaphase**, **metaphase**, **anaphase**, and **telophase**—whose principal features are described in

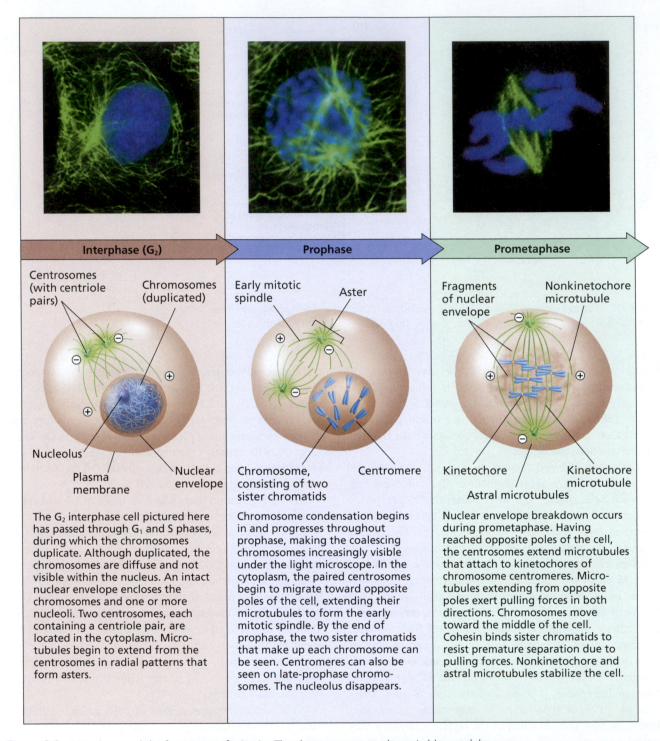

Figure 3.2 Interphase and the five stages of mitosis. The chromosomes are shown in blue, and the centrosomes, asters, and spindle fibers are shown in green.

Figure 3.2. These five substages accomplish two important functions of cell division—(1) the equal partitioning of the chromosomal material into the nuclei of the two daughter cells, a process called **karyokinesis**, and (2) the partitioning of the cytoplasmic contents of the parental cell into the daughter cells, a process known as **cytokinesis**.

During interphase chromosomes are diffuse and cannot be clearly seen by light microscopy. Chromosome condensation, a process that progressively condenses chromosomes into more compact structures, begins in early prophase. Chromosomes become visible in midprophase, and the process continues until chromosomes reach their maximum level of condensation in metaphase. Nuclear envelope breakdown also occurs in prophase, and chromosome centromeres become visible as do the sister chromatids of each chromosome. The **centromere** is a specialized DNA

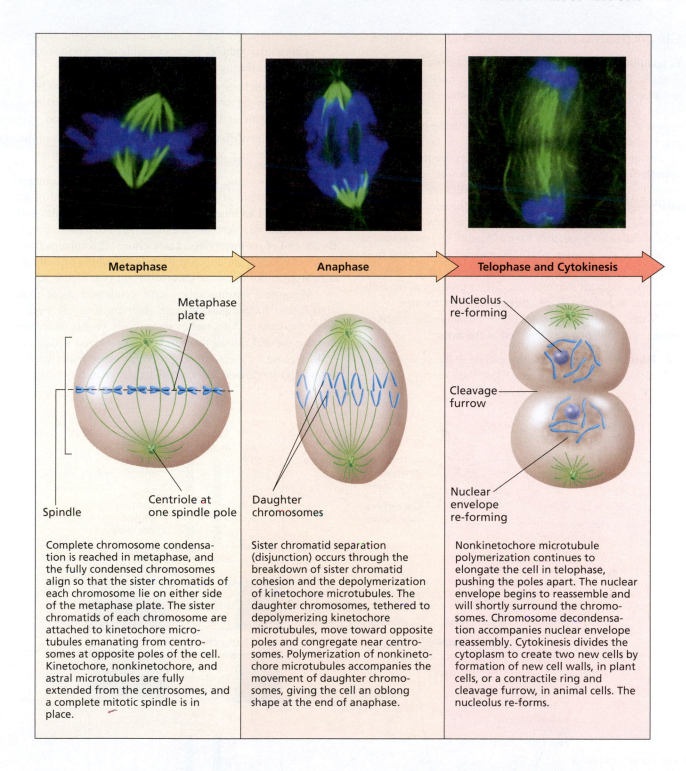

Metaphase

Metaphase plate

Spindle

Centriole at one spindle pole

Complete chromosome condensation is reached in metaphase, and the fully condensed chromosomes align so that the sister chromatids of each chromosome lie on either side of the metaphase plate. The sister chromatids of each chromosome are attached to kinetochore microtubules emanating from centrosomes at opposite poles of the cell. Kinetochore, nonkinetochore, and astral microtubules are fully extended from the centrosomes, and a complete mitotic spindle is in place.

Anaphase

Daughter chromosomes

Sister chromatid separation (disjunction) occurs through the breakdown of sister chromatid cohesion and the depolymerization of kinetochore microtubules. The daughter chromosomes, tethered to depolymerizing kinetochore microtubules, move toward opposite poles and congregate near centrosomes. Polymerization of nonkinetochore microtubules accompanies the movement of daughter chromosomes, giving the cell an oblong shape at the end of anaphase.

Telophase and Cytokinesis

Nucleolus re-forming

Cleavage furrow

Nuclear envelope re-forming

Nonkinetochore microtubule polymerization continues to elongate the cell in telophase, pushing the poles apart. The nuclear envelope begins to reassemble and will shortly surround the chromosomes. Chromosome decondensation accompanies nuclear envelope reassembly. Cytokinesis divides the cytoplasm to create two new cells by formation of new cell walls, in plant cells, or a contractile ring and cleavage furrow, in animal cells. The nucleolus re-forms.

sequence on each chromosome, and its location is identified as a constriction where the sister chromatids are joined together. Centromeric DNA sequence binds a specialized protein complex called the **kinetochore** that facilitates chromosome movement and division later in M phase.

The meaning and usage of the terms *chromosome, chromatid,* and *sister chromatid* sometimes cause confusion, and this is a good time to provide functional definitions. The term chromosome is used throughout the cell cycle to identify each DNA-containing structure that has a centromere. At the end of G_1, a chromosome consists of a single DNA duplex (double helix) with associated proteins. After the completion of S phase, a chromosome consists of two replicated DNA duplexes with associated proteins. The two DNA molecules making up this chromosome are identical. Individually, these DNA molecules are identified as chromatids, and together they are identified as the sister chromatids.

Chromosome Movement and Distribution

In addition to visible changes to chromosomes, extranuclear changes (changes occurring outside the nucleus) are also apparent in prophase. In animal cells, although not in most plants, fungi, or algae, two organelles called **centrosomes** appear that migrate during M phase to form the two opposite poles of the dividing cell. Each centrosome contains a pair of subunits called centrioles. Centrosomes are the source of **spindle fiber microtubules** that emanate from each centrosome **(Figure 3.3)**. Spindle fiber microtubules are polymers of tubulin protein subunits that elongate by the addition of tubulin subunits and shorten by the removal of tubulin subunits. Microtubules are polar; they have a "minus" (−) end anchored at the centrosome and a "plus" (+) end that grows away from the centrosome. Specialized proteins called motor proteins are associated with microtubules. Motor proteins move chromosomes and other cell structures along microtubules.

Three kinds of spindle fibers emanate from centrosomes in a 360° pattern identified as the **aster**:

1. **Kinetochore microtubules** embed in the protein complex called the kinetochore (described shortly) that assembles at the centromere of each chromatid. Kinetochore microtubules are responsible for chromosome movement during cell division.

2. **Nonkinetochore microtubules** extend toward each other from the two polar centrosomes and overlap to help elongate and stabilize the cell during division.

3. **Astral microtubules** grow toward the membrane of the cell, where they attach and contribute to cell stability.

The kinetochore is a protein complex that assembles on each chromatid at the centromere. It is composed of an outer plate and an inner plate and is attached to the plus end of a kinetochore microtubule extending from a centrosome. By the end of prometaphase, kinetochore microtubules from each centrosome are attached to the kinetochore of a different chromatid of the sister chromatid pair (see Figure 3.3).

Metaphase chromosomes have condensed more than 10,000-fold in comparison with their form at the beginning of prophase. This makes them easily visible under the microscope and allows them to be easily moved within the cell. Because they are tethered to kinetochore microtubules from opposite centrosomes, the sister chromatids experience

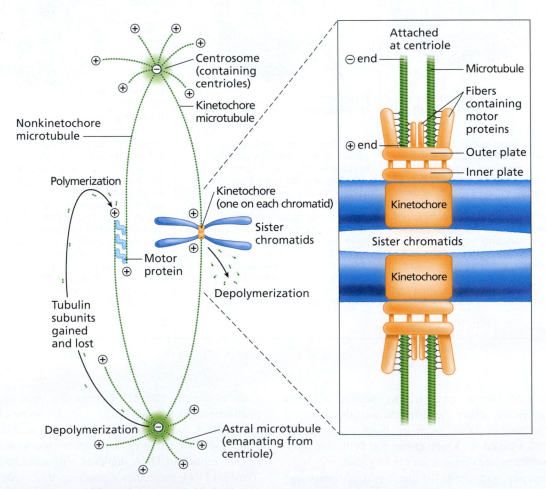

Figure 3.3 Microtubules in dividing cells emanate from centrosomes. Astral microtubules and nonkinetochore microtubules control and stabilize cell shape during division. Kinetochore microtubules attach to chromosome kinetochores to move chromosomes.

opposing forces that are critical to the positioning of chromosomes along an imaginary midline at the equator of the cell. This imaginary line is called the **metaphase plate**.

The tension created by the pull of kinetochore microtubules is balanced by a companion process known as **sister chromatid cohesion**. Sister chromatid cohesion is produced by the protein cohesin that localizes between the sister chromatids and holds them together to resist the pull of kinetochore microtubules (**Figure 3.4**). Cohesin is a four-subunit protein; its central component is a polypeptide produced by the gene *Scc1* for "sister chromatid cohesion." Cohesin coats sister chromatids along their entire length but is most concentrated near centromeres, where the pull of microtubules is greatest. As microtubules move chromosomes toward the midline of the cell, cohesin helps keep the sister chromatids together, to ensure proper chromosome positioning and to prevent their premature separation.

Anaphase is the part of M phase during which sister chromatids separate and begin moving to opposite poles in the cell. Anaphase includes two distinct events tied to microtubule action: anaphase A, characterized by the separation of sister chromatids, and anaphase B, characterized by the elongation of the cell into an oblong shape.

Anaphase A begins abruptly with two simultaneous events. First, the enzyme separase initiates cleavage of polypeptides in cohesin, thus breaking down the connection between sister chromatids. Second, kinetochore microtubules begin to depolymerize at their (+) ends to initiate chromosome movement toward the centrioles. The separation of sister chromatids in anaphase A is called chromosome **disjunction**. As anaphase progresses, sister chromatids complete their disjunction and eventually congregate around the centrosomes at the cell poles.

The next part of anaphase, anaphase B, is characterized by the polymerization of polar microtubules that extends their length and causes the cell to take on an oblong shape. The oblong shape facilitates cytokinesis at the end of telophase, which leads to the formation of two daughter cells.

Completion of Cell Division

In telophase, nuclear membranes begin to reassemble around the chromosomes gathered at each pole, eventually enclosing the chromosomes in nuclear envelopes. Chromosome decondensation begins and ultimately returns chromosomes to their diffuse interphase state. At the same time, microtubules disassemble. As telophase comes to an end, two identical nuclei are observed within a single elongated cell that is about to be divided into two daughter cells by the process of cytokinesis.

In animal cells, a contractile ring composed of actin microfilaments creates a cleavage furrow around the circumference of the cell; the contractile ring pinches the cell in two (**Figure 3.5**). In plant cells, cytokinesis entails the

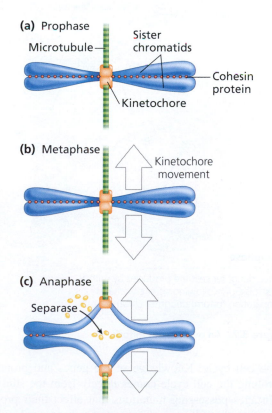

Figure 3.4 **Sister chromatid cohesion and separation.** Cohesin protein induces cohesion between sister chromatids **(a)** and **(b)**. At anaphase **(c)**, separase protein digests cohesin and allows sister chromatids to separate.

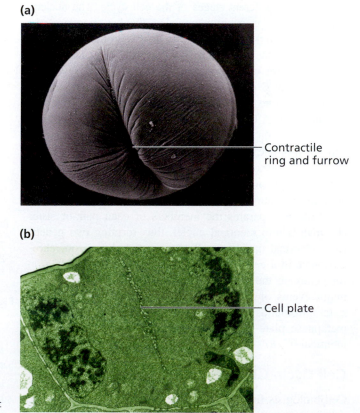

Figure 3.5 **Cytokinesis in animal cells (a) and plant cells (b).**

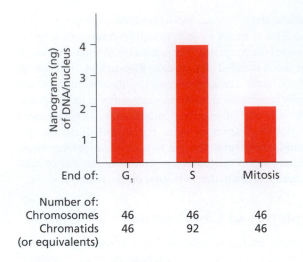

Figure 3.6 A profile of the nuclear contents of a cell through the mitotic cell cycle.

Ⓠ Name the event that causes the doubling of the amount of DNA by the end of S phase.

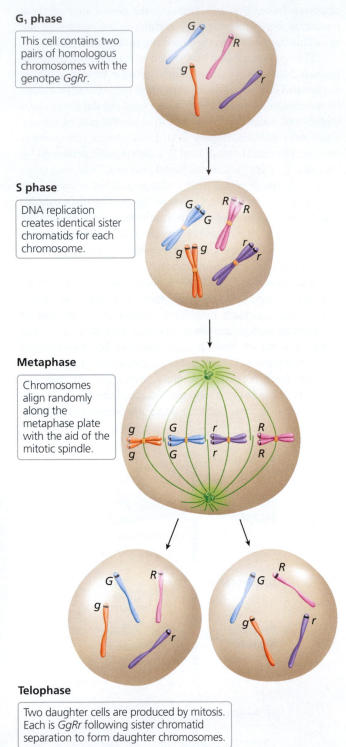

G₁ phase

This cell contains two pairs of homologous chromosomes with the genotpe *GgRr*.

S phase

DNA replication creates identical sister chromatids for each chromosome.

Metaphase

Chromosomes align randomly along the metaphase plate with the aid of the mitotic spindle.

Telophase

Two daughter cells are produced by mitosis. Each is *GgRr* following sister chromatid separation to form daughter chromosomes.

Figure 3.7 An overview of mitosis.

construction of new cell walls near the cellular midline. In both plant and animal cells, cytokinesis divides the cytoplasmic fluid and organelles.

Figure 3.6 presents a profile of the contents of a single nucleus that identifies the amounts of DNA, the number of chromosomes, and the number of chromatids (DNA duplexes) at the end of different stages of the cell cycle. The nucleus depicted is similar to a human nucleus that has approximately 2 nanograms (ng) of DNA in G₁, with 46 chromosomes, each composed of one DNA duplex. DNA amount and the number of duplexes double (forming sister chromatids) with the completion of S phase, and the separation of sister chromatids into separate daughter cell nuclei in anaphase reduces the amount of DNA by one-half. At the end of mitotic M phase, the nucleus again contains 2 ng of DNA and 46 chromosomes composed of one duplex each, at which point the cell is ready to enter G₁ stage of the following cell cycle. Notice that despite changes in the amount of DNA and chromatid number, the chromosome number remains at 46 throughout the cell cycle.

Mitosis separates the members of each pair of sister chromatids into identical nuclei, thus forming two genetically identical daughter cells. **Figure 3.7** shows four chromosomes in a cell of an organism that is dihybrid (*GgRr*) for genes on the chromosomes shown. The figure follows major events of the cell cycle, showing the generation of sister chromatids in S phase, chromosome alignment on the metaphase plate in metaphase, and the production of two identical (*GgRr*) daughter cells at the end of telophase.

Cell Cycle Checkpoints

Cell biologists find that no matter what the duration of the cell cycle, most cells follow the same basic program; this suggests that common, genetically controlled signals drive

the cell cycle. Knowledge of the genes and proteins controlling the cell cycle comes largely from the study of cell lineages possessing mutations that affect their progression through the cell cycle. These studies have produced important insights into genetic control of the cell cycle, and in recent decades, biologists have discovered the identities and functions of many genes responsible for cell cycle control.

What has been learned about genetic control of the cell cycle can be applied to the study of normal cell division as well as to the study of cell division abnormalities such as those displayed in cancer.

As cells move through the cell cycle, their readiness to progress from one stage to the next is regularly assessed. The numerous **cell cycle checkpoints**, four of which are illustrated in **Figure 3.8**, are times during the cell cycle when cells are monitored by protein interactions that assess the status of the cell and its readiness to progress to the next stage. Such controls on cell division are essential for normal growth and development. Mutations that alter the normal control of the cell cycle are linked to a number of cell growth abnormalities. For example, loss of cell cycle control is a fundamental mechanism leading to cancer development. Indeed, cancer is often characterized by out-of-control cell proliferation that leads to tumor formation and the overgrowth of cancerous cells that invade and displace normal cells. We explore mutations altering cell cycle control and other gene mutations associated with cancer development and progression in Application Chapter C titled "The Genetics of Cancer."

3.2 Meiosis Produces Cells for Sexual Reproduction

Reproduction is a basic requirement of living organisms. In more than three centuries of observation, biologists have identified a dizzying array of reproductive methods, mechanisms, and behaviors in animals, plants, and microbes. Even so, reproduction can be divided into two broad categories: (1) asexual reproduction, in which organisms reproduce without mating, giving rise to progeny that are genetically identical to their parent; and (2) sexual reproduction, in which cells called reproductive cells or gametes are produced by cell division and unite during fertilization.

Bacteria and Archaea reproduce exclusively by asexual reproduction. These organisms are haploid; they usually have just a single chromosome. Cell division follows shortly after the completion of chromosome replication; each cell produces two genetically identical daughter cells.

Single-celled eukaryotes, such as yeast, have multiple chromosomes and may be either haploid or diploid, and these organisms can reproduce either sexually or asexually. Asexual reproduction in yeast is similar to cell division in bacteria. A haploid yeast cell undergoes DNA replication and distributes a copy of each chromosome to identical daughter cells. Although yeast spend most of their life cycle in a haploid state and actively reproduce as haploids, it is also common for two haploid yeast cells to fuse and form a diploid cell that produces haploid spores by meiosis.

In contrast to single-celled eukaryotes, multicellular eukaryotes reproduce predominantly by sexual means. In most animal species and dioecious plants, males and females

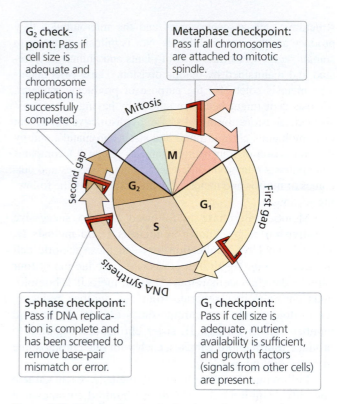

G₂ checkpoint: Pass if cell size is adequate and chromosome replication is successfully completed.

Metaphase checkpoint: Pass if all chromosomes are attached to mitotic spindle.

S-phase checkpoint: Pass if DNA replication is complete and has been screened to remove base-pair mismatch or error.

G₁ checkpoint: Pass if cell size is adequate, nutrient availability is sufficient, and growth factors (signals from other cells) are present.

Figure 3.8   Major cell cycle checkpoints. Genetic mechanisms monitor cell cycle checkpoints to ensure the cell's readiness to progress to the next stage.

carry distinct reproductive tissues and structures. Mating requires the production of haploid gametes from both male structures and female structures. The union of haploid gametes produces diploid progeny. In monoecious plant species, including the *Pisum sativum* that Mendel worked with, male and female reproductive tissues are present in each plant, and self-fertilization is the common mode of reproduction, although fertilization involving pollen from one plant fertilizing the flower of another also occurs.

In sexually reproducing animals, specialized germ-line cells undergo meiosis to produce haploid gametes, or reproductive cells. Female gametes are produced by the ovary in female animals or by the ovule in plants. Male germ-line cells are located in testes in animals, where they produce sperm. In the anthers of flowering plants, pollen containing two sperm cells is produced. These descriptions are broadly true for most plants and animals, but there are many exceptions, including the observation of asexual reproduction in several species of fish, rotifers (small aquatic organisms), and salamanders. In addition, male ants, bees, and wasps have haploid somatic cells, and their processes of gamete production are distinctive.

Meiosis Features Two Cell Divisions

Interphase of the germ-line cell cycle contains stages G_1, S, and G_2 that are indistinguishable from those in somatic cells. Similarly, the actions and functions of subcellular structures such as centrosomes and the microtubules they produce are the same in all cells. Nor is mitosis exclusive to somatic cells. Germ-line cells of plants and animals are created and maintained by mitotic division. These cells undertake meiosis solely for the purpose of producing gametes. Meiosis is distinguished from mitosis by having two successive cell divisions during M phase, by distinctive movement of homologous chromosomes and sister chromatids, and by the production of four haploid gametes. **Table 3.1** compares and contrasts numerous differences in the processes and outcomes of mitosis and meiosis that are described in the following sections.

Meiotic interphase is followed by two successive cell-division stages known as **meiosis I** and **meiosis II**. There is no DNA replication between these meiotic cell divisions, so the result of meiosis is the production of four haploid daughter cells (**Figure 3.9**). In meiosis I, homologous chromosomes separate from one another, reducing the diploid number of chromosomes ($2n$) to the haploid number (n). In meiosis II, sister chromatids separate to produce four haploid gametes, each with one chromosome of every diploid pair.

Following the completion of meiosis, each gamete contains a single nucleus holding a haploid chromosome set. The gametes of the two sexes are often dramatically different in size and morphology, however. Female gametes are generally much larger than male gametes and have a haploid nucleus, a large amount of cytoplasm, and a full array of organelles. In contrast, male gametes contain a haploid nucleus but very little cytoplasm and virtually no organelles. As the fertilized ovum begins mitotic division, the organelles and cytoplasmic structures provided by the maternal gamete support its early zygotic growth.

Meiosis I

Three hallmark events take place during meiosis I:

1. Homologous chromosome pairing
2. Crossing over between homologous chromosomes
3. Segregation (separation) of the homologous chromosomes that reduces chromosomes to the haploid number

Meiosis I is divided into four stages: prophase I, metaphase I, anaphase I, and telophase I. Homologous chromosome pairing, called chromosome synapsis, and recombination take place in prophase I; thus, this stage is subdivided into five substages—leptotene stage, zygotene stage, pachytene stage, diplotene stage, and diakinesis stage—to more accurately trace the interactions and recombination of homologous chromosomes. **Figure 3.10** describes these stages and prophase I substages in detail.

Chromosome condensation begins during leptotene, when the meiotic spindle is formed by microtubules emanating from the centrosomes, which are moving to positions at opposite ends of the cell. The nuclear membrane begins to break down in zygotene, and the first hallmark feature of meiosis occurs—homologous chromosome **synapsis**, the alignment of homologous chromosome pairs. Synapsis initiates formation of a protein bridge called the **synaptonemal complex**, a trilayer protein structure that maintains synapsis by tightly binding *nonsister chromatids* of homologous chromosomes to one another (**Figure 3.11**).

Nonsister chromatids are chromatids belonging to different members of a homologous pair of chromosomes. The binding of nonsister chromatids by a synaptonemal complex draws the homologs into close contact (synapsis). The synaptonemal complex contains two lateral elements, each consisting of proteins adhered to a chromatid from a

Table 3.1	Comparison of Mitosis and Meiosis	
Characteristic	**Mitosis**	**Meiosis**
Purpose	Produce genetically identical cells for growth and maintenance	Produce gametes for sexual reproduction that are genetically different
Location	Somatic cells	Germ-line cells
Mechanics	One round of division following one round of DNA replication	Two rounds of division (meiosis I and meiosis II) following a single round of DNA replication The mechanical basis of Mendel's laws of heredity
Homologous chromosomes	Do not pair Rarely undergo recombination	Synapsis during prophase I Crossing over during prophase I Separation at anaphase I
Sister chromatids	Attach to spindle fibers from opposite poles in metaphase Separate and migrate to opposite poles at anaphase	Attach to spindle fibers from the same pole in metaphase I Migrate to the same pole in anaphase I Attach to spindle fibers from opposite poles in metaphase II Separate and migrate to opposite poles in anaphase II
Product	Two genetically identical diploid daughter cells that continue to divide by mitosis	Four genetically different haploid cells that mature to form gametes and unite to form diploid zygotes

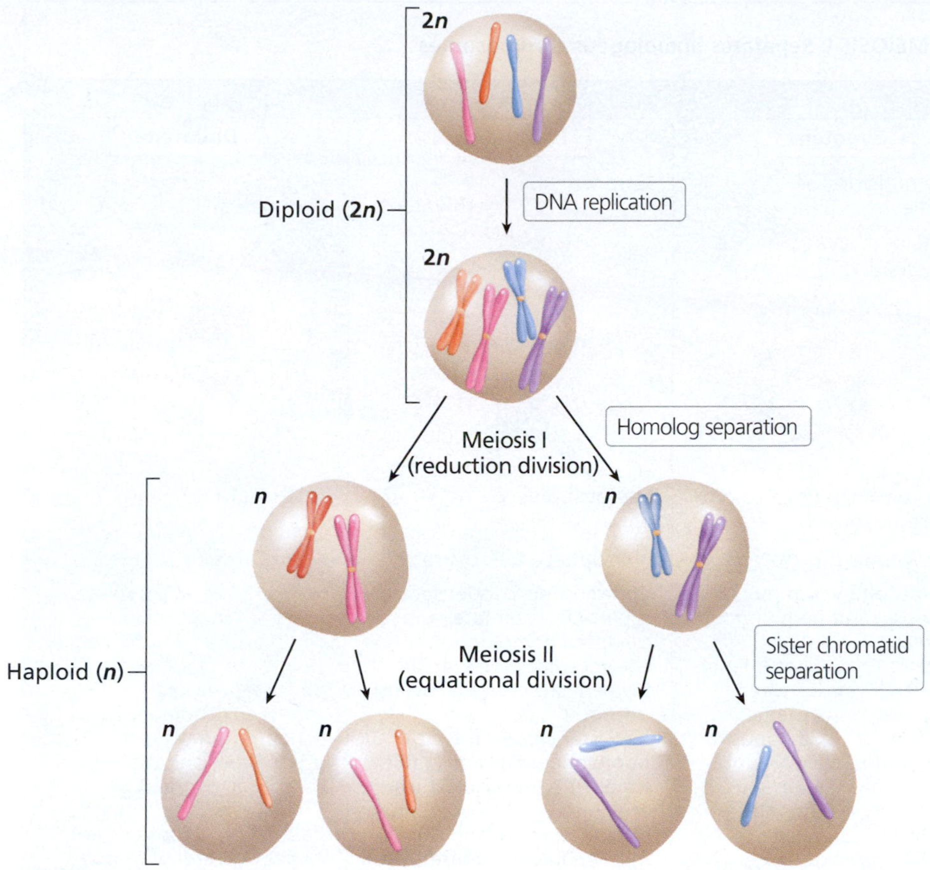

Figure 3.9   An overview of meiosis.

different member of a pair of homologous chromosomes, as well as a central element that joins the lateral elements. The function of the synaptonemal complex is to properly align homologous chromosomes before their separation and then to facilitate recombination between homologous chromosomes.

Chromosome condensation continues in pachytene, and sister chromatids of each chromosome can be visually distinguished by light microscopy. At this stage, the paired homologs are called a tetrad in recognition of the four chromatids that are microscopically visible in each homologous pair. Within the central element of the synaptonemal complex, new structures called **recombination nodules** appear at intervals.

Recombination nodules play a pivotal role in **crossing over** of genetic material between nonsister chromatids of homologous chromosomes. The number of recombination nodules correlates closely with the average number of crossover events along each homologous chromosome arm. Two important observations have been made about recombination nodules. First, their appearance and location within the synaptonemal complex is coincident with the timing and location of crossing over; and second, recombination nodules seem to be present in organisms that undergo crossing over and absent in those that do not. Cell biologists have concluded that recombination nodules are aggregations of enzymes and proteins that are needed to

carry out genetic exchange between the nonsister chromatids of homologous chromosomes during pachytene. Later chapters discuss the genetic consequences of crossing over (Chapter 5) and the molecular processes of crossing over (Chapter 11).

The chromosomes continue to condense in diplotene as the synaptonemal complex begins to dissolve. The dissolution allows homologs to pull apart slightly, revealing contact points between nonsister chromatids. These contact points are called **chiasmata** (singular: **chiasma**), and they are located along chromosomes where crossing over has occurred. Chiasmata mark the locations of DNA-strand exchange between nonsister chromatids of homologous chromosomes.

Cohesin protein is present between sister chromatids to resist the pulling forces of kinetochore microtubules (**Figure 3.12**). In diakinesis, kinetochore microtubules actively move synapsed chromosome pairs toward the metaphase plate, where the homologs will align side by side.

The chiasmata between homologous chromosomes are resolved in late prophase I so that the homologs can be aligned in metaphase I. This process of resolving the contacts between homologs is critical to the completion of recombination between homologous chromosomes.

Homologous chromosomes align on opposite sides of the metaphase plate in metaphase I. Kinetochore microtubules from one centrosome attach to the kinetochores of

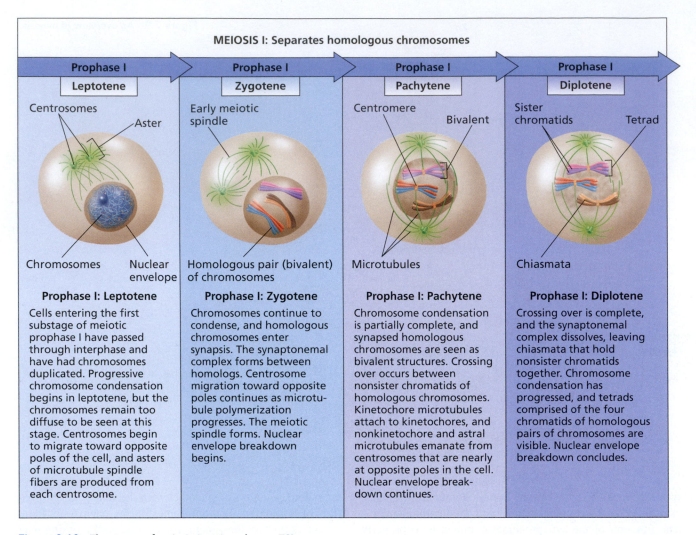

MEIOSIS I: Separates homologous chromosomes

Prophase I
Leptotene

Centrosomes
Aster
Chromosomes   Nuclear envelope

Prophase I: Leptotene

Cells entering the first substage of meiotic prophase I have passed through interphase and have had chromosomes duplicated. Progressive chromosome condensation begins in leptotene, but the chromosomes remain too diffuse to be seen at this stage. Centrosomes begin to migrate toward opposite poles of the cell, and asters of microtubule spindle fibers are produced from each centrosome.

Prophase I
Zygotene

Early meiotic spindle

Homologous pair (bivalent) of chromosomes

Prophase I: Zygotene

Chromosomes continue to condense, and homologous chromosomes enter synapsis. The synaptonemal complex forms between homologs. Centrosome migration toward opposite poles continues as microtubule polymerization progresses. The meiotic spindle forms. Nuclear envelope breakdown begins.

Prophase I
Pachytene

Centromere
Bivalent

Microtubules

Prophase I: Pachytene

Chromosome condensation is partially complete, and synapsed homologous chromosomes are seen as bivalent structures. Crossing over occurs between nonsister chromatids of homologous chromosomes. Kinetochore microtubules attach to kinetochores, and nonkinetochore and astral microtubules emanate from centrosomes that are nearly at opposite poles in the cell. Nuclear envelope breakdown continues.

Prophase I
Diplotene

Sister chromatids
Tetrad

Chiasmata

Prophase I: Diplotene

Crossing over is complete, and the synaptonemal complex dissolves, leaving chiasmata that hold nonsister chromatids together. Chromosome condensation has progressed, and tetrads comprised of the four chromatids of homologous pairs of chromosomes are visible. Nuclear envelope breakdown concludes.

Figure 3.10   The stages of meiosis *(continued on p. 79).*

both sister chromatids of one chromosome. Meanwhile, kinetochore microtubules from the other centrosome attach to the kinetochores of the sister chromatids of the homolog. Karyokinesis takes place in anaphase I as homologous chromosomes separate from one another and are dragged to opposite poles of the cell (see **Figure 3.10**). The sister chromatids of each chromosome remain firmly joined by cohesin. Nuclear membrane re-formation takes place in telophase I, when a haploid set of chromosomes are enclosed at each pole of the cell. Cytokinesis follows the completion of telophase I.

Homologous chromosome disjunction (separation) in meiosis I reduces the number of chromosomes at each pole to the haploid number, so that one representative of each homologous pair of chromosomes is present. The first meiotic division is known as the *reduction division,* to signify the reduction of chromosome number from diploid to haploid.

Sex chromosomes differ from pairs of autosomal chromosomes in that the X chromosome and Y chromosome

have very few genes in common. Even so, the X and Y chromosomes of males align as homologs in prophase I. This synapsis is accomplished with the aid of **pseudoautosomal regions (PARs)** on the two types of sex chromosomes. The term *pseudoautosomal* means "false autosomal"; a PAR is a segment of homology between otherwise different chromosomes. PARs are like homologous sequences carried on authentic autosomes. The pattern of inheritance of a pseudoautosomal region would be indistinguishable from the pattern of autosomal inheritance, as a consequence of the homology.

Human X and Y chromosomes each contain two pseudoautosomal regions, PAR1 and PAR2, that are located at opposite ends of the chromosomes (**Figure 3.13**). PAR1 is located on the short arms of the X and Y chromosomes and contains about 2.7 Mb (millions of base pairs) of DNA. PAR2 is located on the long arms of the chromosomes and is shorter than PAR1—about 300,000 base pairs. Crossing over during chromosome synapsis occurs regularly between PAR1 regions. Studies estimate the rate of recombination to be as

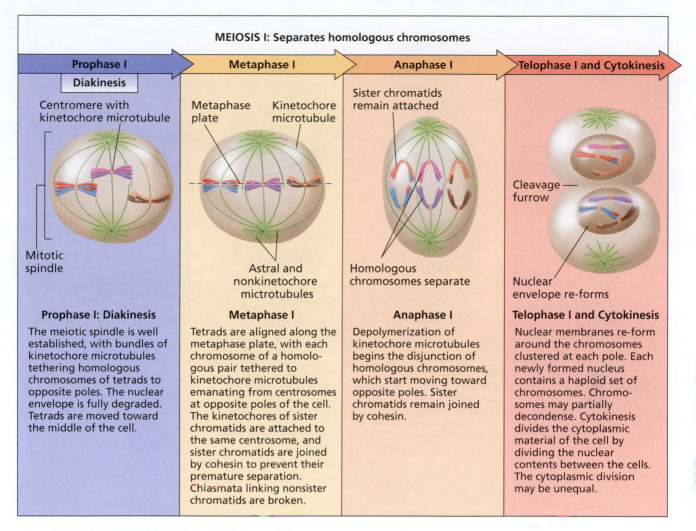

MEIOSIS I: Separates homologous chromosomes

Prophase I	Metaphase I	Anaphase I	Telophase I and Cytokinesis

Prophase I: Diakinesis

The meiotic spindle is well established, with bundles of kinetochore microtubules tethering homologous chromosomes of tetrads to opposite poles. The nuclear envelope is fully degraded. Tetrads are moved toward the middle of the cell.

Metaphase I

Tetrads are aligned along the metaphase plate, with each chromosome of a homologous pair tethered to kinetochore microtubules emanating from centrosomes at opposite poles of the cell. The kinetochores of sister chromatids are attached to the same centrosome, and sister chromatids are joined by cohesin to prevent their premature separation. Chiasmata linking nonsister chromatids are broken.

Anaphase I

Depolymerization of kinetochore microtubules begins the disjunction of homologous chromosomes, which start moving toward opposite poles. Sister chromatids remain joined by cohesin.

Telophase I and Cytokinesis

Nuclear membranes re-form around the chromosomes clustered at each pole. Each newly formed nucleus contains a haploid set of chromosomes. Chromosomes may partially decondense. Cytokinesis divides the cytoplasmic material of the cell by dividing the nuclear contents between the cells. The cytoplasmic division may be unequal.

Figure 3.10   The stages of meiosis *(continued on p. 80).*

much as 20-fold higher than for an equivalently sized region in autosomes.

Meiosis II

The second meiotic division divides each haploid product of meiosis I by separating sister chromatids from one another in a process that is reminiscent of mitosis, except that the number of chromosomes in each cell is one-half the number observed in mitosis. The products of meiosis II mature to form the gametes that contain a haploid set of chromosomes. The four stages of meiosis II—prophase II, metaphase II, anaphase II, and telophase II—are shown and described in Figure 3.10.

Meiosis II bears a general resemblance to mitosis in that kinetochore microtubules from opposite centrosomes attach to the kinetochores of sister chromatids. Also, as in mitosis, in meiosis II the chromosomes align randomly along the metaphase plate. Furthermore, sister chromatid separation is accompanied by cohesin breakdown, the action of motor proteins, and depolymerization of microtubules. Cytokinesis takes place at the end of telophase II. There are, however,

only a haploid number of chromosomes present in each cell during meiosis II. Four genetically distinct haploid cells, each carrying one chromosome that represents each homologous pair, are the products of meiosis II.

Figure 3.14a shows the profile of the content of a nucleus that begins G_1 with 2 ng of DNA and 46 chromosomes composed of one chromatid each. As we discussed for somatic cell nuclei, the amount of DNA and the number of duplexes double during S phase. These values are maintained until homologous chromosomes are separated in anaphase I. The end of meiosis I leaves the nucleus with one-half the DNA, chromosomes, and chromatids it contained at the end of S phase. Anaphase II brings the separation of sister chromatids and a further reduction by one-half in DNA amount and in the numbers of chromosomes and chromatids. The products of meiosis II, containing 1 ng of DNA and 23 chromosomes composed of one chromatid each, are gametes. The union of a sperm and an egg with this nuclear profile produces a fertilized egg with 2 ng of DNA and 46 chromosomes (**Figure 3.14b**). This is the profile of a cell ready to initiate its first somatic cell cycle.

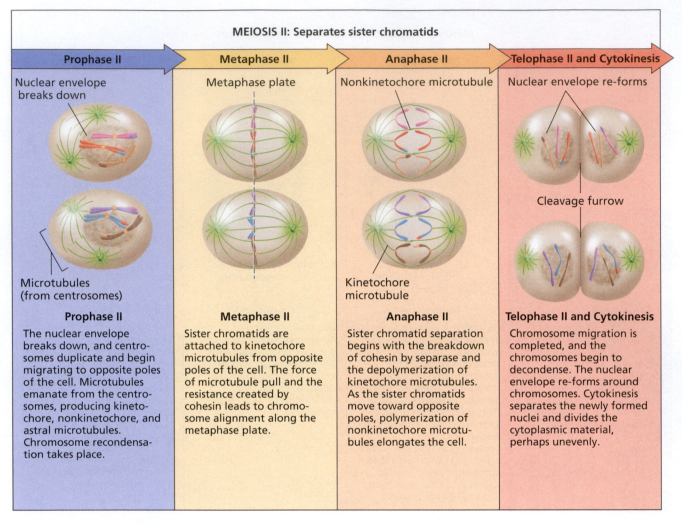

MEIOSIS II: Separates sister chromatids

Prophase II	Metaphase II	Anaphase II	Telophase II and Cytokinesis
Nuclear envelope breaks down	Metaphase plate	Nonkinetochore microtubule	Nuclear envelope re-forms
Microtubules (from centrosomes)		Kinetochore microtubule	Cleavage furrow

Prophase II

The nuclear envelope breaks down, and centrosomes duplicate and begin migrating to opposite poles of the cell. Microtubules emanate from the centrosomes, producing kinetochore, nonkinetochore, and astral microtubules. Chromosome recondensation takes place.

Metaphase II

Sister chromatids are attached to kinetochore microtubules from opposite poles of the cell. The force of microtubule pull and resistance created by cohesin leads to chromosome alignment along the metaphase plate.

Anaphase II

Sister chromatid separation begins with the breakdown of cohesin by separase and the depolymerization of kinetochore microtubules. As the sister chromatids move toward opposite poles, polymerization of nonkinetochore microtubules elongates the cell.

Telophase II and Cytokinesis

Chromosome migration is completed, and the chromosomes begin to decondense. The nuclear envelope re-forms around chromosomes. Cytokinesis separates the newly formed nuclei and divides the cytoplasmic material, perhaps unevenly.

Figure 3.10 The stages of meiosis.

Meiosis Generates Mendelian Ratios

The separation of homologous chromosomes and sister chromatids in meiosis constitutes the mechanical basis of Mendel's laws of segregation and independent assortment. The connection between meiosis and Mendelian hereditary principles was first suggested, independently, by Walter Sutton and Theodor Boveri in 1903. Based on microscopic observations of chromosomes during meiosis, Sutton and Boveri proposed two important ideas. First, meiosis was the process generating Mendel's rules of heredity; and second, genes were located on chromosomes. Over the next 2 decades, work on numerous species proved these hypotheses to be correct.

We can understand segregation by following a pair of homologous chromosomes through meiosis in a heterozygous organism. **Figure 3.15** illustrates meiosis in a pea plant with the heterozygous *Gg* genotype Recall that Mendel's law of segregation predicts that one-half (50%) of the gametes produced by a heterozygote will contain *G* and the remaining one-half will contain *g*. How does meiosis generate this outcome?

DNA replication in S phase creates identical sister chromatids for each chromosome. At metaphase I, the homologs align on opposite sides of the metaphase plate; and at anaphase I, the homologs separate from one another. This movement segregates the chromosome composed of two *G*-bearing chromatids from the chromosome bearing the two *g*-containing chromatids. Following these cells through to the separation of sister chromatids in meiosis II, we find that among the four gametes are two containing the *G* allele and two containing *g*. This outcome explains the 1:1 ratio of alleles that the law of segregation predicts for gametes of a heterozygous organism.

The mechanistic basis of Mendel's law of independent assortment is illustrated in **Figure 3.16** for a *GgRr* dihybrid pea plant. Recall that this law of heredity predicts that a dihybrid organism should produce four genetically different gametes at a frequency of one-quarter (25%) each.

Once again, S phase creates two identical sister chromatids for each chromosome. In metaphase I, however, two equally likely arrangements of the two homologous pairs shown in Figure 3.15 can occur. In each arrangement, the homologous chromosomes are on opposite sides of the metaphase plate.

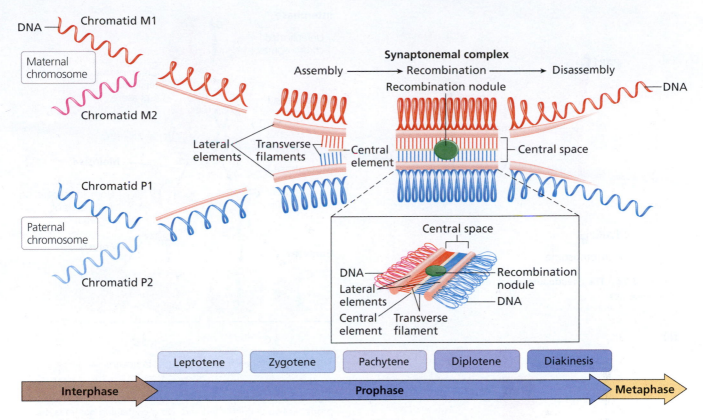

Figure 3.11   The synaptonemal complex. From electron micrograph analysis, the synaptonemal complex is thought to be a three-layer structure that assembles during prophase. Associated recombination nodules are sites of crossing over between homologous chromosomes.

◉ **Does the synaptonemal complex form between sister chromatids or chromatids of homologous chromosomes? Draw a chromosome pair consisting of two sister chromatids each and indicate where the synaptonemal complex is found.**

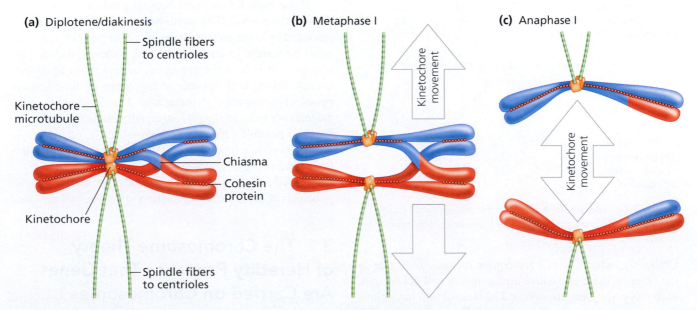

Figure 3.12   Homolog separation in meiosis I. (a) In diplotene and diakinesis of prophase I, crossing over between homologs is complete, and contacts between homologs (chiasmata) are resolved. **(b)** Spindle fibers pull chromosomes to align them on the metaphase plate. Cohesin protein adheres sister chromatids against the pull of spindle fibers. **(c)** Homologous chromosomes separate at anaphase I.

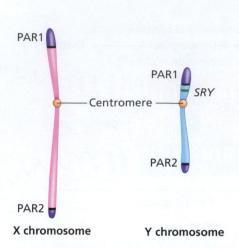

Figure 3.13 **The pseudoautosomal regions of the X and Y chromosomes.**

(a)

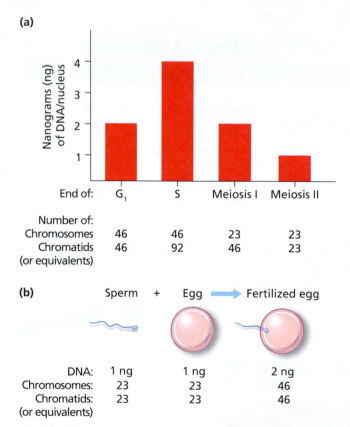

Number of:				
End of:	G$_1$	S	Meiosis I	Meiosis II
Chromosomes	46	46	23	23
Chromatids (or equivalents)	46	92	46	23

(b)

Sperm   +   Egg ➡ Fertilized egg

DNA:	1 ng	1 ng	2 ng
Chromosomes:	23	23	46
Chromatids (or equivalents)	23	23	46

Figure 3.14 **Meiosis. (a)** A profile of the nuclear contents of a cell through the phases of meiosis. **(b)** Gametic contributions to fertilization.

Obviously, when the cell undergoes meiosis, only one or the other of these alternative arrangements will occur; thus, each cell undergoing metaphase I of meiosis will have either "arrangement I" or "arrangement II." Over a large number of meiotic divisions, arrangement I and arrangement II are equally frequent. Arrangement I in Figure 3.15 has chromosomes carrying dominant alleles on one side of the metaphase

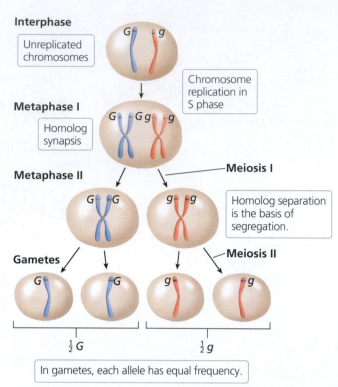

Figure 3.15 **Meiosis and the law of segregation.** This *Gg* cell produces two *G*-containing and two *g*-containing gametes, the ratio predicted by the law of segregation.

plate, and chromosomes carrying recessives on the opposite side. Arrangement II has a dominant-bearing and a recessive-bearing chromosome on each side of the metaphase plate. The first meiotic division segregates *G* from *g* and *R* from *r* to create the haploid products of meiosis I division.

If we now follow each haploid product of meiosis I through the meiosis II division, we see that the four gametes produced by arrangement I have the genotypes *GR* and *gr* in equal frequency. In contrast, the four gametes produced by arrangement II have the genotypes *Gr* and *gR* in equal frequency. Taking both possible arrangements of these homologous chromosomes at metaphase I into account, eight gametes are generated with four equally frequent genotypes. The four possible gamete genotypes—*GR, Gr, gR,* and *gr*—are produced in a frequency of 25% each as predicted by the law of independent assortment.

Genetic Analysis 3.1 gives you practice identifying the principles of Mendelian transmission in meiotic cell division.

3.3 The Chromosome Theory of Heredity Proposes That Genes Are Carried on Chromosomes

The early 20th century was a time of rapid expansion of genetic knowledge, fueled in large part by the rediscovery of Mendel's hereditary principles in 1900 and by the

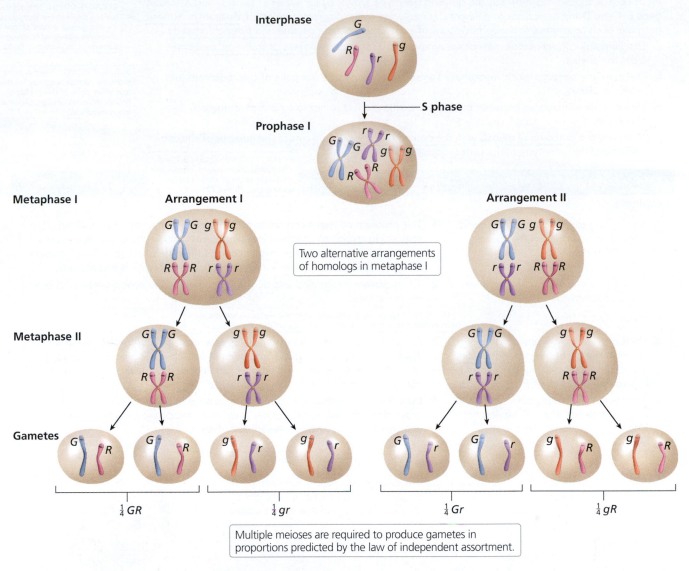

Figure 3.16 **Meiosis and the law of independent assortment.** Assessing the results of meiosis in numerous cells with the *GgRr* genotype, four genetically different gametes, *GR*, *Gr*, *gR*, and *gr* are produced at frequencies of 25% each.

What event reduces the amount of DNA by one-half during meiosis I? What event reduces DNA amount by an additional one-half in meiosis II?

independent discoveries of Sutton and Boveri that chromosome segregation in meiosis mirrored the hereditary transmission of genes. Many biologists turned their work toward testing the new "gene hypotheses" of segregation and independent assortment in an array of organisms.

Thomas Hunt Morgan, initially skeptical of the gene hypothesis, began working on the tiny fruit fly *Drosophila melanogaster* shortly after 1900. Morgan intended to rigorously test Mendel's rules in a natural species, not a domesticated one like *Pisum sativum*. Unlike Mendel, however, Morgan had no readily available phenotypic variants to examine. So, he and his students set out from their laboratory at Columbia University in New York City to the then-rural landscape of Long Island to attract fruit flies by

hanging buckets of rotting fruit on trees. Once captured and transported back to the laboratory, the flies were examined under the microscope to identify phenotypic variants. Flies captured from the wild were easily sexed by their morphology, and they almost invariably had the same phenotype for each trait examined. Morgan's group referred to these phenotypes as the "wild type." We use the term **wild type** today to signify the phenotype that is the most common in a population.

Morgan found *Drosophila* an easy organism to maintain and reproduce in small glass bottles filled with a semisolid mixture of cornmeal, sugar, and water. The life cycle of *Drosophila* is between 12 and 14 days depending on growth conditions, so 25 to 30 generations could be raised in a year.

PROBLEM A diploid organism has the dihybrid genotype $D_1D_2E_1E_2$ for alleles of gene D and alleles of gene E. Gene D and gene E are on different chromosomes. In the diagrams requested, illustrate only these two pairs of chromosomes and label each copy of each allele on chromosomes and sister chromatids.

> **BREAK IT DOWN:** This organism is a dihybrid (heterozygous for two genes). A total of four chromosomes—two homologous pairs—must be illustrated (p. 83).

   a. Diagram *any correct* mitotic metaphase arrangement for these two pairs of chromosomes and label the alleles.

   b. Diagram *any correct* meiotic metaphase I arrangement for these two pairs of chromosomes and label the alleles.

> **BREAK IT DOWN:** There is more than one correct response for this and other parts of this problem. Follow the rules of segregation and independent assortment (p. 83).

   c. Describe the differences between the diagrams with respect to homolog and chromosome alignment.

   d. Compare the outcome of mitosis with the outcome of meiosis in terms of the number of chromosomes and the genotype of the cells produced.

> **BREAK IT DOWN:** Figures 3.7 and 3.9 provide overviews of mitosis and meiosis in terms of chromosome division (pp. 75 and 77).

Solution Strategies	Solution Steps
Evaluate	
1. Identify the topic of this problem and the kind of information the answer should contain.	1. This problem concerns comparisons of mitosis and meiosis. Parts (a) and (b) require illustration of chromosome alignments at metaphase in mitosis and in meiosis I. Part (c) requires an explanation of the differences in those alignments, and part (d) requires comparison of the outcomes of mitosis and meiosis.
2. Identify the critical information given in the problem.	2. The organism is identified as a dihybrid for a pair of autosomal genes on different chromosomes.
Deduce	TIP: Heterozygous organisms carry different alleles on homologous chromosomes, but the alleles on sister chromatids are identical.
3. DNA duplicates in S phase. Identify the distribution of the different alleles on homologous chromosomes following completion of S phase.	3. Sister chromatids carry identical alleles as a result of DNA replication in S phase. Thus, for example, the sister chromatids of one chromosome will each carry a copy of D_1. In each of the other three chromosomes, the sister chromatids will be identical for one of the other alleles.
4. Review the overall patterns of chromosome alignment along the metaphase plate during mitotic and meiotic divisions.	4. During mitotic metaphase, chromosomes align in single file and in an arbitrary order along the metaphase plate. In meiotic metaphase I, homologs align opposite one another along the metaphase plate.
Solve	Answer a
5. Diagram chromosome alignment during mitotic metaphase.	5. Any order of the four chromosomes in single file along the metaphase plate is a correct order. One example is shown. 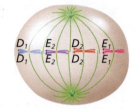
	Answer b
6. Diagram any correct chromosome alignment during meiotic metaphase I.	6. Homologous chromosomes align opposite one another along the metaphase plate in meiotic metaphase I. The two correct arrangements of order of homologous chromosomes are shown. 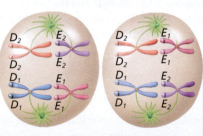
	Answer c
7. Describe the diagram differences with respect to homologs.	7. Homologous chromosomes synapse in meiosis, but not in mitosis. The consequence of synapsis is that homologs align next to one another and on opposite sides of the metaphase plate in metaphase I. The absence of synapsis in mitosis leads chromosomes to align in any order along the metaphase plate in mitotic metaphase.
	Answer d
8. Describe the different outcomes of mitosis and meiosis.	8. Mitosis produces two diploid daughter cells that are genetically identical to one another and to the parental cell they are derived from. Meiosis produces four haploid daughter cells that are genetically different.

For more practice, see Problems 1, 5, and 32.	Visit the Study Area to access study tools.	**Mastering** Genetics

Morgan took advantage of this rapid reproduction to raise large numbers of flies over many generations. His screening of flies from the wild and from his laboratory-raised stocks yielded occasional flies with a phenotype different from the wild type. Morgan set up crosses between these suspected mutant flies and wild-type flies to examine the inheritance of mutations.

Over several years, Morgan found many phenotypic variants that were due to the inheritance of gene mutations. Most of these hereditary mutants followed the same inheritance pattern Mendel described for traits in pea plants, but a few did not. The gene mutations causing the latter group of mutant traits are inherited on the X chromosome, and this section describes both Morgan's work on X chromosome inheritance and the contributions he and his students made confirming that genes are carried on chromosomes.

X-Linked Inheritance

While Sutton and Boveri were observing chromosome movements during meiosis, a researcher named Nettie Stevens, who in 1903 became one of the first women in the United States to receive a Ph.D., was beginning a microscopic study to determine whether differences in chromosomes were evident between males and females of a species of beetles, *Tenebrio molitor*. In her study of *T. molitor*, Stevens discovered sex chromosomes, finding that diploid cells of female beetles contained 20 large chromosomes (18 autosomal chromosomes and 2 X chromosomes), but diploid cells of males contained only 19 large chromosomes and 1 small chromosome (18 autosomes plus an X and a Y chromosome). Stevens's studies of the chromosomes in somatic cells and gametes of *T. molitor* and other insects led her to conclude that sex-dependent hereditary differences are due to the presence of two large X chromosomes in females and one X chromosome and a much smaller Y chromosome in males.

In 1910, Morgan began a series of experiments in *Drosophila* that would validate Stevens's proposal that X and Y chromosomes help determine sex and would also provide evidence suggesting that genes are carried on chromosomes. Morgan's work identified **sex-linked inheritance**, the inheritance of genes on sex chromosomes, and specifically focused on **X-linked inheritance**, the inheritance of genes on the X chromosome. The experiments began when Lilian Morgan, Thomas Hunt Morgan's wife and an important contributor to the laboratory group, found a mutant male *Drosophila* with white eyes in a bottle of wild-type flies that had been maintained in the lab for about a year. This white-eyed male stood out as a mutant because in *Drosophila*, wild-type flies have eyes the color of red bricks (**Figure 3.17**).

The mutant white-eyed male was crossed to a wild-type, red-eyed female. The cross produced 1237 F_1 flies, all with red eyes—a result indicating dominance of the wild type over the mutant. The F_1 were crossed to one another to produce an F_2 generation. Among the F_2 were 2459 red-eyed females, 1011 red-eyed males, and 782 white-eyed males (Cross A in **Figure 3.18**). No white-eyed females appeared in the F_2. Morgan correctly interpreted that these

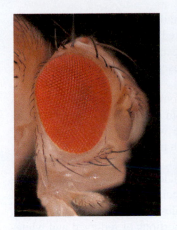
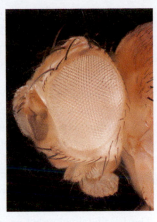

Figure 3.17   X-linked eye-color phenotypes in *Drosophila melanogaster*. Red eyes (left) are produced by a dominant wild-type allele. White eyes (right) are produced by a recessive X-linked mutant allele.

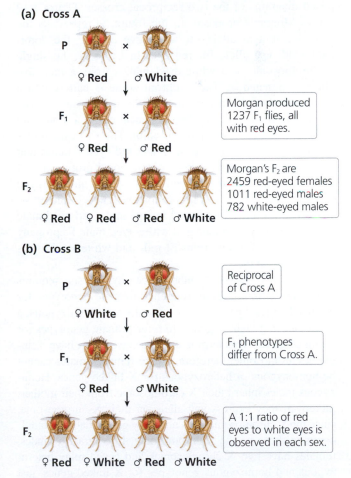

(a) Cross A

P   ♀ Red × ♂ White

Morgan produced 1237 F_1 flies, all with red eyes.

F_1 ♀ Red × ♂ Red

F_2 ♀ Red   ♀ Red   ♂ Red   ♂ White

Morgan's F_2 are
2459 red-eyed females
1011 red-eyed males
782 white-eyed males

(b) Cross B

P   ♀ White × ♂ Red

Reciprocal of Cross A

F_1 ♀ Red × ♂ White

F_1 phenotypes differ from Cross A.

F_2 ♀ Red   ♀ White   ♂ Red   ♂ White

A 1:1 ratio of red eyes to white eyes is observed in each sex.

Figure 3.18   Two reciprocal *Drosophila* crosses performed by Morgan to determine X-linkage of the gene for eye color. (a) Cross A produces F_1 flies that all have red eyes. In the F_2 all female flies have red (wild-type) eye color. The F_2 males are about one-half red-eyed and one-half white-eyed. (b) Cross B is the reciprocal of Cross A and produces different result in the F_1 and F_2 generations.

F_2 results differed significantly from expectation in that white eyes seemed to be linked to male sex. On the basis of Mendel's experiments, Morgan expected to see about a 3:1 ratio of red eyes to white eyes, and to see both eye colors in each sex.

The unexpected result from this cross prompted Morgan to test eye-color inheritance in a reciprocal cross of his first cross. After perpetuating the white-eye lineage for several generations, Morgan had both males and females with white eyes in his possession, and he mated a white-eyed female with a wild-type, red-eyed male as a reciprocal to his original cross. The F_1 of the reciprocal cross were red-eyed females and white-eyed males (Cross B in Figure 3.18). The F_2 contained equal proportions of red-eyed and white-eyed males and females.

The differences between the results of the reciprocal crosses confirmed for Morgan that eye color was inherited differently from other traits he had studied and from traits Mendel had studied. Suspecting that eye-color inheritance was linked to sex and to sex chromosomes, Morgan proposed diagrams of the two reciprocal crosses. **Figure 3.19** shows Morgan's proposal. In the figure, w represents the recessive mutant allele for white eye and w^+ the dominant wild-type allele for red eye. In Cross A, the single X chromosome of a white-eyed male carries a recessive allele designated w. The X chromosome is paired with a Y chromosome in the genome of the male fruit fly. The X chromosomes of the female each carry a dominant allele w^+ that produces red eye color. The F_1 of this cross are red-eyed males that are w^+Y and red-eyed females that are w^+w. The F_2 of this cross contain equal proportions of white-eyed (wY) and red-eyed (w^+Y) males and red-eyed females that are, in equal proportions, w^+w^+ and w^+w. Cross B between a white-eyed female and a red-eyed male produces red-eyed female and white-eyed male F_1 progeny as well as equal proportions of red- and white-eyed males and females in the F_2.

Morgan's X-linked inheritance hypothesis requires some new terminology in reference to male genotypes for X-linked genes. Specifically, we use the term **hemizygous**, a word meaning "half zygous," to refer to male genotypes for X-linked genes. This term is used because males have a single X chromosome; therefore, unlike females, males cannot be homozygous or heterozygous for X-linked genes. Hemizygous males inherit their X chromosome from their mother; moreover, they express any allele on their X chromosome, since the Y chromosome does not carry genes that are homologous to those on the X chromosome. In contrast to males, females have two X chromosomes and can display heterozygous and homozygous genotypes for X-linked genes, just as they can for autosomal genes. Note also that males can transmit either the X chromosome or the Y chromosome, but that the X chromosome is passed exclusively to female progeny and the Y chromosome exclusively to male progeny. In contrast, females can transmit either X chromosome to any of their offspring.

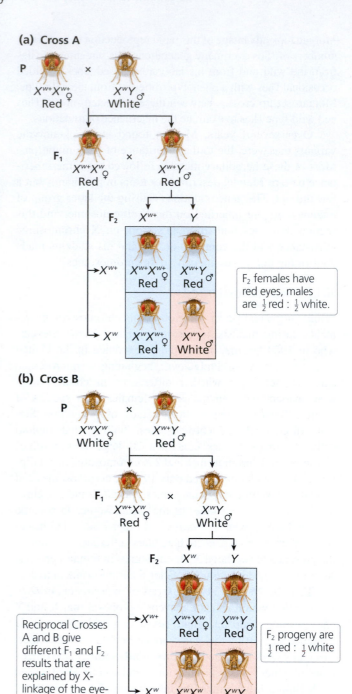

Figure 3.19 **The X-linked genetic model of Morgan's eye-color inheritance experiments in *Drosophila*.** X and Y chromosome segregation in **(a)** Cross A and **(b)** Cross B from Figure 3.18.

Q Observing different outcomes in the F_1 of Cross A versus Cross B is a hallmark of X-linked inheritance. Why are differences not seen in the F_1 of reciprocal crosses involving autosomal genes?

Testing the Chromosome Theory of Heredity

Morgan's observations on the inheritance pattern of *Drosophila* eye color implied that the gene for eye color is on the X chromosome. To verify this proposal required an independent experiment. Calvin Bridges, a student of Morgan, provided this validation in an experiment that studied fruit flies with unexpected eye-color phenotypes and abnormal chromosome numbers. This experiment confirmed that genes are carried on chromosomes, proving the "chromosome theory of heredity."

Bridges focused his study on progeny of crosses that replicated Morgan's Cross B (see Figures 3.18 and 3.19), between a white-eyed female (*ww*) and a red-eyed male (*w⁺Y*). Nearly all the progeny from this cross had the expected phenotype and were either red-eyed females (w^+w) or white-eyed males (*wY*), but about 1 in every 2000 F$_1$ flies had an "exceptional phenotype"—a term used to identify progeny with unexpected characteristics. Specifically, the exceptional flies were either white-eyed *females* or red-eyed *males*. Bridges's detection of exceptional progeny left him with two questions to answer: (1) how could the exceptional progeny be explained, and (2) did the appearance of exceptional progeny provide information that could validate the hypothesis that genes are on chromosomes?

The answer to the first question came when Bridges looked at chromosomes of the exceptional progeny under the microscope. He saw the exceptional females had a total of nine chromosomes, including three sex chromosomes—two X chromosomes and one Y chromosome (XXY)—along with six autosomal chromosomes. As we discuss in the next section, fruit flies with two X chromosomes are females, even if there happens to be a Y chromosome as well, as there is in this case. Bridges also observed an abnormal number of chromosomes in exceptional males. They carried a total of seven chromosomes. These males have a single X chromosome but no Y chromosome (XO), along with six autosomal chromosomes. Fruit flies with one X chromosome are male, regardless of whether they carry a Y chromosome. Based on his observations, Bridges proposed that the Y chromosome carried by exceptional females came from the male parent, the only source of a Y chromosome in the cross, and that both X chromosomes in these exceptional females came from the mother, giving the exceptional females two copies of the *w* allele and white eye color (**Figure 3.20**). Bridges used similar logic to suggest that the single X chromosome in exceptional males came from the male parent that passed the *w⁺* allele. The exceptional males with a single X chromosome expressed the *w⁺* allele as red eyes.

According to Bridges's proposal, the exceptional phenotypes and abnormal numbers of chromosomes were the result of rare mistakes in meiosis caused by the failure of X chromosomes to separate properly in either the first or second meiotic division in females. Failed chromosome separation is called **nondisjunction**. Notice in Figure 3.20 that nondisjunction also produces XXX or YO progeny. Bridges never saw these progeny, however, because YO progeny fail to develop, and XXX is usually lethal. Bridges's observations provide conclusive proof of the chromosome theory of heredity by showing that the white (*w*) allele segregates with the X chromosome during normal meiosis and during

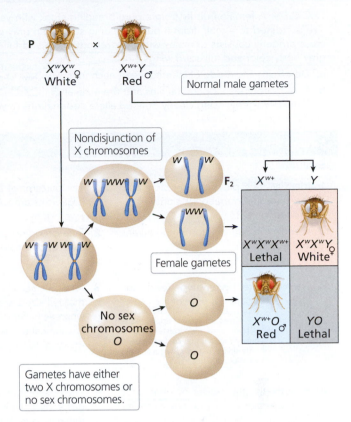

Figure 3.20   Exceptional progeny observed by Calvin Bridges result from X-chromosome nondisjunction during female meiosis.

nondisjunction. Genetic Analysis 3.2 gives you some practice spotting X-linked inheritance.

3.4 Sex Determination Is Chromosomal and Genetic

The term **sex determination** encompasses the genetic and biological processes that produce the male and female characteristics of a species. The sex of most animals is identified on two levels: (1) chromosomal sex, the presence of sex chromosomes associated with male and female sex in a species; and (2) phenotypic sex, the internal and external morphology found in each sex. Chromosomal sex is determined at the moment of fertilization and is controlled by the sex chromosomes contributed by the parents. In contrast, phenotypic sex is determined by gene expression and the development of sex characteristics during gestation or growth. In this section, we examine the patterns and processes of chromosomal and phenotypic sex determination in several organisms.

Sex Determination in *Drosophila*

In *Drosophila*, the number of X chromosomes in relation to the number of haploid sets of autosomal chromosomes is a critical component in determining sex. In this species, flies with the sex-chromosome constitutions XY, XYY, and XO

PROBLEM A female fruit fly from a pure-breeding stock with yellow body color and full wing size is crossed to a male from a pure-breeding stock with gray body and vestigial wings. The cross progeny consists of males with yellow body color and full-sized wings and females with gray body color and full-sized wings.

> **BREAK IT DOWN:** Pure-breeding females and males are homozygous for autosomal alleles. Pure-breeding females are homozygous for X-linked alleles, but males are hemizygous (p. 86).

a. Determine the mode of inheritance of each trait.

> **BREAK IT DOWN:** All male and female progeny have full-sized wings, but they differ in body color, suggesting possible X-linkage for that trait (p. 86).

b. Give genotypes for parental flies and the male and female progeny, using clearly defined allele designations of your choice.

Solution Strategies	Solution Steps
Evaluate	
1. Identify the topic of this problem and the kind of information the answer should contain.	1. The patterns of transmission of two *Drosophila* traits and the genotypes of organisms are to be determined based on the phenotypes of male and female F_1 progeny.
2. Identify the critical information given in the problem.	2. Pure-breeding parental phenotypes are given along with the phenotypes of male and female progeny in the F_1.
Deduce	
3. Consider the F_1 phenotype results in light of the parental phenotypes. TIP: Cross results that appear equally in both sexes are consistent with autosomal inheritance. Sex-dependent differences in a cross suggest X-linked inheritance.	3. All F_1 progeny have full-sized wings and none have vestigial wings, suggesting that full-sized wing is dominant. The F_1 males are exclusively yellow-bodied, whereas F_1 females are exclusively gray-bodied. The F_1 male body color is identical to that of the parental female, whereas the F_1 females' body color is identical to that in the male parent.
4. Hypothesize the modes of inheritance of body color and wing form from the F_1 data. TIP: Test the hypothesized mode of inheritance by comparing the predicted and observed F_1 progeny ratios.	4. The observation of one body color in F_1 males and another in females suggests this is an X-linked trait. Since hemizygous males have yellow body and females have gray body, it is likely that gray body is dominant and yellow body is recessive. The F_1 results for wing form are the same for both sexes, suggesting that this trait is autosomal.
Solve	**Answer a**
5. Test the proposed mode of transmission of wing form.	5. The F_1 of both sexes have full-sized wings, consistent with an autosomal trait. The pure-breeding full-winged parent transmits the dominant alleles to all progeny, and the pure-breeding vestigial parent transmits the recessive allele. The F_1 are predicted to be heterozygous and display the dominant trait.
6. Test the mode of transmission of body color. TIP: Compare observed and expected F_2 progeny to test the hypothesized mode of inheritance. PITFALL: Remember that males are hemizygous for X-linked traits. Describing their genotype as homozygous or heterozygous is incorrect.	6. The sex-dependent difference in body color among F_1 males and females strongly suggests this trait is X-linked. The F_1 males inherit the maternal recessive allele for yellow body color and express the trait because they are hemizygous. F_1 females inherit a recessive allele on the maternal X chromosome and a dominant allele on the paternal X and are heterozygous, thus displaying the dominant phenotype.
	Answer b
7. Determine genotypes for parental and F_1 flies. Use X^{y+} for yellow body, X^y for gray body, v^+ for full wing, and v for vestigial wing.	7. The genotypes of pure-breeding parents are $X^y/X^y;$, v^+/v^+ for yellow-bodied, full-winged females; and $X^{y+}/Y;$, v/v for gray-bodied, vestigial-winged males. The F_1 females are $X^y/X^{y+};$, $v^+/v;$ and the F_1 males are $X^y/Y;$, v^+/v.

are all male, whereas flies that are XX or XXY are female. In *Drosophila,* flies that are XXX are very rarely observed, and those that are YO are never seen.

A ratio of one X chromosome to the number of haploid sets of autosomes—that is, 1X:2A (as in XY)—is seen in males. Flies in which the ratio is 2X:2A (as in XX) are females. Bridges called this the **X/A ratio**, or the **X/autosome ratio**. At the molecular level, we now know that *Drosophila* sex is determined by regulatory proteins that relay the number of X chromosomes present in nuclei of cells in *Drosophila* embryos. These proteins control expression of the *sex-lethal (Sxl)* gene in XX flies. As we discuss in the Case Study at the end of Chapter 8, Sxl protein controls the expression of additional genes that drive sex development.

Mammalian Sex Determination

Like *Drosophila,* placental mammals, including humans, have two kinds of sex chromosomes, identified as X and Y. Unlike *Drosophila,* however, sex determination in placental mammals depends on the presence or absence of the Y chromosome. A single gene on the Y chromosome called either *SRY* (sex-determining region of Y) or, alternatively, *TDF* (testis-determining factor) initiates a series of events that lead to male sex-phenotype development in the embryo. Consequently, mammalian embryos that have one or more Y chromosomes (XY, XXY, and XYY, for example) and therefore express *SRY* will develop as males. Conversely, embryos carrying only X chromosomes (XX, XO, and XXX, for example) and lacking *SRY* expression will develop as females.

As in other placental mammals, human male sex phenotype development is initiated by *SRY* expression. The protein produced by *SRY* is a transcription factor protein that elicits a cascade of gene transcription and developmental events that ultimately produce male internal and external structures. Early mammalian embryos contain undifferentiated gonadal tissue that can develop into either ovaries or testes. Two different sets of tissues, called the Wolffian ducts and the Müllerian ducts, are associated with the undifferentiated gonadal tissue (**Figure 3.21**). Wolffian ducts can develop to form male sexual and reproductive structures. In contrast, Müllerian ducts can develop to form female sexual and reproductive structures. In male embryos, *SRY* expression initiates development of the undifferentiated gonadal tissue into testicles. This is accompanied by the synthesis of male androgenic hormones that help drive Wolffian duct development. Separately during male development, specialized cells produce a Müllerian-inhibitory factor (MIF) that degrades Müllerian ducts to prevent development of female sexual structures. On the other hand, female embryos carry two X chromosomes and do not have a copy of the Y-linked *SRY* gene. The current model suggests that the absence of expression of *SRY* allows the undifferentiated gonad tissue to develop into ovaries and cause Müllerian ducts to develop into female sexual and reproductive structures.

Although *SRY* is necessary for male sex development, it alone is not sufficient; nor is the simple absence of *SRY*

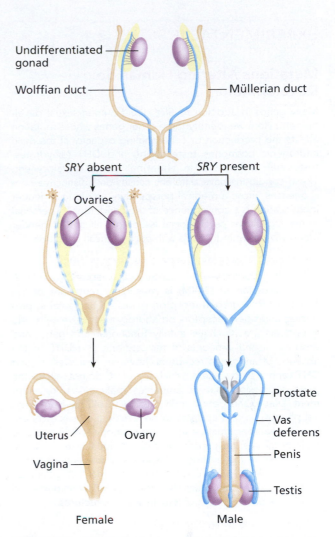

Figure 3.21 Mammalian male sex determination is initiated by the Y-linked *SRY* gene.

🅾 If at fertilization an X and a Y chromosome are present but the *SRY* gene is nonfunctional, what sex phenotype will develop? If at fertilization there are two X chromosomes present but one carries a fully functional copy of *SRY*, what sex phenotype will develop?

sufficient for female sex development. Mutations of various other X-linked and autosomal genes are also known to generate a discordance between chromosomal sex (i.e., XX or XY) and phenotypic sex. **Experimental Insight 3.1** identifies some of these conditions and the genes that are responsible for them.

Diversity of Sex Determination

You are now familiar with the mammalian XX and XY chromosome designation signifying that females carry two X chromosomes (XX) and males carry an X chromosome and a Y chromosome (XY). In many bird species, some reptiles, certain fish, and moths and butterflies, however, females carry two different sex chromosomes, and males carry two

Mutations Altering Human Sex Development

Many genes in addition to *SRY* direct human sexual development. Here we identify three other genes whose mutation affects the production or cell-signaling capacity of the male androgenic hormones testosterone and DHT (dihydrotestosterone) and results in abnormal sexual development. These conditions have different causes and distinctive consequences. From a medical perspective, ambiguous gender identification is a consequence of the conditions. In personal terms, significant psychosocial issues of self and of gender identity confront individuals with each of these conditions.

ANDROGEN INSENSITIVITY SYNDROME (AIS)

AIS (OMIM 300068; see the Case Study in Chapter 2, pp. 57–59, for a discussion of OMIM) is caused by mutations of the X-linked *AR* (androgen receptor) gene. *AR* is pivotal in producing androgen receptors on androgen-sensitive cells. AIS individuals are XY, have a fully functional *SRY* gene, and produce normal amounts of testosterone and DHT. In the absence of androgen receptors, however, testosterone and DHT cannot bind to cells, which therefore do not initiate the gene expression that accompanies male sexual development. Due to this deficit, individuals with AIS have an external phenotype that appears to be female (i.e., sex reversal); but internal reproductive structures do not develop as either male or female, thus rendering AIS individuals sterile. At the same time as the androgen insensitivity prevents development of male sexual structures, the functional *SRY* gene initiates MIF production, which degrades the Müllerian ducts and blocks the development of female sexual structures.

PSEUDOHERMAPHRODITISM

When genes operating in the biochemical pathway controlling testosterone and DHT are mutated, improper androgen levels occur, and individuals can exhibit *pseudohermaphroditism*—a term referring to the appearance of nonfunctional forms of both male and female structures in a single person. Pseudohermaphrodites are sterile. The autosomal recessive disorder 5-alpha-reductase deficiency (OMIM 607306) produces a form of pseudohermaphroditism due to mutation of the steroid 5-alpha-reductase-2 gene (*SRD5A2*). *SRD5A2* produces 5-alpha-reductase enzyme that helps convert testosterone to DHT. Individuals with 5-alpha-reductase deficiency are XY, have a wild-type *SRY* gene, undergo Wolffian duct development, and express MIF. Wolffian duct development produces male internal structures, but the inability to convert testosterone to DHT results in the absence of external male structures. At birth, individuals with 5-alpha-reductase deficiency appear to be female. At puberty, however, the adrenal glands begin testosterone production that leads to secondary male sexual characteristics, such as deepening of the voice, facial hair growth, and development of a masculine physique.

CONGENITAL ADRENAL HYPERPLASIA (CAH)

Mutation of *CYP21*, a gene producing the enzyme 21-hydroxylase, causes the most common form of autosomal recessive congenital adrenal hyperplasia (CAH; OMIM 201910). Functional 21-hydroxylase participates in depletion of testosterone and DHT; thus, its mutation leads to accumulation of testosterone and DHT. *CYP21* mutation produces pseudohermaphroditism in males and females due to high androgen levels. Boys with CAH enter puberty as early as 3 years of age and display male musculature, enlarged penis, and testes growth. Girls with CAH are born with an enlarged clitoris that can be mistaken for a small penis. While normal internal female reproductive anatomy is present, CAH females experience male-like facial hair growth and deepening voice at puberty. Menstruation does not occur, due to excessive androgen levels.

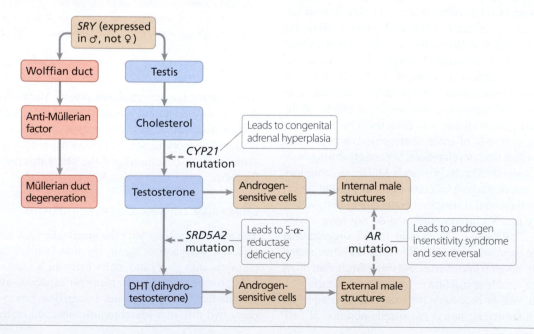

sex chromosomes that are the same. To avoid confusion with the XX/XY system, a different lettering system called the **Z/W system** is used in these cases. In the Z/W system, the letters Z and W are used to highlight the different sex-chromosome compositions associated with each sex. Males are identified as having two Z sex chromosomes, or a sex chromosome composition of ZZ. In contrast, females have two different sex chromosomes and are identified as ZW.

The sex-chromosome differences in the Z/W system cause reciprocal crosses involving Z-linked genes to produce different results, just as there are reciprocal cross differences for X-linked genes. **Figure 3.22** shows reciprocal crosses between

pure-breeding hens (female) and roosters (male) involving a Z-linked dominant allele for barred feathers (Z^B) and its recessive counterpart for nonbarred feathers (Z^b). The F_1 results of the reciprocal crosses reveal differences consistent with sex-linked inheritance. Cross A produces barred hens (Z^BW) and barred roosters (Z^BZ^b) in the F_1, whereas Cross B produces nonbarred hens (Z^bW) and barred roosters (Z^BZ^b). The F_2 results of these crosses also yield differences consistent with sex-linked inheritance. We can conclude that the mechanism of transmission of Z-linked genes in the Z/W system is analogous to that of X-linked genes in the XX/XY system except that the patterns are the reverse of those in placental mammals.

Sex chromosome content is even more unusual in monotremes, like the platypus, an egg-laying mammal that is native to Australia. Male platypus sex chromosomes are represented as $X_1Y_1X_2Y_2X_3Y_3X_4Y_4X_5Y_5$ and female platypus sex chromosomes as $X_1X_1X_2X_2X_3X_3X_4X_4X_5X_5$. Multiple sets of sex chromosomes have also been documented in some plant species, termites, and spiders. In dioecious plants (those with male plants and female plants), sex chromosomes are often not obvious at all, and they are therefore difficult to study. And, in certain reptiles and fishes, sex is dependent on environmental variables such as temperature. In other words, the sex of an individual can change during its lifetime, even though its chromosomes do not.

3.5 Human Sex-Linked Transmission Follows Distinct Patterns

Sex chromosomes differ between males and females of a species and have very few DNA sequences in common outside the pseudoautosomal regions. This means that the number of copies of sex-linked genes usually varies between males and females, and it leads to patterns of inheritance of sex-linked genes that differ from those seen for autosomal genes. With respect to X-linked genes in animal species, two inheritance patterns are common. **X-linked recessive** inheritance is the hereditary pattern that determines white eye color in *Drosophila,* for example. With this mode of inheritance, females homozygous for the recessive allele and hemizygous males whose X chromosome carries the recessive allele display the recessive phenotype. The alternative mode of X-linked transmission is **X-linked dominant** inheritance, in which heterozygous females and males hemizygous for the dominant allele express the dominant phenotype. Genes on the Y chromosome are exclusively transferred patrilineally (i.e., from father to son), since the Y chromosome is male-specific. In species such as chickens where the W chromosome is found exclusively in females, the transmission of W-linked genes is exclusively matrilineal.

Three features of X-linked dominant and X-linked recessive inheritance make them distinct from inheritance of autosomal traits. First, although autosomal dominant and recessive gene expression are generally the same in males and females, the terms *recessive* and *dominant* for X-linked

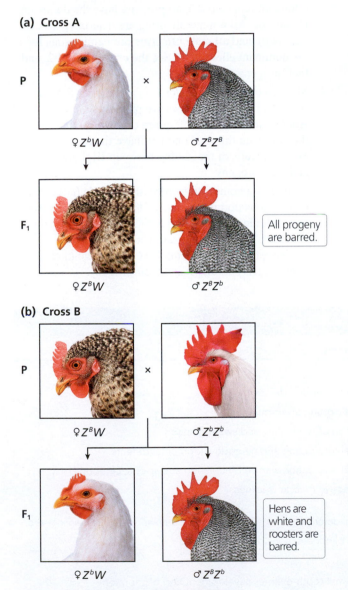

(a) Cross A

P ♀ Z^bW × ♂ Z^BZ^B

F_1 ♀ Z^BW ♂ Z^BZ^b

All progeny are barred.

(b) Cross B

P ♀ Z^BW × ♂ Z^bZ^b

F_1 ♀ Z^bW ♂ Z^BZ^b

Hens are white and roosters are barred.

Figure 3.22   Z/W inheritance of feather form in poultry is revealed by analysis of reciprocal crosses. (a) A hemizygous female (hen) with recessive nonbarred (white) feathers crossed to a pure-breeding male (rooster) with dominant barred feathers produces F_1 progeny that are all barred. **(b)** The reciprocal cross produces barred roosters and nonbarred (white) hens.

gene transmission refer specifically to the expression of traits in females. For X-linked alleles, females can be homozygous or heterozygous, but males are hemizygous and express the allele on their X chromosome regardless of the hereditary pattern in females. Second, the probability of transmission of X-linked alleles to offspring is not the same for the two sexes as it is for autosomal alleles. Female X-linked transmission is identical to autosomal transmission, but hemizygous males always transmit their X chromosome to female offspring and their Y chromosome to male offspring. Lastly, whereas females receive one copy of X-linked alleles from each parent, males receive their X-linked alleles from their mother and their Y chromosome from their father. This means that **Y-linked inheritance**, the inheritance of genes on the Y chromosome, is an exclusively patrilineal (father to son) pattern of hereditary transmission. From an evolutionary perspective, this pattern suggests that only those genes that play a role in male fertility, male-specific metabolism, or other male-specific features are inherited on the Y chromosome.

Expression of X-Linked Recessive Traits

X-linked recessive traits are expressed in hemizygous males who carry the recessive allele and in females who are homozygous for the recessive allele. Because hemizygous males express the single copy of a recessive X-linked allele in their phenotype, one of the hallmarks of X-linked recessive inheritance is the observation that many more males than females express the traits. Table 3.2 lists several human X-linked disorders, including three that we use as examples in this section: color blindness that affects perception of red and green color, hemophilia A (a blood-clotting disorder),

and congenital generalized hypertrichosis (CGH, characterized by excessive hair growth all over the body). Five common features characterizing X-linked recessive inheritance are illustrated in Figure 3.23, which features the inheritance of red–green color blindness.

1. As a result of male hemizygosity, more males than females have the recessive phenotype. The pedigree has six recessive males and one recessive female.

2. Often, the transmission of the recessive allele from grandfather to daughter to grandson gives the appearance of generation skipping. See the transmission of *c* from I-1 to II-2 to III-1.

3. If a recessive male (*cY*) mates with a homozygous dominant female (*CC*), all progeny have the dominant phenotype. All female offspring are heterozygous carriers (*Cc*), and all male offspring are hemizygous for the dominant allele (*CY*). See the cross I-1 × I-2. and their progeny.

4. Matings of recessive males (*cY*) and carrier females (*Cc*) can produce the recessive phenotype in females. About one-half of the offspring of these matings have the dominant trait and one-half have the recessive trait. See the results of the mating between III-4 and III-5 and their progeny.

5. Mating of a homozygous recessive female (*cc*) and a hemizygous dominant male (*CY*) produces male progeny with the recessive trait (*cY*) and female offspring who have the dominant trait who are heterozygous carriers of the recessive allele (*Cc*). See the mating between III-4 and III-5 and their progeny.

Table 3.2	A Short List of Human X-Linked Recessive and X-Linked Dominant Traits[a]
Disease	**Symptoms**
X-Linked Recessive Disorders	
Color blindness (red–green) (OMIM 303800)	Color-perception deficiency
Hemophilia A (OMIM 306700)	Blood-clotting abnormality
Anhidrotic ectodermal dysplasia (OMIM 305100)	Absence of teeth, hair, and sweat glands
Fragile X syndrome (OMIM 300624)	Mental retardation and neurodevelopmental defects
Lesch–Nyhan syndrome (OMIM 300322)	Mental retardation with self-mutilation and spastic cerebral palsy
Muscular dystrophy (Becker type, OMIM 300376; and Duchenne type, OMIM 310200)	Progressive muscle weakness
Ornithine transcarbamylase deficiency (OMIM 311250)	Mental deterioration due to ammonia accumulation with protein ingestion
Retinitis pigmentosa (OMIM 300029)	Night blindness, constricted visual field
X-Linked Dominant Disorders	
Amelogenesis imperfecta (OMIM 301200)	Abnormal tooth-enamel development and distribution
Congenital generalized hypertrichosis (OMIM 307150)	Extensive hair distribution on the face and body
Hypophosphatemia (OMIM 307800)	Phosphate deficiency causing rickets (bowleggedness)
Rett syndrome (OMIM 312750)	Mental retardation and neurodevelopmental defects

[a] OMIM = Online Mendelian Inheritance of Man (see Chapter 2 Case Study for discussion).

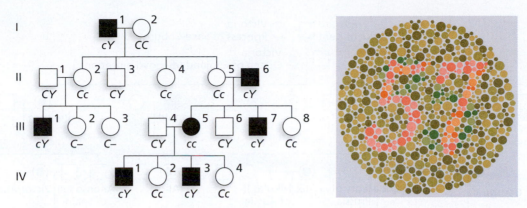

Figure 3.23 **X-linked recessive inheritance of red-green color blindness in a family.** **(a)** See the text for key features of this pattern of inheritance. **(b)** The number 57 is seen by those with full color vision, whereas those with red-green color blindness do not see a number.

Q **Explain how you know with certainty that II-4 is a heterozygous carrier of the recessive *c* allele.**

Hemophilia A, a serious blood-clotting disorder, is caused by mutation of an X-linked gene called *factor VIII (F8)* that produces a blood-clotting protein called factor VIII protein. Hemophilia A is transmitted in an X-linked recessive manner, most often by a carrier mother who passes the mutant allele to an affected son. In typical X-linked recessive fashion, approximately one-half of the sons of carrier mothers have the disease. Also as is common for X-linked recessive conditions, hemophilia often appears to "skip" a generation because the mutant allele is passed from affected father to carrier daughter and on to an affected grandson.

In some families, a de novo (newly occurring) mutation of the *F8* gene is responsible for the appearance of hemophilia. An example occurred in the royal families of England and Europe: An apparent de novo mutation of the *F8* gene affected Queen Victoria of England (**Figure 3.24**). Victoria had five sons, one of whom had hemophilia, along with four daughters, two of whom were known carriers. Victoria's carrier daughters had normal blood clotting but introduced the mutation to the royal families of Russia, Germany, and Spain through intermarriage. These daughters passed the mutation to their sons who had hemophilia and to their daughters who were carriers like their mothers. Genetic Analysis 3.3 analyzes the hereditary transmission of hemophilia A.

X-Linked Dominant Trait Transmission

Transmission of traits such as CGH (see Table 3.2) that are controlled by X-linked dominant alleles has two distinctive characteristics, one indicating transmission from a female and one indicating transmission from a male. A family with CGH is illustrated in **Figure 3.25**. When the transmitting parent is a heterozygous female with the dominant trait (*Hh*) and her mate is a male with the recessive trait (*Yh*), about half

the progeny of each sex have the dominant condition. (See the nine combined progeny of I-1 and I-2 and II-3 and II-4. Five of the nine children—three males and two females—have the dominant condition.) When the transmitting parent is a hemizygous male with the dominant trait (*HY*) and his mate is a female with the recessive trait (*hh*), we see a hallmark that distinguishes autosomal dominant transmission from X-linked dominant transmission. In these matings, the dominant trait appears in *all daughters,* who are *Hh,* and in *no sons,* who are *hY.* (See the nine progeny of II-5 and II-6.)

Y-Linked Inheritance

The key to Y-linked inheritance is that the Y chromosome is found only in males. This means Y-linked genes are transmitted in a male-to-male pattern. In mammals, fewer than 50 genes are found on the Y chromosome; and like *SRY,* those genes are likely to play a role in male sex determination or development. The genes on the human Y chromosome do not have counterparts on the X chromosome, although the DNA sequences in the pseudoautosomal regions are shared by the X and Y chromosomes to facilitate synapsis of the chromosomes during meiosis. There is crossing over between the pseudoautosomal regions, but this does not involve expressed genes.

Females never carry Y chromosomes, so from an evolutionary perspective it makes sense that the genes carried on a Y chromosome should be male-specific, having either to do with male sex determination or reproduction. Indeed, the most recent genomic evidence suggests that the mammalian Y chromosome has rapidly evolved over the past 300 million to 350 million years, undergoing multiple changes in structure but preserving a handful of genes that are essential to male fertility and survival. The fascinating evolution of the mammalian Y chromosome is the subject of the Case Study at the end of this chapter.

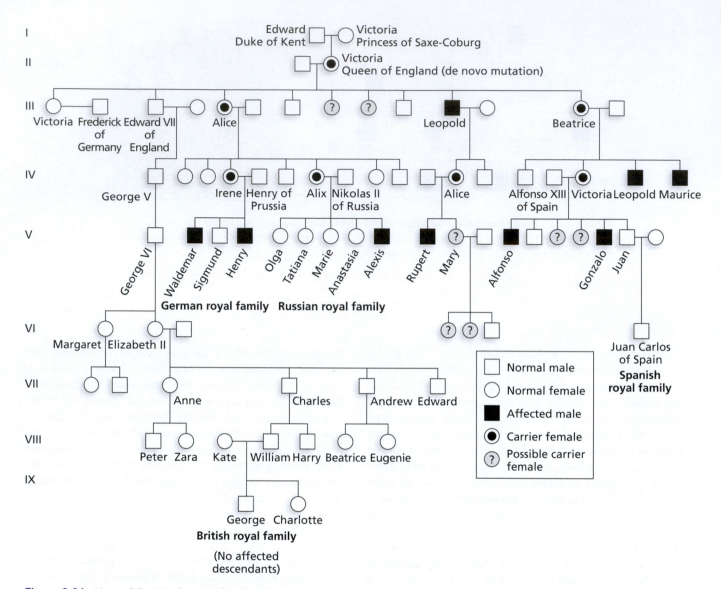

Figure 3.24 Hemophilia A in the royal families of Europe. The disease in these families originated with a de novo mutation in Queen Victoria. Note that some parents are omitted from the pedigree for clarity. In all cases, these individuals carry and contribute wild-type alleles.

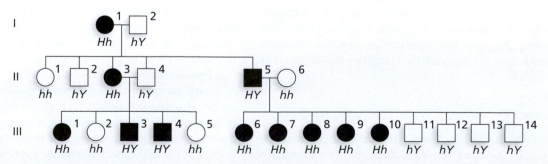

Figure 3.25 X-linked dominant congenital generalized hypertrichosis (CGH) in a family. See the text for key features of this pattern of inheritance.

PROBLEM Hemophilia A is an X-linked recessive blood-clotting disorder caused by mutation of the *factor VIII* gene. Suppose a heterozygous woman with normal blood clotting has children with a man who also has normal blood clotting. Determine the probability of each of the following outcomes.

> **BREAK IT DOWN:** The information given about the pattern of inheritance of hemophilia A and the status of the woman and the man allows identification of their genotypes (p. 92).

a. The probability of a son having hemophilia A.

b. The probability of a child of either sex having normal blood clotting.

> **BREAK IT DOWN:** The woman can transmit the recessive allele to a child of either sex, but the man transmits his X-linked allele to daughters and his Y chromosome to sons (p. 92).

c. The probability of having three children, each of whom has hemophilia A.

d. The probability of having four children, two of whom have hemophilia A and two of whom have normal blood clotting.

> **BREAK IT DOWN:** Parts (a) and (b) can be predicted using a Punnett square (p. 36); part (c) uses the product rule and part (d) is an application of binomial probability (p. 48).

Solution Strategies	Solution Steps
Evaluate	
1. Identify the topic this problem addresses and describe the nature of the required answers.	1. This problem addresses inheritance probabilities of an X-linked recessive trait for the parental genotype and phenotypes given. The answers should be stated as fraction, decimal, or percentage probabilities.
2. Identify the critical information given in the problem.	2. The inheritance pattern of the trait in question is identified as X-linked recessive, the phenotype of each parent is given, and the woman is identified as a heterozygote.

Deduce

3. Identify the genotypes of the woman and the man.

> **TIP:** Remember that males are hemizygous for X-linked traits.

> **TIP:** Use a Punnett square to assist you in accurately predicting the possible outcomes of mating.

4. Determine the possible phenotypes and phenotype probabilities for children of this couple.

3. The woman is described as being heterozygous and so her genotype is $X^H X^h$, where the uppercase and lowercase superscripts represent the dominant and recessive alleles, respectively. The man has normal blood clotting, so he is hemizygous for the wild-type allele. His genotype is $X^H Y$.

4. The Punnett square predicts four different genotypes among the possible children of this couple.

	X^H	Y
X^H	$X^H X^H$ Healthy	$X^H Y$ Healthy
X^h	$X^H X^h$ Healthy	$X^h Y$ Hemophilia A

Solve

5. Determine the probability of a son of this couple having hemophilia A.

Answer a

5. Taking sex into account, we find that approximately one-half the offspring are male and one-half are female. The Punnett square shows two possible male genotypes, one healthy and one a hemizygous male with hemophilia A. The probability that a son will have hemophilia A is therefore one-half, or 50%.

6. Determine the probability of a child with normal blood clotting being produced by this couple.

Answer b

6. The Punnett square shows that three of the four possible offspring genotypes would produce normal blood clotting. The probability that a child of this couple has normal blood clotting is 0.75, or 75%.

7. Calculate the probability that if the couple has three children, each of them will have hemophilia A.

Answer c

7. The risk that each child will have hemophilia A is 25%. For three children with hemophilia A, the probability is $(.25)(.25)(.25) = 0.0156$, or $\left(\frac{1}{4}\right)\left(\frac{1}{4}\right)\left(\frac{1}{4}\right) = \frac{1}{64}$.

8. Calculate the probability that if the couple has four children, two will have hemophilia A and two will have normal blood clotting.

> **TIP:** Use binomial probability to calculate the likelihood of consecutive outcomes.

Answer d

8. The chance the couple has four children, two of whom have hemophilia A and two of whom are healthy, is predicted by the binomial expansion. There are six different ways (birth orders) in which to produce two healthy and two affected children. The probabilities are $\frac{3}{4}$ for a healthy child and $\frac{1}{4}$ for a child with hemophilia A, so the requested probability is $6\left[\left(\frac{3}{4}\right)\left(\frac{3}{4}\right)\left(\frac{1}{4}\right)\left(\frac{1}{14}\right)\right] = \left(\frac{54}{256}\right)$, or 0.2109.

For more practice, see Problems 12, 13, and 25. Visit the Study Area to access study tools. **Mastering Genetics**

3.6 Dosage Compensation Equalizes the Expression of Sex-Linked Genes

In this final section of the chapter, we turn our attention to mechanisms that carry out the essential function of balancing the amount of gene expression of sex-linked genes. In animals there is an imbalance between the sexes in the copy number of genes on the sex chromosomes. Specifically, females are generally XX, and have two copies of each X-linked gene, whereas males are generally XY, and have just one copy of each X-linked gene. This is a potential problem because animals are extraordinarily sensitive to gene dosage imbalance such as could be caused by the presence of the "extra" X chromosome in females if all X chromosomes were to express genes at the same level. The expression of the right number of genes in the correct amounts is essential for normal embryonic development and normal biological processes. If the gene dosage balance is off, the consequences can be severe or even fatal for the animal.

Evolution has provided multiple mechanisms that compensate for differences in the number of copies of genes due to the different chromosome constitutions of males and females. There are at least four major mechanisms to balance X-linked gene expression in placental and marsupial mammals, fruit flies, and nematode worms (Table 3.3). Collectively, these are called **dosage compensation mechanisms**.

Placental mammals, including humans, use *random X inactivation* as their dosage compensation mechanism. Early in mammalian gestational development, about 2 weeks after fertilization in humans, when the female early embryo consists of a few hundred cells, one of the two X chromosomes in each somatic cell of a female is randomly inactivated. This idea was first proposed in 1961 by Mary Lyon in her **random X inactivation hypothesis**, also known as the **Lyon hypothesis**. In approximately one-half of the somatic cells in a female embryo, the maternally derived X chromosome is inactivated; and in the other half of the somatic cells, inactivation silences the paternally derived X chromosome. At the end of this process, each somatic cell

of a female has one active X chromosome that is equally likely to be the maternal X or the paternal X.

Random X inactivation takes place in every cell with two or more X chromosomes. Following inactivation, the inactive chromosome can be seen as a tightly condensed mass adhering to the nuclear wall. The inactive X chromosome is known as a **Barr body**, having first been visualized by Murray Barr in 1949.

X inactivation is a permanent feature of somatic cells of placental mammalian females. Because some cells have an active maternal X chromosome and an inactive paternal X chromosome and other cells have the opposite pattern, normal placental mammalian females are, in terms of X chromosomes, a mosaic of two kinds of cells (Figure 3.26). One cell type (pink in the figure) expresses the maternally derived X chromosome, and the other (blue) expresses the paternally derived X chromosome. Each individual cell expresses the allelic information of only one of those chromosomes, with all descendant cells maintaining the same inactivation pattern as the original ancestral cell.

In most cases, the silencing of one X chromosome in each cell of a female has no detectable effect on the function of a tissue or on the phenotype. Occasionally, however, female carriers of X-linked recessive traits display a phenotypic manifestation of the recessive allele. Calico and tortoiseshell coat-color patterning in female cats is a product of mosaicism created by random X inactivation (Figure 3.27). Females with an allele for black coat color on one X chromosome and orange coat color on the homologous X chromosome have black and orange patches of fur corresponding to portions of skin where each X chromosome is active. The sizes and the distribution of the orange and black sectors of these cats reflect the locations of the clonal descendants of the cells in which each X chromosome was originally inactivated. The specific pattern of X inactivation is unique to each female cat embryo, and the patterns of cellular migration are variable as well. As a result, each adult female calico or tortoiseshell cat has a unique pattern of black and orange sectors marking its coat.

Table 3.3	Mechanisms of Dosage Compensation in Animals		
Animal	**Sex Chromosomes**		**Dosage Compensation Mechanism**
	Males	**Females**	
Fruit fly	XY	XX	Expression of X-linked genes in males is doubled relative to female X-linked gene expression.
Roundworm	XO	XX[a]	Gene expression of each X chromosome in the hermaphrodite ("female") is decreased to one-half that of the X chromosome in the male.
Marsupial mammals	XY	XX	The paternally derived X chromosome is inactivated in all female somatic cells.
Placental mammals	XY	XX	One X chromosome is randomly inactivated in each female somatic cell.

[a] XX worms are hermaphrodites.

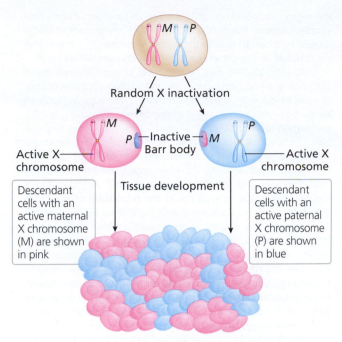

Figure 3.26   Random X inactivation in female mammals. One X chromosome is randomly inactivated in each nucleus. Descendant cells maintain the initial inactivation, leading to clusters of descendant cells with the same X chromosome. M represents the maternally derived X chromosome and P the paternally derived X chromosome.

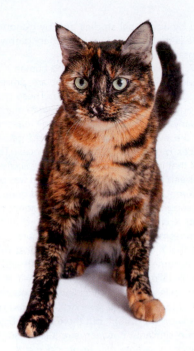

Figure 3.27   Calico coat, produced by X inactivation in female cats. Coat color patches are the result of gene expression from the one active X chromosome in each cluster of cells.

Not all genes on the "inactivated" X chromosome are transcriptionally silent. A 2005 study of 624 X-linked genes showed that about 15% of the genes on the inactivated chromosome escape complete silencing. On average, transcription of those genes is reduced by about 50–85% in comparison to transcription on the active X chromosome. The genes that escape inactivation are largely clustered on the short arm of the chromosome near PAR1.

Random X inactivation requires a gene on the X chromosome called the *X-inactivation–specific transcript (XIST)* that encodes a large RNA molecule. *XIST* RNA spreads out from the gene, "painting" the X chromosome as it accumulates. X chromosomes that are painted with *XIST* RNA have all, or nearly all, of their genes silenced. The *XIST* gene is expressed on only one of the two X chromosomes, and its RNA accumulates only on the chromosome transcribing the gene; it does not spread to the homologous X chromosome. In other words, *XIST* acts only in cis (on the same chromosome) but not in trans (on the homologous chromosome). Examination of inactivated chromosomes in the nucleus detects *XIST* RNA coating the Barr body in a nucleus.

CASE STUDY

The (Degenerative) Evolution of the Mammalian Y Chromosome

Mammalian X and Y chromosomes are the "odd couple" of homologous chromosomes. They are very different from each other in size and are only homologous in their pseudoautosomal regions. Further, because the Y chromosome is exclusively found in males, the genes it contains are, naturally enough, only expressed in males. For example, the human Y chromosome contains only about one-third as many base pairs as the X chromosome. Whereas the human X chromosome carries more than 2000 genes, the Y chromosome contains just a few dozen.

The small pseudoautosomal regions of the X and Y chromosomes make up just a few percent of the total sequence of either chromosome. The PARs are sufficient for synapsis in prophase I, and recombination between X and Y is frequent in these regions, but only about 5% of the Y chromosome participates in recombination. The other 95% of the chromosome experiences no crossing over. Studies in evolutionary genetics reveal that the mammalian Y chromosome has evolved very rapidly over the past 300 million years or so, shrinking in size and genetic content as essential genes have been shifted to other chromosomes, leaving just a handful of genes behind.

A STORY OF DEGENERATION Beginning with the work of Bruce Lahn and David Page in 1999, the composition and evolution of the mammalian Y chromosome have been subjects of active investigation. The view of Y chromosome evolution first proposed by Lahn and Page has been supported and verified by additional studies and by genome sequencing, and it tells the story of an evolutionary pathway that features progressive degeneration.

In 1999, Lahn and Page studied the human X and Y chromosomes and identified 19 genes that are present on both chromosomes, called X–Y shared genes. These genes are left over from a time when the chromosomes were much more similar and regularly recombined. Lahn and Page reasoned that they could trace the evolution of the X–Y shared genes by studying differences between their DNA sequences. Their starting premise was that in general more differences accrue the longer genes have been separated. What they found was quite surprising: The differences between the X–Y shared genes followed a distinct and suggestive pattern. X–Y shared genes nearest each other on the X chromosome short arm were most similar to their Y-chromosome counterparts, but X–Y shared genes on the long arm of the X chromosome were the most different from their Y-chromosome counterparts. In all, Lahn and Page identified four well-defined "strata" among the X–Y shared genes, each stratum having its own distinct level of sequence similarity. Within each of the strata, the level of X–Y shared-gene similarity was remarkably consistent, but there were substantial differences in gene similarity between strata. This suggested four major evolutionary events that reshaped the Y chromosome, resulting in structural changes that progressively restricted recombination between the X and the Y chromosomes.

MAJOR RESTRUCTURING EVENTS By comparing DNA sequences across species, Lahn and Page determined that the autosomal precursors of X and Y were very similar at the time reptiles diverged from mammals, about 350 million years ago (mya). The monotremes (such as the platypus and echidna) separated from the placental mammals 240–320 mya, but not before the *SRY* gene evolved in their common ancestor. Both monotremes and mammals have *SRY*, but reptiles do not. This implies that *SRY* developed about 350 mya (**Figure 3.28**). The *SRY* gene produces TDF, the protein that initiates a cascade of events that produces males. With the acquisition of *SRY*, the Y chromosome became different from the X chromosome, and

the region surrounding *SRY*—the first of Lahn and Page's four strata—became the first region of the Y chromosome to be unable to recombine with the X chromosome. This event also contributed to the shrinkage of the Y chromosome.

About 130–170 mya, a structural change altered the Y chromosome and produced a second stratum that was unable to recombine with the X chromosome. Marsupials (such as kangaroos) retain the old Y-chromosome structure, so the generation of the second stratum demarcates the separation of marsupial and placental mammals. Another structural change to the Y chromosome, between 80 and 130 mya, created a third stratum of divergence, further restricting recombination with the X chromosome and shrinking the Y chromosome. This change marks the separation of the monkeys from nonsimian placental mammals. Most recently, about 30–50 mya, the fourth stratum was created by another structural change to the Y chromosome. This change—present in the human lineage that includes our great ape relatives but not present in monkeys—limited recombination to the end of the Y chromosome and reduced its size. In humans, recombination between X and Y chromosomes is limited to PAR1 (on the short arm), the largest of the remaining regions of X–Y homology. Little if any recombination occurs in PAR2.

The functioning of genes remaining on the Y chromosome was directly affected by the events that prevented X–Y recombination. Without recombination, Y-linked genes were subject to mutational degradation that would eventually render them nonfunctional. Strong natural selection operated to prevent this by moving essential genes off the Y chromosome to other chromosomes. The genes that remain on the human Y chromosome are almost exclusively important in male development or sperm production, but even these remain subject to mutational degradation.

What will be the ultimate fate of the human Y chromosome? Is it destined to be lost? Scientists don't know what will happen, but recent genomic data may provide a clue. The Y chromosome, it seems, has backup copies of its genes. These duplicated copies are also on the Y chromosome, and they may serve to protect the Y chromosome from the loss of critical information.

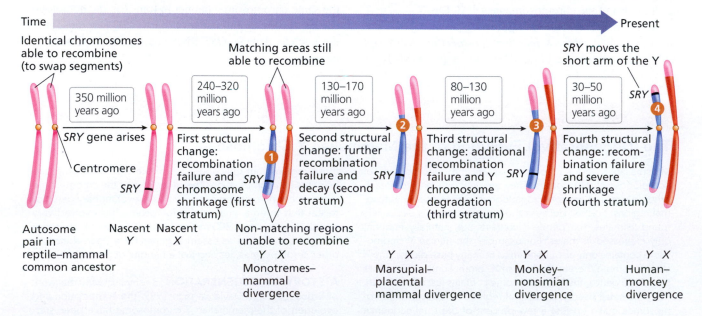

Figure 3.28 **The proposed evolutionary development of the mammalian Y chromosome through four major structural rearrangements.**

SUMMARY   **Mastering Genetics**   For activities, animations, and review quizzes, go to the Study Area.

3.1 Mitosis Divides Somatic Cells

▌ The cell cycle has two principal phases: interphase, whose stages are G_1, S, and G_2; and M phase, during which cell division occurs.

▌ Mitosis is the process of division for somatic cells. Mitosis contains five substages: prophase, prometaphase, metaphase, anaphase, and telophase.

▌ Mitosis contains a single cell division and separates sister chromatids into diploid daughter cells that are genetically identical to one another and to the parental cell they are derived from.

▌ The cell cycle is under tight genetic control. Regulatory molecules control the transition from one stage of the cycle to the next by acting at genetically controlled checkpoints to monitor cell cycle transitions.

▌ Mutation of cell cycle control genes is associated with cancer development.

3.2 Meiosis Produces Cells for Sexual Reproduction

▌ Meiosis contains two cell divisions, designated meiosis I and meiosis II.

▌ During meiosis I (the "reduction division"), homologous chromosomes are separated to produce haploid daughter cells that carry one chromosome from each homologous pair of chromosomes.

▌ The meiosis II division separates sister chromatids and produces four genetically different haploid daughter cells that form gametes.

▌ During prophase I, homologous chromosomes synapse with the aid of the synaptonemal complex. Homologous chromosomes can cross over to exchange genetic material during this substage.

▌ Mendel's laws of segregation and independent assortment find their mechanical basis in the patterns of separation of chromosomes and sister chromatids during meiosis.

3.3 The Chromosome Theory of Heredity Proposes That Genes Are Carried on Chromosomes

▌ The chromosome theory of heredity proposes that genes are carried on chromosomes and are faithfully transmitted through gametes to successive generations.

▌ Thomas Hunt Morgan's identification of X-linked transmission of white eye color in *Drosophila* and Calvin Bridges's analysis of exceptional phenotypes produced by X-chromosome nondisjunction demonstrated the validity of the chromosome theory of heredity.

3.4 Sex Determination Is Chromosomal and Genetic

▌ Mechanisms of sex determination take many forms in animals. *Drosophila* sex is determined by the ratio of expression of X-linked and autosomal genes, whereas human sex is determined by the presence of *SRY* on the Y chromosome.

▌ Sex-chromosome patterns are diverse among organisms. Birds, fishes, and some insects have Z and W sex chromosomes, and monotremes have multiple sets of sex chromosomes.

3.5 Human Sex-Linked Transmission Follows Distinct Patterns

▌ Human X-linked dominant inheritance and X-linked recessive inheritance are identifiable, respectively, by the pattern of male transmission and the pattern of male expression of traits.

▌ Genes on the Y chromosome are transmitted exclusively from male to male.

3.6 Dosage Compensation Equalizes the Expression of Sex-Linked Genes

▌ Dosage compensation balances the level of expression of sex-linked genes and is critical for normal animal development. Mechanisms for achieving dosage compensation vary among species.

▌ Random inactivation of one X chromosome in each cell of placental mammalian females is controlled by an X-inactivation center on the X chromosome.

PREPARING FOR PROBLEM SOLVING

In addition to the list of problem-solving tips and suggestions given here, you can go to the Study Guide and Solutions Manual that accompanies this book for help at solving problems.

1. The terminology of cell division is important for understanding and communicating during problem solving. Be able to define terms such as *chromosome* and *sister chromatid* in the context of mitosis and meiosis.

2. From the perspective of genetics, meiotic cell division provides the mechanism for transmission of genes and alleles from one generation to the next. Be sure you have a clear picture of how and when homologous chromosomes and sister chromatids separate and how these events lead to segregation and independent assortment.

3. Be prepared to analyze hereditary transmission of genes on autosomal chromosomes and on sex chromosomes.

4. Remember that for X-linked genes females are either "homozygous" or "heterozygous" but males are "hemizygous." Be careful to use these terms correctly and also to indicate the corresponding genotypes correctly.

5. Understand the chromosomal basis of sex determination and the mechanisms of gene dosage compensation for X-linked genes in mammals.

6. As with problem solving in Chapter 2 ("Transmission Genetics"), the use of Punnett squares and the forked-line method will aid you in finding solutions to problems concerning heredity.

PROBLEMS

Mastering Genetics Visit for instructor-assigned tutorials and problems.

Chapter Concepts

For answers to selected even-numbered problems, see Appendix: Answers

1. Examine the following diagrams of cells from an organism with diploid number $2n = 6$, and identify what stage of M phase is represented.

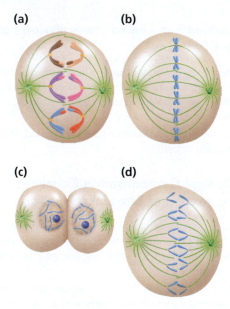

(a) (b)

(c) (d)

2. Our closest primate relative, the chimpanzee, has a diploid number of $2n = 48$. For each of the following stages of M phase, identify the number of chromosomes present in each cell.

   a. end of mitotic telophase   b. meiotic metaphase I
   c. end of meiotic anaphase II   d. early mitotic prophase
   e. mitotic metaphase   f. early prophase I

3. In a test of his chromosome theory of heredity, Morgan crossed an F_1 female *Drosophila* with red eyes to a male with white eyes. The F_1 females were produced from Cross A shown in Figure 3.19. Predict the offspring Morgan would have expected under his hypothesis that the gene for eye color is on the X chromosome in fruit flies.

4. Cohesion between sister chromatids, as well as tension created by the pull of kinetochore microtubules, is essential to ensure efficient separation of chromatids at mitotic anaphase or in meiotic anaphase II. Explain why sister chromatid cohesion is important, and discuss the role of the proteins cohesin and separase in sister chromatid separation.

5. The diploid number of the hypothetical animal *Geneticus introductus* is $2n = 36$. Each diploid nucleus contains 3 ng of DNA in G_1.

   a. What amount of DNA is contained in each nucleus at the end of S phase?
   b. Explain why a somatic cell of *Geneticus introductus* has the same number of chromosomes and the same amount of DNA at the beginning of mitotic prophase as one of these cells does at the beginning of prophase I of meiosis.
   c. Complete the following table by entering the number of chromosomes and amount of DNA present per cell at the end of each stage listed.

End of Cell Cycle Stage	Number of Chromosomes	Amount of DNA
Telophase I		
Mitotic telophase		
Telophase II		

6. An organism has alleles R_1 and R_2 on one pair of homologous chromosomes, and it has alleles T_1 and T_2 on another pair. Diagram these pairs of homologs at the end of metaphase I, the end of telophase I, and the end of telophase II, and show how meiosis in this organism produces gametes in expected Mendelian proportions. Assume no crossover between homologous chromosomes.

7. Explain how the behavior of homologous chromosomes in meiosis parallels Mendel's law of segregation for autosomal alleles D and d. During which stage of M phase do these two alleles segregate from one another?

8. Suppose crossover occurs between the homologous chromosomes in the previous problem. At what stage of M phase do alleles D and d segregate?

9. Alleles *A* and *a* are on one pair of autosomes, and alleles *B* and *b* are on a separate pair of autosomes. Does crossover between one pair of homologs affect the expected proportions of gamete genotypes? Why or why not? Does crossover between both pairs of chromosomes affect the expected gamete proportions? Why or why not?

10. How many Barr bodies are found in a normal human female nucleus? In a normal male nucleus?

11. Describe the role of the following structures or proteins in cell division:
    a. microtubules
    b. cohesin protein
    c. kinetochores
    d. synaptonemal complex

Application and Integration

For answers to selected even-numbered problems, see Appendix: Answers.

12. A woman's father has ornithine transcarbamylase deficiency (OTD), an X-linked recessive disorder producing mental deterioration if not properly treated. The woman's mother is homozygous for the wild-type allele.
    a. What is the woman's genotype? (Use *D* to represent the dominant allele and *d* to represent the recessive allele.)
    b. If the woman has a son with a man who does not have OTD, what is the chance the son will have OTD?
    c. If the woman has a daughter with a man who does not have OTD, what is the chance the daughter will be a heterozygous carrier of OTD? What is the chance the daughter will have OTD?
    d. Identify a male with whom the woman could produce a daughter with OTD.
    e. For the instance you identified in part (d), what proportion of daughters produced by the woman and the man are expected to have OTD? What proportion of sons of the woman and the man are expected to have OTD?

13. In humans, hemophilia A (OMIM 306700) is an X-linked recessive disorder that affects the gene for factor VIII protein, which is essential for blood clotting. The dominant and recessive alleles for the *factor VIII* gene are represented by *H* and *h*. Albinism is an autosomal recessive condition that results from mutation of the gene producing tyrosinase, an enzyme in the melanin synthesis pathway. *A* and *a* represent the tyrosinase alleles. A healthy woman named Clara (II-2), whose father (I-1) has hemophilia and whose brother (II-1) has albinism, is married to a healthy man named Charles (II-3), whose parents are healthy. Charles's brother (II-5) has hemophilia, and his sister (II-4) has albinism. The pedigree is shown below.

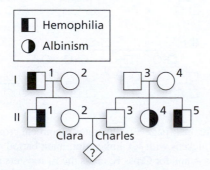

Clara   Charles

a. What are the genotypes of the four parents (I-1 to I-4) in this pedigree?
b. Determine the probability that the first child of Clara and Charles will be a
   i. boy with hemophilia
   ii. girl with albinism

iii. healthy girl
iv. boy with both albinism and hemophilia
v. boy with albinism
vi. girl with hemophilia

c. If Clara and Charles's first child has albinism, what is the chance the second child has albinism? Explain why this probability is higher than the probability you calculated in part (b).

14. A wild-type male and a wild-type female *Drosophila* with red eyes and full wings are crossed. Their progeny are shown below.

Males	Females
$\frac{3}{8}$ full wing, red eye	$\frac{3}{4}$ full wing, red eye
$\frac{3}{8}$ miniature wing, red eye	$\frac{1}{4}$ purple eye, full wing
$\frac{1}{8}$ purple eye, full wing	
$\frac{1}{8}$ miniature wing, purple eye	

a. Using clearly defined allele symbols of your choice, give the genotype of each parent.
b. What is/are the genotype(s) of females with purple eye? Of males with purple eye and miniature wing?

15. A woman with severe discoloration of her tooth enamel has four children with a man who has normal tooth enamel. Two of the children, a boy (B) and a girl (G), have discolored enamel. Each has a mate with normal tooth enamel and produces several children. G has six children—four boys and two girls. Two of her boys and one of her girls have discolored enamel. B has seven children—four girls and three boys. All four of his daughters have discolored enamel, but all his boys have normal enamel. Explain the inheritance of this condition.

16. In a large metropolitan hospital, cells from newborn babies are collected and examined microscopically over a 5-year period. Among approximately 7500 newborn males, six have one Barr body in the nuclei of their somatic cells. All other newborn males have no Barr bodies. Among 7500 female infants, four have two Barr bodies in each nucleus, two have no Barr bodies, and the rest have one. What is the cause of the unusual number of Barr bodies in a small number of male and female infants?

17. In cats, tortoiseshell coat color appears in females. A tortoiseshell coat has patches of dark brown fur and patches of orange fur that each in total cover about half the body but have a unique pattern in each female. Male cats can be either dark brown or orange, but a male cat with

tortoiseshell coat is rarely produced. Two sample crosses between males and females from pure-breeding lines produced the tortoiseshell females shown.

Cross I	P: dark brown male × orange female
	F₁: orange males and tortoiseshell females
Cross II	P: orange male × dark brown female
	F₁: dark brown males and tortoiseshell females

a. Explain the inheritance of dark brown, orange, and tortoiseshell coat colors in cats.
b. Why are tortoiseshell cats female?
c. The genetics service of a large veterinary hospital gets referrals for three or four male tortoiseshell cats every year. These cats are invariably sterile and have underdeveloped testes. How are these tortoiseshell male cats produced? Why do you think they are sterile?

18. The gene causing Coffin–Lowry syndrome (OMIM 303600) was recently identified and mapped on the human X chromosome. Coffin–Lowry syndrome is a rare disorder affecting brain morphology and development. It also produces skeletal and growth abnormalities, as well as abnormalities of motor control. Coffin–Lowry syndrome affects males who inherit a mutation of the X-linked gene. Most carrier females show no symptoms of the disease but a few carriers do. These carrier females are always less severely affected than males. Offer an explanation for this finding.

19. Four eye-color mutants in *Drosophila*—apricot, brown, carnation, and purple—are inherited as recessive traits. Red is the dominant wild-type color of fruit-fly eyes. Eight crosses (A through H) are made between parents from pure-breeding lines.

Cross	Parents		F₁ Progeny	
	Female	Male	Female	Male
A	Apricot	Red	Red	Apricot
B	Brown	Red	Red	Red
C	Red	Purple	Red	Red
D	Red	Apricot	Red	Red
E	Carnation	Red	Red	Carnation
F	Purple	Red	Red	Red
G	Red	Brown	Red	Red
H	Red	Carnation	Red	Red

a. Which of these eye-color mutants are X-linked recessive and which are autosomal recessive? Explain how you distinguish X-linked from autosomal heredity.
b. Predict F₂ phenotype ratios of Crosses A, B, D, and G.

20. For each pedigree shown,
   a. Identify which simple pattern of hereditary transmission (autosomal dominant, autosomal recessive, X-linked dominant, or X-linked recessive) is most likely to have occurred. Give genotypes for individuals involved in transmitting the trait.

b. Determine which other pattern(s) of transmission is/are possible. For each possible mode of transmission, specify the genotypes necessary for transmission to occur.
c. Identify which pattern(s) of transmission is/are impossible. Specify why transmission is impossible.

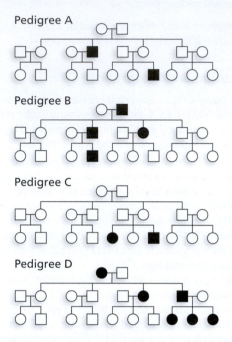

Pedigree A

Pedigree B

Pedigree C

Pedigree D

21. Use the blank pedigrees provided to depict transmission of (a) an X-linked recessive trait and (b) an X-linked dominant trait, by filling in circles and squares to represent individuals with the trait of interest. Give genotypes for each person in each pedigree. Carefully design each transmission pattern so that pedigree (a) cannot be confused with autosomal recessive transmission and pedigree (b) cannot be confused with autosomal dominant transmission. Identify the transmission events that eliminate the possibility of autosomal transmission for each pedigree.

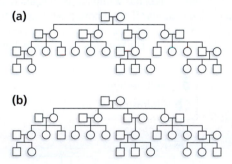

(a)

(b)

22. Figure 3.22 (page 89) illustrates reciprocal crosses involving chickens with sex-linked dominant barred mutation. For Cross A and for Cross B, cross the F₁ roosters and hens and predict the feather patterns of roosters and hens in the F₂.

23. In fruit flies, yellow body (*y*) is recessive to gray body (*y⁺*), and the trait of body color is inherited on the X chromosome. Vestigial wing (*v*) is recessive to full-sized wing (*v⁺*), and the trait has autosomal inheritance. A cross of a male with yellow body and full wings to a female with

gray body and full wings is made. Based on an analysis of the progeny of the cross shown below, determine the genotypes of parental and progeny flies.

Phenotype	Number of Males	Number of Females
Yellow body, full wing	296	301
Yellow body, vestigial wing	101	98
Gray body, full wing	302	298
Gray body, vestigial wing	101	103
	800	800

24. In a species of fish, a black spot on the dorsal fin is observed in males and females. A fish breeder carries out a pair of reciprocal crosses and observes the following results.

Cross I   Parents: black-spot male × nonspotted female

Progeny: 22 black-spot males

24 black-spot females

25 nonspotted males

21 nonspotted females

Cross II   Parents: nonspotted male × black-spot female

Progeny: 45 black-spot males

53 nonspotted females

a. Why does this evidence support the hypothesis that a black spot is sex linked?

b. Identify which sex is heterogametic. Give genotypes for the parents in each cross, and explain the progeny proportions in each cross.

25. Lesch–Nyhan syndrome (OMIM 300322) is a rare X-linked recessive disorder that produces severe mental retardation, spastic cerebral palsy, and self-mutilation.

a. What is the probability that the first son of a woman whose brother has Lesch–Nyhan syndrome will be affected?

b. If the first son of the woman described in (a) is affected, what is the probability that her second son is affected?

c. What is the probability that the first son of a man whose brother has Lesch–Nyhan syndrome will be affected?

26. In humans, *SRY* is located near a pseudoautosomal region (PAR) of the Y chromosome, a region of homology between the X and Y chromosomes that allows them to synapse during meiosis in males and is a region of crossover between the chromosomes. The diagram below shows *SRY* in relation to the pseudoautosomal region.

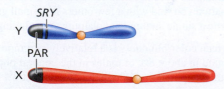

About 1 in every 25,000 newborn infants is born with sex reversal; the infant is either an apparent male, but with two X chromosomes, or an apparent female, but with an X and a Y chromosome. Explain the origin of sex reversal

in human males and females involving the *SRY* gene. (*Hint*: See Experimental Insight 3.1 for a clue about the mutational mechanism.)

27. In an 1889 book titled *Natural Inheritance* (Macmillan, New York), Francis Galton, who investigated the inheritance of measurable (quantitative) traits, formulated a law of "ancestral inheritance." The law stated that each person inherits approximately one-half of his or her genetic traits from each parent, about one-quarter of the traits from each grandparent, one-eighth from each great grandparent, and so on. In light of the chromosome theory of heredity, argue either in favor of Galton's law or against it.

28. In *Drosophila*, the X-linked echinus eye phenotype disrupts formation of facets and is recessive to wild-type eye. Autosomal recessive traits vestigial wing and ebony body assort independently of one another. Examine the progeny from the three crosses shown below, and identify the genotype of parents in each cross.

Parental Phenotype		Progeny Phenotype	Proportion	
Female	Male		Female	Male
a. Wild type	Echinus	Wild type	$\frac{3}{8}$	$\frac{3}{8}$
		Echinus	$\frac{3}{8}$	$\frac{3}{8}$
		Vestigial	$\frac{1}{8}$	$\frac{1}{8}$
		Echinus, vestigial	$\frac{1}{8}$	$\frac{1}{8}$
b. Wild type	Wild type	Vestigial, ebony	$\frac{2}{32}$	$\frac{1}{32}$
		Vestigial	$\frac{6}{32}$	$\frac{3}{32}$
		Ebony	$\frac{6}{32}$	$\frac{3}{32}$
		Wild type	$\frac{18}{32}$	$\frac{9}{32}$
		Echinus, vestigial, ebony	0	$\frac{1}{32}$
		Echinus, vestigial	0	$\frac{3}{32}$
		Echinus, ebony	0	$\frac{3}{32}$
		Echinus	0	$\frac{9}{32}$
c. Ebony	Echinus	Echinus, vestigial, ebony	$\frac{1}{32}$	$\frac{1}{32}$
		Echinus, vestigial	$\frac{3}{32}$	$\frac{3}{32}$
		Echinus, ebony	$\frac{3}{32}$	$\frac{3}{32}$
		Echinus	$\frac{9}{32}$	$\frac{9}{32}$
		Vestigial, ebony	$\frac{1}{32}$	$\frac{1}{32}$
		Vestigial	$\frac{3}{32}$	$\frac{3}{32}$
		Ebony	$\frac{3}{32}$	$\frac{3}{32}$
		Wild type	$\frac{9}{32}$	$\frac{9}{32}$

29. A wild-type *Drosophila* male and female are crossed, producing 324 female progeny and 161 male progeny. All their progeny are wild type.

a. Propose a genetic hypothesis to explain these data.

b. Design an experiment that will test your hypothesis, using the wild-type progeny identified above. Describe the results you expect if your hypothesis is true.

30. *Drosophila* has a diploid chromosome number of $2n = 8$, which includes one pair of sex chromosomes (XX in females and XY in males) and three pairs of autosomes. Consider a *Drosophila* male that has a copy of the A_1 allele on its X chromosome (the Y chromosome is the homolog) and is heterozygous for alleles B_1 and B_2, C_1 and C_2, and D_1 and D_2 of genes that are each on a different autosomal pair. In the diagrams requested below, indicate the alleles carried on each chromosome and sister chromatid. Assume that no crossover occurs between homologous chromosomes.

    a. What is the genotype of cells produced by mitotic division in this male?

    b. Diagram *any correct* alignment of chromosomes at mitotic metaphase.

    c. Diagram *any correct* alignment of chromosomes at metaphase I of meiosis.

    d. For the metaphase I alignment shown in (c), what gamete genotypes are produced at the end of meiosis?

    e. How many different metaphase I chromosome alignments are possible in this male? How many genetically different gametes can this male produce? Explain your reasoning for each answer.

Collaboration and Discussion

For answers to selected even-numbered problems, see Appendix: Answers.

31. The cell cycle operates in the same way in all eukaryotes, from single-celled yeast to humans, and all share numerous genes whose functions are essential for the normal progression of the cycle. Discuss why you think this is the case.

32. From a piece of blank paper, cut out three sets of four cigar-shaped structures (a total of 12 structures). These will represent chromatids. Be sure each member of a set of four chromatids has the same length and girth. In set one, label two chromatids "A" and two chromatids "a." Cut each of these chromatids about half way across near their midpoint and slide the two "A" chromatids together at the cuts, to form a single set of attached sister chromatids. Do the same for the "a" chromatids. In the second set of four chromatids, label two "B" and two "b." Cut and slide these together as you did for the first set, joining the "B" chromatids together and the "b" chromatids together. Repeat this process for the third set of chromatids, labeling them as "D" and "d." You now have models for three pairs of homologous chromosomes, for a total of six chromosomes.

    a. Give the genotype of the cell with six chromosomes.
    b. Align the chromosomes as they might appear at metaphase of mitosis.
    c. Are there any alternative alignments of the chromosomes for this cell division stage? Explain.
    d. Separate the chromosomes and chromatids as though mitotic anaphase and telophase have taken place.
    e. What are the genotypes of the daughter cells?
    f. Align the chromosomes as they might appear at metaphase I of meiosis.
    g. Are there any alternative alignments of the chromosomes for this cell division stage? Explain.
    h. Separate the chromosomes as though meiotic anaphase I and telophase I have taken place.
    i. Align the chromosomes of each daughter cell as they might appear in metaphase II of meiosis.
    j. Are there any alternative alignments of the chromosomes for this cell division stage? Explain.
    k. Separate the chromosomes as though anaphase II and telophase II have taken place.
    l. What are the genotypes of the daughter cells?
    m. Repeat steps (h) through (l) for the alternative alignment of chromosomes you identified in step (g).

    n. Combining your work in steps (f) through (m), provide a written explanation of the connection between meiotic cell division and Mendel's law of independent assortment.

33. Form a small discussion group and decide on the most likely genetic explanation for each of the following situations;

    a. A man who has red–green color blindness and a woman who has complete color vision have a son with red–green color blindness. What are the genotypes of these three people, and how do you explain the color blindness of the son?

    b. Cross A performed by Morgan and shown in Figure 3.18 is between a mutant male fruit fly with white eyes and a female fruit fly from a pure-breeding, red-eye stock. The figure shows that 1237 F1 progeny were produced, all of them with red eyes. In reality, this isn't entirely true. Among the 1237 F1 progeny were 3 male flies with white eyes. Give two possible explanations for the appearance of these white-eyed males.

34. Duchenne muscular dystrophy (DMD; OMIM 310200) and Becker muscular dystrophy (BMD; OMIM 300376) are both X-linked recessive conditions that result from different mutations of the same gene, known as *dystrophin*, on the long arm of the chromosome. BMD and DMD are quite different clinically. DMD is a very severe disorder that first appears at a young age, progresses rapidly, and is often fatal in the late teens to 20s. BMD, on the other hand, is much milder. Often symptoms don't first appear until the 40s or 50s, the progression of the disease is slow, and fatalities due to BMD are infrequent. Go to http://www.ncbi.nlm.nih/omim and survey the information describing the gene mutations causing these two conditions. Discuss the information you find with a few others in a small group, and write a single summary explaining your findings.

35. Red–green color blindness is a relatively common condition found in about 8% of males in the general population. From this, population, biologists estimate that 8% is the frequency of X chromosomes carrying a mutation of the gene encoding red and green color vision. Based on this frequency, determine the approximate frequency with which you would expect females to have red–green color blindness. Explain your reasoning.

Gene Interaction

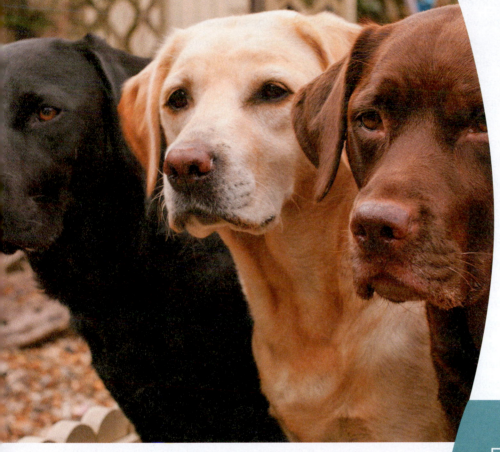

Coat colors in Labrador retrievers, black (left), yellow (center), and choco-late (right), are determined by the interaction of two genes, one deter-mining the production of coat color pigment and the other, pigment distribution.

CHAPTER OUTLINE

4.1 Interactions between Alleles Produce Dominance Relationships

4.2 Some Genes Produce Variable Phenotypes

4.3 Gene Interaction Modifies Mendelian Ratios

4.4 Complementation Analysis Distinguishes Mutations in the Same Gene from Mutations in Different Genes

ESSENTIAL IDEAS

▌ Dominance relationships between alleles have a molecular basis. The biological effects of gene products determine what type of dominance is observed.

▌ Gene expression can be affected by nongenetic (environmental) factors and also as a consequence of factors related to sex.

▌ Gene expression can be affected by interactions with other genes, causing characteristic changes in Mendelian ratios.

▌ Mutation of different genes can produce the same effect on phenotype. The number of genes causing mutation of a phenotype is discovered by genetic complementation analysis.

Mendel's laws of segregation and independent assortment encapsulate the basic rules of genetic transmission in diploid organisms. We see the results of these rules in the relative proportions of progeny with dif-ferent phenotypes from crosses. By assessing the molecular basis for the phenotypic variation, we can also glimpse the connection between hereditary transmission of phenotypic traits and DNA, RNA, and protein sequence variability.

Mendel's success in identifying and describing the law of segregation and the law of independent assortment was partly because of his use of traits whose phenotypic characteristics are determined exclusively by inheritance of alleles for single genes. In interpreting the inheritance of these traits, he did not have to contend with phenotypic variation introduced by other genes or by environmental (nongenetic) factors. In Mendel's experiments, each of the seven traits was decided by a single pair of alleles, one fully dominant and one fully recessive, for a gene determining that particular trait; and environmental factors played a minimal role in the phenotypic variation he observed.

The simple case in which just two alleles influence a trait and environment plays no meaningful role is relatively rare in nature. Although a diploid organism can have no more than two alleles for a given gene—because such individuals have just two copies of each chromosome—there may be more than two alleles for a single gene within a population, and these different alleles may produce different phenotypic effects. In addition, alleles can exhibit dominance relationships other than the simple dominance and recessiveness we saw in Chapters 2 and 3; and a few alleles are expressed differently in males and females. Two other phenomena influencing phenotype development are important to consider as well. First, many phenotypes are the consequence of two or more genes interacting with one another, and second, the phenotypic expression of some genes is influenced by environmental factors. Taken together, these circumstances impart a further dimension to the way geneticists view the function of genes in determining phenotypes. The phrase "extensions of Mendelian inheritance" is frequently used to include these gene–gene and gene–environment interactions.

These interactions, detectable in all organisms, are particularly relevant to humans when medical conditions are considered. As we discuss in later chapters, numerous common human diseases, including heart disease, diabetes, and cancers, can have an inherited component that increases disease risk. Environmental factors play a major role in producing these diseases, however, and interactions between genes and the environment can be critically important in the disease process.

In this chapter, we examine several examples of allele interactions that are different from those described by Mendel and we also examine interactions between genes and between genes and

environmental factors. The concepts presented here include the following:

▎ There may be more than two alleles for a given gene within the population.
▎ Dominance of one allele over another may not be complete.
▎ Two or more genes may affect a single trait.
▎ The expression of a trait may be dependent on the interaction of two or more genes, on the interaction of genes with nongenetic factors, or both.

4.1 Interactions between Alleles Produce Dominance Relationships

Mendel wisely chose to examine traits presenting in one of two easily distinguishable forms. One form of each trait he studied displayed complete dominance over the other form. Complete dominance makes the phenotype of a heterozygous organism indistinguishable from that of an organism homozygous for the dominant allele; thus, only organisms homozygous for the recessive allele display the recessive phenotype. The complete dominance of one allele also results in the exclusive expression of the dominant phenotype among the heterozygous F_1 progeny of a cross between pure-breeding homozygous parents, while the F_2 progeny display a 3:1 ratio of dominant to recessive phenotypes. We now know that the phenotypes of the seven traits that Mendel studied are controlled by two alternative alleles at seven different genes. For the four traits of Mendel that have been described at the molecular level (see Section 2.6), the dominant alleles produce full function of the gene, while the recessive alleles encode gene products with reduced or no functional activity.

Questions concerning the molecular basis of dominant and recessive alleles drove genetic research in the early and mid-20th century. Questions such as how dominance of an allele could be ascertained, why certain mutations are recessive whereas others are dominant, and whether mutations always cause genes to lose function or whether mutations can impart new or additional functions to alleles were commonly asked.

The Molecular Basis of Dominance

A character is called dominant if the same phenotype is seen in organisms with the homozygous and heterozygous genotypes. The correlative character is called recessive if it is observed only in a single homozygous genotype. In this sense, dominance and recessiveness have a phenotypic basis. The phenotypes are, however, a consequence of the characteristics of proteins produced by the alleles of a gene. In this sense, dominance and recessiveness also have a molecular basis. The dominance of one allele over another is determined by the protein products of the allele—by the manner in which the protein products of alleles work to produce the phenotype.

Let's compare two examples to illustrate the molecular basis of dominance and recessiveness. In both examples, a wild-type allele produces an enzyme with full activity and a mutant allele produces either very little enzyme activity or none at all. In the first example the mutant allele is recessive, but in the second example the mutant allele is dominant. Recall from our discussion at the beginning of Section 3.3 that the term *wild type* derives from the work of Thomas Hunt Morgan, who determined that most flies in his wild populations had the same phenotype. The wild-type trait or allele is the most common allele in a natural (wild) population.

Haplosufficient Wild-Type Allele Is Dominant In the first example, gene R has a dominant wild-type allele R^+ and a recessive mutant allele r. Gene R produces an enzyme that must generate 40 or more units of catalytic activity to drive a critical reaction step. Successful completion of this step produces the wild-type phenotype, whereas failure to complete the step generates a mutant phenotype. Each copy of allele R^+ produces 50 units of enzyme activity. The mutant allele r produces no functional enzyme and leads to 0 units of activity. Homozygous R^+R^+ organisms produce 100 units of enzyme activity (50 units from each copy of R^+), far exceeding the minimum required to achieve the wild-type phenotype. Heterozygous organisms (R^+r) produce a total of 50 units of enzyme activity, which is sufficient to produce the wild-type phenotype. Homozygous rr organisms produce no enzymatic action, however, and display the mutant phenotype. Based on its ability to catalyze the critical reaction step and produce the wild-type phenotype in either a homozygous (R^+R^+) or heterozygous (R^+r) genotype, R^+ is dominant over r. Dominant wild-type alleles of this kind are identified as **haplosufficient** since one (haplo) copy is sufficient to produce the wild-type phenotype in the heterozygous genotype.

Haploinsufficient Wild-Type Allele is Recessive The second example involves gene T, for which the wild-type allele is recessive to a mutant allele. Gene T produces an enzyme required to catalyze a critical reaction step that produces a wild-type phenotype if it is completed. The inability to complete the reaction step results in a mutant phenotype. For the reaction step in question, 18 units of enzyme activity are required. The wild-type allele T_1 produces 10 units of activity. A mutant allele, T_2, generates 5 units of enzyme activity. Homozygous T_1T_1 organisms generate 20 units of catalytic enzyme activity, enough to catalyze the critical reaction step and produce the wild-type phenotype. Heterozygous organisms, on the other hand, produce only 15 units of enzymatic activity and have the mutant phenotype because they fall short of the 18 units required to catalyze the reaction step. Similarly, homozygous T_2T_2 organisms, which produce 10 units of enzyme activity, also have a mutant phenotype. In this case, the mutant allele T_2 is dominant over the wild-type allele T_1 since both the heterozygous (T_1T_2) and homozygous (T_2T_2) organisms have a mutant phenotype. In cases like this, the wild-type allele is identified as **haploinsufficient** because a single copy is not sufficient to produce the wild-type phenotype in the heterozygous genotype.

Functional Effects of Mutation

The study of mutations and their consequences is a central tool of genetic analysis. In many instances, the study of mutations provides clues to the production of the wild type and to the underlying causes of abnormal outcomes. In the study of mutations, a central question concerns the mechanism through which the mutation disrupts normal (wild-type) gene function and leads to the mutant phenotype.

From a functional perspective, organisms with two copies of the wild-type allele have the wild-type phenotype (**Figure 4.1a**). The same would be true if an organism had a single copy of a fully dominant wild-type allele. Using the level of activity of the protein products of the wild-type allele as the basis for comparison, mutant alleles can often be placed into either a *loss-of-function* or a *gain-of-function* category. A **loss-of-function mutation** results in a significant decrease or in the complete loss of the functional activity of a gene product. This common mutational category includes mutations like those described in the R-gene and T-gene examples. Loss-of-function mutant alleles are usually recessive, but under certain circumstances, they may be dominant, depending on whether the wild-type allele is haplosufficient or haploinsufficient.

Gain-of-function mutations identify alleles that have acquired a new function or have their expression altered in a way that gives them substantially more activity than the wild-type allele. Gain-of-function mutations are almost always dominant and usually produce dominant mutant phenotypes in heterozygous organisms. As a consequence of their newly acquired functions, certain gain-of-function mutations are lethal in a homozygous state.

Loss-of-Function Mutations As the previous discussion suggests, mutations resulting in a loss of function vary in the extent of loss of normal activity of the gene product. A loss-of-function mutation that results in a complete loss of gene function in comparison with the wild-type gene product is identified as a **null mutation**, also known as an **amorphic mutation** (**Figure 4.1b**). The word *null* means "zero" or "nothing," and the word *amorphic* means "without form." These mutant alleles produce no functional gene product and are often lethal in a homozygous genotype. The elimination of functional gene products can result from various types of mutational events, including those that block transcription, produce a gene product that lacks activity, or result in deletion of all or part of the gene.

Alternatively, a mutation resulting in partial loss of gene function may be identified as a **leaky mutation**, also known

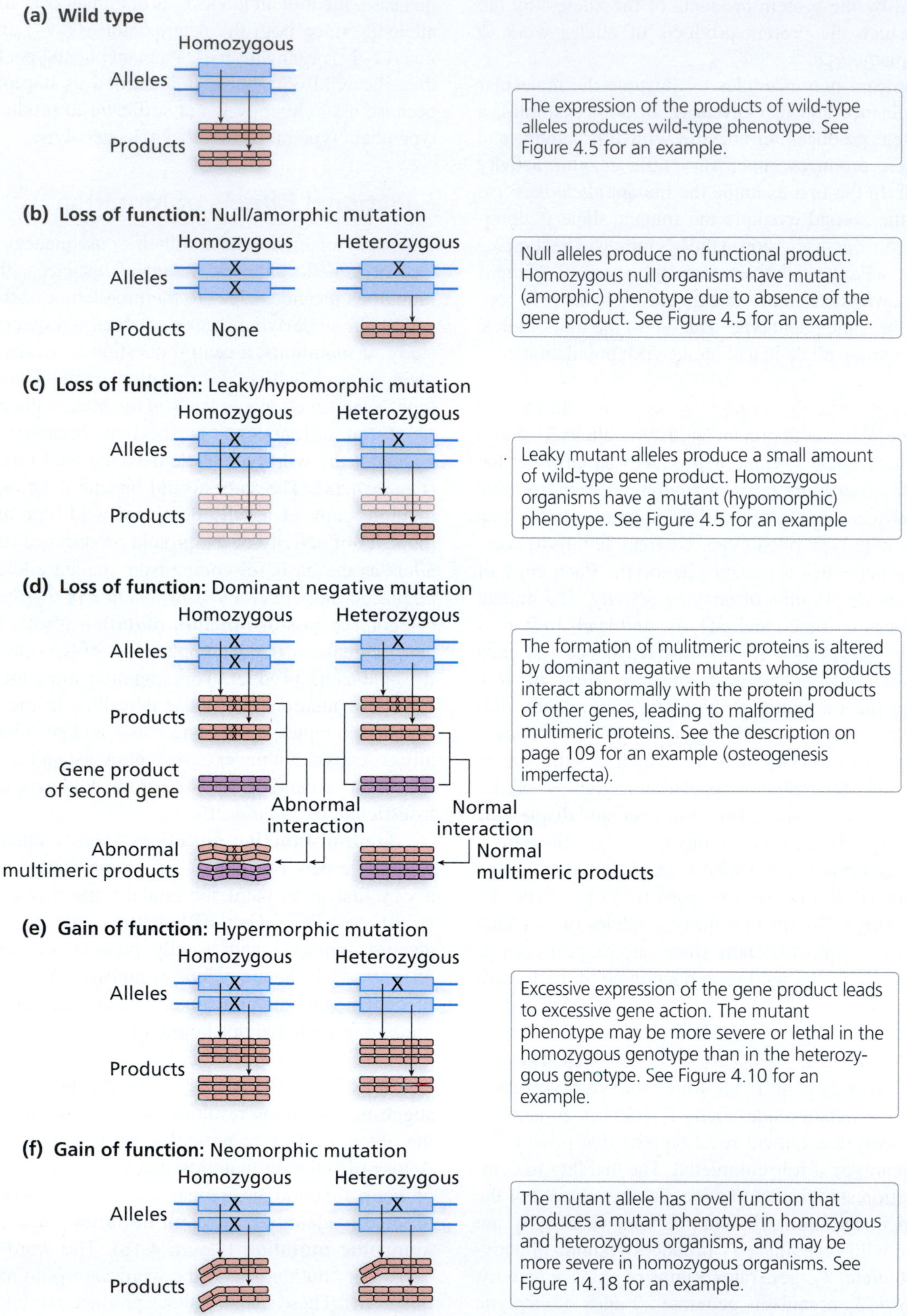
(a) Wild type
Homozygous
Alleles
Products
The expression of the products of wild-type alleles produces wild-type phenotype. See Figure 4.5 for an example.
(b) Loss of function: Null/amorphic mutation
Homozygous
Heterozygous
Alleles
Products
None
Null alleles produce no functional product. Homozygous null organisms have mutant (amorphic) phenotype due to absence of the gene product. See Figure 4.5 for an example.
(c) Loss of function: Leaky/hypomorphic mutation
Homozygous
Heterozygous
Alleles
Products
Leaky mutant alleles produce a small amount of wild-type gene product. Homozygous organisms have a mutant (hypomorphic) phenotype. See Figure 4.5 for an example
(d) Loss of function: Dominant negative mutation
Homozygous
Heterozygous
Alleles
Products
Gene product of second gene
Abnormal interaction
Normal interaction
Abnormal multimeric products
Normal multimeric products
The formation of mulitmeric proteins is altered by dominant negative mutants whose products interact abnormally with the protein products of other genes, leading to malformed multimeric proteins. See the description on page 109 for an example (osteogenesis imperfecta).
(e) Gain of function: Hypermorphic mutation
Homozygous
Heterozygous
Alleles
Products
Excessive expression of the gene product leads to excessive gene action. The mutant phenotype may be more severe or lethal in the homozygous genotype than in the heterozygous genotype. See Figure 4.10 for an example.
(f) Gain of function: Neomorphic mutation
Homozygous
Heterozygous
Alleles
Products
The mutant allele has novel function that produces a mutant phenotype in homozygous and heterozygous organisms, and may be more severe in homozygous organisms. See Figure 14.18 for an example.

Figure 4.1 The functional consequences of mutation. **(a)** Wild type. **(b)**, **(c)**, and **(d)** Loss-of-function mutations. **(e)** and **(f)** Gain-of-function mutations. The "X" indicates the presence of a mutation in a copy of a gene.

as a **hypomorphic mutation** (**Figure 4.1c**). *Hypomorphic* means "reduced form"; like the term *leaky,* it implies that a small percentage of normal functional capability is retained by the mutant allele but at a lower level than is found for the wild-type allele. The severity of the phenotypic abnormality depends on the residual level of activity from the leaky mutant allele. A greater percentage of activity from a leaky allele results in a less severely affected phenotype than when the mutation incurs a more substantial loss of function. Both null and hypomorphic loss-of-function mutations are often recessive and homozygous lethal.

Dominant loss-of-function mutations are also known to occur. Some of these produce dominant mutant phenotypes through alterations in the function of a multimeric protein of which the mutant polypeptide forms a part (**Figure 4.1d**). Multimeric proteins, composed of two or more polypeptides that join together to form a functional protein, are particularly subject to **dominant negative mutations** as a consequence of some change that prevents the polypeptides from interacting normally to produce a functional protein. A multimeric protein that contains an abnormal polypeptide may suffer a reduction or total loss of functional capacity. Mutations of this kind are dominant due to the substantial loss of function of the multimeric protein (as illustrated in the following paragraph). These mutations are characterized as "negative" due to the spoiler effect of the abnormal polypeptide on the multimeric protein.

An example of dominant negative mutation is seen in the human hereditary disorder osteogenesis imperfecta (OMIM 116200, 116210, and 116220), which is caused by defects in the bone protein collagen and has multiple forms with different severity. Collagen protein is composed of three interwoven polypeptide strands—two polypeptides from the *COL1A1* gene and one polypeptide from the *COL1A2* gene. The trimeric collagen protein is subject to dominant negative mutation as a consequence of *COL1A1* mutations that produce a defective polypeptide. The trimeric structure of collagen and the 2:1 ratio of incorporation of COL1A1 polypeptide over COL1A2 polypeptide means that in individuals who are homozygous wild type for *COL1A2* and heterozygous for *COL1A1* mutation, most collagen protein contains one or two mutant COL1A1 proteins. As a result, most collagen protein is defective, and osteogenesis imperfecta develops.

Gain-of-Function Mutations Mutations resulting in a gain of function fall into two categories that depend on the functional behavior of the new mutation. **Hypermorphic** ("greater than wild-type form") **mutations** produce more gene activity per allele than the wild type (**Figure 4.1e**) and are usually dominant. The gene product of a hypermorphic allele is indistinguishable from that of the wild-type allele, but it is present in a greater amount and thus induces a higher level of activity. The excess concentration is the functional equivalent of overdrive, pushing processes forward more rapidly, at the wrong time, in the wrong place, or for a longer time than normal. Hypermorphic mutants often result

from regulatory mutations that increase gene transcription, block the normal response to regulatory signals that silence transcription, or increase the number of gene copies by gene duplication. The phenotypic effect may be more severe in mutation homozygotes than in heterozygotes, but often, particularly in humans, mutant homozygotes are not seen because homozygosity is lethal.

Gain-of-function mutations resulting from **neomorphic** ("new form") **mutations** acquire novel gene activities not found in the wild type (**Figure 4.1f**) and are usually dominant. The gene products of neomorphic mutants are functional but have structures that differ from the wild-type gene product. The altered structures lead the mutant protein to function differently than the wild-type protein. Homozygotes for a neomorphic allele may exhibit a more severely affected phenotype than do heterozygotes.

Notational Systems for Genes and Allele Relationships

Our description of the molecular basis of dominance and of loss-of-function and gain-of-function mutations provides a conceptual basis for understanding how different patterns of dominance relationships can develop among alleles of a gene. These concepts apply to all diploid organisms, but the various notational systems used to identify genes and alleles in different species do not all depict these relationships in the same ways. Historically, these different gene notation systems developed along species lines due to the propensity of early 20th-century biology to study one species in isolation from other species. Biology today is far more interdisciplinary. For example, in discussing Mendel's work in Chapter 2, we mostly used a notational system in which an uppercase letter (for example, *A*) indicates a dominant allele and the same letter in lowercase (*a*) designates a recessive allele. When the dominance of one allele is not complete, however, a different notational system—one that avoids implying dominance or recessiveness—is used. In this nomenclature system, alleles can be symbolized with either upper- or lowercase letters plus a suffix that may be a number or a letter. Examples of how pairs of alleles with incomplete dominance can be designated are $A1$ and $A2$, B^1 and B^2, d_1 and d_2, and w^a and w^b. We apply some of these notational systems in the following section.

It is not surprising that there are a number of different notational systems employed in genetics, involving various uses of italics, capital letters, and symbols such as "+" for wild-type alleles and "−" for mutant alleles. They developed in the early years of genetics research when genetic experiments were being carried out by experts in widely divergent fields of biology with little intercommunication. Geneticists studying fruit flies developed one notation system for identifying wild-type and mutant alleles, geneticists studying yeast developed another, and geneticists studying plants developed another. As the table inside the back cover illustrates, each model organism has its own unique style of gene description and nomenclature. These various styles are the conventions we follow throughout this book for discussing the genetics of different model organisms.

Incomplete Dominance

Mendel's description of inheritance of traits controlled by single genes having a dominant and a recessive allele is a simple hereditary process that is relatively rare in nature. More commonly with single-gene traits, the dominance of one allele over another is not complete but instead is described as **incomplete dominance**, also known as **partial dominance**. When incomplete dominance exists among alleles, the phenotype of the heterozygous organism is distinctive; it falls somewhere on a phenotypic continuum between the phenotypes of the homozygotes and is typically more similar to one homozygous phenotype than the other. When traits display incomplete dominance, two pure-breeding parents with different phenotypes produce F_1 heterozygotes having a phenotype different from that of either parent.

One of the many traits displaying incomplete dominance is the trait described as flowering time in Mendel's pea plants (*Pisum sativum*). In peas, the first appearance of flowers is under the genetic control of a gene that we will call *T,* for flowering *time*. The earliest-flowering strain of pea plants has the homozygous genotype T_1T_1; the flowering time of this strain is described as day 0.0. The latest-flowering strain is homozygous T_2T_2, and it flowers 5.2 days later on average than T_1T_1 plants. A cross of pure-breeding early-flowering and late-flowering strains produces T_1T_2 heterozygous progeny that begin to flower 3.7 days later on average than the earliest-flowering strain (**Figure 4.2a**).

Genetic crosses show that flowering time is controlled by a single locus. Self-fertilization of T_1T_2 plants produces a 1:2:1 ratio of early-, intermediate-, and late-flowering progeny (**Figure 4.2b**). We say the T_2 allele is partially dominant, but not completely dominant, to T_1 because the heterozygous phenotype is distinct from either homozygous phenotype but more closely resembles the late-flowering strain.

Codominance

Codominance, like incomplete dominance, leads to a heterozygous phenotype different from the phenotype of either homozygous parent. Unlike incomplete dominance, however, codominance is characterized by the detectable

expression of both alleles in heterozygotes. Codominance is most clearly identified when the protein products of both alleles are detectable in heterozygous organisms, typically by means of some sort of molecular analysis or a biochemical assay that can distinguish between the different proteins. An example of codominance is presented in the following discussion of ABO blood type.

Dominance Relationships of ABO Alleles

More than one pattern of dominance between the alleles of a gene can occur under certain circumstances. Here we examine the codominance of two alleles and the recessiveness of a third allele of the gene determining human ABO blood type.

All of us have one of the four common blood types—type O, type A, type B, or type AB—that result from our genotype at the ABO blood group gene located on chromosome 9 (OMIM 110300).

The three alleles of the ABO gene are identified as I^A, I^B, and i, and the four blood groups are phenotypes produced by six genotypes. On the basis of genotype–phenotype (i.e., blood type) correlation, geneticists have concluded that I^A and I^B have complete dominance over i, and that I^A and I^B are codominant to one another. The complete dominance of I^A and I^B to i is indicated by the identification of blood type A in individuals whose genotype is I^AI^A or I^Ai, and of blood type B in individuals whose genotype is I^BI^B or I^Bi. The completely recessive nature of the i allele is confirmed by the observation that only ii homozygotes have blood type O. Lastly, codominance of I^A and I^B to one another is confirmed by the observation that blood type AB occurs only in individuals who have the heterozygous genotype I^AI^B.

Determining ABO Blood Type ABO blood type is identified by an antigen–antibody reaction on a microscope slide. The test involves placing a drop of blood into a drop of anti-A antiserum in one well of a microscope slide and placing another drop of blood into anti-B antiserum in the other well of the slide. The two antisera contain antibodies, molecules produced by the immune system that bind to a specific antigen (for each kind of antibody there is a specific antigen). Each antigen in the case of ABO blood type is a carbohydrate group (sugar) embedded on the surface of red blood cells. A positive reaction occurs when an antibody

(a)

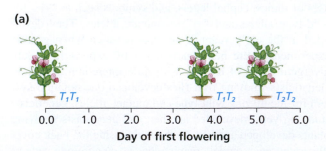

Day of first flowering

(b)

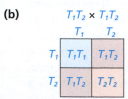

$\frac{1}{4}$ T_1T_1 Early flowering (Day 0.0)
$\frac{1}{2}$ T_1T_2 Intermediate flowering (Day 3.7)
$\frac{1}{4}$ T_2T_2 Late flowering (Day 5.2)

Figure 4.2 Incomplete dominance in flowering time of pea plants.
(a) Allele T_2 is incompletely dominant over allele T_1 as indicated by the late flowering time of T_1T_2 plants.
(b) Segregation of alleles T_1 and T_2.

detects its antigen target. The antibody binds the antigen and also attaches to other antigen-bound antibodies, causing red blood cells to form visible clumps. Clumping indicates that the antibody has detected its antigen target, whereas an absence of clumping indicates that the blood does not contain the antigen target of the antibody.

Blood from a person with blood type A shows clumping with anti-A antiserum but not with anti-B (**Figure 4.3**). Conversely, blood type B is identified when clumping occurs with anti-B but not with anti-A. If clumping occurs with both antisera, the blood type is AB. Clumping with neither antiserum identifies blood type O.

The antibodies anti-A and anti-B develop in humans from birth, but people do not carry an antibody if they also carry the corresponding antigen. Thus people with blood type A, who have the A antigen, also carry the anti-B antibody. People with blood type B have the B antigen and the anti-A antibody. Those with blood type AB have both antigens and neither anti-A nor anti-B antibody. Finally, people with blood type O have neither A nor B antigen and have both anti-A and anti-B antibody.

The ABO system is one of several blood types that must be tested before blood transfusion to ensure the safety of the procedure. The general rule for safe blood transfusion is that the recipient blood must not contain an antibody that reacts

Table 4.1	Donor-Recipient Compatibility for ABO Blood Types			
Donor blood type	Recipient blood type			
	A	B	AB	O
A	√	X	√	X
B	X	√	√	X
AB	X	X	√	X
O	√	√	√	√

√ = Safe transfusion
X = Clumping, unsafe transfusion

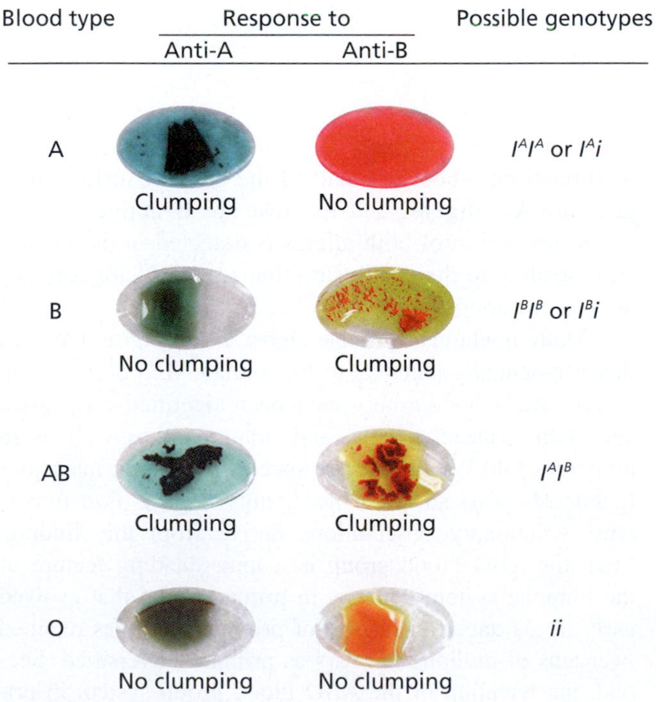

with an antigen in the donated blood. When such a reaction occurs, blood clots produced by clumping blood cells form at the site of transfusion. These adverse reactions can potentially cause life-threatening complications. **Table 4.1** lists safe and unsafe matches for ABO blood transfusions. Notice that people with blood type O are "universal donors" who can donate to people of any blood type. This is because type O contains neither A nor B antigens. Notice also that people with blood type AB are "universal recipients" who can receive blood from any blood type. This is because their blood contains neither anti-A nor anti-B antibodies.

The Molecular Basis of Dominance and Codominance of ABO Alleles The two ABO blood group antigens on the surfaces of red blood cells each have a slightly different molecular structure. The antigens are glycolipids that contain a lipid component and an oligosaccharide component. The lipid portion of the antigen is anchored in the red blood cell membrane, and the segment protruding outside the cell contains the oligosaccharide. Initially, the oligosaccharide is composed of five sugar molecules and is called the H antigen. It results from the activity of an enzyme produced by the H gene (**Figure 4.4**). The H antigen is present on the surfaces of all red blood cells, but it can be further modified, in two alternative ways, by the addition of a sixth sugar, or it can be left unmodified. The final modification of the H antigen depends on the enzymatic activity of the protein product of the ABO blood group locus.

Either of two alternative sugars can be added to the H antigen by the respective gene products of the I^A or I^B allele. If the I^A allele is present in the genotype, it produces the gene product α-3-N-acetyl-d-galactosaminyltransferase, or simply, "A-transferase." A-transferase catalyzes the addition of the sugar N-acetylgalactosamine to the H antigen, producing a six-sugar oligosaccharide known as the A antigen. The I^B allele, on the other hand, produces α-3-d-galactosyltransferase, commonly called "B-transferase," which catalyzes the addition of

Blood type	Response to		Possible genotypes
	Anti-A	Anti-B	
A	Clumping	No clumping	$I^A I^A$ or $I^A i$
B	No clumping	Clumping	$I^B I^B$ or $I^B i$
AB	Clumping	Clumping	$I^A I^B$
O	No clumping	No clumping	ii

Figure 4.3 ABO blood type. Blood type is determined by mixing a drop of blood with a drop of anti-A or anti-B antiserum. Clumping indicates that the antibody has detected the corresponding antigen in the blood.

Q Is it possible for a child with blood type O to be born to a mother with blood type A and a father with blood type B? Explain why or why not.

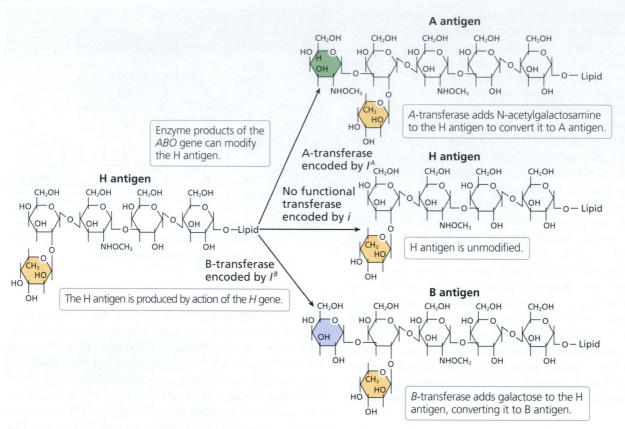

Figure 4.4   Production of ABO blood group antigens.

a different sugar, galactose, and produces a six-sugar oligosaccharide known as the B antigen. Molecular analysis reveals that the A and B alleles differ in several nucleotides, causing four amino acids of the resulting transferase enzymes to differ and leading to differences in enzymatic activity. In contrast, the i allele is due to a single base-pair deletion and is a null allele that does not produce a functional gene product capable of adding a sixth sugar to the H antigen.

At the cellular level, anti-A antibody recognizes the N-acetylgalactosamine addition mediated by I^A, and anti-B antibody identifies the galactose addition produced by the action of I^B. Neither of these antibodies has any reactivity with the unmodified H antigen, so unmodified H antigen, present in individuals with blood type O, is not recognized by either antibody. One copy of the I^A or the I^B allele in a genotype is sufficient to produce an ABO antigen detectable by the corresponding antibody; and both I^A and I^B are dominant to i, since I^A and I^B produce enzymes that modify the H antigen but i does not. When the $I^A I^B$ genotype is present, on the other hand, both A-transferase and B-transferase are produced, resulting in the addition of N-acetylgalactosamine to some H antigens and the addition of galactose to other H antigens. In this case, all red blood cells carry both types of H-antigen

modifications; about one-half of the red cell surface antigens are A antigens, and the rest are B antigens. As a result, the action of both alleles is detected in the phenotype, leading to the conclusion that I^A and I^B are codominant to one another.

Many nonhuman primates have a blood group system that is essentially identical to the human ABO blood group system. ABO blood groups have been identified in the great apes (chimpanzee, gorilla, and orangutan) as well as in numerous Old World monkey species, including macaques (genus *Macaca*) and baboons (genus *Papio*). Two important evolutionary observations derive from this finding. First, the ABO blood group is a long-standing feature of the immune system genetics in primates, one that evolved early in the ancestral history of primates and was retained over tens of millions of years as primates diversified. Second, the retention of the ABO blood group system in primates demonstrates the importance of this immune system response in protecting primates from infectious and foreign antigens. Natural selection has played a preeminent role in maintaining this system. The ABO blood group genes are one example of the shared evolutionary history that can be identified through the examination of the taxonomic distribution of genes in lineages. **Genetic Analysis 4.1** examines

PROBLEM The MN blood group in humans is an autosomal codominant system with two alleles, *M* and *N*. Its three blood group phenotypes, M, MN, and N, correspond to the genotypes *MM*, *MN*, and *NN*. The ABO blood group assorts independently of the MN blood group.

A male with blood type O and blood type MN has a female partner with blood type AB and blood type N. Identify the blood types that might be found in their children, and state the proportion for each type.

> **BREAK IT DOWN:** The discussion on p. 113 about the relationships among ABO alleles will help you to identify the parental genotypes from the phenotypes given here.

> **BREAK IT DOWN:** Alleles of the ABO system have both dominant-recessive and codominant relationships (p. 114).

Solution Strategies	Solution Steps
Evaluate	
1. Identify the topic of this problem and the kind of information the answer should contain.	1. The problem concerns the inheritance of two blood types. The gene determining ABO blood type carries three alleles: I^A and I^B are codominant to one another and dominant to i. The MN blood group gene carries two alleles that are codominant. The answer requires finding the possible blood types, and their expected proportions, of the children of parents whose blood types are given.
2. Identify the critical information given in the problem.	2. The blood types of the parents are given.
Deduce	
3. Deduce the blood group genotypes of the male parent.	3. The male has blood types O and MN. Type O results from homozygosity for the recessive i allele, whereas MN is produced in heterozygotes carrying both alleles. The male genotype is ii MN.
4. Deduce the blood group genotypes of the female parent.	4. The female has blood groups AB and N. The AB blood type is found in heterozygotes, and blood type N in homozygotes. The female blood group genotype is $I^A I^B$ NN.
Solve	
5. Identify the gamete genotypes and their frequencies for the male.	5. Independent assortment predicts two gamete genotypes for the male: All gametes contain i, half carry M, and half carry N.
6. Identify the female gamete genotypes and their frequencies.	6. Independent assortment predicts two gamete genotypes for the female: All gametes contain N, half contain I^A, and half contain I^B.
7. Predict the progeny genotypes and phenotypes.	7. Blood types A and B are each expected in 50% of the offspring of this cross, as are blood types MN and N. Four different blood group phenotypes, each with an expected frequency of 25% are predicted.

TIP: Blood type O is the recessive phenotype, and blood type MN is due to codominance of alleles.

TIP: Blood type AB is due to codominance, and blood type N is due to homozygosity.

TIP: Use a Punnett square to evaluate this cross.

♂ / ♀	Mi	Ni
NI^A	MNI^Ai Blood types: **MN** and **A**	NNI^Ai Blood types: **N** and **A**
NI^B	MNI^Bi Blood types: **MN** and **B**	NNI^Bi Blood types: **N** and **B**

For more practice, see Problems 6, 9, and 31.   Visit the Study Area to access study tools.   **Mastering Genetics**

---

the inheritance of blood group phenotypes, where alleles have a variety of dominance relationships.

Allelic Series

Diploid genomes contain pairs of homologous chromosomes; thus, each individual organism can possess at most two alleles at a locus. In populations, however, the number of alleles is theoretically unlimited, and some genes have scores of alleles. At the population level, a locus possessing three or more alleles is said to have multiple alleles; and like the ABO gene, many multiallelic genes display a variety of dominance relationships among the alleles. Commonly, an

order of dominance emerges among the alleles, based on the activity of each allele's protein product, forming a sequential series known as an **allelic series**. Alleles in an allelic series can be completely dominant or completely recessive, or they can display various forms of incomplete dominance or codominance.

The C-Gene System for Mammalian Coat Color

Genetic analysis of coat color in mammals reveals that many genes are required to produce and distribute pigment to the hair follicles or skin cells, where they are displayed as coat color or skin color. Although various interactions among these genes can modify color expression, we focus here on just one gene, the *C* (color) gene that is responsible for coat color in mammals such as cats, rabbits, and mice. This gene has dozens of alleles that have been identified over nearly a century of genetic analysis, but we limit our discussion to just four alleles that form an allelic series. The *C* gene produces the enzyme tyrosinase, which is active in the first two steps of a multistep biochemical pathway that synthesizes the pigment melanin, which imparts coat color in furred mammals and skin color in humans. In the initial melanin pathway steps, tyrosinase is responsible for the breakdown (catabolism) of the amino acid tyrosine.

The *C*-gene alleles form an allelic series that is revealed by the phenotypes of offspring of various matings. Allele *C* is dominant to all other alleles of the gene, and any genotype with at least one copy of *C* produces wild-type coat color. These genotypes are written as *C*– to indicate that regardless of the second allele in the genotype, the phenotype is dominant. Three other alleles, producing tyrosinase enzymes with reduced or no tyrosinase activity, form an allelic series with *C* (**Figure 4.5**). The allele c^{ch} in homozygotes produces a phenotype called chinchilla, a diluted coat color. This allele is hypomorphic and generates reduced coat color as a result of the reduced level of activity of the gene product. The c^h allele in homozygotes produces the Himalayan phenotype, characterized by fully pigmented extremities (paws, tail, nose, and ears) but virtually absent pigmentation on other parts of the body. This allele is temperature sensitive, as we describe momentarily. Finally, the *c* allele produces a protein product with no enzymatic activity. This is a fully recessive null (amorphic) allele that does not produce a functional gene product. Homozygosity for this allele produces an albino phenotype.

Crosses between animals with different genotypes at the *C* gene indicate the dominance relations of the alleles. For example, in Crosses A, B, and C in **Figure 4.6**, complete dominance of *C* over other alleles in the series is demonstrated by the finding that all of the progeny of an animal with the genotype *CC* have full color, regardless of the genotype of the mate. The dominance order of alleles in the series is revealed by the pattern of 3:1 ratios obtained from crosses of various heterozygous genotypes shown in Figure 4.6. Cross D shows that chinchilla is completely dominant over albino. Himalayan, too, is completely dominant over albino (Cross E). Cross F shows that the chinchilla allele (c^{ch}) is partially dominant over the Himalayan allele (c^h). Note the F_2 of this cross have a 1:2:1 ratio of phenotypes, with the heterozygous F_2 displaying Himalayan markings and dilute coat color over the rest of the body that are both somewhat lighter than in their homozygous counterparts. The dominance relationships within this allelic series locus can be expressed as $C > c^{ch} > c^h > c$.

The Molecular Basis of the C-Gene Allelic Series Tyrosinase enzymes produced by different *C*-gene alleles have distinctive levels of catabolic activity that are the basis for the dominance relationships between the alleles. The allele *C* is a dominant wild-type allele producing fully active tyrosinase that is defined as 100% activity. The percentage of wild-type tyrosinase activity produced by each allele explains the order observed for the allelic series. Biochemical examination reveals that the enzyme produced by the c^{ch} hypomorphic allele has much less activity than the wild-type enzyme. In the homozygous $c^{ch}c^{ch}$ genotype or heterozygous genotypes $c^{ch}c^h$ or $c^{ch}c$, only a small amount of melanin is synthesized. This leads to a decreased amount of pigment, and it has the effect of muting the coat color, more so in heterozygous genotypes, where just one c^{ch} allele is present, than in the $c^{ch}c^{ch}$ homozygous genotype, where two alleles are present.

The tyrosinase enzyme produced by the hypomorphic c^h (Himalayan) allele is unstable and is inactivated at a temperature very near the normal body temperature of most mammals. This type of gene product is an example of a **temperature-sensitive allele**. Cats with the Siamese

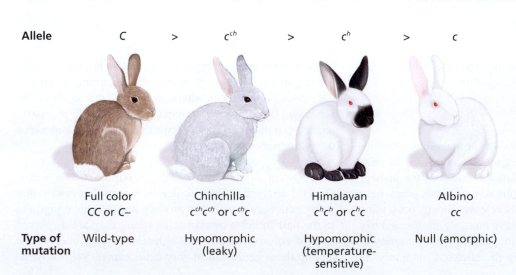

Allele	C	>	c^{ch}	>	c^h	>	c
	Full color		Chinchilla		Himalayan		Albino
	CC or C–		$c^{ch}c^{ch}$ or $c^{ch}c$		$c^h c^h$ or $c^h c$		cc
Type of mutation	Wild-type		Hypomorphic (leaky)		Hypomorphic (temperature-sensitive)		Null (amorphic)

Figure 4.5 Allelic series for coat-color determination in mammals.

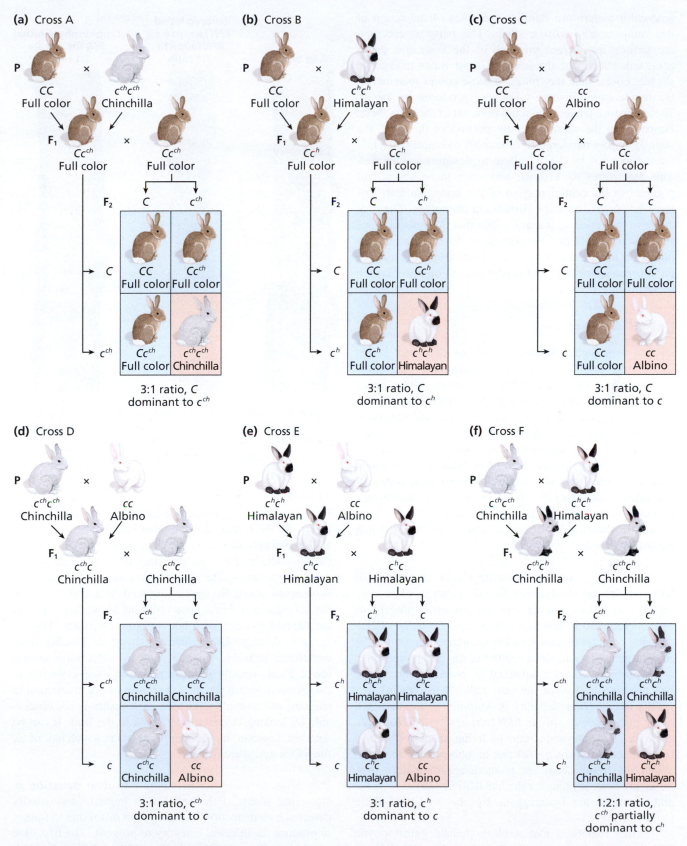

(a) Cross A

3:1 ratio, C dominant to c^{ch}

(b) Cross B

3:1 ratio, C dominant to c^h

(c) Cross C

3:1 ratio, C dominant to c

(d) Cross D

3:1 ratio, c^{ch} dominant to c

(e) Cross E

3:1 ratio, c^h dominant to c

(f) Cross F

1:2:1 ratio, c^{ch} partially dominant to c^h

Figure 4.6 The genetics of C gene dominance. Crosses A to F illustrate the complete dominance of C, the recessiveness of c, and the incomplete dominance of c^{ch} over c^h. Dominance in this allelic series is $C > c^{ch} > c^h > c$.

🔵 Based on the activities of C gene alleles described in this chapter, explain why one-half of the F_2 progeny shown in Cross F have chinchilla fur and dark paws, nose, and ears.

coat-color pattern are familiar examples of the action of this temperature-sensitive allele. The parts of cats that are farthest away from the core of the body (the paws, ears, tail, and tip of the nose) at most times tend to be slightly cooler than the trunk. At these cooler extremities, the temperature-sensitive tyrosinase produced by the c^{ch} allele remains active, producing pigment in the hairs there. However, in the warmer central portion of the body, the slightly higher temperature is enough to cause the tyrosinase produced by the c^{ch} allele to denature, or unravel. This inactivates the enzyme and leads to an absence of pigment in the central portion of the body. Animals that are $c^{ch}c^{ch}$ or $c^{ch}c$ have the Himalayan phenotype. The final allele in the series, c, is a null allele that does not produce functional tyrosinase. Homozygotes for this allele are unable to initiate the catabolism of tyrosine. This leads to an absence of melanin and produces the condition known as albinism.

Lethal Alleles

Certain single-gene mutations are so detrimental that they cause death early in life or terminate gestational development. These life-ending mutations affect genes whose products are essential to life. Homozygosity for mutation of these essential genes is lethal, and the mutations are identified as **lethal alleles**. As a rule, recessive lethal alleles have low frequencies in populations, although they may persist in some populations over a long period of time. Natural selection can eliminate copies of the allele when they occur in homozygous genotypes; however, recessive lethal alleles are "hidden" by dominant wild-type alleles in heterozygous genotypes, thus evading natural selection.

Detection in Plants In flowering plants, the effects of lethal alleles can be observed directly either as embryonic lethals that fail to produce homozygous lethal progeny or as gametophytic lethals that fail to generate lethal allele–carrying gametes (**Figure 4.7**). For example, mutation of the *RPN1a* gene that encodes a subunit of the 26S proteosome, a multiprotein complex involved in protein degradation, has produced a loss-of-function null allele (*rpn1a*) that results in embryonic lethality in *Arabidopsis thaliana* and other plant species. In an *RPN1a/rpn1a* × *RPN1a/rpn1a* cross, a 3:1 segregation ratio of living seeds (*RPN1a/_*) to dead seeds (*rpn1a/rpn1a*) can be observed in the fruit. When the living seeds are planted, approximately two-thirds are heterozygous for the lethal allele (*RPN1a/rpn1a*) and one-third are homozygous for the wild-type allele (*RPN1a/RPN1a*).

Lethal mutations that result in female gametophytic lethality are also detectable in flowering plants. Consider a plant heterozygous for a female gametophytic allele, *FER/fer*, in which the wild-type *FER* allele was derived from

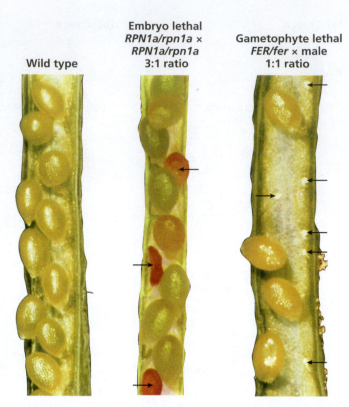

Figure 4.7 Evidence of lethal mutations in plants. Embryonic lethality is detected by observing a 3:1 ratio of viable to nonviable seeds, and gametophytic lethality is detected by observing a 1:1 ratio. Arrows indicate undeveloped seeds.

its mother and the mutant *fer* allele came from its father. During megasporogenesis, one-half of all megaspores will inherit the *FER* allele and the other half will inherit the *fer* allele. Embryo sacs derived from megaspores inheriting the *fer* allele will die, so that only one-half of all ovules develop into seeds. The alleles segregate in a 1:1 ratio that is observed among the developing seeds in a fruit. Note that the 1:1 ratio is a direct observation of Mendelian ratios in the haploid gametes of a heterozygous organism. Thus, a 1:1 ratio distinguishes female gametophytic lethality from embryonic lethality, which results in a 3:1 ratio among seeds. Plants usually produce pollen in excess, similar to the excess of sperm production relative to egg production in animals, and so male gametophytic lethality is not observable by looking at developing seeds in the fruit. It can be detected, however, by looking for plants in which half of all the pollen grains are dead.

Detection in Animals In contrast to their detection in flowering plants, lethal alleles in animals are usually detected by a distortion in segregation ratios due to failure to produce the affected category of progeny. The first case of a lethal allele was identified in 1905 by Lucien Cuenot, who studied a lethal mutation in mice carrying a dominant mutation for yellow coat color. In mice, wild-type

(a) Agouti coat color

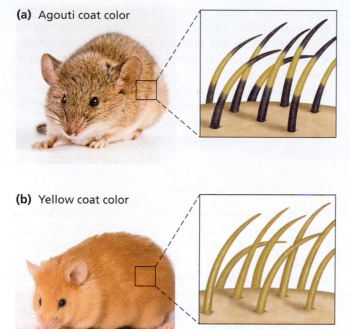

(b) Yellow coat color

Figure 4.8   Coat color in mice. (a) Wild-type agouti coat color is a mixture of black and yellow pigment in hair shafts. **(b)** Yellow coat occurs when yellow pigment produced by the overly active mutant allele A^Y displaces black pigment.

coat color is a brown color, called "agouti" (*a-GOO-tee*), produced by the presence of yellow and black pigments in each hair shaft (**Figure 4.8a**). Agouti hairs are black at the base and tip, with yellow pigment in the central portion of the shaft. Yellow coat color is seen when yellow pigment is deposited along the entire length of the hair shaft, not just in the middle portion as it is in agouti (**Figure 4.8b**). The *Agouti* gene is one of the pigment-producing genes found in mammals with furry coats. It produces a yellow pigment called pheomelanin that is found in the hairs of mammalian coats. An independently assorting gene produces the black pigment that is also visible in the hair shafts in Figure 4.8a. The wild-type allele for agouti coat color is designated *A,* and its normal activity leads to the production of a moderate amount of yellow pigment. The mutant allele, designated A^Y, is a hypermorphic allele. It is a dominant gain-of-function mutation that produces substantially more yellow pigment than does the wild-type allele.

The A^Y mutation is dominant, but true-breeding yellow mice cannot be produced. From a genetic perspective, this means that all mice with yellow coat color are heterozygous (AA^Y) and that the A^YA^Y genotype is lethal in embryonic development due to its interference with an essential gene, as we explain momentarily. From this

information, two important observations about the genetics of the yellow allele can be made. First, mating an agouti mouse and a yellow mouse will *always* result in a 1:1 ratio of agouti and yellow among progeny (**Figure 4.9a**). Second, crosses between two yellow mice (both of which are necessarily heterozygous) produce evidence of the recessive lethal nature of the A^Y allele (**Figure 4.9b**). The outcome of these crosses is a 2:1 ratio of yellow to agouti, rather than the 3:1 ratio that is anticipated when heterozygotes expressing a dominant allele are crossed. The genetic interpretation of this observation is that alleles of heterozygous yellow mice segregate normally in gamete formation and unite at random to produce a 1:2:1 ratio at conception, but that A^YA^Y zygotes do not survive gestation. Recessive lethality of A^Y prevents embryonic development of homozygotes, eliminating that class among progeny and resulting in the 2:1 ratio seen among progeny of heterozygous parents.

Nearly a century after Cuenot first identified homozygous lethality of the mutant A^Y allele, the molecular basis of the lethality was identified. Much to the surprise of geneticists, the lethality had little to do with yellow coat color itself; instead, yellow coat was an almost inadvertent consequence of a mutation that deleted part of a gene near the coat-color gene.

The mutation producing the A^Y allele results from a deletion that affects two genes, the *Agouti* gene and a neighboring gene identified as *Raly*. *Raly* produces a protein that is essential for mouse embryo development. Each of these genes has its own promoter. The wild-type *Raly* promoter

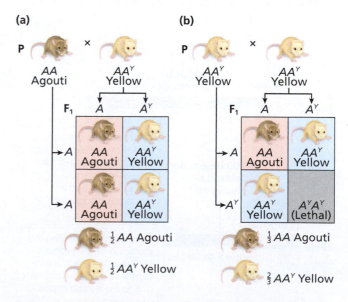

Figure 4.9   Dominance and lethality of A^Y. (a) A 1:1 ratio identifies A^Y as a dominant mutant allele. **(b)** The recessive lethality of A^Y in the homozygous genotype results in a 2:1 ratio of yellow to agouti in the cross of yellow-coated heterozygous mice.

drives a high level of transcription, whereas the *Agouti* gene promoter is considerably less actively transcribed (**Figure 4.10**). The dominant mutation producing yellow coat color comes about by a deletion of approximately 120,000 base pairs that deletes the entire *Raly* gene and the *Agouti* gene promoter, thus bringing the *Agouti* gene under the control of the *Raly* promoter, leading to a mutant hypermorphic agouti allele. The *Raly* promoter drives a high level of *Agouti* gene transcription that results in excess yellow pigment that displaces black pigment in hair shafts and leads to the mutant yellow phenotype. At the same time the absence of the *Raly* gene means the mutant allele fails to produce the Raly protein. Heterozygotes with the AA^Y genotype have yellow coats and survive due to haplosufficiency of the single copy of *Raly*. Homozygous A^YA^Y mice are unable to produce the essential protein product from the *Raly* gene and fail to develop, resulting in the skewed 2:1 Mendelian ratio that characterizes the progeny of two heterozygous yellow-coated mice.

An Allele That Is Both Dominant and Recessive The A^Y allele is an example of an allele that can be classified as both dominant and recessive. This may sound confusing and contradictory, but it is based on the phenotypes produced by genotypes of the *Agouti* gene. We refer to the mutant allele as dominant or as recessive depending on the particular phenotype we happen to be examining.

When we look at the ratio of agouti versus yellow coat color among the progeny produced by a yellow mouse mating with an agouti mouse, we see a 1:1 ratio that indicates dominance of the mutant allele over the wild-type allele. Dominance in this instance is due to the gain-of-function of yellow pigment by the mutant allele. If, on the other hand, we look at the ratio of progeny with yellow versus agouti coat color in the cross of two yellow mice, we see a 2:1 ratio that is the result of the homozygous lethality of the mutant allele. In this context, lethality only affects homozygotes, and the mutant allele is recessive to the wild type. This relationship is due to the loss of function of the *Raly* gene caused by its deletion. We have, therefore, the odd circumstance of one mutant allele that is both dominant and recessive, depending on how its phenotypic effect is examined.

Delayed Age of Onset

From an evolutionary perspective, it is easy to understand that a dominant lethal allele can be efficiently eliminated by the action of natural selection when it is expressed during gestation or very early in life. Even so, there are numerous examples of dominant lethal hereditary conditions, and a pertinent evolutionary genetic question concerns how these mutations persist in populations. One reason, in the case of a small number of dominant lethal alleles, is that they sidestep natural selection by having a **delayed age of onset**; the abnormalities they produce do not appear until after affected organisms have had an opportunity to reproduce and transmit the mutation to the next generation.

One well-characterized human hereditary disorder displaying delayed age of onset of a dominant lethal allele is the condition called Huntington disease (HD). This progressive neuromuscular disorder, usually fatal within 10 to 15 years of diagnosis, is caused by mutation of a gene near one end of chromosome 4. The HD mutant allele persists in the population because symptoms do not begin in about half of all cases until the person's late thirties or early forties, well after most people have begun having children (**Figure 4.11**).

Functionally, the onset of symptoms of HD is delayed because the symptoms are due to neuron death, which usually takes place over an extended period of time that often stretches over several decades.

4.2 Some Genes Produce Variable Phenotypes

To interpret phenotype ratios and identify the distribution of genotypes among phenotypic classes, geneticists make the assumption that phenotypes differ because their underlying genotypes differ. This assumption is valid only to the extent that a particular genotype always produces the same phenotype. If the correspondence between genotype and phenotype holds true in every case, the trait is identified as having **complete penetrance**. When the correspondence between genotype and phenotype does not consistently hold true—if instead the same genotype can produce different phenotypes—the usual reasons are gene–environment

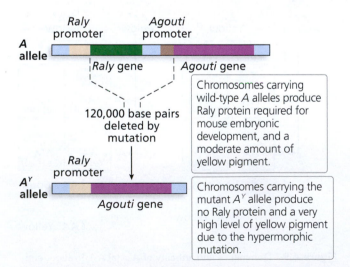

Figure 4.10   **Mutation of *Raly* and *Agouti* producing yellow coat.**

🔍 Refer back to Figure 4.1. Using the letters (a) through (f) in that figure, identify the type of mutation causing yellow coat color and the type of mutation producing lethality.

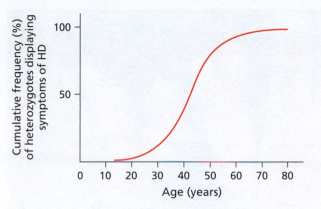

Figure 4.11 The age-of-onset curve for Huntington disease (HD).

interaction or interactions with alleles of other genes in the genome.

In this section, we describe four phenomena in which a certain genotype does not always produce the same phenotype. We first discuss *sex-limited traits* and *sex-influenced traits,* two categories of traits in which the sex of the organism influences how certain genotypes are expressed. In these cases, the hormonal environment is the critical factor influencing phenotypic expression of the genotypes. The other two phenomena, referred to as *incomplete penetrance* and *variable expressivity*, are circumstances in which phenotypic variation among organisms with the same genotype is due to some sort of unspecified or unknown genetic or environmental interaction.

Sex-Limited Traits

The sex of an organism can exert an influence on its gene expression, due to the differences in hormone profiles that characterize males and females of a species. These sex-dependent differences amount to expressing genes in different environments. One form such influence can take is described as **sex-limited traits**. Both sexes typically carry the genes for sex-limited traits, but the genes produce a phenotype in just one sex.

In mammals, for example, the development of breasts and the ability to produce milk are traits limited to females. Horn development is a trait limited to males in some species of sheep, cows, and other hoofed animals. Behavioral traits in some species, particularly traits related to mating, are also strongly influenced by sex. For example, the courtship behavior of crowned cranes includes an elaborate display of body positioning, neck intertwining, and vocalization that is performed differently by males and females of the species. In the case of male canary vocalization, changes in male singing patterns are initiated in late winter by an increase in male hormones released by the brain in response to increased day length and warmer temperatures. In this case, male hormones are thought to stimulate enlargement of the testes and increased production of

testosterone. This stimulates the development of neurons in the brain that elaborate the song center, induces the development of muscles in the vocalization area of the throat, and allows males to produce sex-limited vocalization to attract mates.

Sex-Influenced Traits

Sex-influenced traits are those in which the inheritance pattern for a trait in one sex differs from the inheritance pattern for the trait in the other sex, even when the genotype is the same. As with sex-limited traits, hormones influence this pattern of differential gene expression between the sexes.

The appearance of a chin beard versus the absence of a beard, the beardless phenotype, in certain goat breeds is an example of a sex-influenced trait. Bearding is inherited as an autosomal trait determined by two alleles, B_1 and B_2, which are present in three genotypes in each sex. In both sexes, B_1B_1 homozygotes are beardless, and homozygotes of either sex with the B_2B_2 genotype are bearded. It is thought that androgenic hormones are a principal factor influencing the bearded phenotype. The effect of different levels of androgenic hormones on bearding in the sexes is seen by comparing females and males with the heterozygous genotype (B_1B_2). Heterozygous males have a beard, whereas heterozygous females are beardless. **Figure 4.12** illustrates the results of a cross between two heterozygotes that produces different ratios of bearded to beardless males and females. Mendelian inheritance occurs, but as a consequence of sex-influenced expression, the cross yields a 3:1 ratio of bearded to beardless males and a 3:1 ratio of beardless to bearded females. In short, the dominance relationship of these alleles varies with sex. Allele B_1 is dominant to B_2 in females, since females that are heterozygous B_1B_2 have the same beardless phenotype as do B_1B_1 females. On the other hand, allele B_2 is dominant over B_1 in males since heterozygotes are bearded just like B_2B_2 homozygotes. Analogous to the classification of the

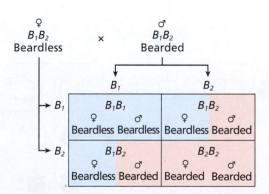

Figure 4.12 **Sex-influenced inheritance of beard appearance in goats.** Dominance of the B_1 and B_2 alleles is expressed differently in males and females.

A^Y allele we discussed earlier, the B_1 and B_2 alleles exhibit flexibility of dominance, in this case depending on the sex of the bearer.

Incomplete Penetrance

When the phenotype of an organism is consistent with the organism's genotype, the organism is said to be **penetrant** for the trait. In such a case, if the organism carries a dominant allele for the trait in question, the dominant phenotype is displayed. Sometimes an organism with a particular genotype fails to produce the corresponding phenotype, in which case the organism is **nonpenetrant** for the trait. Traits for which a genotype is *always* expressed in the phenotype are identified as **fully penetrant**. In contrast, traits that are nonpenetrant in some individuals are characterized as displaying **incomplete penetrance**.

The human condition known as polydactyly ("many digits") is an autosomal dominant condition that displays incomplete penetrance. Individuals with polydactyly have more than five fingers and toes—the most common alternative number is six (**Figure 4.13**). Polydactyly occurs in hundreds of families around the world, and in these families the dominant allele is nonpenetrant in about 25–30% of individuals who carry it. Most people who carry the dominant mutant polydactyly allele have extra digits; but at least one in four people with the mutant allele do not have extra digits and instead express the normal five digits. The gene mutated to produce polydactyly was recently identified (see Chapter 18).

Figure 4.14 shows a family in which polydactyly segregates as a dominant mutation. Nine individuals in the family carry a copy of the polydactyly allele. Six of them are penetrant for the phenotype (meaning that they express the phenotype), but at least three family members—II-6, II-10, and III-10—are nonpenetrant. Each of these individuals has a child or grandchild with polydactyly; thus, each carries the dominant allele for polydactyly but is nonpenetrant for the condition. When nonpenetrant individuals are relatively common, the magnitude of frequency

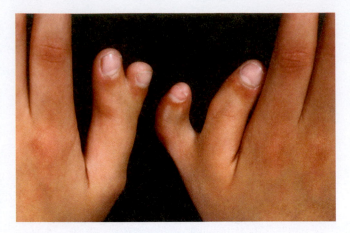

Figure 4.13 Polydactyly is an autosomal dominant trait with incomplete penetrance.

of penetrance can be quantified. Penetrance values vary between families, but for the family shown in Figure 4.14, the penetrance of polydactyly is $\frac{6}{9}$, or 66.7%, which is about the average seen worldwide among hundreds of families with polydactyly.

Variable Expressivity

Sometimes the discrepancy between genotype and phenotype is a matter of the degree or specific manifestation of expression of a trait rather than presence or absence of the trait altogether. In the phenomenon of **variable expressivity**, the same genotype produces phenotypes that vary in the degree or form of expression of the allele of interest.

Waardenburg syndrome is a human autosomal dominant disorder displaying variable expressivity. Individuals with Waardenburg syndrome may have any or all of four principal features of the syndrome: (1) hearing loss, (2) different-colored eyes, (3) a white forelock of hair, and (4) premature graying of hair. In the pedigree shown in **Figure 4.15**, notice that the circles and squares representing

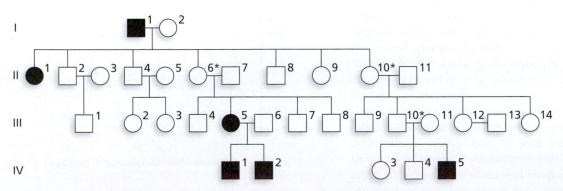

* Nonpenetrant individual

Figure 4.14 Incomplete penetrance for polydactyly. Three nonpenetrant individuals (II-6, II-10, and III-10) are seen in this family.

family members with Waardenburg syndrome may be entirely or only partly colored. Each quadrant of the symbols represents one of the principal features of the syndrome. The diversity of symbol darkening demonstrates the variation in expressivity of Waardenburg syndrome in this family. Molecular genetic analysis tells us that each family member with Waardenburg syndrome carries exactly the same dominant allele, yet among the six affected members of the family, there are five different patterns of phenotypic expression.

Pinpointing the cause of incomplete penetrance or variable expressivity is a challenging task. Three kinds of interactions may be responsible: (1) other genes that act in ways that modify the expression of the mutant allele, (2) environmental or developmental (i.e., nongenetic) factors that interact with the mutant allele to modify its expression, or (3) some combination of other genes and environmental factors interacting to modify expression of the mutation. Indeed, the characterization of a trait as having incomplete penetrance or variable expressivity is an acknowledgment that an as yet unknown factor is interacting with gene expression to produce variability in expressivity or to reduce penetrance.

Gene–Environment Interactions

Genes control innumerable differences between species. The genome of an organism lays out the body plan and biochemical pathways of the organism, and it controls the progress of development from conception to death. But genes alone are not responsible for all the variation seen between organisms. The environment—the myriad of physical substances, events, and conditions an organism encounters at different stages of life—is the other essential contributor to observable variation between organisms. **Gene–environment interaction** is the term describing the influence of environmental factors (i.e., nongenetic factors) on the expression of genes and on the phenotypes of organisms.

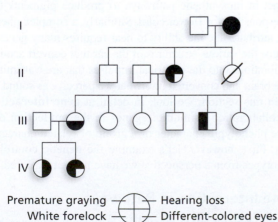

Figure 4.15 Variable expressivity of Waardenburg syndrome.

Premature graying — Hearing loss
White forelock — Different-colored eyes

What are the phenotypes of the two females in generation IV?

As an example, consider the tall and short pure-breeding lines of pea plants studied by Mendel. Inherited genetic variation dictates that one line will produce tall plants and the other line will produce short plants, but the environment in which the individual plants are grown also has a significant influence on plant height. Environmental factors such as variations in water, light, soil nutrients, and temperature each influence plant growth. It is not hard to imagine that genetically identical plants of a type adapted to temperate zones might grow to different heights if one plant has an ideal growth environment while the other faces a hot, arid environment with poor soil.

Phenotypic expression of genotypes can also depend on the interaction of genetically controlled developmental programs and external factors operating on organisms. For example, the seasonal change in coat color observed in arctic mammals that are nearly white in winter but have darker coats in spring and summer results from an interaction between numerous genes and external environmental cues such as day length and temperature. Similarly, environmental cues that induce plants to bloom in the spring trigger changes in gene expression that stimulate the growth and development of multiple plant structures, including flowers and reproductive structures. Such capacities to make seasonal changes evolved by aiding the survival of these organisms, and they suggest that gene–environment interaction is pivotal in understanding and interpreting phenotypic variation.

Environmental Modification to Prevent Hereditary Disease In some cases, the expression of a given gene is entirely dependent on the presence of certain environmental conditions. An example of this kind of gene–environment interaction—or, more precisely, an example of the manipulation of this relationship to achieve a desired outcome—is found in an element of the medical management that prevents development of the human autosomal recessive condition known as phenylketonuria (PKU) (OMIM 261600). PKU is caused by the absence of the enzyme phenylalanine hydroxylase (PAH), which catalyzes the first step of the pathway that breaks down the amino acid phenylalanine, a common component of dietary protein.

At one time, PKU accounted for thousands of cases of severe mental retardation every year. PKU occurred in 1 out of 10,000 to 1 out of 20,000 newborns in most populations around the world. Infants with PKU are normal at birth, but over the first several months of life the body's inability to carry out the normal breakdown of phenylalanine leads to the buildup of a compound that is toxic to developing neurons. As neurons die, mental and motor capacities are irretrievably lost, making full manifestation of PKU inevitable. In the 1960s, a simple blood test became available to detect PKU in the first days of life. The test identifies the disease before the disease has had a chance to manifest itself and begin to damage the body. PKU was among the first, and is now one of dozens of rare hereditary disorders for which newborn infants are routinely screened in U.S. hospitals and in hospitals around the world. The key feature shared by all of the hereditary diseases screened by newborn genetic testing is that the disease symptoms can be prevented or substantially reduced in severity by strict and consistent dietary management. Dietary control either prevents individuals from consuming compounds that allow the disease to develop, or it provides the essential compound missing in those with the disease. Application Chapter B (Human Genetic Screening) discusses newborn genetic testing.

The key dietary control for management of PKU is elimination of the amino acid phenylalanine from the diet. Phenylalanine is a component of almost all proteins, but a diet consisting of specially selected and processed proteins that have had phenylalanine removed is started as soon as PKU is diagnosed. This usually happens in the first hours or days after birth. An infant who is started on the phenylalanine-free diet soon after birth and kept on it through adolescence avoids the complications of PKU and will develop and function normally despite having PKU. Thousands of people with PKU are living fully normal and productive lives today, thanks to this simple environmental modification that prevents the expression of the devastating PKU phenotype. In this case, people who are homozygous recessive for the mutant PKU allele do not express the trait if they are raised in a largely phenylalanine-free environment.

Dietary hazards abound for children and young adults with PKU, particularly in the form of the artificial sweetener known as aspartame. This sweetener is made by a chemical reaction that fuses the amino acids phenylalanine and aspartic acid to form a compound we perceive to taste sweet. Once consumed, aspartame is quickly broken down into its two constituent amino acids, and phenylalanine is released. Regular intake of aspartame is dangerous for those with PKU; for this reason, a dietary caution reading "Phenylketonurics: Contains phenylalanine" appears on the packaging of food products containing aspartame. Look for it on the next artificially sweetened product you pick up!

Pleiotropic Genes

Pleiotropy is a phenomenon describing the alteration of multiple features of the phenotype by the presence of one mutation. It is distinguished from variable expressivity by the fact that variable expressivity affects one trait, whereas pleiotropy alters several aspects of the phenotype. Most mutations displaying pleiotropy do so either by altering the development of phenotypic features through the direct action of the mutant protein or as a secondary result of a cascade of problems stemming from the mutation.

Pleiotropy through the direct action of a mutant protein product is frequently encountered in studies of development. One example is the activity of the *Drosophila* hormone called juvenile hormone (JH), which is active throughout the *Drosophila* life cycle and influences numerous attributes of development and reproduction. Increased production or increased activity of JH has been shown to prolong developmental time, decrease adult body size, promote early sexual maturity, raise fecundity (the ability to produce offspring), and decrease life span. An evolutionary tradeoff is associated with changes in JH level or activity. On the one hand, producing more JH can lead to production of more offspring through earlier sexual maturity and higher fecundity. On the other hand, body size decreases and life span is shortened because of increased JH activity.

Pleiotropy in the human hereditary condition sickle cell disease (SCD) is an example of the phenotypically diverse secondary effects that can occur due to a mutant allele. SCD (OMIM 603903) is an autosomal recessive condition caused by mutation of the β-globin gene that, in turn, affects the structure and function of hemoglobin, the main oxygen-carrying molecule in red blood cells. Many of the red blood cells of people with SCD take on a sickle shape and cause numerous physical problems and complications (**Figure 4.16**).

4.3 Gene Interaction Modifies Mendelian Ratios

No gene operates alone to produce a phenotypic trait. Rather, genes work together to build the complex structures and organ systems of plants and animals. What we see as a phenotype is the physical manifestation of the action of many genes that have each played a role and have worked in complex but coordinated ways to produce a trait or structure. At the cellular and molecular levels, the mutual reliance of genes on one another requires each gene to carry out its activity in the right place, at the right time, and at the appropriate level.

Think of this process as analogous to a symphony orchestra playing a piece of classical music. The orchestra has many instruments and players, each with their own notes, tones, keys, and volume. If the players use their instruments as directed by the sheet music, the result will be smooth and harmonious. If, however, one musician is playing off-time or off-key, the error might disrupt the entire performance. The same can be said of genes: Each must play its part correctly— that is, give a wild-type performance—or the integrity of the trait will be at risk. For example, the products of several genes interact in biosynthetic pathways to produce pigments that are responsible for flower color. Similarly, a complex phenotypic attribute like the ability to hear requires many genes to produce the various structures of the ear that convert acoustical vibrations into the electrical impulses that are transmitted to the brain and converted into what we perceive as sound.

In this section, we look in detail at **gene interaction**, the collaboration of multiple genes in the production of a single phenotypic character or a group of related characteristics. First, however, let's examine the genetic control of phenotypes from a perspective we have not yet explored.

Gene Interaction in Pathways

Genes commonly work together in pathways, multistep biochemical processes that operate either as biosynthetic pathways, synthesizing complex compounds such as amino acids,

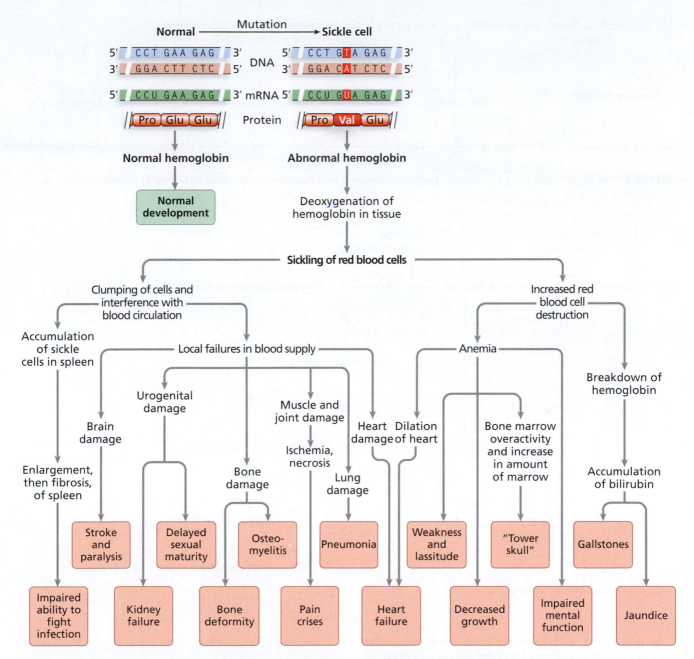

Figure 4.16 **Pleiotropy in sickle cell disease.** The sickling of red blood cells has a range of phenotypic consequences, due primarily to excessive red blood cell destruction and the reduced oxygen-delivery capacity in those with the disease.

or as degradation pathways, breaking complex compounds down into simpler or elemental constituents. Biosynthetic pathways result from the expression of genes whose products help build complex compounds or molecules that are the end product of the pathway. Through successive reaction steps that produce a series of intermediate compounds, these pathways—known broadly as anabolic pathways—lead ultimately to the production of an end product such as a pigment, amino acid, hormone, or nucleotide. The opposite process, the breakdown of compounds into intermediate compounds and often into elemental constituents, is undertaken by catabolic pathways.

An anabolic pathway that synthesizes the amino acid methionine is shown in **Figure 4.17a**. The production of methionine, the end product of the pathway, requires the expression of four genes that each produce an enzyme catalyzing a distinct step of the pathway. Homozygosity for a mutant allele of any of these genes can block the pathway and would prevent methionine synthesis.

The catabolic pathway that breaks down the amino acid phenylalanine is shown in **Figure 4.17b**. It, too, utilizes the enzyme products of multiple genes. The figure identifies several steps of the pathway that are blocked by mutations of

(a) In anabolic pathways the sequential action of gene products catalyzes steps of a biosynthesis.

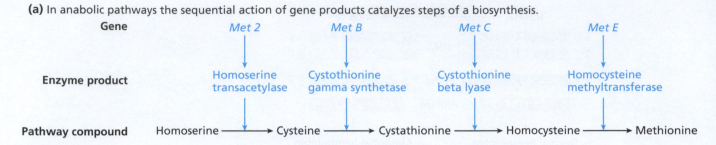

Gene   *Met 2*   *Met B*   *Met C*   *Met E*

Enzyme product   Homoserine   Cystothionine   Cystothionine   Homocysteine
                                        transacetylase   gamma synthetase   beta lyase   methyltransferase

Pathway compound   Homoserine ⟶ Cysteine ⟶ Cystathionine ⟶ Homocysteine ⟶ Methionine

(b) The action of gene products in catabolic pathways breaks down complex compounds into simpler compounds.

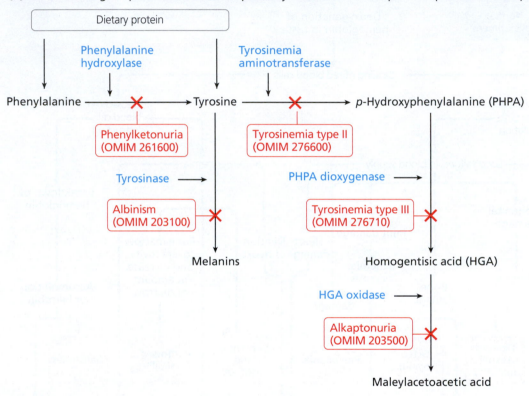

Figure 4.17   Gene action in pathways.

certain genes. Each of these mutations causes a distinct human hereditary disorder, including PKU that we just described.

In addition to biosynthetic (anabolic) pathways and catabolic pathways, other pathways such as *signal transduction pathways* and *developmental pathway* also feature the interaction of multiple genes in the production of a trait or characteristic. Signal transduction pathways are responsible for receiving a variety of chemical signals generated outside a cell and initiating a response inside a cell. Operating by way of hormones and other compounds, signal transduction pathways culminate in the activation or repression of gene expression in response to an intracellular or extracellular signal.

Developmental pathways direct the growth, development, and differentiation of body parts and structures. Researchers have discovered the functions of genes in numerous developmental pathways through experimental analyses of mutant phenotypes.

The One Gene–One Enzyme Hypothesis

The concept of pathways requiring gene action originated with Archibald Garrod's suggestion in 1902 that the inability to produce the enzyme homogentisic acid oxidase (HGA oxidase) is the cause of the autosomal recessive human hereditary condition known as alkaptonuria (see Figure 4.17b). It was not until the middle of the 20th century, however, that details of specific genetic pathways began to emerge. George Beadle and Edward Tatum were among the first to investigate biosynthetic pathways, in research that laid the groundwork for the later definition and examination of signal transduction and developmental pathways.

Beadle and Tatum's experiment studied growth variants of the fungus *Neurospora crassa,* and its details are described in **Experimental Insight 4.1**. The idea behind their experiment was simple—to generate single-gene growth mutations in *Neurospora* and interpret the normal function of genes by observing the phenotypic consequences of their mutation. The famous hereditary proposal known as the **one gene–one enzyme hypothesis** came out of this experiment. It says that each gene produces an enzyme, and each enzyme has a specific functional role in a biosynthetic pathway. Beadle and Tatum observed that single-gene mutations block the completion of biosynthetic pathways and lead to the production of mutant fungi that are deficient in their ability to grow without specific nutritional supplementation. Their hypothesis proposed that each mutant phenotype was attributable to the loss or defective function of a specific enzyme. The consequence of these enzyme losses or defects was the blockage of a biosynthetic pathway and the absence of the end product of the pathway. Since each enzyme defect was inherited as a single-gene defect, the one gene–one enzyme hypothesis identifies the direct connection between genes, proteins,

and phenotypes. Two new terms that are used multiple times in this section appear in Experimental Insight 4.1. The term **prototroph**, or **protrophic**, means "wild type" and derives from *prototype*, meaning "the original version." In contrast, the term **auxotroph**, or **auxotrophic**, means "mutant."

The one gene–one enzyme concept has undergone modifications since it was first proposed. These changes take account of three observations: (1) many protein-producing genes do not produce enzymes but produce transport proteins, structural proteins, regulatory proteins, or other non-enzyme proteins; (2) some genes produce RNAs rather than proteins; and (3) some proteins (e.g., β-globin) must join with other proteins to acquire a function. Despite these modifications, Beadle and Tatum's fundamental conclusion linking each gene to a particular product is valid and forms the basis for understanding gene function.

EXPERIMENTAL INSIGHT 4.1

The One Gene–One Enzyme Hypothesis

George Beadle and Edward Tatum's experiments had the goal of describing gene function. Their work took place at about the time DNA was being identified as the hereditary molecule, and more than a decade before DNA structure was identified. To provide information for analysis, Beadle and Tatum devised an experiment that would induce single-gene mutations in the filamentous fungus *Neurospora crassa* and then studied the mutants to determine how mutations altered *Neurospora* growth. They made use of the ability of *Neurospora* to either grow as a haploid or, alternatively, to propagate as two haploid cells that fuse to form and grow as diploids that undergo meiosis.

CREATION OF MUTANTS

To begin, Beadle and Tatum grew numerous genetically identical cultures of haploid wild-type fungi that were irradiated to induce random mutations (see step **1** of the accompanying illustration). The irradiated conidia (asexually produced fungal spores) were mated with wild-type haploids. The resulting diploids underwent meiosis to produce haploid spores that were grown in a two-step process to identify mutants. Irradiated diploids could also be tested to confirm the presence of a single-gene mutation by observation of a 1:1 ratio of wild types to mutants among their haploid spores. Beadle and Tatum started their screen for mutants by first growing fungi on a *complete growth medium* that contains a rich mixture of nutrients and supplements and is capable of supporting the growth of wild-type and mutant fungi **2**. Next, samples of the growing fungi were picked from colonies on the complete medium and transferred to a *minimal growth medium* that supplies only the minimal constituents needed to support the growth of wild-type fungi **3**. Mutant fungi are identified by the inability to grow on a minimal medium. Although they grow on complete medium containing many nutritional and other supplements that support the growth of mutant as well as wild-type fungi, their mutation prevents them from growing on a minimal growth medium that supplies only elemental constituents and supports the growth of wild-type fungi only.

ANALYSIS OF MUTANTS

With numerous mutants in hand, Beadle and Tatum were able to address questions of which genes were mutated by first identifying the biochemical category of the compound that the mutants could not produce and then determining the specific missing compound. An example of this analysis is illustrated in steps **4** and **5**, where growth analysis tests a mutant for its ability to grow on various kinds of *supplemented minimal media*. These are growth media that have had one or more compounds added to them to support the growth of specific kinds of mutants. Step **4** shows one mutant that grows only on medium that has been supplemented with all 20 of the common amino acids; this result indicates that the strain lacks the ability to synthesize one or more amino acids. The specific defect in this mutant strain is tested in step **5** using 20 different supplemented minimal media, each supplemented with one amino acid. The mutant grows on minimal medium supplemented with methionine (met), thus identifying the strain as one that is unable to synthesize methionine. This strain is described as being *met−* ("met minus" or "methionine minus"), to identify the defective pathway as the one synthesizing methionine. The wild type is able to synthesize methionine and is identified as *met+* ("met plus" or "methionine plus").

HYPOTHESIS OF GENE FUNCTION

By testing hundreds of independent mutants in this way, Beadle and Tatum discovered that most mutants carried single mutations that could be overcome by supplementing minimal growth media with one particular compound. In the above case, supplementing a minimal medium with methionine supports the growth of *met-* fungi. This finding led them to posit that single-gene mutations prevented mutants from completing a specific step of a biochemical pathway. Based on this outcome, they proposed that single-gene mutations altered the ability of mutants to produce one enzyme critical in a particular biosynthetic pathway. The correlation between single-gene mutations and single defects in biosynthetic pathways is the basis of the one gene–one enzyme hypothesis.

(continued)

EXPERIMENTAL INSIGHT 4.1 Continued

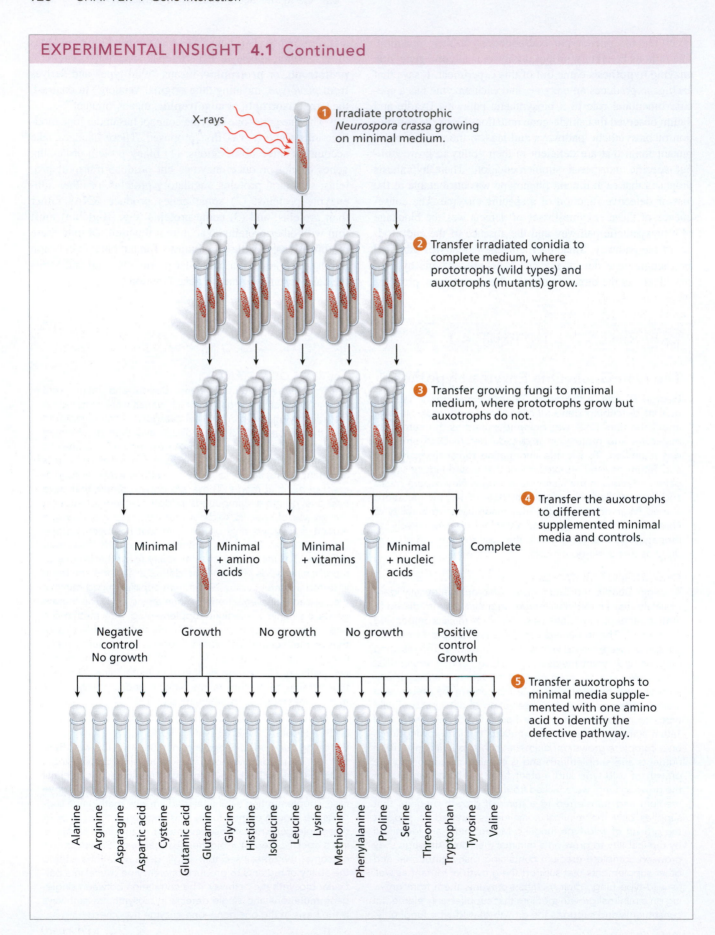

X-rays

1 Irradiate prototrophic *Neurospora crassa* growing on minimal medium.

2 Transfer irradiated conidia to complete medium, where prototrophs (wild types) and auxotrophs (mutants) grow.

3 Transfer growing fungi to minimal medium, where prototrophs grow but auxotrophs do not.

4 Transfer the auxotrophs to different supplemented minimal media and controls.

Minimal

Minimal + amino acids

Minimal + vitamins

Minimal + nucleic acids

Complete

Negative control No growth

Growth

No growth

No growth

Positive control Growth

5 Transfer auxotrophs to minimal media supplemented with one amino acid to identify the defective pathway.

Alanine
Arginine
Asparagine
Aspartic acid
Cysteine
Glutamic acid
Glutamine
Glycine
Histidine
Isoleucine
Leucine
Lysine
Methionine
Phenylalanine
Proline
Serine
Threonine
Tryptophan
Tyrosine
Valine

Genetic Dissection to Investigate Gene Action

Beadle and Tatum's experiments opened the way to investigation of the roles of individual-gene mutations in biosynthetic pathways. These investigations began with three assumptions about biosynthetic pathways that have proven to be correct: (1) Biosynthetic pathways consist of sequential steps, (2) completion of one step generates the substrate for the next step in the pathway, and (3) completion of every step is necessary for production of the end product of the pathway. These assumptions support the conclusion that wild-type strains are able to complete each pathway step, and that mutant strains are unable to complete a pathway because one or more pathway steps are blocked by mutation.

Genetic dissection in this context is an experimental approach that separately tests the ability of a mutant to execute each step of a biosynthetic pathway and assembles the steps of a pathway by determining the point at which the pathway is blocked in each mutant. The strategy of genetic dissection is illustrated for *met-* strain in **Figure 4.18** using experimental data collected in 1947 by Norman Horowitz on four independently isolated *Neurospora crassa met–* mutants.

The goals of Horowitz's genetic dissection analysis were to (1) determine the number of intermediate steps within the methionine biosynthetic pathway, (2) determine the order of steps in the pathway, and (3) identify the step affected by each mutation. In designing his experiment, Horowitz relied on previous biochemical work identifying homoserine as the first compound in the methionine biosynthetic pathway and identifying cysteine, homocysteine, and cystathionine as later intermediates in the pathway. Horowitz tested the control prototroph (*met+*) and four methionine-requiring auxotrophs (Met 1 to Met 4) for their ability to grow on (1) minimal medium, (2) minimal medium plus cysteine only, (3) minimal medium plus cystathionine only, (4) minimal medium plus homocysteine only, and (5) minimal medium plus methionine only. Figure 4.18a shows growth (+) or no growth (−) of the four *met−* mutants and the wild-type strain (*met+*) on each of the experimental media. The wild-type strain grows on all media, since supplementation of minimal medium with any

of the intermediates has no effect on its growth. Each methionine mutant grows on minimal medium plus methionine, the end product of the biosynthetic pathway, but they show different growth patterns with other supplemented media. The following is an analysis of each mutant:

1. Met 1 grows only on minimal medium plus methionine, thus indicating that a mutation in the last step of the pathway prevents conversion of the final intermediate product to methionine. Only the addition of methionine to minimal medium bypasses the pathway block.

2. Met 2 exhibits growth with supplementation by either methionine or homocysteine, thus indicating a block at the step that produces homocysteine. This result also tells us that homocysteine is the substrate converted to methionine in the biosynthetic pathway.

3. Met 3 grows on minimal medium supplemented with either methionine, homocysteine, or cystathionine, but not on minimal medium plus cysteine. This tells us that Met 3 is blocked at the step that produces cystathionine and that cystathionine precedes homocysteine in the pathway.

4. Met 4 grows with any supplementation of minimal medium. This tells us that Met 4 is defective at a step that precedes the production of cysteine.

Figure 4.18b shows the steps of the biosynthetic pathway for methionine as determined by analysis of these mutants. The pathway step that is blocked in the mutant is identified based on the logic that supplementation by a compound needed *after* the blockage will permit growth, whereas adding a compound used *before* the blockage will not aid growth. The blocked step is also identified by the substance that accumulates in the auxotroph: In each mutant, a different intermediate substance builds up because the step that would convert it to the next intermediate in the pathway is defective. Accumulation of cysteine by Met 3, cystathionine by Met 2, and homocysteine by Met 1 supports the assignment of these mutants to specific steps in the pathway. Genetic Analysis 4.2 illustrates genetic dissection of a biosynthetic pathway by assessment of the growth habits of auxotrophs.

(a) Experimental data

Mutant strain	Minimal medium	Minimal + cysteine	Minimal + cystathionine	Minimal + homocysteine	Minimal + methionine	Compound accumulating in mutant
Control prototroph	+	+	+	+	+	None
Met 1	−	−	−	−	+	Homocysteine
Met 2	−	−	−	+	+	Cystathionine
Met 3	−	−	+	+	+	Cysteine
Met 4	−	+	+	+	+	Homoserine

Growth Medium

(b) Order of intermediates in pathway

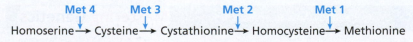

Figure 4.18 Genetic dissection of methionine biosynthesis pathway. (a) Growth of a wild-type strain and four independent *met−* mutant strains on minimal medium and various supplemented minimal media. For each mutant, the compound that accumulates is the one that immediately precedes the point of blockage. (b) The order of intermediate compounds in the methionine biosynthesis pathway and the step blocked in each *met−* mutant strain.

Why does homocysteine accumulate in Met 1, and why does only the addition of methionine lead to growth?

PROBLEM Four *zmt⁻* bacterial mutants (*zmt-1* to *zmt-4*), each with a single-gene mutation, are available for study. Five intermediates in the zmt-synthesis pathway have been identified (D, F, M, R, and S), but their order in the pathway is not known. Each mutant is tested for its ability to grow on minimal medium supplemented with one of the intermediate compounds. All mutants grow when zmt is added to minimal medium, and the wild-type strain grows under all growth conditions tested. Find the order of intermediates in the zmt-synthesis pathway, and identify the step that is blocked in each mutant strain. In the growth table at right, "+" indicates growth and "−" indicates no growth.

> **BREAK IT DOWN:** zmt is the pathway end product, and compounds D, F, M, R, S are intermediate compounds that precede zmt (p. 127).

Mutant Strain	Added to Minimal Medium						
	D	F	M	R	S	Nothing	zmt
Wild type	+	+	+	+	+	+	+
zmt-1	−	−	−	−	+	−	+
zmt-2	−	+	+	+	+	−	+
zmt-3	−	+	−	−	+	−	+
zmt-4	−	+	+	−	+	−	+

> **BREAK IT DOWN:** Growth on a supplemented minimal medium occurs if the medium provides a compound the mutant is unable to produce (p. 125).

Solution Strategies	Solution Steps
Evaluate	
1. Identify the topic of this problem and the kind of information the answer should contain.	1. This problem deals with mutants of the zmt-synthesis pathway and requires an analysis of the defect in each mutant as well as ordering of the intermediates in the zmt-synthesis pathway.
2. Identify the critical information given in the problem.	2. The problem provides growth information for wild-type *zmt⁺* bacteria as well as four *zmt⁻* mutant strains when plated on minimal medium and on media individually supplemented with zmt or one of five intermediates in the zmt-synthesis pathway.
Deduce	
3. Compare and evaluate the patterns of growth supported by the supplements. [TIP: A supplement that supports growth of all or most mutants is likely to be near the end of the pathway.]	3. All mutants grow with zmt supplementation and with supplementation by compound S. None grows without any supplementation, and none obtains growth support from compound D. Compounds F, M, and R each support growth of one or more mutants.
4. Identify the final product of the pathway and next-latest pathway intermediate compound.	4. The compound zmt is the final product of the pathway. Compound S also supports the growth of all mutants and is likely the immediate precursor of zmt.
Solve [TIP: A supplement supporting growth of the fewest mutants is likely to be at the beginning of the pathway.]	
5. Identify the first compound synthesized in the pathway.	5. Compound D does not support growth of any of the *zmt⁻* mutants and likely occurs before any of the synthesis steps affected by mutations. Compound D is the first compound shown in the pathway.
6. Identify the second, third, and fourth compounds synthesized in the pathway. [TIP: Medium supplemented with an intermediate compound that occurs after the pathway step blocked by a mutation will support growth.]	6. Compound R supports the growth of only one mutant, *zmt-2*, indicating the compound bypasses the step blocked in *zmt-2*. Compound R likely follows compound D in the pathway, and *zmt-2* is defective in its ability to convert D to R. *zmt-2* grows on intermediate compounds that occur after its point of pathway blockage, but not on compound D that comes before the *zmt-2* blockage.
	Compound M supports growth of *zmt-2* and *zmt-4*, bypassing the blockage in both mutants. Growth of *zmt-4* is not supported by compounds D or R that occur before the conversion step blocked in *zmt-4*. The conclusion is that compound M follows R and that *zmt-4* is unable to convert R to M. Compounds F, M, and S each support growth of *zmt-4*, so each bypasses the blockage.
[TIP: To confirm this solution, verify that growth of each mutant is supported by supplementation with compounds that follow the blockage but not by supplementation with compounds that precede the blockage.]	Compound F supports growth of *zmt-3* and follows compound M in the pathway. *zmt-3* is unable to convert M to F. Compound S supports new growth of *zmt-1*, indicating that it follows compound F in the pathway and that *zmt-1* fails to convert compound F to S.
7. Assemble the zmt-synthesis pathway, and identify the mutants at each pathway step.	7. zmt-2 zmt-4 zmt-3 zmt-1 D ⟶ R ⟶ M ⟶ F ⟶ S ⟶ zmt

For more practice, see Problems 4, 18 and 19.   Visit the Study Area to access study tools.   **Mastering Genetics**

Gene interaction:	None	Complementary	Duplicate	Dominant	Recessive epistasis	Dominant epistasis	Dominant supression
Phenotype ratio:	9:3:3:1	9:7	15:1	9:6:1	9:3:4	12:3:1	13:3
Genotype ratio $\frac{1}{16}$ AABB $\frac{2}{16}$ AaBB $\frac{2}{16}$ AABb $\frac{4}{16}$ AaBb	$\frac{9}{16}$ A–B–	$\frac{9}{16}$ A–B–	A–B–	$\frac{9}{16}$ A–B–	$\frac{9}{16}$ A–B–	A–B– $\frac{12}{16}$	$\frac{9}{16}$ A–B–
$\frac{1}{16}$ AAbb $\frac{2}{16}$ Aabb	$\frac{3}{16}$ A–bb	A–bb	$\frac{15}{16}$ A–bb	A–bb $\frac{6}{16}$	$\frac{3}{16}$ A–bb	A–bb	$\frac{3}{16}$ A–bb
$\frac{1}{16}$ aaBB $\frac{2}{16}$ aaBb	$\frac{3}{16}$ aaB–	$\frac{7}{16}$ aaB–	aaB–	aaB–	aaB– $\frac{4}{16}$	$\frac{3}{16}$ aaB–	aaB– $\frac{4}{16}$
$\frac{1}{16}$ aabb	$\frac{1}{16}$ aabb	aabb	$\frac{1}{16}$ aabb	$\frac{1}{16}$ aabb	aabb	$\frac{1}{16}$ aabb	aabb

FIGURE 4.19 Phenotype patterns in the F$_2$ of a dihybrid cross that result from epistatic gene interaction.

Epistasis and Its Results

Genes contributing to different steps of a multistep pathway work together to produce the pathway end product or outcome. Each gene is required to produce its normal product to achieve the wild-type (normal) outcome; thus, a mutation of any gene in the pathway can result in a failure of the pathway to be complete. Mutant phenotypes are the result of these pathway breakdowns. All the genes but one involved in a pathway can be normal, but the one mutant gene results in a mutation. In this context, gene interaction is the result of one gene influencing whether and how other pathway genes are expressed or how they function.

The discussion that follows describes certain alterations of the 9:3:3:1 phenotype ratios that may be seen in F$_2$ generations of dihybrid crosses when the mutant alleles belong to one or more multistep pathways. These patterns of altered phenotype ratios result from gene interaction phenomena known collectively as **epistasis**. We describe and illustrate six distinct patterns of **epistatic interactions** that result from different ways gene products may interact in pathways.

All six altered ratios resulting from epistatic interactions have been seen in plants or animals. **Figure 4.19** gives an overview of these patterns, showing the modification of dihybrid ratios that characterizes each form of epistasis. **Foundation Figure 4.21** provides a summary of the gene interactions, using the examples we explore below. In these six examples, each of the two interacting genes has a dominant and a recessive allele. As we describe the patterns, and as you examine Figure 4.21, notice that the epistatic ratios result from the merging of two or more of the F$_2$ phenotype categories as a consequence of the epistatic gene interaction.

First, however, we describe a dihybrid cross in which there is *no interaction* between the two genes in question, genes that both contribute to feather color in budgerigar parakeets (popularly known as "budgies"). The result is the 9:3:3:1 phenotypic ratio expected for the independent assortment of alleles of two genes.

No Interaction (9:3:3:1 Ratio) Epistasis is most easily identified through specific deviations from the expected 9:3:3:1 ratio

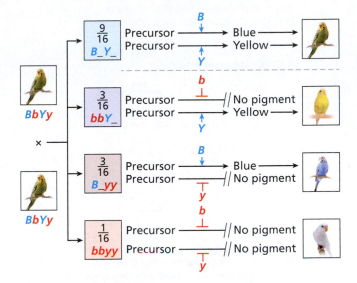

Figure 4.20 **No gene interaction in the production of feather color in budgerigar parakeets.** A 9:3:3:1 ratio results from the independent assortment of alleles in a dihybrid cross of green-feathered budgies with the dihybrid genotype *BbYy*.

among the F$_2$ progeny of a dihybrid cross involving dominant and recessive alleles. This "expected" F$_2$ ratio results from the action of two independently assorting genes *in the absence of epistasis*. Specific types of epistasis can be identified by the characteristic change in phenotypic ratio each produces.

As an example of no interaction between two genes, consider the feather color of the budgie. Two genes, *B* and *Y*, contribute to separate pigment-producing biosynthetic pathways that produce a blue pigment and a yellow pigment. Wild-type budgies have feathers that are green, a mixture of blue and yellow. Budgies are also found to have blue feathers (due to the absence of yellow pigment), yellow feathers (due to the lack of blue pigment), and white feathers (the absence of both pigments). Consider the mating of a pure-breeding blue budgie (*BByy*) to a pure-breeding yellow budgie (*bbYY*). The F$_1$ progeny have wild-type green feather color and are dihybrid (*BbYy*), and they are shown at the left in **Figure 4.20**, across from the F$_2$ progeny that have all

Epistatic Ratios in the F₂ Generation of Dihybrid Crosses.

❶ Complementary gene interaction

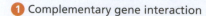

9:7

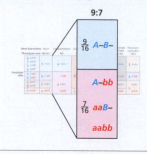

$\frac{9}{16}$ A–B–

A–bb

$\frac{7}{16}$ aaB–

aabb

Complementary gene interaction occurs when genes must act in tandem to produce a phenotype. The wild-type action from both genes is required to produce the wild-type phenotype. Mutation of one or both genes produces a mutant phenotype.

Example: sweet pea flower color

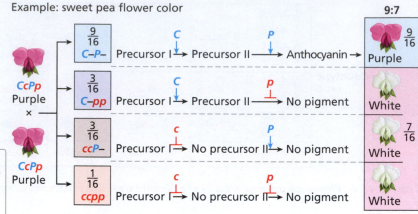

9:7

CcPp Purple × CcPp Purple

Genotype	Pathway	Phenotype	Ratio
$\frac{9}{16}$ C–P–	Precursor I $\xrightarrow{C}$ Precursor II $\xrightarrow{P}$ Anthocyanin →	Purple	$\frac{9}{16}$
$\frac{3}{16}$ C–pp	Precursor I $\xrightarrow{C}$ Precursor II $\xrightarrow{p}$ No pigment	White	
$\frac{3}{16}$ ccP–	Precursor I $\xrightarrow{c}$ No precursor II $\xrightarrow{P}$ No pigment	White	$\frac{7}{16}$
$\frac{1}{16}$ ccpp	Precursor I $\xrightarrow{c}$ No precursor II $\xrightarrow{p}$ No pigment	White	

❷ Duplicate gene action

15:1

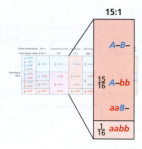

A–B–

$\frac{15}{16}$ A–bb

aaB–

$\frac{1}{16}$ aabb

Duplicate gene action allows dominant alleles of either duplicate gene to produce the wild-type phenotype. Only organisms with homozygous mutations of both genes have a mutant phenotype.

Example: bean flower color

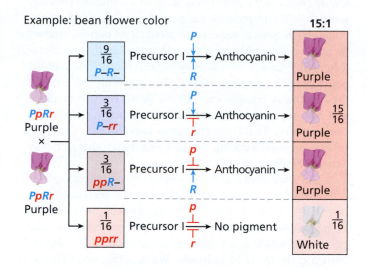

15:1

PpRr Purple × PpRr Purple

Genotype	Pathway	Phenotype	Ratio
$\frac{9}{16}$ P–R–	Precursor I $\xrightarrow[R]{P}$ Anthocyanin →	Purple	
$\frac{3}{16}$ P–rr	Precursor I $\xrightarrow[r]{P}$ Anthocyanin →	Purple	$\frac{15}{16}$
$\frac{3}{16}$ ppR–	Precursor I $\xrightarrow[R]{p}$ Anthocyanin →	Purple	
$\frac{1}{16}$ pprr	Precursor I $\xrightarrow[r]{p}$ No pigment	White	$\frac{1}{16}$

❸ Dominant gene interaction

9:6:1

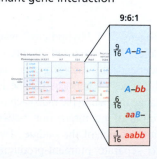

$\frac{9}{16}$ A–B–

A–bb

$\frac{6}{16}$ aaB–

$\frac{1}{16}$ aabb

Dominant gene interaction occurs between genes that each contribute to a phenotype, producing one phenotype if dominant alleles are present at each gene, a second phenotype if recessive alleles are homozygous for either gene, and a third phenotype if recessive homozygosity occurs at both genes.

Example: squash fruit shape

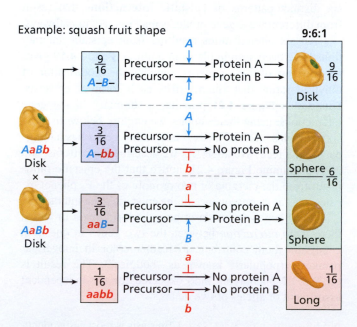

9:6:1

AaBb Disk × AaBb Disk

Genotype	Pathway	Phenotype	Ratio
$\frac{9}{16}$ A–B–	Precursor $\xrightarrow{A}$ Protein A → Precursor $\xrightarrow{B}$ Protein B →	Disk	$\frac{9}{16}$
$\frac{3}{16}$ A–bb	Precursor $\xrightarrow{A}$ Protein A → Precursor $\xrightarrow{b}$ No protein B	Sphere	$\frac{6}{16}$
$\frac{3}{16}$ aaB–	Precursor $\xrightarrow{a}$ No protein A Precursor $\xrightarrow{B}$ Protein B →	Sphere	
$\frac{1}{16}$ aabb	Precursor $\xrightarrow{a}$ No protein A Precursor $\xrightarrow{b}$ No protein B	Long	$\frac{1}{16}$

4 **Recessive epistasis**

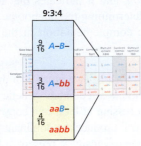

Recessive epistasis occurs when recessive alleles at one gene mask or reduce the expression of alleles at the interacting locus.

Example: labrador retriever coat color

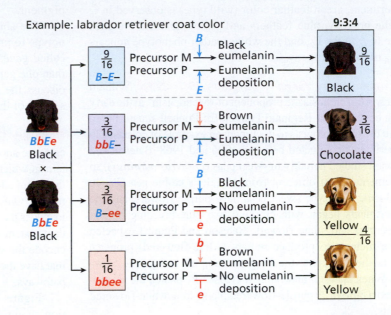

5 **Dominant epistasis**

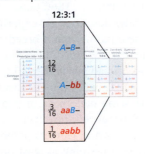

In dominant epistasis, a dominant allele of one gene masks or reduces the expression of alleles of a second gene.

Example: summer squash color

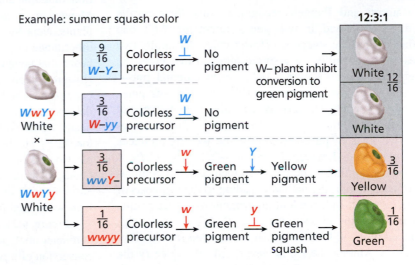

6 **Dominant suppression**

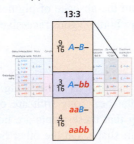

Dominant suppression occurs when the dominant allele of one gene suppresses the expression of alleles of a second gene.

Example: blue pimpernel flower color

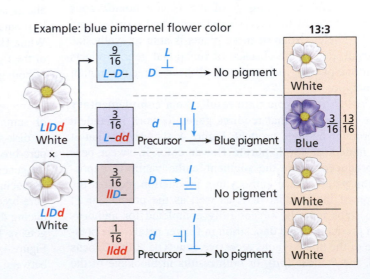

four feather-color phenotypes. As predicted by independent assortment, green feather color (wild type) is observed in $\frac{9}{16}$ of the progeny, blue feathers and yellow feathers are each seen in $\frac{3}{16}$ of the F_2, and the white-feather phenotype appears in $\frac{1}{16}$ of the F_2 progeny.

Complementary Gene Interaction (9:7 Ratio) William Bateson (an enthusiastic proponent of "Mendelism" in the early 20th century) and Reginald Punnett (of Punnett square fame) were the first biologists to document an example of epistasis, in experiments conducted between 1906 and 1908. Bateson and Punnett studied heredity in sweet peas (*Lathyrus odoratus*), an ornamental plant different from Mendel's edible pea (*Pisum sativum*). Wild-type sweet peas have purple flowers, and the experiments began with crossing two pure-breeding mutant plants that had white flowers. Bateson and Punnett expected these mutants to produce mutant (white-flowered) progeny, but to their surprise, the F_1 generation all had purple flowers. When Bateson and Punnett crossed F_1 plants, the F_2 produced a ratio of $\frac{9}{16}$ purple-flowered plants to $\frac{7}{16}$ white-flowered plants.

Bateson and Punnett recognized that their results could be explained if two genes interacted with one another to produce sweet pea flower color. Assuming two genes are responsible for a single pigment that gives the sweet pea flower its purple color, each parental line—represented by the genotypes *ccPP* and *CCpp*—is pure-breeding for white flowers as a result of homozygosity for recessive alleles at one of the genes. The cross of these two lines of pure-breeding white parents produces dihybrid purple-flowered F_2 plants—genotype *CcPp*—because the dominant allele at each locus enables completion of each step of the pathway leading to the synthesis of purple pigment. Independent assortment of alleles results in four genotypic classes, *C–P–*, *ccP–*, *C–pp*, and *ccpp*, produced in the 9:3:3:1 ratio that is expected from a dihybrid cross. Among the F_2, however, only the $\frac{9}{16}$ carry the *C–P–* genotype that confers the ability to produce purple pigment. The remaining $\frac{7}{16}$ of the F_2 are homozygous either for one of the recessive alleles *c* and *p* or for both sets of alleles. None of these plants is able to synthesize pigment, due to the absence of functional gene products from one or both loci, and they all have the same mutant phenotype.

A 9:7 phenotypic ratio results from **complementary gene interaction** that requires genes to work in tandem to produce a single product. Figure 4.21 ❶ shows that at the molecular level, purple flower color in sweet peas is produced when the pigment anthocyanin is deposited in petals. Since anthocyanin production requires the action of the product of *C* as well as the product of *P*, both steps must be successfully completed for anthocyanin production and deposition in flower petals. The presence of the homozygous recessive genotype at the *C* locus (*cc*), the *P* locus (*pp*), or both results in blockage of the

pathway and production of white flowers containing no pigment.

The ability of two mutants with the same mutant phenotype to produce progeny with the wild-type phenotype is called *genetic complementation*, and it indicates that more than one gene is involved in determining the phenotype. We discuss the details of genetic complementation in the last section of this chapter.

Duplicate Gene Action (15:1 Ratio) Two genes that duplicate one another's activity constitute a redundant genetic system in which any genotype possessing at least one copy of a dominant allele at *either* locus will produce the dominant phenotype. Only when recessive homozygosity is present at both loci does the recessive phenotype appear. The genes in a redundant system are said to have **duplicate gene action**; they either encode the same gene product, or they encode gene products that have the same effect in a single pathway or compensatory pathways.

Figure 4.21 ❷ provides an illustration and explanation of duplicate gene action identified inadvertently by Mendel in an experiment involving flower color in bean plants. Near the end of his famous 1866 paper describing inheritance in peas, Mendel described an experiment with beans that began with the cross of a pure-breeding purple-flowered bean plant to a pure-breeding white-flowered bean plant. The F_1 plants all had purple flowers, and Mendel probably assumed that flower color determination in beans would follow the same pattern as in peas. Among the 32 F_2 plants Mendel produced, however, 31 had purple flowers and only 1 had white flowers. Among the F_2 plants, $\frac{15}{16}$ have a genotype containing at least one copy of either *P* or *R*, and only $\frac{1}{16}$ have the genotype *pprr* and the white-flowered phenotype.

Figure 4.21 ❷ shows that the protein product of the dominant allele of either gene is capable of catalyzing the conversion of a precursor to anthocyanin and producing the dominant phenotype. Conversely, if homozygous recessive alleles are present at both loci, no functional gene product is produced, and the synthesis pathway is not completed. White flowers result from the absence of pigment in the $\frac{1}{16}$ of the F_2 progeny that are homozygous recessive for alleles of both genes.

Dominant Gene Interaction (9:6:1 Ratio) The shape of summer squash is classified as either long, spherical, or disk-shaped. Plants that bear long fruit are consistently pure-breeding, indicating that these plants are homozygous for genes controlling fruit shape. On the other hand, plants producing disk-shaped fruit or spherical fruit are sometimes pure-breeding and sometimes not, indicating that plants producing disk-shaped or spherical fruit can be either homozygous or heterozygous for the genes controlling their shape. Figure 4.21 ❸ illustrates and describes **dominant interaction** between two genes controlling squash fruit shape. Dominant interaction is characterized by a 9:6:1 ratio of phenotypes in the progeny of a dihybrid cross.

A cross of pure-breeding disk plants (*AABB*) to pure-breeding long plants (*aabb*) produces dihybrid F_1 plants with disk-shaped fruit. The F_2 progeny of these dihybrids are $\frac{9}{16}$ disk, $\frac{6}{16}$ spherical, and $\frac{1}{16}$ long, a 9:6:1 ratio. The phenotype of an F_2 plant depends on whether a dominant allele is present for both genes, one gene, or neither gene. The molecular model of fruit shape production assumes that each gene produces a distinct protein that contributes to fruit shape.

Recessive Epistasis (9:3:4 Ratio) Black, chocolate, and yellow coat colors in Labrador retrievers result from the interaction of two genes, one that produces pigment and another that distributes the pigment to hair follicles. This form of gene interaction, in which homozygosity for a recessive allele at one locus can mask the phenotypic expression of a second gene, is called **recessive epistasis** and has the characteristic 9:3:4 ratio of phenotypes illustrated by Figure 4.21 ❹.

Crossing pure-breeding chocolate to pure-breeding yellow dogs produces F_1 progeny with black coats. That the F_1 progeny are dihybrid is revealed by the F_2 generation, in which $\frac{9}{16}$ of the progeny carry the genotypes in the *B–E–* class and have black coats, $\frac{3}{16}$ have a genotype that is *bbE–*, resulting in chocolate-colored coats, and $\frac{4}{16}$ carry genotypes that are either *B–ee* or *bbee* and have yellow coats.

The molecular explanation for this genetic system is tied to production of the hair pigment melanin. Dogs can produce eumelanin that gives hair a black or brown color and pheomelanin that gives hair a reddish or yellowish tone. The *E* gene is *TYRP1* that controls eumelanin distribution. A single copy of the wild-type allele *E* yields full eumelanin deposition, but allele *e* homozygosity blocks deposition. Gene *B* is *MC1R* that controls eumelanin synthesis, with *B* producing a large amount of eumelanin that overwhelms the pheomelanin present to produce a black coat color. The alternative allele *b* produces a reduced amount of eumelanin. When mixed with pheomelanin in the coat, the resulting color is brown, sometimes called "chocolate." Dogs that are *B–E–* produce, transport, and deposit large amounts of eumelanin and have black coats. Dogs that are *bbE_* produce less eumelanin due to their *bb* genotype and have chocolate (brown) coats. Dogs that are homozygous *ee* are unable to transport and deposit eumelanin and instead deposit only pheomelanin. These dogs have yellow coat color.

Dominant Epistasis (12:3:1 Ratio) Determination of fruit color in summer squashes provides an example of **dominant epistasis**. In this type of epistatic interaction, the dominant allele of one gene blocks the expression of alleles of the second gene. Summer squash occur in three colors: white, yellow, and green. In Figure 4.21 ❺, the cross of dihybrid *WwYy* (white) plants yields a 12:3:1 ratio of white:yellow:green plants. Plants with one or two copies of *W*—that is, *W–Y–* (9/16) and *W–yy* (3/16)—produce white

squash due to the inhibition of conversion of the colorless precursor compound to green pigment. The protein products of the *Y* gene require a pigment substrate for their action, and because plants that are *W–* do not produce a substrate, the action of the protein products of alleles of the *Y* gene does not occur. Plants that are homozygous *ww* are able to convert the colorless precursor to green pigment, yielding substrate for *Y* gene activity. The dominant allele of the *Y* gene produces an enzyme that converts green pigment to yellow pigment. Homozygosity for the recessive allele (*yy*) leaves the green pigment unaltered and green squash are produced. Notice that in *ww* plants, segregation of *Y* gene alleles in a cross of *Yy* monohybrids produces a 3:1 ratio of *Y–* (yellow) and *yy* (green) squash. This ratio can be seen by looking at plants that are *wwY–* $\left(\frac{3}{16}\right)$ and *wwyy* $\left(\frac{1}{16}\right)$.

Dominant Suppression (13:3 Ratio) Our final example of epistatic gene interaction is **dominant suppression**, illustrated in Figure 4.21 ❻. In dominant suppression, the dominant allele of one gene suppresses expression of the other gene. In the blue pimpernel plant, production of the blue flower pigment is controlled by the *L* gene. Plants that are *L–* are capable of producing blue pigment, whereas those that are *ll* produce no pigment and are white. A second gene, *D*, has a dominant allele that suppresses the expression of the *L* gene; thus, plants that are *D–* are white regardless of the *L* gene genotype, because the *D* allele controls *L* gene expression. Plants that are *dd* allow *L* gene expression. Crosses between pure-breeding blue-flowered plants (*LLdd*) and pure-breeding white flowered plants (*llDD*) produce white-flowered F_1 that are dihybrid (*LlDd*), and the F_2 have a 13:3 ratio that is characteristic of dominant suppression. Flowers that are *L–D–* are white because the dominant *D* allele suppresses *L* gene expression. Plants that are *L–dd* are blue because the *L* gene is not suppressed and the *L* allele catalyzes pigment production. Plants that are *llD–* are white due to the presence of *D* and the inability of recessive *ll* plants to produce pigment. Lastly, plants that are *lldd* are white due to the inability of *ll* plants to produce pigment.

Genetic Analysis 4.3 tests your ability to analyze crosses involving epistatic gene interaction.

4.4 Complementation Analysis Distinguishes Mutations in the Same Gene from Mutations in Different Genes

Suppose you are a geneticist working in California and you have identified a recessive mutation causing petunia flowers to be white rather than the wild-type purple color. A friend of yours, also a geneticist, is working on petunias in the Netherlands and contacts you because she has also

PROBLEM Dr. Ara B. Dopsis, a famous plant geneticist, decides to try his hand at iris propagation. He selects two pure-breeding irises, one red and the other blue, and crosses them. To his surprise, all F1 plants have purple flowers. He decides to create more purple irises by self-fertilizing the F_1 irises. Dr. Dopsis produces 320 F_2 plants consisting of 182 with purple flowers, 59 with blue flowers, and 79 with red flowers.

> BREAK IT DOWN: Neither red nor blue is dominant (p. 135).

> BREAK IT DOWN: Examine the ratio of progeny phenotypes carefully to propose a mechanism of inheritance (p. 133).

a. From the information available, identify the genetic phenomenon that produces the phenotypic ratio observed in the F_2 plants. Include the number of genes that are involved in this trait.

b. Using clearly defined symbols of your own choosing, identify the genotypes of parental and F_1 plants.

Solution Strategies	Solution Steps
Evaluate	
1. Identify the topic this problem addresses and describe the nature of the required answer.	1. This problem concerns the interpretation of F_1 and F_2 results; it requires identification of the genetic mechanism responsible for the observed results, and the assignment of genotypes to parental and F_1 plants in a manner consistent with the genetic mechanism.
2. Identify the critical information given in the problem.	2. The problem states that the blue- and red-flowered parents are pure-breeding and that their F_1 are exclusively purple flowered. Among the F_2, purple is predominant, but red and, to a lesser extent, blue are also observed.
Deduce	
3. Deduce the potential genetic mechanisms that could account for producing purple-flowered F_1 plants from the pure-breeding red and blue parental plants.	3. Two potential mechanisms are suggested by these data. First, a single gene with incomplete dominance might generate a phenotype in F_1 heterozygous plants that is different from that of either homozygous parent. Second, two genes displaying an epistatic interaction might account for a phenotype in an F_1 dihybrid that is distinct from either pure-breeding parent.
4. Determine the relative phenotype proportions predicted by the possible genetic mechanisms and compare them with the observed phenotype ratio.	4. A single-gene model predicts that the self-fertilization of an F_1 heterozygote will result in a 1:2:1 (25%:50%:25%) ratio in the F_2. A two-gene epistasis model producing three F_2 phenotypes could be dominant gene interaction (9:6:1 ratio), dominant epistasis (12:3:1 ratio), or recessive epistasis (9:4:3 ratio). Recessive epistasis predictions are a closer match to the observations than dominant epistasis predictions. Recessive epistasis predicts phenotype percentages of approximately 56%:25%:19%. The observed ratio of F_2 phenotypes is $\frac{182}{320} = 56.8\%$ purple, $\frac{79}{320} = 24.7\%$ red, and $\frac{59}{320} = 18.4$ blue.

TIP: Compare the relative percentages of each phenotype to see which genetic model most closely predicts the observed percentages.

Solve	Answer a
5. Identify the genetic mechanism most likely to account for the outcomes of these crosses.	5. Comparison of the F_2 predictions of the single-gene incomplete dominance model and the two-gene recessive epistasis model determines that recessive epistasis is a better match with the relative progeny proportions. The likely genetic model explaining these data is recessive epistasis. (For confirmation, the number of F_2 observed in each category can be compared with the number expected by chi-square analysis.)

TIP: See Foundation Figure 4.21 for the phenotype ratios characteristic of each type of epistatic interaction.

Answer b

6. Assign genotypes to parental and F_1 plants.

TIP: Foundation Figure 4.21 identifies genotypes associated with each phenotype.

6. Using symbols A and a for one gene and B and b for the second gene, the genotypes of plants are

Parents: $aaBB$ (red) and $AAbb$ (blue)

F_1: $AaBb$ (purple).

For more practice, see Problems 5, 10, and 22.   Visit the Study Area to access study tools.   **Mastering** Genetics

identified a recessive mutation resulting in white-flowered petunias. Since there has been no contact between California petunias and Netherland petunias, the mutations have arisen independently. When geneticists encounter organisms with the same mutant phenotype, two initial questions are (1) do these organisms have mutations on the same gene or on different genes, and (2) how many genes are responsible for the mutations observed?

Mutations of different genes can produce the same, or very similar, abnormal phenotypes. This phenomenon is known as **genetic heterogeneity**, and several examples have been seen in this chapter. For example, in a multistep pathway whose end point is the production of a pigment that colors flower petals, it is possible that a mutation of any of the genes in the pathway could block production of the pigment and produce mutant flower color. In this section, we discuss **genetic complementation analysis**, an experimental analysis of crosses designed to test alternative genetic explanations of an abnormal phenotype. The results of genetic complementation analysis can determine whether mutant organisms carry mutations of different genes that produce the abnormal phenotype or if the abnormal phenotype occurs due to allelic mutations on the same gene.

Genetic complementation testing is done by crossing pure-breeding mutants for a recessive mutation and observing the phenotype of F_1 progeny. If the F_1 progeny have the wild-type phenotype, genetic complementation has occurred, and the conclusion is that the mutant alleles are of different genes. On the other hand, if the mutant alleles are of the same gene, the progeny of two pure-breeding mutants will have a mutant phenotype. This result indicates that no genetic complementation has taken place.

Let's look at an example using two genes we identified in Figure 4.21. In discussing complementary gene interaction, we described production of the purple-colored pigment anthocyanin as requiring the action of dominant alleles of the C gene and the P gene. **Figure 4.22** shows three crosses involving four pure-breeding white-flower mutants. Cross 1, between mutant A and mutant B, produces F_1 progeny that have wild-type purple flowers. The genetic interpretation of this result is that genetic complementation is observed. Genotypes given for each

mutant indicate homozygosity for recessive alleles on different genes in the parents and a dihybrid genotype in the F_1. In contrast to this result, Cross 2 and Cross 3 are also made using pure-breeding white-flower parentals. In both crosses, however, the F_1 have the mutant phenotype. This indicates that there is no genetic complementation and that the mutant parents in the respective crosses carry mutations on the same gene. Cross 2 illustrates mutant parental plants that are homozygous for the C gene ($ccPP$), and cross 3 illustrates mutant parental plants for gene P ($CCpp$).

Genetic complementation analyses using numerous crosses of different pure-breeding mutants can determine which mutants represent mutations of a certain gene, which represent mutations of certain other genes, and how many different mutant genes are represented in a group of mutants. A genetic complementation table organizing each of the crosses made to test genetic complementation of nine different mutations of eye color in the fruit fly *Drosophila* is shown in **Figure 4.23**. Crosses of pure-breeding parental eye color mutants that produce wild-type eye color in F_1 progeny are indicated by plus symbols ($+$), signaling genetic complementation (i.e., mutations in different genes). Parental crosses producing mutant F_1 are indicated by minus symbols ($-$), signaling no genetic complementation (i.e., mutations in the same gene).

Complementation analysis of this type initially focuses on crosses that indicate *no complementation*, as this is a sign of mutations that are in the same gene. Mutations that mutually fail to complement one another are identified as a **complementation group**, which can consist of one or more mutant alleles of a single gene. All members of a complementation group will fail to complement other members of the group, but they will complement members of other complementation groups that represent mutations of other genes. In the genetic context, a "complementation group" is synonymous with a "gene" because the mutant alleles of each complementation group all affect the same phenotypic characteristic. Thus, in genetic complementation analysis, the number of complementation groups equals the number of genes.

Assessment of the complementation testing data in Figure 4.23 finds that apricot, buff, cherry, coral, and white

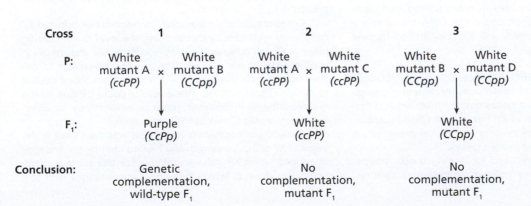

Cross	1		2		3	
P:	White mutant A ($ccPP$)	× White mutant B ($CCpp$)	White mutant A ($ccPP$)	× White mutant C ($ccPP$)	White mutant B ($CCpp$)	× White mutant D ($CCpp$)
F₁:		Purple ($CcPp$)		White ($ccPP$)		White ($CCpp$)
Conclusion:		Genetic complementation, wild-type F₁		No complementation, mutant F₁		No complementation, mutant F₁

Figure 4.22 Genetic complementation analysis. Four pure-breeding white flower mutants (A–D) are crossed in three crosses (1–3) to test genetic complementation. Cross 1 shows genetic complementation, whereas Crosses 2 and 3 do not.

Mutation	Apricot	Brown	Buff	Carnation	Cherry	Claret	Coral	Vermilion	White
Apricot	−	+	−	+	−	+	−	+	−
Brown		−	+	+	+	+	+	+	+
Buff			−	+	+	−	+	+	−
Carnation				−	+	+	+	+	+
Cherry					−	+	−	+	−
Claret						−	+	+	+
Coral							−	+	−
Vermilion								−	+
White									−

Complementation group	Mutant (allele)
I	Apricot (w^a), buff (w^b), cherry (w^{ch}), coral (w^{co}), white (w)
II	Carnation (c)
III	Claret (cl)
IV	Brown (b)
V	Vermilion (v)

Figure 4.23 Genetic complementation analysis of *Drosophila* eye color mutants. Genetic complementation testing among nine distinct *Drosophila* eye color mutants reveals five complementation groups corresponding to five genes. Five mutant alleles of *white* mutually fail to complement and are assigned to the same gene. The other four mutants each complement one another and the *white* gene mutants and are assigned to their own gene. Complementation is indicated by "+" and no complementation by "−."

If a tenth eye color mutation fails to complement carnation but complements the other eight mutations, into which group is it placed?

all exhibit a mutual failure to complement. This result identifies the five mutations as occurring in the same gene. The conclusion is that apricot, buff, cherry, coral, and white are mutant alleles of the *white* (*w*) gene in *Drosophila*. These mutations form complementation group I. In contrast, the mutations brown, carnation, claret, and vermilion each complement all other mutations. This observation tells investigators that each of these mutant alleles represents a separate gene. In other words, because each of these mutants complements mutants of group I (gene *w*), they are not mutations of gene *w*. Further, the mutations carnation, claret, brown, and vermillion all complement one another, thus each represents

a mutation of a gene of its own (i.e., complementation groups II through V). Therefore, among the nine *Drosophila* eye color mutants examined, five genes (five complementation groups) are identified. One gene is represented by five mutants, and the other four genes are represented by one mutation each.

Genetic complementation analysis is an important tool of genetic analysis. The rare human cancer-prone disorder xeroderma pigmentosum (various OMIM designations) can result from inherited mutations of any of seven genes that were originally identified by genetic complementation analysis. The following Case Study outlines this analysis.

CASE STUDY

Complementation Groups in a Human Cancer-Prone Disorder

In this case study, we examine the use of genetic complementation analysis to identify the number of genes involved in a rare human cancer-prone condition called xeroderma pigmentosum (XP). XP is characterized by severe sensitivity to ultraviolet (UV) irradiation from sunlight and by an increase of up to a thousandfold in the rate of sun-induced skin cancer.

People with XP are deficient in a type of DNA damage repair called nucleotide excision repair (NER), one of the normal processes the body uses to repair UV-induced damage in DNA. In NER, a short section of DNA containing a UV-induced lesion is removed, and the gap is filled by new DNA (see Section 11.5).

COMPLEMENTATION GROUPS Research work that began in the late 1970s identified seven complementation groups representing seven different genes that are mutated in different forms of XP. Each form of XP has its own OMIM number, and the forms differ in their severity and clinical presentation as a result of these different mutant genes.

Two approaches were used to identify these groups. Anthony Andrews and his colleagues obtained cultured

skin cells from XP patients and from normal controls and tested the ability of the cells to grow after exposure to measured doses of UV irradiation (**Figure 4.24**). The cells were exposed to UV light for different amounts of time, and their growth was measured as the percentage of original cells able to form colonies after UV exposure. These researchers identified five distinct patterns of response to UV exposure that are designated as complementation groups A to E.

Other researchers measured the response of cultured XP cells to UV exposure by determining the level of NER taking place in XP cell cultures taken from different XP individuals in comparison with normal cells. The results showed that XP cell lines vary in their levels of NER from less than 5% of normal to about 50% of normal. These results could be due to the mutations being in different genes or, alternatively, to different hypomorphic alleles of the same gene.

Genetic complementation analysis was then used in the study of XP cell cultures with low NER to identify cell lineages carrying different XP gene mutations. For this analysis, many tests were done in which two cells from lineages with low

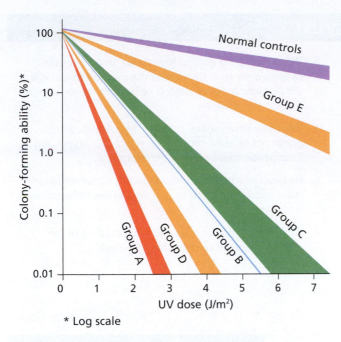

Figure 4.24 **Growth of cultured cells from patients with xeroderma pigmentosum (XP).** Five XP complementation groups are identified based on growth ability.

NER were fused to form a heterokaryon, a hybrid cell with two nuclei. A heterokaryon contains all the genetic information from both contributing cells. The experimental rationale is that if the two cells contain mutations of different genes, the heterokaryon will experience genetic complementation that would be detected as normal or near normal levels of NER; but if the mutations are in the same gene, NER will be about the same in the heterokaryon as in the individual cell lines. This analysis of NER levels in XP heterokaryons ultimately indicated seven complementation groups of XP genes.

ASSOCIATED GENE FUNCTIONS In the last decade or so, each of the seven XP-associated genes has had its function identified and its position mapped in the human genome. Four of the genes produce proteins that are required to remove a segment of the strand of DNA damaged by UV irradiation as part of the DNA repair process. Proteins from two other XP-associated genes are required to recognize UV-induced DNA damage, and the seventh gene produces a protein that binds to the DNA lesion once it is located. This information concerning the identities of seven XP-associated genes has led in turn to the discovery that other cancer-associated hereditary diseases also involve mutations of one or another of the XP-associated genes.

SUMMARY   Mastering Genetics   For activities, animations, and review quizzes, go to the Study Area.

4.1 Interactions between Alleles Produce Dominance Relationships

- Loss-of-function mutations decrease or eliminate gene activity. Gain-of-function mutations can cause overexpression or result in new functions.
- Incomplete dominance produces heterozygotes with phenotypes that differ from those of either homozygote but are closer to one homozygous phenotype than the other.
- Codominant alleles are both detected in the heterozygous phenotype.
- The levels of activities of allelic products and their effects on phenotypes determine the dominance relationship between alleles.
- ABO blood types are produced by alleles whose protein products produce dominance or codominance depending on the genotype.
- Multiple alleles of a single gene can display a variety of dominance relationships that establish an allelic series.
- Lethal alleles can kill gametes, can prevent the gestational development of certain classes of progeny, or can have their lethal effect later in life.

4.2 Some Genes Produce Variable Phenotypes

- Sex-limited and sex-influenced traits are expressed differently in the sexes due to the influences of hormones.
- In incomplete penetrance, a genotype does not always have the expected corresponding phenotype.

- In variable expressivity, organisms with the same genotype have different degrees of phenotypic expression.
- Pleiotropic mutations affect two or more distinct and seemingly independent attributes of the phenotype.

4.3 Gene Interaction Modifies Mendelian Ratios

- Epistasis is revealed by six alternative ratios that are modifications of the 9:3:3:1 ratio expected among the progeny of a dihybrid cross.
- The types of epistasis and their ratios are complementary gene interaction (9:7), duplicate gene action (15:1), dominant gene interaction (9:6:1), recessive epistasis (9:3:4), dominant epistasis (12:3:1), and dominant suppression (13:3).

4.4 Complementation Analysis Distinguishes Mutations in the Same Gene from Mutations in Different Genes

- Genetic complementation produces progeny with the wild-type phenotype from parents that are pure-breeding for similar mutant phenotypes. The detection of genetic complementation means the mutations occur in different genes.
- The failure to detect genetic complementation from the cross of two similar mutant organisms identifies the mutant alleles as being carried by the same gene.

PREPARING FOR PROBLEM SOLVING

In addition to the list of problem-solving tips and suggestions given here, you can go to the Study Guide and Solutions Manual that accompanies this book for help at solving problems.

1. Dominance relationships between the alleles of a gene are determined by the activity of the allelic gene products. Do not assume the mutations are always recessive. Instead, use the transmission pattern to determine the dominance relationships of alleles to one another.

2. Genes determine phenotypes by the sequential action of their gene products in multistep pathways. Usually, one step must be completed before the next step can occur. Fit genetic data to molecular models of pathways.

3. When building a genetic hypothesis, use the results of genetic crosses. Begin with the simplest model and devise more complex models only when the data do not fit a simpler model.

4. Once you have formed a genetic hypothesis, assign genotypes or make predictions about phenotypes and their frequencies based on the hypothesis.

5. Be familiar with the ratios commonly observed in epistatic interactions, and be prepared to use those ratios to interpret the results of crosses.

6. Be familiar with the rules and interpretation of the results of genetic complementation analysis.

PROBLEMS

Mastering **Genetics** Visit for instructor-assigned tutorials and problems.

Chapter Concepts

For answers to selected even-numbered problems, see Appendix: Answers.

1. Define and distinguish *incomplete penetrance* and *variable expressivity*.

2. Define and distinguish *epistasis* and *pleiotropy*.

3. When working on barley plants, two researchers independently identify a short-plant mutation and develop homozygous recessive lines of short plants. Careful measurements of the height of mutant short plants versus normal tall plants indicate that the two mutant lines have the same height. How would you determine if these two mutant lines carry mutation of the same gene or of different genes?

4. Fifteen bacterial colonies growing on a complete medium are transferred to a minimal medium. Twelve of the colonies grow on minimal medium.
   a. Using terminology from the chapter, characterize the 12 colonies that grow on minimal medium and the 3 colonies that do not.
   b. The three colonies that do not grow on minimal medium are transferred to minimal medium supplemented with the amino acid serine (min + Ser), and all three colonies grow. Characterize these three colonies.
   c. The serine biosynthetic pathway is a three-step pathway in which each step is catalyzed by the enzyme product of a different gene, identified as enzymes A, B, and C in the diagram below.

3-Phosphoglycerate $\xrightarrow{\text{Enzyme A}}$ 3-Phospho-hydroxypyruvate $\xrightarrow{\text{Enzyme B}}$
(3-PHP)

3-Phosphoserine $\xrightarrow{\text{Enzyme C}}$ Serine
(3-PS)   (Ser)

Mutant 1 grows only on min + Ser. In addition to growth on min + Ser, mutant 2 also grows on min + 3-PHP and min + 3-PS. Mutant 3 grows on min + 3-PS and min + Ser. Identify the step of the serine biosynthesis pathway at which each mutant is defective.

5. In a type of parakeet known as a "budgie," feather color is controlled by two genes. A yellow pigment is synthesized under the control of a dominant allele Y. Budgies that are homozygous for the recessive y allele do not synthesize yellow pigment. At an independently assorting gene, the dominant allele B directs synthesis of a blue pigment. Recessive homozygotes with the bb genotype do not produce blue pigment. Budgies that produce both yellow and blue pigments have green feathers; those that produce only yellow pigment or only blue pigment have yellow or blue feathers, respectively; and budgies that produce neither pigment are white (albino).
   a. List the genotypes for green, yellow, blue, and albino budgies.
   b. A cross is made between a pure-breeding green budgie and a pure-breeding albino budgie. What are the genotypes of the parent birds?
   c. What are the genotype(s) and phenotype(s) of the F_1 progeny of the cross described in part (b)?
   d. If F_1 males and females are mated, what phenotypes are expected in the F_2, and in what proportions?
   e. The cross of a green budgie and a yellow budgie produces offspring that are 12 green, 4 blue, 13 yellow, and 3 albino. What are the genotypes of the parents?

6. The ABO and MN blood groups are shown for four sets of parents (1 to 4) and four children (a to d). Recall that the ABO blood group has three alleles: I^A, I^B, and i. The MN blood group has two codominant alleles, M and N. Using

your knowledge of these genetic systems, match each child with every set of parents who might have conceived the child, and exclude any parental set that could not have conceived the child.

	Mother		Father	
	ABO	MN	ABO	MN
1	O	M	B	M
2	B	N	B	N
3	AB	MN	B	MN
4	A	N	B	MN

	Children	
	ABO	MN
a	B	M
b	O	M
c	AB	MN
d	B	N

7. The wild-type color of horned beetles is black, although other colors are known. A black horned beetle from a pure-breeding strain is crossed to a pure-breeding green female beetle. All of their F_1 progeny are black. These F_1 are allowed to mate at random with one another, and 320 F_2 beetles are produced. The F_2 consists of 179 black, 81 green, and 60 brown. Use these data to explain the genetics of horned beetle color.

8. Two genes interact to produce various phenotypic ratios among F_2 progeny of a dihybrid cross. Design a different pathway explaining each of the F_2 ratios below, using hypothetical genes R and T and assuming that the dominant allele at each locus catalyzes a different reaction or performs an action leading to pigment production. The recessive allele at each locus is null (loss-of-function). Begin each pathway with a colorless precursor that produces a white or albino phenotype if it is unmodified. The ratios are for F_2 progeny produced by crossing wild-type F_1 organisms with the genotype $RrTt$.
   a. $\frac{9}{16}$ dark blue : $\frac{6}{16}$ light blue : $\frac{1}{16}$ white
   b. $\frac{12}{16}$ white : $\frac{3}{16}$ green : $\frac{1}{16}$ yellow
   c. $\frac{9}{16}$ green : $\frac{3}{16}$ yellow : $\frac{3}{16}$ blue : $\frac{1}{16}$ white
   d. $\frac{9}{16}$ red : $\frac{7}{16}$ white
   e. $\frac{15}{16}$ black : $\frac{1}{16}$ white
   f. $\frac{9}{16}$ black : $\frac{3}{16}$ gray : $\frac{4}{16}$ albino
   g. $\frac{13}{16}$ white : $\frac{3}{16}$ green

9. The ABO blood group assorts independently of the Rhesus (Rh) blood group and both assort independently of the MN blood group. Three alleles, I^A, I^B, and i, occur at the ABO locus. Two alleles, R, a dominant allele producing Rh+, and r, a recessive allele for Rh−, are found at the Rh locus, and codominant alleles M and N occur at the MN locus. Each gene is autosomal.
   a. A child with blood types A, Rh−, and M is born to a woman who has blood types O, Rh−, and MN and a

man who has blood types A, Rh+, and M. Determine the genotypes of each parent.
   b. What proportion of children born to a man with genotype $I^A I^B\ Rr\ MN$ and a woman who is $I^A i\ Rr\ NN$ will have blood types B, Rh−, and MN? Show your work.
   c. A man with blood types B, Rh+, and N says he could not be the father of a child with blood types O, Rh−, and MN. The mother of the child has blood types A, Rh+, and MN. Is the man correct? Explain.

10. In rats, gene B produces black coat color if the genotype is $B-$, but black pigment is not produced if the genotype is bb. At an independent locus, gene D produces yellow pigment if the genotype is $D-$, but no pigment is produced when the genotype is dd. Production of both pigments results in brown coat color. If neither pigment is produced, coat color is cream. Determine the genotypes of parents of litters with the following phenotype distributions.
   a. 4 brown, 4 black, 4 yellow, 4 cream
   b. 3 brown, 3 yellow, 1 black, 1 cream
   c. 9 black, 7 brown

11. In the rats identified in Problem 10, a third independently assorting gene involved in determination of coat color is the C gene. At this locus, the genotype $C-$ permits expression of pigment from genes B and D. The cc genotype, however, prevents expression of coat color and results in albino rats. For each of the following crosses, determine the expected phenotype ratio of progeny.
   a. $BbDDCc \times BbDdCc$
   b. $BBDdcc \times BbddCc$
   c. $bbDDCc \times BBddCc$
   d. $BbDdCC \times BbDdCC$

12. Using the information provided in Problems 10 and 11, determine the genotype and phenotype of parents that produce the following progeny:
   a. $\frac{9}{16}$ brown : $\frac{3}{16}$ black : $\frac{4}{16}$ albino
   b. $\frac{3}{8}$ black : $\frac{3}{8}$ cream : $\frac{2}{8}$ albino
   c. $\frac{27}{64}$ brown : $\frac{16}{64}$ albino : $\frac{9}{64}$ yellow : $\frac{9}{64}$ black : $\frac{3}{64}$ cream
   d. $\frac{3}{4}$ brown : $\frac{1}{4}$ yellow

13. Total cholesterol in blood is reported as the number of milligrams (mg) of cholesterol per 100 milliliters (mL) of blood. The normal range is 180–220 mg/100 mL. A gene mutation altering the function of cell-surface cholesterol receptors restricts the ability of cells to collect cholesterol from blood and draw it into cells. This defect results in elevated blood cholesterol levels. Individuals who are heterozygous for a mutant allele and a wild-type allele have levels of 300–600 mg/100 mL, and those who are homozygous for the mutation have levels of 800–1000 mg/100 mL. Identify the genetic term that best describes the inheritance of this form of elevated cholesterol level, and justify your choice.

14. Flower color in snapdragons results from the amount of the pigment anthocyanin in the petals. Red flowers are produced by plants that have full anthocyanin production, and ivory-colored flowers are produced by plants that lack the ability to produce anthocyanin. The allele

An1 has full activity in anthocyanin production, and the allele *An2* is a null allele. Dr. Ara B. Dopsis, a famous genetic researcher, crosses pure-breeding red snapdragons to pure-breeding ivory snapdragons and produces F_1 progeny plants that have pink flowers. He proposes that this outcome is the result of incomplete dominance, and he crosses the F_1 to test his hypothesis. What phenotypes does Dr. Dopsis predict will be found in the F_2, and in what proportions?

15. A plant line with reduced fertility comes to the attention of a plant breeder who observes that seed pods often contain a mixture of viable seeds that can be planted to produce new plants, and withered seeds that cannot be sprouted. The breeder examines numerous seed pods in the reduced fertility line and counts 622 viable seeds and 204 nonviable seeds.
    a. What single-gene mechanism best explains the breeder's observation?
    b. Propose an additional experiment to test the genetic mechanism you propose. If your hypothesis is correct, what experimental outcome do you predict?

16. In cattle, an autosomal mutation called *Dexter* produces calves with short stature and short limbs. Embryos that are homozygous for the *Dexter* mutation have severely stunted development and either spontaneously abort or are stillborn. What progeny phenotypes do you expect from the cross of two *Dexter* cows? What are the expected proportions of the expected phenotypes?

Application and Integration

For answers to selected even-numbered problems, see Appendix: Answers.

17. The coat color in mink is controlled by two codominant alleles at a single locus. Red coat color is produced by the genotype R_1R_1, silver coat by the genotype R_1R_2, and platinum color by R_2R_2. White spotting of the coat is a recessive trait found with the genotype *ss*. Solid coat color is found with the *S–* genotype.
    a. What are the expected progeny phenotypes and proportions for the cross $SsR_1R_2 \times ssR_2R_2$?
    b. If the cross $SsR_1R_2 \times SsR_1R_1$ is made, what are the progeny phenotypes, and in what proportions are they expected to occur?
    c. Two crosses are made between mink. Cross 1 is the cross of a solid, silver mink to one that is solid, platinum. Cross 2 is between a spotted, silver mink and one that is solid, silver. The progeny are described in the table below. Use these data to determine the genotypes of the parents in each cross.

Cross	Offspring					
	Spotted, platinum	Spotted, silver	Spotted, red	Solid, platinum	Solid, silver	Solid, red
1	2	3	0	6	5	0
2	3	7	2	4	5	3

18. Strains of petunias come in four pure-breeding colors: white, blue, red, and purple. White petunias are produced when plants synthesize no flower pigment. Blue petunias and red petunias are produced when plants synthesize blue or red pigment only. Purple petunias are produced in plants that synthesize both red *and* blue pigment (the mixture of red and blue makes purple). Flower-color pigments are synthesized by gene action in two separate pigment-producing biochemical pathways. Pathway I contains gene *A* that produces an enzyme to catalyze conversion of a colorless pigment designated white$_1$ to blue pigment. In Pathway II, the enzymatic product of gene *B* converts the colorless pigment designated white$_2$ to red pigment. The two genes assort independently.

$$\text{Pathway I: White}_1 \xrightarrow{\text{gene } A} \text{Blue}$$
$$+ \quad = \quad \text{Purple}$$
$$\text{Pathway II: White}_2 \xrightarrow{\text{gene } B} \text{Red}$$

a. What are the possible genotype(s) for pure-breeding red petunias?
b. What are the possible genotype(s) for true-breeding blue petunias?
c. True-breeding red petunias are crossed to pure-breeding blue petunias, and all the F_1 progeny have purple flowers. If the F_1 are allowed to self-fertilize and produce the F_2, what is the expected phenotypic distribution of the F_2 progeny? Show your work.

19. Feather color in parakeets is produced by the blending of pigments from two biosynthetic pathways shown below. Four independently assorting genes (*A, B, C,* and *D*) produce enzymes that catalyze separate steps of the pathways. For the questions below, use an uppercase letter to indicate a dominant allele producing full enzymatic activity and a lowercase letter to indicate a recessive allele producing no functional enzyme. Feather colors produced by mixing pigments are green (yellow + blue) and purple (red + blue). Red, yellow, and blue feathers result from production of one colored pigment, and white results from absence of pigment production.

$$\text{Pathway I: Compound I} \xrightarrow{\text{Enzyme A}} \text{Compound II} \xrightarrow{\text{Enzyme B}} \text{Compound III}$$
$$\text{(colorless)} \qquad \text{(red)} \qquad \text{(yellow)}$$
$$\text{Pathway II: Compound X} \xrightarrow{\text{Enzyme C}} \text{Compound Y} \xrightarrow{\text{Enzyme D}} \text{Compound Z}$$
$$\text{(colorless)} \qquad \text{(colorless)} \qquad \text{(blue)}$$

a. What is the genotype of a pure-breeding purple parakeet strain?
b. What is the genotype of a pure-breeding yellow strain of parakeet?
c. If a pure-breeding blue strain of parakeet (*aa BB CC DD*) is crossed to one that is pure-breeding purple, predict the genotype(s) and phenotype(s) of the F_1. Show your work.
d. If F_1 birds identified in part (c) are mated at random, what phenotypes do you expect in the F_2 generation? What are the ratios among phenotypes? Show your work.

20. Brachydactyly type D is a human autosomal dominant condition in which the thumbs are abnormally short and broad. In most cases, both thumbs are affected, but occasionally just one thumb is involved. The accompanying pedigree shows a family in which brachydactyly type D is segregating. Filled circles and squares represent females and males who have

involvement of both thumbs. Half-filled symbols represent family members with just one thumb affected

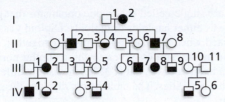

a. Is there any evidence of variable expressivity in this family? Explain.
b. Is there evidence of incomplete penetrance in this family? Explain.

21. A male and a female mouse are each from pure-breeding albino strains. They have a litter of 10 pups, all of which have normal pigmentation. The F_1 pups are crossed to one another to produce 56 F_2 mice, of which 31 are normally pigmented and 25 are albino.
    a. Using clearly defined allele symbols of your own choosing, give the genotypes of parental and F_1 mice. What genetic phenomenon explains these parental and F_1 phenotypes?
    b. What genetic phenomenon explains the F_2 results? Use your allelic symbols to explain the F_2 results.

22. Xeroderma pigmentosum (XP) is an autosomal recessive condition characterized by moderate to severe sensitivity to ultraviolet (UV) light. Patients develop multiple skin lesions on UV-exposed skin, and skin cancers often develop as a result. XP is caused by deficient repair of DNA damage from UV exposure.
    a. Many genes are known to be involved in repair of UV-induced DNA damage, and several of these genes are implicated in XP. What genetic phenomenon is illustrated by XP?
    b. A series of 10 skin-cell lines was grown from different XP patients. Cells from these lines were fused, and the heterokaryons were tested for genetic complementation by assaying their ability to repair DNA damage caused by a moderate amount of UV exposure. In the table below, + indicates that the fusion cell line performs normal DNA damage mutation repair, and – indicates defective DNA repair. Use this information to determine how many DNA-repair genes are mutated in the 10 cell lines, and identify which cell lines share the same mutated genes.

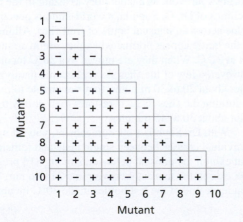

23. Three strains of green-seeded lentil plants appear to have the same phenotype. The strains are designated G_1, G_2, and G_3. Each green-seeded strain is crossed to a pure-breeding yellow-seeded strain designated Y. The F_1 of each cross are yellow; however, self-fertilization of F_1 plants produces F_2 with different proportions of yellow- and green-seeded plants as shown below.

Parental Strain		F1 Phenotype	F2 Phenotype	
Green	Yellow		Green	Yellow
G_1	Y	All yellow	$\frac{1}{4}$	$\frac{3}{4}$
G_2	Y	All yellow	$\frac{7}{16}$	$\frac{9}{16}$
G_3	Y	All yellow	$\frac{37}{64}$	$\frac{27}{64}$

a. For what number of genes are variable alleles segregating in the $G_1 \times Y$ cross? The $G_2 \times Y$ cross? In the $G_3 \times Y$ cross? Explain your rationale for each answer.
b. Using the allele symbols A and a, B and b, and D and d to represent alleles at segregating genes, give the genotypes of parental and F_1 plants in each cross.
c. For each set of F_2 progeny, provide a genetic explanation for the yellow : green ratio. What are the genotypes of yellow and green F_2 lentil plants in the $G_2 \times Y$ cross?
d. If green-seeded strains G_1 and G_3 are crossed, what are the phenotype and the genotype of F_1 progeny?
e. What proportion of the F_2 are expected to be green? Show your work.
f. If strains G_2 and G_3 are crossed, what will be the phenotype of the F_1?
g. What proportion of the F_2 will have yellow seeds? Show your work.

24. Blue flower color is produced in a species of morning glories when dominant alleles are present at two gene loci, A and B. (Plants with the genotype A–B– have blue flowers.) Purple flowers result when a dominant allele is present at only one of the two gene loci, A or B. (Plants with the genotypes A–bb and aaB– are purple.) Flowers are red when the plant is homozygous recessive for each gene (i.e., $aabb$).
    a. Two pure-breeding purple strains are crossed, and all the F_1 plants have blue flowers. What are the genotypes of the parental plants?
    b. If two F_1 plants are crossed, what are the expected phenotypes and frequencies in the F_2?
    c. If an F_1 plant is backcrossed to one of the pure-breeding parental plants, what is the expected ratio of phenotypes among progeny? Why is the phenotype ratio the same regardless of which parental strain is selected for the backcross?

25. The crosses shown on the following page are performed between morning glories whose flower color is determined as described in Problem 24. Use the segregation data to determine the genotype of each parental plant.

Parental Phenotypes	Offspring Phenotypes
a. blue × blue	$\frac{3}{4}$ blue : $\frac{1}{4}$ purple
b. purple × purple	$\frac{1}{4}$ blue : $\frac{1}{2}$ purple : $\frac{1}{4}$ red
c. blue × red	$\frac{1}{4}$ blue : $\frac{1}{2}$ purple : $\frac{1}{4}$ red
d. purple × red	$\frac{1}{2}$ purple : $\frac{1}{2}$ red
e. blue × purple	$\frac{3}{8}$ blue : $\frac{1}{2}$ purple : $\frac{1}{8}$ red

26. Two pure-breeding strains of summer squash producing yellow fruit, Y_1 and Y_2, are each crossed to a pure-breeding strain of summer squash producing green fruit, G_1, and to one another. The following results are obtained:

Cross	P	F_1	F_2
I	Y_1 (yellow) × G_1 (green)	All yellow	$\frac{3}{4}$ yellow : $\frac{1}{4}$ green
II	Y_2 (yellow) × G_1 (green)	All green	$\frac{3}{4}$ green : $\frac{1}{4}$ yellow
III	Y_1 (yellow) × Y_2 (yellow)	All yellow	$\frac{13}{16}$ yellow : $\frac{3}{16}$ green

  a. Examine the results of each cross and predict how many genes are responsible for fruit-color determination in summer squash. Justify your answer.
  b. Using clearly defined symbols of your choice, give the genotypes of parental, F_1, and F_2 plants in each cross.
  c. If the F_1 of Crosses I and II are mated, predict the phenotype ratio of the progeny.

27. Marfan syndrome is an autosomal dominant disorder in humans. It results from mutation of a gene on chromosome 15 that produces the connective tissue protein fibrillin. In its wild-type form, fibrillin gives connective tissues, such as cartilage, elasticity. When mutated, however, fibrillin is rigid and produces a range of phenotypic complications, including excessive growth of the long bones of the leg and arm, sunken chest, dislocation of the lens of the eye, and susceptibility to aortic aneurysm, which can lead to sudden death in some cases.

  Different sets of symptoms are seen among various family members, as shown in the pedigree below. Each quadrant of the circles and squares represents a different symptom, as the key indicates.

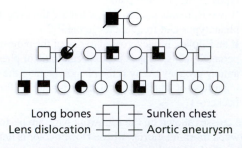

Long bones ─┬─ Sunken chest
Lens dislocation ─┴─ Aortic aneurysm

All cases of Marfan syndrome are caused by mutation of the fibrillin gene, and all family members with Marfan syndrome carry the same mutant allele. What do the differences shown in the phenotypes of family members say about the expression of the mutant allele?

28. Yeast are single-celled eukaryotic organisms that grow in culture as either haploids or diploids. Diploid yeast are generated when two haploid strains fuse together. Seven haploid mutant strains of yeast exhibit similar normal growth habit at 25°C, but at 37°C, they show different growth capabilities. The table below displays the growth pattern

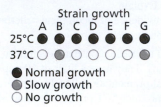

Strain growth
A B C D E F G
25°C ● ● ● ● ● ● ●
37°C ○ ◐ ○ ○ ○ ○ ◐
● Normal growth
◐ Slow growth
○ No growth

  a. Hypothesize about the nature of the mutation affecting each of these mutant yeast strains, including why strains B and G display different growth habit at 37°C than the other strains.
  b. Researchers induce fusion in pairs of haploid yeast strains (all possible combinations), and the resulting diploids are tested for their ability to grow at 37°C. The results of the growth experiment are shown below.

37°C growth data

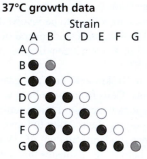

How many different genes are mutated among these seven yeast strains? Identify the strains that represent each gene mutation.

29. During your work as a laboratory assistant in the research facilities of Dr. O. Sophila, a world-famous geneticist, you come across an unusual bottle of fruit flies. All the flies in the bottle appear normal when they are in an incubator set at 22°C. When they are moved to a 30°C incubator, however, a few of the flies slowly become paralyzed; and after about 20 to 30 minutes, they are unable to move. Returning the flies to 22°C restores their ability to move after about 30 to 45 minutes.

  With Dr. Sophila's encouragement, you set up 10 individual crosses between single male and female flies that exhibit the unusual behavior. Among 812 progeny, 598 exhibit the unusual behavior and 214 do not. When you leave one of the test bottles in the 30°C incubator too long, you discover that more than 2 hours at high temperature kills the paralyzed flies. When you tell this to Dr. Sophila, he says, "Ah ha! I know how to explain this condition." What is his explanation?

30. Dr. Ara B. Dopsis and Dr. C. Ellie Gans are performing genetic crosses on daisy plants. They self-fertilize a blue-flowered daisy and grow 100 progeny plants that consist of 55 blue-flowered plants, 22 purple-flowered plants, and 23 white-flowered plants. Dr. Dopsis believes this is the result of segregation of two alleles at one locus and that the progeny ratio is 1:2:1. Dr. Gans thinks the progeny phenotypes are the result of two epistatic genes and that the ratio is 9:3:4.

    The two scientists ask you to resolve their conflict by performing chi-square analysis on the data for *both* proposed genetic mechanisms. For each proposed mechanism, fill in the values requested on the form the researchers have provided for your analysis.

    a. Use the form below to calculate chi square for the 1:2:1 hypothesis of Dr. Sophila.

Phenotype	Observed	Expected
Blue	55	_____
Purple	22	_____
White	23	_____
Chi-square value: _____ df: _____ p value > _____		

    b. Use the form below to calculate chi square for the 9:3:4 hypothesis of Dr. Gans.

Phenotype	Observed	Expected
Blue	55	_____
Purple	22	_____
White	23	_____
Chi-square value: _____ df: _____ p value > _____		

    c. What is your conclusion regarding these two genetic hypotheses?

    d. Using any of the 100 progeny plants, propose a cross that will verify the conclusion you proposed in part (c). Plants may be self-fertilized, or one plant can be crossed to another. What result will be consistent with the 1:2:1 hypothesis? What result will be consistent with the 9:3:4 hypothesis?

31. Human ABO blood type is determined by three alleles, two of which (I^A and I^B) produce gene products that modify the H antigen produced by protein activity of an independently assorting *H* gene. A rare abnormality known as the "Bombay phenotype" is the result of epistatic interaction between the gene for the ABO blood group and the *H* gene. Individuals with the Bombay phenotype appear to have blood type O based on the inability of both anti-A antibody and anti-B antibody to detect an antigen. The apparent blood type O in Bombay phenotype is due to the absence of H antigen as a result of homozygous recessive mutations of the *H* gene. Individuals with the Bombay

phenotype have the *hh* genotype. Use the information above to make predictions about the outcome of the cross shown below.

$$I^A I^B \, Hh \times I^A I^B \, Hh$$

32. In rabbits, albinism is an autosomal recessive condition caused by the absence of the pigment melanin from skin and fur. Pigmentation is a dominant wild-type trait. Three pure-breeding strains of albino rabbits, identified as strains 1, 2, and 3, are crossed to one another. In the table below, F_1 and F_2 progeny are shown for each cross. Based on the available data, propose a genetic explanation for the results. As part of your answer, create genotypes for each albino strain using clearly defined symbols of your own choosing. Use your symbols to diagram each cross, giving the F_1 and F_2 genotypes.

	Cross	F_1 Progeny	F_2 Progeny
Cross A	strain 1 × strain 2	56 albino	192 albino
Cross B	strain 1 × strain 3	72 pigmented	181 pigmented, 139 albino
Cross C	strain 2 × strain 3	34 pigmented	89 pigmented, 72 albino

33. Dr. O. Sophila, a close friend of Dr. Ara B. Dopsis, reviews the F_2 results Dr. Dopsis obtained in his experiment with iris plants described in Genetic Analysis 4.3. Dr. Sophila thinks the F_2 progeny demonstrate that a single gene with incomplete dominance has produced a 1:2:1 ratio. Dr. Dopsis insists his proposal of recessive epistasis producing a 9:4:3 ratio in the F_2 is correct. To test his proposal, Dr. Dopsis examines the F_2 data under the assumptions of the single-gene incomplete dominance model using chi-square analysis. Calculate and interpret this chi-square value. Can Dr. Dopsis reject the single-gene incomplete dominance model on the basis of this analysis? Explain why or why not.

34. In a breed of domestic cattle, horns can appear on males and on females. Males and females can also be hornless. The following crosses are performed with parents from pure-breeding lines.

Cross I	Cross II
Parents: horned male × hornless female	Parents: hornless male × horned female
F_1: males horned, females hornless	F_1: males horned, females hornless
F_2: males are $\frac{3}{4}$ horned, $\frac{1}{4}$ hornless	F_2: males are $\frac{3}{4}$ horned, $\frac{1}{4}$ hornless
females are $\frac{1}{4}$ horned, $\frac{3}{4}$ hornless	females are $\frac{1}{4}$ horned, $\frac{3}{4}$ hornless

Explain the inheritance of this phenotype in cattle, and assign genotypes to all cattle in each cross.

Collaboration and Discussion

For answers to selected even-numbered problems, see Appendix: Answers.

35. Cross 1 shown in Figure 4.22 illustrates genetic complementation of flower-color mutants. The F_1 produced from this cross of two pure-breeding mutant parental plants are dihybrid ($CcPp$) and have wild-type flower color. If these F_1 are allowed to self-fertilize, what phenotypes are expected in the F_2 and what are the expected ratios of the phenotypes?

36. The wild-type allele of a gene has an A–T base pair at a particular location in its sequence, and a mutant allele of the same gene has a G–C base pair at the same location. Otherwise, the sequences of the two alleles are identical. Does this information tell you anything about the dominance relationship of the alleles? Explain why or why not.

37. Epistatic gene interaction results in a modification of the F_2 dihybrid ratio.

    a. What is the expected F_2 ratio?

    b. What genetic principle is the basis of this expected F_2 ratio?

    c. Give two examples of modified F_2 ratios produced by epistatic gene interactions and describe how gene interaction results in the ratios.

38. Draw a pedigree containing two parents and four children. Both of the parents have AB blood type. The first child is type A, the second child is type AB, and the third child is type B.

    a. Assign the genotypes to these five people.

    b. The fourth child tests as having blood type O, which is not possible given the parental genotypes. Look at Figure 4.4 and read the description of the molecular process that generates ABO blood group antigens. What other mutation could account for this observation?

    c. What is the name of the genetic phenomenon producing this observation?

Genetic Linkage and Mapping in Eukaryotes

5

CHAPTER OUTLINE

5.1 Linked Genes Do Not Assort Independently

5.2 Genetic Linkage Mapping Is Based on Recombination Frequency between Genes

5.3 Three-Point Test-Cross Analysis Maps Genes

5.4 Multiple Factors Cause Recombination to Vary

5.5 Human Genes Are Mapped Using Specialized Methods

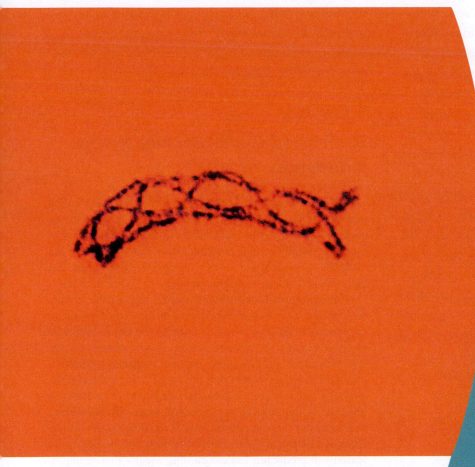

Recombination between homologous chromosomes reshuffles the genetic information in genomes. These two homologs show multiple chiasmata that indicate the locations of crossing over between the chromosomes.

ESSENTIAL IDEAS

■ Genetic linkage occurs between genes that lie so close to one another on a chromosome that alleles are unable to assort independently.

■ Genetic linkage produces significantly more progeny with parental phenotypes and significantly fewer progeny with nonparental phenotypes than are expected by chance.

■ Crossing over between homologous chromosomes results in recombination of alleles on chromosomes in gametes.

■ Geneticists use the frequency of recombination between genes to construct gene maps identifying the relative order of and distance between genes on chromosomes.

■ Cytological evidence demonstrates that recombination results from crossing over between homologous chromosomes.

■ Specialized statistical methods aid in mapping human genes.

■ Recombination creates substantial new genetic diversity that is favored by evolution. It also randomizes the arrangements of alleles of linked genes on chromosomes.

In 1933, Thomas Hunt Morgan won the Nobel Prize for Physiology or Medicine in recognition of his many contributions to genetics. These include his work establishing sex-linked inheritance and the chromosome theory of heredity, which we explored in Chapter 3, and also his role in identifying and explaining *genetic linkage and recombination* and their application to *genetic linkage mapping*, which we discuss in this chapter. Morgan, like all successful scientists, was assisted by dedicated colleagues, including many exceptional students. Among the latter were Calvin Bridges, whose work we discussed in connection with the chromosome theory of heredity, and Alfred Sturtevant, who as an undergraduate researcher in Morgan's laboratory became the first person to use genetic linkage data to assemble a genetic map. A number of less well remembered researchers, including Morgan's wife Lilian, were also important members of the research enterprise.

The work of Morgan, his colleagues, and numerous others led to the validation of three foundational theories in genetics. First, the work validated the chromosome theory of heredity—the idea that genes are carried on chromosomes—and expanded the theory by showing that each chromosome carries many genes in a specific order. Second, the research validated the concept of the gene as a physical entity that is an integral part of a chromosome, and led to work that expanded understanding of gene structure by demonstrating that genes are composed of nucleotides between which recombination may occur. Third, the work validated evolutionary theory by confirming that closely related species have a similar number of chromosomes and a similar arrangement of genes on chromosomes; and it expanded evolutionary theory by suggesting that recombination could be a mechanism through which variation in chromosome number and in the arrangement of genes on chromosomes could accrue as species diverge from a common ancestor.

The investigation of genetic linkage and recombination is a central tool of genetic analysis, and recombination itself is an essential biological process. Along with mutation, recombination generates the raw genetic diversity on which evolution depends. Along with sexual reproduction, recombination operates to increase diversity between generations. In addition, it has an important functional role in mammalian meiosis. Homologous chromosome synapsis and segregation does not occur normally in the absence of recombination. Given its pivotal functions, one might be tempted to think that recombination would be ubiquitous among sexually reproducing organisms and would occur to an equal degree throughout the genome of such an organism. In fact, genome-based analysis of recombination reveals that none of these presumptions is true. Recombination is highly variable within any one genome, and it is highly variable among different organisms. These findings open new avenues for investigating the evolutionary biology of organisms and the role of recombination in genetics.

The detection and analysis of genetic linkage and recombination; the principles of genetic linkage mapping; and the role of recombination in evolution are the topics on which we focus in this chapter. In the process, we explore recent developments in gene mapping, molecular genetic marker mapping, and the investigation of chromosome evolution.

5.1 Linked Genes Do Not Assort Independently

Genes that are located on the same chromosome are called **syntenic genes**. When two syntenic genes are so close to one another that their alleles are unable to assort independently, the genes display **genetic linkage**. Genetic linkage produces a distinctive pattern of gamete genotypes that can be quantified and analyzed to map the locations of genes on chromosomes.

Homologous recombination is the process that occurs as a result of crossing over in prophase I of meiosis in eukaryotic cells. It takes place through the equal exchange of genetic material contained in homologous chromosomes. It is a reciprocal process, meaning that neither of the participating chromosomes has more or less genetic material at the end of the process than at the start. At the end of meiosis the outcome is the generation of **recombinant chromosomes** or nonparental chromosomes that come about by the reshuffling of alleles residing on recombining chromosomes. In sexually reproducing organisms this means that recombinant chromosomes contain a combination of alleles initially carried by the different parents of the organism in which recombination is occurring. In contrast, homologous chromosomes that do not undergo crossing over during meiosis retain all the same alleles they had when they were transmitted from a parent. To distinguish them from recombinant chromosomes, these are called **parental chromosomes** or **nonrecombinant chromosomes**.

Syntenic genes located very near each other on a chromosome tend to recombine less often during crossing over than do genes located farther apart on the chromosome. This creates a distinguishing pattern by which linkage can be recognized and quantified.

On the other hand, syntenic genes located far apart on a chromosome, and genes located on separate chromosomes, always assort independently according to the predictions of Mendel's law of independent assortment. The independent assortment of genes on separate chromosomes is explained by the movement of chromosomes and chromatids in meiosis, as Figure 3.15 illustrates. The independent assortment of syntenic genes is a product of there being sufficient recombination along the homologous chromosomes containing those genes to randomize the allele combinations. Thus, to establish the presence of genetic linkage requires a statistical demonstration of the absence of independent assortment. The chi-square statistic discussed in Section 2.5 is used to compare the observed and expected outcomes of crosses for this purpose. In experimental analysis of genetic linkage, independent assortment is the expected result of crosses; to be indicative of genetic linkage, a cross outcome must have a statistically significant deviation from cross expectations.

In this chapter section and throughout the remainder of the chapter, these basic concepts of genetic linkage and some of the experimental results that support them are elaborated and explained. To help focus the discussion, we offer the following observations and conclusions, all of which are essential to understanding the linkage phenomenon.

1. Linked genes are always syntenic, and they are always located near one another on a chromosome. When syntenic genes are so far apart on the chromosome that crossing over between them generates independent assortment of the alleles, the genes are not linked.

2. Genetic linkage leads to the production of a significantly greater number of gametes containing chromosomes with parental combinations of alleles than would be expected under assumptions of independent assortment, and to a significantly smaller number of gametes containing chromosomes with alleles that are different from the parental combinations.

3. Crossing over is less likely to occur between linked genes that are close to one another than between genes that are farther apart on a chromosome. The frequency of crossing over is roughly proportionate to the distance between genes, a relationship that allows genes to be mapped.

The discovery of genetic linkage, made more than a century ago, opened the door to the development of several applications. The first of these was **genetic linkage mapping**, which plots the positions of genes on chromosomes. Over the ensuing century, new methods for identifying genetic variants and new applications for mapping genes and variants have added to the analytical arsenal of genetics. Genetic linkage and its old and new mapping applications remain a strong central pillar of genetic analysis.

Detecting Genetic Linkage

Genetic linkage can be detected by comparing the observed frequencies of gamete genotypes, or the corresponding progeny phenotypes, with the frequencies expected under the assumptions of independent assortment. If genes are linked, parental gametes—also known as nonrecombinant gametes—that contain parental combinations of the alleles will be produced significantly more often than predicted by chance. The excess parental gametes will also result in progeny in which *parental* phenotypes (or parental combinations of alleles) will be detected significantly more often than predicted by chance.

Figure 5.1 illustrates the consequences of genetic linkage by comparing the frequencies of gamete genotypes for two crosses. In Figure 5.1a, gene *A* and gene *B* are on different chromosomes, and alleles of the genes assort independently. The parental organisms are *AABB* and *aabb*, and their gametes *AB* and *ab* are the parental gametes. The F_1 progeny are dihybrid (*AaBb*), and independent assortment predicts these dihybrids will produce four genetically different gametes in a ratio of 1:1:1:1. Notice that the frequency of parental gametes (*AB* and *ab*) is 50%, and that the frequency of nonparental gametes (*Ab* and *aB*) is also 50%.

Figure 5.1b illustrates gamete-genotype production for syntenic genes *D* and *E* that are linked. The *DDee* parent produces parental gametes that are *De*, and the *ddEE* parent produces *dE* gametes. The dihybrid F_1 progeny are *DdEe*, carrying alleles *D* and *e* on one chromosome and *d* and *E* on the homolog. This arrangement of alleles can be written *De/dE*, with the slash ("/") separating the alleles carried on one member of the homologous chromosome pair from the alleles carried on the other member of the pair. The use of a slash to separate the alleles of homologous chromosomes is usually reserved for linked genes. A genotype designated *De/dE* is the same as *DdEe*, the difference being that in the former case the genes are linked and the alleles on each homolog are known.

A characteristic of genetic linkage is that the rate of recombination between linked genes is low, and parental allele combinations usually stay together during meiosis, leading to the production of parental gametes (*De* and *dE*) at a combined frequency that is significantly greater than 50% ($\gg 50\%$), as in Figure 5.1b. The low frequency of crossing over between closely linked genes results in the production of recombinant, or nonparental, gametes (*DE* and *de*) at a combined frequency that is significantly less than 50% ($\ll 50\%$). Note that the term "parental" refers to the combination of alleles carried by parental organisms and "nonparental" to allele combinations not on the parental chromosomes.

Complete genetic linkage is observed when no recombination at all occurs between linked genes. Complete genetic linkage can be identified, for example, in cases where a dihybrid produces two equally frequent gametes containing only parental allele combinations and no recombinant gametes (**Figure 5.2a**). The absence of recombination between homologs usually has a specific biological basis. Certain organisms, including *Drosophila* males and other males in the insect order *Diptera* (of which *Drosophila* is a member), exhibit complete genetic linkage. There is no recombination between homologous chromosomes in these male flies. The biological basis of the absence of recombination in these organisms remains unknown.

Incomplete genetic linkage is far more common for linked genes. The resulting recombination between the homologs produces a mixture of parental and nonparental gametes. In the F_1 dihybrid shown in **Figure 5.2b**, recombination produces four genetically different gametes, of which two are parental (nonrecombinant) and two are nonparental (recombinant). The two parental gametes each have

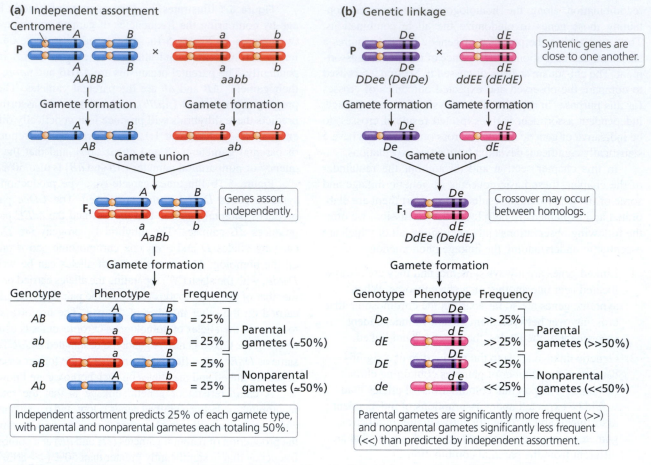

Figure 5.1   Independent assortment versus genetic linkage. (a) For this dihybrid, four genetically different gametes are expected at 25% each when the genes assort independently. **(b)** When genes are linked,
parental gametes are significantly more frequent than expected by chance, and their individual and combined frequencies are much greater than nonparental gametes.

approximately the same frequency, and their total is significantly greater than 50% of all gametes. In this example, the
frequency of each parental gamete (*RT* and *rt*) is 40%, and
the total frequency of parental gametes is 80%. Recombinant gametes, which have nonparental combinations of
alleles, are approximately equal to one another in frequency
and constitute significantly less than 50% of all gametes. In
this case, a total of 20% of gametes are recombinant: 10%
of the gametes are *Rt* and 10% are *rT*.

The proportion of parental to recombinant chromosomes or gametes from a cross depends on the frequency of
crossing over between syntenic genes. This proportion differs among different pairs of genes and is expected to be
greater for syntenic genes that are farther apart and smaller
for genes that are closer together on a chromosome. Note
that the percentages of different gametes obtained for the
cross in **Figure 5.2c** are different from those in Figure 5.2b,
and also notice that the parental alleles on chromosomes in
Figure 5.2c are a dominant and a recessive allele—*Mn/mN*.
Once again, parental chromosomes are defined by the specific combinations of alleles that are present on the homologs of the parents in the cross.

The **recombination frequency**, expressed in the general formula as the variable *r*, identifies the rate of recombination for a given pair of syntenic genes. The value of *r* is
expressed as

$$r = \frac{\text{number of recombinants}}{\text{total number of progeny}}$$

As stated above, recombination frequency varies between
different pairs of syntenic genes, depending roughly on the
distance separating the genes on the chromosome. Comparing Figure 5.2b and Figure 5.2c, for example, we see that
recombination frequency is 20% ($r = 0.20$) in Figure 5.2b
and 40% ($r = 0.40$) in Figure 5.2c. The greater recombination frequency in Figure 5.2c compared with Figure 5.2b is
most likely the consequence of a greater distance between
genes *N* and *M* than between genes *T* and *R*. The correlation
between recombination frequency and gene distance can be
expressed in two equivalent ways: (1) crossing over occurs
at a higher rate between genes that are separated by a greater
distance, and at a lower rate for genes that are closer together;
and (2) linked genes with higher recombination frequencies
are more distant from one another than linked genes with

(a) Complete genetic linkage (no crossover)

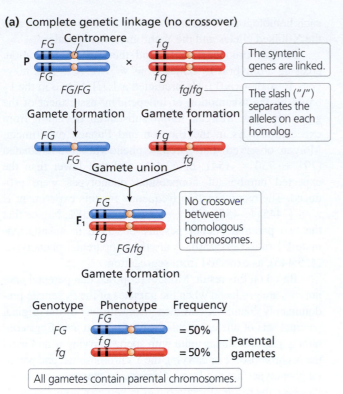

(b) Incomplete genetic linkage (crossover in 20% of gametes)

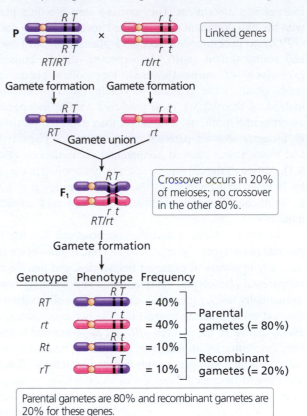

Parental gametes are 80% and recombinant gametes are 20% for these genes.

Figure 5.2   Complete versus incomplete genetic linkage.
(a) Genes exhibiting complete genetic linkage do not recombine, and all gametes are parental. **(b)** Linked genes with a recombination frequency of 20% produce 20% nonparental gametes and 80% parental gametes. **(c)** Linked genes with a recombination frequency of 40% produce 60% parental gametes and 40% nonparental gametes.

⊙ **If a sample of 200 gametes from the F₁ organisms in part (b) were examined, how many would be *rT*?**

(c) Incomplete genetic linkage (crossover in 40% of gametes)

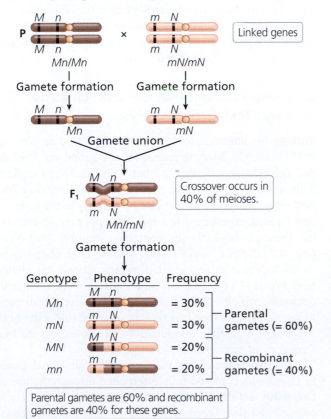

Parental gametes are 60% and recombinant gametes are 40% for these genes.

lower recombination frequencies. There are some caveats to this generalization, however, as we discuss in later sections.

The Discovery of Genetic Linkage

William Bateson, an early champion of Mendelian genetics, and Reginald Punnett, after whom the Punnett square is named, reported a series of experiments on sweet peas in 1905, 1906, and 1908. Those experiments opened a new chapter in genetics by drawing attention to genetic linkage. Bateson and Punnett studied the traits of flower color and the shape of pollen grains in sweet peas, first as independent traits and then together in the same plants.

When the traits were studied separately, the genes for flower color and pollen shape obeyed the rules of segregation—generating 3:1 phenotypic ratios among the F₂, for example. But Bateson and Punnett went on to study both traits in the same plants, intending to test the law of independent assortment. They crossed pure-breeding plants with the two dominant traits, purple flowers and long pollen (*PPLL*), to pure-breeding recessive plants with red flowers and round pollen (*ppll*). As expected, the F_1 consisted exclusively of purple-flowered, long-pollen plants, and these plants were crossed to obtain the F_2. But then, instead of the 9:3:3:1 ratio predicted by the independent assortment hypothesis, a far larger than expected portion of F_2 progeny showed parental combinations of phenotypes, and many fewer showed nonparental combinations (Table 5.1). Although the chi-square test was not applied to the data by Bateson and Punnett, its use today identifies $p < 0.05$, a significant deviation between observed and expected numbers.

In the F_2, Bateson and Punnett observed that the two parental phenotypes—purple, long and red, round—were substantially in excess of expected frequencies, and that the two nonparental phenotypes—purple, round and red, long—were substantially less frequent than expected. This observation led Bateson and Punnett to suggest that the two combinations of alleles carried in the parents—*PL* and *pl*—remained together very frequently, by an unknown mechanism, when they were passed through gametes to subsequent generations. Bateson and Punnett described these alleles as exhibiting "coupling." They described the appearance of new, nonparental phenotypes in the F_2 as indicating "repulsion" of the parental alleles, to produce nonparental phenotypes in progeny.

In 1911, Morgan performed the first of a series of experimental crosses that confirmed genetic linkage, explained the apparent coupling and repulsion identified by Bateson and Punnett, and led to the development of the first genetic linkage map. Morgan had by this time identified several genes on the X chromosome of his wild-caught fruit flies. The X-linked genes identified included *w* (white eye) and *m* (miniature wing). Figure 5.3 illustrates one of Morgan's experimental crosses, this one between a female pure-breeding for white eyes and miniature wings (*wm/wm*) and a hemizygous wild-type male displaying red eye and full wing ($w^+ m^+ /Y$). The F_1 progeny were dihybrid wild-type females ($w^+ m^+ /wm$) and white, miniature (*wm/Y*) hemizygous males. Here the slash ("/") identifies the alleles on

each homologous X chromosome in females and indicates the X-linked alleles and the Y chromosome in males.

Morgan produced an F_1 and then an F_2 generation, crossing a dihybrid F_1 female ($w^+ m^+ /wm$) to a hemizygous F_1 male (*wm/Y*). He predicted a 1:1:1:1 ratio in the F_2 based on the assumption of independent assortment of the genes. Instead, Morgan found substantial deviation from expectations. As in the Bateson and Punnett experiment, Morgan observed that parental phenotypes predominated (791 + 750 = 1541, or 63.1%) and that fewer than the expected number of nonparental phenotypes were produced. The recombination frequency for this experiment is $r = (445 + 455) /2441 = 0.369$, or 36.9%. Notice that the two parental phenotypes are observed in an approximate 1:1 ratio (791:750), as are the nonparental phenotypes (455:445), as expected from segregation.

Based on this result, Morgan proposed that parental phenotypes are produced when the gametes of the F_1 female predominantly contain X chromosomes with one of the original parental sets of alleles, in this case $w^+ m^+$ and *wm*. Eggs containing parental alleles unite with sperm carrying *w* and *m* on the X chromosome or carrying the Y chromosome, and parental phenotypes are produced. Conversely, nonparental phenotypes are the result of recombination between homologous X chromosomes during F_1 female meiosis (Figure 5.4). The production of recombinant chromosomes carrying either $w^+ m$ or wm^+ requires the physical rearrangement (recombination) of homologous X chromosomes. Morgan confirmed this explanation through the examination of many other pairs of linked genes on the fruit fly X chromosome.

Detecting Autosomal Genetic Linkage through Test-Cross Analysis

Turning his attention to autosomal genes and employing 20/20 hindsight, Morgan realized that Bateson and Punnett had detected genetic linkage but were unable to explain it because, with respect to experimental design, *they had performed the wrong cross!* The F_2 progeny in the Bateson and Punnett experiment fell into four phenotypic classes, but three of those classes contained multiple genotypes (e.g., *PPLL*, *PpLL*, and *PPLl* all had the same phenotype), owing to the dominance relationships among the alleles (see Figure 2.11). Bateson and Punnett were unable to determine which alleles in the progeny derived from each F_1 parent because they had no way of ascertaining the high frequency of parental combinations of alleles and the low frequency of recombinants in F_1 gametes.

Morgan realized that the linkage of autosomal genes in *Drosophila* could be fully interpreted through the use of **two-point test-cross analysis** in which a dihybrid F_1 fly is crossed to a pure-breeding mate with the recessive phenotypes. The "two points" in these analyses are the two genes being tested. In two-point test-cross analysis, the homozygous recessive fly contributes only recessive alleles to test-cross progeny. In contrast, the dihybrid fly can contribute

Table 5.1	Bateson and Punnett's Observed and Expected Phenotypes in F_2 Sweet Peas		
Phenotype	Genotype	Number of Progeny	
		Observed	Expected (9:3:3:1 ratio)
Purple, long	*P–L–*	4831	(6952)(9/16) = 3910.5
Purple, round	*P–ll*	390	(6952)(3/16) = 1303.5
Red, long	*ppL–*	393	(6952)(3/16) = 1303.5
Red, round	*ppll*	1338	(6952)(1/16) = 434.5
		6952	6952.0

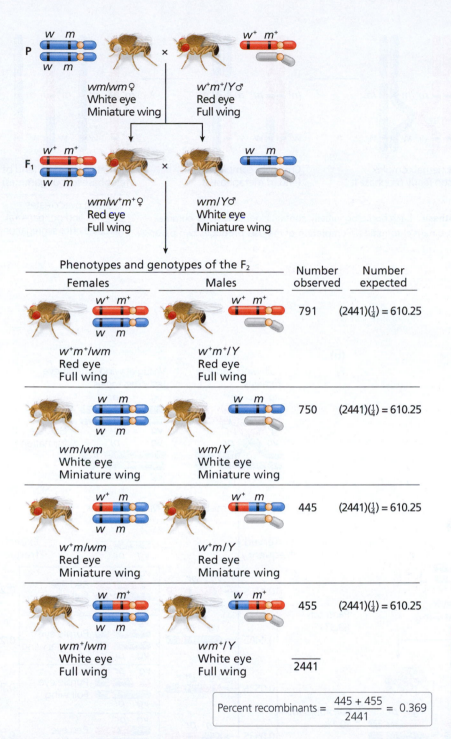

Figure 5.3 Morgan's analysis of genetic linkage of X-linked genes for eye color (*w*) and wing form (*m*). The number of test-cross progeny with each phenotype are compared with expected values that are determined assuming independent assortment of the genes.

either a dominant allele of a gene, in which case the progeny display the dominant phenotype, or the recessive allele, thus producing the recessive form of the trait.

In one experiment, Morgan used test-cross analysis to examine genetic linkage of autosomal genes affecting eye color and wing shape. *Drosophila* eye color is red if an autosomal dominant allele *pr*+ is present, whereas the recessive purple eye color is produced when the only allele present is *pr*. Full-sized wing is the product of an autosomal dominant allele *vg*+, and its recessive counterpart, vestigial wing, is determined by the allele *vg*. Morgan crossed

fruit flies that are pure-breeding for red eyes and full wing with pure-breeding purple-eyed, vestigial-winged flies (**Figure 5.5a**). The F_1 were uniformly red eyed and full winged (*pr*+ *vg*+/*pr vg*). Morgan then test-crossed dihybrid F_1 females to purple-eyed, vestigial-winged males (*pr vg/pr vg*). In this cross, males contributed only recessive alleles (*pr* and *vg*), but females could produce any one of four gamete genotypes. The alleles of the female gamete thus controlled the phenotype of test-cross progeny. If the female contributed a dominant allele to progeny, the phenotype for that trait was dominant; and conversely, if the donated

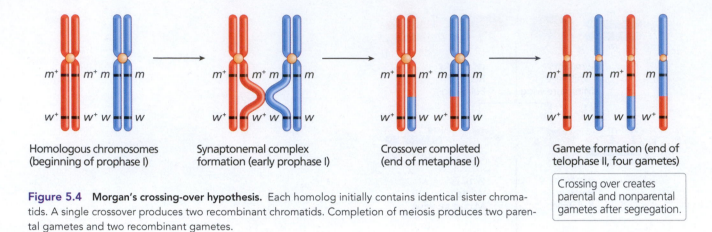

Figure 5.4 Morgan's crossing-over hypothesis. Each homolog initially contains identical sister chromatids. A single crossover produces two recombinant chromatids. Completion of meiosis produces two parental gametes and two recombinant gametes.

Crossing over creates parental and nonparental gametes after segregation.

🔴 **Draw a chromosome pair with *Ab/aB*. Illustrate a crossover between the two genes and identify the resulting parental and recombinant chromosomes.**

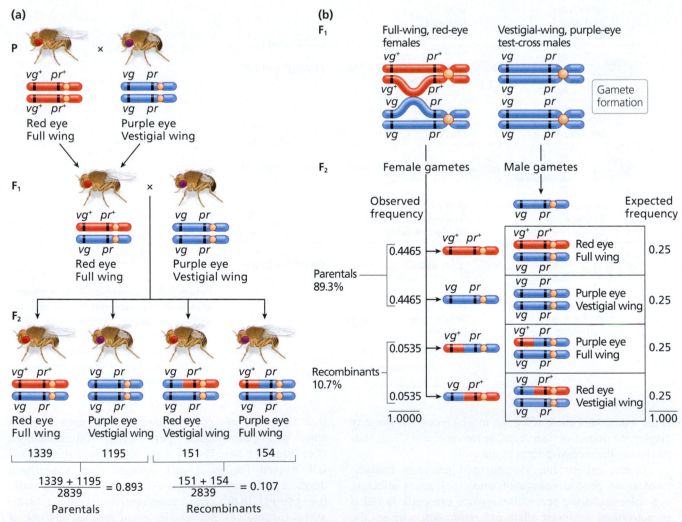

Figure 5.5 Morgan's test-cross analysis of genetic linkage between autosomal genes. (a) Dihybrid F_1 females ($pr^+vg^+/pr\ vg$) are test-crossed to males homozygous for recessive mutant purple eye color and vestigial wing ($pr\ vg/pr\ vg$), permitting identification of progeny as carrying either a parental or a recombinant chromosome. **(b)** Single crossover during female meiosis leads to parental and recombinant gametes at frequencies specified by recombination or by chance, and gamete union produces test-cross progeny.

female allele was recessive, the phenotype was recessive. Test-cross progeny phenotypes corresponded directly to the alleles contributed by F_1 females, thus making it possible to unambiguously identify the allelic content of chromosomes in female gametes.

Under the assumption of independent assortment, dihybrid females should produce four equally frequent gametes, and test-cross progeny are expected to have four phenotypes distributed in a 1:1:1:1 ratio (see Figure 2.12). With genetic linkage however, parental combinations of alleles would occur preferentially in gametes, producing test-cross progeny with a significant excess of parental phenotypes and a significant deficit of nonparental phenotypes.

Morgan's test-cross progeny displayed the four expected phenotypes, but in numbers that deviated dramatically from expected Mendelian proportions. Among test-cross progeny, 89.3% were parental, and just 10.7% were recombinant. The nonrecombinant progeny classes were found in approximately a 1:1 ratio (1339:1195), as were the recombinant classes (154:151); thus, the two parental chromosomes were transmitted equally frequently, as were the two recombinant chromosomes. **Figure 5.5b** shows that among the 89.3% of parental female gametes, one-half, or 44.65%, should be of each parental type. Similarly, among the 10.7% of gametes that are recombinant, each recombinant type should have a frequency of 5.35%.

In the years immediately following Morgan's explanation of genetic linkage, other biologists, working on plant species and animal species, used test-cross analysis to verify Morgan's hypothesis. The collective results of these experimental observations can be summarized as follows:

1. Genetic linkage is a physical relationship between genes that are located near one another on a chromosome.

2. Recombination between linked genes on homologous chromosomes occurs in significantly less than 50% of meiotic divisions. Significantly more than 50% of gametes contain parental combinations of alleles.

3. The recombination frequency varies among linked genes and is roughly proportionate to the distance between genes on a chromosome.

Genetic Analysis 5.1 takes you through the identification of parental and recombinant progeny and the determination of recombination frequency.

Cytological Evidence of Recombination

Morgan's hypothesis that gene recombination required physical exchange between homologous chromosomes was a functional working hypothesis, but direct evidence of exchange was not obtained until 20 years after Morgan proposed it. In 1931, research published by Harriet Creighton and Barbara McClintock on crossing over in corn (*Zea mays*), and a nearly simultaneous report by Curt Stern on crossing over in *Drosophila*, provided direct evidence that

gene recombination and physical exchange between homologous chromosomes went hand in hand.

Creighton and McClintock studied recombination between homologous copies of chromosome 9 in corn that were distinguished by having different alleles for two linked genes—the genes controlling kernel color (*c1*) and starch type (*wx*) in *Zea mays*—and by two cytological, or structural, differences in the homologous copies of chromosome 9 that were observable under the microscope. One copy of chromosome 9 had the normal microscopic appearance and carried alleles *c1* and *Wx*. The homologous copy of chromosome 9 carried alleles *C1* and *wx* and was cytologically altered in two ways. On the end nearer *C1*, the chromosome had a darkly staining region called a "knob"; on the other end, near *wx*, the chromosome carried a fragment of chromosome 8 that had been transferred by a chromosome-rearrangement event called *translocation* (we explore this event in Section 10.5). Creighton and McClintock obtained cytological evidence that recombination involved the physical exchange between homologous chromosomes by detecting genetic recombinants (chromosomes carrying the alleles *C1* and *Wx* or carrying the alleles *c1* and *wx*) that were also cytologically rearranged chromosomes (**Figure 5.6**).

(a) *c1 Wx/C1 wx* heterozygote

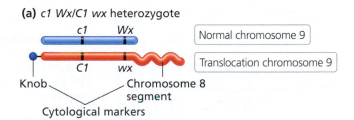

(b) Homologous recombination

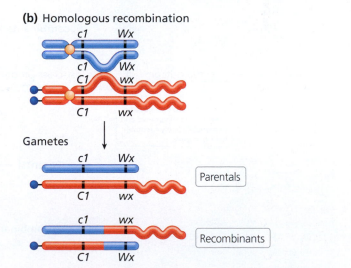

Figure 5.6 **Cytological proof from *Zea mays* that recombination results from crossing over.** Progeny displaying recombinant phenotypes are also seen to carry physically rearranged chromosomes.

🅠 In two or three sentences explain why the results of this experiment confirm that the genetic observation of recombination is the result of physical exchange between homologous chromosomes.

PROBLEM In tomato plants (*Lycopersicon esculentum*), red fruit color (*T*—) is dominant to tangerine color (*tt*), and smooth leaf (*H*—) is dominant to hairy leaf (*hh*). Both genes are located on chromosome 7, and they have a recombination frequency of 20%. A pure-breeding plant producing tangerine-colored fruit and smooth leaves is crossed to a pure-breeding red-fruited, hairy-leaved plant. The F$_1$ are test-crossed to a pure-breeding tangerine-fruited, hairy plant. What are the expected genotypes, phenotypes, and phenotype proportions among test-cross progeny?

> BREAK IT DOWN: A recombination frequency of 20% means that 80% of gametes are parental and 20% are recombinant (p. 148).

> BREAK IT DOWN: Pure-breeding tangerine, smo is *ttHH* and pure-breedin red, hairy is *TThh* (pp. 15 and 152).

> BREAK IT DOWN: The F$_1$ are *TtHh*, and they are test-crosse to *tthh* (pp. 151 and 152).

Solution Strategies	Solution Steps
Evaluate	
1. Identify the topic of this problem and the nature of the required answer.	1. This problem concerns the prediction of inheritance in progeny of a test cross for linked genes. The answer requires that the expected frequency of each possible category of test-cross progeny be predicted from the information given about recombination frequency between the genes.
2. Identify the critical information given in the problem.	2. Dominant and recessive phenotypes, the phenotypes of two pure-breeding parental plants, and the recombination frequency between genes controlling two traits are given in the problem.
Deduce	
3. Identify the alleles in the gametes of the parental plants.	3. Each parent is pure-breeding for a dominant and a recessive trait: Tangerine, smooth = *ttHH* Red, hairy = *TThh* Parental gametes = all *tH* from one parent and all *Th* from the other
4. Identify the genotype and phenotype of F$_1$ plants, and determine the parental arrangements of alleles.	4. F$_1$ are dihybrid (*tH/Th*) and have the two dominant phenotypes (red and smooth). The pure-breeding parents have contributed chromosomes carrying *tH* and *Th*.
Solve	
5. Determine the number and frequency of F$_1$ gametes, given the recombination frequency of 20%. TIP: With genetic linkage, parental combinations of alleles are significantly greater than 50% of the gametes.	5. Four genetically different gametes are possible: *tH*, *Th*, *TH*, and *th*. Among these gametes, 20% will be recombinants and 80% parentals (100% − 20% = 80%). Chance predicts that the two parental gametes (*tH* and *Th*) are produced at equal frequency. Likewise, the two recombinant gametes (*TH* and *th*) are produced at equal frequency. The expected gamete frequencies are Parentals: $tH = (0.80)(1/2) = 0.40$ $Th = (0.80)(1/2) = 0.40$ Recombinants: $TH = (0.20)(1/2) = 0.10$ $th = (0.20)(1/2) = 0.10$
6. Determine the expected outcome of the test cross. TIP: There are two equally likely parental gametes and two equally likely recombinant gametes.	6. Test-cross progeny are expected to be 40% each tangerine, smooth and red, hairy; and 20% each red, smooth and tangerine, hairy.

		th (1.0)		Progeny	
Parental	0.40 *tH*	*tH/th*	0.40	Tangerine, smooth	40%
	0.40 *Th*	*Th/th*	0.40	Red, hairy	40%
Recombinant	0.10 *TH*	*TH/th*	0.10	Red, smooth	10%
	0.10 *th*	*th/th*	0.10	Tangerine, hairy	10%

Just a few weeks after Creighton and McClintock reported their evidence of a link between chromosome rearrangement and genetic recombination, Stern reported similar findings in *Drosophila*. The combined genetic and chromosomal recombination analyses in corn and fruit fly provided convincing evidence that genetic recombination between homologous chromosomes is accompanied by physical exchange between the chromosomes in plants and in animals.

5.2 Genetic Linkage Mapping Is Based on Recombination Frequency between Genes

An important outcome of Morgan's studies of linked genes in *Drosophila* was his recognition that significantly more parental than recombinant progeny occurred and that the proportion of recombinants varied considerably from one pair of linked genes to another. Morgan summarized this idea in 1911, stating, "The proportions that result are not so much the expression of a numerical system as of the relative location of the factors (genes) in the chromosome." Morgan was saying that independent assortment was not determining the relative proportions of all gametes produced by an organism. Instead, the close proximity of linked genes on a chromosome overrode the expected influence of independent assortment on the alleles of those genes. The linkage of genes preferentially retained parental combinations of alleles and led to a much higher proportion of parental gametes and a much lower proportion of nonparental gametes than were expected by chance. Morgan's intuition was correct, and his insight profoundly changed views of hereditary transmission and of the location and organization of genes on chromosomes. In this section, we examine methods for constructing genetic maps from recombination data for two linked genes, and in the next section, we'll move on to consider the mapping of three linked genes.

The First Genetic Linkage Map

In the context of early 20th-century biology, Morgan's idea that genes were on chromosomes was not novel. For example, Sutton, Boveri, and others had noted the parallel between hereditary transmission and chromosome division. But biologists at the time did not know either the structure of genes or how they were encoded on chromosomes (see Section 3.3). Morgan was the first to demonstrate that genes are on chromosomes, and his proposal that the recombination frequency for a linked pair of genes might correspond to the *distance* between those genes on a chromosome was a novel idea.

Morgan viewed genes as inhabiting fixed locations on chromosomes. Like cities along a road, the order of genes could be determined, the locations of genes on a chromosome could be specified, and the distances between genes

could be quantified. If this hypothesis was correct, then recombination frequencies could be used to produce a genetic linkage map depicting gene order along a chromosome and to infer the linear distances between genes. As Morgan discussed his ideas about recombination frequency and gene distances, Alfred Sturtevant, then an undergraduate student working in Morgan's laboratory, had an epiphany. In a 1965 book, Sturtevant recalled the moment:

> In the latter part of 1911, in a conversation with Morgan, I suddenly realized that the variations in strength of linkage, already attributed by Morgan to differences in the spatial separation of genes, offered the possibility of determining sequences in the linear dimension of a chromosome. I went home and spent most of the night (to the neglect of my other undergraduate homework) in producing the first chromosome map.

Sturtevant used the results of numerous two-point testcross experiments on five X-linked genes in *Drosophila* to create the first genetic linkage map. He based his map-building approach on the idea that smaller recombination frequencies indicated genes residing closer to each other on the chromosome, and larger recombination frequencies indicated greater distances between genes on the chromosome. To construct his genetic map, Sturtevant used the data in Table 5.2. His finished recombination map is illustrated in Figure 5.7. In the century since Sturtevant first compiled his map, millions of progeny fruit flies have been analyzed for X-chromosome recombination. The accumulated data have led to slight modifications in Sturtevant's estimated recombination frequencies but have not necessitated any changes in gene order. Sturtevant assembled his map using logic of the kind demonstrated in the following four steps:

1. Of the genes tested, the pair with the smallest recombination frequency, and therefore in closest proximity, are the gene producing white eye (*w*) and the gene carrying yellow (*y*) body. With their recombination frequency of just 1%, they must be at almost the same spot on the chromosome.

Table 5.2	Sturtevant's Recombination Data for Five X-Linked Genes in *Drosophila*
Gene Pairs	**Recombination Frequency (*r*)**
Yellow (*y*) and white (*w*)	214/21,736 = 0.010
Yellow (*y*) and vermilion (*v*)	1464/4551 = 0.322
Vermilion (*v*) and white (*w*)	471/1584 = 0.297
Vermilion (*v*) and miniature (*m*)	17/573 = 0.030
Miniature (*m*) and white (*w*)	2062/6116 = 0.337
White (*w*) and rudimentary (*r*)	406/898 = 0.452
Rudimentary (*r*) and vermilion (*v*)	109/405 = 0.269

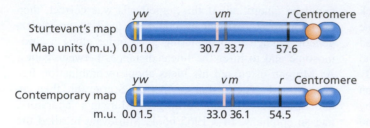

❓ **Consider the relative distances between and recombination frequencies for (1) the *white* and *vermillion* genes and (2) the *yellow* and *white* genes. Make a summary statement about the relationship between the physical distance between two genes and the recombination frequency between them.**

2. Vermilion (*v*) is more distant from yellow (32.2% recombination) than it is from white (29.7% recombination), suggesting the order *y–w–v*.

3. Miniature (*m*) is close to vermilion (3% recombination) but is more distant from white (33.7% recombination) than is vermilion. Adding miniature to the gene map produces the order *y–w–v–m*.

4. Rudimentary (*r*) is very distant from white (45.2% recombination) and also fairly distant from vermilion (26.9% recombination). This information places rudimentary on the opposite side of the map from white, yielding the final map *y–w–v–m–r*.

Map Units

As we examine our map of the *Drosophila* X chromosome, the correlation between recombination frequency and physical distance on chromosomes becomes easier to understand. The recombination frequencies between genes on a chromosome can even be converted into units of physical distance, using the concept of a **map unit (m.u.)**. A map unit is also known as a **centiMorgan (cM)** in honor of Thomas Hunt Morgan's contribution to recombination mapping. It is common (at least in introductory genetics courses) to use the equivalency

1% recombination = 1 m.u. or 1 cM of distance
between linked genes

This is an approximation, and not a very good one for certain regions of particular genomes, as we discuss in a later section. Despite its shortcomings, however, it is accurate enough for our instructional purposes in this textbook.

Chi-Square Analysis of Genetic Linkage Data

In our discussion of genetic linkage data, we have noted that when genes are linked, *significantly* more parental phenotypes than recombinant phenotypes are found among progeny. But how can we tell whether the observed data constitute evidence of genetic linkage rather than a simple case of chance variation from expected values? The question is settled by the use of chi-square analysis of observed

and expected values to identify statistically significant differences. (Section 2.5 describes the chi-square test and demonstrates the calculation and interpretation of chi-square *p*, or probability, values.)

As an example, let's revisit the data obtained by Morgan on the *w* gene affecting eye color and the *m* gene controlling wing form in *Drosophila*, presented in Figure 5.3. The cross of F_1 dihybrid females (wm/w^+m^+) to white-eyed, miniature-winged males (wm/Y) produces an F_2 generation that would have been expected to display a 1:1:1:1 phenotypic ratio. This ratio is based on the assumption that independent assortment determines the alleles contained in female gametes.

The question to answer by chi-square testing is whether the results are consistent with independent assortment or not. In other words, this is a test of a hypothesis of *no genetic linkage* between the genes. Using the observed and expected values, we calculate the chi-square value as follows:

$$\chi^2 = \frac{(791 - 610.25)^2}{610.25} + \frac{(750 - 610.25)^2}{610.25}$$
$$+ \frac{(445 - 610.25)^2}{610.25} + \frac{(455 - 610.25)^2}{610.25} = 169.79$$

For this analysis there are 3 degrees of freedom (df = 3), and the corresponding *p* value is $p < 0.005$ (see Table 2.4). This observed result indicates a significant deviation from expected results, suggesting that chance is not responsible for the observed distribution. Combined with the observation that the two phenotypes that exceed the expected number are parental, these data are consistent with the presence of genetic linkage between the genes.

5.3 Three-Point Test-Cross Analysis Maps Genes

Two-point test-cross analysis is an effective way to calculate the recombination frequency between two linked genes and to infer the distance between the genes, but it is not the most effective way to build genetic maps containing multiple genes. By expanding the idea of test-cross analysis to **three-point test-cross analysis,** however, geneticists can efficiently map three linked genes simultaneously.

Identifying Parental, Single-Crossover, and Double-Crossover Gametes in Three-Point Mapping

Let's consider a three-point test cross between a trihybrid organism ($a^+ab^+bc^+c$) and an organism that is homozygous recessive for the three traits ($aabbcc$). The configuration of alleles in the trihybrid (i.e., which of the alleles are on the same homolog) does not have to be known at the start, since the three-point analysis will deduce the configuration of alleles on parental chromosomes as part of the process.

Incomplete genetic linkage of three genes in a trihybrid produces eight genetically different gamete genotypes. This is the same number of genetically different gametes expected if we assume independent assortment; but, unlike the expectations for independent assortment, the gamete frequencies are unequal if the genes are linked. Among the eight gamete genotypes are two parental genotypes that are significantly more frequent than expected by chance as well as six recombinant genotypes, each detected less often than expected. Assuming, for the purposes of this example, that the three linked genes are in the order a–b–c, we can identify parental and recombinant gametes by the relative frequencies of the corresponding test-cross progeny classes.

Suppose a trihybrid organism, designated trihybrid 1, has the genotype $a^+b^+c^+/abc$ with alleles arranged so that the three dominant alleles are on one chromosome and

the three recessive alleles are on the homologous chromosome (**Figure 5.8a**). A total of eight genetically different chromosomes are expected: two parental, four from single crossovers, and two from double crossover. During meiosis, trihybrid 1 generates parental chromosomes ($a^+b^+c^+$ and abc) when no crossovers occur between the genes. A single crossover occurring between genes a and b produces two recombinant chromosomes, a^+bc and ab^+c^+, and likewise, a single crossover occurring between genes b and c also produces two different recombinant chromosomes, a^+b^+c and abc^+. A double-crossover event that causes crossing over both between a and b and between b and c will produce a pair of double-crossover chromosomes, a^+bc^+ and ab^+c.

Trihybrid 2, shown in **Figure 5.8b**, has a different arrangement of the dominant and recessive alleles on homologous chromosomes. Trihybrid 2 is $a+bc+/ab+c$. Trihybrid 2 produces the same eight chromosome genotypes as trihybrid 1, but since the alleles start out with different configurations on the parental chromosomes, the assignment of chromosomes to parental and recombinant categories differs from those assigned for trihybrid 1. For trihybrid 2, the parental chromosomes are a^+bc^+ and ab^+c. The single-crossover chromosomes are a^+b^+c and abc^+ for crossover between genes a and b. Single crossover between genes b and c produces chromosomes a^+bc and ab^+c^+. A double crossover causing recombination between each pair of genes produces double-crossover chromosomes $a^+b^+c^+$ and abc.

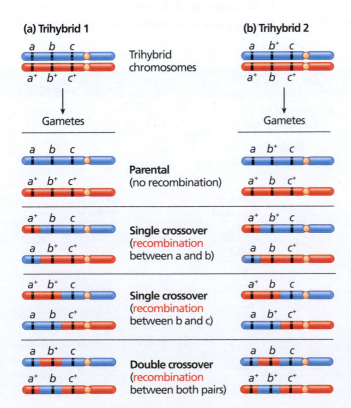

Figure 5.8 Gametes from trihybrid organisms with different allele configurations. (a) Trihybrid 1 is $a^+b^+c^+/abc$. Meiosis in trihybrid 1 produces two chromosomes with parental combinations of alleles, a total of four single-crossover chromosomes in two pairs, and two double-crossover chromosomes. **(b)** Trihybrid 2 is a^+bc^+/ab^+c. Meiosis in this organism also produces parental, single-crossover, and double-crossover chromosomes, but the alleles on these chromosomes differ from those of trihybrid 1 due to different allele configurations of the parental chromosomes.

In evaluating genetic linkage and crossing over, the two most important guidelines to follow are (1) find out what alleles are carried on the parental chromosomes—this information may be given or it may have to be deduced—and (2) expect that each of the six recombinant gametes will be observed at a frequency that is significantly less than predicted by chance. Single-crossover gametes form at frequencies determined by the relative distances between gene pairs. Within each single-crossover class, the two gametes will be equally frequent. Double-crossover gametes will be the least frequent class because *both* crossover events must occur. As within each single-crossover class, the two kinds of double-crossover gametes are produced at equal frequency.

Constructing a Three-Point Recombination Map

To illustrate the evaluation of genetic linkage and recombination for the purpose of mapping gene order and relative distance, we turn to the use of three-point test-cross analysis. The data presented are based on test crosses between an organism that is trihybrid (the allele arrangements may be known or may have to be deduced) and an organism that is homozygous for the three recessive alleles. This cross design ensures that the phenotypes of test-cross progeny will directly reflect the alleles contributed during mating by the trihybrid parent. The triple-recessive parent can contribute only recessive alleles, so if progeny exhibit a dominant trait, the trihybrid parent has contributed the dominant allele, and if progeny exhibit a recessive trait, the trihybrid parent has contributed a recessive allele. The data we describe are from a 1935 study by Rollins Emerson of genetic linkage in maize (*Zea mays*). Emerson tested three genes: the gene producing the phenotypes green seedling (*V−*) and yellow seedling (*vv*), the gene producing rough leaf (*Gl−*) and glossy leaf (*gl gl*), and the gene for normal fertility (*Va−*) and variable fertility (*va va*).

Emerson crossed pure-breeding wild-type plants having the dominant phenotypes green seedling, rough leaves, and normal fertility (which, not knowing the gene order, we will provisionally identify as *V Gl Va/V Gl Va*) to pure-breeding plants having the recessive phenotypes yellow seedling, glossy leaves, and variable fertility (*v gl va/v gl va*). The cross produced F_1 trihybrid plants with the dominant phenotypes and the genotype *V Gl Va/v gl va* that carries three dominant alleles on one chromosome and three recessive alleles on the homolog. The F_1 were then test-crossed to pure-breeding yellow, glossy, variable plants (*v gl va/v gl va*). The test-cross progeny are shown in **Table 5.3**. To create a genetic map that places the three genes in correct relative order and to calculate recombination frequencies between gene pairs, we ask and answer five questions about these data:

1. Are the data consistent with the proposal of genetic linkage?

2. What alleles are on each parental chromosome?

3. What is the gene order on the chromosome?

4. What are the recombination frequencies of the gene pairs?

5. Is the frequency of double crossovers consistent with the independent occurrence of single crossovers?

Table 5.3	Emerson's Three-Point Test-Cross Analysis		
Parental cross:	*V Gl Va/V Gl Va* Green, rough, normal	×	*v gl va/ v gl va* yellow, glossy, variable
Test cross:	*V Gl Va/v gl va* Green, rough, normal	×	*v gl va/v gl va* yellow, glossy, variable

Test-cross progeny:

Phenotype	Number Observed	Number Expected	Genotype (gamete / gamete)
1. Yellow, rough, normal	60	90.75	*v Gl Va/v gl va*
2. Yellow, glossy, normal	48	90.75	*v gl Va/v gl va*
3. Yellow, rough, variable	4	90.75	*v Gl va/v gl va*
4. Yellow, glossy, variable	270	90.75	*v gl va/v gl va*
5. Green, rough, normal	235	90.75	*V Gl Va/v gl va*
6. Green, glossy, normal	7	90.75	*V gl Va/v gl va*
7. Green, rough, variable	40	90.75	*V Gl va/v gl va*
8. Green, glossy, variable	62	90.75	*V gl va/v gl va*
	726	726	

Question 1: Are the Data Consistent with the Proposal of Genetic Linkage? Under the assumptions of independent assortment, trihybrid plants produce eight genetically different gametes at a frequency of 0.125, or 1/8, each, and test-cross progeny are expected in eight equally frequent phenotypic classes. In this experiment, with 726 test-cross progeny, the expected number of progeny in each class would be $(726)(0.125) = 90.75$. Chi-square analysis comparing observed and expected numbers of progeny in each class (Table 5.3) yields a chi-square value in excess of 800. There are $(8 - 1) = 7$ degrees of freedom, and the corresponding p value is $p < 0.005$. From this result, we conclude that the observed distribution of test-cross progeny deviates significantly from expectation, and we reject the independent assortment hypothesis as the explanation of these data.

If the deviation in this experiment is due to genetic linkage, then we would expect the numbers of progeny having parental phenotypes to be excessively high. Comparing the observed and expected values in each test-cross class shows that only two phenotype classes exceed expected numbers: the green, rough, normal class and the yellow, glossy, variable class. These are the two parental phenotypes. From this analysis, we conclude that the data are consistent with genetic linkage: the distribution of test-cross progeny deviates significantly from what would be expected from independent assortment, and only parental phenotypes are seen more often than expected by chance.

Question 2: What Alleles Are on Each Parental Chromosome? We can answer this question in two ways. The simpler approach is to use the phenotype information available about pure-breeding parental plants in the cross. The parent plants were pure-breeding dominant and pure-breeding recessive. From this information, we know that trihybrid F_1 plants have the dominant alleles on one chromosome and the recessive alleles on the homologous chromosome. The genetic structure of the test cross is *V Gl Va/v gl va* × *v gl va/v gl va*, and so the alleles on parental chromosomes must be *V Gl Va* and *v gl va*. Test-cross progeny Classes 4 and 5 in Table 5.3 are parentals.

The second approach is necessary when we do not know the phenotypes of parents or when the alleles on each chromosome are not known. In this approach, test-cross data are used to determine parental chromosomes. The data in Table 5.3 indicate that the test-cross progeny in Class 5—green, rough, normal (*V Gl Va/v gl va*)—and in Class 4—yellow, glossy, variable (*v gl va/v gl va*)—exceed expected frequency and are therefore the parental classes. Both approaches tell us the same story: The parental chromosomes carry alleles *V Gl Va* and *v gl va*.

Question 3: What Is the Gene Order on the Chromosome? With parental chromosomes identified, the six remaining classes must be recombinants: four are single-crossover classes, and two are double crossovers. Double-crossover progeny will be the least frequent of all classes, because *both* crossover events must occur simultaneously to produce **double recombinants**, or **double crossovers**. From progeny numbers, we may presume that the smallest classes, Class 3—yellow, rough, variable—and Class 6—green, glossy, normal—are the probable double recombinants. We can use these predictions to test possible gene orders on parental chromosomes.

For these three genes there are only three possible gene orders: (1) *va–v–gl*, (2) *v–va–gl*, or (3) *va–gl–v*. There are no data to assist us in determining the left-to-right orientation of the chromosome, so the difference between these gene orders is defined entirely by which gene is in the *middle—v, va,* or *gl*—and which two genes flank the middle gene. Each gene order could be written in the opposite direction, since each is a *relative* order of the three genes. For example, *va–v–gl* and *gl–v–va* are equivalent gene orders because each has *v* as the middle gene.

There are two ways to determine the gene order. One procedure is to list each gene order possible for the parental chromosomes, draw the corresponding double-crossover chromosomes, and then determine whether the double-crossover gametes produced by this activity match the predicted double-crossover progeny. If a match is not seen, the gene order is incorrect, but if a match is found, the correct gene order has been identified.

1. Possible gene order *va–v–gl*

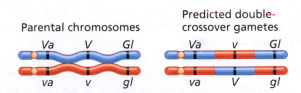

Result: Double-crossover gametes obtained from this gene order are not those predicted from the data (i.e., do not match Class 3 and Class 6 phenotypes).

Conclusion: The proposed gene order is incorrect; *v* is not the middle gene.

2. Possible gene order *v–va–gl*

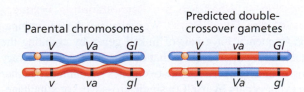

Result: Double-crossover gametes obtained from this gene order are not those predicted from the data (i.e., do not match Class 3 and Class 6 phenotypes).

Conclusion: The proposed gene order is incorrect; *va* is not the middle gene.

3. Possible gene order *v–gl–va*

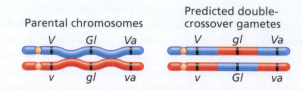

Result: Double-crossover gametes obtained from this gene order match those predicted from the data (i.e., do match Class 3 and Class 6 phenotypes).

Conclusion: This proposed gene order is correct: *gl* is the middle gene, and the gene order may be written as either *v–gl–va* or *va–gl–v*. This analysis confirms that test-cross progeny Classes 3 and 6 are double-crossover progeny.

The second method for determining gene order is a shortcut approach that requires some familiarity with recombination. Looking back at Figure 5.8, note that if we compare parental and double-crossover chromosomes, the alleles of the outside genes appear to remain the same while the middle allele appears to switch. In other words, when we compare one parental chromosome with one double-recombinant chromosome, two alleles match and one does not. The odd one out is the allele in the middle. If a trihybrid parent has alleles arranged as $a^+b^+c^+/abc$, then double crossover produces gametes that are a^+bc^+/ab^+c. Parental alleles a^+ and c^+ match one double recombinant, and alleles b and b^+ are switched. Similarly, the second parental gamete has alleles a and c that match the other double recombinant. Alleles of the middle gene, b and b^+, have switched in the double recombinant compared with the parental chromosome.

Remember, we have already identified the parental and double-crossover phenotypic groups by their numbers. We now look at the double crossovers to see which two alleles match parental phenotypes and to see which allele changes and is therefore the middle gene. In our data set, double-recombinant chromosomes are *V gl Va* and *v Gl va*. In this case, alleles of the *gl* gene have switched, indicating that *gl* is the middle gene. Based on this approach, the gene orders and alleles on parental chromosomes are *V Gl Va* and *v gl va*.

Question 4: What Are the Recombination Frequencies of the Gene Pairs?

We calculate the recombination frequency for a pair of linked genes by counting the total number of crossovers that occur between them. Every crossover event between the two genes is counted, whether the event occurs by itself (a single crossover) or simultaneously with another event (a double crossover). In this case, there are 11 double recombinants, each with one crossover between *v* and *gl* and one crossover between *gl* and *va*, for a total of 22 crossover events. These 22 crossovers must be counted in the determination of recombination frequency, so 11 of these crossovers will be added to the number of

single crossovers between *v* and *gl*, and 11 are also added to the number of single crossovers between *gl* and *va*.

Let's continue with our presumption that the gene order is *v–gl–va*. Between *v* and *gl*, a single crossover produces the following

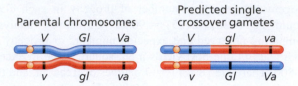

Test-cross progeny carrying recombination between these two genes have the phenotypes yellow, rough, normal (Class 1) and green, glossy, variable (Class 8). The recombination frequency is calculated as the sum of all single crossovers for this gene pair plus the 11 crossovers seen in double recombinants divided by the total number of progeny: $(60 + 62 + 4 + 7)/726 = 0.183$, or 18.3%. Therefore, the distance between *v* and *gl*, is approximately 18.3 cM.

Single crossover between *gl* and *va* produces the following

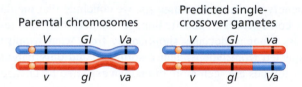

Test-cross progeny carrying recombination between these two genes have the phenotypes yellow, glossy, normal (Class 2) and green, rough, variable (Class 7). Recombination frequency $r = (48 + 40 + 4 + 7)/726 = 0.136$, or 13.6%. The intergenic distance between *gl* and *va* is approximately 13.6 cM.

Recombination between the flanking genes, *va* and *v*, is calculated by counting all crossovers between those genes. Recombination between *v* and *va* is $r = (60 + 62 + 48 + 40 + 22)/726 = 0.320$, or 32%.

Question 5: Is the Frequency of Double Crossovers Consistent with the Independent Occurrence of the Single Crossovers?

In most tests of genetic linkage, the number of double crossovers is *less* than the number expected given the frequencies of the single crossovers. Question 5 allows this common observation to be quantified. The reduction in the observed number of double crossovers relative to the number expected if the two single crossovers happened independently of one another is caused by an effect called **interference** (*I*). Interference indicates the influence of some process or processes that limit the number of crossovers that can occur in a short length of chromosome. Interference is quantified by comparing the number or frequency of observed double-crossover events with the number or frequency expected assuming each crossover event occurs independently. In Emerson's data set, there are 11 double crossovers among test-cross progeny, or $(11/726) = 0.015$ (1.5%). If each crossover were independent, the expected double-crossover frequency would be the product of the two single-crossover frequencies, $(0.183)(0.136) = 0.025$, or 2.5%. The expected number of double-crossover progeny would therefore be $(0.025)(726) = 18.2$. Observed double recombinants are divided by expected double recombinants to produce a value known as the **coefficient of coincidence** (*c*). Either the numbers or the frequencies of observed and expected double recombinants can be used to determine *c*:

$$c = \frac{\text{observed double recombinants}}{\text{expected double recombinants}}$$

$$= 11/18.2 = 0.60 \text{ (using numbers)}$$

or

$$= 0.015/0.025 = 0.60 \text{ (using frequencies)}$$

Interference is defined as $I = 1 - c$, so for this data set $I = 1 - 0.60 = 0.40$. Interference identifies the proportion of double recombinants that are expected but *are not produced* in the experiment (the difference between expectation and actuality). In this case, the number of double recombinants was 40% lower than expected. Interference is a very common observation in most regions of most genomes. On occasion, however, certain regions of some genomes generate *more* double recombinants than expected. In these cases $I < 0$, a situation called **negative interference**. Interference will be zero ($I = 0$) when the observed and expected double crossovers are equal. The molecular basis of interference is not fully understood, but current research suggests that the molecular process of crossing over operates to distribute cross-over events widely on chromosomes and that there is a mechanical limit that restricts the number of recombination events in close proximity on a chromosome. We discuss the molecular process of homologous recombination in Chapter 10.

Determining Gamete Frequencies from Genetic Maps

The same principle used for constructing genetic linkage maps—the relation between relative distances and recombination frequency—can be used for making predictions in the reverse direction, that is, to determine the expected frequencies of recombinant and nonrecombinant gametes on the basis of completed genetic linkage maps.

In **Figure 5.9a**, two linked genes have a recombination frequency of 10%. For the dihybrid organism *AB/ab*, two gametes (*AB* and *ab*) are parental, and two (*Ab* and *aB*) are recombinant. Recombinant gametes equal 10% of total gametes, and each recombinant is expected to occur with the same frequency. The probability is calculated as $(\frac{1}{2})(0.010) = 0.05$ for each recombinant gamete. In this calculation, $\frac{1}{2}$ is the probability of each recombinant chromosome appearing in a gamete, and 0.010 is the probability of recombination between the genes. From this information, we can calculate that, conversely, parental gametes *AB* and

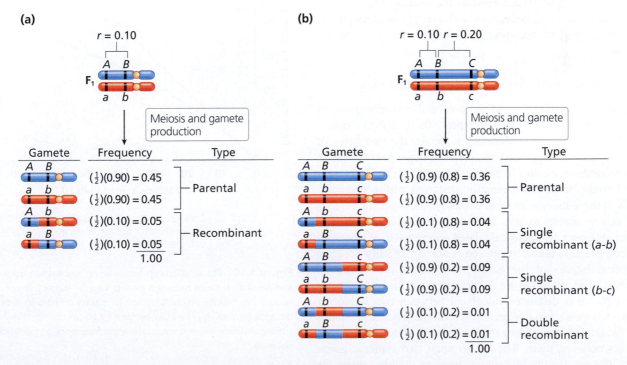

Figure 5.9 **Gamete genotype frequencies calculated from genetic linkage data.** (a) Gamete frequencies predicted from a map of two linked genes. (b) Gamete frequencies predicted from a map of three linked genes assuming interference is zero ($I = 0$).

ab are formed at a frequency equal to 100% minus 10%, or 90% of total gametes. Both of the parental gametes are also expected at equal frequency—in this case $(\frac{1}{2})(0.90)$, or 45% each.

Gamete frequencies for three linked genes are predicted in a similar manner. In **Figure 5.9b**, genes *a* and *b* are shown along with a third gene, *c*, located 20 cM from gene *b*. To predict gamete frequencies, we make the assumption that interference is $I = 0$ to simplify the calculation of the number of recombinants. For the trihybrid organism *ABC/abc*, parental gametes are produced when crossover does not occur in either gene interval. According to the genetic map, the probability of *no crossovers* between genes *a* and *b* is 90% (0.9), and between *b* and *c* it is 80% (0.8). Considering both gene pairs, the proportion of nonrecombinant gametes is $(0.9)(0.8) = 0.72$: there are two equally frequent parental gametes, each with an expected frequency of $(\frac{1}{2})(0.9)(0.8) = 0.36$. Recombination frequency is 10%, or 0.1, between *a* and *b*. The two single recombinants between genes *a* and *b* each have an expected frequency of $(0.1)(0.8)(\frac{1}{2}) = 0.04$ each (the frequency of recombination between *a* and *b* times the frequency of no recombination between *b* and *c* times $\frac{1}{2}$ since there are two such gametes). Similarly, single recombinants between genes *b* and *c* have expected frequencies of $(0.9)(0.2)\frac{1}{2} = 0.09$ each. Each of the double-recombinant gametes, *AbC* and *aBc*, are expected with a frequency of $(0.1)(0.2)(0.5) = 0.01$. The sum of frequencies of the eight predicted gamete genotypes is 1.0, indicating that all gametes have been counted.

Genetic Analysis 5.2 presents the results of test crosses involving three linked genes and takes you through the determination of recombination frequencies between the genes.

Correction of Genetic Map Distances

Many factors affect crossing over and recombination in eukaryotic genomes. As examples, there are (1) differences in genetic recombination maps for the two sexes of a species; (2) age- and temperature-dependent variation in recombination in *Drosophila* females; and (3) hotspots and coldspots of recombination scattered within genomes. Given these diverse and sometimes species-specific effects, it is reasonable to ask whether recombination frequencies and map distances calculated on the basis of observed recombination between gene pairs are in fact fully accurate representations of the actual numbers of recombination events. The answer is no. Experimental evidence indicates that the map distances calculated between two randomly selected genes usually *underestimate* the physical distance between the genes, largely because of undetected crossovers between them. The farther apart two syntenic genes are, the greater the inaccuracy, because double crossovers between a pair of genes are not detected in the progeny phenotype.

A single crossover between genes *A* and *B* in a dihybrid (*AB/ab*) produces two parental gametes (*AB* and *ab*) and two recombinant gametes (*Ab* and *aB*). Double crossover between the same genes, however, produces crossover gametes that are not recombinant for the *A* and *B* genes and so are indistinguishable from parentals. These crossover-nonrecombinant gametes are not counted when recombination frequency between genes is calculated, because they are not observed. Larger distances between genes provide greater opportunity for double crossover and thus greater likelihood of crossover-nonrecombinant gametes.

In theory, the relationship between recombination frequency and map distance is linear, but this is not the case in reality. Line ❶ in **Figure 5.10** depicts a linear relationship between recombination frequency and the distance in map units (cM). In contrast, line ❷ illustrates the correspondence between recombination frequency and actual distance along the map. The lines diverge at about 8 cM, indicating that the relationship between recombination frequency and map distance is linear only for linked genes that are separated by less than 8 cM, and that observed recombination frequencies usually underestimate the physical distance between genes.

The central problem in correlating recombination frequency with the number of recombination events is the difficulty of identifying the number of meioses that produce each possible number of crossovers—zero, one, two, three, four crossovers, and so on. In an attempt to correctly model

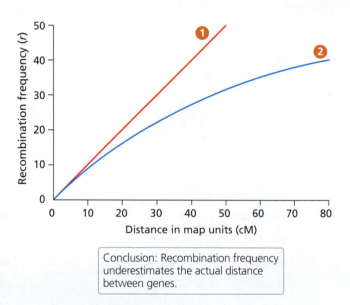

Conclusion: Recombination frequency underestimates the actual distance between genes.

Figure 5.10 **The relationship between recombination frequency and physical distance between genes.** Line ❶ traces a linear relationship between recombination frequency and the physical distance separating linked genes. Line ❷ traces the observed correspondence between recombination frequency and physical distance.

◉ Compare line 1 and line 2 in this chart and identify the map distance over which they match one another, and describe how they differ as map distances increase.

PROBLEM Dr. O. Sophila, a famous geneticist, is evaluating genetic linkage among three X-linked genes in *Drosophila*. At these genes, red eye (v^+) is dominant to vermilion eye (v); full wing (r^+) is dominant to rudimentary wing (r); and gray body color (y^+) is dominant to yellow (y). Dr. Sophila has the results of three test crosses. Help Dr. Sophila identify which pairs of genes are linked, and calculate the recombination frequency between linked genes.

> **BREAK IT DOWN:** Test-cross progeny allow each allele to be assigned to a chromosome (p. 150).

> **BREAK IT DOWN:** If genes are linked, the frequency of progeny with parental phenotypes will be significantly greater than expected by chance (p. 153).

Test Cross I:

♀ *yv*/++ (gray body, red eye) ×
♂ *yv*/Y (yellow body, vermilion eye)

Progeny	Number
Yellow, vermilion	338
Gray, red	332
Yellow, red	160
Gray, vermilion	170
	1000

Test Cross II:

♀ *vr*/++ (red eye, full wing) ×
♂ *vr*/Y (vermilion eye, rudimentary wing)

Progeny	Number
Vermilion, rudimentary	396
Red, full	389
Vermilion, full	110
Red, rudimentary	105
	1000

Test Cross III:

♀ *yr*/++ (gray body, full wing) ×
♂ *yr*/Y (yellow body, rudimentary wing)

Progeny	Number
Yellow, rudimentary	246
Gray, full	252
Yellow, full	259
Gray, rudimentary	243
	1000

Solution Strategies	Solution Steps

Evaluate

1. Identify the topic of this problem and the nature of the required answer.

1. This problem involves the assessment of three test crosses involving X-linked genes. The answer requires determination of genetic linkage versus independent assortment for each gene pair and, for linked genes, the calculation of recombination frequency.

2. Identify the critical information given in the problem.

2. The genotypes and phenotypes of test-cross flies are given, and the number of test-cross progeny in each phenotypic category is also given.

Deduce

3. Determine the test-cross results expected under the assumption of independent assortment.

3. In each cross, the dihybrid female would be expected to produce four genetically different gametes at frequencies of 25% each, and the progeny would be expected to display four phenotypes in a 1:1:1:1 ratio (250 each). In Test cross I, for example, the following results would be expected, and expected results would be similar for the other test crosses as well.

Phenotype	Female	Male	Number
Yellow, vermilion	*yv/yv*	*yv/Y*	250
Gray, red	*yv/y⁺v⁺*	*y⁺v⁺/Y*	250
Yellow, red	*yv/yv⁺*	*yv⁺/Y*	250
Gray, vermilion	*yv/y⁺v*	*y⁺v/Y*	250

> **TIP:** Chi-square analysis could be used to test the statistical significance of deviations between observed and expected outcomes.

Solve

4. Examine each cross and determine if there is evidence of genetic linkage between the gene pairs.

4. Test cross I and Test cross II show clear deviation from the predicted ratio, with parental categories substantially greater than 250 each and nonparental categories substantially less than 250 each. The progeny of Test cross III are distributed in numbers consistent with the independent assortment prediction. These statements are based on chi-squared analysis that is not shown.

5. Calculate the recombination frequencies between linked pairs of genes.

5. In Test cross I, the recombinant progeny are yellow, red and gray, vermilion. $r = (160 + 170)/1000 = 0.330$, indicating that these genes are linked and are separated by 33 m.u.

In Test cross II, the recombinant phenotypes are vermilion, full and red, rudimentary. The recombination frequency is $r = (110 + 105)/1000 = 0.215$, or approximately 21.5 m.u.

For more practice, see Problems 2, 4, and 28.　　Visit the Study Area to access study tools.　**Mastering Genetics**

different recombination classes and to accurately assess the correlation between recombination frequency and crossover, J. B. S. Haldane in 1919 developed a **mapping function** that correlates map distance and recombination frequency between gene pairs. The Haldane mapping function has limitations, and several researchers proposed modifications of it to account for specific conditions affecting recombination in different species.

One consistent concern raised about Haldane's mapping function is that it may overestimate the actual recombination frequency when interference occurs. Damodar Kosambi developed a modified mapping function to correct map distance in species with interference, and it has become one of the most widely applied improvements.

Mapping functions are a quantitative solution to the problem of variability of recombination frequencies across the genome and between species. Mapping functions are largely made obsolete by genomic sequence analysis in gene mapping that allows geneticists to use genome sequences to devise physical maps of the genes on chromosomes. Gene mapping is no less important today than it was when Alfred Sturtevant determined the first genetic map more than 100 years ago, but the methods for constructing maps continue to evolve.

5.4 Multiple Factors Cause Recombination to Vary

Despite the biological and evolutionary importance of recombination, its occurrence is variable among organisms. For example, recombination is a vital component of accurate chromosome segregation in mammalian meiosis, but it is not required for meiotic efficiency in other organisms. Most animal species undergo recombination, but in certain species, such as *Drosophila,* recombination is exclusive to females and does not occur in males. Furthermore, although our discussion of recombination in this chapter is limited to events taking place in meiosis, crossing over between homologous chromosomes also occurs in mitosis in many species, and rates of mitotic crossover are also highly variable.

From an evolutionary perspective, crossing over and recombination contribute to genetic diversity. Experimental evidence supports the idea that homologous recombination is a potent factor in evolution and that recombination is favored by natural selection. A meta-analysis by Sarah Otto and Thomas Lenormand in 2002 examined recombination rates in a large number of artificial selection experiments conducted by other researchers who were studying the evolution of traits that were unrelated to sex or recombination. (A meta-analysis is a study that combines the results of multiple previous studies with similar structure.) Otto and Lenormand determined that in the majority of cases, the rate of recombination had increased significantly as a result of the application of artificial selection to a trait. This result indicates that evolution is enhanced by the occurrence of recombination and that recombination rates increase in response to evolution.

The discussion of mapping functions in Section 5.3 mentioned that age, environment, sex, and other, as yet undetermined, factors may influence recombination frequency and affect the relationship between the genetic recombination map and the physical map of a chromosome. In female fruit flies, advancing age decreases the frequency of crossover between gene pairs, so that more crossovers between a specific pair of genes are seen in younger females than in older ones. Female *Drosophila* crossover frequency is also affected by temperature: Growing a fruit-fly colony at 22°C produces many crossovers between chromosomes. Recombination frequencies change, however, with increases or decreases in temperature. Restricting dietary levels of calcium and magnesium, important cofactors for enzymes that interact with DNA, also decreases crossover frequency in fruit flies.

Several other biological factors affecting recombination and recombination frequency in organisms are identified in the remainder of this section.

Sex Affects Recombination

The sex of an animal can have a dramatic impact on recombination frequency, which differs for males and females of most animal species. In the general pattern, the heterogametic sex, the sex with two different sex chromosomes (most often males), has a lower rate of recombination than the homogametic sex, the sex with two fully homologous sex chromosomes (most often females). The higher recombination frequency in the homogametic sex is a genome-wide phenomenon and *is not* limited to the sex chromosomes.

This difference is seen across the taxonomic spectrum, including in humans. Human females experience more crossing over than human males, resulting in a larger recombination map in females. A detailed recombination and genome sequencing analysis of human chromosome 19 exemplifies this phenomenon. Chromosome 19 is composed of about 65 megabases (Mb), or 65 million base pairs, in both male and female genomes (**Figure 5.11**). However, the length of the chromosome as determined by adding the estimated recombination distances along its entire length is a larger number of map units in females than in males. Also notice that recombination frequencies are greater in regions at the ends of the chromosome in males but are greater in females in central chromosome regions. For the human genome as a whole, the female genetic map contains about 4400 cM, and the male map about 2700 cM. Geneticists studying the human genome usually produce a "sex averaged" human genetic map that is slightly larger than 3500 cM.

Among different species, the number of nucleotide base pairs per map unit varies. For example, the human genome consists of a little less than 3 billion base pairs of DNA, and the sex-averaged genome contains about 830,000 bp/cM. In contrast, the *Arabidopsis* genome contains about 200,000 bp/cM; thus, recombination is about four times as frequent in *Arabidopsis* as it is in humans.

Recombination Is Dominated by Hotspots

Estimates of average numbers of base pairs per centiMorgan, of the average recombination frequency for a species, and of distances in a sex-averaged recombination map such as the one described for humans are just that: averaged estimates. In contrast, genome-based information on organisms has led to the creation of fine-scale genetic maps of species that identify the distribution of recombination across the genome with much greater precision. Detailed assessment of recombination in human, mouse, and yeast genomes reveals a highly variable pattern of recombination within each genome that has led to the identification of **recombination hotspots** and **recombination coldspots**, even while reinforcing the general theme of a rough proportionality between recombination frequencies and the physical maps of chromosomes.

Genetic recombination maps are generated by analysis of recombination information and recombination frequency data. Physical maps of chromosomes, on the other hand, are based on genomic sequence data that identify specific genes within DNA sequence. The proportionality between genetic recombination maps and physical maps of a chromosome makes it possible to generate gene maps that locate the position and approximate distance between genes along a chromosome. This proportionality exists because almost all

regions of DNA are about equally likely to initiate recombination. Nevertheless, as noted above, many genomes do contain hotspots and coldspots of recombination—segments of chromosomes that undergo substantially more or substantially less recombination than the average for a species.

Studies in yeast have examined this phenomenon in detail, and one study of yeast chromosomes has identified hotspots and coldspots side by side. In **Figure 5.12**, the coldspot of recombination between *spo7* and *cdc15* results in mapping data that appear to place the genes closer to one another than they are in the physical map. In contrast, the hotspot between *cdc15* and *FLO1* makes them appear to be farther apart on the genetic recombination map than on the

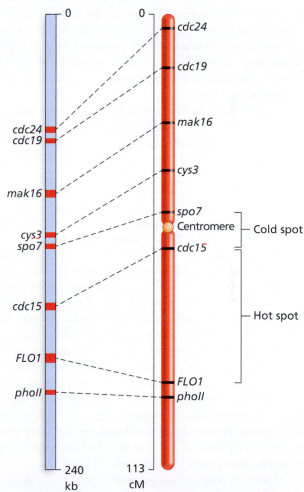

Figure 5.12   Recombination hotspots and coldspots. A comparison of the physical map and recombination map of yeast chromosome 1 identifies a hotspot of recombination between *cdc15* and *FLO1* and a coldspot of recombination between *spo7* and *cdc15*.

🅠 Considering the information in this figure, in Figure 5.11, and in the corresponding discussion in this chapter, why is the generalization that 1% recombination equals 1 map unit of distance between genes not an accurate reflection of the reality of crossing over?

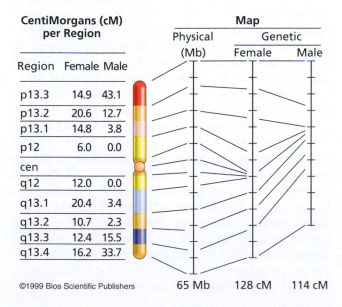

CentiMorgans (cM) per Region		
Region	Female	Male
p13.3	14.9	43.1
p13.2	20.6	12.7
p13.1	14.8	3.8
p12	6.0	0.0
cen		
q12	12.0	0.0
q13.1	20.4	3.4
q13.2	10.7	2.3
q13.3	12.4	15.5
q13.4	16.2	33.7

©1999 Bios Scientific Publishers

Figure 5.11   Physical distance versus recombination distance on human male and female chromosome 19. In most sexually reproducing organisms, the heterogametic sex has fewer recombination events and a shorter recombination map than does the homogametic sex. *Data adapted from J. L. Weber et al. (1993).*

physical map of the chromosome. The other genes in this chromosome region have generally good proportionality between recombination and physical distances.

The reason for the existence of hotspots and coldspots of recombination may have to do with the ability of DNA regions near specific genes to initiate the molecular events associated with the first steps of crossing over. In the case of the coldspot between *spo7* and *cdc15* in yeast, the chromosome centromere is between the genes, which may be an additional factor contributing to the relatively low recombination between them. We discuss more about the molecular process of recombination in Section 11.6.

Genome Sequence Analysis Reveals Recombination Hotspot Distribution

Variability of recombination across the genome appears to be the rule, as verified by recent studies in *Drosophila*, mouse, and humans. These studies show that within the genome, recombination occurs primarily at specific hotspots, punctuated by long stretches in which little or no recombination occurs.

A 2013 study in *Drosophila* by Nadia Singh and colleagues examined more than 6700 crossovers in the X chromosome between the *garnet* gene controlling eye color and the *scalloped* gene controlling wing shape. The authors identified a recombination rate of 7.3% (7.3 cM) between these genes, using the kind of recombination mapping analysis described in the preceding discussion. *Drosophila* genome sequence information indicated that the two genes are separated by approximately 2 million base pairs. To find specifically *where* within the 2 million base pairs recombination occurs, the authors used 451 known sequence variations lying between the two genes to map the location of each recombination event with great precision. The 2 million base pairs between the genes were divided into blocks of 5000 base pairs, and the number of crossovers in each 5000-bp block was tabulated. The results revealed a 90-fold difference in recombination rates for different blocks. Some 5000-bp regions had low recombination rates equivalent to 0.3 cM per million base pairs, whereas other blocks had rates as high as the equivalent of 27 cM per million base pairs. This result indicates that recombinational hotspots are distributed very unevenly within the *Drosophila* genome and that most recombination events are limited to relatively short segments of DNA.

Studies in mammalian genomes, particularly those of mouse and human, produce similar results. In the mouse genome, recombination rates are highly uneven, with hotspots of recombination serving as the predominant locations of crossing over. Mouse results have identified thousands of regions containing a 13-bp sequence—a so-called 13-mer—that appears to be located at the sites of up to 40% of the hotspots in the genome. Strong evidence indicates that a mouse protein designated PRDM9 binds to genome regions containing the 13-mer. It has been proposed that in a large proportion of mouse recombination events, PRDM9

plays an important role in determining the site at which recombination will occur.

Recent studies in humans verify the possible involvement of PRDM9 in recombination at hotspots. In addition, human genome–aided analysis of recombination distribution finds that human recombination hotspots are located in short regions of 1000–2000 bp. The data indicate that there may be 30,000 or so such recombination hotspots in the human genome, spaced about every 50,000 to 100,000 bp.

5.5 Human Genes Are Mapped Using Specialized Methods

Until relatively recently, the human genetic map was rather sparse. Humans cannot be studied through controlled matings and in any case produce much smaller numbers of offspring than do organisms like *Drosophila* and *Zea mays*. Consequently, gene-mapping methods developed and used successfully to map genes in model organisms are difficult to apply to human gene mapping. Historically, X-linked genes, by virtue of their unique patterns of transmission, were the first and easiest human genes to map, whereas progress in mapping human autosomal genes was hampered by a scarcity of known polymorphic genes, such as those for blood group antigens and blood proteins.

Human genome mapping changed significantly in the mid-1980s, facilitated both by the emergence of molecular genetic methods to identify polymorphic DNA sequences and by advances in gene-mapping software. The various DNA sequence polymorphisms are broadly identified as **genetic markers**. This term includes several types of inherited DNA sequence polymorphisms that we describe below. Collectively, these genetic markers provide thousands of signposts on every chromosome to assist in gene mapping and linkage analysis. Combined with sophisticated statistical techniques and modern computer power, the use of these genetic markers has given geneticists the ability to effectively map human genes by genetic linkage analysis.

The availability of large numbers of DNA markers on each chromosome led first to the identification of **linkage groups**, clusters of syntenic genes that are linked to one another, and then to assignment of chromosomal locations to linkage groups. The discovery of genetic linkage between a genetic marker with a known chromosome location and any member of a linkage group assigns the linkage group to a chromosome location near the genetic marker. Different linkage groups on the same chromosome can then be organized into maps of chromosome segments and whole chromosomes.

Mapping with Genetic Markers

An array of different variants of DNA sequence constitute the genetic markers that are located along chromosomes and can be used to study the locations of expressed genes.

These markers are almost always in noncoding regions of the genome, meaning that the sequence variation does not affect the coding or regulatory region of an expressed gene or protein and does not affect the phenotype of the organisms in any way. One kind of genetic marker is the **variable number tandem repeat (VNTR)**. These consist of short sequences of DNA, usually 3 to 20 base pairs. The short sequences are repeated end-to-end in a chromosome region. Since these occur in noncoding regions, natural selection does not put any rigid constraints on their variation; different chromosomes can carry different numbers of repeats of the sequence, and there may be a large number of different repeat lengths among chromosomes in a population.

Each individual is either homozygous or heterozygous for alleles at a VNTR marker. **Figure 5.13a** illustrates the appearance of a VNTR in a pair of homologous chromosomes of a heterozygous individual. **Figure 5.13b** illustrates the observation of VNTRs in a gel and the codominant pattern of transmission of VNTRs on autosomal chromosomes when heterozygous parents each donate one VNTR allele to each child. Transmission of these alleles is codominant because each allele in a heterozygous genotype can be detected, and homozygotes can be distinguished from heterozygotes.

Much more commonly used than VNTRs as genetic markers are **single nucleotide polymorphisms (SNPs;** pronounced "snips"). SNPs are DNA sequence variants in which one base pair is substituted by another base pair; SNPs, too, are usually located in noncoding parts of the genome. **Figure 5.13c** shows a pair of SNP alleles: allele *A1* contains an A–T base pair whereas allele *A2* contains a G–C base pair. As with VNTR genotypes, individuals are either homozygous or heterozygous for SNP alleles, which also are transmitted in a codominant manner. It is estimated that there are approximately 3.3 million SNPs spread throughout the human genome, and they have proven to be enormously useful in mapping analysis of the human genome.

A type of DNA genetic marker related to SNPs is the **restriction fragment length polymorphism (RFLP;** pronounced "riff lip"). RFLPs result from a change in DNA sequence, but they are analyzed in a different way. Instead of sequencing the region containing the sequence variant, geneticists detect RFLPs with the aid of DNA-cutting enzymes known as **restriction endonucleases—restriction enzymes**, for short—that recognize and cut specific sequences of DNA. There are hundreds of different restriction enzymes. Each recognizes a different short sequence of DNA and cuts DNA at that recognition site every time the site is encountered. For example, the restriction enzyme *Eco*RI (pronounced "eco are one") recognizes the double-stranded DNA sequence 5′–GAATTC–3′. *Eco*RI cuts DNA at this sequence, and only at this sequence. (To repeat, other restriction enzymes have their own recognition sequences.) A large genome like the human genome contains hundreds of thousands of the *Eco*RI recognition sequence, and treating human DNA with *Eco*RI produces hundreds of thousands of

(a) VNTR (variable number tandem repeat)

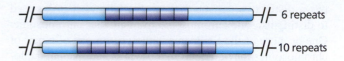

6 repeats
10 repeats

(b) Codominant inheritance of a VNTR

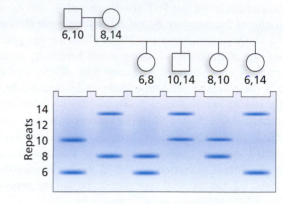

6,10   8,14

6,8   10,14   8,10   6,14

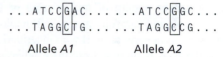

Repeats
14
12
10
8
6

(c) SNP (single nucleotide polymorphism)

...ATCC**G**AC.......ATCC**G**GC...
...TAGG**C**TG.......TAGG**C**CG...

Allele *A1*   Allele *A2*

Figure 5.13 VNTRs and SNPs. Variable number tandem repeats (VNTRs) contain a variable number of repeat-sequence blocks. **(a)** A chromosome pair in which one homolog has 6 repeats and the other has 10 repeats. **(b)** VNTRs are inherited in a codominant manner. **(c)** Single nucleotide polymorphisms (SNPs) are single base-pair sequence variants, also inherited in a codominant manner.

DNA fragments called **restriction fragments**. These restriction fragments are detected by methods that are similar to those used to identify VNTRs. RFLPs on autosomal chromosomes are also transmitted in a codominant manner.

The Inheritance of Disease-Causing Genes Linked to Genetic Markers

The genetic markers used to help map genes usually have known chromosome locations. SNP genes, for example, are identified by detecting variation in DNA sequence at a particular location. Contemporary methods of detecting and recording genome sequences are able to identify these locations with precision, leading to a catalog of SNPs on each chromosome and a map that identifies the location of each of them.

With more than 3 million SNPs in the human genome, tens of thousands of SNPs are located on each chromosome. Syntenic SNPs that are close together in a small region of a chromosome constitute a set of closely linked variants called a **haplotype**. Haplotypes consist of several genetic variants closely packed along a segment of a chromosome.

The term is a contraction of "**haplo**id geno**type**," where *haploid* is used to mean one chromosome. Each haplotype has a distinctive genetic makeup that allows it to be used to distinguish one chromosome from another chromosome: One or more of the SNPs in a haplotype on one of a pair of chromosomes may differ from those in the equivalent haplotype on the other chromosome.

Figure 5.14a shows a haplotype consisting of two SNPs. The alleles of one SNP are designated A_1 and A_2, and the alleles of the other are B_1 and B_2. A gene, gene D, is also shown on these chromosomes. The D allele for this gene is a dominant mutant allele causing a rare hereditary disease inherited as an autosomal dominant trait. Allele d of this gene is the recessive wild-type allele. Individual I-1 in the family tree shown in **Figure 5.14b** has the SNP haplotype containing alleles B_1 and A_1 on one chromosome and alleles B_2 and A_2 on the homologous chromosome. He also has the autosomal dominant disease, suggesting that the disease-causing allele D is carried on one of these chromosomes. His mate, I-2, has the wild-type phenotype and the genotype dd. Her SNP haplotypes are B_2A_1 and B_1A_2.

In generations II and III of the family tree, the autosomal dominant pattern of transmission of the disease is apparent. Looking carefully at the SNP haplotypes, we see that each child in generation II who inherits the disease also inherits the B_1A_1 haplotype from their father, and each child who has the wild-type phenotype has inherited the father's B_2A_2 SNP haplotype. This is consistent with the D allele being on the chromosome with the B_1A_1 haplotype and the

d allele being on the chromosome with the B_2A_2 haplotype. This pattern holds true for individuals III-1 through III-4.

Individuals III-5 and III-6 display different patterns of the haplotype and disease gene alleles. The mother of each child (II-6) has donated the B_2A_1 haplotype along with a copy of her d allele. Individual III-5 has the wild-type phenotype, has received the father's B_1A_1 haplotype, and has received the d allele. This is the result of crossing over between his father's chromosomes, as illustrated in **Figure 5.14c**. By similar analysis, we see that III-6 has the disease allele D inherited on her father's chromosome that contains the B_2A_1 haplotype. This is also the result of crossing over between the father's chromosomes as shown in Figure 5.14c.

Allelic Phase

Suppose the chromosome location of a disease-causing gene is unknown. What research strategy should be used by researchers seeking to map the gene? Often, the answer is to use genetic linkage analysis to establish linkage between genetic markers of haplotypes with known chromosome locations and the disease-causing genes whose chromosome location is sought. Determining that genetic linkage exists identifies the location of the unmapped gene.

To map genes by this approach, it is essential that parental and recombinant chromosomes be identified. Thus, one of the first challenges researchers encounter in the effort to map human genes is to determine the **allelic phase**—the particular combination of alleles of linked genes—on each

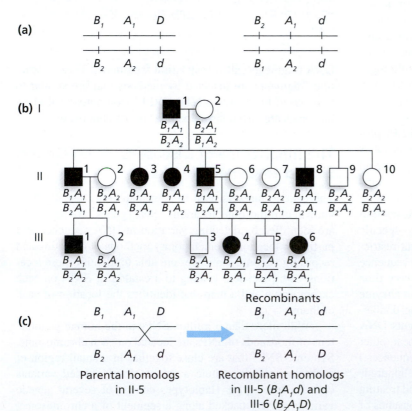

Figure 5.14 Haplotype inheritance. (a) Syntenic alleles for two SNPs (*A* and *B*) and a disease gene (*D*) that form a haplotype. **(b)** Haplotype inheritance in a family is used to identify recombinant and nonrecombinant chromosomes. **(c)** Recombination between the homologs of II-5 produces two recombinant chromosomes that are identified by haplotype changes.

parental chromosome. The simplest approach to determining the allelic phase is to consider the alleles of two linked genes. Knowing, for example, the allelic phase of a marker gene and a gene at which a mutant allele causes a genetic disease of interest improves the statistical power of genetic linkage estimates used to map the location of the disease-causing gene. **Figure 5.15** illustrates how allelic phase is identified in a family in which an autosomal dominant disease is present. The two pedigrees in the figure are identical in structure and in the distribution of the autosomal dominant disease that is indicated by shaded symbols. Notice, however, that individuals I-1 and I-2 are alive and so could be genotyped for the genetic marker in Family A, which is not the case in Family B. The alleles of the gene determining the disease phenotype are D and d. In addition to allelic information for the disease locus, the pedigrees show allelic information for a closely linked polymorphic DNA marker that has six alleles identified as P_1 to P_6.

Allelic phase for the disease allele and the genetic marker is known to be P_1D in Family A because the affected woman in generation I (I-2) transmits marker allele P_1 along with the dominant disease allele (D) to her son, II-1. The unaffected man in generation I (I-1) is homozygous for the recessive wild-type allele (dd) at the disease locus and heterozygous for DNA marker alleles P_2 and P_5. Allelic phase in II-1 is P_1D/P_2d; the chromosome on the left of the solidus (/) is maternal, the chromosome on the right paternal. Considering that his mate (II-2) is P_3d/P_4d, we can identify the transmission of parental and recombinant gametes from II-1 to his children in generation III. Children III-1, III-3, and III-4 inherited a paternal chromosome carrying P_1D to produce their disease and either the P_3 or P_4 allele along with d on their maternal chromosome. On the other hand, III-2, III-5, III-7, and III-8 inherited alleles P_2 and d on their paternal chromosome and either P_3 or P_4 along with d on their maternal chromosome. Child III-6 has apparently inherited a recombinant chromosome carrying alleles P_2 and D from her father along with P_3 and d on the maternal chromosome.

The pedigree for Family B does not allow identification of allelic phase. In this family, there is no marker

information for generation I, and thus allelic phase for II-1 is unknown. He could either be P_1D/P_2d or P_1d/P_2D. For the purposes of genetic linkage analysis, each possible phase must be treated as equally likely. With allelic phase in II-1 unknown, we cannot be certain which of his children have inherited parental chromosomes and which carry recombinants. If II-1 is P_1D/P_2d, his children III-1 to III-5, and III-7 and III-8 are parental, and III-6 is recombinant. Alternatively, if he is P_1d/P_2D, then III-1 to III-5 and III-7 and III-8 are recombinant and III-6 is parental.

Lod Score Analysis

The unique genetic challenges presented by the study of heredity in humans have also led to investigatory methods that rely heavily on statistics. A statistical method developed by Newton Morton in 1955 and refined and expanded since then is one of the central methods for analyzing genetic linkage in humans. Morton's method determines whether genetic linkage exists between genes for which allelic phase is unknown by comparing the likelihood of obtaining the genotypes and phenotypes observed in a pedigree if two genes are linked versus the likelihood of getting the same pedigree outcomes if the genes assort independently. The ratio of these two likelihoods gives the "odds" of genetic linkage, and the logarithm of the **od**ds ratio generates the **lod score,** a statistical value representing the probability of genetic linkage between the genes.

The numerator of the odds ratio that yields the lod score is the likelihood that the distribution of phenotypes and genotypes in the pedigree is produced by genetic linkage between the genes. The denominator is the likelihood of the same pedigree outcomes assuming independent assortment between the genes (i.e., no genetic linkage). Lod score analysis evaluates each pedigree and determines the likelihood of genetic linkage for many different recombination frequencies, each expressed as a variable called the θ **value** ("theta value"). Using input data on each family member that identifies presence or absence of the disease and the genotype at a potentially linked marker gene, software programs calculate the likelihoods of genetic linkage

(a)

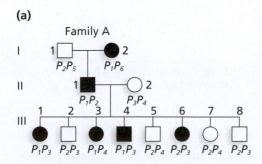

Allelic phase is known in family A by tracing the transmission of the disease allele (D) and the P_1 genetic marker allele from I-2 to II-1 and to III-1, III-3 and III-4; III-6 is a probable recombinant.

(b)

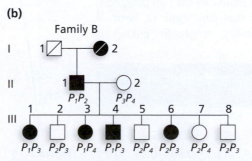

Allelic phase is not known in family B because the disease allele carried by II-1 could be on either the chromosome carrying genetic marker allele P_1 or the chromosome carrying P_2.

Figure 5.15 Allelic phase analysis in human families A and B.

versus no linkage and compute lod scores for each θ value specified by the investigator. The θ values are any recombination frequency between θ = 0 (complete genetic linkage) and θ = 0.50 (independent assortment). The programs determine lod scores, and because they are log values, the lod scores for a given θ value in different families can be added together. After analyzing all available family data, the lod scores for each θ value are summed, and the highest lod score value obtained in a study is designated Z_{max}. The Z_{max} corresponds to the θ value that is the most likely recombination frequency between the genes tested.

For each θ value tested, the lod score will be positive if the likelihood of genetic linkage is greater than the likelihood of independent assortment, because in that case, the numerator value (likelihood assuming genetic linkage) is greater than the denominator value (likelihood assuming independent assortment). Conversely, if the pedigree is more likely to be produced by independent assortment than by genetic linkage, the independent assortment likelihood will be larger than the genetic linkage likelihood, and the lod score will be negative.

Lod scores are calculated using the assumption that if two genes have a recombination frequency equal to θ, the probability that a particular gamete is recombinant is also equal to θ, and the probability that a gamete is nonrecombinant is 1 − θ. **Table 5.4** shows calculated lod score values for the two families shown in Figure 5.15. Notice that the lod scores are higher for Family A than for Family B. This is because, with allelic phase known in Family A, the likelihood estimate for genetic linkage between the disease gene and the marker gene is more accurate and leads to a higher probability of genetic linkage in this case. For each child in generation III, the probability that the gamete from the mother is parental is 1 − θ, and the probability that a recombinant gamete is transmitted from mother to child is θ. Since allelic phase is known for Family A, only the known phase is tested. In contrast, Family B does not have a known allelic phase; thus, each possible phase is assumed to be equally likely. In the Family B lod score computation, each phase is tested and is part of the numerator. A known allelic phase produces more genetic linkage information, so in the context of lod score analysis, the pedigree for Family A is identified as the more informative of the two pedigrees.

A lod score is a statistic that can argue in favor of genetic linkage, if the probability of genetic linkage is

sufficiently greater than the probability of independent assortment; or it can argue against genetic linkage, if the probability of independent assortment is sufficiently greater than the linkage probability. Lod scores can be interpreted for individual families, or they can be added together for as many families as are analyzed. In either case, lod score significance is interpreted by the following parameters:

1. A lod score of 3.0 or greater is considered significant evidence *in favor* of genetic linkage. Such a score indicates significant odds of genetic linkage at each θ value at which it occurs. The θ values identified as significant indicate the most likely number of centiMorgans between linked genes.

2. Lod score values of less than −2.0 represent significant evidence *against* genetic linkage. Any lod score values for single or multiple families less than −2.0 reject genetic linkage at each θ value with that result.

3. Lod score values between 3.0 and −2.0 are inconclusive, neither affirming nor rejecting genetic linkage between the genes examined. Inconclusive results can be revised as additional data are collected.

The three lod score curves shown in **Figure 5.16** illustrate that lod score results may produce different patterns

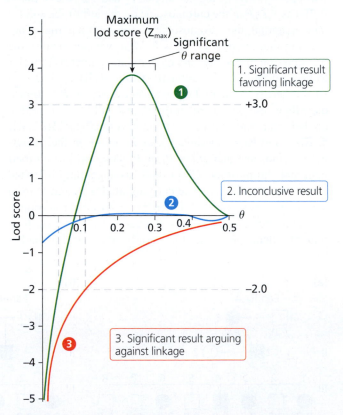

Figure 5.16 Sample lod score curves. Lod score values (vertical axis) are plotted against recombination frequencies (θ values, horizontal axis) for three hypothetical lod score analyses.

Q In a sentence or two, contrast the meaning and interpretation of a lod score of −3.2 versus a lod score of +3.2.

Table 5.4	Lod Score Values for the Families in Figure 5.15					
Family A (Phase Known)						
θ value	0	0.1	0.2	0.3	0.4	0.5
Lod score	−∞	1.09	1.03	0.80	0.46	0.0
Family B (Phase Unknown)						
θ value	0	0.1	0.2	0.3	0.4	0.5
Lod score	−∞	0.79	0.73	0.50	0.19	0.0

EXPERIMENTAL INSIGHT 5.1

Mapping a Gene for Breast and Ovarian Cancer Susceptibility

Most cases of cancer develop through the acquisition of multiple mutations in somatic cells, with no inherited mutation increasing the likelihood of cancer development. In some families, however, the frequent occurrence of a particular kind of cancer in a pattern consistent with single-gene inheritance can strongly suggest the hereditary transmission of a mutant allele that increases the susceptibility of individuals to the cancer. The identity, indeed the very existence of these genes, is not known until they are conclusively shown to contribute to cancer development. One research strategy for identifying cancer-susceptibility genes looks for genetic linkage of susceptibility genes to genetic markers that have a known chromosome location.

In the late 1970s, Mary-Claire King and several collaborators conducted a search for a gene whose mutation could increase susceptibility to breast and ovarian cancer in families. The strategy devised by King and her colleagues to maximize their chance of finding such a cancer-susceptibility gene was to carefully select families in which multiple cases of breast and ovarian cancers appeared at young ages, and in which occasional cases of bilateral cancer occurred (affecting both breasts or both ovaries in a single patient) in patterns consistent with an autosomal dominant inheritance of disease susceptibility.

King initially looked for genetic linkage between inherited cancer susceptibility and biochemical markers such as polymorphic blood proteins and enzymes. None of the dozens of biochemical markers screened produced significant evidence of genetic linkage to a breast and ovarian cancer susceptibility gene. In the early 1990s, however, King and her colleagues turned to the use of DNA genetic markers. In 1994, they identified genetic linkage between a group of tightly clustered DNA markers on human chromosome 17 and a gene named *Breast Cancer 1* (*BRCA1*). Lod score analysis of chromosome 17, as summarized in the following table, revealed that the candidate gene has a Z_{max} value of 21.68 at $\theta = 0.13$.

Five genetic markers that are part of a multipoint linkage analysis are shown. *BRCA1* is most likely close to the middle of this linkage group, near the DNA marker gene *D17S588*.

Subsequent studies have identified and cloned the *BRCA1* gene and determined that it participates with a second gene called *BRCA2* in DNA mutation repair. A large number of mutations of *BRCA1* have been identified, and some of them dramatically increase the likelihood that a woman will develop breast or ovarian cancer. Other mutations of *BRCA1* do not appear to significantly increase breast or ovarian cancer risk. A good deal of work remains to be done to clarify the role of this gene in breast and ovarian cancer development, but the research strategy designed by King demonstrates the power of genetic linkage analysis for locating genes of interest. (We discuss more about *BRCA1* and cancer in Application Chapter C).

Lod Score Data for Linkage of *BRCA1* to Chromosome 17q in Humans

Genetic Marker	Lod Scores at Recombination (θ) Values						Z_{max}	θ_{max}
	0.001	0.01	0.05	0.10	0.20	0.30		
D17S250	−11.98	−8.96	−1.20	3.81	7.30	6.65	7.42	0.23
D17S579	−1.43	1.62	8.55	12.08	12.55	9.17	13.02	0.16
D17S588	8.23	11.39	18.35	21.33	20.15	14.79	21.68	0.13
NME1	−1.41	0.75	6.01	8.70	9.13	6.76	9.45	0.16
D17S74	−39.15	−31.73	−13.34	−2.73	6.32	7.50	7.67	0.27

Source: Data from J. Hall et al. (1994).

depending on the level of information available for the pedigree and on the actual relationship between the genes tested. Curve ❶ displays data with a maximum lod score value (Z_{max}) of about 4.0 at $\theta = 0.23$, suggesting the two genes are separated by 23 cM. The lod scores are significantly positive in the range of 18 to 30 map units. The curve provides significant evidence against genetic linkage at $\theta < 0.5$. Curve ❷ results from a situation in which very little genetic linkage information is available, and its lod scores are inconclusive at all distances. Curve ❸ rejects genetic linkage at θ values less than 0.12 but is inconclusive through the rest of the linkage range.

A number of more comprehensive software programs permitting multipoint linkage analysis have been developed to analyze genetic linkage data for multiple genes and genetic markers simultaneously. Multipoint linkage analysis tests all possible gene orders to identify the most likely order of linked genes.

Experimental Insight 5.1 discusses the application of lod score analysis in the mapping of *BRCA1*, a gene whose mutation can increase susceptibility to breast and ovarian cancer in women. **Genetic Analysis 5.3** guides you through the interpretation of lod score values for linkage between a disease-causing gene and a linked DNA genetic marker.

PROBLEM In a study of human families with an autosomal dominant disease caused by a gene whose location is unknown, geneticists use lod score analysis to test linkage between the disease gene and a variable DNA genetic marker. Provide a complete interpretation of the lod score data displayed in the following table, and identify the most likely distance between the marker gene and the disease gene.

> **BREAK IT DOWN:** The lod score is a statistical value that allows identification of the most likely recombination distance between genes and, by extension, rejection of linkage (p. 169).

> **BREAK IT DOWN:** Lod score values greater than +3.0 indicate statistically significant evidence in favor of genetic linkage, and values less than −2.0 significant evidence against linkage, at specified θ values (p. 170).

						θ Value							
0.0	0.01	0.02	0.03	0.04	0.05	0.06	0.08	0.10	0.15	0.20	0.30	0.40	0.50
$-\infty$	−6.95	−1.10	0.20	1.22	2.25	7.23	7.02	5.11	4.23	−2.01	−6.84	−9.91	0.0

Solution Strategies	Solution Steps
Evaluate	
1. Identify the topic of this problem and the nature of the required answer.	1. This problem concerns lod score analysis assessing genetic linkage between a variable DNA genetic marker and a gene carrying a dominant mutation producing a disease. The answer requires interpretation of the lod score values, identification of potential genetic linkage, and determination of the most likely distance between the DNA marker gene and the disease gene.
2. Identify the critical information given in the problem.	2. Lod score values are given for 14 θ values (map units between genes).
Deduce	
TIP: Survey the entire lod score table to identify significant and nonsignificant lod score values.	
3. Identify significant lod score values in the lod score table and locate Z_{max}.	3. Significant evidence against genetic linkage occurs at θ ≤ 0.01 and at θ ≥ 0.20. Conversely, significant results in favor of genetic linkage are seen at θ = 0.06 to θ = 0.15. The Z_{max} value is 7.23 and corresponds to θ = 0.06 (6 m.u.).
Solve	
4. Interpret the meaning of the lod scores for genetic linkage.	4. The data support genetic linkage between the marker gene and the disease gene at recombination distances of between 6 m.u. and 15 m.u. Linkage between the genes is rejected at less than 2 m.u. and at more than 20 m.u. The lod score results between 2 m.u. and 5 m.u. are inconclusive.
TIP: Note the θ values corresponding to significant lod score values.	
5. Identify the most likely distance between the DNA marker gene and the disease gene.	5. The Z_{max} value is 7.23 at θ = 0.06, thus identifying the most likely distance between the disease gene and the marker gene as 6 m.u.
TIP: The maximum lod score value corresponds to a specific distance between genes that is identified by its θ value.	

For more practice, see Problems 18, 28, and 29. Visit the Study Area to access study tools. **Mastering Genetics**

Genome-Wide Association Studies

The genetic mapping approach that links alleles for phenotypic traits to molecular markers is built on one-to-one relationships. This means that one genetic marker is linked to another genetic marker, and that a series of linked markers along a chromosome constitutes a genetic map of the chromosome. Tens of thousands of genes have been mapped by this approach in the genomes of organisms commonly used for genetic study, including fruit flies, corn, mice, and humans.

Another method of analysis known as **genome-wide association studies (GWAS)** takes a different approach.

GWAS is designed to detect and locate the genes that as a group influence the form or appearance of traits produced by multiple genes. The multiple genes contributing to a particular trait or condition are likely to be scattered throughout the genome. GWAS helps identify where in the genome the genes influencing a trait are located.

GWAS does not create a gene map along a chromosome. Instead, it looks for *associations* between traits and groups of alleles in *populations* of organisms to spot where on different chromosomes influential genes are located. In the context of GWAS, the term "association" means that a trait co-occurs with a group of alleles more often than expected by chance. The alleles used in GWAS are usually SNPs, as these are the most frequent type of molecular marker in most genomes. The statistical analysis that identifies associations between a SNP marker and a disease-susceptibility gene identifies the strength or level of significance of the association as a *P* value (probability value).

GWAS uses small haplotypes consisting of very closely linked SNPs. Many such groups of SNPs can be identified on all chromosomes throughout the genome. These groups of SNPs have known chromosome locations, usually as a result of genome sequence mapping (see Chapter 16). Because these haplotypes are most often used for purposes of GWAS, each chromosome of a homologous pair can be conveniently described by a particular haplotype. As an example, the same DNA region of two homologous chromosomes can be compared as shown here (each chromosome is represented by only one strand of its DNA duplex):

Chromosome 1: AT**T**CATG**C**TC**G**A
Chromosome 2: AT**A**CATG**A**TC**T**A

The third, eight, and eleventh nucleotides of these sequences differ, thus there are three SNP variants detected. Each chromosome can also be said to carry a distinct haplotype for this region of the genome.

In populations, alleles for different genes are expected to be found in genotypes in random combinations. Generally, no allele for any one gene is associated with a given allele for any other gene in a genotype more frequently than would be expected by chance. This is a common state that is known as **linkage equilibrium**. For example, if allele *A* has a frequency of 70 percent in a population (0.70), with allele *A'*, the other allele of the gene, having a frequency of 30 percent (0.30), and if allele *B* has a frequency of 20 percent (0.20), with allele *B'* having a frequency of 80 percent (0.80), then linkage equilibrium is in place when the frequency of each genotype is the product of the two allele frequencies. In other words, linkage equilibrium predicts the following frequencies for the combinations of alleles of these two genes in haplotypes:

$$
\begin{aligned}
AB &= (0.70)(0.20) = 0.14 \\
AB' &= (0.70)(0.80) = 0.56 \\
A'B &= (0.30)(0.20) = 0.06 \\
A'B' &= (0.30)(0.80) = \underline{0.24} \\
&\qquad\qquad\qquad\qquad 1.00
\end{aligned}
$$

The close proximity of SNP variants in a haplotype can severely limit the occurrence of crossing over between the variants. This delays the attainment of linkage equilibrium for many generations, since the alleles of a haplotype are passed together during reproduction. Crossing over will eventually randomize the combinations of alleles in genotypes, but until that time, alleles of any other genes in close proximity to the haplotype genes will also tend to remain syntenic to the haplotype. This relationship is called **linkage disequilibrium.** It reflects the nonrandom relationship between alleles of very closely linked genes. Linkage disequilibrium indicates that one particular allele

of a gene is preferentially associated with the haplotype on the same chromosome. This can lead to particular alleles of the gene contributing to the trait of interest being found more frequently than expected with a particular haplotype. For example, an allele contributing to the development of a particular condition might be more commonly found on a chromosome with a certain haplotype than expected by chance. The detection of linkage disequilibrium between an allele of a gene that contributes to the development of a particular trait or condition can help researchers locate the contributing gene by genetic linkage to the haplotype. GWAS analysis assesses linkage disequilibrium between alleles of genes potentially involved in generating phenotypic variation and closely linked haplotypes to map the locations of the potential contributory genes. The potential significance of associations is assessed by determining *P* (probability) values. Significant *P* values indicate the likely presence of a gene influencing the appearance of a trait or condition.

In recent years, GWAS has been used to analyze the human genome and other eukaryotic genomes in the search for genes that influence many kinds of traits to which multiple genes make a contribution. This is done by using GWAS to show that significant associations exist between an inherited trait or condition and haplotypes on multiple chromosomes. GWAS results of this kind suggest that there are multiple genes contributing to the condition or trait of interest.

One large GWAS analysis of common conditions in humans is a 2007 meta-analysis that tested for linkage disequilibrium between several thousand SNPs and seven common disease conditions in humans. The genomes of more than 14,000 patients and more than 3000 condition-free control individuals were part of the analysis. The study identified more than two dozen regions where a gene likely to contribute to the development of one of the conditions may occur. **Figure 5.17** shows a "Manhattan plot" that indicates the locations of genes contributing to the development of each of these conditions in humans. Manhattan plots are so named because their high-rise profile is reminiscent of the Manhattan (New York City) skyline. The profile is scattered with green dots and bars representing locations of chromosomes where linkage disequilibrium has been detected between a SNP haplotype and a potential contributing gene. The higher the green bar, the stronger the association between a potential contributing gene and a chromosome location as determined by the *P* value.

Additional molecular genetic investigation is required to identify the potential contributing genes associated with each SNP haplotype. Twelve likely contributing genes are identified in the figure. To determine that a gene actually contributes to the development of a condition, it is necessary to first locate all the genes in the chromosome region showing linkage disequilibrium to a SNP haplotype. The activities of identified genes are then determined to see if

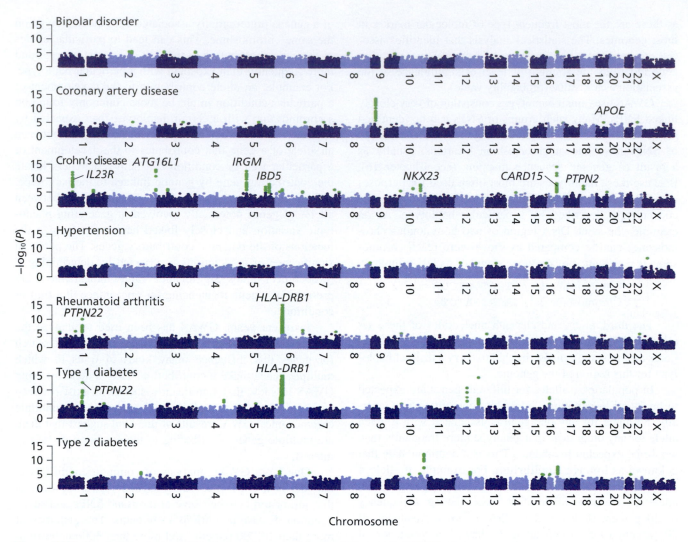

Figure 5.17 **Manhattan plots resulting from a genome-wide association study (GWAS) of seven common human diseases.** The vertical axes show the *P* value for each SNP–disease association along 22 autosomes and the X chromosome. Green dots and bars mark the locations of regions yielding significant associations. Known genes mapping to these regions are shown.

their action might potentially contribute to the development of a condition.

One example shown in Figure 5.17 is the gene *CARD15* on human chromosome 16 that contributes to the development of the intestinal condition Crohn's disease (CD). CD is an inflammatory condition that affects the intestines. GWAS first identified a specific region of chromosome 16 as likely to contain a gene contributing to the development of CD. Researchers subsequently screened expressed genes in that region of chromosome 16 and identified *CARD15* and several other genes. Additional screening searched for variants of these genes that co-occurred with the appearance of CD, and the researchers indeed found that certain *CARD15* variants correlated with the appearance of CD. This led to investigations of the action of *CARD15*. It was determined that expression of the *CARD15* variant alleles associated with CD increased the inflammatory response of intestinal tissue, thus contributing to the development of CD.

To date, GWAS has identified numerous genes contributing to traits and conditions in humans and other eukaryotes, and it has the potential to be instrumental in the discovery of genes contributing to some very complex conditions, including psychiatric disorders, heart disease, and diabetes. We discuss GWAS more fully and give additional examples of its application in Chapter 19.

Linkage Disequilibrium and Evolutionary Analysis

In addition to its usefulness in GWAS analysis, linkage disequilibrium can also be analyzed in an evolutionary context. Two evolutionary scenarios are observed to cause linkage disequilibrium. First, the migration of individuals into established populations can produce linkage disequilibrium by introducing haplotypes into a population. The generations that immediately follow this introduction of new haplotypes are in linkage disequilibrium since it takes multiple generations for crossing over to randomize (establish linkage equilibrium between) the introduced haplotypes and linked alleles already present in the population. A second evolutionary mechanism generating linkage disequilibrium is the operation of natural selection in favor of a particular allele that is very closely linked to a haplotype. The effect of natural selection can be to increase the frequency both of the favored allele and of the haplotype in the population. In most cases, the alleles in the haplotype are passengers that are favored because of their close proximity to the favored allele.

Evolutionary analysis involving haplotypes takes advantage of such retention of linkage disequilibrium to study the origins of alleles that have been subject to natural selection. One example of the application of this research strategy in the assessment of human evolution concerns a specific mutation known as the β^S mutation, caused by a base-pair substitution at position 6 in the wild-type allele, β^A, of the human β-*globin* gene. The DNA base-pair substitution is shown in Figure 4.16 (p. 123). The base substitution leads to an amino acid change in the β-globin protein,

altering the function of the oxygen-carrying protein hemoglobin in red blood cells and producing the autosomal recessive condition known as sickle cell disease. Pleiotropy in sickle cell disease is the subject of Figure 4.16.

Sickle cell disease exists in several human populations, notably in populations of east and central Africa, southern Europe, and the Middle East. Evolutionarily, the question is whether the β^S alleles in these populations have a common evolutionary origin—that is, did they originate with a mutation in a single ancestral population—or are they independent mutations that have risen to high frequency in certain populations due to natural selection. The analysis of haplotypes surrounding the β-globin gene on chromosome 11 holds the answer. The results of extensive genotyping of chromosomes carrying the β^S mutation in populations in Africa, southern Europe, and the Middle East conclusively show that the chromosome 11 haplotypes are substantially different from one another. The differences are not the result of recombination and could only occur if independent β^S mutations occurred on these chromosomes. This evidence clearly indicates that the human β^S mutation has occurred and evolved independently at least three times.

CASE STUDY

Mapping the Gene for Cystic Fibrosis

Cystic fibrosis (CF; OMIM 219700) is an autosomal recessive disorder caused by a defect in the *cystic fibrosis transmembrane conductance regulator* (*CFTR*) gene that is located on chromosome 7 in humans. The protein product of *CFTR* spans the membrane of cells, regulating the flow of chloride ions in and out of the cell. Mutations of *CFTR* primarily affect glands producing mucus, digestive enzymes, and sweat.

First identified in the late 1930s, CF proved to be a relatively common disorder, particularly in Caucasian populations, where it occurs at a frequency of 1 in 2500 infants, according to the American Lung Association. It is much less common in Hispanics (1 in 15,000), African Americans (1 in 30,000), and Native Pacific Islanders (1 in 100,000). In Caucasians, the frequency of heterozygous carriers of the recessive allele is approximately 4%. Numerous family studies identified CF as being caused by mutation of a single gene, although the gene was not identified until the 1980s. Many mutant alleles of the gene are known, although one mutation is very common.

The principal clinical difficulty in CF is very thick mucus that clogs the airways in the lungs and obstructs the ducts that transport digestive enzymes from the pancreas to the small intestine. Chronic and severe respiratory infections are a hallmark of CF, as are digestive difficulties that can result in chronic malnutrition, even with adequate food intake. Awareness of these complications has led to better management and improved survival. In the 1950s, CF patients rarely survived long enough to enter elementary school. By 1985, the average age of survival stood at about 25 years. By 2007, mean survival had improved to approximately 28 years. CF patients with less severe forms of the disease survive even longer.

With family studies indicating that a single autosomal gene was responsible for CF, researchers used genetic linkage mapping and lod score analysis to locate the CF gene. All 22 autosomes were studied, and initially a great deal of negative genetic linkage information was obtained. These data identified chromosomes where the gene *was not* located. The first important piece of positive gene mapping evidence came in 1985 when Hans Eiberg and colleagues identified the close linkage of the CF gene to the *PON* gene that produces the blood serum enzyme paraoxonase. Unfortunately, *PON* did not have a known chromosome location at the time, so despite the finding that the CF gene was near *PON*, the identity of the chromosome carrying the genes remained a mystery.

A few months later, however, Lap-Chee Tsui and colleagues identified a DNA RFLP marker known as *D7S15* that was linked to both the CF gene and to *PON* (see Section 5.5). *D7S15* was known to reside near the middle of the long arm of chromosome 7. Like almost all RFLPs, *D7S15* is not part of an expressed gene, and it has nothing to do with causing CF. It is merely a DNA sequence variant that is detected in a noncoding segment of chromosome 7. As **Table 5.5** shows, however, lod score values for *D7S15*–CF and *D7S15*–*PON* linkage as reported by Tsui et al. (1985) for 39 families with CF clearly demonstrated close genetic linkage between the genes and the RFLP. Lod score values greater than +3.0 are seen for *D7S15*–CF linkage in the range $\theta = 0.10$ to 0.20, with a maximum θ value of 3.96 at $\theta = 0.14$. For the *D7S15*–*PON* analysis, significantly positive lod scores are seen in the range $\theta = 0.01$ to 0.20, with a Z_{max} value of 5.01 at $\theta = 0.05$. Taken together, these lod score analyses indicated the order *D7S15*-*PON*-CF with a distance of approximately 5 cM from *D7S15* to *PON* and 14 cM from *PON* to CF.

With the segment of chromosome 7 containing the CF gene identified, researchers examined that chromosome 7 region and found additional DNA genetic markers that were linked even more closely to the CF gene. Using these markers, they identified a segment of about 500,000 bp of DNA as the likely location of the CF gene. By examining DNA sequences for the probable presence of expressed genes and by testing for the presence of genes that were known to be expressed in sweat glands, a group of investigators led by Tsui and Francis Collins cloned and sequenced the CF gene in 1989. Investigators soon determined that the protein product of the CF gene is a transmembrane conductance regulatory protein, at which point the gene acquired its *CFTR* designation.

One mutation known to delete three consecutive DNA base pairs and alter one amino acid of the CFTR protein accounts for almost 50% of the known *CFTR* mutant alleles. Numerous other *CFTR* mutant alleles have also been identified, but none of these has a frequency of more than a few percent. The various *CFTR* mutant alleles produce different levels of functionality in the transmembrane protein, to some extent allowing clinical variation in CF patients to be attributed to particular mutant alleles. Knowing the frequency of the one common mutation and having identified many other *CFTR* mutations, medical geneticists are able to offer prenatal genetic testing to CF families and to accurately identify the mutant alleles and probable disease severity in patients.

The process of first mapping, then cloning, then sequencing *CFTR* to identify its function is a genetic strategy known as *positional cloning* or *reverse genetic analysis*. We discuss this investigative strategy more completely in Chapter 14.

Table 5.5	Linkage Data from 39 Families with Cystic Fibrosis								
	Lod Scores at Various Recombination Distances (θ)								
Marker–Gene	**0.01**	**0.05**	**0.10**	**0.15**	**0.20**	**0.25**	**0.30**	**0.35**	**0.40**
D7S15–CF	−5.88	1.67	3.63	3.95	3.62	2.97	2.18	1.38	0.67
D7S15–PON	4.27	5.01	4.78	4.28	3.66	2.97	2.25	1.51	0.81

SUMMARY   Mastering Genetics   For activities, animations, and review quizzes, go to the Study Area.

5.1 Linked Genes Do Not Assort Independently

▮ Genetic linkage identifies genes that are so close to one another on a chromosome that their alleles do not assort independently.

▮ With genetic linkage, parental combinations occur at frequencies that are significantly greater than those predicted by chance, and nonparental combinations are much less frequent than expected.

▮ William Bateson and Reginald Punnett first observed genetic linkage when they noticed high numbers of parental phenotypes in F_2 progeny.

▮ Thomas Hunt Morgan performed test-cross analysis of linked genes to demonstrate that linkage violates independent assortment and that crossover between homologous chromosomes is responsible for the production of recombinant gametes.

▮ Crossover frequency between linked genes is correlated with the distance between genes on a chromosome. Crossover occurs less often between genes that are close together than between genes that are farther apart.

▮ In crosses involving linked genes, the two parental phenotypes are observed in progeny in approximately equal frequencies. The two recombinant phenotypes also occur at approximately equal frequency.

▮ Studies correlating genetic recombination with the visible recombination of distinctive physical structures on chromosomes support the idea that crossing over causes recombination.

5.2 Genetic Linkage Mapping Is Based on Recombination Frequency between Genes

▮ The correlation between physical map distance and recombination frequency permits gene mapping based on recombination frequency.

5.3 Three-Point Test-Cross Analysis Maps Genes

▮ Three or more genes can be mapped by test-cross analysis. In a three-point cross, parental phenotypes are most frequent, double recombinants are least frequent, and the four phenotypes resulting from two single-recombination events are of intermediate frequency that depends on the actual distance between genes.

▮ Genetic linkage maps are constructed in five steps:

  1. Find significantly higher proportions of parental phenotypes than predicted by chance.

  2. Identify the alleles on parental chromosomes (the most common classes).

3. Identify double recombinants (the least frequent classes), comparing them with parental chromosomes to determine gene order.
4. Calculate recombination frequencies between genes.
5. Calculate interference in the occurrence of double crossovers.

■ Recombination frequency usually underestimates the physical distance between genes. Mapping functions are used to correct these estimates.

5.4 Multiple Factors Cause Recombination to Vary

■ Several biological properties of organisms affect recombination. In animals, the heterogametic sex experiences less recombination genome-wide than the homogametic sex.

■ Recombination between homologs adds substantially to the genetic diversity produced through sexual reproduction.

■ Hotspots and coldspots of recombination are found in many genomes, reflecting the uneven distribution of homologous recombination.

■ Mammalian genome analysis reveals potential sequences and mechanisms associated with recombinational hotspots.

5.5 Human Genes Are Mapped Using Specialized Methods

■ Statistical approaches such as lod score analysis detect evidence of linkage in small families.

■ Lod score analysis determines the likelihood of genetic linkage between genes at specified recombination values (θ values). A cumulative lod score of $+3.0$ or more is statistically significant evidence in favor of genetic linkage between two genes. Lod scores of -2.0 or less represent significant evidence against genetic linkage.

■ Genome-wide association studies (GWAS) locate genes affecting phenotypes that are the result of the action of several genes.

PREPARING FOR PROBLEM SOLVING

In addition to the list of problem-solving tips and suggestions given here, you can go to the Study Guide and Solutions Manual that accompanies this book for help at solving problems.

1. Be sure you have a clear understanding of the rules, computation, and expected outcomes of crosses involving independently assorting genes. You cannot assess genetic linkage without understanding what is expected as a result of independent assortment.

2. Be prepared to evaluate and interpret genetic maps by understanding the relationship between recombination frequencies and the distance between genes on a map.

3. Be prepared to deduce genetic maps from genetic-cross data by identifying the occurrence of genetic linkage and calculating recombination frequencies.

4. Practice solving three-point test-cross analysis using the five steps illustrated in the chapter in the order in which they are presented.

5. Be ready to propose and construct genetic tests based on a hypothesis of genetic linkage.

6. Understand the interpretation of lod scores in the assessment of human genetic linkage analysis.

PROBLEMS

Mastering Genetics Visit for instructor-assigned tutorials and problems.

Chapter Concepts

For answers to selected even-numbered problems, see Appendix: Answers.

1. For parts (a), (b), and (c) of this problem, draw a diagram illustrating the alleles on homologous chromosomes for the genotypes given, assuming in each case that the genes reside on the chromosome in the order written. For parts (d) and (e), give the information requested.
   a. *AB/ab*
   b. *aBc/abC*
   c. *DFg/DFG*
   d. the gametes produced by an organism with the genotype *Rt/rT*
   e. progeny of the cross *Rt/rT* × *rt/rt*

2. In a diploid species of plant, the genes for plant height and fruit shape are syntenic and separated by 18 m.u. Allele *D* produces tall plants and is dominant to *d* for short plants, and allele *R* produces round fruit and is dominant to *r* for oval fruit.

   a. A plant with the genotype *DR/dr* produces gametes. Identify gamete genotypes, label parental and recombinant gametes, and give the frequency of each gamete genotype.
   b. Give the same information for a plant with the genotype *Dr/dR*.

3. A pure-breeding tall plant producing oval fruit as described in Problem 2 is crossed to a pure-breeding short plant producing round fruit.
   a. The F_1 are crossed to short plants producing oval fruit. What are the expected proportions of progeny phenotypes?
   b. If the F_1 identified in part (a) are crossed to one another, what proportion of the F_2 are expected to be short and produce round fruit? What proportion are expected to be tall and produce round fruit?

4. Genes E and H are syntenic in an experimental organism with the genotype EH/eh. Assume that during each meiosis, one crossover occurs between these genes. No homologous chromosomes escape crossover, and none undergo double crossover. Are genes E and H genetically linked? Why or why not? What is the proportion of parental gametes produced by meiosis?

5. In tomato plants, purple leaf color is controlled by a dominant allele A, and green leaf by a recessive allele a. At another locus, hairy leaf H is dominant to hairless leaf h. The genes for leaf color and leaf texture are separated by 16 m.u. on chromosome 5. On chromosome 4, a gene controlling leaf shape has two alleles: a dominant allele C that produces cut-leaf shape and a recessive allele c that produces potato-shaped leaf.

   a. The cross of a purple, hairy, cut plant heterozygous at each gene to a green, hairless, potato plant produces the following progeny:

Phenotype	Frequency %
Purple, hairy, cut	21
Purple, hairy, potato	21
Green, hairless, cut	21
Green, hairless, potato	21
Purple, hairless, cut	4
Purple, hairless, potato	4
Green, hairy, cut	4
Green, hairy, potato	4
	100

   Give the genotypes of parental and progeny plants in this experiment.

   b. Fully explain the number and frequency of each phenotype class.

6. In *Drosophila*, the map positions of genes are given in map units numbering from one end of a chromosome to the other. The X chromosome of *Drosophila* is 66 m.u. long. The X-linked gene for body color—with two alleles, y^+ for gray body and y for yellow body—resides at one end of the chromosome at map position 0.0. A nearby locus for eye color, with alleles w^+ for red eye and w for white eye, is located at map position 1.5. A third X-linked gene, controlling bristle form, with f^+ for normal bristles and f for forked bristles, is located at map position 56.7. At each locus the wild-type allele is dominant over the mutant allele.

   a. In a cross involving these three X-linked genes, do you expect any gene pair(s) to show genetic linkage? Explain your reasoning.

   b. Do you expect any of these gene pair(s) to assort independently? Explain your reasoning.

   c. A wild-type female fruit fly with the genotype y^+w^+f/ywf^+ is crossed to a male fruit fly that has yellow body, white eye, and forked bristles. Predict the frequency of each progeny phenotype class produced by this mating.

   d. Explain how each of the predicted progeny classes is produced.

7. Genes A, B, and C are linked on a chromosome and found in the order A-B-C. Genes A and B recombine with a frequency of 8%, and genes B and C recombine at a frequency of 24%. For the cross $a^+b^+c/abc^+ \times abc/abc$, predict the frequency of progeny genotypes. Assume interference is zero.

8. Gene G recombines with gene T at a frequency of 7%, and gene G recombines with gene R at a frequency of 4%.

   a. Draw two possible genetic maps for these three genes, and identify the recombination frequencies predicted for each map.

   b. Assuming that organisms with any desired genotype are available, propose a genetic cross whose result could be used to determine which of the proposed genetic maps is correct.

9. Genes A, B, C, D, and E are linked on a chromosome and occur in the order given.

   a. The test cross $Ae/aE \times ae/ae$ indicates the genes recombine with a frequency of 28%. If 1000 progeny are produced by this test cross, determine the number of progeny in each outcome class.

   b. Previous genetic linkage crosses have determined that recombination frequencies are 6% for genes A and B, 4% for genes B and C, 10% for genes C and D, and 11% for genes D and E. The sum of these frequencies between genes A and E is 31%. Why does the recombination distance between these genes as determined by adding the intervals between adjacent linked genes differ from the distance determined by the test cross?

10. Syntenic genes can assort independently. Explain this observation.

11. Define linkage disequilibrium. What is the physical basis of linkage, and what causes linkage equilibrium? Explain how crossing over eliminates linkage disequilibrium.

12. On the *Drosophila* X chromosome, the dominant allele y^+ produces gray body color, and the recessive allele y produces yellow body. This gene is linked to one controlling full eye shape by a dominant allele lz^+ and lozenge eye shape with a recessive allele lz. These genes recombine with a frequency of approximately 28%. The Lz gene is linked to gene F controlling bristle form, where the dominant phenotype is long bristles and the recessive one is forked bristles. The Lz and F genes recombine with a frequency of approximately 32%.

    a. Using any genotypes you choose, design two separate crosses, one to test recombination between genes Y and Lz and the second between genes Lz and F. Assume 1000 progeny are produced by each cross, and give the number of progeny in each outcome category. (In setting up your crosses, remember that *Drosophila* males do not undergo recombination.)

    b. Can any cross reveal genetic linkage between gene Y and gene F? Why or why not?

    c. Why is "independent assortment" the genetic term that best describes the observations of a genetic cross between gene Y and gene F?

Application and Integration

For answers to selected even-numbered problems, see Appendix: Answers.

13. Researchers cross a corn plant that is pure-breeding for the dominant traits colored aleurone (*C1*), full kernel (*Sh*), and waxy endosperm (*Wx*) to a pure-breeding plant with the recessive traits colorless aleurone (*c1*), shrunken kernel (*sh*), and starchy (*wx*). The resulting F₁ plants were crossed to pure-breeding colorless, shrunken, starchy plants. Counting the kernels from about 30 ears of corn yields the following data.

Kernel Phenotype	Number
Colored, shrunken, starchy	116
Colored, full, starchy	601
Colored, full, waxy	2538
Colored, shrunken, waxy	4
Colorless, shrunken, starchy	2708
Colorless, full, starchy	2
Colorless, full, waxy	113
Colorless, shrunken, waxy	626
	6708

a. Why are these data consistent with genetic linkage among the three genes?
b. Perform a chi-square test to determine if these data show significant deviation from the expected phenotype distribution.
c. What is the order of these genes in corn?
d. Calculate the recombination frequencies between the gene pairs.
e. What is the interference value for this data set?

14. Nail–patella syndrome is an autosomal disorder affecting the shape of nails on fingers and toes as well as the structure of kneecaps. The pedigree below shows the transmission of nail–patella syndrome in a family along with ABO blood type.

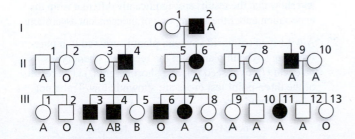

a. Is nail–patella syndrome a dominant or a recessive condition? Explain your reasoning.
b. Does this family give evidence of genetic linkage between nail–patella syndrome and ABO blood group? Why or why not?
c. Using *N* and *n* to represent alleles at the nail–patella locus and I^A, I^B, and *i* to represent ABO alleles, write the genotypes of I-1 and I-2 as well as their five children in generation II.
d. Explain why III-6 has nail–patella syndrome and III-8 does not. Give genotypes for these two individuals.

e. Explain why III-11 has nail–patella syndrome and III-12 does not. Give genotypes for these two individuals.

15. Three dominant traits of corn seedlings, tunicate seed (*T−*), glossy appearance (*G−*), and liguled stem (*L−*), are studied along with their recessive counterparts, nontunicate (*tt*), nonglossy (*gg*), and liguleless (*ll*). A trihybrid plant with the three dominant traits is crossed to a nontunicate, nonglossy, liguleless plant. Kernels on ears of progeny plants are scored for the traits, with the following results:

Phenotype	Number
Tunicate, glossy, liguled	102
Tunicate, glossy, liguleless	106
Tunicate, nonglossy, liguled	18
Tunicate, nonglossy, liguleless	20
Nontunicate, glossy, liguled	22
Nontunicate, glossy, liguleless	23
Nontunicate, nonglossy, liguled	99
Nontunicate, nonglossy, liguleless	110
	500

a. Is there evidence of genetic linkage among any of these gene pairs? If so, identify the evidence.
b. Is there evidence of independent assortment among any of these gene pairs? If so, identify the evidence.
c. Using the gene symbols given above, write the genotypes of F₁ and F₂ plants.
d. If evidence of linkage is present, calculate the recombination frequency or frequencies from the data presented.
e. Could all three genes be carried on the same chromosome? Discuss why or why not.

16. In a diploid plant species, an F₁ with the genotype *Gg Ll Tt* is test-crossed to a pure-breeding recessive plant with the genotype *gg ll tt*. The offspring genotypes are as follows:

Genotype	Number
Gg Ll Tt	621
Gg Ll tt	3
Gg ll Tt	64
Gg ll tt	109
gg Ll Tt	103
gg Ll tt	67
gg ll Tt	7
gg ll tt	626
	1600

a. What is the order of these three linked genes?
b. Calculate the recombination frequency between each pair of genes.
c. Why is the recombination frequency for the outside pair of genes not equal to the sum of recombination frequencies between the adjacent gene pairs?

d. What is the interference value for this data set?

e. Explain the meaning of this I value.

17. The table given here lists the arrangement of alleles of linked genes in dihybrid organisms, the recombination frequency between the genes, and specific gamete genotypes. Using the information provided, determine the expected frequency of the listed gametes. Assume one map unit equals 1% recombination and, when three genes are involved, interference is zero.

Dihybrid Genotype	Recombination Frequency	Gamete Genotype
A. *DE/de*	8%	*De*
B. *AD/ad*	28%	*ad*
C. *DEF/def*	E–F 24%	*dEf*
	D–E 8%	
D. *BdE/bDe*	B–D 18%	*Bde*
	D–E 8%	

18. The Rh blood group in humans is determined by a gene on chromosome 1. A dominant allele produces Rh+ blood type, and a recessive allele generates Rh−. Elliptocytosis is an autosomal dominant disorder that produces abnormally shaped red blood cells that have a short life span resulting in hereditary anemia. A large family with elliptocytosis is tested for genetic linkage of Rh blood group and the disease. The lod score data below are obtained for the family.

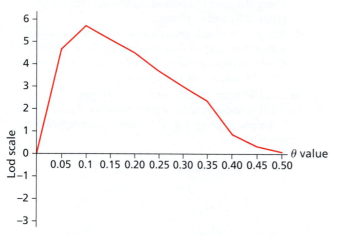

a. From these data, can you conclude that Rh and elliptocytosis loci are genetically linked in this family? Why or why not?

b. What is Z_{max} for this family?

c. Over what range of θ do lod scores indicate significant evidence in favor of genetic linkage?

19. Genetic linkage mapping for a large number of families identifies 4% recombination between the genes for Rh blood type and elliptocytosis (see Problem 18). At the Rh locus, alleles R and r control Rh+ and Rh− blood types. Allele E producing elliptocytosis is dominant to the wild-type recessive allele e. Tom and Terri each have elliptocytosis, and each is Rh+. Tom's mother has elliptocytosis and is Rh− while his father is healthy and has

Rh+. Terri's father is Rh+ and has elliptocytosis; Terri's mother is Rh− and is healthy.

a. What is the probability that the first child of Tom and Terri will be Rh− and have elliptocytosis?

b. What is the probability that a child of Tom and Terri who is Rh+ will have elliptocytosis?

20. A group of families in which an autosomal dominant condition is present are studied to determine lod scores for possible genetic linkage between three RFLP markers (R1, R2, and R3) and the disease gene. The chart shows lod scores at each of the recombination distances (θ values) tested. Provide an interpretation of the lod score results for each RFLP. Be specific about any significant evidence of genetic linkage.

RFLP	θ values							
	0.05	0.10	0.15	0.20	0.25	0.30	0.35	0.40
R1	0.5	0.8	1.8	2.2	1.9	0.7	0.2	0.1
R2	1.1	3.1	3.8	3.0	2.1	1.0	0.8	0.1
R3	0.2	0.3	0.1	0.3	0.4	0.6	0.8	0.7

21. Gene R and gene T are genetically linked. Answer the following questions concerning a dihybrid organism with the genotype Rt/rT:

a. If $r = 0.20$, give the expected frequencies of gametes produced by the dihybrid.

b. If two crossover events occur between these two genes, what are the genotypes of the recombinant chromosomes?

c. Can you make a general statement about how the occurrence of two crossover events between a given pair of linked genes affects the estimate of recombination frequency? (Hint: Think about this problem for a gene pair with a small recombination frequency versus a gene pair with a much higher recombination frequency. See also Figure 5.10.)

22. T. H. Morgan's data on eye color and wing form, shown in Figures 5.3 and 5.5, reveal genetic linkage between the two genes. Test this genetic linkage data with chi-square analysis, and show that the results are significantly different from the expectation under the assumption of independent assortment.

23. A wild-type trihybrid soybean plant is crossed to a pure-breeding soybean plant with the recessive phenotypes pale leaf (l), oval seed (r), and short height (t). The results of the three-point test cross are shown below. Traits not listed are wild type.

Phenotype	Number
Pale	648
Pale, oval	64
Pale, short	10
Pale, oval, short	102
Oval	6
Oval, short	618
Short	84
Wild type	98
	1630

a. What are the alleles on each homologous chromosome of the parental wild-type trihybrid soybean plant? Place the alleles in their correct gene order. Use L, R, and T to represent dominant alleles and l, r, and t for recessive alleles.

b. Calculate the recombination frequencies between the adjacent genes.

c. Calculate the interference value for these data.

24. The boss in your laboratory has just heard of a proposal by another laboratory that genes for eye color and the length of body bristles may be linked in *Drosophila*. Your lab has numerous pure-breeding stocks of *Drosophila* that could be used to verify or refute genetic linkage. In *Drosophila*, red eyes (c^+) are dominant to brown eyes (c), and long bristles (d^+) are dominant to short bristles (d). Your lab boss asks you to design an experiment to test the genetic linkage of eye color and bristle-length genes, and to begin by crossing a pure-breeding line homozygous for red eyes and short bristles to a pure-breeding line that has brown eyes and long bristles.

a. Give the genotypes of the pure-breeding parental flies, and the genotype(s) and phenotype(s) of the F_1 progeny they produce.

b. In your experimental design, what are the genotype and phenotype of the line you propose to cross to the F_1 to obtain the most useful information about genetic linkage between the eye color and bristle-length genes? Explain why you make this choice.

c. Assume the eye color and bristle-length genes are separated by 28 m.u. What are the approximate frequencies of phenotypes expected from the cross you proposed in part (b)?

d. How would the results of the cross differ if the genes are not linked?

25. In rabbits, chocolate-colored fur (w^+) is dominant to white fur (w), straight fur (c^+) is dominant to curly fur (c), and long ear (s^+) is dominant to short ear (s). The cross of a trihybrid rabbit with straight, chocolate-colored fur and long ears to a rabbit that has white, curly fur and short ears produces the following results:

Phenotype	Number
White, short, straight	13
Chocolate, long, straight	165
Chocolate, long, curly	13
White, long, straight	82
Chocolate, short, straight	436
Chocolate, short, curly	79
White, short, curly	162
White, long, curly	450
	1400

a. Determine the order of the genes on the chromosome, and identify the alleles that are present on each of the homologous chromosomes in the trihybrid rabbits.

b. Calculate the recombination frequencies between each of the adjacent pairs of genes.

c. Determine the interference value for this cross.

26. The following progeny are obtained from a test cross of a trihybrid wild-type plant to a plant with the recessive phenotypes compound leaves (c), intercalary leaflets (i), and green fruits (g). (Traits not listed are wild type.) The test-cross progeny are as follows:

Phenotype	Number
Compound leaves	324
Compound leaves, intercalary leaflets	32
Compound leaves, green fruits	5
Compound leaves, intercalary leaflets, green fruits	51
Intercalary leaflets	3
Intercalary leaflets, green fruits	309
Green fruits	42
Wild type	49
	815

a. Determine the order of the three genes, and construct a genetic map that identifies the correct order and the alleles carried on each chromosome in the trihybrid parental plant.

b. Calculate the frequencies of recombination between the adjacent genes in the map.

c. How many double-crossover progeny are expected among the test-cross progeny? Calculate the interference for this cross.

27. In tomatoes, the allele T for tall plant height is dominant to dwarf allele t, the P allele for smooth skin is dominant to the p allele for peach fuzz skin, and the allele R for round fruit is dominant to the recessive r allele for oblong fruit. The genes controlling these traits are linked on chromosome 1 in the tomato genome, and the genes are arranged in the order and with the recombination frequencies shown.

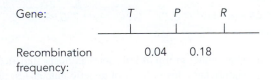

Gene: T P R

Recombination frequency: 0.04   0.18

a. A pure-breeding tall, peach fuzz, round plant is crossed to a pure-breeding plant that is dwarf, smooth, oblong. What are the gamete genotypes produced by each of these plants?

b. What are the genotype and phenotype of the F_1 progeny of this cross?

c. What are the genotypes of gametes produced by the F_1, and what is the predicted frequency of each gamete?

d. The F_1 are test-crossed to dwarf, peach fuzz, oblong plants, and 1000 test-cross progeny are produced. What are the phenotypes of test-cross progeny, and what number of progeny is expected in each class?

28. Neurofibromatosis 1 (NF1) is an autosomal dominant disorder inherited on human chromosome 17. Part of the analysis mapping the *NF1* gene to chromosome 17 came from genetic linkage studies testing segregation of *NF1* and DNA genetic markers on various chromosomes.

A DNA marker with two alleles, designated *1* and *2*, is linked to *NF1*. The pedigree below shows segregation of *NF1* (darkened symbols) and gives genotypes for the DNA marker for each family member.

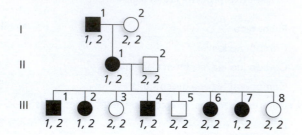

a. Determine the alleles for the *NF1* gene and the DNA marker gene on each chromosome carried by the four family members in generation I and generation II. Use *N* for the dominant *NF1* allele and *n* for the recessive allele and assume I-1 is heterozygous for the disease allele (*Nn*).
b. Based on the phase of alleles on chromosomes in generation II, is there any evidence of recombination among the eight offspring in generation III? Explain.
c. What is the estimated recombination frequency between the *NF1* gene and the DNA marker?

29. A 2006 genetic study of a large American family *(Ikeda et al., 2006)* identified genetic linkage between DNA markers on chromosome 11 and the gene producing the autosomal dominant neuromuscular disorder spinocerebellar ataxia type 5 (*SCA5*). The following lod score data are taken from the 2006 study:

	Theta (θ) Value					
	0.01	0.05	0.10	0.20	0.30	0.40
SCA5 and DNA marker *A*	11.02	12.26	11.94	10.04	7.26	3.77
SCA5 and DNA marker *B*	0.35	0.94	1.07	0.99	0.75	0.43

a. Does either group of lod scores indicate statistically significant odds in favor of genetic linkage? Explain your answer.
b. What is the maximum value for each set of lod scores?
c. Based on the available information, is DNA marker *A* linked to the gene producing SCA5? Explain your answer.
d. Based on available information, is DNA marker *B* linked to the gene for SCA5? Explain your answer.

30. A *Drosophila* experiment examining potential genetic linkage of X-linked genes studies a recessive eye mutant (echinus), a recessive wing-vein mutation (crossveinless), and a recessive bristle mutation (scute). The wild-type phenotypes are dominant. Trihybrid wild-type females (all have the same genotype) are crossed to hemizygous males displaying the three recessive phenotypes. Among the 20,765 progeny produced from these crosses are the phenotypes and numbers listed in the table. Any phenotype not given is wild type.

Phenotype	Number
1. Echinus	8576
2. Scute	977
3. Crossveinless	716
4. Echinus, scute	681
5. Scute, crossveinless	8808
6. Scute, crossveinless, echinus	4
7. Echinus, crossveinless	1002
8. Wild type	1
	20,765

a. Determine the gene order and identify the alleles on the homologous X chromosomes in the trihybrid females.
b. Calculate the recombination frequencies between each of the gene pairs.
c. Compare the recombination frequencies and speculate about the source of any apparent discrepancies in the recombination data.
d. Use chi-square analysis to demonstrate that the data in this experiment are not the result of independent assortment.

31. A genetic study of an early onset form of heart disease identifies 10 families containing members with the condition. No clear dominant or recessive pattern of inheritance is evident, but an analysis of SNP markers for five families detects a strong association with a marker on chromosome 12, and genetic linkage analysis for the marker produces a lod score of 2.2.

a. What do the association and lod score results suggest about this genetic marker?
b. What next step do you recommend for this genetic analysis?

32. In experiments published in 1918 that sought to verify and expand the genetic linkage and recombination theory proposed by Morgan, Thomas Bregger studied potential genetic linkage in corn (*Zea mays*) for genes controlling kernel color (colored is dominant to colorless) and starch content (starchy is dominant to waxy). Bregger performed two crosses. In Cross 1, pure-breeding colored, starchy-kernel plants (*C1 Wx/C1 Wx*) were crossed to plants pure-breeding for colorless, waxy kernels (*c1 wx/c1 wx*). The F$_1$ of this cross were test-crossed to colorless, waxy plants. The test-cross progeny were as follows:

Phenotype	Number
Colored, waxy	310
Colored, starchy	858
Colorless, waxy	781
Colorless, starchy	311
	2260

In Cross 2, plants pure-breeding for colored, waxy kernels (*C1 wx/C1 wx*) and colorless, starchy kernels (*c1 Wx/c1*

Wx) were mated, and their F_1 were test-crossed to color-less, waxy plants. The test-cross progeny were as follows:

Phenotype	Number
Colored, waxy	340
Colored, starchy	115
Colorless, waxy	92
Colorless, starchy	298
	845

Collaboration and Discussion

33. DNA sequences for 10 individuals are

	Nucleotide Position		
	1	5	10
Person 1	...GACCTATTGC...		
Person 2	...GAACTATTGC...		
Person 3	...GACCTTTTGC...		
Person 4	...GACCTATTGC...		
Person 5	...CAACTATTGC...		
Person 6	...GACCTTTTGC...		
Person 7	...CAACTATTGC...		
Person 8	...GACCTATTGC...		
Person 9	...CAACTATTGC...		
Person 10	...GAACTATTGC...		

    a. Identify the nucleotide positions of all SNPs (single nucleotide polymorphisms).
    b. How many different SNP haplotypes are represented in the data?
    c. What is the sequence of each haplotype?
    d. Identify the haplotype carried by each person.

34. The accompanying pedigree below shows a family in which an autosomal recessive disorder is present. Family members I-2 and II-2 are affected by the disorder and have the genotype *dd*. A pregnancy involving II-4 has just undergone genetic testing for a VNTR that is linked to the disease gene. The VNTR has a recombination frequency of $r = 0.20$ with the disease gene. The VNTR has two alleles, V_1 and V_2. The gel electrophoresis patterns for each family member are shown, including the VNTR genotype for II-4. Based on the information given, answer the following questions about the family.
    a. Excluding II-4, what is the genotype of each family member for the disease gene?

a. For each set of test-cross progeny, determine whether genetic linkage or independent assortment is more strongly supported by the data. Explain the rationale for your answer.
b. Calculate the recombination frequency for each of the progeny groups.
c. Taken together, are the results of these two experiments compatible with the hypothesis of genetic linkage? Explain why or why not.
d. Merge the two sets of progeny data and determine the combined recombination frequency.

For answers to selected even-numbered problems, see Appendix: Answers.

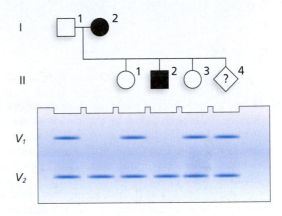

    b. What is the genotype of each family member, including II-4, for the VNTR?
    c. What are the syntenic disease gene and VNTR alleles in I-1 and I-2?
    d. What is the chance II-4 has the disease?

35. Based on previous family studies, an autosomal recessive disease with alleles *A* and *a* is suspected to be linked to an RFLP marker. The RFLP marker has four alleles, R_1, R_2, R_3, and R_4. The accompanying pedigree shows a three-generation family in which the disease is present. The gel shows the RFLP alleles for each family member directly below the pedigree symbol for that person. After determining the genotypes for the RFLP and disease gene for each family member, answer the following questions.
    a. What is the most likely arrangement of syntenic alleles for the RFLP and the disease gene in I-1 and I-2?
    b. Is there any evidence of recombination in this pedigree? If so, identify the recombinant individuals and illustrate the recombination that has occurred.
    c. Based on your analysis, what is the recombination frequency in this family? Explain how you obtained your answer.

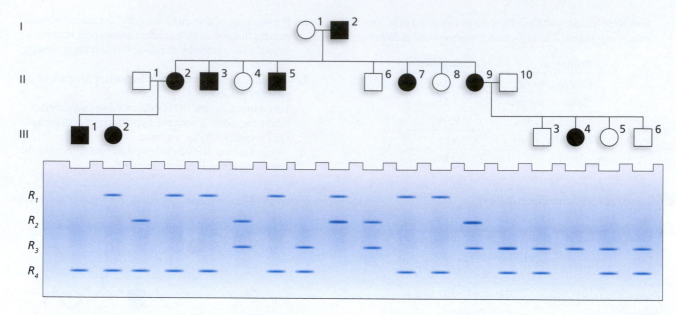

36. Divide a clean sheet of paper into four quadrants and draw one pair of homologous chromosomes in each quadrant. Draw the chromosomes with two sister chromatids each. The four sets of homologous pairs are identical. Label one chromosome of each pair with alleles A_1 and B_1 and the other member of each pair with the alleles A_2 and B_2. You are to illustrate a single crossover between the homologs in each quadrant, and list the parental and recombinant chromosomes, but you are to illustrate four different ways the crossover can occur by involving *different chromatids* in each illustration.

37. For six genes known to be linked on chromosome 10 of corn (*Zea mays*), the recombination frequencies between various pairs have been determined in a series of genetic crosses. Use the recombination frequency data in the table below to determine the order of and distance between the genes on a genetic map. The gene *lc1* is known to be closest to the telomere of the chromosome.

GENE	du1	mgs1	ms10	tp2	wsm3	lc1
du1		7		19		41
mgs1			5			34
ms10	14				19	
tp2		12	7		12	22
wsm3	31	24				
lc1			29		10	

Genetic Analysis and Mapping in Bacteria and Bacteriophages

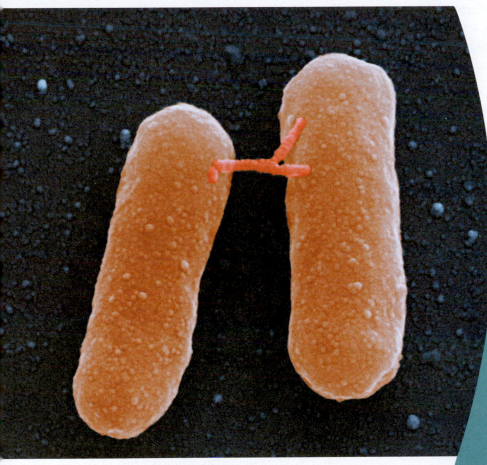

Bacterial conjugation is a process by which genetic material is transferred from one bacterial cell (the donor) to another bacterial cell (the recipient) by way of a hair-like pilus shown in the center of the photo.

Here's a surprising little secret of human life: Your body contains approximately 100 trillion cells, but only about 10 trillion of them are yours! The other 90% of the cells you carry around are bacteria, fungi, and other forms of microscopic life. Many of these biological hitchhikers perform useful, even essential, functions. For example, you carry hundreds of species of bacteria in your gut that collectively have a mass of more than 3 pounds. Without these intestinal bacteria, your digestion of carbohydrates would be impaired, and your ability to manufacture essential nutrients such as vitamin B_{12} and vitamin K would be disabled. The bacteria teeming in your digestive tract also help keep potentially harmful bacteria at bay by vigorously competing for available nutrients. Similarly,

CHAPTER OUTLINE

6.1 Specialized Methods Are Used for Genetic Analysis of Bacteria

6.2 Bacteria Transfer Genes by Conjugation

6.3 Bacterial Transformation Produces Genetic Recombination

6.4 Bacterial Transduction Is Mediated by Bacteriophages

6.5 Bacteriophage Chromosomes Are Mapped by Fine-Structure Analysis

6.6 Lateral Gene Transfer Alters Genomes

ESSENTIAL IDEAS

▌ Bacteria are propagated in liquid growth media or on semisolid growth plates.

▌ Bacterial genotypes are identified by ability to grow on plates containing various compounds.

▌ Bacterial conjugation is a one-way transfer of genetic material from a donor cell to a recipient cell. Three types of donor cells can conjugate with recipient cells to transfer DNA.

▌ Donor bacterial genetic maps are derived from conjugation analysis.

▌ A particular type of bacterial conjugation can produce bacteria with genomes that are partially diploid.

▌ Transformation is the absorption of extracellular DNA across the cell wall and membrane of a recipient bacterial cell, and its analysis leads to mapping of donor bacterial genes.

▌ Transduction, mediated by bacteriophages, transfers DNA from a donor bacterial cell to a recipient cell, and its analysis leads to mapping of donor bacterial genes.

▌ Fine-structure genetic analysis of a bacteriophage genome demonstrated that DNA nucleotide base pairs are the fundamental units of mutation and recombination.

▌ Lateral gene transfer is a prevalent mechanism for the exchange of genes among bacteria and for the evolution of genomes.

the millions of bacteria that currently reside on your skin (yes, even though you showered recently!) help keep your skin healthy by competing with infectious bacteria. Despite this normal and healthy competition, harmful bacteria can gain access to our bodies. Occasionally even our normally helpful microbial passengers turn against us and cause illness, infection, or, in extreme cases, death.

Given the biological, medical, and technological importance of bacteria and other microorganisms, it is no wonder they are studied intensively in modern genetics, using the bacterium *Escherichia coli* and the yeast *Saccharomyces cerevisiae* as model genetic organisms. The relative ease of studying microorganisms fueled revolutionary change in genetics in the latter half of the 20th century. Much of the initial knowledge of molecular genetics and many of the methods of genetic analysis were acquired in the study of bacteria and have proven valuable in the study of more complex organisms.

In this chapter, we investigate how genetic analysis is applied to the study of gene transfer and mapping in bacterial and bacteriophage genomes. We take a historical genetic approach in our discussion, focusing on the applications of genetic analysis that were used to map genes in bacterial genomes in the decades before genome sequencing was developed. Genome sequences of thousands of bacterial species are now published, and their analysis verifies the accuracy and validity of the conclusions reached through use of the approaches described in this chapter.

6.1 Specialized Methods Are Used for Genetic Analysis of Bacteria

Bacteria are a highly diverse taxonomic group essential for genetic study. Among the features that make bacteria so useful to geneticists are the following:

■ **Relative genomic simplicity.** Most bacterial genomes contain fewer genes and fewer base pairs in their haploid genomes than do the genomes of eukaryotes, making bacterial genomes less complex by comparison.

■ **Haploid genomes.** The haploid genomes of most bacteria allow all mutations to be observed directly,

without interference from dominance interactions between alleles.

■ **Short generation times.** Bacteria can reproduce rapidly, with generation times measured in minutes. Rapid doubling of the number of bacterial cells can produce millions of cells from a few dozen original cells within hours.

■ **Large numbers of progeny.** Enormous numbers of clonal progeny can be examined, increasing the likelihood that statistically rare events will be observed.

■ **Ease of propagation.** Microbes may be grown either in liquid culture or on culture plates. The cultures are easy and inexpensive to maintain, and they require little laboratory space.

■ **Numerous heritable differences.** Mutants are easily created, identified, isolated, and manipulated for examination.

The techniques used to study bacteria are essentially the same as those used to study all single-celled organisms, whether bacteria, archaea, yeast, or fungi. We briefly outline these methods in this section and introduce essential terminology for discussing them.

Bacterial Culture and Growth Analysis

Bacteria are haploid organisms that have one copy of each gene. These genes are usually carried on a single bacterial chromosome. A few bacterial species have their genome divided into more than one chromosome, but no bacteria (or archaea, for that matter) have homologous chromosome pairs.

Bacteria propagate by **binary fission**, a process in which the bacterial chromosome replicates and a copy is distributed to each of the progeny cells. During rapid growth, each fission cycle lasts 20 to 30 minutes and more than one copy of the chromosome may be present. Bacterial fissioning is clonal, meaning that the two daughter cells of an original bacterial cell are genetically identical to one another and to the original cell. In a matter of hours, this growth can generate a bacterial **colony**, a cluster of millions of bacterial cells all derived from a single cell.

Bacteria can be grown in either a liquid growth medium or on a growth plate containing a semisolid growth medium (**Figure 6.1**). Both kinds of growth media contain the same nutritional ingredients. The difference is that the medium in growth plates contains agar that congeals when cooled.

Because they are haploid organisms with only one copy of each gene, wild-type bacteria rely on the normal functioning of all their genes that are essential for growth. With these genes functioning properly, the bacteria are able to synthesize all the compounds they require from elements and compounds in their growth environment. The most important of these are a carbon source—usually the simple sugar glucose—and sources of nitrogen and certain other elements—usually supplied in inorganic salts. They also need water, which is present in the growth medium, and oxygen, which is readily available from the atmosphere. Glucose is the raw material that supplies

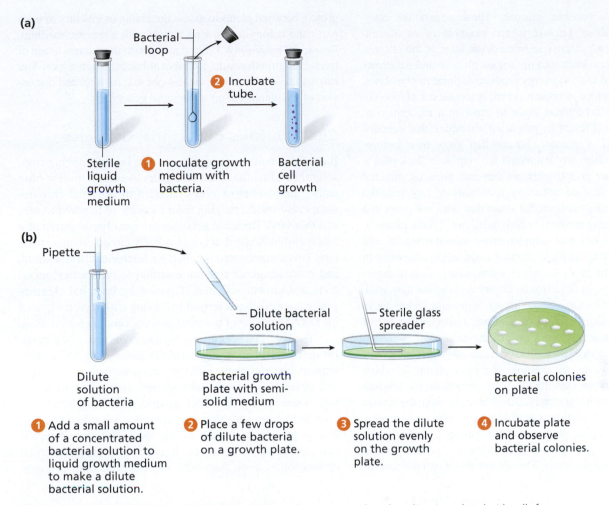

(a)

Bacterial loop

Sterile liquid growth medium

1 Inoculate growth medium with bacteria.

2 Incubate tube.

Bacterial cell growth

(b)

Pipette

Dilute bacterial solution

Sterile glass spreader

Dilute solution of bacteria

Bacterial growth plate with semi-solid medium

Bacterial colonies on plate

1 Add a small amount of a concentrated bacterial solution to liquid growth medium to make a dilute bacterial solution.

2 Place a few drops of dilute bacteria on a growth plate.

3 Spread the dilute solution evenly on the growth plate.

4 Incubate plate and observe bacterial colonies.

Figure 6.1   Bacterial growth methods. (a) Bacteria can be grown in a liquid medium inoculated with cells from another culture. In liquid, dense growth occurs making the medium appear cloudy. **(b)** Bacteria can be grown on a plate of semisolid growth medium on which a few drops of a dilute bacterial-cell solution have been spread. On the semisolid medium, bacteria grow as colonies.

the important energy-producing process known as glycolysis that operates in most organisms, including humans.

A **minimal medium** is one containing glucose as the sugar source along with a nitrogen source, some inorganic material, and water. Wild-type cells of many bacterial species are able to grow in minimal medium and are called **prototrophs**, or **prototrophic strains**. Prototrophic bacteria produce all the compounds required for their metabolism, growth, and reproduction using the energy provided by glycolysis. Another way of saying this is that prototrophs do not carry any mutations that block their ability to produce a compound that is required for growth. For this reason, a prototrophic strain is defined by its ability to grow in a minimal medium.

Bacteria that are mutant for one or more genes lack the ability to produce an essential compound or perform a required growth function. These bacteria are unable to grow in a minimal medium. Mutant bacteria are called **auxotrophs** or **auxotrophic strains**. Auxotrophic species also include many bacterial species with more complex growth requirements, such as those living symbiotically

with other organisms. These auxotrophs lack some of the genes required to grow on minimal medium and instead obtain essential nutrients from their hosts.

Auxotrophs are able to grow on a **complete medium**. This is a medium containing glucose and a nitrogen source along with all the other compounds required for growth and reproduction, such as amino acids and DNA and RNA nucleotides. An auxotroph will also be able to grow on the right **supplemented minimal medium**. This is a minimal medium to which has been added the specific compound the auxotrophic strain is unable to produce on its own. Say, for example, that an auxotrophic bacterial strain is unable to synthesize the amino acid leucine. Such a strain is designated as being *leu*⁻ (spoken "leucine minus"). If all the other essential compounds can be produced by this strain, then supplementing a minimal medium with leucine will permit the growth of a *leu*⁻ strain on that medium.

Certain bacterial strains are able to grow in a growth medium that does not contain glucose but rather a sugar that is more complex than glucose, or a sugar that requires metabolism to generate glucose. These sugars are alternatives to glucose. Lactose is one example of an alternative sugar. As we discuss in more detail later in the chapter, lactose is broken down into the sugars glucose and galactose. Glucose is used to drive energy production through glycolysis, and once galactose is broken down, it too drives glycolysis. The ability of a bacterial strain to grow in a medium containing lactose is tested by preparing a medium that contains lactose instead of glucose. Strains that grow in a lactose-containing medium are designated lac^+ (spoken "lack plus"). Such strains are prototrophic, as they can grow on minimal medium and they do not carry mutations of any required genes. A prototrophic bacterial strain that does not grow in a lactose-containing medium is designated lac^- ("lack minus").

Complete, minimal, supplemented minimal media, and media prepared using an alternative sugar are instrumental in bacterial genetic analysis, where a frequent goal is to determine the genotypes of strains by observing whether they grow or fail to grow on various media. An important technique in these investigations is **replica plating**, a simple process of transferring some cells from each of the bacterial colonies on an original growth plate to one or more other growth plates. Figure 6.2 illustrates an example of replica plating in which two auxotrophs are identified by their growth on the original plate with complete medium but their absence from the replica minimal medium plate where only prototrophs will grow. A key feature of replica plating is that it transfers bacterial colonies from the original growth plate to the new growth plate in the *same relative positions*. This allows direct comparisons of

growth between plates to assess the ability or inability of each particular colony to grow on a plate with a specific medium. Research Technique 6.1 introduces you to the interpretation of microbial growth results to discover bacterial genotypes. You can also review Experimental Insight 4.1, for a related discussion of the identification of bacterial genotypes.

Characteristics of Bacterial Genomes

Bacterial genomes are highly variable in size, ranging from several hundred thousand base pairs to several million base pairs. The number of genes encoded by bacterial chromosomes also varies, ranging from a couple of hundred to several thousand. Bacterial genomes are usually composed of a *single* chromosome that is a covalently closed circular structure. This chromosome is called the **bacterial chromosome**, and it carries genes that are essential to the species' metabolic and growth activities (**Figure 6.3**). Bacterial chromosomes are also characterized by having a high proportion of the DNA sequence of bacterial genomes coding for proteins.

The bacterial species *Escherichia coli* is one of a handful of so-called model genetic organisms that are so designated because their biology, reproduction, metabolism, and genetics are well characterized and suited to scientific research. These model genetic organisms have been used in biology and genetics experiments for decades. The *E. coli* genome is typical of the most common characteristics of bacterial genomes. It contains a single, circular chromosome, more than 90% of which encodes proteins.

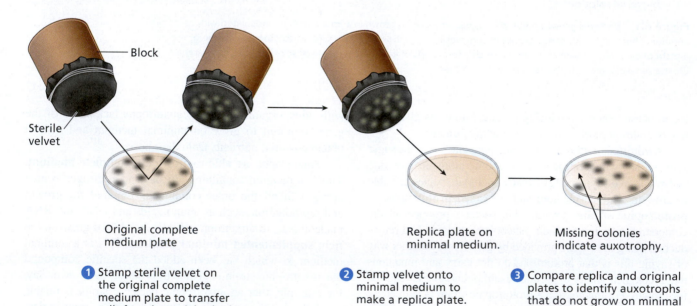

Figure 6.2 **Replica plating.** Sterile velvet is used as a stamp that is first pressed upon the colonies on the original, complete-medium plate and then pressed onto a new, minimal-medium plate, transferring cells from all the colonies of the original plate to the new plate. After an interval to allow continued growth, the original and replica plates are compared. The absence of growth of a colony on the replica plate indicates auxotrophy.

Q Consider a growth plate containing complete medium with 200 growing colonies on it. If you wanted to determine which of these colonies were auxotrophic, what would you do? How does replica plating make this task easier?

The *E. coli* chromosome is made up of approximately 4.6 million base pairs and contains about 4200 genes.

Although most bacterial species have genomes composed of a single, circular chromosome, there are some exceptions. *Vibrio cholerae*, the species that causes the disease cholera, contains two circular chromosomes, one of them much larger than the other. *Rhizobium meliloti*, a species that grows on plant roots and helps make nitrogen available to the plants, contains three chromosomes. A handful of species have linear chromosomes.

Plasmids in Bacterial Cells

In addition to the main bacterial chromosome, most bacteria also carry multiple copies of **plasmids**, small double-stranded circular DNA molecules containing nonessential genes that are used infrequently or under specialized conditions not ordinarily encountered by the species (see Figure 6.3). Plasmids vary widely in their number of genes and their total number of base pairs, but they are always considerably smaller than bacterial chromosomes. Plasmids

RESEARCH TECHNIQUE 6.1

Genotyping Using Microbial Growth

The results of the experiments on microbes described in this chapter have shaped our understanding of how genes work, including how they are organized and how they are expressed. A basic set of common laboratory techniques and analyses assessing growth or failure to grow in liquid or semisolid media made up of different components can be used to determine the genetic makeup of microorganisms. Proper interpretation of the genotype of a microbe based on its pattern of growth on different media is an essential skill of genetic analysis that is easy to master once you understand a few key concepts.

ANABOLIC AND CATABOLIC PATHWAYS Compounds that influence the growth of microbes on growth media fall into two broad categories. In the first are compounds synthesized by prototrophic (wild-type) microbes in biosynthetic pathways that are often described as *anabolic pathways*. In anabolic pathways, *energy is used to synthesize* complex compounds from simpler ones through sequential reaction steps. Figure 4.17 and the accompanying discussion of the anabolic pathway that synthesizes the amino acid methionine (pages 123–124) provide an example. In contrast, *catabolic pathways* are pathways through which *energy is produced* by the *breakdown* of complex compounds into simpler ones. Catabolic pathways also follow sequential steps. Our discussion of phenylketonuria (PKU; pages 122–123) highlights the catabolic pathway that breaks down the amino acid phenylalanine. Similarly, polysaccharide sugars like lactose and other carbohydrates are broken down in catabolic pathways.

VISUALIZING MICROBIAL GROWTH When microbial growth occurs on a semisolid growth plate in a petri dish, individual colonies may appear on the plate. Each colony is actually hundreds of thousands to millions of individual microbes that are all descended from a single microbial cell among those originally spread on the plate in a very dilute solution. Depending on microbe genotypes and the composition of the growth medium, it is possible that more than one microbial genotype is growing on a particular plate. In addition, although each bacterial colony on a growth plate consists of cells with virtual genetic identity, a colony of millions of cells can be expected to contain some cells with mutations. In a liquid growth medium, microbial growth produces cloudiness—the result of the presence of so many living cells in the growth vessel that they impede the passage of light through the medium. There are no colonies in liquid media.

Identifying the genotype of a microbe often requires assessing the growth of a particular colony on different growth media. This is accomplished by the replica plating technique described in Figure 6.2. An alternative method of replica plating is to simply touch a colony growing on one growth medium with a sterile toothpick or a similar instrument to gather some cells of the colony and then touch a spot on a different growth plate. Systematic use of a grid pattern on the new plate and care in the recording of growth results permit comparison of growth results on these different plates so as to identify colony genotypes.

ALLELIC IDENTIFICATION Distinguishing between compounds produced by anabolic pathways (anabolism builds compounds from elemental building blocks) and those broken down in catabolic pathways (catabolism breaks down compounds into elements) is a critical aspect of interpreting microbial growth and identifying microbial genotype that requires knowledge of growth media and their constituents.

In a convention you saw employed in Experimental Insight 4.1, the ability to synthesize an essential compound by completion of an anabolic pathway is indicated in genetic notation by a "+" (plus) symbol and identifies a wild-type allele; thus, a microbe capable of biosynthesizing the amino acid methionine is identified as *met*$^+$ (spoken "met plus"). In contrast, the "−" (minus) symbol indicates the organism is an auxotroph (mutant) that is unable to synthesize a particular compound due to mutation. The control prototroph shown in Figure 4.18 (page 127) is *met*$^+$, whereas the four other strains are each *met*$^-$.

The convention is similar for catabolic pathways: allelic symbols identify the ability of a strain to complete a catabolic pathway with a superscript "+" and the inability to complete a catabolic pathway with the "−" symbol. For example, microbes that are able to grow on a medium containing the milk sugar lactose instead of glucose are *lac*$^+$. The ability to grow on lactose requires production of the enzymes that break lactose down into simpler compounds. In contrast, microbes that are unable to grow on lactose-containing media are *lac*$^-$. These strains are unable to produce one or more of the enzymes required for lactose metabolism.

The accompanying figure guides you through the identification of prototrophs and auxotrophs for the amino acids alanine (*ala*) and proline (*pro*) among 10 microbial colonies and also for the ability of the colonies to break down lactose. Genotype identification is accomplished by comparing growth on plates of media containing different constituents. The accompanying table summarizes the genotype of each colony and the reasoning used to identify the genotype.

(continued)

RESEARCH TECHNIQUE 6.1 Continued

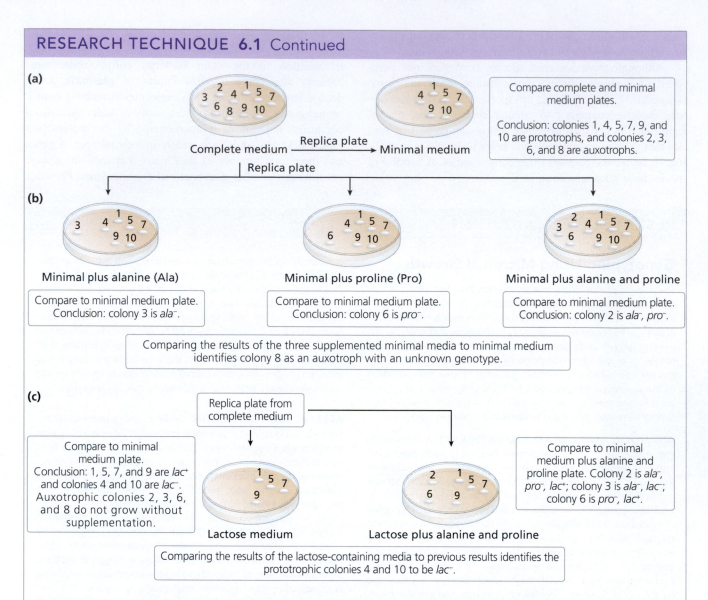

(a)

Complete medium — Replica plate → Minimal medium

Replica plate

Compare complete and minimal medium plates.

Conclusion: colonies 1, 4, 5, 7, 9, and 10 are prototrophs, and colonies 2, 3, 6, and 8 are auxotrophs.

(b)

Minimal plus alanine (Ala)

Compare to minimal medium plate.
Conclusion: colony 3 is *ala*⁻.

Minimal plus proline (Pro)

Compare to minimal medium plate.
Conclusion: colony 6 is *pro*⁻.

Minimal plus alanine and proline

Compare to minimal medium plate.
Conclusion: colony 2 is *ala*⁻, *pro*⁻.

Comparing the results of the three supplemented minimal media to minimal medium identifies colony 8 as an auxotroph with an unknown genotype.

(c)

Replica plate from complete medium

Compare to minimal medium plate.
Conclusion: 1, 5, 7, and 9 are *lac*⁺ and colonies 4 and 10 are *lac*⁻. Auxotrophic colonies 2, 3, 6, and 8 do not grow without supplementation.

Lactose medium

Lactose plus alanine and proline

Compare to minimal medium plus alanine and proline plate. Colony 2 is *ala*⁻, *pro*⁻, *lac*⁺; colony 3 is *ala*⁻, *lac*⁻; colony 6 is *pro*⁻, *lac*⁺.

Comparing the results of the lactose-containing media to previous results identifies the prototrophic colonies 4 and 10 to be *lac*⁻.

Colony	Genotype	Explanation
1, 5, 7, and 9	*ala*⁺ *pro*⁺ *lac*⁺	These are prototrophs: they grow on minimal (glucose-containing) medium. Also grow on lactose (lactose-containing) medium.
2	*ala*⁻ *pro*⁻ *lac*⁺	Auxotroph: does not grow on minimal medium. Grows on minimal medium supplemented with both alanine and proline. Also grows on lactose medium supplemented with alanine and proline.
3	*ala*⁻ *pro*⁺ *lac*⁻	Auxotroph: does not grow on minimal medium. Grows on minimal medium supplemented with alanine. Does not grow on lactose medium supplemented with alanine and proline.
4 and 10	*ala*⁺ *pro*⁺ *lac*⁻	Prototroph: grows on minimal medium. Does not grow on lactose medium.
6	*ala*⁺ *pro*⁻ *lac*⁺	Auxotroph: does not grow on minimal medium. Grows on minimal medium plus proline and grows on lactose medium plus alanine and proline.
8	Unknown genotype	Auxotroph: does not grow on minimal medium.

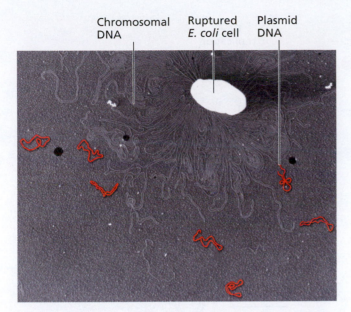

Chromosomal DNA   Ruptured *E. coli* cell   Plasmid DNA

Figure 6.3 **Bacterial chromosome and plasmids.** This electron micrograph shows a ruptured *E. coli* cell that has released its bacterial chromosomal DNA (gray) along with multiple plasmids (red).

are described as extrachromosomal DNA, meaning they are generally separate from the bacterial chromosome. As such, they are not part of the bacterial genome. There are, however, certain circumstances under which plasmid DNA can be inserted into the bacterial chromosome. We discuss some of these events later in the chapter.

Many different kinds of naturally occurring plasmids are found in bacteria, and each contains several genes. One plasmid we are about to discuss, called an **F (fertility) plasmid**, contains genes that promote its own transfer from a donor bacterium to a recipient. Another type of plasmid we discuss, known as an **R (resistance) plasmid**, carries **antibiotic resistance** genes that can be transferred from donors to recipients. Plasmids are easily modified in the laboratory to produce specific characteristics or to carry particular genes that are useful in a wide range of recombinant DNA applications (see Chapter 15). In most of our discussions in this chapter, we portray all antibiotic resistance genes as being carried on an R plasmid. In other words, we describe a strain resistant to an antibiotic as carrying an R plasmid (a plasmid containing the resistance gene), and we describe a strain susceptible to the antibiotic as carrying no R plasmid. This pretense simplifies our discussion and explanation of experimental results, but in reality, numerous bacterial strains carry antibiotic resistance genes on the bacterial chromosome. The transfer of both plasmid-borne and chromosome-borne antibiotic resistance genes between bacterial strains is a major contributing factor to the rapid spread of antibiotic resistant strains of infectious bacteria.

Plasmids generally replicate autonomously. Consequently, up to several dozen copies of a plasmid can be found in a single bacterial cell. Such plasmids are identified as "high-copy-number" plasmids. Alternatively, low-copy-number plasmids

are generally unable to replicate on their own because their replication is tied to that of the bacterial chromosome. These plasmids are present in one or two copies per bacterial cell.

6.2 Bacteria Transfer Genes by Conjugation

The ability of bacteria to produce colonies of clones does not mean that bacteria never recombine genetically. In fact, a characteristic of great usefulness to microbial geneticists is the propensity of bacteria to transfer genetic material from one individual bacterium to another. Bacterial gene transfer is a one-way process in which replicated DNA is donated by one bacterium, called the **donor** to another bacterium called the **recipient**. The donated DNA can be a plasmid, a fragment of the donor bacterial chromosome, or a combination of the two. At the same time, the transferred DNA is often a newly replicated copy of DNA in the donor cell. Thus the donor does not lose any genetic information. Rather, the recipient gains information by the donation. Successful gene transfer requires that donor DNA be incorporated into the genome of the recipient. Transfer occurs by three processes:

1. **Conjugation**, the transfer of replicated DNA from a donor bacterium to a recipient bacterium through temporary contact. Conjugation requires the donor cell to make physical contact with the recipient cell, establish a bridge between the two cells, and initiate DNA transfer across the bridge. Inside the recipient cell the donated genetic material re-forms as a plasmid, if that is what has been transferred; or, if a fragment of the donor chromosome is what has been copied and transferred, the donated DNA recombines into the homologous region of the recipient chromosome. This event is illustrated in **Figure 6.4a**.

2. **Transformation**, the uptake of DNA, derived from a donor cell, from the growth medium of the recipient. The donated DNA comes from a donor cell that has died and ruptured, and whose bacterial chromosome has fragmented. One or more of these donor DNA fragments cross the cell membrane of the recipient and are recombined into the recipient chromosome. An overview of transformation is illustrated in **Figure 6.4b**.

3. **Transduction**, the transfer of DNA from a donor bacterium to a recipient bacterium by way of a bacterial virus known as a bacteriophage. Bacteriophages carry DNA containing genetic information that drives their infection of host bacterial cells. Part of the infection cycle is the rupture of the host bacterium and the release of new progeny bacteriophages. Occasionally new progeny phages can carry a segment of the infected host cell's chromosome instead of the normal phage DNA. In these cases, the chromosome fragment from the host—the

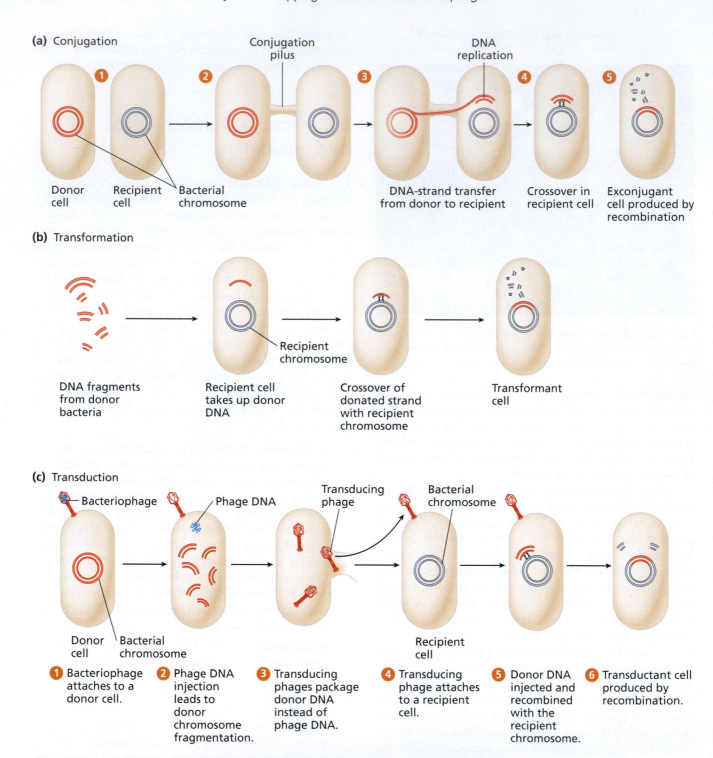

(a) Conjugation

① Donor cell | Recipient cell | Bacterial chromosome

② Conjugation pilus

③ DNA-strand transfer from donor to recipient | DNA replication

④ Crossover in recipient cell

⑤ Exconjugant cell produced by recombination

(b) Transformation

DNA fragments from donor bacteria

Recipient cell takes up donor DNA | Recipient chromosome

Crossover of donated strand with recipient chromosome

Transformant cell

(c) Transduction

Bacteriophage | Phage DNA | Transducing phage | Bacterial chromosome

Donor cell | Bacterial chromosome

Recipient cell

① Bacteriophage attaches to a donor cell.

② Phage DNA injection leads to donor chromosome fragmentation.

③ Transducing phages package donor DNA instead of phage DNA.

④ Transducing phage attaches to a recipient cell.

⑤ Donor DNA injected and recombined with the recipient chromosome.

⑥ Transductant cell produced by recombination.

Figure 6.4 **Gene-transfer processes in bacteria. (a)** Conjugation. A single DNA strand transferred during DNA replication in the donor is used to replicate a second strand in the recipient. Subsequent crossing over recombines DNA to form the exconjugant cell. **(b)** Transformation. A single strand of donor DNA taken across the membrane of the recipient cell recombines with recipient DNA to form the transformant cell. **(c)** Transduction. A donor DNA fragment encapsulated in a transducing phage is injected into the recipient cell, where it recombines to form the transductant cell.

donor in this process—can be inserted into a new bacterial cell—the recipient—where it can recombine into the recipient chromosome. Transduction is illustrated in **Figure 6.4c**, and it is discussed in the following section.

Each of these processes is an example of *lateral gene transfer*, a nonreproductive process through which bacteria and archaea actively exchange genetic material. Lateral gene transfer also takes place between bacteria and eukaryotes. The impact of these events on genomes and on the evolution of life are topics for discussion later in this chapter.

Conjugation Identified

Conjugation was first identified by Joshua Lederberg and Edward Tatum in 1946. They used two triple-auxotrophic strains of *E. coli* that had different nutritional requirements for growth. The researchers first established three separate bacterial cultures growing, initially, in a complete medium (**Figure 6.5**). In culture ❶, they grew an auxotrophic strain called Y-24, which has the genotype $met^- \ bio^- \ leu^+ \ cys^- \ phe^- \ thr^+ \ thi^+$. Because of its genotype, the Y-24 strain requires addition of the vitamin biotin

(*bio*) and the amino acids methionine (*met*), cysteine (*cys*) and phenylalanine (*phe*) to a minimal medium for growth. In culture ❷, they placed an auxotrophic strain called Y-10, which has the genotype $met^+ \ bio^+ \ leu^- \ cys^+ \ phe^+ \ thr^- \ thi^-$. The Y-10 strain requires addition of the vitamin thiamine (*thi*) and the amino acids leucine (*leu*) and threonine (*thr*) for growth. Culture ❸ contained an equal mixture of both Y-10 and Y-24.

Each culture was allowed to grow, and cells from each culture were plated on minimal medium. Lederberg and Tatum saw no growth on Plates 1 and 2, which contained cells transferred from culture ❶ and culture ❷, respectively. These results were consistent with the nutritional requirements of Y-24 and Y-10 and indicated that all the cells transferred to those plates were auxotrophs. Plate 3, however, developed about 100 growing colonies! These colonies grew from bacterial cells that had somehow acquired the prototrophic genotype ($met^+ \ bio^+ \ leu^+ \ cys^+ \ phe^+ \ thr^+ \ thi^+$).

Lederberg and Tatum were certain that this outcome did not result from the reversion (reverse mutation) of auxotrophs to prototrophs. Instead of reversion, the researchers proposed the transfer of genetic information. Lederberg and Tatum hypothesized that physical contact between bacteria was necessary for gene transfer, but their original experiment did not provide direct evidence that this might be so. Four years later, Bernard Davis replicated the work and showed the necessity of contact between bacterial cells for gene transfer to take place. For his experiment, Davis constructed a U-tube with a fine glass filter separating one arm from the other (**Figure 6.6**). The filter was a glass disk with very small

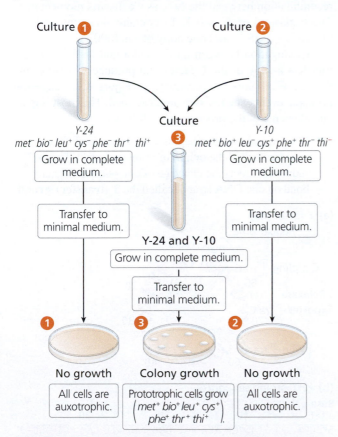

Figure 6.5 Lederberg and Tatum's detection of recombination between auxotrophic *E. coli* cells. Auxotrophic bacterial strains ❶ (Y-24) and ❷ (Y-10) each contain multiple mutations and grow on complete medium but not on minimal medium. ❸ Mixing the strains leads to the formation of prototrophic bacteria that grow on minimal medium.

Q Why do you think it is highly unlikely that the prototrophic colonies detected in this experiment came about by mutation?

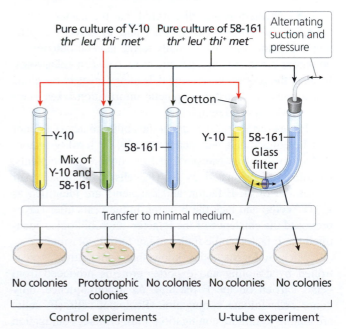

Figure 6.6 Davis's U-tube experiment, showing that genetic recombination requires cell-to-cell contact. Auxotrophic bacterial strains Y-10 and 58-161 are unable to grow on minimal medium but produce some prototrophs that grow on minimal medium when they make contact following mixing. Prototrophs are not produced when the auxotrophs are placed in a U-tube, indicating that direct contact is required to generate prototrophic bacteria.

pores that allowed passage of small molecules such as nutrients but not bacterial cells. A cotton ball plugging one end of the U-tube and a rubber stopper connected to an air line at the other allowed Davis to move the material in the tube by alternating suction and pressure. The tube contained a culture of *E. coli* strain Y-10 on one side of the glass disk and a culture of strain 58-161, auxotrophic for methionine synthesis (*met⁻*), on the other side of the disk, and the glass disk prevented direct contact between the two bacterial strains.

Based on Lederberg and Tatum's experiments, Davis hypothesized that direct contact between the auxotrophic strains was needed to produce prototrophic bacteria. After alternating suction and pressure for several hours, Davis plated bacterial samples from each side of the U-tube onto minimal medium and found no growth from either side of the U-tube. This lack of growth was an indication that cells on either side of the disk retained their auxotrophy. Davis concluded that physical contact between bacterial cells is required for gene transfer to take place.

Lederberg, Tatum, and Davis were correct in their proposal that direct contact between bacteria is required for conjugation. The genetic information is conveyed by way of a hollow tube known as a **conjugation pilus** or that physically connects donor and recipient. Conjugation is pictured in the chapter-opening photo on page 185. The conjugation pilus is the thread-like structure in the center of the photo, connecting the donor and recipient bacterial cells.

Transfer of the F Factor

In 1953, William Hayes discovered that the bacteria interacting in Lederberg and Tatum's and in Davis's experiments did not contribute equally to the genetic outcome as do parent organisms in a genetic cross between eukaryotes. Instead, the process was unequal, leading Hayes to conclude that a one-way transfer of genetic information takes place between donors and recipients.

Hayes further proposed that the ability to act as a donor was hereditary and was determined by a "fertility factor" (F factor) that was transferable from donors to recipients. Donors are designated as F^+ (F^+**cells**) to indicate their possession of an F factor, and recipients are identified as F^- (F^-**cells**) and lack the F factor. In the years after Hayes proposed the existence of the F factor, microbiologists identified the F factor as the F plasmid, or fertility plasmid.

Microbiologists today know that conjugation is controlled by coupling and exporter proteins produced from genes carried on the F plasmid. As a consequence, only donor cells initiate conjugation. Recipient cells (F^- cells) are unable to initiate conjugation. Furthermore, conjugation occurs between a donor cell and a recipient but not between two donor cells. F factor genes direct the construction of an **exporter structure** formed from coupling proteins that link the donor and recipient cells and from exporter proteins that form the bridge through which a single strand of F factor DNA will pass from the donor to the recipient. A protein complex known as the **relaxosome** is responsible for cutting

one strand of F factor DNA. This leads to DNA replication that along with proteins moves one strand of F factor DNA into the recipient cell, where separate DNA replication forms a double-stranded F factor.

Three kinds of cells are seen in conjugation: a donor cell that contains an F plasmid and donates genetic information, a recipient cell that receives DNA from a donor cell but does not contain a functional F factor, and the **exconjugant cell** that is produced by conjugation. An exconjugant cell is essentially a recipient cell that has had its genetic content modified by receiving DNA from a donor cell.

The F factor of the *E. coli* strain is the most extensively mapped F plasmid. It consists of some 100 kb of DNA, and about 35% of its sequence is devoted to 36 genes that control conjugation and gene transfer (**Figure 6.7**). The F plasmid genes that play a role in *E. coli* conjugation are given four-letter designations consisting of the prefix *tra* or *trb* followed by a capital letter. Much of the remainder of the F factor consists of four **insertion sequence (IS) elements**. IS elements are DNA sequences that when shared by an F plasmid and a bacterial chromosome are locations for recombination between the two, as we discuss momentarily. The F plasmid of *E. coli* K-12 contains one copy of IS-2, two copies of IS-3, and one copy of Tn-1000.

Conjugation between an F^+ donor and an F^- recipient transfers a copy of the F factor and produces exconjugants that are F^+ donors, as illustrated in **Figure 6.8**, where the principal events at each step are described. The most important elements of the process are as follows:

1. DNA transfer always begins at a specialized F factor sequence called the **origin of transfer (*oriT*)**. The *oriT* sequence directs the cleavage of one phosphodiester bond on one DNA strand, called the **T (transfer) strand**.

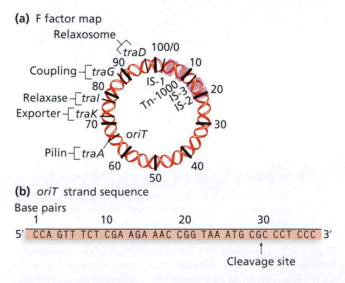

(a) F factor map

(b) *oriT* strand sequence

Base pairs

5′ CCA GTT TCT CGA AGA AAC CGG TAA ATG CGC CCT CCC 3′

↑
Cleavage site

Figure 6.7 F plasmid structure. (a) Selected genes important in donor–recipient cell conjugation and F factor transfer are shown along with the origin of transfer (*oriT*) and four insertion sequences (IS) around the 100-kb map of the F plasmid of the *E. coli* K-12 strain. **(b)** The 36-base sequence of *oriT*, including the cleavage site on the T strand.

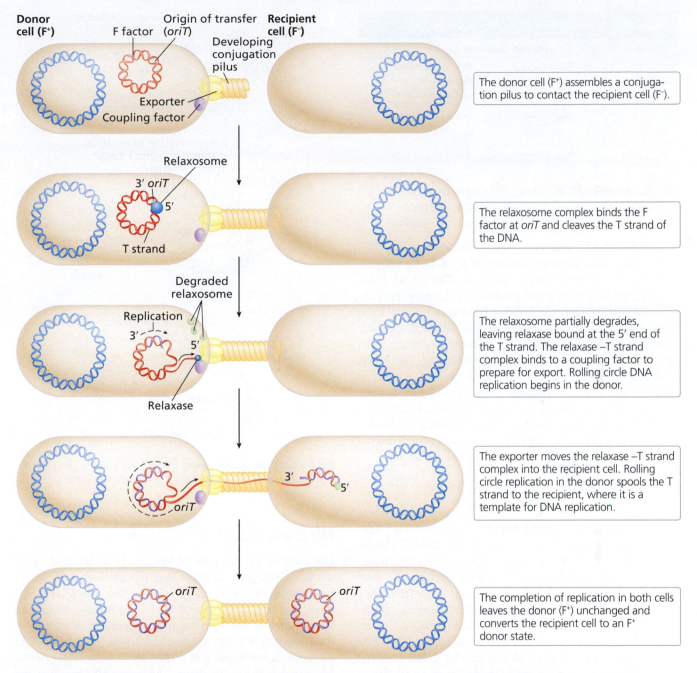

Figure 6.8 Conjugation of F⁺ and F⁻ cells. Rolling circle replication transfers a single strand of the F factor, beginning at *oriT*, from a donor cell to a recipient cell, where it is replicated to convert the recipient cell (F⁻) to an F⁺ donor.

2. A protein complex composed of exporter proteins and pilin protein forms a conjugation pilus between the donor and recipient cells. The conjugation pilus contains a narrow channel that only allows passage of a single DNA strand.

3. The protein complex called the relaxosome binds at *oriT* and makes a single-stranded cut to the T strand. The relaxosome then partially degenerates, leaving relaxase attached to the free 5′ end of the T strand.

4. Facilitated by the action of relaxase, the T strand enters the conjugation pilus and passes into the recipient cell.

Inside the recipient it is used as a template to produce a second plasmid DNA strand and thus generate a double-stranded F factor. The F⁻ recipient is converted to an F⁺ donor by this process.

5. Within the donor, T strand transfer is accompanied by a specialized process of DNA replication, known as **rolling circle replication** that uses the remaining strand as a template. Rolling circle replication is a specialized unidirectional process different from the more common process of bidirectional replication that we describe in Chapter 7.

Table 6.1	Outcomes of Bacterial Conjugation	
	Conjugation Outcome	
	Exconjugant Converted to Donor State?	Donor Bacterial Genes Transferred to Exconjugant?
$F^+ \times F^-$	Yes, $F^+ \rightarrow F^-$	No
Hfr $\times$ F^-	No	Yes
$F' \times F^-$	Yes, $F' \rightarrow F^-$	Yes

6. The completion of rolling circle replication in the donor cell restores the donor's double-stranded F factor, leaving that cell's F^+ donor state intact.

Table 6.1 identifies two pivotal outcomes of $F^+ \times F^-$ conjugation. First, complete transfer of the F factor converts the F^- recipient cell to an F^+ donor cell. Second, no donor bacterial chromosomal genes are transferred during this conjugation process. Only the F factor DNA is transferred to an F^- recipient cell by an F^+ donor cell. You will recall that Lederberg and Tatum provided clear evidence of chromosomal gene transfer from one bacterial strain to another, and Davis showed that conjugation was required for the transfer to occur. However, $F^+ \times F^-$ conjugation *is not responsible* for the observations of Lederberg and Tatum; the logical conclusion is that there must be some other type of conjugation, involving different kinds of bacterial donor cells, to transfer bacterial chromosomal genes from a donor cell to a recipient cell.

Formation of an Hfr Chromosome

An experiment in 1953 by Luigi Luca Cavalli-Sforza provided critical new insight that eventually explained Lederberg and Tatum's observations. Using careful genetic analysis, Cavalli-Sforza identified donor strains that transferred donor bacterial genes to recipient bacteria at a very high rate. He called these donor bacteria **high-frequency recombination**, or **Hfr**, bacteria. Cavalli-Sforza also determined that conjugation involving Hfr donors and F^- recipients virtually never converted the recipients to F^+ or Hfr donors. Since most donors do not transfer donor bacterial genes and always convert the F^- recipient to an F^+ donor, Cavalli-Sforza's description of Hfr bacterial strains suggested that Hfr strains differ from F^+ strains in structure and relationship of the bacterial chromosome and the F factor.

Examination of Cavalli-Sforza's Hfr strain revealed that instead of being an extrachromosomal plasmid, the F factor in Hfr strains is integrated into the bacterial chromosome, forming an **Hfr chromosome** (**Figure 6.9**). The formation of Hfr chromosomes is rare: Only about 1 in every 100,000 F^+ cells converts to an Hfr cell. The integration event takes place at IS elements that are shared by F plasmids and bacterial chromosomes. Because there are multiple IS elements shared by plasmids and bacterial chromosomes, many different Hfr chromosomes can potentially form. Once an Hfr chromosome forms, it does not change to an alternative Hfr form.

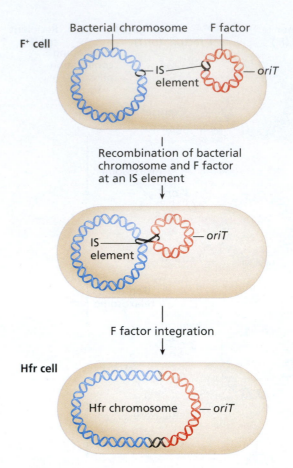

Figure 6.9 Hfr chromosomes. Hfr cells carry an Hfr chromosome that is created when an F factor integrates at an insertion sequence (IS) in the bacterial chromosome.

Hfr Gene Transfer

Hfr bacteria transfer genetic material to recipient cells by the same rolling circle replication process seen in $F^+ \times F^-$ conjugation. As in $F^+ \times F^-$ conjugation, the relaxosome binds and cuts the T strand at *oriT* to initiate unwinding and transfer of the T strand to the recipient. A portion of the integrated F factor is transferred first, followed by the bacterial chromosome and finally by the remainder of the integrated F factor. In theory the entire Hfr chromosome could be transferred during Hfr $\times$ F^- conjugation, but in reality this is impossible. The normal movement of bacteria will break the conjugation pilus long before Hfr transfer is completed. Thus, only a portion of the F factor sequence is transferred from the donor to the recipient, along with a portion of the donor bacterial chromosome containing genes located near the IS site of insertion. In conjugation experiments, the duration of conjugation is variable. Some conjugation events are very short, others quite long, and others of intermediate duration.

The segment of T strand DNA that is successfully transferred into the recipient cell is used as template DNA to generate a double-stranded linear fragment. At whatever point the conjugation pilus ruptures, conjugation is interrupted, and

T strand transfer and replication cease. **Figure 6.10** illustrates conjugation between an Hfr with the genotype *thr⁺ leu⁻ strˢ* and an F⁻ with the genotype *thr⁻ leu⁺ strᴿ* (the function of *strᴿ* and *strˢ* is explained momentarily). Within the recipient cell, the donor DNA is a linear double-stranded DNA fragment containing a portion of the F factor and a segment of donor bacterial DNA that was adjacent to *oriT*. Without the complete *oriT* sequence, the linear DNA cannot circularize; and since only a portion of the F factor is transferred, Hfr donors cannot convert F⁻ recipient cells to a donor state (see Table 6.1). However, before the linear segment of donated donor DNA undergoes enzymatic degradation in the recipient cell, it can undergo homologous recombination with the recipient chromosome. The new exconjugant cell, formerly the recipient cell, may thus acquire one or more genes from the donor bacterial chromosome.

Conjugation experiments mix one strain of donor bacteria in a culture vessel with a different strain of recipient bacteria. Exconjugants produced within the vessel can be identified by their acquisition of donor genes that give them genotypes distinct from those of either the donor strain or recipient strain. These exconjugants can be recognized by their growth on a **selective growth medium**, a medium containing compounds that permit only exconjugants with specific genotypes to grow and that also prevent the growth of donor cells and recipient cells.

In experiments of this kind, antibiotic sensitivity and resistance is used as a tool to control growth of bacteria. In the recipient cells, resistance to the antibiotic streptomycin (*strᴿ*) comes from a gene carried on an extrachromosomal R plasmid. The donor cell is streptomycin sensitive (*strˢ*), but this is due to the *absence of an R plasmid,* not to the presence of an allele for streptomycin sensitivity. Streptomycin resistance is therefore a genotypic attribute of recipient and exconjugant cells but not of donor cells, and the presence of streptomycin in the selective growth medium will kill donor cells so they do not grow and potentially confuse the analysis.

As an example, consider again a conjugation experiment involving an Hfr strain that is susceptible to streptomycin (*strˢ*) and carries the alleles *thr⁺* and *leu⁻* (for biosynthesis of the amino acid threonine and the inability to synthesize leucine). Imagine that the F⁻ strain is unable to synthesize threonine (*thr⁻*) but capable of leucine synthesis (*leu⁺*) and resistant to streptomycin (*strᴿ*). The selective medium necessary to grow and isolate exconjugants in this case is a minimal medium plate with added streptomycin. The streptomycin in the selective medium kills *strˢ* donor cells, and the absence of threonine prevents growth of nonrecombinant recipient cells. All growing cells on the selection plate are *thr⁺ leu⁺ strᴿ*, a genotype that could occur only in exconjugants.

In Figure 6.10, a segment of donor DNA containing *thr⁺ leu⁻* is shown aligning with its homologous counterpart in the recipient bacterial chromosome, containing *thr⁻ leu⁺*. Homologous recombination can replace a segment of the

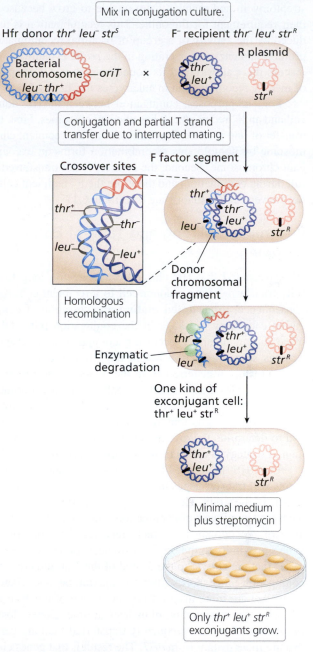

Figure 6.10   Hfr conjugation and exconjugant detection. An Hfr chromosome fragment transferred during interrupted mating between an Hfr donor cell to an F⁻ recipient cell can undergo homologous recombination with the recipient chromosome. Exconjugants are detected on selective growth media, such as the minimal medium shown here.

🔘 **Explain why the statement in the last message box of this figure that "only *thr⁺ leu⁺ strᴿ* exconjugants grow" is correct.**

recipient chromosome with a homologous segment of DNA from the donor chromosome. In the case shown here, two crossovers transfer *thr⁺* from the donor DNA into the recipient chromosome, so that the resulting exconjugants have the genotype *thr⁺ leu⁺ strᴿ*. Only these cells are able to grow on the plate containing minimal medium plus streptomycin shown in Figure 6.10, since donors are killed by streptomycin and recipients are unable to grow because of their requirement for threonine. This recombination is produced by the activity of a group of bacterial recombination proteins and enzymes operating in the *recBCD* pathway. We discuss this pathway and its counterpart in our description of meiotic recombination in eukaryotes in Chapter 11.

For our purposes, conjugation between an Hfr donor cell and an F⁻ recipient cell has two key outcomes. First, the transfer of one or more donor alleles into the recipient chromosome by homologous recombination forms an exconjugant chromosome. Second, the F factor is not transferred in full during conjugation, and therefore the F⁻ recipient cell is not converted to a donor state (see Table 6.1).

Interrupted Mating and Time-of-Entry Mapping

We have noted that Hfr chromosomes are too long to be fully transferred from a donor cell to a recipient cell. As a consequence, **interrupted mating**, the cessation of conjugation caused by breakage of the conjugation pilus, takes place during naturally occurring conjugation. Interrupted matings stop conjugation before the Hfr chromosome can be completely transferred from the donor to the recipient. Several decades ago, researchers realized that if experimental conjugation was tested for gene transfer at timed intervals, it would be possible to map the order of donor genes, and to determine the distances between genes. This experimental strategy is called **time-of-entry mapping**.

Each Hfr strain used in time-of-entry mapping experiments will transfer genes in a specific order that is a characteristic of the strain. The *order* of gene transfer and the *time*, measured in minutes of conjugation time, to the first appearance of recombinants for each gene are functions of the gene's proximity to the origin of transfer (*oriT*). As a result, genes that are closest to the 5′ end of the T strand cross the conjugation pilus shortly after conjugation begins, whereas genes that are more distant from the 5′ end of the T strand will cross the conjugation pilus later in time. Genes closest to *oriT* are also more frequently transferred than are genes that are more distant from *oriT*. The result is that genes closest to *oriT* recombine into exconjugant chromosomes at earlier times and in greater numbers than genes distant from *oriT*. The number of minutes between the beginning of conjugation and the appearance of a particular recombinant is identified as the "time of entry" of the gene of interest. This measure can be used to determine the order of genes on the Hfr chromosome in a time-of-entry map.

Time-of-Entry Mapping Experiments

In 1956, Ellie Wollman, Francois Jacob, and William Hayes used conjugation data from the F⁻ strain P678 and the Hfr strain HfrH to demonstrate the utility of interrupted mating for time-of-entry mapping. In this experiment, P678 is str^R, resistant to the antibiotic streptomycin, and HfrH is str^S, streptomycin sensitive. The donor and recipient genotypes

Table 6.2	Genotypes of *E. coli* Strains F⁻ P678 and HfrH
HfrH	**F⁻ P678**
thr⁺ (prototrophic for threonine)	*thr⁻* (auxotrophic for threonine)
leu⁺ (prototrophic for leucine)	*leu⁻* (auxotrophic for leucine)
azi^R (resistant to sodium azide)	*azi^S* (susceptible to sodium azide)
tonA^R (resistant to phage T1 infection)	*tonA^S* (sensitive to phage T1 infection)
lac⁺ (able to utilize lactose)	*lac⁻* (unable to utilize lactose)
galB⁺ (able to utilize galactose)	*galB⁻* (unable to utilize galactose)

for six genes studied are given in **Table 6.2**. Two of these genes had known locations: the genes for threonine and leucine synthesis (*thr* and *leu*), which are closer to the origin of transfer in HfrH than any of the other genes tested. The goal of this experiment was to map the positions of *azi, tonA, lac,* and *galB* relative to *thr* and *leu* and to determine the distance between genes in minutes of conjugation.

The experiment begins by mixing donor and recipient bacterial strains to initiate conjugation. Every few minutes, a small sample of the culture is removed and agitated to break any conjugation pili, interrupt the mating, and stop the process of DNA transfer. The sample bacteria are then plated on growth plates containing different supplemental compounds in the medium to determine if exconjugants have formed by recombination between the recipient chromosome and homologous donated DNA. The first recombinant alleles in exconjugants are, as expected, *thr⁺* and *leu⁺*. The researchers select for these exconjugants by plating cells on a medium that lacks leucine and threonine but contains streptomycin and therefore will permit the growth of only *leu⁺ thr⁺ str^R* exconjugants. The order of the other four genes is determined using these *leu⁺ thr⁺ str^R* exconjugants.

Samples continue to be taken from the conjugation mixture every few minutes and plated on the selective medium that identifies those with the *leu⁺ thr⁺ str^R* genotype. Exconjugants with this genotype are then placed on a second plate to determine which other donor alleles have undergone recombination.

Figure 6.11a shows the results of this experiment, which are interpreted in **Figure 6.11b**: Exconjugants carrying the donor *azi* allele appear 8 minutes after conjugation begins, *tonA* recombinants appear at 10 minutes, *lac* recombinants appear at 16 minutes, and *galB* recombinants are the last to appear, at 25 minutes. The order of these four genes and the distances in minutes between them are combined to produce the time-of-entry genetic map for HfrH (Figure 6.8c). Genetic Analysis 6.1 guides you through time-of-entry mapping for an Hfr conjugation experiment.

PROBLEM An interrupted mating experiment is carried out in *E. coli* to map genes for biosynthesis of the amino acids threonine (*thr*), leucine (*leu*), glutamic acid (*glu*), and alanine (*ala*). An Hfr strain that is *his⁺ thr⁺ leu⁺ glu⁺ ala⁺ str^S* transfers *his* very early and is sensitive to the antibiotic streptomycin. It is mated to an F⁻ strain with the genotype *his⁻ thr⁻ leu⁻ glu⁻ ala⁻ str^R*. A time-of-entry profile for *thr*, *leu*, *glu*, and *ala* is shown at right.

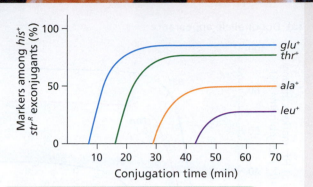

> **BREAK IT DOWN:** A time-of-entry map gives the order of genes on the donor chromosome based on their successive appearance in exconjugants. The gene closest to the origin of transfer appears first and is followed, in order, by additional genes (p. 198).

a. Exconjugants that are *his⁺* and *str^R* are initially selected for additional experimental analysis. What compounds must be present or absent in growth plates to allow exconjugants containing these selected markers to grow?

> **BREAK IT DOWN:** These initial exconjugants must be able to biosynthesize histidine and must be resistant to streptomycin. Genotypes for the other genes are not tested in initial screening, but they are tested in the time-of-entry experiment (p. 198).

b. Use the data provided to deduce the order of genes transferred in this Hfr strain and to identify the distances in minutes. Draw a map showing the order of genes on the donor chromosome and indicate the approximate location of the *his* gene.

> **BREAK IT DOWN:** See Research Technique 6.1 (pp. 189–190) for assistance determining bacterial growth on plates.

Solution Strategies	Solution Steps
Evaluate	
1. Determine the topic this problem addresses and the nature of the required answer.	1. The problem concerns conjugation between an Hfr donor and an F⁻ recipient. Answer (a) requires identification of growth medium constituents for a *his⁺*, *str^R* exconjugant; answer (b) requires a map of the donor genes based on their time of entry.
2. Identify the critical information given in the problem.	2. Donor and recipient genotypes are given. A time-of-entry profile identifies the minutes of conjugation needed to transfer each donor gene to the recipient.
Deduce	
3. Consider the significance of the very early transfer of *his⁺* in the context of developing a time-of-entry map.	3. Very early transfer of *his⁺* indicates the gene is close to *oriT* and for this reason is the first of the genes in the experiment to cross the conjugation tube.

> **TIP:** Genes that are closer to *oriT* have earlier and more frequent opportunities to transfer to the recipient and to appear as recombinants in exconjugants than do genes that are distant from *oriT*.

Solve

4. Identify the compounds needed to allow growth of exconjugants with the selected markers *his⁺* and *str^R*, irrespective of the genotypes for the other genes.

> **TIP:** To select exconjugants that are *his⁺* and *str^R*, growth plates must provide conditions in which only the exconjugants that are resistant to streptomycin and able to synthesize histidine can grow.

Answer a

4. The growth plate used to select these markers would contain streptomycin and the amino acids threonine, leucine, glutamic acid, and alanine. The plate would lack histidine, thus requiring the growing strain to be *his⁺*.

Answer b

5. Construct a time-of-entry map based on the conjugation data.

5. Given that *his* transfers first, and that gene order and distances are identified by the time at which recombinants appear in exconjugants, the Hfr map for this strain is as follows:

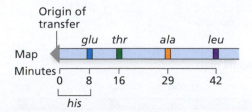

(a) Donor allele appearance

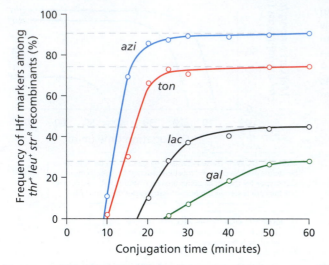

(b) Conjugation progression

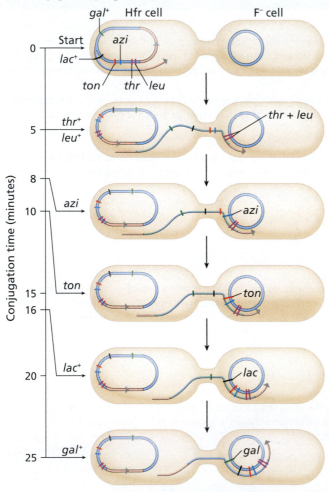

(c) Hfr chromosome map

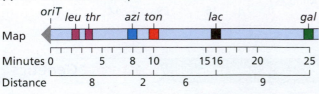

Figure 6.11 Time-of-entry mapping. (a) Recombinants are identified by screening exconjugants for donor allele acquisition at regular intervals and plotting their time of entry into the exconjugant chromosome. **(b)** Donor alleles *leu*+ and *thr*+ appear in exconjugants within 4 minutes of conjugation initiation. Other donor alleles follow according to their order on the chromosome. **(c)** The Hfr chromosome time-of-entry map is assembled from the recombinant data.

Consolidation of Hfr Maps

Time-of-entry mapping is an effective approach for mapping genes near the 5′ end of the T strand. However, the genetic mapping information obtainable from a single Hfr strain is limited. First, because the conjugation pilus is soon broken, causing mating to be interrupted, the likelihood of gene transfer drops off quickly with distance from *oriT*. Second, each Hfr strain can transfer genes in just one direction. On the other hand, different Hfr strains, having F factors integrated at different insertion sequences, have different orders of gene transfer. Furthermore, an F factor can be integrated into an Hfr chromosome in either of two orientations, creating the possibility that two Hfr strains will transfer the same genes but in *opposite* orders. In other words, one Hfr might transfer genes in the order A–B–C, and a different Hfr might transfer the same genes in the opposite order C–B–A. These two distinctive features of each Hfr strain—the starting point of gene transfer and the orientation of gene transfer—are used to join the information of multiple Hfr strains together to produce consolidated gene maps of entire bacterial chromosomes.

Using this method, more than 4300 genes were mapped in the genome of the model genetic organism *E. coli* before genomic sequencing became a reality. A simplified version of the time-of-entry map of the *E. coli* chromosome is shown in **Figure 6.12a**. The chromosome is measured as 100 minutes in length, the approximate length of time it would take to transfer the entire chromosome from a donor to a recipient.

With the advent of genomic sequencing, it became possible to identify every nucleotide base pair, and every gene, in a genome, and therefore to evaluate the accuracy and validity of Hfr mapping. **Figure 6.12b** compares a small segment of *E.coli* genomic sequence with the corresponding segment of the *E. coli* time-of-entry map. The comparison spans about 2.5 minutes of conjugation time, more than 160,000 base pairs of DNA, and dozens of genes, a few of which are shown. Comparison of the Hfr and genome sequence maps in the figure reveals exact correlation of gene placement and gene order for the genes the two maps have in common, attesting to the accuracy of Hfr mapping.

Let's practice consolidating time-of-entry maps into a larger map of a circular chromosome using the following data on gene transfer from four different Hfr strains. For each strain, the genes are listed in order of transfer. The first gene transferred is at the top and the last gene transferred is at the bottom, and the minutes of conjugation are given in parentheses for each gene. The genes mentioned in the following discussion are indicated with color.

Hfr Strain			
Hfr1	**Hfr2**	**Hfr3**	**Hfr4**
serR (2)	*nadB* (8)	*tyrT* (4)	*serR* (4)
leuY (10)	*proL* (17)	*fumC* (12)	*pheR* (12)
asnB (15)	*fumC* (29)	*proL* (24)	*cysE* (25)
serC (20)	*tyrT* (37)	*nadB* (33)	*leuU* (37)
tyrT (27)	*serC* (44)	*leuU* (46)	*nadB* (50)
fumC (35)	*asnB* (49)	*cysE* (58)	*proL* (59)

The data set from each Hfr strain is used to generate a partial map showing gene order, the distance in minutes between genes, and the orientation of the integrated F factor. The individual Hfr maps are then laid out so that the genes in the different maps align. We anticipate that the minutes of conjugation between a given pair of genes will be the same in each Hfr strain transferring the gene pair. For example, Hfr strains 1, 2, and 3 each transfer the gene pair *tyrT-fumC,* and in each strain those two genes are 8 minutes apart, no matter their orientation in the Hfr chromosome.

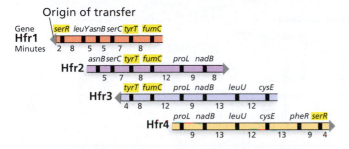

Next, the maps are arranged in partial concentric circles by overlapping the segments that have the same genes. Placing the maps one by one into such an arrangement will gradually reveal the organization of the circular *E. coli* chromosome of the donor strain. The Hfr gene map arrangement shown here indicates the location of each integrated fragment on the circular chromosome, its orientation, and the gene order and distances in minutes:

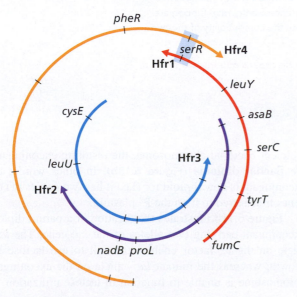

Continuation of this overlap process leads eventually to closure of the circle and completion of the chromosome map. In the table of Hfr strains, for example, notice that Hfr1 and Hfr4 share *serR* as the gene nearest the site of insertion. This is the connection that allows us to close the circular map. To begin construction of the circular map, we arbitrarily assumed that Hfr1 transfers genes in a clockwise direction, in other words, *serR* is first and, on that fragment, *fumC* is last.

Once completed, the consolidated Hfr map identifies gene order, the cumulative number of minutes, the site of each transferred fragment, and the orientation of each transferred fragment.

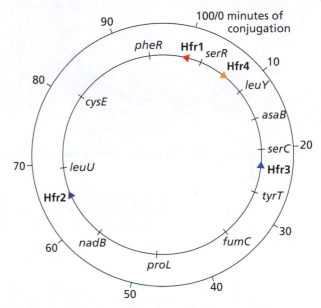

Conjugation with F′ Strains Produces Partial Diploids

Table 6.1 lists a third configuration of the F factor in donor bacteria, that of the so-called **F′ ("F prime") donor**, which contains a functional but altered F factor derived from imperfect excision of the F factor out of the Hfr chromosome. The integration event that creates an Hfr chromosome depends on interactions between matching IS elements of the F factor and of the bacterial chromosome, and when this process is reversed, the F factor can once again become an extrachromosomal F⁺ factor. Occasionally, however, the excision event is imprecise, and the excised F factor—in this case called an **F′ factor**—contains all of its own DNA plus a segment of bacterial chromosomal DNA from the region adjacent to the integration site (**Figure 6.13a**). An F′ factor can carry a variable length of bacterial DNA. Donor cells carrying an F′ factor are called **F′ cells**.

Like the other forms of conjugation described above, conjugation between an F′ donor and an F⁻ recipient follows the by-now-familiar process of cleavage of the T strand at *oriT* and movement of the T strand across the conjugation pilus with its 5′ end leading the way. DNA replication using the transferred strand takes place inside the recipient cell.

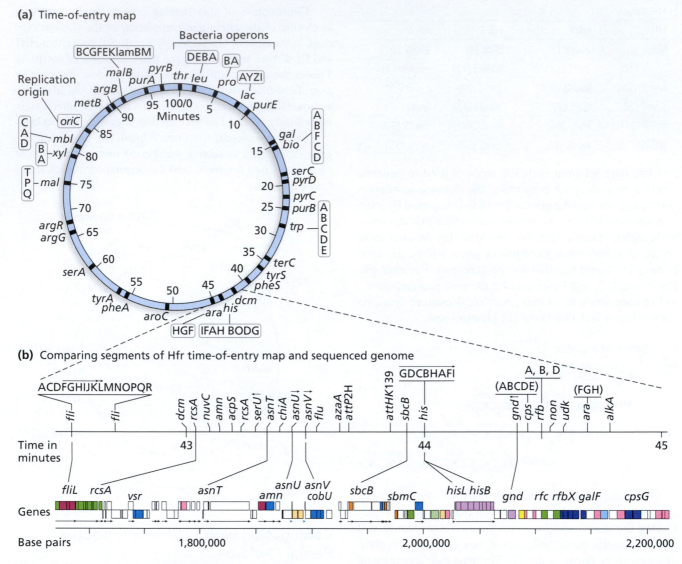

Figure 6.12 Consolidated Hfr map of *E. coli*. (a) The 100-minute genetic map of *E. coli*. Genes of bacterial operons (discussed in Section 12.2) are boxed. The origin of replication (*oriC*) is seen at 84 minutes. **(b)** A 2.5-minute segment (minutes 42.5–45) of the *E. coli* time-of-entry map in comparison with a segment of approximately 500,000 base pairs of the *E. coli* genome derived from *E. coli* genomic sequencing. Selected genes between 42.5 minutes and 45 minutes on the time-of-entry map (upper) are aligned with their positions in the genome sequence map (lower) to illustrate the compatibility of the two mapping approaches.

Q About how many nucleotide base pairs are there in a DNA segment that spans one minute of conjugation time?

If the entire F′ chromosome is transferred, both parts of *oriT* are transferred, allowing the F′ factor to circularize in the recipient cell. At the completion of F′ factor transfer in such cases, the exconjugant cell, now containing a complete F′ factor, is converted to an F′ donor (see Table 6.1). In this process the exconjugant has also acquired copies of the donor chromosomal genes carried on the F′ factor. Because the newly received chromosomal genes are homologs of genes already present on the recipient bacterial chromosome, the resulting exconjugants are **partial diploids** (**Figure 6.13b**). In other words, the exconjugant is now diploid for (i.e., it has two copies of) the genes transferred to it on the F′ plasmid.

Figure 6.11b illustrates the creation of a partial diploid exconjugant carrying two alleles of the *lac* gene. The *lac*+ allele on the F′ factor enables the cell to use lactose for growth, whereas the mutant *lac*− allele on the exconjugant chromosome is unable to function in lactose utilization. In

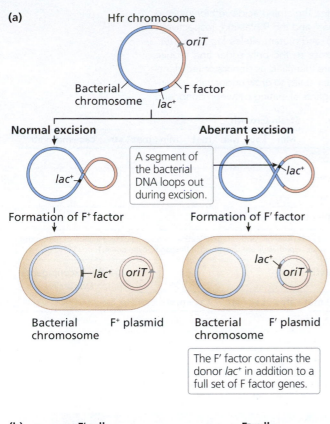

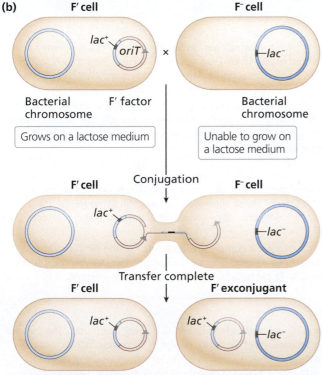

The exconjugant is a *lac⁺/lac⁻* partial diploid and has acquired the ability to grow on a lactose medium. Because F′ plasmid transfer was complete, the exconjugant can act as an F′ donor.

Figure 6.13 F factor excision from Hfr integration. (a) Normal excision (left) restores an Hfr to an F⁺, whereas aberrant excision (right) forms an F′ plasmid in an F′ donor cell. **(b)** F′ × F⁻ conjugation produces an exconjugant that is a partial diploid *lac⁺/lac⁻*.

this partial diploid, the *lac⁺* allele is dominant over the *lac⁻* allele. Partial diploids of this type have been used in genetic studies to examine the mode of action of genes in bacteria and to dissect the regulation of coordinated gene action in bacterial metabolism and growth (see Section 12.3).

Genetic Analysis 6.2 guides you through an analysis of donor and recipient bacterial strains and the identification of donor types through the analysis of three conjugation experiments.

Plasmids and Conjugation in Archaea

Research on archaea species is still in its infancy in comparison with the many decades of research that exist on bacteria. Despite this short research history, a number of significant observations have been made with regard to archaeal plasmids and conjugation among archaeal cells.

Like bacteria, archaea are single-celled haploid organisms, usually with a single chromosome and various plasmids. All of the genes that are essential for the normal metabolic and physiologic activities of the cell are carried on the archaeal chromosome. Ongoing research on archaea plasmids that began in the early 1990s has identified dozens of different plasmids among archaeal species. Although much more study is needed, the information available at present indicates that most archaeal plasmids replicate by rolling circle replication. The data further identify numerous instances of plasmid-driven conjugation between archaeal donor and recipient cells. The genetic composition of archaeal conjugative plasmids has not been well characterized, nor is there enough information to be able to describe the details of the archaeal conjugation apparatus. To date there is evidence of some similarities to bacterial conjugation, but there is also evidence that some aspects of archaeal conjugation may be substantially different from bacterial conjugation.

6.3 Bacterial Transformation Produces Genetic Recombination

Transformation occurs when a recipient cell takes up a fragment of donor cell DNA from the surrounding growth medium. The DNA fragment passes through the wall and membrane of the recipient cell and is incorporated into the recipient cell chromosome by homologous recombination. A recipient cell that is able to take up transforming DNA is described as "competent."

Transformation is a naturally occurring mechanism that can be used to produce accurate maps of bacterial genes, including those that are closely linked and not readily mapped by conjugation experiments. Transformation is also used as a laboratory technique by molecular biologists seeking to introduce DNA into microbial cells, plant cells, or animal cells as part of the process of creating recombinant DNA or transgenic organisms (see Sections 15.1 and 15.2).

PROBLEM In *E. coli*, the abilities to utilize the sugar lactose, synthesize the amino acid methionine, and resist the antibiotic streptomycin are conferred by alleles *lac*⁺ and *met*⁺ and the R plasmid, respectively. Bacteria without the R plasmid are susceptible to streptomycin (*str*ˢ), and mutant alleles *lac*⁻ and *met*⁻ produce bacteria that are unable to grow on media containing lactose as the only sugar and require methionine supplementation for growth, respectively. *E. coli* strains are identified as donors or recipients in the first table presented here, which also contains information on their ability to grow under various conditions. The second table contains growth information for the exconjugants of mating between donor and recipient strains. In each table, "+" indicates growth and "−" indicates no growth. "Min" signifies a minimal medium, and supplemented minimal medium plates are indicated by, for example, "Min+met" (minimal medium plus methionine). "Lac" indicates a plate containing only lactose as the sugar.

Strain	Type	Strain Growth				
		Min	Lac	Min+met	Min+met+str	Lac+met+str
A	Donor	+	+	+	−	−
B	Donor	+	+	+	−	−
C	Donor	+	+	+	−	−
D	Recipient	−	−	+	+	−

a. Use the growth information in the first table to determine the genotype of each strain at the *lac* and *met* genes and for resistance or susceptibility to streptomycin.

> **BREAK IT DOWN:** Anabolic and catabolic pathways and the determination of genotypes for alleles in these pathways are described in Research Technique 6.1, pp. 189–190.

b. Use the growth information in the second table to determine the genotypes of exconjugants produced by each mating.

c. Compare the genotypes and mating behavior of donors, recipient, and exconjugants to determine whether each donor is F⁺, Hfr, or F'. Explain your rationale for each donor identification.

Mating	Exconjugant Growth				Are the Exconjugants Donors?
	Min+str	Min+met+str	Lac+str	Lac+met+str	
A × D	+	A × D	−	−	Yes
B × D	A × D	+	−	−	Yes
C × D	−	+	−	+	No

> **BREAK IT DOWN:** Table 6.1, p. 196, summarizes the potential conversion of and bacterial gene transfer to exconjugants by donors.

Solution Strategies	Solution Steps

Evaluate

1. Identify the topic this problem addresses and the nature of the required answer.

1. This is a conjugation problem in which genotypes of donors and a recipient are determined by growth characteristics. Donor types (F⁺, Hfr, F') are to be identified by growth characteristics of exconjugants. The answers require identifying genotypes for *lac, met,* and *str* for the recipient and each donor and exconjugant.

2. Identify the critical information given in the problem.

2. The two tables identify growth characteristics. The first table contains growth information on three donors (A, B, and C) and a recipient (D). The second table contains growth information on the exconjugants of mating between each donor and the recipient.

Deduce

3. Compare the growth characteristics of donors and the recipient in the first table, and deduce which genotypes are likely the same.

3. The growth characteristics of the three donor strains (A, B, and C) are identical on each kind of medium. These three strains have the same genotype. The recipient, strain D, has a different set of growth characteristics and therefore a different genotype.

4. Examine the exconjugants in the second table and determine which have been converted from recipients to donors.

4. Donor A and donor B transfer a complete F sequence to the recipient and convert the exconjugant to a donor. Donor C does not transfer the complete F sequence, so the C × D exconjugant is not converted to a donor.

> **TIP:** When an exconjugant has been converted to a donor state, we know it has received a complete copy of the F factor.

Solve

Answer a

5. Determine the genotypes of the donor and recipient strains from growth information in the first table.

5. The genotype shared by donor strains A, B, and C is *met*⁺ *lac*⁺ *str*ˢ. The minimal medium contains glucose. Growth of donor strains in this medium indicates their prototrophy for methionine (*met*⁺). Growth in the lactose–containing medium indicates they are *lac*⁺. The inability of donors to grow in media containing streptomycin indicates they are *str*ˢ.

The recipient genotype is *met*⁻ *lac*⁻ *str*ᴿ. It is unable to grow on the minimal (glucose-containing) medium, but it can grow on glucose plus methionine, indicating it is *met*⁻. It also grows on the minimal medium plus methionine and streptomycin, indicating that it is *str*ᴿ. Lactose utilization is tested on the medium containing lactose plus methionine and streptomycin. Here it fails to grow, indicating it is *lac*⁻.

6. Determine the genotypes of exconjugants from growth information in the second table.

TIP: Compare the genotypes of exconjugants to the recipient genotype to determine if one or more donor alleles have been transferred during conjugation. Use Table 6.1 for help in categorizing each donor.

7. Identify each donor by donor type and explain the rationale for each identification.

Answer b

6. Using analysis similar to that employed above, we conclude that the exconjugant genotypes are

A × D met^+ lac^- str^R, conversion to donor

B × D met^- lac^- str^R, conversion to donor

C × D met^- lac^+ str^R, no conversion

Answer c

7. A × D exconjugants have acquired met^+ and have undergone conversion to a donor state. F′ donors can transfer an allele and convert the recipient, so we conclude that strain A is an F′ donor. Exconjugants of the B × D mating retain the recipient genotype, but they are converted to a donor state. F⁺ donors produce this result, so strain B is an F⁺ donor. The C × D conjugation produces exconjugants that have acquired lac^+ but have not undergone conversion. This is a characteristic of Hfr donors, so we conclude that strain C is Hfr.

For more practice, see Problems 19 and 23.   Visit the Study Area to access study tools. **Mastering** Genetics

Steps in Transformation

Transformation is a four-step process, as illustrated in **Figure 6.14**. It is preceded by the **lysis**, or breakage, of a donor cell and the release of fragmented DNA from the donor chromosome. The transforming DNA is double-stranded and can be taken up by a competent recipient bacterial cell.

The passage of double-stranded transforming DNA across the recipient cell wall and cell membrane is accompanied by degradation of one of the strands (step ❶). The remaining strand of transforming DNA aligns with, or "invades," a complementary region of the recipient chromosome ❷. The alignment triggers the action of several enzymes that excise one strand of the recipient chromosome and replace it with the transforming strand. This recombination event forms heteroduplex DNA: One strand is derived from the recipient cell, and the approximately complementary transforming strand is derived from the bacterial donor ❸. After the subsequent DNA replication and cell-division cycle ❹, one daughter cell is a transformed cell, also called the **transformant**. It contains a chromosome carrying the transforming strand and its newly synthesized complementary strand. The other daughter cell retains the recipient chromosome and is not genetically altered.

Mapping by Transformation

Transforming DNA is usually shorter than about 100,000 bp (100 kb) in length. For a bacterial species like *E. coli*, which has a genome of 4×10^6 bp of DNA and approximately 5000 genes, the transforming DNA may have 1, 2, or as many as 50 genes. This means that even at maximum lengths, transforming DNA from the donor cell represents only 1 to 2% of the total genome of the recipient cell. Consequently, transformation is useful for mapping genes that are closely linked. In mapping by transformation,

geneticists look for two or more genes that are transferred into the recipient on the same fragment of transforming DNA. Thus, genetic analysis focuses on **cotransformation**, the simultaneous transformation of two or more genes. For cotransformation to occur, the crossover events must incorporate closely linked genes on a single fragment of transforming DNA.

6.4 Bacterial Transduction Is Mediated by Bacteriophages

In *transduction*, the transfer of genetic material from a donor bacterial cell to a recipient cell occurs by means of a bacteriophage (bacterial virus) acting as a vector to carry donor DNA to the recipient cell. A **transductant** is formed when the donated DNA is integrated into the recipient cell's chromosome by homologous recombination.

In this section, we review the life cycles of bacteriophages (*phages,* for short) that infect *E. coli*. We then consider *cotransduction mapping*—a powerful technique for mapping bacterial genomes—and the role of *generalized transduction* in this process. We conclude the section with a discussion of *specialized transduction*.

Bacteriophage Life Cycles

Bacteriophages are tiny viral particles that infect bacterial host cells. The bacteriophage has an outer proteinaceous structure consisting of an icosahedral head, a hollow protein sheath, and in some phages, a set of appendages called tail fibers (**Figure 6.15**). The phage's head houses its tiny genome, composed of a single DNA molecule ranging in size from about 5000 to 100,000 base pairs. The replication of phage DNA, the transcription of phage genes, and the translation that produces phage proteins are dependent on

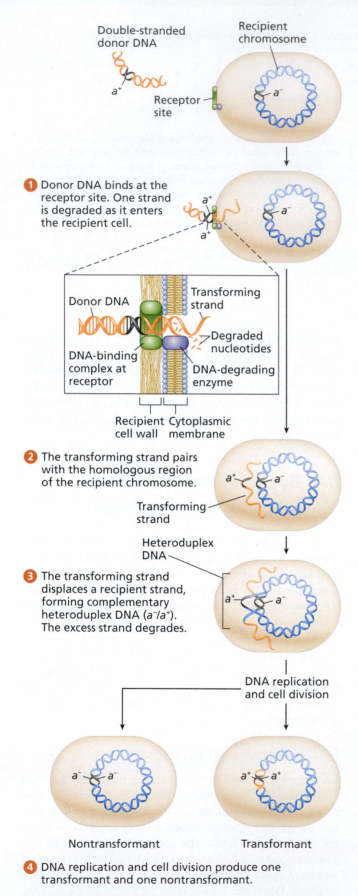

① Donor DNA binds at the receptor site. One strand is degraded as it enters the recipient cell.

Donor DNA

DNA-binding complex at receptor

Transforming strand

Degraded nucleotides

DNA-degrading enzyme

Recipient cell wall

Cytoplasmic membrane

② The transforming strand pairs with the homologous region of the recipient chromosome.

Transforming strand

Heteroduplex DNA

③ The transforming strand displaces a recipient strand, forming complementary heteroduplex DNA (a^-/a^+). The excess strand degrades.

DNA replication and cell division

Nontransformant

Transformant

④ DNA replication and cell division produce one transformant and one nontransformant.

Figure 6.14 **Transformation of a competent bacterium (a^-) by donor DNA (a^+).**

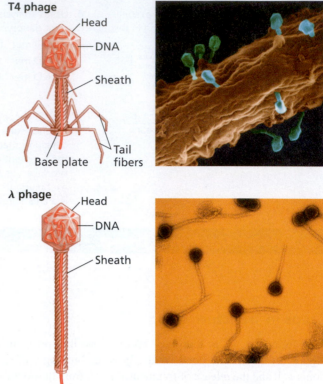

Figure 6.15 **T4 bacteriophage and λ phage structures.** Bacteriophages consist of a proteinaceous head filled with DNA, a sheath, and, in some phages, tail fibers.

Ⓠ Bacteriophages, like other viruses, cannot replicate autonomously, do not have an energy metabolism, and produce no waste products. They can only reproduce and express their genetic content by invading host cells and using numerous host proteins and other host compounds and components. Most biologists classify viruses as nonliving acellular particles. Do you agree or disagree?

numerous enzymes and other compounds found in the host bacterial cells, as bacteriophages are incapable of autonomous DNA replication, transcription, and translation.

Bacteriophages employ a variety of mechanisms to attack bacteria. By whatever specific mechanism they may use, however, bacteriophages actively seek out and attach to host cells, commencing a six-step process called the **lytic cycle**, in which infection by a bacteriophage leads to the lysis (rupture) of the host cell and the release of up to 200 new progeny phage particles. The steps composing the lytic cycle are depicted in **Figure 6.16**.

❶ Attachment of the phage particle to the host cell.

❷ Injection of the phage chromosome into the host cell. Injection is quickly followed by circularization of the phage chromosome, to protect it from enzymatic degradation.

❸ Replication of phage DNA, using numerous host enzymes and other proteins. A copy of the phage chromosome is required for each of the eventual

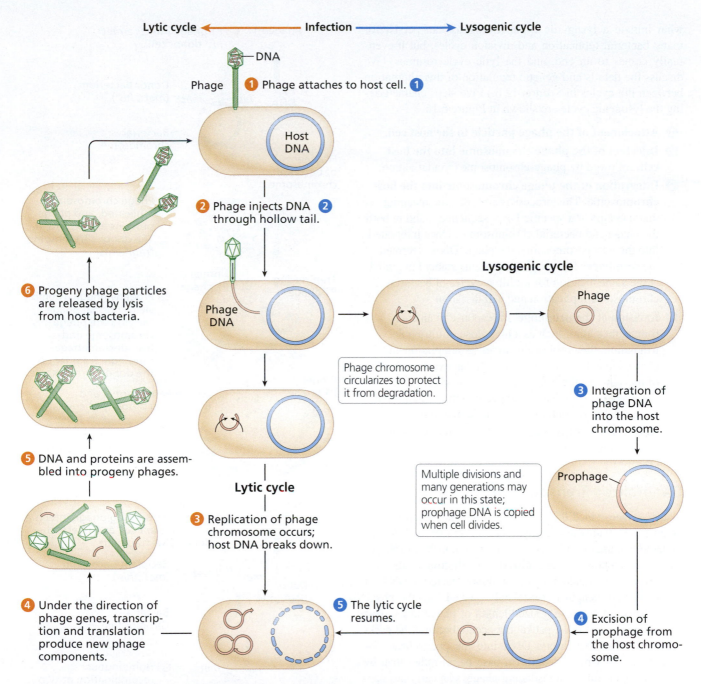

Figure 6.16   The lytic and lysogenic life cycles of a temperate bacteriophage. The lytic cycle progresses directly from infection through phage reproduction to lysis. The lysogenic cycle features the integration of the phage into the host chromosome, where it resides until excision and resumption of the lytic cycle.

progeny phage particles, which generally number between 50 and 200.

❹ **Transcription and translation of phage genes,** using numerous host enzymes, other proteins, and ribosomes. Heads, sheaths, and tail fibers for all progeny particles must be synthesized and assembled.

❺ **Packaging of phage chromosomes into phage heads.** This step is commonly accompanied by fragmentation of the host chromosome. Occasional mispackaging of

a fragment of the host chromosome into a phage head can follow chromosome fragmentation.

❻ **Lysis of the host cell,** resulting in the death of the host and the release of progeny phage particles.

Bacteriophages called **temperate phages** are capable of a temporary alternative life cycle that leads to the temporary integration of the phage chromosome into the bacterial host chromosome. The integration process is termed **lysogeny**. Environmental and growth conditions are largely what initiate a **lysogenic cycle**. Lysogeny can persist for many bacterial replication and division cycles, but it eventually comes to an end, and the lytic cycle resumes. (We discuss the details and genetic regulation of this alternation between life cycles in Section 12.6.) Five steps characterizing the lysogenic cycle are shown in Figure 6.16.

1. **Attachment of the phage particle to the host cell.**
2. **Injection of the phage chromosome into the host cell,** followed by phage-chromosome circularization.
3. **Integration of the phage chromosome into the host chromosome.** This process is site specific, meaning that it occurs at a specific DNA sequence found in both the phage and bacterial chromosomes. Once integrated into the host chromosome, the phage DNA is termed the **prophage**. The prophage remains stably integrated at the same location for multiple cycles of bacterial chromosome replication and cell division.
4. **Excision of the prophage.** In response to an environmental signal, such as a high dose of ultraviolet irradiation, the prophage reverses its integration and is excised intact. This event is usually an exact reversal of the site-specific integration, but rare mistakes in prophage excision lead to a specific kind of abnormal phage that may contain host genetic material.
5. **Resumption of the lytic cycle,** beginning with phage-chromosome replication.

Generalized Transduction

In the decades since the 1952 discovery and description of **generalized transduction** by Norman Zinder and Joshua Lederberg, numerous kinds of generalized transducing phages have been identified. **Generalized transducing phages** are formed when a random piece of donor bacterial DNA of the appropriate length is mistakenly packed into the phage head instead of a similarly sized length of phage DNA. This occasional error in DNA packaging occurs because the packing mechanism that inserts DNA into the phage head discriminates DNA by its length (in base pairs) rather than by sequence. Generalized transducing phages can carry any segment of donor DNA, since the process of mistaken packaging is random.

The phage P1 is a well-studied bacteriophage that infects *E. coli* and is a prolific producer of generalized transducing phages. This phage was initially chosen for intensive study of its transduction ability because it has a large genome of nearly 100,000 bp (100 kb). To produce progeny that are generalized transducing phages, P1 must capture segments of donor bacterial DNA that are almost exactly 100 kb, a length that is about 2% of the *E. coli* chromosome. Analysis of P1 infections tells us that about 1 in 50 progeny of a P1 infection are generalized transducing phages.

Figure 6.17 illustrates generalized transduction in seven steps (combining attachment and injection into a single first step). The outcome of transduction, as noted at the start

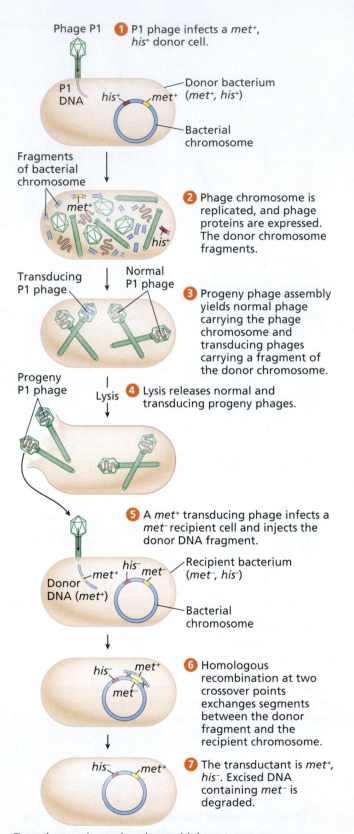

Phage P1 ① P1 phage infects a *met⁺*, *his⁺* donor cell.

P1 DNA

his⁺ *met⁺* Donor bacterium (*met⁺*, *his⁺*)

Bacterial chromosome

Fragments of bacterial chromosome

met⁺

② Phage chromosome is replicated, and phage proteins are expressed. The donor chromosome fragments.

his⁺

Transducing P1 phage Normal P1 phage

③ Progeny phage assembly yields normal phage carrying the phage chromosome and transducing phages carrying a fragment of the donor chromosome.

Progeny P1 phage Lysis ④ Lysis releases normal and transducing progeny phages.

⑤ A *met⁺* transducing phage infects a *met⁻* recipient cell and injects the donor DNA fragment.

Donor DNA (*met⁺*) *met⁺* *his⁻* *met⁻* Recipient bacterium (*met⁻*, *his⁻*)

Bacterial chromosome

his⁻ *met⁺* ⑥ Homologous recombination at two crossover points exchanges segments between the donor fragment and the recipient chromosome.

met⁻

his⁻ *met⁺* ⑦ The transductant is *met⁺*, *his⁻*. Excised DNA containing *met⁻* is degraded.

Transductant bacterium (*met⁺*, *his⁻*)

Figure 6.17 An example of transduction by P1 phage. Transducing phages are generated by the mistaken packaging of a fragment of the donor bacterium's DNA into a phage head. Transductant bacteria are produced by homologous recombination between the introduced fragment of donor DNA and the recipient bacterial chromosome.

of this section, is the production of a *transductant*, a bacterium that has acquired one or more donor genes through transduction:

❶ A normal P1 phage attaches to a donor bacterial cell and injects its chromosome into the cell.

❷ Replication of the phage chromosome is followed by transcription and translation to produce phage proteins. Fragmentation of the bacterial chromosome precedes the packaging of phage chromosomes into phage heads.

❸ Assembly of progeny phages, including packing of phage heads, is largely normal, but a few progeny phages receive a random fragment of the donor bacterial chromosome that is approximately the same length as the phage chromosome. These abnormal progeny phages are *generalized transducing phages*.

❹ Host-cell lysis releases normal and generalized transducing phages.

❺ Generalized transducing phages attach to new recipient cells and inject the fragment of donor DNA.

❻ In each recipient cell, homologous recombination occurs between the fragment of donor DNA and the recipient chromosome. Pairs of crossover events are required to splice the donor fragment into the recipient chromosome and excise a homologous segment of the chromosome. The excised chromosome fragment is degraded by enzymes.

❼ A stable transductant strain results.

Cotransduction

The donor cell in the transduction experiment shown in Figure 6.17 has the genotype $met^+ his^+$, and the recipient is $met^- his^-$. The bacterial culture in which this experiment takes place will contain millions of bacteria, most of which are not transduced. In addition, many cells may be transduced with donor alleles that are not tested for in the experiment. The transductants detected in this particular experiment are those in which either the met^+ or his^+ allele or both are transduced.

Transductants having either the genotype $met^+ his^-$ or the genotype $met^- his^+$ offer evidence that each allele can be individually transduced. In addition, a certain number of transductants will undergo simultaneous transduction of both genes to produce $met^+ his^+$ transductants. These cells have undergone **cotransduction** of both donor alleles. The frequency of cotransduction, called **cotransduction frequency**, depends on how close the two genes are to one another on the donor chromosome. The closer the genes are, the higher the probability of cotransduction (thus, the higher the cotransduction frequency), and the farther apart the genes are, the lower the cotransduction probability. If, for example, an experimenter carried out the transduction cross in Figure 6.17 and identified 200 transductants for met^+, the experimenter could determine the frequency of cotransduction by then identifying how many of those met^+ transductants were also transduced (i.e., were cotransduced)

for his^+. If the analysis determined that 28 of the 200 met^+ transductants were also transduced for his^+, the cotransduction frequency for those genes would be 14% $\left(\frac{28}{200}\right)$.

To succeed in finding cotransductants in an experiment, researchers may have to genotype large numbers of colonies. To reduce the number of colonies that must be genotyped in such experiments, a two-step strategy is used that first identifies cells transduced with one donor allele and then screens those transductants for the acquisition of additional donor alleles. The first step employs a **selected marker screen**, or selection, to identify transductants for one of the donor alleles of interest. Transductants that are selected are then screened a second time, for a second donor allele, in an **unselected marker screen**. The goal is to determine the percentage of transductants for the selected marker that are also transduced for the unselected marker, while reducing unnecessary colony genotyping.

Cotransduction Mapping

Genetic map construction in bacteria uses cotransduction frequencies to determine the relative order of three or more genes. **Cotransduction mapping** makes use of the fact, described above, that the frequency of cotransduction is greater for genes that are close together and is lower for genes that are farther apart. Any two genes on the donor chromosome have two chances to be separated by a chromosomal event. The first separation chance comes when the donor chromosome is broken into fragments. Genes that are close together are more likely to end up on the same donor chromosome fragment than genes that are far apart. The second chance for separation comes during homologous recombination, when genes that are close together on the donor fragment are less likely to be separated by a crossover event than genes that are far apart on the fragment.

Let's look at two studies that test the order of the same four genes in *E. coli*. **Figure 6.18** provides cotransduction

(a) Cotransduction frequencies

Donor genotype	Recipient genotype	Selected marker	Unselected marker	Percent cotransduction of unselected marker with cys^+
$cys^+ trpE^+$	$cys^- trpE^-$	cys^+	$trpE^+$	63
$cys^+ trpC^+$	$cys^- trpC^-$	cys^+	$trpC^+$	53
$cys^+ trpB^+$	$cys^- trpB^-$	cys^+	$trpB^+$	47
$cys^+ trpA^+$	$cys^- trpA^-$	cys^+	$trpA^+$	46

(b) *trp* operon map

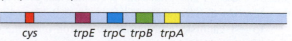

cys   trpE trpC trpB trpA

Figure 6.18 Yanofsky's cotransduction frequency analysis and mapping of *trp* operon genes in *E. coli*. (a) Cotransduction frequencies of cys^+ and a gene of the *trp* operon are determined in separate selected marker–unselected marker experiments. **(b)** Yanofsky's proposed map of the *trp* operon.

data for experiments performed in 1959 by Charles Yanofsky on genes that are part of the *tryptophan operon*, a cluster of genes involved in the synthesis of the amino acid tryptophan that share a single promoter. (We discuss this operon in detail in Section 12.2). For the current discussion, you only need to know that genes in an operon are transcribed under the control of a single promoter and are much closer to one another than genes that have their own promoters.

Yanofsky used the selected–unselected marker approach to determine cotransduction frequencies for each of four genes in the tryptophan operon (*trpA, trpB, trpC,* and *trpE*) and a gene outside the operon, *cys*. Yanofsky performed four crosses, each with a donor strain that was *cys*⁺ and also prototrophic for one *trp* gene. His recipient strains were each *cys*⁻ and also auxotrophic for the *trp* gene being tested. At the time he began his experiments, Yanofsky knew that *cys* lies outside the tryptophan operon, and he constructed his experiments to measure the cotransduction frequency between *cys* and the *trp* gene of interest. In each experiment, *cys*⁺ was the selected marker used to identify informative transductants. The unselected marker was the *trp* allele from the donor. Yanofsky acquired data to determine the cotransduction frequency of *cys*⁺ and the unselected *trp* marker.

In his first experiment for the first study, he determined that among *cys*⁺ transductants, 63% are cotransduced for *trpE*⁺. In his second experiment, he found 53% cotransduction between *cys*⁺ and *trpC*⁺. Yanofsky concluded that *trpE* is closer to *cys* than is *trpC* based on the higher cotransduction frequencies for *cys* and *trpE* than for *cys* and *trpC*. Cotransduction frequencies for *cys* and *trpB* and for *cys* and *trpA* are not sufficiently different to determine gene order, but based on cotransduction frequencies, *trpA* and *trpB* are each more distant from *cys* than are *trpE* and *trpC*. Yanofsky proposed a genetic map of the tryptophan operon with the order *cys-trpE-trpC-trpB-trpA*.

The second study was conducted to test the order of these genes and either corroborate or refute Yanofsky's proposed gene map. In this study the donor bacterial genotype is *cys*⁺ *trpC*⁻ *trpB*⁻, and the recipient genotype is *cys*⁻ *trpC*⁺ *trpB*⁺. Transductants are selected for *cys*⁺ transduction, and the transductants are then screened to determine their genotypes for *trpC* and *trpB*. The genotypes of 302 *cys*⁺ transductants are shown in **Table 6.3**. Cotransductants for the donor *cys* and *trpC* alleles have the genotype *cys*⁺ *trpC*⁻ and are found in Class 1, which has 139 cotransductants, and Class 2, which has 18. The *cys–trpC* cotransduction frequency is therefore $\frac{139}{302} + \frac{18}{302} = 0.52$, or 52%. Similarly, cotransduction of *cys* and *trpB* is identified by the genotype *cys*⁺ *trpB*⁻. Transductant Classes 1 and 4 have this cotransductant genotype, and the cotransduction frequency is $\frac{139}{302} + \frac{4}{302} = 0.47$, or 47%.

To test Yanofsky's proposed *trp* operon map, the crossover events required to produce each cotransductant class were identified. **Figure 6.19** illustrates the locations of four crossover points at which different combinations of crossovers would produce each cotransductant class. Transductants acquiring *cys*⁺ must undergo crossover at point 1 plus at least

Table 6.3	Test of Yanofsky's Proposed *trp* Operon Gene Order	
Transductant Class	Transductant Genotype	Number
1	*cys*⁺ *trpC*⁻ *trpB*⁻	139
2	*cys*⁺ *trpC*⁻ *trpB*⁺	18
3	*cys*⁺ *trpC*⁺ *trpB*⁺	141
4	*cys*⁺ *trpC*⁺ *trpB*⁻	4
TOTAL		302

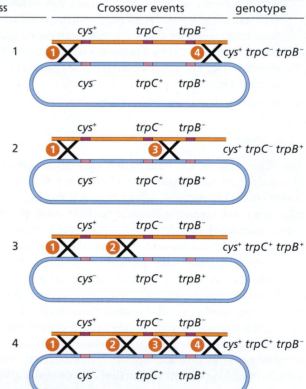

Figure 6.19   A test of Yanofsky's proposed *trp* operon gene map. The approximate locations of possible crossovers are numbered 1 through 4. For each cotransductant genotype, the required crossover sites are identified.

one additional point. The precise location of crossover point 1 can vary over a large expanse of the chromosome to the left of *cys*. The second crossover point must occur to the right of *cys* in any of three locations: at location 2, within a relatively large distance between *cys,* which is outside the operon, and *trpC* within the operon; at point 3, a very small space in the operon between *trpC* and *trpB*; or at point 4, a large region to the right of *trpB*. Three different double-crossover combinations generate transductant Classes 1, 2, and 3, respectively, and transductant Class 4 is produced by a quadruple recombination requiring crossover at all four points. The quadruple crossover is expected to be the least frequent of the combinations producing cotransductants. This study verifies Yanofsky's proposed *trp* operon map for two reasons. First, cotransduction frequencies for *cys–trpC* and for *cys–trpB* are almost identical in the two studies (53% versus 52% for *cys–trpC,* and 46% versus 47% for *cys–trpB*), placing *trpC* closest to *cys* in both. Second, the quadruple recombination event is expected to occur less frequently than any of the double crossover events.

Genetic Analysis 6.3 guides you through an analysis of a transduction to determine gene order in a donor strain.

Specialized Transduction

As described above, temperate bacteriophages have the ability to lysogenize their host by integrating into the host chromosome to create a prophage. The site of integration is a DNA sequence called the ***att*** **site** (for "attachment") that is identical in the bacterial chromosome and the phage chromosome. The shared 15-bp sequences are called *attP* in temperate bacteriophage (the *P* stands for phage) and *attB* (*B* for bacteria) in its host *E.coli* bacterium. There is just one *att* site in each bacterial genome possessing one. A specialized phage enzyme recognizes the *att* sites and makes a staggered cut there. The complementary single-stranded ends of cleaved *att* DNA reanneal as the prophage integrates, to create an *att* sequence at each end of the integrated prophage.

Because the *attB* and *attP* sequences are identical, the excision of a prophage is almost always the exact reversal of prophage integration. Occasionally, however, excision is inaccurate: Aberrant excision removes much of the integrated prophage but along with it a small segment of the transductant chromosome that is immediately adjacent to the *att* site of integration. Aberrant excision of a prophage forms what is called a **specialized transducing phage** because the chromosomal material of the transductant that is removed in error is limited to regions immediately to the right or immediately to the left of the *att* site. Thus, rather than transductants carrying random pieces of donor DNA, as in generalized transduction, specialized transductants can only carry donor DNA located immediately around the *att* site.

6.5 Bacteriophage Chromosomes Are Mapped by Fine-Structure Analysis

Before DNA was identified as the hereditary material, many biologists regarded genes as indivisible units of heredity that could not be subdivided by recombination. This idea derives

from Mendel's original description of "particulate inheritance" of traits. Before knowing the molecular structure of DNA, biologists had difficulty describing how recombination within a gene could occur. Geneticists knew that different mutations could affect a single gene, and had data showing that different mutations can occupy unique locations within a gene. But what remained lacking was a refined understanding of the internal structure, or fine structure, of genes.

Beginning in the early 1950s, Seymour Benzer helped define how biologists view the structure of genes with a series of experiments that revealed the existence of a **genetic fine structure**, a phrase referring to the composition of genes at the level of their molecular building blocks. Benzer demonstrated that the building blocks of genes (later determined to be DNA nucleotide base pairs) were responsible for both mutation and recombination. The publication of his principal conclusions coincided with the identification of the molecular structure of DNA. When the functional subunits of DNA were revealed to be nucleotides, it was impossible to miss the connection between them and Benzer's fine structure.

Benzer focused on two questions. First, was the gene the fundamental unit of mutation, or could components of genes be mutated? Second, was recombination a process occurring only between genes, or did recombination also occur between the components of genes? Benzer studied these questions using the *rII* region of the T4 bacteriophage. Genes in the *rII* region determine whether and how the phage will lyse its *E. coli* host.

Lysis is examined using a bacterial lawn, a solid coating of bacteria on the surface of a growth medium. If the growing bacteria are exposed to a bacteriophage, infected cells lyse and progeny phages are released. Progeny phages infect new host cells, and as the infection-lysis-infection cycle continues, a bacteria-free spot called a plaque—a hole in the bacterial lawn—appears on the growth medium.

Benzer showed that two genes, *rIIA* and *rIIB*, control the ability of T4 phages to lyse *E. coli* host cells. Those T4 phages carrying wild-type copies of *rIIA* and *rIIB* lyse multiple strains of *E. coli,* leading to the production of small plaques (**Figure 6.20**). On the other hand, phages with

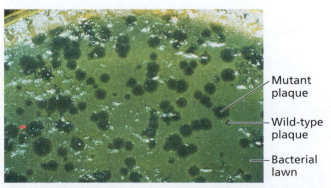

Mutant plaque

Wild-type plaque

Bacterial lawn

Figure 6.20 **Plaque formation by *rII* wild types and mutants.** On a bacterial lawn of *E. coli* B strain, small, circular wild-type plaques are formed by T4 phages with a wild-type *rII* region. Large, irregular mutant plaques are formed by T4 phages with *rII* mutations.

PROBLEM In *E. coli*, *thr⁺* and *leu⁺* are prototrophic alleles that control synthesis of the amino acids threonine and leucine. The auxotrophic alleles are defective in their ability to synthesize these amino acids. Bacteria carrying the *aziᴿ* allele are resistant to the effects of the compound azide that inhibits protein transport, and those carrying *aziˢ* are susceptible to the inhibitory effects of azide. *E. coli* with the genotype *thr⁺ leu⁺ aziᴿ* are infected with the P1 phage. Progeny phages are collected and used to infect bacteria with the genotype *thr⁻ leu⁻ aziˢ*, and the cells are then placed on media selective for one or two of the donor markers in a transduction experiment. The table identifies the selected markers and gives the frequency of cotransduction of unselected

> **BREAK IT DOWN:** Carefully note the genotypes of the donor and recipient strains and remember that transductant genotypes are the former recipient genotypes that have acquired one or more donor genes (p. 209).

Experiment	Selected Marker(s)	Unselected Marker(s)
1	*leu⁺*	*aziᴿ* = 50%, *thr⁺* = 4%
2	*thr⁺*	*aziᴿ* = 0%, *leu⁺* = 4%
3	*leu⁺* and *thr⁺*	*aziᴿ* = 2%

markers for each experiment. From the information provided, determine the order of the three genes on the donor chromosome.

Solution Strategies	Solution Steps
Evaluate	
1. Identify the topic this problem addresses and the nature of the required answer.	1. This is a cotransduction problem in which cotransduction frequencies are to be used to determine the order of three genes in the donor.
2. Identify the critical information given in the problem.	2. The results of three transduction experiments are given. Each experiment has a different gene or a gene combination as the selected marker(s).
Deduce	
3. Keep in mind the advantage of using the selected–unselected marker experimental approach.	3. Selecting for transduction of one of the genes of interest and then evaluating transductants for the other gene(s) reduces the number of plates that must be evaluated and simplifies the experimental analysis.
4. Interpret the results of each experiment.	4. Experiment 1 indicates close proximity of *leu* and *azi*, and a greater distance between *leu* and *thr*. Experiment 2 suggests the same more-distant relationship between *thr* and *leu* but also shows no cotransduction between *thr* and *azi*. Experiment 3 informs us that cotransduction of all three donor alleles occurs, though at a low frequency. We can interpret this to mean that the segment of chromosome containing these genes is small enough to form a single fragment for transduction.
> **TIP:** Cotransduction frequencies are highest for genes that are closest together on the bacterial chromosome.	
Solve	
5. Combine your observations to identify the order of these three genes.	5. Putting the results of these experiments together, we can identify cotransduction of *thr* and *azi* (shown at 0% in Experiment 2) as the quadruple-crossover cotransductant. All other events are a result of double crossover. The quadruple crossover event is expected to be least frequent among the cotransductants. On this basis, *leu* can be identified as the middle gene of the three tested. The gene map is shown below, and the four crossover intervals are identified.
> **TIP:** Crossovers occur in pairs during the homologous recombination that accompanies transduction. When three genes are involved, a quadruple crossover is less frequent than any of the double crossovers.	

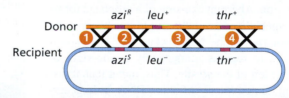

The crossover events accounting for each cotransduction detected in the experiments are shown below.

Cotransduction	Crossovers
aziᴿ and *leu⁺*	1 and 3
leu⁺ and *thr⁺*	2 and 4
aziᴿ, *leu⁺*, and *thr⁺*	1 and 4

For more practice, see Problems 9, 20, and 24. Visit the Study Area for a Video Tutor solution. **Mastering** Genetics

mutation of either *rIIA* or *rIIB* form large, irregularly shaped plaques on *E. coli* strain B, but they are unable to form any plaques on *E. coli* K-12 (λ).

Benzer used several different mutagens to produce almost 20,000 *rII* mutants that he studied in three ways. First, he used *genetic complementation analysis,* which showed that there are two genes in the *rII* region. Second, he mapped different mutations of *rIIA* and different mutations of *rIIB*, thus showing that *intragenic recombination* (within the gene) was possible and could be used to establish the locations of different mutations in each gene. Finally, Benzer developed *deletion mapping* to refine the genetic map. The following discussions explain each of these achievements individually.

Genetic Complementation Analysis

To identify the number of genes in the *rII* region, Benzer performed genetic complementation analysis, coinfecting K-12 (λ) bacteria with different pairs of *rII* mutants (see Section 4.4). When two *rII* mutants exhibiting genetic complementation coinfect K-12 (λ) bacteria, plaques form on the bacterial lawn, indicating that wild-type lysis has been restored. This result identifies the mutants as mutations of different genes. Coinfections by *rII* mutants that did not lead to plaque formation on K-12 (λ) represented a failure to complement, identifying these pairs as different mutations of the same gene—in other words, alleles of one another. Benzer identified two genetic complementation groups, which he designated A and B, and these led him to identify two genes in the *rII* region: *rIIA* and *rIIB*.

Subsequent analysis revealed that each gene produces a protein and that both proteins are required for lysis. **Figure 6.21a** illustrates genetic complementation for one pair of *rII* mutants. One mutant produces functional A protein and the other produces functional B protein, thus providing all the protein components necessary to carry out lysis. Genetic complementation produces a large number of plaques in infected bacterial lawns, but the individual progeny phages released following lysis remain mutant. **Figure 6.21b** illustrates a failure of mutants to complement. In this example, both mutants carry a mutation of *rIIB*.

Intragenic Recombination Analysis

On rare occasions, Benzer observed that two lysis mutants that fail to complement (i.e., mutants of the same gene) nonetheless produce a few plaques of K-12 (λ). He proposed that these plaques were produced by wild-type phage that resulted from rare intragenic recombination between two mutants whose chromosomes carry mutations in different locations in a single gene (**Figure 6.22**). One of the resulting recombinant chromosomes carries a double mutation, and the other is wild type. Wild-type chromosomes are found in progeny phages that carry out wild-type lysis.

Based on a determination of the number of cells in an experimental flask and counting the number of K-12 (λ)

(a) Complementation of mutations in different genes

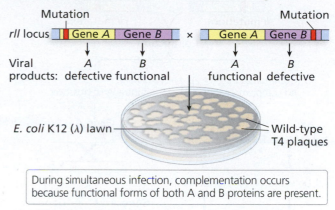

During simultaneous infection, complementation occurs because functional forms of both A and B proteins are present.

(b) No complementation of mutations in the same genes

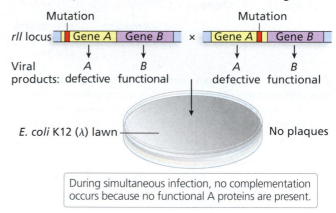

During simultaneous infection, no complementation occurs because no functional A proteins are present.

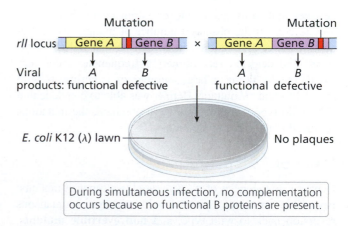

During simultaneous infection, no complementation occurs because no functional B proteins are present.

Figure 6.21 Genetic complementation analysis for *rII* lysis.
(a) Genetic complementation of two lysis-defective phage mutants occurs when the mutants carry mutations of different genes. Genetic complementation is revealed by the formation of many wild-type plaques on K12 (λ) bacteria. **(b)** No complementation occurs in lysis-defective mutants that carry mutations of the same gene.

plaques subsequently produced, Benzer was able to calculate the intragenic recombination frequency within the *rII* gene for a given pair of mutations. Reasoning that reciprocal recombination was more likely to occur between two mutations that are distant within a gene, and less likely

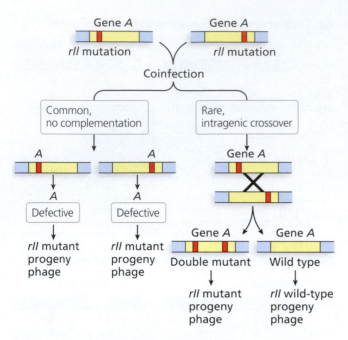

Figure 6.22 **Simultaneous coinfection of a host cell by two noncomplementing *rIIA* mutants.** No complementation (left) is the common and expected outcome. Rarely, however, intragenic recombination (right) produces wild-type and double-mutant progeny phages.

Genetic complementation produces many plaques but recombination produces single plaques. Why is the number of plaques produced so different between these mechanisms?

between mutations that are closer within a gene, Benzer was able to convert the observed number of plaques into a frequency of recombination with which he mapped *rII* mutations. The detected recombination frequencies were very small, but by doing a large number of experiments with many different *rII* mutants, Benzer was able to conclude that if no wild-type recombinants were obtained, the mutations occurred in the same nucleotide.

Deletion-Mapping Analysis

Benzer's mutagenesis of *rII* generated two types of mutants: **revertible mutants**, which could undergo spontaneous reversion back to wild type, and **nonrevertible mutants**, which *never* reverted. Revertible mutations, also known as **reversions**, are caused by DNA base-sequence substitutions (point mutations), which can be changed back to wild-type sequence by a subsequent point mutation that reverts back to the original nucleotide. On the other hand, nonrevertible mutations are partial deletion mutations, in which part of the gene sequence is lost. A deleted DNA sequence cannot be restored by reversion (see Chapter 11 for more discussion of reversions).

Using a technique called **deletion mapping**, Benzer took advantage of this difference between revertible and nonrevertible mutants to map the position of individual *rII* mutations. Deletion mapping relies on the production of wild-type phage

by intragenic recombination between a revertible mutant and nonrevertible mutant. When one mutant is revertible and the other is nonrevertible, the ability to form wild-type intragenic recombinants depends on the locations of the mutations. **Figure 6.23a** illustrates reversion to wild type through intragenic recombination between a point mutation and a deletion mutation whose locations *do not overlap*. In contrast, **Figure 6.23b** shows that if the locations of the point mutation and the deletion mutation *overlap* one another, the production of wild-type intragenic recombinants is impossible. Wild-type recombinants are not formed in this case, because the deletion mutant cannot provide the wild-type sequence to replace the mutated sequence in the point mutant.

In research published between 1955 and 1962, Benzer conducted deletion mapping of almost 20,000 *rII* mutants. He infected bacteria with phage carrying individual revertible mutations (point mutations), paired one at a time with phage carrying different nonrevertible mutations (deletion mutations).

In 1961, Benzer published a fine-structure map containing 1612 point mutations of *rIIA* and *rIIB* (**Figure 6.24**). Two features of this map are of interest. First, the mutations are scattered throughout *rIIA* and *rIIB*, suggesting the genes are composed of subunits that are individually mutable. Second, the distribution of the mutations is nonrandom. More than 100 point mutations aggregate in region A6c, and region B4 is the site of more than 500 independent point mutations. These sites are *mutational hotspots* that can be brought about by several circumstances (see Section 11.1).

6.6 Lateral Gene Transfer Alters Genomes

The genetic maps created by analysis of data from conjugation, transduction, and transformation experiments were extraordinarily important for understanding the content and organization of bacterial genomes. Contemporaneous with the identification of DNA structure (the early 1950s) and with descriptions of the molecular basis of DNA replication, transcription, and translation (the late 1950s and early 1960s), these genetic maps served as the foundation for DNA-sequence–based maps of bacterial and archaeal genomes that have been produced by the thousands since the late 1990s. By conveying the precise order and relative positions of most genes in commonly investigated genomes such as that of *E.coli*, the early genetic maps jump-started the process of identifying genes and their functions in the sequenced genomes of bacteria and archaea, a process known as *annotation*. Chapter 16 contains a detailed discussion of genome sequencing strategies, genome structures, evolutionary genomics, and genome annotation. Here we provide a brief overview of the *lateral gene transfer* that has contributed substantially to the content of many genomes.

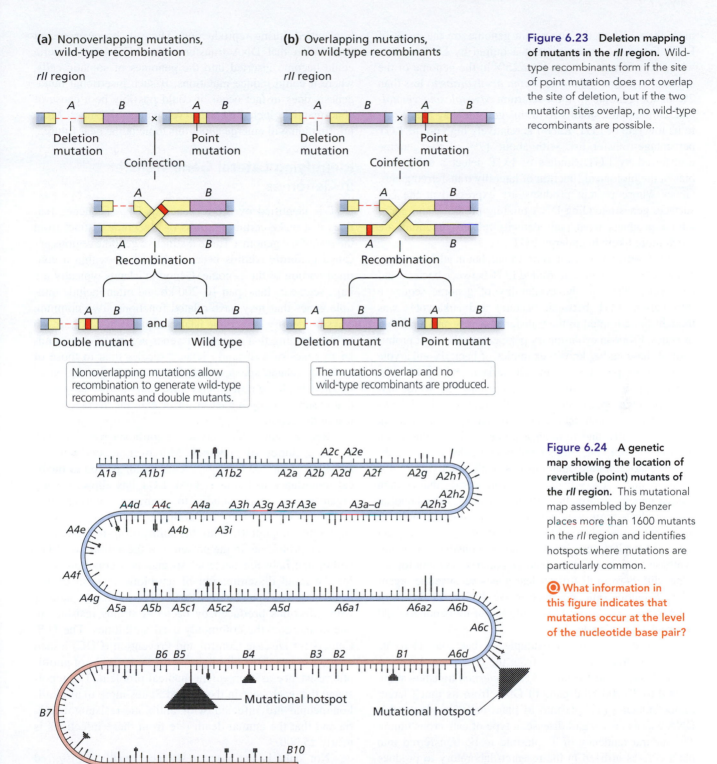

(a) Nonoverlapping mutations, wild-type recombination

(b) Overlapping mutations, no wild-type recombinants

Nonoverlapping mutations allow recombination to generate wild-type recombinants and double mutants.

The mutations overlap and no wild-type recombinants are produced.

Figure 6.23 Deletion mapping of mutants in the *rII* region. Wild-type recombinants form if the site of point mutation does not overlap the site of deletion, but if the two mutation sites overlap, no wild-type recombinants are possible.

Figure 6.24 A genetic map showing the location of revertible (point) mutants of the *rII* region. This mutational map assembled by Benzer places more than 1600 mutants in the *rII* region and identifies hotspots where mutations are particularly common.

Q What information in this figure indicates that mutations occur at the level of the nucleotide base pair?

Lateral Gene Transfer and Genome Evolution

Lateral gene transfer (LGT), also known as horizontal gene transfer (HGT), is the transfer of genetic material between individual bacteria or archaea and other organisms. The participating organisms are sometimes members of the same species, but they can also be members of different species or even distinct taxonomic groups. Common examples of LGT are the three bacterial transfer processes discussed in this chapter: conjugation, transformation, and transduction. Each of these processes occurs readily in and between species. Extensive studies of LGT across a wide range of bacterial and archaeal species find that on average more than 12% of the genes in a genome are the result of LGT. The range in the amount acquired by LGT is quite wide, from a high of more than 25% in the genome of the archaeal organism *Methanosarcina acetivorans* to less than 2% of the genome in the bacterium *Mycoplasma genitalium*, although the small size of this genome may play a role in its low rate of LGT. *E. coli* is relatively high on the LGT percentage-transfer list, with about 17% of the genome transferred by LGT. Studies of LGT detect a substantial bias in the biological function of laterally transferred genes. Genes whose protein products are expressed at the cell surface, genes encoding DNA-binding proteins, and genes whose products have pathogenicity-related functions are much more likely to undergo LGT.

LGT between bacteria is prevalent, but in addition, there has long been evidence of limited LGT between bacteria and eukaryotes. Prior to the availability of genome sequence information, LGT between bacteria and eukaryotes was thought to be limited to the transfer of a very small number of genes. From an evolutionary perspective, the most prominent of these earlier known examples of bacteria–eukaryote LGT are the presence of mitochondria in eukaryotic cells and the presence of chloroplasts in plant cells. Mitochondria and chloroplasts are essential organelles in eukaryotic cells. Millennia ago, ancient bacteria invaded ancient eukaryotic cells, and through a process of coevolution on the part of both cells, mitochondria and chloroplasts established endosymbiotic relationships with eukaryotic cells. Both organelles carry their own chromosomes that contain unique genetic information. In animal cells, mitochondrial gene products work with nuclear gene products to produce adenosine triphosphate (ATP) used for energy; and in plant cells, chloroplast gene products are responsible for photosynthesis. The inheritance of mitochondrial and chloroplast genes differs from that of nuclear genes because the organelles are cytoplasmic, not nuclear. We discuss the details of cytoplasmic heredity and the evolution of mitochondria and chloroplasts in Chapter 17.

Another well-known example of bacteria–eukaryote LGT is the transfer of DNA from the bacterium *Agrobacterium tumefaciens* to plants. *Agrobacterium* transfers about 10,000 to 30,000 base pairs of DNA from its much larger tumor-inducing (Ti) plasmid to plant cells. In plants, this DNA causes crown gall disease, a type of cancerous tumor. The natural tendency of Ti plasmid to be transferred into plant cells is utilized in the research laboratory to produce transgenic plants, as we discuss in Chapter 15.

In 2007, genome sequencing information demonstrated extensive LGT between the bacterium *Wolbachia* and a large number of insects. The data indicate that roughly one-third of all arthropod genomes contain *Wolbachia* DNA transferred by LGT. Researchers speculate that LGT between bacteria and animals may be much more common than previously thought. Only some of the transferred genes appear to actually enter the germ line, where they can be transmitted during reproduction. There is, however, recent speculation that DNA transferred by LGT from bacteria could become inserted into the genomes of somatic cells, where it could induce mutations. If such insertional mutagenesis does in fact occur, it could possibly be a cause of abnormalities, including the development of cancer. More information will emerge about this topic in the near future.

Identifying Lateral Gene Transfer in Genomes

LGT is identified by the presence of DNA-sequence features that make certain portions of a genome distinct from the rest of the genome. These distinctive genome regions are called **genomic islands** because they occur within a confined portion of the genome. Genomic islands typically are large segments that span 10–200 kb and often include multiple genes that may have related functions. Two common ways to identify a genomic island acquired by LGT are (1) by determining that a group of genes are much more similar to genes of a distantly related species than to those of a closely related species, and (2) by detecting a region of genome that has a ratio of G–C base pairs to A–T base pairs that is substantially higher or lower than the average in the rest of the genome.

Recent evidence points to a significant role for LGT in the evolution of genomes. Moreover, in two particular ways, some LGT-driven events are of profound medical importance to humans. First, LGT has allowed many organisms to adapt rapidly to changing environmental conditions by acquiring the ability to resist one or more antibiotic compounds. With this ability, drug-resistant bacteria can proliferate in the presence of the antibiotics. LGT within and between bacterial species is a common route for the rapid dissemination of antibiotic resistance, and medical practitioners today routinely encounter patients with infections produced by bacterial strains resistant to one or more of the commonly used antibiotics. The U.S. Centers for Disease Control and Prevention (CDC) issued a report in late 2013 highlighting the seriousness of antibiotic resistance as a prevalent medical problem. The report stated that each year in the United States more than 2 million people are infected with antibiotic-resistant bacteria and that the annual death rate from these infections is nearly 25,000.

Not only is antibiotic resistance readily transferred between bacteria by LGT, but the prevalence of resistance genes is increased by the extensive use, and misuse, of antibiotics. The 2013 CDC report attributes a substantial portion of the increase in antibiotic-resistant strains to the pervasive use of antibiotics in animal agriculture, where they are often used to promote growth in animals with no signs of infection. These circumstances and the impact of this phenomenon on the practice of medicine are the subject of the Case Study at the end of this chapter.

The second medically relevant consequence of LGT in bacteria is the acquisition of **pathogenicity islands**, a subtype of genomic islands, containing multiple genes for proteins that promote the ability of the bacteria to invade the body of a host and also containing genes that produce toxic compounds.

Among the various strains of the common, and usually friendly, intestinal bacterium *E. coli* are some strains that are pathogenic. The most common strains of *E. coli* are commensal bacteria that inhabit our intestinal tract and provide benefits without doing harm. Certain strains, however, have acquired pathogenicity islands and cause illnesses such as diarrhea and meningitis. The recently identified pathogenic strain *E. coli* O157:H7 contains a pathogenicity island

acquired by transduction. *E. coli* O157:H7 is found in some contaminated beef and on some fresh produce, including lettuce. Thorough rinsing can, but does not always, remove the pathogen from lettuce, and undercooking contaminated beef does not raise its temperature high enough to kill pathogens that may be present. The pathogenicity island in *E. coli* O157:H7 contains genes that promote the adhesion of the pathogen to intestinal cells and a toxin gene that acts similarly to, although not as dramatically as, the *Vibrio cholera* toxin. Infection with *E. coli* O157:H7 produces diarrhea that can be severe in immune-compromised individuals or in infants and the elderly. The island also contains a gene producing a toxin that blocks translation in cells. This toxin particularly affects kidney and intestinal cells and contributes to bloody diarrhea.

CASE STUDY

The Evolution of Antibiotic Resistance and Its Impact on Medical Practice

Alexander Fleming got a little sloppy with his sterile technique one day in 1929 and made a mistake that has since saved millions of lives. Fleming was working with *Staphylococcus*, a common bacterial strain that causes a serious and potentially fatal "staph" infection when it enters the body through a cut or abrasion. On the fateful day, Fleming unknowingly contaminated his *Staphylococcus* culture with a fungus.

Normally, fungal cells reproduce in culture along with bacterial cells and are noticed when the culture is spread on plates. Fleming's contaminating fungus was different, however, because when Fleming spread his contaminated culture on plates, only fungal colonies grew—there were no bacterial colonies! The fungus had killed the bacterial cells in the culture. Recognizing this as an important, if inadvertent, discovery, Fleming quickly identified the fungus as *Penicillium* and gave the compound that killed *Staphylococcus* the name penicillin.

In the 1930s, Howard Florey showed that penicillin was an effective antibiotic against a broad spectrum of infectious bacteria. At the beginning of World War II, Florey directed a major "scale–up" project to put penicillin into mass production. Penicillin proved tremendously effective at preventing what otherwise might have been fatal bacterial infections.

Today, although penicillin and other antibiotics continue to save lives, antibiotic-resistant strains of bacteria are increasingly the cause of difficult-to-treat infections and even death. This is quickly becoming an acute problem in modern medicine. For example, at present more than 95% of *Staphylococcus* strains found in hospitals are resistant to penicillin, and some strains carry resistance alleles to multiple antibiotics. One such strain is methicillin-resistant *Staphylococcus aureus* (MRSA). What happened to bring about this shift? The answer has two parts. One component we have already mentioned—the evolution of antibiotic resistance and the acquisition of pathogenicity by bacteria through lateral gene transfer. Antibiotic resistance can be readily transferred within a species and between bacterial species by conjugation, transduction, or transformation, and by LGT.

The second factor is the use and misuse of antibiotics themselves that establishes an environment in which resistant strains proliferate at the expense of sensitive strains. Exposing bacteria to antibiotics, which generally leads to killing antibiotic-sensitive bacteria, can at the same time allow the survival of antibiotic-resistant bacteria. Even when they are properly used, antibiotics can act as an agent of artificial selection that fosters the survival of resistant strains at the expense of sensitive strains. When antibiotics are misused (as when they are used to encourage growth in livestock), when they are not taken for the prescribed period of time by a patient, or when they are used to treat nonbacterial infections, they eliminate great numbers of antibiotic-sensitive bacteria and promote the proliferation of resistant bacteria.

A part of the challenge to physicians dealing with these changing circumstances is that resistance and sensitivity to antibiotics are not absolute characteristics. A "resistant" strain is just that—*resistant* to an antibiotic but not necessarily *impervious* to it. It takes more antibiotic to kill a resistant strain than to kill a sensitive strain. With regard to treating an infected person or animal, the medical question is: At what dosage is the benefit of the antibiotic outweighed by the harm that might be done to the patient by toxicity of the antibiotic or by too many of the body's beneficial bacteria being destroyed? Antibiotic resistance is a rapidly growing problem that has already changed practices in medical treatment of infectious disease. The future holds more changes, both in patient treatment and in other uses of antibiotics.

At present, and increasingly in the future, physicians must be acutely aware of the events and behaviors that can lead to bacterial infection, be hypervigilant in spotting potential infections by resistant strains, and be prepared to quickly adapt medical treatments and protocols to manage resistant strains of bacteria. Physicians must understand how and why antibiotic resistance has evolved if they are going to be successful in dealing with its ramifications for their patients.

6.1 Specialized Methods Are Used for Genetic Analysis of Bacteria

▌ Bacteria can be propagated in liquid growth media or on semisolid growth media.

▌ Replica plating allows the bacterial colonies on one plate to be transferred to additional plates in the same relative positions, thus facilitating genetic analysis of individual colonies.

6.2 Bacteria Transfer Genes by Conjugation

▌ Bacteria transfer genetic material in a unidirectional process (donor cell to recipient cell) called conjugation. Experimental analysis found that conjugation requires direct contact between donor and recipient.

▌ Conjugation is controlled by genes on a plasmid known as an F factor. Donor bacteria that carry an extrachromosomal F factor are F^+ cells, and bacteria without an F factor are F^-, or recipient, cells.

▌ F factor transfer begins with the binding of a relaxosome protein complex at the transfer origin (*oriT*) of F factor DNA, where they cleave one strand, the T strand. Rolling circle DNA replication then transfers the T strand of the F factor from the donor cell to the recipient cell across a conjugation pilus.

▌ Conjugation between an F^+ donor and an F^- recipient transfers the F factor only. The F^- cell is converted to an F^+ cell but receives no genetic material from the donor bacterial chromosome.

▌ F factor integration into the donor chromosome takes place by recombination at insertion sequences (IS) found in both the F factor and the donor chromosome. F factor integration creates an Hfr (high-frequency recombination) chromosome.

▌ Many different kinds of Hfr chromosomes can occur in a single bacterial species. These differences arise from the two possible orientations and various possible sites of F factor integration into the chromosome.

▌ Conjugation between an Hfr donor and an F^- recipient transfers a portion of the F factor and a segment of donor DNA. The donor segment undergoes homologous recombination with the recipient chromosome. Exconjugants receive donor bacterial genes but are not converted to a donor state.

▌ Time-of-entry maps are created for each Hfr strain by interrupted mating studies that identify the order of entry of donor genes and determine the distance (in minutes) between transferred genes.

▌ Hfr maps for a given bacterium are consolidated to form a genetic map of the donor chromosome as a whole.

▌ F′ donor strains are created when excision of an F factor from Hfr integration removes F factor DNA along with adjacent donor chromosome DNA.

▌ Conjugation between an F′ donor and an F^- recipient generates partial diploidy in exconjugants.

6.3 Bacterial Transformation Produces Genetic Recombination

▌ Extracellular fragments of DNA released when a donor bacterial cell lyses can be absorbed across the cell membrane of a competent recipient cell as transforming DNA.

▌ Transforming DNA undergoes homologous recombination with the recipient chromosome to produce transformants that have acquired donor DNA.

6.4 Bacterial Transduction Is Mediated by Bacteriophages

▌ Bacteriophage infection of a host bacterial cell can lead to lysis of the host cell.

▌ Temperate bacteriophages can undergo site-specific integration into the host chromosome by lysogeny.

▌ Generalized transducing phages are created when a phage particle mistakenly packages a segment of a bacterial chromosome during lysis of the host cell.

▌ Recipient cells undergo generalized transduction when donor DNA introduced by a generalized transducing phage recombines with the recipient chromosome. Any donor genes can be transduced during generalized transduction.

▌ Cotransduction mapping determines the order of genes on the donor chromosome.

▌ Specialized transducing phages are produced by the aberrant excision of a lysogenic prophage that removes a portion of the prophage and an adjacent segment of host DNA. Specialized transduction is limited to transduction of genes adjacent to the site of prophage integration.

6.5 Bacteriophage Chromosomes Are Mapped by Fine-Structure Analysis

▌ Seymour Benzer used genetic complementation analysis to determine that two genes make up the *rII* region controlling T4 bacteriophage lysis of *E. coli*.

▌ Analysis of intragenic recombination, and deletion mapping of more than 1600 *rIIA* and *rIIB* mutants, led to the conclusion that DNA nucleotides are the fundamental unit of recombination.

6.6 Lateral Gene Transfer Alters Genomes

▌ LGT is common within species and also between diverse species.

▌ LGT usually involves multiple genes in genomic islands.

▌ Bacteria commonly acquire pathogenicity and antibiotic resistance through LGT.

▌ LGT between bacterial and eukaryotic genomes is well documented and may be more common than was previously thought.

PREPARING FOR PROBLEM SOLVING

In addition to the list of problem-solving tips and suggestions given here, you can go to the Study Guide and Solutions Manual that accompanies this book for help at solving problems.

1. Be able to describe or diagram the chromosomes and plasmids of F$^+$, Hfr, and F$'$ bacteria.

2. Be able to describe the differences between conjugation, transformation, and transduction.

3. Be familiar with basic microbiological laboratory methods for growing and replica plating bacterial cells.

4. Be familiar with Table 6.1 (p. 196) and be ready to use the outcomes listed in it to identify types of donor bacterial strains.

5. Be prepared to assess bacterial genotypes based on growth ability in media of various compositions and to apply those assessments in analyzing conjugation and transduction experiments.

6. Be prepared to use the results of time-of-entry experiments to determine gene order and map distance in donor bacterial strains.

7. Be prepared to calculate cotransduction frequencies and to apply those calculations to gene order determination.

8. Understand genetic complementation analysis of bacteriophages and how to distinguish the results of genetic complementation from those of recombination.

PROBLEMS

Mastering Genetics Visit for instructor-assigned tutorials and problems.

Chapter Concepts

For answers to selected even-numbered problems, see Appendix: Answers.

1. For bacteria that are F$^+$, Hfr, F$'$, and F$^-$, perform or answer the following.
   a. Describe the state of the F factor.
   b. Which of these cells are donors? Which is the recipient?
   c. Which of these donors can convert exconjugants to a donor state?
   d. Which of these donors can transfer a donor gene to exconjugants?
   e. Describe the results of conjugation (i.e., changes in the recipient and the exconjugant) that allow detection of the state of the F factor in a donor strain.
   f. Describe a "partial diploid" and how it originates.

2. The flow diagram identifies relationships between bacterial strains in various F factor states. For each of the four arrows in the diagram, provide a description of the events involved in the transition.

$$F^- \xrightarrow{1} F^+ \underset{3}{\overset{2}{\rightleftarrows}} Hfr \xrightarrow{4} F'$$

3. Conjugation between an Hfr cell and an F$^-$ cell does not usually result in conversion of exconjugants to the donor state. Occasionally however, the result of this conjugation is two Hfr cells. Explain how this occurs.

4. Bacteria transfer genes by conjugation, transduction, and transformation. Compare and contrast these mechanisms. In your answer, identify which if any processes involve homologous recombination and which if any do not.

5. Explain the importance of the following features in conjugating donor bacteria:
   a. the origin of transfer
   b. the conjugation pilus
   c. homologous recombination
   d. the relaxosome
   e. relaxase
   f. T strand DNA
   g. pilin protein

6. Describe the difference between the bacteriophage lytic cycle and lysogenic cycle.

7. Describe what is meant by the term *site-specific recombination* as used in identifying the processes that lead to the integration of temperate bacteriophages into host bacterial chromosomes during lysogeny or to the formation of specialized transducing phage.

8. What is a prophage, and how is a prophage formed?

9. How is the frequency of cotransduction related to the relative positions of genes on a bacterial chromosome? Draw a map of three genes and describe the expected relationship of cotransduction frequencies to the map.

10. Describe the differences between genetic complementation and recombination as they relate to the detection of wild-type lysis by a mutant bacteriophage.

11. Among the mechanisms of gene transfer in bacteria, which one is capable of transferring the largest chromosome segment from donor to recipient? Which process generally transfers the smallest donor segments to the recipient? Explain your reasoning for both answers.

Application and Integration

For answers to selected even-numbered problems, see Appendix: Answers.

12. What is lateral gene transfer? How might it take place between two bacterial cells?

13. Lateral gene transfer is thought to have played a major role in the evolution of bacterial genomes. Describe the impact of LGT on bacterial genome evolution.

14. Seven deletion mutations (1 to 7 in the table below) are tested for their ability to form wild-type recombinants with five point mutations (a to e). The symbol "+" indicates that wild-type recombination occurs, and "−" indicates that wild types are not formed. Use the data to construct a genetic map of the order of point mutations, and indicate the segment deleted by each deletion mutation.

Point Mutation	Deletion Mutation						
	1	2	3	4	5	6	7
a	−	+	−	−	+	+	−
b	+	+	+	−	+	−	−
c	+	+	+	+	−	−	−
d	−	+	+	−	+	−	−
e	+	−	−	−	+	+	−

15. A 2013 CDC report identified the practice of routinely adding antibiotic compounds to animal feed as a major culprit in the rapid increase in the number of antibiotic-resistant strains. Agricultural practice in recent decades has encouraged the addition of antibiotics to animal feed to promote growth rather than to treat disease.
    a. Speculate about the process by which feeding antibiotics to animals such as cattle might lead to an increase in the number of antibiotic-resistant strains of bacteria.
    b. How might the increase in antibiotic-resistant strains of bacteria in cattle be a threat to human health?

16. Hfr strains that differ in integrated F factor orientation and site of integration are used to construct consolidated bacterial chromosome maps. The data below show the order of gene transfer for five strains.

Hfr Strain	Order of Gene Transfer (First →Last)
Hfr A	oriT – thr – leu – azi – ton – pro – lac – ade
Hfr B	oriT – mtl – xyl – mal – str – his
Hfr C	oriT – ile – met – thi – thr – leu – azi – ton
Hfr D	oriT – his – trp – gal – ade – lac – pro – ton
Hfr E	oriT – thi – met – ile – mtl – xyl – mal – str

    a. Identify the overlaps between Hfr strains. Identify the orientations of integrated F factors relative to one another.
    b. Draw a consolidated map of the bacterial chromosome. (*Hint:* Begin by placing the insertion site for Hfr A at the 2 o'clock position and arranging the genes *thr-leu-azi-* . . . in clockwise order.)

17. Five Hfr strains from the same bacterial species are analyzed for their ability to transfer genes to F⁻ recipient bacteria. The data shown below list the origin of transfer (*oriT*) for each strain and give the order of genes, with the first gene on the left and the last gene on the right. Use the data to construct a circular map of the bacterium.

Hfr Strain	Genes Transferred
Hfr 1	oriT met ala lac gal
Hfr 2	oriT met leu thr azi
Hfr 3	oriT gal pro trp azi
Hfr 4	oriT leu met ala lac
Hfr 5	oriT trp azi thr leu met

18. An interrupted mating study is carried out on Hfr strains 1, 2, and 3 identified in Problem 17. After conjugation is established, a small sample of the mixture is collected every minute for 20 minutes to determine the distance between genes on the chromosome. Results for each of the three Hfr strains are shown below. The total duration of conjugation (in minutes) is given for each transferred gene.

Hfr strain 1	oriT	met	ala	lac	gal
Duration (min)	0	2	8	13	17
Hfr strain 2	oriT	met	leu	thr	azi
Duration (min)	0	2	7	10	17
Hfr strain 3	oriT	gal	pro	trp	azi
Duration (min)	0	3	8	14	19

    a. For each Hfr strain, draw a time-of-entry profile like the one in Figure 6.11a.
    b. Using the chromosome map you prepared in answer to Problem 17, determine the distance in minutes between each gene on the map.
    c. Explain why *azi* is the last gene of strain 2 to transfer in the 20 minutes of conjugation time. How many minutes of conjugation time would be needed to allow the next gene on the map to transfer from Hfr strain 2?
    d. Write out the interrupted mating results you would expect after 20 minutes of conjugation for Hfr strains 4 and 5. Use the format shown at the beginning of this problem.
    e. In minutes, what is the total length of the chromosome in the donor species?

19. An Hfr strain with the genotype *cys⁺ leu⁺ met⁺ str*ˢ is mated with an F⁻ strain carrying the genotype *cys⁻ leu⁻ met⁻ str*ᴿ. In an interrupted mating experiment, small samples of the conjugating bacteria are withdrawn every 3 minutes for 30 minutes. The withdrawn cells are shaken vigorously to stop conjugation and then placed on three different selection media, composed as follows:

Medium 1: Minimal medium plus leucine, methionine, and streptomycin

Medium 2: Minimal medium plus cysteine, methionine, and streptomycin

Medium 3: Minimal medium plus cysteine, leucine, and
   streptomycin
a. What donor gene is the selected marker in each
   medium?
b. List all possible bacterial genotypes growing on each
   medium.
c. What is the purpose of adding streptomycin to each
   selection medium?

The following table shows the number of colonies growing on each selection medium. The sampling time indicates how many minutes have passed since conjugation
began.

Sampling Time (minutes)	Number of Colonies		
	Plate 1	Plate 2	Plate 3
3	0	0	0
6	0	0	0
9	0	62	0
12	0	87	0
15	51	124	0
18	79	210	62
21	109	250	85
24	144	250	111
27	152	250	122
30	152	250	122

d. Determine the order of donor genes *cys, leu,* and *met*
   from the interrupted mating data.
e. Suppose a fourth selection medium containing leucine
   and streptomycin is prepared. At what sampling time
   do you expect the first-growing colonies to appear?
   Explain your reasoning.

20. A triple-auxotrophic strain of *E. coli* having the genotype
   phe⁻ met⁻ ara⁻ is used as a recipient strain in a transduction experiment. The strain is unable to synthesize its own
   phenylalanine or methionine, and it carries a mutation that
   leaves it unable to utilize the sugar arabinose for growth.
   The recipient is crossed to a prototrophic strain with the
   genotype *phe⁺ met⁺ ara⁺*. The table below shows the
   selected marker and gives cotransduction frequencies for
   the unselected markers.

Selected Marker	Selected Colonies Containing the Unselected Marker (%)		
	phe⁺	*met⁺*	*ara⁺*
met⁺	4	–	7
phe⁺	–	2	51
met⁺, phe⁺	–	–	79
ara⁺	68	5	–

a. Identify the compounds present in each of the selective
   media.
b. Use the cotransduction data to determine the order of
   these genes.

21. Penicillin was first used in the 1940s to treat gonorrhea
   infections produced by the bacterium *Neisseria gonorrhoeae*. In 1984, according to the CDC, fewer than 1% of
   gonorrhea infections were caused by penicillin-resistant
   N. gonorrhoeae. By 1990, more than 10% of cases were
   penicillin-resistant, and a few years later the level of
   resistance was at greater than 95%. Almost every year the
   CDC issues new treatment guidelines for gonorrhea that
   identify the recommended antibiotic drugs and dosages.
a. Why is the CDC so active in making these
   recommendations?
b. What are the short-term implications of these frequent
   changes for physicians and clinics that treat sexually
   transmitted diseases like gonorrhea and for individuals
   infected with gonorrhea?
c. What are the long-term implications of these frequent
   changes in treatment recommendations for the patient
   population?

22. An attribute of growth behavior of eight bacteriophage
   mutants (1 to 8) is investigated in experiments that establish coinfection by pairs of mutants. The experiments
   determine whether the mutants complement one another
   (+) or fail to complement (−). These eight mutants are
   known to result from point mutation. The results of the
   complementation tests are shown below.

Mutations								
	1	2	3	4	5	6	7	8
1	–	+	+	+	–	+	+	–
2		–	+	+	+	+	+	+
3			–	+	+	+	–	+
4				–	+	–	+	+
5					–	+	+	–
6						–	+	+
7							–	+
8								–

a. How many genes are represented by these mutations?
b. Identify the mutants of each gene.
c. In each coinfection identified as a failure to complement (−) in the table, researchers see evidence of
   recombination producing wild-type growth. How do
   the researchers distinguish between wild-type growth
   resulting from complementation and wild-type growth
   that is due to recombination?
d. A new mutation, designated 9, fails to complement
   mutants 1, 3, 5, 7, and 8. Wild-type recombinants form
   between mutant 9 and mutations 3, 5, and 8; however,
   no wild-type recombinants form between mutant 9 and
   mutations 1 and 7. What kind of mutation is mutant 9?
   Explain your reasoning.
e. New mutation 10 fails to complement mutants 1, 4, 5,
   6, 8, and 9. Mutant 10 forms wild-type recombinants
   with mutants 1, 5, and 6, but not with mutants 4 and 8.
   Mutant 9 and mutant 10 form wild-type recombinants.
   What kind of mutation is mutant 10? Explain your
   reasoning.

f. Gene mapping information identifies mutations 2 and 3 as the flanking markers in this group of genes. Assuming these mutations are on opposite ends of the gene map, determine the order of mutations in the region of the chromosome.

23. Synthesis of the amino acid histidine is a multistep anabolic pathway that uses the products of 13 genes (*hisA* to *hisM*) in *E. coli*. Two independently isolated *his⁻ E. coli* mutants, designated *his1⁻* and *his2⁻*, are studied in a conjugation experiment. A *his⁺* F′ donor strain that carries a copy of the *hisJ* gene on the plasmid is mated with a *his1⁻* recipient strain in Experiment 1 and with a *his2⁻* recipient in Experiment 2. The exconjugants are grown on plates lacking histidine. Growth is observed among the exconjugants of Experiment 2 but not among those of Experiment 1.

    a. Why is growth observed in Experiment 2 but not in Experiment 1?
    b. What is the genotype of exconjugants in Experiment 2?

24. The phage P1 is used as a generalized transducing phage in an experiment combining a donor strain of *E. coli* of genotype *leu⁺ phe⁺ ala⁺* and a recipient strain that is *leu⁻ phe⁻ ala⁻*. In separate experiments, transductants are selected for *leu⁺* (Experiment A), for *phe⁺* (Experiment B), and for *ala⁺* (Experiment C). Following selection, transductant genotypes for the unselected markers are identified. The selection experiment results below show the frequency of each genotype.

Experiment A		Experiment B		Experiment C	
phe⁻ ala⁻	26%	*leu⁻ ala⁻*	65%	*leu⁻ phe⁻*	71%
phe⁺ ala⁻	50%	*leu⁺ ala⁻*	48%	*leu⁺ phe⁻*	21%
phe⁻ ala⁺	19%	*leu⁻ ala⁺*	0%	*leu⁻ phe⁺*	0%
phe⁺ ala⁺	3%	*leu⁺ ala⁺*	4%	*leu⁺ phe⁺*	3%

a. What compound or compounds are added to the minimal medium to select for transductants in Experiments A, B, and C?
b. Determine the order of genes on the donor chromosome.
c. Diagram the crossover events that form each of the transductants in Experiment A.
d. In Experiment B, why are there no transductants with the genotype *leu⁻ ala⁺*?

Collaboration and Discussion

For answers to selected even-numbered problems, see Appendix: Answers.

25. Define the term *genetic complementation*.
    a. Describe how the term applies to an experiment in which two lysis-defective bacteriophages are able to coinfect a bacterial cell and produce lysis.
    b. Locate another example of genetic complementation in this book and describe how genetic complementation works in that case.
    c. Does the term *genetic complementation* have the same meaning in both cases? Explain.

26. Devise an experiment to identify bacteria that are auxotrophic and unable to produce two amino acids, lysine (lys) and valine (val). The auxotrophic bacteria are in a pool of bacteria in which all the other bacteria are prototrophic. The genotype of the auxotrophs is *lys⁻ val⁻*. Describe each step in the experiment, identify the constituents in any growth media or growth plates you propose, and identify the results that will conclusively identify bacteria that are *lys⁻ val⁻*.

27. Look closely at the consolidated Hfr map and the data used to build the map on page 201. Suppose a fifth Hfr strain had the F factor inserted exactly halfway between *cysE* and *leuU* and had an orientation that was the same as that of Hfr 1. List the order of gene transfer for the first six genes transferred by this Hfr and the number of minutes of conjugation at which each gene is expected to be seen.

28. Fifty bacterial colonies are on a complete-medium growth plate. The colonies are replica plated to a minimal medium plate, and 46 colonies grow. What can you say about the bacteria from the four colonies that do not grow? Design an experiment and describe the methods you would use to determine if any of these four colonies are *leu⁻*, *arg⁻*, or *val⁻*.

Human Hereditary Disease and Genetic Counseling

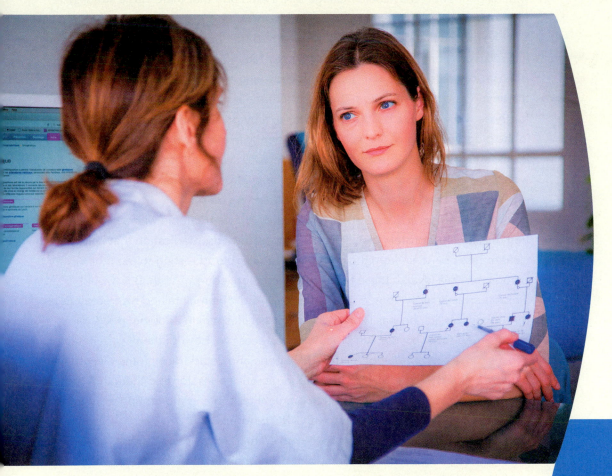

Genetic counseling, a central activity in medical genetics, seeks to provide individuals, couples, and families with medical and genetic information they can use to make informed decisions about genetic testing and medical treatment, in person-to-person meetings involving physicians, genetic counselors, and consultands.

When B.K. was born in San Francisco, California, in July 2015, he appeared to be a healthy baby boy. Among the myriad forms B.K.'s parents signed at the hospital was one informing them that B.K. would undergo mandated newborn genetic testing for almost four dozen different hereditary conditions within 24 hours of his birth. All the conditions tested are rare, but each can be treated to eliminate or substantially reduce the symptoms and complications of the disease. California, like all U.S. states and many other countries, mandates tests for several dozen rare genetic diseases of all newborns. We discuss this testing again later in the chapter and more fully in Application Chapter B: Human Genetic Screening.

Parents almost never hear about the results of these newborn genetic tests because a positive result is rare. But B.K.'s parents were told of a result indicating that B.K. had argininemia, commonly abbreviated ARG. B.K.'s parents had never heard of ARG and were naturally very upset to learn that their first child had a genetic disease. In a rapid series of meetings over the next two days, B.K.'s parents met with a pediatrician, a medical geneticist, a dietician, and a genetic counselor. What they learned brought them considerable relief and assurance that with diligent effort they could manage B.K.'s ARG and that there was a strategy for monitoring future pregnancies for the risk of ARG.

Over those first days, B.K.'s parents learned that ARG is a very rare autosomal recessive condition. Only 1 in 350,000 to 1 in 1,000,000 newborns have the disease. It is caused by a deficiency of the enzyme arginase that helps break down the amino acid arginine during the digestion of dietary protein. The main problem for those with ARG is a buildup of ammonia, a by-product of protein breakdown, in the blood because of the inability to efficiently break down arginine. At high levels, ammonia is toxic, especially to the nervous system. Without treatment, B.K. would experience poor growth that would be evident in his first year or two, poor muscle control and balance, and significant learning delays.

Fortunately, as B.K.'s parents also learned, ARG is treatable with a combination of a very low protein diet, specially prepared foods, medication that helps clear excess ammonia from the blood, and regular blood testing to monitor B.K.'s blood ammonia level. If these treatments were applied from birth, B.K. would almost certainly grow up normal and healthy. And if he maintained his treatment throughout his life, he was likely to live a normal lifespan. In addition, B.K.'s parents learned that because ARG is autosomal recessive, both of them were heterozygous carriers of a mutation of the *ARG1* gene and could transmit the disease to a future child. Their medical geneticist and genetic counselor told them that the risk of this occurring was 25% but that prenatal testing and monitoring were available to identify any future children with ARG before birth.

Since B.K.'s birth, his parents have worked hard to maintain his diet, administer his medication, and monitor his blood ammonia level. They received a great deal of counseling and referral assistance from their genetic counselor, and they have been in regular contact with their medical geneticist, their pediatrician (who has had to learn about ARG herself), and their dietician. They also found a support group for parents of children with medical conditions. To date, B.K. has hit all of his motor and mental milestones. He began to babble and form words on schedule and likes to go to the park where he can run on the grass.

Medical genetics, the area of human medicine aimed at diagnosing and managing the medical, psychological, and social aspects of diseases caused by gene mutations or influenced by genetics, has developed and expanded substantially in the past several decades. It is an enterprise involving not only clinicians but also diagnostic scientists, researchers, genetic counselors, and a range of other allied health professionals. Like all branches of human medicine, it focuses on the patient, but more than any other field of medicine, it also focuses on the family of the patient. This family focus takes two directions. One is medical, addressing the family's role in care of the patient and management of the case. The second is a more forward-looking consideration: the use of genetic information derived from the patient or family to address the risks that future children in the immediate or extended family will have a genetic condition.

A comprehensive overview of medical genetics would fill a book at least, and is a topic more likely to be covered in medical, nursing, pharmacological, or allied health professional programs. Here we offer a brief introduction to two elements of medical genetics that demonstrate the broad relevance of the principles presented in this textbook. The first is the identification and classification of various types of hereditary disease, and the second is the role genetic counseling plays in medical genetics.

A.1 Hereditary Disease and Disease Genes

In some cases there is a one-to-one correlation between a hereditary disease and a gene whose mutation causes the disease. In other cases, the disease phenotype can be caused by a mutation of any one of multiple genes; and in still other cases, disease onset is influenced by genes along with environmental or developmental factors.

Typically, the first job of the medical geneticist is to correctly diagnose the condition so that genetic information can be used appropriately. But correctly diagnosing a genetic disease can be challenging. Hereditary diseases vary widely in their onset, their severity, and the frequencies with which they occur in populations. This means that the likelihood of encountering certain genetic diseases can be influenced by the population frequency of gene mutations, the population of origin of the patient, the degree of genetic relationship between the parents, and the occurrence of other factors that contribute to or modify the appearance of a disease.

The list of hereditary diseases and of genes whose mutations cause or contribute to hereditary disease grows almost by the day. In the Case Study at the end of Chapter 2, we discussed the cataloging of hereditary diseases and genes in the online human genetic database known as the Online Mendelian Index of Man (OMIM) and also looked at estimated rates of human gene mutations. You may refer to that case study for details on OMIM and its contents when OMIM is mentioned in the discussion below.

Types of Hereditary Disease

Hereditary disease has three major classifications. Within each of these classifications the conditions differ widely in onset, diagnosis, and management, and also in the probabilities of their recurrence in families.

Mendelian Conditions Conditions that are caused by the mutation of a single gene are Mendelian conditions. Among them, six patterns of inheritance are observed: autosomal dominant, autosomal recessive, X-linked dominant, X-linked recessive, Y-linked inheritance, and mitochondrial inheritance. Up to this point in the text, we have discussed the first five of these inheritance patterns (see Sections 2.6 and 3.5 for a review). Mitochondrial inheritance and human mitochondrial diseases are discussed in Chapter 17, and we will not address them here.

Mendelian conditions either can be inherited through alleles carried by one or both parents or can be the result of a new mutation. Whether the mutation is new or inherited has no effect on the condition itself; but it does influence the risk that the condition could recur in a subsequent child. We discuss this difference momentarily.

When the population as a whole is considered, it is common to find that a disease-producing gene has more than one mutant allele. Since these alleles differ from one another, they may have different effects on the phenotype. In other words, the phenotypic abnormalities or complications that develop may differ somewhat from case to case as the result of different mutations of a particular gene. For this reason, it is common to refer to Mendelian conditions as "syndromes," a term referring to a set of abnormalities, some or all of which may appear in a specific patient.

Chromosomal Conditions The presence of an extra chromosome, the absence of a chromosome, the duplication or deletion of a chromosome segment, and certain structural rearrangements of chromosomes can each lead to developmental and physical abnormalities. These conditions and their production are topics of discussion in Chapter 10. Humans are especially sensitive to changes in the number of copies of their genes, requiring two copies of each autosomal gene and one expressed copy of each X-linked, and in males, each Y-linked gene for normal development. The presence of three copies of genes, as happens in chromosome trisomy, when there are three copies of a chromosome instead of the normal homologous pair of chromosomes, or as occurs when a portion of a chromosome is duplicated, disrupts normal development and can produce substantial abnormalities.

Most of the conditions associated with chromosome numerical or structural changes are also classified as syndromes, since the specific characteristics can vary somewhat in different patients. For example, individuals with trisomy 21, or Down syndrome, collectively display a wide range of intellectual deficits and physical complications. One syndrome caused by chromosomal insufficiency is cri-du-chat syndrome (the French term means "cat's cry"), resulting from the deletion of a small segment of one copy of chromosome 5. The deletion creates a partial monosomy (one copy of a portion of a chromosome pair). Cri-du-chat syndrome, like most chromosomal conditions, produces a number of abnormalities, but it is recognized by the cat-like cry of newborn infants with the condition.

Similar to autosomal gains and losses, the gain or loss of all or part of the X or the Y chromosome also results in abnormal development. Changes in the number of sex chromosomes, such as sex chromosome trisomies XXY and XXX or the sex chromosome monosomy XO (one X chromosome and no second sex chromosome), each produce their own unique set of developmental anomalies.

For the most part, chromosomal conditions are the result of new mutations. Aberrations of chromosome number are most often caused by errors during meiotic cell division that lead to sperm or eggs whose nuclei contain the wrong number of chromosomes. Recall from Chapter 3 that normal human sperm and egg cells carry one chromosome from each homologous chromosome pair. The normal chromosome content of sperm or egg is the human haploid chromosome number $n = 23$. Errors during meiotic cell division can, for example, generate sperm or egg cells with an extra copy of a chromosome, such as $n + 1 = 24$ chromosomes. When such a cell is united at fertilization with a cell containing 23 chromosomes, the result is $n + n + 1 = 47$ chromosomes. This is the usual way trisomy 21 is produced.

Because chromosome aberrations are usually the result of spontaneous errors during meiotic cell division, their recurrence risk is generally low. There are certain exceptions, however. As we discuss in Chapter 10, maternal age at conception (or, in *in vitro* fertilization techniques, the age of the ovum) affects the likelihood of the occurrence of a meiotic cell division error that is strongly correlated with the chance of having a child with trisomy 21. This means that determining the recurrence risk of trisomy 21 must take the mother's age (or condition of the ovum) into account.

Multifactorial Conditions A number of human diseases and conditions occur through the influence of multiple genes along with nongenetic (environmental) factors. Conditions of this type, that include diabetes, many kinds of heart disease, certain types of cancer, and several other conditions, are called multifactorial conditions. This name indicates that inherited genetic variation may play a role in making some individuals more likely than others to develop particular conditions or diseases. It is common to refer to an "inherited susceptibility" to certain diseases in referring to individuals whose genotype puts them at higher risk for a disease than an average member of the general population.

Inherited susceptibilities to certain diseases vary between populations. This is often due to different frequencies of certain mutant alleles in different populations. Determining the risk of a multifactorial disease recurring in a family must take into account the incidence of diseases associated with particular susceptibility genotypes. A more detailed discussion of multifactorial disease is presented in Chapter 17.

Genetic Testing and Diagnosis

Clinical observations and examinations are the information-gathering step for diagnosing any condition, including genetic disease. Many genetic diseases first manifest symptoms in infants or children, so it is common for an obstetrician or a pediatrician to be the first clinician to note an unusual finding. On the other hand, a number of genetic conditions are very subtle and symptoms may not appear until later in life; some are even delayed until adulthood. In these cases, internists and general practitioners may be the medical personnel who first notice an abnormality. Often, owing to the large number of different genetic conditions and the relative rarity of many of them, personal physicians feel the need to refer their patients to larger regional hospitals where medical staff members include clinical

geneticists, genetic scientists, and genetic counselors. Even clinicians with a specialty in genetics may need assistance from medical personnel with expertise in particular body systems to accurately diagnose and counsel individuals who may have inherited certain rare genetic conditions.

Today, accurate clinical diagnosis of genetic diseases and conditions is greatly aided by the availability of molecularly based genetic tests that use blood and tissues as the source of DNA and RNA for the identification of gene mutations. These tissues can also be sources of proteins for biochemical analysis and of material used to culture cells and examine chromosomes. There are three general categories of genetic testing: molecular analysis, biochemical analysis, and chromosome analysis. Molecular analysis of DNA or RNA is very useful when there is the suspicion of a specific Mendelian condition. This type of analysis is best applied when specific genes known to be involved in the condition can be tested, and especially when specific gene mutations can be targeted for examination. Molecular analysis can be effective in identifying both newly occurring mutations and mutations passed from parents to affected children.

Biochemical analysis takes blood or tissues from affected body organs or systems and assays them for the absence or presence of particular proteins, studies them to determine whether levels of particular proteins are within normal ranges, or examines them for the presence of protein variants associated with disease. This approach is used in diagnosing many kinds of disease, including many genetic diseases.

Chromosome analysis can be used in the diagnosis of a fetus or a newborn infant affected by malformations associated with a chromosomal condition. It also aids in diagnosing patients of any age who have otherwise unexplained mental impairment or physical abnormalities and in cases of long-term infertility in adults.

In addition to their diagnostic applications, these three approaches to genetic analysis have other applications as well. The molecular details of these testing approaches are discussed in Application Chapter B: Human Genetic Screening. All three forms of testing can be made use of in the following assessment strategies.

Carrier Testing Carrier testing is the use of a molecular, biochemical, or chromosomal analysis to identify individuals who do not have a genetic condition but who are heterozygous and carry recessive alleles for autosomal or X-linked conditions in their genotype that might be passed to a child, or who carry a chromosome abnormality that could produce a chromosome condition in a future child. Carrier testing can be done as part of a genetic assessment of a family or it can be done on a population or community-wide basis as part of a public health effort to identify carriers.

Population-based carrier testing, or community-based carrier testing, usually focuses on individuals of specific backgrounds in which the frequency of a certain genetic disease is high and where a large proportion of the population are carriers. An example is Tay–Sachs disease (OMIM 272800), a fatal autosomal recessive condition that manifests in infants. Tay–Sachs disease, caused by the absence of the enzyme hexosaminidase A (hexA), is a progressive neuromuscular disorder that is usually fatal in childhood. The mutant allele of hexA is particularly frequent in Ashkenazi Jewish populations originating in Eastern Europe. Carrier testing programs targeting teenagers and young adults of Ashkenazi descent are designed to identify carriers and to provide information about the disease and about reproductive options if two prospective parents are both carriers of the mutant allele.

Presymptomatic Testing Presymptomatic testing is carried out for genetic conditions that have a late age of onset. Huntington disease (HD), discussed in Chapter 4 (see Figure 4.11), is one example of a genetic disease that appears later in life and has a variable age of onset. By age 40, only about 50% of people who carry the autosomal dominant mutant allele for HD have symptoms of the disease. Many people who have a parent with HD wish to know definitively whether or not they carry the mutation. Presymptomatic testing can make that determination by testing DNA to identify a mutation of the affected gene.

Newborn Testing Newborn testing consists of a set of mandated genetic tests that together require only a few drops of blood taken by "heel stick" from a newborn infant. (A heel stick is, quite literally, the pricking of a newborn's heel with a small lancet to collect a small amount of blood.) Every state in the United States, and many foreign countries as well, requires this collection of a newborn's blood, which is then tested for three dozen or more rare genetic diseases that are preventable or can have their symptoms greatly ameliorated by early and ongoing treatment, as the case of ARG described at the beginning of this chapter exemplifies. Treatment regimens include replacing missing or defective enzymes or other substances, dietary supplementation or dietary restriction, removal of toxic byproducts, or blocking of a pathogenic process. (See Application Chapter B: Human Genetic Screening for more details on newborn genetic testing.)

Prenatal Testing Prenatal testing is performed during pregnancy for the purpose of determining whether a fetus has a particular condition or disorder. Prenatal testing most commonly either collects a biopsy of tissue from the placental chorion through chorionic villus sampling (CVS) or collects a small amount of amniotic fluid from the amniotic sac through amniocentesis. Other methods of collecting either fetal tissue for DNA analysis or fluids for biochemical analysis can also be used.

In decades past, the principal focus of prenatal testing was to identify chromosome abnormalities. Chromosome analyses are performed by culturing cells collected by CVS or amniocentesis and then visualizing the chromosomes using microscopy. Conditions such as trisomy 21 and other chromosomal conditions can be identified *in utero* by these methods. More frequently today, prenatal testing is performed to determine whether a fetus has a particular genetic disorder. This can involve tissue collection by CVS, amniocentesis, or another method, isolation of DNA from the collected tissues, and testing the DNA for mutations of specific genes involved in producing a genetic disease or condition.

A.2 Genetic Counseling

Genetic counseling is an integral part of medical genetics. It is provided by specially trained professionals who have strong practical skills and knowledge both in genetics and in counseling. A genetic counselor may be the first point of contact a patient or family has with clinical genetics services, and there may be multiple contacts with the genetic counselor during and after the process of genetic testing. This individual is responsible for communicating all relevant information about upcoming genetic tests or the results of genetic tests. Genetic counselors in the United States and Canada complete a training program accredited, in the United States, by the American Board of Genetic Counseling, and in Canada, by the Canadian Board of Genetic Counselling. Europe also has a number of genetic counseling organizations that certify counselors in various countries. At the end of 2016 there were three dozen accredited genetic counseling programs in the United States and three additional programs in Canada. At that time there were more than 4000 certified genetic counselors in the United States and smaller numbers in Canada, European countries, and other countries around the world. The field is expected to grow over the next decade as the need for genetic counselors increases.

Genetic counselors are, most frequently, part of a large medical group that provides genetic services or are on the staff of hospitals that offer clinical genetics. Increasingly, however, genetic counselors are sole practitioners or work in small groups with business models and structures similar to those of psychologists in private practice. The daily work of genetic counselors includes a great deal of counseling to help individuals, identified as **consultands**, manage their concerns and the personal, familial, and social issues related to the genetic condition in question. In contrast to the large amount of time invested in counseling, it is fair to say that the genetic component of genetic counseling is an important but secondary activity.

Indicators and Goals of Genetic Counseling

There are many reasons to seek genetic counseling. Table A.1 lists the most common situations in which genetic counseling may be sought or recommended. Typically, the consultand

Table A.1	Common Indicators for Genetic Counseling Referral

1. A previous child with a genetic or chromosome condition
2. A family history of a genetic or chromosome condition
3. Advanced maternal age or other indicator of elevated risk in pregnancy
4. Fetal exposure to a toxic or harmful compound
5. Prolonged infertility or repeated pregnancy loss
6. New diagnosis of a genetic or chromosome condition
7. Consultation for pre- or -postgenetic or chromosome test risk assessment

Table A.2	Goals of Genetic Counseling

1. Provide comprehensive information before or after a genetic or chromosomal test or diagnosis, including test results, available particulars about the course of the condition, and available medical management options.
2. Explain risk recurrence, the meaning of the recurrence risk estimate, and the role genetics plays in the condition.
3. Identify the beliefs, values, and relationships that are affected by the presence of a current or future genetic or chromosomal condition.
4. Identify and determine the course of action most appropriate for the consultand given the information available.
5. Provide referrals to support groups or services.

is an adult, couple, or family who either has a child with a genetic or chromosomal condition or has a family history of a condition. The genetic counselor will be asked to provide detailed, complete, and understandable information about the case and will be called upon to provide nondirective counseling that permits and encourages the consultand to understand and review the possible courses of action, and to facilitate the decision-making process. Providing genetic counseling is rarely a one-time event. Rather, genetic counseling is an ongoing process of communication designed to help the consultand address the complex personal, familial, and social issues associated with a genetic or chromosomal condition.

Genetic counseling has several goals as enumerated in Table A.2. Achieving these goals is aided by the active participation of the genetic counselor in the clinical team managing the case. For this reason, genetic counselors usually work closely with medical geneticists, treating physicians, medical laboratory personnel, and social service agencies or groups to coordinate a comprehensive, team-based plan for aiding the consultand in the near and long term.

Assessing and Communicating Risks and Options

A principal goal of genetic counseling is to provide the consultand with comprehensive, understandable medical information about a current condition or, where appropriate, about the risk of recurrence of a condition in a future pregnancy. With this information in hand, the consultand and the genetic counselor can talk through the consultand's options, and the consultand can reach a decision regarding immediate needs or begin to prepare for situations that may arise in the future.

Immediate Decision Making To illustrate the kind of information and discussion that might occur in a case requiring immediate decision making, let's look at a hypothetical situation.

Example Case 1: The consultand in this case is C.R., who is 40 years old. She has two healthy children, ages 8 and 12, and is in her 14th week of an unplanned pregnancy. As a consequence of her age, C.R. has been offered and has

taken a maternal serum screen (MSS), in which maternal blood is drawn and tested to establish the circulating levels of four compounds. These can indicate the possibility of elevated risk for chromosome conditions, including trisomy 21 (Down syndrome) and trisomy 18 (Edward syndrome), as well as two neural tube defects, spina bifida (a serious condition that causes permanent paralysis) and anencephaly (a fatal condition of abnormal brain development). An MSS result indicating the possibility of any of these conditions can be followed up with ultrasound to examine the fetus for visual evidence of a neural tube defect, or with amniocentesis or CVS to collect fetal cells for chromosome inspection.

At age 40, the risk of Down syndrome is the highest of the four conditions. It increases with maternal age, especially after age 35, and at age 40 is nearly 1 in 100. This risk of Down syndrome was the reason for recommending MSS testing to C.R. We discuss this risk and its possible causes in Chapter 10.

Unfortunately, the MSS result indicates an increased possibility of Down syndrome, and C.R. is referred to a genetic counselor for follow-up discussion. When MSS indicates an increased chance of Down syndrome, it is correct in about 80% of cases. The false-positive rate, the rate at which the MSS results indicate the possibility of Down syndrome when the condition is not present, is about 9%.

The medical information collected by C.R.'s team would include her medical history and information on her current pregnancy, along with her MSS test results. At the meeting with the genetic counselor, C.R. and her partner hear about the results of MSS, are told about the test's predictive accuracy and the rate of false-positive results, and are informed that they have the option of additional follow-up with either amniocentesis or CVS. The genetic counselor explains that the results of these tests take about 2 weeks to complete and that counseling services would be available to C.R. and her partner during the wait. The results would be explained as soon as they become available, and the options at that point would be discussed. The couple are also told that they can opt not to have additional follow-up testing.

C.R. and her partner decide to have CVS performed to assess the fetal chromosomes. They have two counseling sessions while they wait for the test results, to talk about their concerns and about ways to manage their stress. C.R. and her partner are very happy when C.R.'s obstetrician tells them that the result of CVS testing indicates the normal diploid count of 46 chromosomes in the fetus. C.R.'s child does not have Down syndrome and her MSS result was apparently a false-positive. C.R. and her partner have one final visit with the genetic counselor at which the CVS test result is confirmed, they are shown a karyotype (see Chapter 11 for discussion) of the fetal chromosomes, and they are able to express their relief that the fetus is healthy. C.R. is closely followed for the rest of her pregnancy and delivers a healthy baby girl after 39 weeks of gestation.

Assessment of Future Risk Estimating the likelihood that a future fetus will have a genetic condition is a central aim of genetic counseling. The approaches required to estimate the chance of a genetic condition appearing or to estimate the likelihood of any particular genotype occurring depend on the pattern of inheritance of the trait, the structure of the family, and the information available about the genotypes of family members.

If the genotypes of parents can be identified directly by molecular or biochemical testing, that is the surest way to determine the risk of a genetic condition occurring in an individual or of determining carrier status for a condition. When direct testing is not available, probability estimates can be made using a methodology first described by Reverend Thomas Bayes in 1763. Known as **Bayesian analysis**, this method of determining the probability of a certain genotype occurring in a certain family member uses known or inferred genotype information along with other information available from the offspring previously produced by a set of parents.

Bayesian analysis begins by establishing the **prior probability** of a genotype. This is often the Mendelian probability, but more formally it is the likelihood that the hypothesis that an individual has a certain genotype is true. The Bayesian analysis sets prior probabilities for each possible genotype for the individual of interest. The analysis then identifies other available information, such as the traits of other offspring of the same parents who were born before the individual of interest, and uses it to calculate a **conditional probability**. (See the discussion of conditional probability in Chapter 2, Section 2.4, for a review). The next step is to determine the **joint probability** of the genotype of an individual. This is the product of the prior probability and the conditional probability. In many cases, this serves as the estimate of the likelihood of an individual having a certain genotype (i.e., a disease genotype) or phenotype (i.e., the disease phenotype) given all the information available in the family.

Bayesian calculations of an individual's genotype can be considerably simplified by information known or inferred from the available family data. Let's consider two example

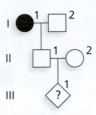

Figure A.1   The family described in Example Case 2. The diamond-shaped symbol with the question mark is a future child.

cases involving families in which an autosomal recessive condition occurs for which 1 in 25 people in the general population, or 4% of the general population, are heterozygous carriers of the condition.

Example Case 2: The consultands are II-1 and II-2 in **Figure A.1.** They plan to have a family in the future but are concerned about the risk that a child of theirs will have the autosomal recessive condition that occurs in I-1, the mother of II-1. Given the pedigree shown in Figure A.1, the matter at hand is to determine the probability that a future child (III-1, symbolized by a diamond shape with a question mark) will have the recessive condition. The required equation can be stated as

(carrier probability of parent 1) $\times$
(carrier probability of parent 2) $\times$
(probability the child inherits both recessive alleles if both parents are carriers) $= x.$

An examination of the pedigree and interpretation of the genotypes of family members tells us that II-1 is a heterozygous carrier with a probability of 1.0. He does not have the condition, but his mother (I-1) has the recessive condition and his father (I-2) does not. II-1 has received a recessive allele from his mother and a dominant allele from his father. This is a conditional probability based on analysis of the pedigree. The prior probability that II-1 is a heterozygous carrier is 4%, or 0.04, which is the 1 in 25 population frequency of carriers. If both II-1 and II-2 are carriers, there is a 25% chance (0.25) that III-1 will have the recessive condition. In this case the joint probability that III-1 has the recessive condition is $(0.04)(0.25) = 0.01$, or 1% (1 in 100).

The discussion between the genetic counselor and the consultands will inform the couple of the 1% chance a future child of theirs will have the recessive condition. The counselor can, and very likely will, contrast that probability with two other probabilities. One is the corresponding 99% chance that a child of theirs *will not* have the recessive condition. The second contrasting probability is the chance that two individuals selected at random from the general population will have a child with the recessive condition. This chance is $(0.04)(0.04)(0.25) = 0.0004$, or about 1 in 2500. In that equation, each 0.04 value is the chance a person is a heterozygous carrier, and 0.25 is the chance two heterozygotes will have a child with the recessive

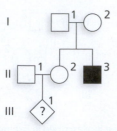

Figure A.2 The family described in Example Case 3.

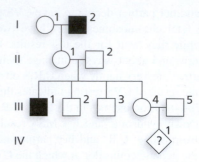

Figure A.3 The family described in Example Case 4.

condition. Due to the family history, the consultands have about a 25-fold increased risk of having a child with the recessive condition compared to random members of the population at large.

Example Case 3: **Figure A.2** shows the occurrence in a different family of the same autosomal recessive condition seen in Example Case 2. In this family there is less information about the genotypes of family members than in the previous case. In this case, the consultands are II-1 and II-2 who are planning a family in the future. Their question concerns the probability that a future child (identified as III-1) will have the recessive condition. In this case, we know that both I-1 and I-2 must be heterozygous carriers since their child II-3 has the recessive condition. The chance that his sister II-2 is a heterozygous carrier requires a conditional probability estimate. In this case, II-2 is produced by two heterozygous carriers, but she has the dominant phenotype. Assuming there is no molecular test for carrier status, and thinking back to our discussion of conditional probability in Section 2.4 (see page 47 for details), we calculate the conditional probability that II-2 is heterozygous as 2/3, or 0.66. As in the previous family, the chance II-1 is a heterozygous carrier is 0.04, the population average, and if both II-1 and II-2 are carriers there is a 25% chance their child III-1 will have the recessive condition. Taking all this into account, the chance of III-1 having the condition is $(0.66)(0.04)(0.25) = 0.0066$, about 1 in 170. The consultands can therefore be told that there is less than a 1% chance a child of theirs will have the recessive condition and, in contrast, about a 99.3 percent chance the child will be free of the condition.

Similar kinds of estimates are made for X-linked traits. As an example, let's look at two families in which a female is at risk for being a carrier of an X-linked recessive condition and is concerned about having a child with the condition.

Example Case 4: The consultands, shown as III-4 and III-5 in **Figure A.3**, are concerned about a future child of theirs, shown as IV-1, having a rare X-linked recessive condition that affected I-2, the grandfather of III-4. In this family, II-1 is an obligate carrier of the X-linked recessive condition since her father (I-2) had the condition and must have passed his X-chromosome to his daughter. An *obligate carrier* is someone who does not have the condition

but according to the family pedigree must be a carrier based on the transmission pattern observed in the pedigree. Female III-4 has received the X chromosome from her father, II-2, and has a 50% chance of having received the X chromosome carrying the recessive allele from her mother, II-1. Since III-5 does not have the condition, his X chromosome carries the dominant wild-type allele.

For IV-1 to have the recessive condition, the child must be a boy. This probability is 50%. Male III-5 will pass his Y chromosome to his son, and if III-4 is a carrier and passes her recessive-bearing X chromosome to the child, IV-1 would be a hemizygous male with the recessive condition. If IV-1 were a girl, she could not be homozygous for the X-linked recessive condition since the father's X chromosome carries the dominant allele. If III-4 is a carrier and if she has a son, there is a 50% chance he will inherit his mother's recessive-bearing X chromosome and a 50% chance he will inherit her dominant-bearing X chromosome. The Bayesian calculation multiplies the 50% chance of III-4 being a carrier, times the 50% chance the couple has a boy times the 50% chance the boy inherits the recessive-bearing maternal X chromosome. The probability of III-4 and III-5 having a child with the X-linked recessive condition is $(0.50)(0.50)(0.50) = 0.125$, or 12.5%.

The consultands can be told of this joint probability of having a child with the X-linked recessive condition. The overall estimate can be broken down further by the sex of the child. The genetic counselor can say that if the child is a girl there is a zero probability of the condition appearing and if it is a boy there is a 1 in 4 chance he will have the condition. This is the 50% chance that II-4 is a heterozygous carrier times the 50% chance that the boy inherits the recessive allele from III-4. If this couple has boys who are not affected by the condition, Bayes's theorem dictates that each time a male child is born with the dominant phenotype, the chance of the couple producing a boy with the recessive condition will be reduced. The final example case illustrates how this calculation is applied to family analysis.

Example Case 5: The family shown in **Figure A.4** presents a complex Bayesian analysis. The consultands are III-4 and III-5, and as with the previous family they are concerned

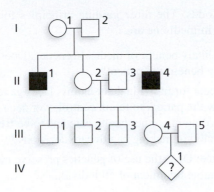

Figure A.4 The family described in Example Case 5.

about the risk that a child of theirs has the X-linked recessive condition that affects II-1 and II-4, the uncles of III-4. I-1 is an obligate heterozygous carrier of the X-linked condition who has passed the recessive allele to her two sons (II-1 and II-4). Male II-3 is hemizygous for the dominant allele, but the genotype of II-2 is not certain. She could be a heterozygous carrier or she could be homozygous dominant. This uncertainty regarding genotype requires determining two values for III-4, one for the chance she is a carrier and the other for the chance she is not a carrier.

Female III-4 is the youngest of four children. Each of her older siblings is a brother. Had any one of them exhibited the recessive condition, it would be certain that II-2 is a carrier, and the calculation of risk for a child of III-4 and III-5 would be made as shown in the previous example. None of the three brothers have the recessive X-linked condition, however, so the genotype of II-2 remains uncertain. The prior probability that II-2 is a carrier is 50%. This is the one-half chance that she has inherited her mother's recessive-bearing X chromosome. That three sons with the dominant phenotype have been born to II-2, however, impacts the determination that III-4 is a carrier because the Bayesian probability estimate is reduced for each male sibling of III-4 who has the dominant phenotype.

The first step in answering the question from III-4 and III-5 is to estimate the genotype probabilities for II-2. **Table A.3** shows the Bayesian calculation for two genotype hypotheses for II-2. Hypothesis 1 calculates the chance that II-2 is a carrier and hypothesis 2 the chance that she is not a carrier. The prior probability that she is a carrier is $\frac{1}{2}$ (hypothesis 1). Similarly, there is a $\frac{1}{2}$ chance she is not a carrier (hypothesis 2). If she is not a carrier, the conditional probability that she passes the dominant-bearing X chromosome is 1.0, since she has no other allele to pass. If she is a carrier, however, the conditional probability is $\frac{1}{2}$ for each of her three sons. This is calculated as $\left(\frac{1}{2}\right)^3 = \frac{1}{8}$ The joint probability for hypothesis 2 is the $\frac{1}{2}$ chance, whereas for the hypothesis that she is a carrier, the joint probability is $\frac{1}{2} \times \frac{1}{8} = \frac{1}{16}$, or 0.0625. The posterior probability for each hypothesis is calculated as the joint probability for the hypothesis divided by the sum of the two joint probabilities. These values are 0.111 as the estimate of the likelihood II-2 is a carrier and 0.889 as the probability she is not a carrier.

With these genotype estimates in hand, the chance III-4 is a carrier is one-half her mother's chance, or $(0.50)(0.111) = 0.055$, about 5.5%. From this value the genetic counselor can calculate that for III-4 and III-5 to have a child with the X-linked recessive phenotype the child must be a boy (probability 50%) who inherits the recessive-bearing X chromosome (probability 50%). The chance of this outcome is $(0.055)(0.50)(0.50) = 0.01375$, or just a little less than 1.4%. This is the estimated chance of having a child with the X-linked recessive condition that the genetic counselor will report to the consultands along with the statement that there is a greater than 98% chance that a child of the couple will not have the X-linked condition.

The use of Bayesian analysis is a fundamental element of the genetic analysis a genetic counselor will employ in determining the risk of particular genotype or phenotype outcomes for his or her consultands. Applying Bayesian analysis requires a clear understanding of patterns of hereditary transmission for genetic conditions and comprehension of the transmission probabilities of alleles under various scenarios. Determining and delivering these estimates is part of the initial discussion between a genetic counselor and his or her consultands, and it is followed up with all necessary explanations and by counseling to help the consultands understand the estimate and make any decisions that follow from it.

Ethical Issues in Genetic Medicine

Genetic science and the practice and application of genetics in a medical context has advanced more quickly than the public debate over the ethical guidelines and rules that should govern the use of human genetic information. The privacy of personal genetic and genomic information is an important part of the practice of genetic medicine, just as all personal information is important in medical practice as a whole. Because the availability of genetic information is new, however, it has merited special study. Part

Table A.3	Bayesian Analysis of the Genotype of II-2 in Figure A.4	
	Hypothesis 1	**Hypothesis 2**
	(II-2 is a carrier)	(II-2 is not a carrier)
Prior probability	$\frac{1}{2}$	$\frac{1}{2}$
Conditional probability	$\left(\frac{1}{2}\right)^3 = \frac{1}{8}$	1
Joint probability	$\frac{1}{2} \times \frac{1}{8} = \frac{1}{16} = 0.0625$	$\frac{1}{2} \times 1 = \frac{1}{2}$

of the funding for the Human Genome Project was earmarked for an initiative supporting research and education concerning the Ethical, Legal, and Social Implications (ELSI) of the project. The workshops, research, pre- and postdoctoral support, and yearly conferences sponsored by ELSI focused on four specific areas of investigation that are affected by the collection of personal genetic or genomic information:

1. **Genetic Research:** Examining the design, conduct, and analysis of research and the dissemination of personal genetic or genomic information, especially with regard to detailed health information.

2. **Genetic Health Care:** Studying the uses of genetic or genomic information and the influence this information has on health care. In addition, examining the implications of this use for individuals, families, and society.

3. **Societal Issues of Genetics and Genomics:** Investigation of the beliefs, practices, and policies surrounding the collection and use of genetic and genomic information. Additionally, studying how information can be understood with respect to health, disease, and individual responsibility.

4. **Legal, Regulatory, and Public Policy Issues:** Examining the impact of current policies and regulations on genetic and genomic information collection and use, and recommending new regulations and policies as needed.

Beyond this effort, United States federal public policy has addressed some elements of the use and sharing of personal genetic information through two laws. In 2008, Congress passed the Genetic Information Nondiscrimination Act (GINA) that severely restricts the use of personal genetic information in issuing health insurance and life insurance, and in employment decisions. This protection was bolstered in 2010 with passage of the Affordable Care Act (ACA) that excluded the use of personal genetic information in issuing health insurance as part of the clause eliminating preexisting conditions as a basis for rejection.

Genetic Counseling and Ethical Issues

These GINA and ACA regulations help ease the concern that personal genetic or genomic information might be used by external entities to make decisions about an individual's employment or insurance coverage, but they do not address other ethical issues stemming from medical genetics. Three fundamental principles guide medical genetics, and ethical dilemmas often arise when these principles are perceived to be in conflict. One important role for genetic counseling is to help individuals and families make decisions in situations where these principles seem

to be at odds. The three guiding principles for the use of genetics in medicine are:

1. The likely benefit of medical genetics: Does genetic study benefit the patient?

2. Respect for individual autonomy: Does genetic study allow the patient to retain control over decisions regarding his or her health care and to be free from coercion in making health care decisions?

3. Justice: Does the use of genetics preserve the fair and equitable treatment of all individuals?

Ethical dilemmas presented by genetic testing are a frequent topic of discussion between genetic counselors and consultands. Three areas where dilemmas commonly arise are prenatal genetic and chromosome testing, newborn genetic screening, and testing for genetic predisposition.

Prenatal Genetic and Chromosome Testing Prenatal genetic testing is performed for a variety of reasons and for a wide range of genetic and chromosome conditions. Results pointing to the absence of a condition are a welcome outcome, although if the condition runs in the family, counseling may be indicated to help individuals deal with "survivor guilt." Chromosome conditions are very unlikely to be treatable, so a result indicating the presence of such a condition in a fetus may well trigger ethical conflicts about keeping or terminating an affected pregnancy. Or the degree of physical or mental impairment or the prognosis may be variable, which can also trigger ethical concerns and present difficult choices that require sorting out and discussing with a counselor.

A number of genetic conditions are amenable to treatment that can dramatically prolong and improve the quality of life. Cystic fibrosis, an autosomal recessive condition that affects respiration and causes chronic and serious respiratory infections, and severe combined immunodeficiency syndrome are examples of genetic diseases for which effective symptomatic treatments are routine. It is an open debate as to whether or not such conditions are good candidates for prenatal genetic testing. Detecting one of these conditions is very unlikely to lead to pregnancy termination. Aside from facilitating treatment early in infancy, there may be little to gain from performing such tests. On the other hand, with a genetic condition such as Tay–Sachs disease that is invariably fatal and for which no effective treatment is known, a good case can be made for prenatal genetic testing.

Newborn Genetic Screening Much like mandated vaccination programs, newborn genetic screening is a public policy intended to save lives, reduce medical costs to society, and support the well-being of families. Identification of a targeted genetic condition prompts immediate initiation of treatment, such as permanent dietary restrictions or dietary supplements, administration of medication, or other kinds of biochemical or physical therapies. Few if any ethical discussions take place around newborn testing, but consultands and families often benefit from counseling to manage the personal and family dynamics affected by a sick child.

Testing for Genetic Predisposition Genetic testing may also be done to detect the presence of a genetic variant that is likely to produce disease in the future (presymptomatic genetic testing) or the presence of a variant that confers additional risk of disease under particular conditions (testing for inherited susceptibility to a disease). The ethical issues surrounding both of these types of testing can be profound.

The autosomal dominant condition Huntington disease (HD) is an example of a condition with a delayed age of onset that is virtually certain to manifest devastating symptoms during the person's life. The average age of onset is nearly 40 years (see Section 4.1 and Figure 4.11). Currently there is no effective treatment for HD. Among the challenges HD presents is that, often, because of its dominant nature, a person inheriting the disease has dealt with the disease in a parent. Further, the average age of onset is old enough that a person can pass the mutant allele to his or her child before beginning to experience any of the symptoms. Both of these can be important factors in the decision to undergo presymptomatic genetic testing. For young people, the implications of finding out that the disease allele is present can have a profound effect on life choices. Beyond the concern about when symptoms might appear and how rapidly they will progress are lifestyle choices such as decisions about going to college, marrying, and saving for retirement. An additional issue raised by genetic testing for a condition like HD is that if the disease allele is detected in a consultand, then the consultand's siblings, too, each have a 50% risk of having inherited the mutant allele, and they may not yet be aware or may not wish to be informed of their risk.

A thorough consideration of all of the implications of presymptomatic test results, both personal and familial, by both the consultand and by family members, is required before the decision is made to go forward with the testing. Counseling is provided again by a genetic counselor both after the test is performed (to allow a reconsideration of the consequences of the result) and after the results are made available (to facilitate decision making in response to the test result).

Conditions such as familial breast and ovarian cancer present a different set of challenges. Certain mutations of the *BRCA1* or *BRCA2* genes can increase a woman's lifetime risk of breast or ovarian cancer. For the general population, this risk is about 11% (about 1 in 9). For women who carry certain *BRCA1* mutations, the lifetime risk of breast cancer can be 60 to 70%. Not all mutations of these genes produce the same level of increased risk, and some appear not to increase the lifetime risk of cancer at all. In this case, even the most severe mutation in the most at-risk population leaves about a 30 to 40% chance of no cancer developing.

Cases of breast or ovarian cancer that result from *BRCA1* or *BRCA2* mutations tend to cluster in families and to have an age of onset in the 30s or 40s. Women in these families are frequently aware of the potential risk and may pursue genetic testing to discover if they have such a mutation. The decision to undergo genetic testing requires careful consideration under the guidance of a genetic counselor who will explain the meaning of a positive result (indicating a mutation is present) and a negative (no mutation) test result. The counselor will also lead the consultand through the medical options should the test result be positive for a mutation, both before testing and after the result is known. These options include regular and intensive monitoring to detect cancer at its early stages, and prophylactic mastectomy (surgical removal of the breasts) or oophorectomy (surgical removal of the ovaries) to eliminate the risk of disease in those organs. We discuss more about cancer genetics in Application Chapter C: The Genetics of Cancer.

In Closing

The explosion of knowledge in genetics over the past 50 years has had profound impacts on the understanding of human heredity and genetic diseases and on the practice of medical genetics. In particular, the Human Genome Project has been instrumental in identifying and locating human genes, including genes whose mutations lead to genetic disease. Human medicine relies much more heavily on genetics and genomics today than it did just a decade or so ago, and the level of reliance is bound to increase in the next decade. The concept of "personalized medicine," in which the genetic profile of a patient or of the disease in a patient is used to help select the most effective treatment regimen, is already beginning to affect the practice of medicine. The scope of this personalization of medicine will likely reduce the notion that "one size fits all" when it comes to the treatment of many diseases and conditions.

As in recent decades, genetic counselors will continue to play a pivotal role in genetic medicine. In fact, most experts in the field expect the need for genetic counselors to increase in the future. Despite the vast increase in knowledge about human genetics, the goal of genetic medicine is not to acquire knowledge for its own sake but instead to use the acquired knowledge to improve the health and well-being of patients, to relieve suffering, and to ensure the fair treatment and dignity of all individuals who come into contact with the field of genetic medicine and its practitioners.

PROBLEMS

For answers to selected even-numbered problems, see Appendix: Answers.

1. Match each statement (a–e) with the best answer from the following list: consultand, 50%, prior probability, 66.7%, obligate carrier, 100%.

   a. The Mendelian risk that a person is a heterozygous carrier of a recessive condition.

   b. A person who on the basis of family history must be a heterozygous carrier of a recessive mutant allele.

   c. The probability that the healthy brother of a woman with an autosomal recessive condition is a heterozygous carrier.

   d. The person receiving genetic counseling.

   e. The probability that the son of a woman with an autosomal recessive condition is a heterozygous carrier.

2. Go online to the Mendelian Index of Man (OMIM) website. Look up the following genetic conditions and answer the questions posed about them.

   a. Look up Tay–Sachs disease (TSD), OMIM number 272800, and give the name and abbreviation of the affected gene and the chromosome location of the gene.

   b. Go to the "Population Genetics" section discussing the TSD gene. In a few sentences, summarize the human population in which TSD is most frequently found and give the approximate frequency of heterozygous carriers for the TSD mutation in North American Jews.

   c. Look up cystic fibrosis (CF), OMIM 602421, and give the gene name and abbreviation and the chromosome location of the gene.

   d. Go to the "Molecular Genetics" section and describe the most common mutation of the CF gene.

3. A couple comes into your genetic counseling practice with a question about the chance a future child of theirs might have a genetic disease. Three or four men in the woman's family, including her father, had a condition that might be genetic. Although her father is still alive, she has had little contact with him for much of her life and cannot describe or name the condition. Her partner is a healthy man whose family has no history indicating the presence of a genetic condition. To provide more information about this possible genetic condition for the couple, what is the first step you recommend?

4. A man, J.B., has a sister with autosomal recessive galactosemia (OMIM 230400), and his partner, S.B., has a brother with galactosemia. Galactosemia is a serious condition caused by an enzyme deficiency that prevents the metabolism of the sugar galactose. Neither J.B. nor S.B. has galactosemia, but they are concerned about the risk that a future child of theirs will have the condition. What is the probability their first child will have galactosemia?

5. A woman, S.R., had a maternal grandfather with hemophilia A (OMIM 306700), an X-linked recessive condition that reduces blood clotting. S.R.'s maternal grandmother and paternal grandparents are free of the condition, as is her partner, his parents, and his grandparents. S.R. has no siblings. She wants to know the chance that a son of hers will have the condition. What is that probability?

6. A 40-year-old woman whose father had Huntington disease currently shows no symptoms of the disease. She is newly pregnant with her first child and seeks your best estimate of the chance her child will inherit the disease. What is your estimate and how did you arrive at it? (*Hint:* See Figure 4.11)

DNA Structure and Replication

7

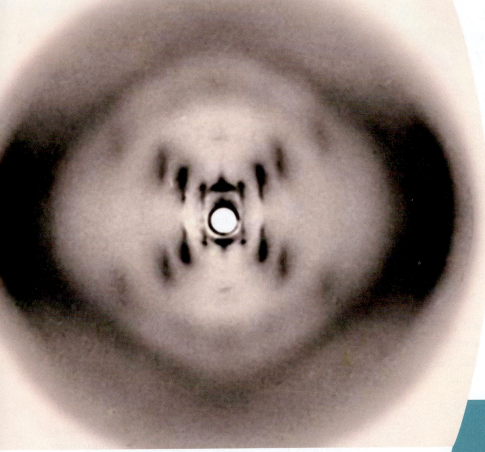

Rosalind Franklin used the X-ray diffraction method to produce this image of double-stranded DNA that is known as *Photo 51*. Photo 51 is the first visual experimental evidence supporting the model that DNA contains two strands twisted around one another.

he central dogma of biology identifies DNA as the repository of genomic information for organisms and describes its key role in the production of RNA transcripts of genes leading to the production of polypeptides (see Figure 1.9). DNA's ongoing role in these processes requires its faithful replication in each cell cycle, and that is the subject of this chapter.

In Chapter 1, we reviewed the primary and secondary structures of DNA and RNA and the fundamentals of DNA replication. In this chapter, we discuss the structure of DNA in greater detail and extend the earlier description to include the molecular processes occurring in DNA replication. We also examine two analytical methodologies—polymerase chain reaction (PCR) and DNA sequencing techniques—that were

CHAPTER OUTLINE

7.1 DNA Is the Hereditary Molecule of Life

7.2 The DNA Double Helix Consists of Two Complementary and Antiparallel Strands

7.3 DNA Replication Is Semiconservative and Bidirectional

7.4 DNA Replication Precisely Duplicates the Genetic Material

7.5 Methods of Molecular Genetic Analysis Make Use of DNA Replication Processes

ESSENTIAL IDEAS

▌ Seventy-five years of observations and analysis culminated in the identification of DNA as the hereditary molecule.

▌ DNA is a double-stranded molecule consisting of four kinds of nucleotides, abbreviated A, T, C, and G, that is held together by a mechanism of complementary base pairing.

▌ DNA replication faithfully duplicates the genome by a semiconservative process that progresses bidirectionally from each origin of replication.

▌ Origins of replication are defined by their nucleotide sequence. Numerous proteins and enzymes act in concert to produce two identical DNA duplexes.

▌ Laboratory techniques based on a molecular understanding of DNA replication perform targeted replication of short DNA sequences and sequence DNA.

235

developed as an outcome of the understanding of replication. The Case Study at the end of the chapter discusses some human hereditary conditions caused by mutations of genes for critically important proteins involved in DNA replication.

7.1 DNA Is the Hereditary Molecule of Life

DNA (deoxyribonucleic acid) is the hereditary molecule of life. Our contemporary understanding of hereditary transmission and the evolution of species is rooted in this fact. Long before the hereditary role of DNA was established, however, research had identified five essential characteristics of hereditary material. The hereditary material must be

1. Localized to the nucleus, and a component of chromosomes
2. Present in a stable form in cells
3. Sufficiently complex to contain the genetic information required to direct the structure, function, development, and reproduction of organisms
4. Able to accurately replicate itself so that daughter cells contain the same information as parental cells
5. Mutable, undergoing mutation at a low rate that introduces genetic variation and serves as a foundation for evolutionary change

Chromosomes Contain DNA

The weakly acidic substance known today as DNA was first noticed in 1869, when Friedrich Miescher isolated it from the nuclei of white blood cells in a mixture of nucleic acids and proteins he called "nuclein". At the same time Miescher was isolating nuclein, microscopic studies were identifying the fusion of male and female nuclei during reproduction. In addition, microscopic analysis of cells and reproduction identified chromosomes in cell nuclei and also determined that the nuclei of different species contain different numbers of chromosomes. Furthermore, biologists determined that the chromosome contributions of males and females to fertilization were equal in terms of chromosome number.

These and other observations led to the earliest suggestion that DNA was the hereditary material. The suggestion came from Edmund Beecher Wilson in 1895. After accurately documenting that sperm and egg cells contribute the same number of chromosomes during reproduction, Wilson speculated,

> The precise equivalence of the chromosomes contributed by the sexes is a physical correlative of the fact that the two sexes play, on the whole, equal parts in hereditary transmission, and it seems to show that the chromosomal

substance, the chromatin, is to be regarded as the physical basis of inheritance. Now, chromatin is known to be closely similar to, if not identical with[,] a substance known as nuclein ($C_{29} H_{49} N_9 P_3 O_{22}$, according to Miescher), which analysis shows to be a tolerably definite chemical composed of nucleic acid (a complex organic acid rich in phosphorus) and albumin. And thus we reach the remarkable conclusion that inheritance may, perhaps, be effected by the physical transmission of a particular chemical compound from parent to offspring.

In 1900, Mendel's hereditary principles were rediscovered, and their predictions were widely disseminated in biology (see Section 2.3). Shortly thereafter, in 1903, Wilson's student Walter Sutton and, independently, Theodor Boveri accurately described the parallels between, on the one hand, homologous chromosome and sister-chromatid separation during meiotic cell division and, on the other hand, the inheritance of genes.

Over the next 20 years, the nucleus and chromosomes were a focus of biological investigations of heredity. By 1920, the principal constituent of nuclein was identified as DNA, and the basic chemistry of DNA was deciphered. The molecule was determined to be a polynucleotide consisting of four repeating subunits—the four DNA nucleotides—held together in a series by covalent bonds. The four DNA nucleotides are adenine (A), thymine (T), cytosine (C), and guanine (G).

In 1923, conclusive evidence that DNA resides in chromosomes made DNA a candidate for the hereditary material. However, DNA is not the sole constituent of chromosomes. Proteins are in high concentration in chromosomes, and RNA is present in the nucleus and around chromosomes, along with lipids and carbohydrates. The presence of all these compounds meant that they each had to be considered potential candidates for the hereditary material. In fact, some early researchers, including, eventually, Edmund B. Wilson himself, thought protein was potentially a better candidate for the hereditary material than DNA. The proponents of this idea pointed out that protein is composed of 20 different amino acids, whereas DNA has only 4 kinds of nucleotides. The protein proponents suggested that the "20-letter alphabet" of protein could contain more information than the "4-letter alphabet" of DNA. It was against this backdrop that the results of three experiments conducted between 1928 and 1952 combined to identify DNA—not RNA, protein, or another chemical constituent of cells—as the hereditary material of organisms.

A Transformation Factor Responsible for Heredity

Frederick Griffith, a British physician, studied pneumonia infection in mice and published a lengthy research report in 1928 describing his findings. Modern biology focuses on just the last few pages of Griffith's long report, where he describes infecting mice with different combinations of treated and untreated pneumonia bacteria. Through his experiments, Griffith provided indirect evidence that DNA is the hereditary molecule.

Griffith studied strains of the bacterium *Pneumococcus* that cause fatal pneumonia in mice but do not infect humans. He found that strains of the bacterium that cause pneumonia in mice grow in colonies that have a smooth (S) appearance, whereas the *Pneumococcus* strains that do not cause disease are identifiable by their rough (R) appearance (**Figure 7.1**). It was later determined that rough bacterial strains have a mutation affecting a polysaccharide gene. The mutation results in a weak bacterial capsule that leaves R bacteria vulnerable to attack by the mouse immune system.

The S and R strains of *Pneumococcus* occur in four types, identified as I, II, III, and IV. Each type elicits the production of a different group of antibodies from the mouse immune system to attack the invading bacteria. The differences in antibody production are a result of several genetic differences between the four *Pneumococcus* types. A single mutation of a polysaccharide gene can convert an S strain to an R strain *of the same type*—for example, it can change an SII strain to an RII strain—but the bacterial type cannot be changed by a single mutation. In other words, mutation alone cannot change RII bacteria into SIII.

Griffith's most important observations are derived from four experiments he performed using S and R bacterial strains of different types (**Figure 7.2**). In these experiments, either he injected a single type of bacteria or he injected two types of bacteria simultaneously into individual mice. Following each injection test, he drew blood from injected mice and cultured the blood to identify the type of bacteria growing, if any, in the mouse. Two of Griffith's injection experiments involved

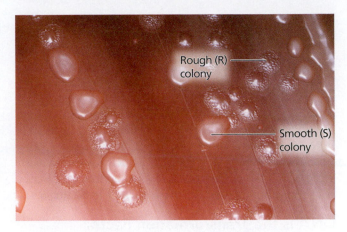

Figure 7.1 Smooth and rough colonies of *Pneumococcus.*

the use of "heat-killed" bacteria. These bacteria were grown normally in culture, but before their use in an injection experiment the cultures were subjected to treatment in a high-heat, high-pressure environment. These conditions are essentially those used today in an autoclave where scientific and medical tools and equipment are sterilized. Autoclave treatment sterilizes by bursting the bacterial cells, causing their death.

Griffith's first three injection results show that ❶ injecting mice with S-strain bacteria produces illness and death, ❷ injection of heat-killed S-strain bacteria does not induce illness, and ❸ injection of an R strain does not produce illness. Griffith's most significant result ❹ came when he injected a mixture of heat-killed SIII strain and living RII strain. He found that most of the mice became ill and died from

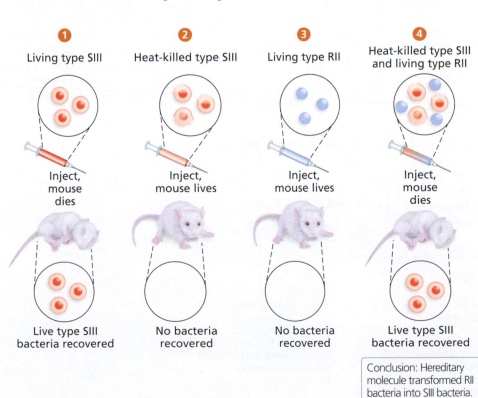

Figure 7.2 Frederick Griffith's experiment identifying a "transformation factor" responsible for heredity. ❶ Injection of living SIII bacteria kills mice. ❷ Heat-killed SIII do not kill mice, nor do living RII bacteria ❸. ❹ Coinjection of a mixture of heat-killed SIII and living RII bacteria results in mouse death by SIII infection.

pneumonia. His tests of blood cultures from the dead mice revealed living SIII bacteria. Knowing that this outcome could not have been the result of a simple mutational event, Griffith proposed that a molecular component he called the "transformation factor" was responsible for transforming RII into SIII.

In Griffith's proposal, the transforming factor was a compound that carried hereditary information. He was unable to identify his transformation factor, but today we know that it is DNA. Today biologists also know that the biological process responsible for the conversion of living RII bacteria by heat-killed SIII is the process of transformation that we describe as a mechanism for gene transfer in bacteria in Section 6.4.

DNA Is the Transformation Factor

Shortly after Griffith published his report on the transformation factor, Martin Dawson, working with Oswald Avery, developed an in vitro transformation procedure to mix living R cells with a purified extract of cellular material derived from heat-killed SIII cells containing the transformation factor. Translated from Latin, *in vitro* means "in glass." Commonly, this means either an experiment conducted in a test tube or a procedure that takes place outside the body of an organism. Biochemical assays indicated that the SIII extract used in the Dawson–Avery in vitro transformation consisted mostly of DNA, along with a small amount of RNA and trace amounts of proteins, lipids, and polysaccharides.

Direct evidence that DNA was the transformation factor came from an experiment performed by Avery and his colleagues Colin MacLeod and Maclyn McCarty in 1944 (**Figure 7.3**). This experiment identified the role of DNA in transformation by eliminating lipids, polysaccharides, protein, RNA, and DNA one at a time from the SIII extract. In each experimental trial, the SIII extract was treated to remove a different component or set of components, and the treated extract was then mixed with RII cells. After time was allowed for an in vitro transformation reaction to take place, the occurrence or absence of transformation was assessed.

Figure 7.3 shows that in vitro transformation takes place in the control experiment ❶ and when lipids and polysaccharides ❷, proteins ❸, or RNA ❹ is removed from the extract. In contrast to the other results, the fifth experiment, which uses DNase to specifically degrade DNA, does not result in transformation ❺—a clear indication that transformation is blocked by the destruction of DNA. Based on these observations, Avery, MacLeod, and McCarty correctly concluded that DNA is the transformation factor and the probable hereditary material.

DNA Is the Hereditary Molecule

Avery, MacLeod, and McCarty's work convinced most biologists that DNA was the long-sought hereditary material, and a great deal of research in the late 1940s and early 1950s was devoted to deducing the physical structure of DNA. Biologists

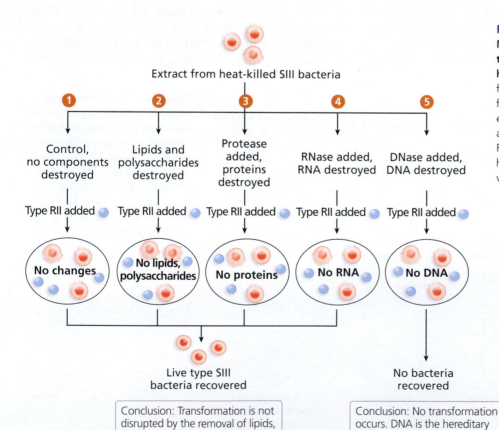

Figure 7.3 Avery, MacLeod, and McCarty's use of in vitro transformation to identify DNA as the most likely hereditary molecule. A purified extract from heat-killed SIII bacteria successfully transforms RII cells in the control experiment ❶. Destruction of lipids and polysaccharides ❷, proteins ❸, or RNA ❹ does not affect transformation; however, destruction of DNA ❺ prevents transformation.

realized that once the structure of DNA was known, the chemical nature of genes would be identified, and biological research would move into the realm of genetic molecular biology. As clear and convincing as the work of Avery and his colleagues seems in retrospect, however, there were several unanswered questions about the role of DNA in heredity. There was also a need to demonstrate directly that the presence of a specific DNA molecule induces the appearance of a particular phenotype. That evidence came in a 1952 report by Alfred Hershey and Martha Chase, who showed that DNA, but not protein, is responsible for bacteriophage infection of bacterial cells.

Bacteriophages, also known as **phages**, are viruses that infect bacteria. Phages such as T2, for example, consist of a protein shell with a tail segment that attaches to a host bacterial cell and a head segment that contains DNA. T2 phages are among the many bacteriophages that do not carry any RNA. Like other phages, T2 must infect host bacterial cells

to reproduce. Infection by a phage proceeds as illustrated in Figure 6.17 and culminates in the lysis of the host cell and the release of dozens of progeny phages.

In their experiment, Hershey and Chase took advantage of an essential difference between the chemical composition of DNA and protein to confirm the hereditary role of DNA (**Figure 7.4**). Proteins contain large amounts of sulfur but almost no phosphorus; conversely, DNA contains a large amount of phosphorus but no sulfur. Hershey and Chase initially grew phage cultures in different growth media. One growth medium contained ^{35}S, the radioactive form of sulfur, to label protein ❶ ; the other contained radioactive phosphorus, ^{32}P, to label DNA ❶. In parallel experiments, the researchers used radioactively labeled phages—from the radioactive sulfur medium in one experiment and from the radioactive phosphorus medium in the other—to infect unlabeled host bacterial cells ❷ ❷.

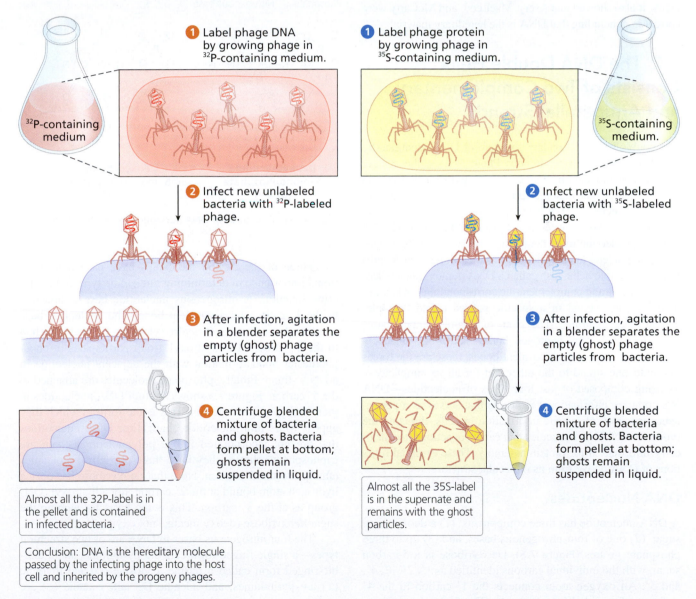

❶ Label phage DNA by growing phage in ^{32}P-containing medium.

^{32}P-containing medium

❶ Label phage protein by growing phage in ^{35}S-containing medium.

^{35}S-containing medium.

❷ Infect new unlabeled bacteria with ^{32}P-labeled phage.

❷ Infect new unlabeled bacteria with ^{35}S-labeled phage.

❸ After infection, agitation in a blender separates the empty (ghost) phage particles from bacteria.

❸ After infection, agitation in a blender separates the empty (ghost) phage particles from bacteria.

❹ Centrifuge blended mixture of bacteria and ghosts. Bacteria form pellet at bottom; ghosts remain suspended in liquid.

❹ Centrifuge blended mixture of bacteria and ghosts. Bacteria form pellet at bottom; ghosts remain suspended in liquid.

Almost all the 32P-label is in the pellet and is contained in infected bacteria.

Almost all the 35S-label is in the supernate and remains with the ghost particles.

Conclusion: DNA is the hereditary molecule passed by the infecting phage into the host cell and inherited by the progeny phages.

Figure 7.4   The Hershey-Chase experiment. Experimental results show that DNA is the molecule in bacteriophages that is transferred by infection of bacterial cells.

After a short time, each mixture was agitated in a blender to separate bacterial cells from the now empty phage shells. Such empty phage shells are called "ghosts" ❸ ❸. The relatively large bacterial cells were easily separated from the ghosts by centrifugation. The heavier bacteria collect in a pellet at the bottom of the centrifuge tube, while the lighter ghosts remain suspended in the supernatant. Testing each fraction for radioactivity revealed that virtually all the ^{32}P label was associated with newly infected bacterial cells and almost none with ghost particles ❹. On the other hand, the ^{35}S label was found in the ghost-particle fraction, and only trace amounts were found associated with the bacterial pellet ❹. This result demonstrates that phage DNA, but not phage protein, is transferred to host bacterial cells and directs the synthesis of phage DNA and proteins, the assembly of progeny phage particles, and ultimately the lysis of infected cells. The experiment demonstrated that the transformation factor identified previously by Griffith was DNA; it also showed that Avery, MacLeod, and McCarty were correct in concluding that DNA is the hereditary material.

7.2 The DNA Double Helix Consists of Two Complementary and Antiparallel Strands

The double helical secondary structure of DNA identified by Rosalind Franklin in her famous Photo 51 (see the chapter opener) and modeled by James Watson and Francis Crick in 1963 indicates that in some respects, DNA is a simple molecule (see Section 1.2). It is composed of four kinds of DNA nucleotides joined covalently by phosphodiester bonds that link one nucleotide to its neighbors in polynucleotide chains. Two polynucleotide chains come together along their lengths to form a double helix, also called a DNA duplex. The nucleotides in one strand complement the corresponding nucleotides in the partner strand in a specific pattern called "complementary base pairing." The pairs of complementary bases are held together by hydrogen bonds; and while relatively weak in comparison with covalent bonds, these are the forces that bind one strand to the other. Yet for all its simplicity—its being composed of just four types of nucleotides—DNA is a complex informational molecule that serves as a permanent repository of genetic information in cells, directing the production of RNA molecules that carry out actions in cells or carry information for protein assembly. These essential functions of DNA derive from its molecular structure.

DNA Nucleotides

A DNA nucleotide has three components: (1) a deoxyribose sugar, (2) one of four nitrogenous bases, and (3) up to three phosphate groups (**Figure 7.5**). Deoxyribose is a 5-carbon sugar, with the individual carbons identified as 1', 2', 3', 4', and 5'. An oxygen atom connects the 1' carbon to the 4' to form a five-sided (pentose) ring. The 5' carbon projects outward from the 4' carbon (and from the ring).

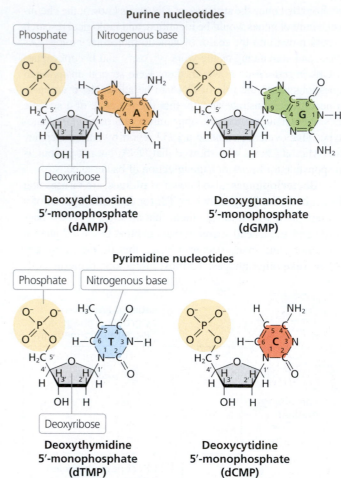

Figure 7.5   Structures of DNA nucleotide monophosphates.

Three of the carbon molecules have particular functional importance in determining nucleotide type and nucleotide function. A nitrogenous nucleotide base is attached to the 1' carbon by a covalent bond. The nucleotide base is either A, G, T, or C. A hydroxyl group (OH) is attached to the 3' carbon. The hydroxyl group participates in phosphodiester bond formation with the adjacent nucleotide in a DNA strand. Finally, phosphate molecules are attached to the 5' carbon. Figure 7.5 shows the four DNA nucleotides in their monophosphate forms. This is the form in which they appear while in a nucleotide chain. Free DNA nucleotides that are not incorporated into a polynucleotide chain are triphosphates; that is, they have three phosphate molecules attached to the 5' carbon. Note that deoxyribose has only a hydrogen atom bound at the 2' carbon, not a hydroxyl (OH) group as at the 3' carbon. This is the basis for naming the sugar *deoxy*ribose (deoxy means "not oxygenated").

The four nitrogenous bases in DNA are of two structural types—a single-ringed form called a pyrimidine, and a double-ringed form called a purine. Cytosine (C) and thymine (T) are pyrimidines, and adenine (A) and guanine (G) are purines. In their monophosphate configurations, the nucleotides that carry the purine bases adenine and guanine are designated, respectively, deoxyadenosine 5'-monophosphate (dAMP) and deoxyguanosine 5'-monophosphate (dGMP); and the nucleotides that carry the pyrimidine bases cytosine and thymine are deoxycytidine 5'-monophosphate (dCMP) and deoxythymidine 5'-monophosphate (dTMP). Collectively, these are identified as the **deoxynucleotide monophosphates**, or **dNMPs**, where N can refer to any of the four nucleotide bases. In contrast, free (reactive) DNA nucleotides in their triphosphate configurations are identified as dATP, dGTP, dCTP, and dTTP. Collectively, these are the **deoxynucleotide triphosphates (dNTPs)**.

DNA strand formation is catalyzed by the enzyme DNA polymerase. The enzyme catalyzes the formation of a phosphodiester bond between the 3' hydroxyl group of one nucleotide and the 5' triphosphate group of an adjacent nucleotide (**Figure 7.6**). Two of the three phosphates of the dNTP are removed during phosphodiester bond formation, leaving the nucleotides of a polynucleotide chain in their monophosphate form. The two discarded phosphates are called the pyrophosphate group. As mentioned before, the resulting strand is a polynucleotide chain composed of nucleotides joined by covalent bonds. The pattern of phosphodiester bond formation gives each strand a **sugar-phosphate backbone** consisting of alternating sugar and phosphate groups along its length.

The DNA Duplex

DNA is stable as a double helix. The two polynucleotide strands that make up the duplex have a specific relationship that follows two rules: (1) the arrangement of the nucleotides is such that the nucleotide bases of one strand are *complementary* to the corresponding nucleotide bases on the second strand (A pairs with T, and G pairs with C), and (2) the two strands are *antiparallel* in orientation (see the opposite-pointing arrows on each side of the diagrams in Figure 7.6). If one strand is, for example 5'-ATCG-3', then the complementary strand is 3'-TAGC-5'.

Complementary base pairing joins a purine nucleotide on one strand to its complementary pyrimidine nucleotide on the other. The chemical basis of such pairing is the formation of a stable number of hydrogen (H) bonds between the bases of the different strands. Hydrogen bonds are noncovalent bonds that form between the partial charges that are associated with hydrogen, oxygen, and nitrogen atoms of the nucleotide bases. As Figure 7.6 shows, two stable hydrogen bonds form for each A-T base pair, and three hydrogen bonds are formed by each G-C base pair (see also Figure 1.6).

Antiparallel strand orientation is essential to the formation of stable hydrogen bonds. In Figure 7.6, notice that the nucleotides in one strand are oriented with their 3' carbon toward the top and their 5' carbon toward the bottom. The complementary nucleotides in the other strand are antiparallel to these; that is, their 5'-to-3' orientations run in the *opposite* direction.

A key observation made from Franklin's research was the recognition of two slightly different forms of DNA. These were designated A-form DNA and B-form DNA. B-form

DNA was much more common than A-form DNA, and it is now known to predominate in all organisms. A third type of DNA is also known, as we describe at the end of this section.

The molecular dimensions of DNA are measured using the unit called an angstrom (Å) or in nanometers (nm). One angstrom is equal to 10^{-10} meters, or 1 ten-billionth of a meter, and 1 nm equals one-billionth of a meter, or 10^{-9} meters. In B-form DNA, the distance from the axis of symmetry to the outer edge of either sugar-phosphate backbone is 10 Å (1 nm), and the molecular diameter is 20 Å (2 nm) at any point along the length of the helix (**Figure 7.7a**). The 20-Å molecular symmetry of the double helix was the key observation that told Watson and Crick that DNA structure results from pairing of a purine (A or G) with its complementary pyrimidine (T or C). The purine–pyrimidine base-pair pattern gives each base pair the same dimension.

A second key observation derived from Franklin's Photo 51 is that nucleotide base pairs are spaced at intervals of 3.4 Å along DNA duplexes. This tight packing of DNA bases in the duplex leads to **base stacking**, the slight rotation of adjacent base pairs around the axis of symmetry so that their planes are parallel, imparting a twist to the double helix. Figure 7.7a shows that one complete helical turn spans 34 Å. This span is occupied by approximately 10.5 base pairs. **Figure 7.7b** is a space-filling model that illustrates base-pair stacking and the twisting of the sugar-phosphate backbones. **Figure 7.7c** is a ball-and-stick model illustrating how base pairs twist around the axis of symmetry to create the helical spiral.

Base-pair stacking creates two grooves in the double helix, gaps between the spiraling sugar-phosphate backbones that partially expose the nucleotides. The alternating grooves, known as the **major groove** and **minor groove**, are highlighted in Figures 7.7b and 7.7c. The major groove is approximately 12 Å wide, and the minor groove is approximately 6 Å wide. The major and minor grooves are regions where DNA-binding proteins can most easily make direct contact with nucleotides along one or both strands of the double helix. In this chapter and in later chapters, we discuss many of the important functions DNA-binding proteins perform, such as regulating the initiation of transcription and controlling the onset and progression of DNA replication. Most of these functions depend on the presence of characteristic sequences of DNA nucleotides. DNA-binding proteins gain access to DNA nucleotides in major and minor grooves of the molecule.

B-form DNA, overwhelmingly the most common DNA structure in organisms, has a right-handed twisting of the sugar-phosphate backbone. A-form DNA also has a right-handed twist to the helix. It is more compact than B-form DNA, with about 11 base pairs per complete helical twist, although its diameter is a little greater than that of B-form DNA (**Table 7.1**). A-form DNA is occasionally detected in cells, and it appears to be particularly common in bacteriophage, where its more compact size makes it functional for packaging of bacteriophage DNA. A-form DNA may be less amenable to binding by DNA-binding regulatory proteins, due to alterations of the major and minor grooves in comparison

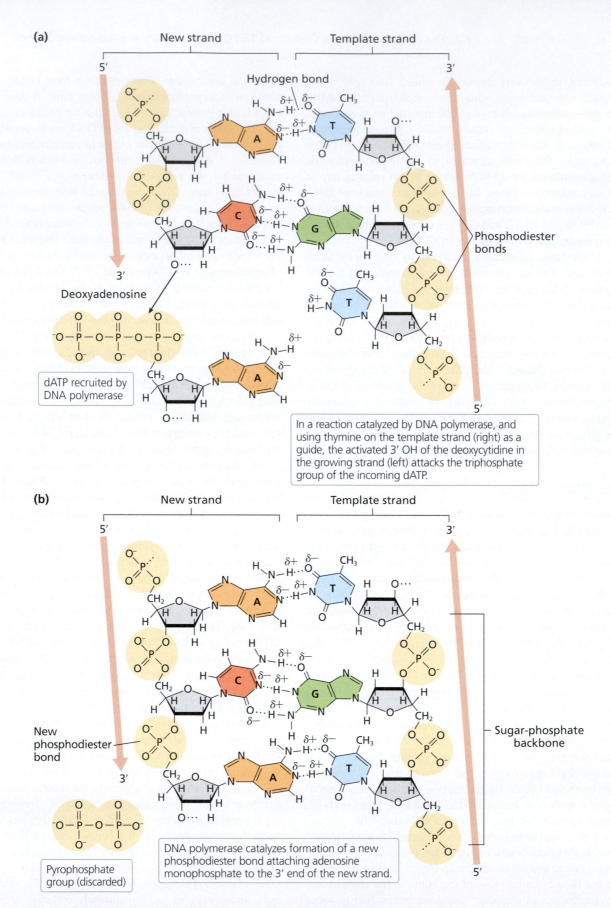

Figure 7.6 DNA strand elongation. (a) Complementary nucleotides form hydrogen bonds by the attraction of positive and negative charges. The nucleotide triphosphate complementary to the template strand nucleotide is recruited by DNA polymerase. **(b)** DNA polymerase catalyzes the addition of the new nucleotide to the 3′ end of the growing strand by removing two phosphates (the pyrophosphate group) and forming a new phosphodiester bond.

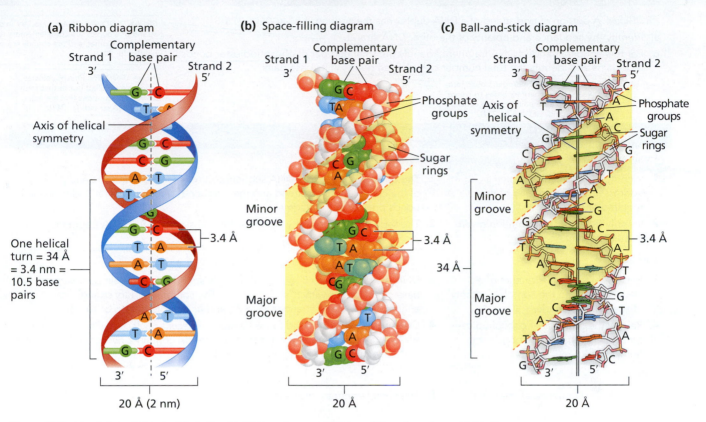

Figure 7.7 **The B-form DNA double helix.** (a) Ribbon diagram, (b) space-filling diagram, and (c) ball-and-stick diagram show the sugar-phosphate backbones, base pairs, major and minor grooves, and dimensions of the DNA duplex.

Table 7.1	Characteristics of Three Forms of DNA		
	A-Form	**B-Form**	**Z-Form**
Helical twist	Right-handed	Right-handed	Left-handed
Rotation per base pair	32.7°	34.3°	60.2°
Base-pair spacing	2.6 Å	3.4 Å	3.7 Å
Base pairs per turn	11	10.5	12
Helix diameter	23 Å	20 Å	18 Å

with B-form DNA. A-form DNA major grooves are deeper and narrower than those of B-form DNA, and its minor grooves are wider and shallower than those of B-form DNA. Research subsequent to Franklin's initial discovery of A-form DNA identifies the level of hydration of DNA as the principal factor determining its formation. Dehydration converts B-form DNA to the A form, and it is thought that by assuming the A form, DNA is better protected from damage under desiccation conditions. Such conditions occur in certain bacterial species.

The third form of DNA, Z-form DNA, was discovered by Robert Wells and colleagues in 1970, and its structure was determined by Andrew Wang, Alexander Rich, and colleagues in 1979. Z-form DNA is quite different from A-form and B-form DNA in that it has a left-handed twist that gives

the sugar-phosphate backbone a zigzag appearance—hence the name Z-form—and other structural differences as well (see Table 7.1). No definitive biological significance has been identified for Z-form DNA; however, it occurs in cells and is particularly common near the start sites for gene transcription. Studies of Z-form DNA have identified certain DNA sequences that are associated with Z-form DNA formation. These too occur most frequently near the starting points of gene transcription. Study of the human genome reveals numerous such sequences where Z-form DNA is detected. Human chromosome 22 appears to have a number of transcription start sequences where Z-form DNA can occur.

Two questions about DNA frequently come up in discussions of DNA molecular structure. Why do complementary base pairs consist of one purine and one pyrimidine? Why are the strands of the double helix antiparallel and not parallel? The presence of one purine and one pyrimidine per base pair is a matter of molecular symmetry. Were the molecule to be composed of two paired purines (both double-ringed) the base pair would measure more than 20 Å across. Conversely, if the base pair was two pyrimidines (both single-ringed), the measurement would be much less than 20 Å. This would give the molecule an irregular diameter that might make it more difficult to package in cells and nuclei, or might make the binding of DNA-binding regulatory proteins more difficult. The reason why DNA strands are antiparallel to one another and not parallel is a matter of hydrogen bond formation. For hydrogen bonds

GENETIC ANALYSIS 7.1

PROBLEM A portion of one strand of a DNA duplex has the sequence 5'-ACGACGCTA-3'.
a. Identify the sequence and polarity of the other DNA strand.
b. For this double-stranded DNA fragment, identify the total number of phosphodiester bonds it contains and identify the total number of hydrogen bonds in its base pairs.

> **BREAK IT DOWN:** DNA nucleotides in one strand of a duplex are complementary to those in the other, and the strands are anti-parallel (p. 241).

> **BREAK IT DOWN:** Phosphodiester bonds are covalent bonds that form between nucleotides that are adjacent in DNA strands (p. 241).

> **BREAK IT DOWN:** Hydrogen bonds form between complementary bases to create A–T and G–C base pairs and join complementary strands of DNA (p. 241).

Solution Strategies	Solution Steps
Evaluate	
1. Identify the topic this problem addresses, and the nature of the required answer.	1. The question concerns a DNA sequence. It asks for the sequence and polarity of the complementary strand and the number of phosphodiester and hydrogen bonds present in the fragment.
2. Identify the critical information given in the problem.	2. The sequence and polarity are given for one strand of the DNA fragment.
Deduce	
3. Review the general structure of a DNA duplex and the complementarity of specific nucleotides.	3. DNA is a double helix composed of single strands that contain complementary base pairs (A pairs with T, and G with C). The complementary strands are antiparallel (i.e., one strand is 5' to 3', and its complement is 3' to 5').
4. Review the patterns of phosphodiester bond and hydrogen bond formation in DNA.	4. One phosphodiester bond forms between adjacent nucleotides on each strand of DNA. A–T base pairs (joining the two strands) contain 2 hydrogen bonds, and G–C base pairs contain 3 hydrogen bonds.
Solve	
5. Identify the sequence of the complementary strand.	5. The complementary sequence is TGCTGCGAT.
6. Give the polarity of the complementary strand.	6. The polarity of the complementary strand is 3'-TGCTGCGAT-5'.
7. Count the number of phosphodiester bonds in this DNA fragment.	7. Between the adjacent nucleotides of this fragment there are eight phosphodiester bonds per strand for a total of 16 phosphodiester bonds.
8. Count the number of hydrogen bonds between the two strands of this DNA fragment.	8. There are four A–T bases pairs containing 2 hydrogen bonds each, and five G–C base pairs containing 3 hydrogen bonds each, for a total of 8 + 15 = 23 hydrogen bonds in this DNA fragment.

For more practice, see Problems 5, 8, 9, 16, and 17. Visit the Study Area to access study tools. **Mastering Genetics**

to form, the negative charge of an oxygen or nitrogen must occur opposite the positive charge of a hydrogen. This occurs when complementary base pairs align in antiparallel strands. If a purine and a pyrimidine were aligned in parallel strands, positively charged hydrogens would be opposite one another, as would negatively charged nitrogens and oxygens. These repelling forces would prevent hydrogen bond formation.

Review **Genetic Analysis 7.1** to explore complementary base pairing and the formation of bonds creating single and double strands of DNA.

7.3 DNA Replication Is Semiconservative and Bidirectional

Given the role of DNA as an information repository and an information transmitter, the integrity of the nucleotide sequence of DNA is of paramount importance. Each time DNA is copied, the new version must be a precise duplicate of the original version. The high fidelity of DNA replication is essential to reproduction and to the normal development of biological structures and functions. Without faithful DNA replication, the information of life would become hopelessly garbled by rapidly accumulating mutations that would threaten survival.

Considering the importance of DNA throughout the biological world, it was no surprise to discover that the general mechanism of DNA replication is the same in all organisms. This universal process evolved in the earliest life-forms and has been retained for billions of years. As organisms diverged and became more complex, however, an array of differences did develop among DNA replication proteins and enzymes. Despite the diversification of these specific components of DNA replication, three attributes of DNA replication are shared by all organisms:

1. Each strand of the parental DNA molecule remains intact during replication.
2. Each parental strand serves as a template directing the synthesis of a complementary, antiparallel daughter strand.

3. Completion of DNA replication results in the formation of two identical daughter duplexes, each composed of one parental strand and one daughter strand.

As we describe DNA replication in bacteria, archaea, and eukaryotes in this and the following section, we will point out similarities and differences in DNA replication among the domains. The three domains share the features they do because all life evolved from a common origin. At the same time, the differences in DNA replication between the domains are also the result of evolution, which favored specific adaptations.

Three Competing Models of Replication

In their 1953 paper describing the structure of DNA, Watson and Crick concluded with the following observation:

> It has not escaped our notice that the specific base-pairing we have proposed immediately suggests a possible copying mechanism for the genetic material.

Specifically, Watson and Crick recognized that a consequence of complementary base pairing was that nucleotides on one strand of the duplex could be used to guide the ordering of nucleotides on the other strand. Watson and Crick presumed that DNA replication used the nucleotide sequence of each strand to form a new pair of DNA duplexes, hypothesizing that each DNA strand of the original duplex would act as a template for the synthesis of a new daughter strand. Watson and Crick did not know the precise mechanism by which template-based replication took place, however, raising the crucial question of what the exact mechanism of replication might be.

Almost immediately after the structure of DNA was identified, three competing models of DNA replication emerged

(Figure 7.8). The ❶ **semiconservative DNA replication** model—which proved to be correct—proposed that each daughter duplex contains one original parental strand of DNA and one complementary, newly synthesized daughter strand. The ❷ **conservative DNA replication** model predicts that one daughter duplex contains the two strands of the parental molecule and the other contains two newly synthesized daughter strands. Lastly, the ❸ **dispersive DNA replication** model predicts that each daughter duplex is a composite of interspersed parental duplex segments and daughter duplex segments.

The Meselson–Stahl Experiment

In 1958, Matthew Meselson and Franklin Stahl took advantage of the newly developed method of high-speed cesium chloride (CsCl) density gradient ultracentrifugation to decipher the mechanism of DNA replication in an experiment of beautiful simplicity. In this analytical method, a tube filled with a CsCl mixture is subjected to high ultracentrifuge speeds that exert thousands of gravities of separating force, creating a graded variation in density—a density gradient—throughout the CsCl mixture. When substances are placed in the CsCl gradient and ultracentrifugation takes place, the substances migrate until they reach the point in the density gradient where their molecular density is matched by that of the gradient. Migration stops at that point. This technique is capable of separating molecules that have only slightly different molecular weights.

Meselson and Stahl began their experiment by growing *Escherichia coli* in a growth medium containing the rare heavy isotope of nitrogen, ^{15}N, for many generations. Under these growth conditions, the bacteria produce DNA that is fully saturated with the heavy isotope. In other words, all

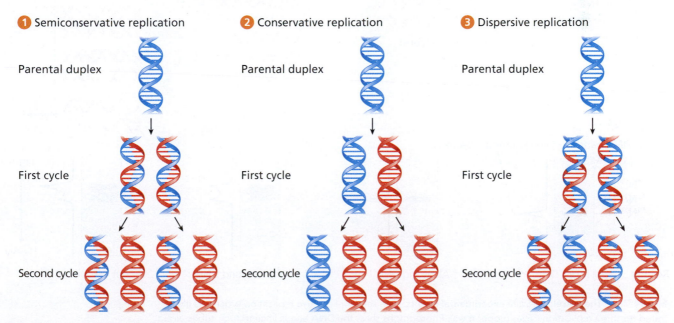

❶ Semiconservative replication   ❷ Conservative replication   ❸ Dispersive replication

Parental duplex   Parental duplex   Parental duplex

First cycle   First cycle   First cycle

Second cycle   Second cycle   Second cycle

Figure 7.8 Three proposed mechanisms of DNA replication tested by Meselson and Stahl. The results expected for two cycles of DNA replication are shown for each model.

🔴 **Using the same red and blue color scheme, draw a third cycle of DNA replication for the semiconservative replication model.**

the nitrogen in these DNA duplexes is ^{15}N. The duplexes are designated ^{15}N/^{15}N to signify the incorporation of ^{15}N throughout both strands. (By the same token, a DNA duplex composed of two strands containing only ^{14}N, the normal isotope of nitrogen, is designated ^{14}N/^{14}N, and a duplex with one strand containing each isotope is designated ^{15}N/^{14}N.) DNA collected for CsCl gradient analysis from this starting generation, designated generation 0, was exclusively ^{15}N/^{15}N.

Next, some of these ^{15}N-labeled *E. coli* were transferred to a new growth medium containing only the normal light isotope of nitrogen, ^{14}N. Growth in this medium leads to the incorporation of DNA nucleotides containing the light isotope into newly synthesized strands. At the end of each successive DNA replication cycle, DNA was collected from a few cells growing on the ^{14}N medium and was subjected to CsCl analysis.

Figure 7.9 shows the results of CsCl gradient analysis of DNA collected from three replication cycles, beginning

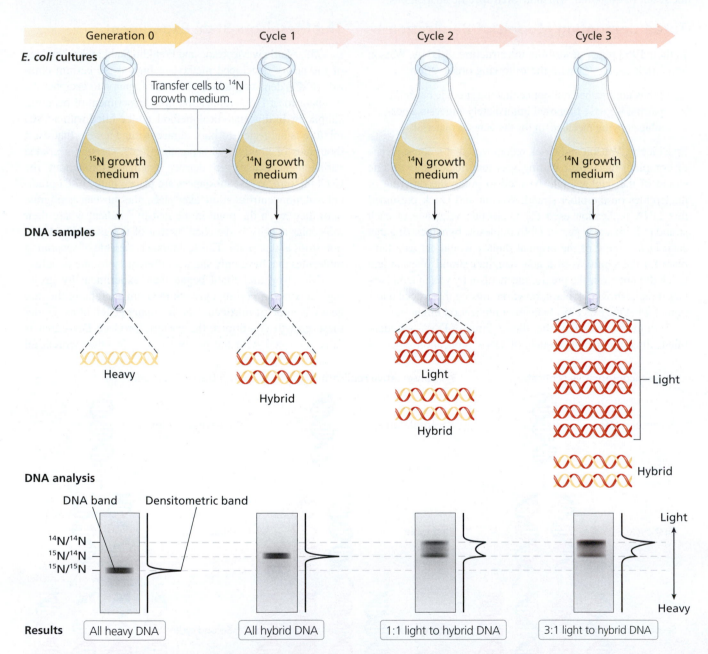

Figure 7.9 **The Meselson–Stahl experimental results.** The semiconservative replication process is illustrated for three replication cycles (upper rows). Photographs show the DNA bands in centrifuge tubes along with densitometry scans in which the amplitudes of peaks indicate the relative concentrations of material in each centrifuge band (lower rows). These results are consistent only with semiconservative DNA replication.

 If a fourth cycle of DNA replication takes place, what is the expected ratio of light to hybrid DNA duplexes?

with generation 0. The experimental results are consistent with the semiconservative model only. The conservative model predicted DNA molecules with two distinct densities after generation 1 ($^{15}N/^{15}N$ and $^{14}N/^{14}N$). The results reject this model. Similarly, the dispersive model predicted a single DNA density in all generations. The generation 2 results reject this replication model. The data are consistent with the predictions of the semiconservative model of DNA replication through generation 3 shown and beyond. Within a few years of Meselson and Stahl's identification of semiconservative replication in bacteria, the mechanism was identified experimentally in eukaryotes as well, solidifying the idea that all life shares the same general process of DNA replication, as a consequence of life's single origin and the evolutionary connections among living things.

Origin and Directionality of Replication in Bacterial DNA

Solving the riddle of the basic mechanism of DNA replication introduced new questions about how replication is initiated and how it progresses. Does replication commence at specific points on each chromosome? If so, how many such points does a chromosome have? Does DNA replication progress in one direction or in both directions from a replication origin? Experimental evidence clearly demonstrates that DNA replication is most often **bidirectional**, progressing in both directions from a single **origin of replication** in bacterial chromosomes and from multiple origins of replication in eukaryotic chromosomes.

In 1963, John Cairns reported the first evidence of a single origin of DNA replication in *E. coli*. Based on Cairn's evidence, it appeared that once replication gets underway in bacteria, there is expansion around the origin of replication, forming a **replication bubble** (**Figure 7.10**). The image shown in the figure is similar to the type of result Cairns obtained, and shows two regions known as **replication forks** at either end of the replication bubble.

Cairns experiment did not determine whether replication takes place in one direction away from the origin (unidirectional) or in both directions (bidirectional). This remaining question held important implications. If DNA replicated bidirectionally, the time required to replicate a bacterial chromosome would be, give or take, about half that required if replication were unidirectional.

Evidence suggesting that bidirectional replication was the mechanism by which the chromosomal DNA of organisms was replicated accumulated during the 1960s, but it was not until 1973 that the matter was resolved. In that year, Raymond Rodriguez and his colleagues performed an experiment in which the origin of replication of an *E. coli* chromosome and the terminus of replication of the same chromosome were identified by a radioactive

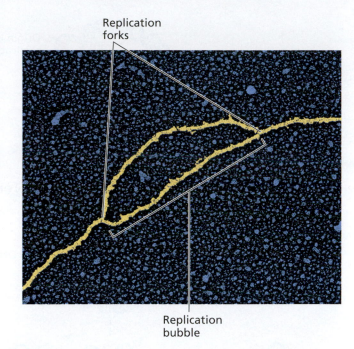

Replication forks

Replication bubble

Figure 7.10 **Color-enhanced electron micrograph of a DNA replication bubble and replication forks.** A replication bubble expands bidirectionally from an origin of replication, and active DNA synthesis takes place at each replication fork.

compound. The origin and terminus of DNA replication were found to be on opposite sides of the chromosome almost exactly 180 degrees apart (**Figure 7.11**). If DNA replicated in a unidirectional manner, the origin and terminus would overlap, since the process would begin and end at the same point on the circular chromosome. Figure 7.11 illustrates the progression of bidirectional replication from its origin to its completion and shows the replication bubble and replication forks that develop during the process.

Part of the evidence suggesting the bidirectionality of DNA replication came in 1968 when Joel Huberman and Arthur Riggs used a technique called pulse–chase labeling to study the directionality of replication in mammalian chromosomes. In pulse–chase labeling experiments, cells are exposed for a time to high levels of a radioactive compound that they then incorporate into the DNA they are synthesizing. This is the "pulse." Following each pulse, the radioactive compound is temporarily removed to allow replication to proceed without radioactive labeling of newly synthesized DNA. This is the "chase." The pulse–chase method results in the incorporation of radioactivity into DNA replicated during a pulse but the absence of incorporated radioactivity during a chase. If replication is bidirectional, moving outward in both directions from an origin of replication, Huberman and Riggs predicted that it would result in a symmetrical pattern of alternating labeled and nonlabeled segments of newly replicated DNA moving outward from an origin of replication, consistent with the pattern of pulses and chases.

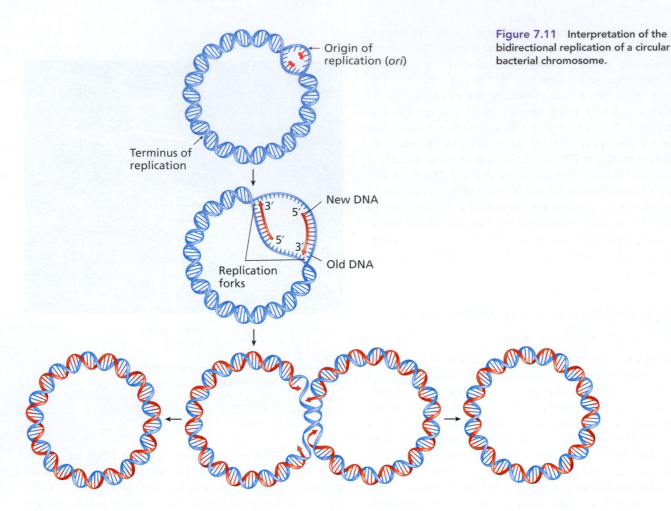

Huberman and Riggs's results, depicted in **Figure 7.12**, show exactly what was predicted for bidirectional DNA replication. Dark regions indicating incorporation of radioactivity during a pulse alternate with light regions indicating DNA replication during a chase. The alternation is symmetrical on both sides of replication origins, demonstrating that replication moves away from replication origins in both directions at once.

Multiple Replication Origins in Eukaryotes

Replication evidence from Cairns and from Rodriguez and colleagues demonstrates that the *E. coli* chromosome has a single origin of replication, and studies of archaeal species generally indicate a single replication origin, but what about the chromosomes of eukaryotes? Certainly each eukaryotic chromosome must have its own origin or origins of replication, but are there one, two, dozens, or thousands of DNA replication origins on each chromosome? Electron micrograph evidence shown in **Figure 7.13** shows multiple DNA replication origins in a single *Drosophila melanogaster* chromosome. The best evidence indicates hundreds to thousands of replication origins in eukaryotic species. Yeast genomes contain about 400 origins, *Drosophila* genomes about 10,000, and the human genome may have as many as 50,000 origins of replication.

Figure 7.13a is a snapshot of a moment during DNA replication, but notice that the replication bubbles in the micrograph are of different sizes. This indicates that replication was initiated in them at different times. Large replication bubbles appear to extend from origins that started replication earlier than those belonging to the smaller replication bubbles in this micrograph. Cell biologists have determined that among different types of cells, the length of S phase is variable. This means that the rate of progression of DNA replication varies among cells of different types. Rapidly dividing cells replicate their DNA more quickly (i.e., have a shorter S phase) than do slowly dividing cells. In addition, experimental evidence identifies "early-replicating" (i.e., early in S phase) and "late-replicating" (late in S phase) segments of large eukaryotic genomes. Early-replicating genome segments appear to contain many expressed genes, whereas late-replicating regions contain many fewer expressed genes. In *Drosophila*, for example, late-replicating regions include chromosome segments immediately surrounding centromeres, where few expressed genes are located.

Regardless of differences in the timing of initiation at the multiple origins of replication on a eukaryotic chromosome, each of the replication bubbles emanating from an origin of replication expands toward the others to eventually

(a) Result of pulse-labeling experiment

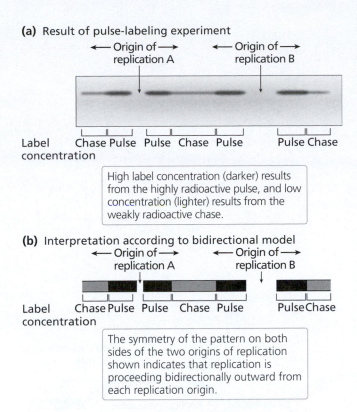

Label concentration

High label concentration (darker) results from the highly radioactive pulse, and low concentration (lighter) results from the weakly radioactive chase.

(b) Interpretation according to bidirectional model

Label concentration

The symmetry of the pattern on both sides of the two origins of replication shown indicates that replication is proceeding bidirectionally outward from each replication origin.

Figure 7.12 Pulse–chase labeling evidence of bidirectional DNA replication in mammalian chromosomes. (a) Alternating dark and light banding of replicating DNA and **(b)** diagram illustrating pulse–chase results are consistent with the bidirectional model of replication.

merge, resulting in the replication of all of the DNA in each eukaryotic nucleus by the end of S phase (Figure 7.13b). The end products of replication of each eukaryotic chromosome are a pair of identical DNA duplexes that are sister chromatids. The sister chromatids will remain joined through G_2 and will be separated at anaphase of the upcoming M phase.

7.4 DNA Replication Precisely Duplicates the Genetic Material

A great deal of what molecular biologists know about DNA replication comes from the study of bacteria, particularly *E. coli*, but increasingly the processes of DNA replication in archaeal and eukaryotic genomes are also becoming clear. Chapter 1 presents a general overview of some of the basic steps of DNA replication, gleaned primarily from bacterial species. The present section provides additional details of this process and also offers comparative information on DNA replication in archaea and eukaryotes. What is revealed by comparisons of DNA replication between species representative of the three domains is the overall similarity of the process in all the domains, combined with differences that belong uniquely to each one. These observations conform to a common theme in evolutionary biology: the presence of

a high proportion of shared genes and functions as a result of the common ancestry of life, along with a great deal of modification and specialization that accumulates over the millennia of evolution and diversification.

Foundation Figure 7.14 serves as a starting point and as a touchstone for this discussion by providing an overview of the major steps in bacterial DNA replication. At each step, the activities of the principal molecular players are identified. You can refer back to this foundation figure as you make your way through the following pages.

DNA Sequences at Replication Origins

Origins of DNA replication contain sequences that attract replication enzymes. The best-characterized origin-of-replication sequence is from *E. coli* and is designated *oriC*. This sequence, which contains approximately 245 bp of DNA, is AT-rich (i.e., has a preponderance of adenine and thymine base pairs). DNA regions containing AT richness require less energy for their denaturation, a process we will see happening at *oriC* early in the initiation of replication.

OriC is subdivided by three 13-bp sequences, so-called 13-mers, followed by four 9-bp sequences, called 9-mers (**Figure 7.15**). Other bacterial species have origin-of-replication sequences that are similar to *oriC*. This similarity is a product of common ancestry and strong evolutionary conservation of the function of these DNA sequences. Natural selection has acted to maintain sequence similarity because the function of the conserved sequence region is essential to the survival of the organism.

Comparisons of evolutionarily conserved sequences within and among related species can lead to the identification of **consensus sequences**. Consensus sequences have similar functions, similar overall length, and similarity of the pattern of base pairs. They feature nucleotides occurring frequently at the same positions in the DNA sequences of many species. Consensus sequences are not, however, identical to one another. Instead, consensus sequences are defined by the nucleotides that occur *most often* at particular positions in the sequence. The sequence making up a consensus sequence is determined by recognizing the similar sequences in several related species and identifying the most common nucleotide at each position. Table 7.2 illustrates this process for the 9-mer segment of the origin of replication for eight bacterial species. Notice the overall sequence similarity and that the nucleotides at six positions are identical among the species whereas the nucleotides at three positions—2, 3, and 5—vary among the species. Based on the 9-mer sequences for the bacterial species listed in Table 7.2, the consensus sequence is TTATCCACA. Consensus sequences are not unique to DNA replication. They are common features identified by comparative genomics in the study of numerous regulatory processes. You will see the term used again in subsequent chapters.

Some archaeal species have single origins of replication, but others have up to four origins. The DNA sequences at archaeal origins are termed *origin recognition boxes*

(a)

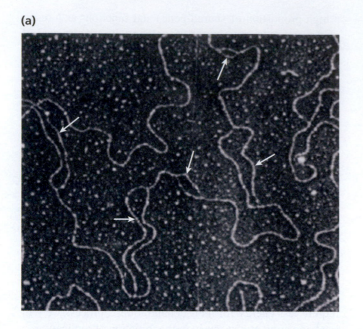

(b)

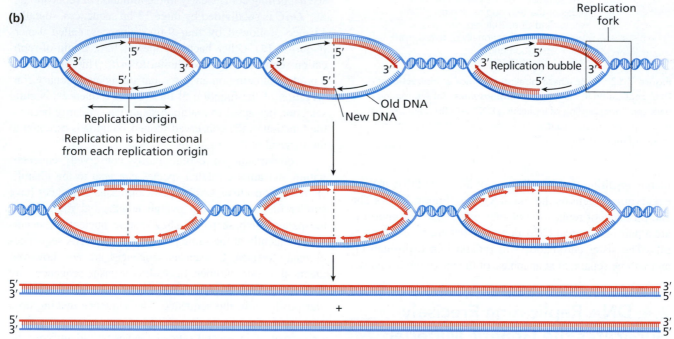

Figure 7.13 **Multiple origins of replication on a single chromosome from *Drosophila melanogaster*.**
(a) The arrows indicate replication bubbles, which are expanding bidirectionally. Different-sized replication bubbles indicate different replication start times. **(b)** Replication bubbles from multiple origins (upper) expand bidirectionally (middle) and merge, ultimately forming two sister chromatids (lower).

(ORBs), and they are of two types. Long ORB sequences are 22 to 35 nucleotides in length and may be present at two or more origins in species with multiple replication origins. Shorter, so-called miniORB, sequences are 12 to 13 nucleotides in length and may occur one or more times in archaeal genomes. Long ORBs and miniORBs may also be found in the same genome.

Among eukaryotic organisms, the yeast *Saccharomyces cerevisiae* has the most fully characterized origin-of-replication

sequences. In yeast, the multiple origins of replication are known as *autonomously replicating sequences* (ARSs). There is general conservation of DNA sequence in ARSs, and their organization is similar throughout the genome of *S. cerevisiae*. ARS1 in yeast has been fully sequenced (**Figure 7.16**). Within the 95 bp of ARS1 is an 11-bp consensus sequence and three other regions (B_1, B_2, and B_3) of conserved DNA sequences that differ somewhat from one another and from the 11-bp consensus sequence region.

DNA replication in bacteria

1 Helicase breaks hydrogen bonds. Topoisomerase relaxes supercoiling.

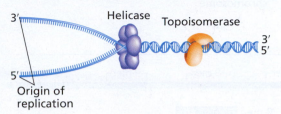

2 Single-stranded binding (SSB) protein prevents reannealing.

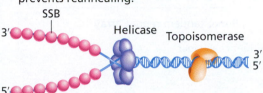

3 Primase synthesizes RNA primers.

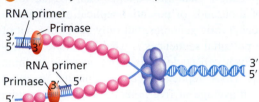

4 DNA polymerase III synthesizes daughter strand.

Leading strand (SSB has been deleted for clarity)

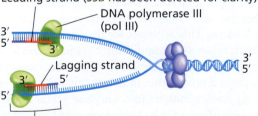

Okazaki fragment 1

5 DNA polymerase III elongates the leading strand continuously and the lagging strand discontinuously.

Leading strand

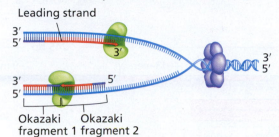

Okazaki fragment 1 Okazaki fragment 2

6 DNA polymerase I removes and replaces nucleotides of the RNA primer.

DNA polymerase I (pol I)

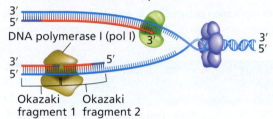

Okazaki fragment 1 Okazaki fragment 2

7 DNA ligase joins Okazaki fragments.

DNA ligase Primase

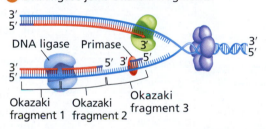

Okazaki fragment 1 Okazaki fragment 2 Okazaki fragment 3

Protein						
DNA topoisomerase	Helicase (DnaB)	SSB	Primase	DNA pol III	DNA pol I	DNA ligase
Icon						
Role Relaxes supercoiling	Unwinds the double helix	Prevents reannealing of separated strands	Synthesizes RNA primers	Synthesizes DNA	Removes and replaces RNA primer with DNA	Joins DNA segments

251

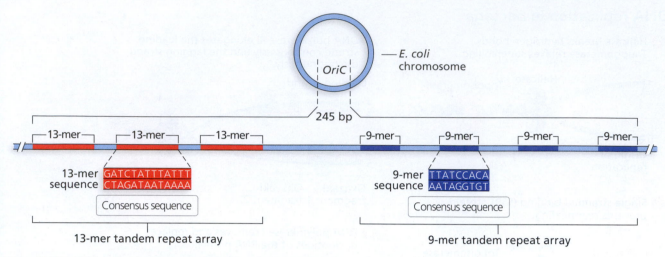

Figure 7.15 **Origin of replication sequence in *E. coli.*** *OriC* in *E. coli* contains three 13-mer and four 9-mer consensus sequences in a region of 245 base pairs of conserved sequence.

Table 7.2	Bacterial Origin-of-Replication Consensus Sequences
Species	**9-mer Sequence**
Escherichia coli	TTATCCACA
Bacillus subtilis	TTATCCACA
Pseudomonas putida	TTATCCACA
Vibrio cholerae	TTATCCACA
Caulobacter crescentus	T**G**ATCCACA
Mycobacterium tuberculosis	TT**G**TCCACA
Streptomyces coelicolor	TT**G**TCCACA
Helicobacter pylori	T**CAT**TCACA
Consensus sequence	TTATCCACA

DNA sequences denote origins of replication, multicellular eukaryotes use a less sequence-dependent process to initiate DNA replication. Genome sequence analysis has identified tens of thousands of potential replication origins in many large eukaryotic genomes, but only about one out of five of these potential sequences is used to initiate replication in any given cell cycle. It is more accurate to think of eukaryotic DNA replication as originating in zones that contain an average of five potential replication origin sequences, with just one of these sequences being used in a given cell cycle.

In a second level of organization in multicellular eukaryotes, the replication zones can be categorized according to whether they are initiated at an early, intermediate, or late point in S phase. This accounts for the observation that DNA replication is not synchronous throughout the eukaryotic genome. It appears that the state of the chromosome organization plays a pivotal role in determining the sites at which DNA replication initiates in eukaryotic genomes. We discuss this aspect of eukaryotic chromosomes in Chapter 10 and provide additional molecular details of eukaryotic organization in those discussions.

Less is known about the DNA sequences at replication origins in other eukaryotic species, particularly in multicellular species. What *is* known, however, suggests that the sequence of the origin of replication is flexible. This means that unlike bacteria, archaea, and yeast, in which specific

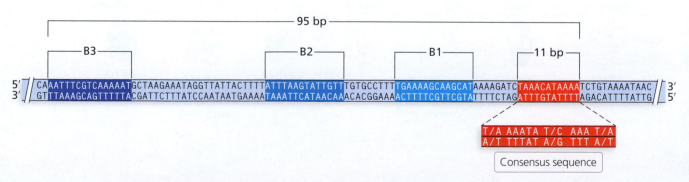

Figure 7.16 **The yeast ARS1 origin of replication.** The origin of replication in yeast contains a consensus 11-bp segment and regions B₁, B₂, and B₃, spanning 95 base pairs of conserved sequence. A solidus (/) between nucleotides of consensus sequences (e.g., A/T) indicates that the two nucleotides are equally common at this position.

Molecular Biology of Replication Initiation

DNA replication in *E. coli* requires that replication-initiating enzymes locate and bind to the consensus sequences in *oriC*. In *E. coli,* three enzymes, DnaA, DnaB, and DnaC, bind at *oriC* and initiate DNA replication (**Figure 7.17**). The protein DnaA binds to the 9-mer components of *oriC* and bends the DNA, breaking hydrogen bonds in the AT-rich 13-mer region of *oriC*. This creates an open origin complex, a short region where the DNA strands are separated. A DnaB then binds to *oriC*, and replication initiates. The DnaB is a **helicase** protein that breaks hydrogen bonds to separate the DNA strands and unwinds the double helix ahead of advancing DNA replication. The unwound strands are bound by **single-stranded binding protein (SSB)**, which prevents them from

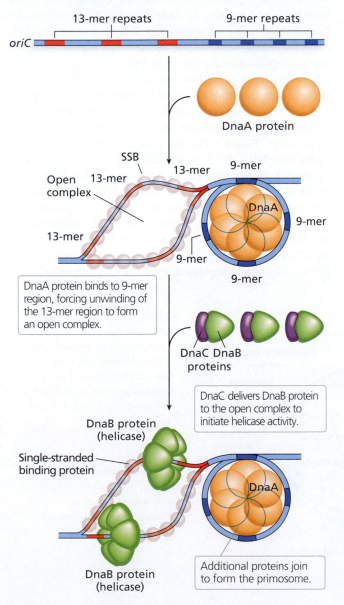

DnaA protein binds to 9-mer region, forcing unwinding of the 13-mer region to form an open complex.

DnaC delivers DnaB protein to the open complex to initiate helicase activity.

Additional proteins join to form the primosome.

Figure 7.17   Replication initiation at *oriC*, requiring DnaA, DnaB, and DnaC proteins.

reforming a DNA duplex and thus keeps them available to serve as templates for new DNA synthesis (see Figure 7.14, steps ❶ and ❷).

The first steps in DNA replication initiation are similar in archaea and eukaryotes. In archaea, a protein complex identified as Orc1/Cdc6 binds to ORB and miniORB sequences. Orc1/Cdc6 has helicase activity that separates the DNA strands at those sequences. The protein Mcm then binds to the separated strands, followed by additional proteins and enzymes that bind to the region, and synthesis begins. In eukaryotes, helicase recruitment and activity is best understood in yeast, where four protein subcomplexes are involved. At eukaryotic replication origins, a prereplication complex (preRC) of 14 proteins assembles. An aggregation of six of these proteins form a subunit identified as the *origin replication complex* (ORC) that acts as the initiator of eukaryotic DNA replication by identifying the origin site. ORC is then bound by the proteins Cdc6 and Cdt1. This is followed by binding of another eight proteins. The resulting complex separates the DNA strands at the replication origin, and DNA replication gets under way.

In all organisms, DNA polymerase enzymes that are responsible for synthesizing new DNA strands use a template strand to direct the addition of nucleotides to daughter strands in a complementary and antiparallel manner. These new nucleotides are added to the 3′ end of the growing daughter strand, and the overall direction of daughter strand elongation is 5′ to 3′. Curiously, however, DNA polymerases are unable to *initiate* DNA strand synthesis on their own. To perform its catalytic activity, a DNA polymerase requires the presence of a primer sequence, a short single-stranded segment that begins a daughter strand and provides an OH end to which a new DNA nucleotide can be added by DNA polymerase. To satisfy the requirement for a primer, DNA replication in bacteria is initiated by **primase**, a specialized enzyme that synthesizes a short **RNA primer** (see step ❸ of Figure 7.14).

Measuring just one dozen to two dozen nucleotides in length, RNA primers provide the 3′ OH needed for DNA polymerase activity. RNA primers contain the nucleotide base uracil (U) in place of thymine. Consequently, RNA primers cannot remain as part of fully replicated DNA. Thus, although they are essential for allowing DNA polymerase to begin its DNA synthesis, RNA primers are temporary and are removed from newly synthesized DNA strands before replication is completed. Primase enzymes also operate in the initial stages of archaeal and eukaryotic DNA replication. As in bacterial replication, primases in archaea and eukaryotes synthesize a short RNA primer that functions identically to bacterial RNA primers.

Continuous and Discontinuous Strand Replication

Each strand of parental DNA acts as a template for the synthesis of a new daughter strand of DNA. In *E. coli,* daughter DNA strands are synthesized at the replication fork by

DNA polymerase III (DNA pol III), the principal DNA-synthesizing enzyme (see Figure 7.14, step ❹). DNA pol III begins its work at the 3'-OH end of an RNA primer and rapidly synthesizes new DNA by adding one nucleotide at a time in a sequence that is complementary and antiparallel to the template-strand nucleotides. Pol III requires a template nucleotide to add a new nucleotide to a daughter strand. Enzymes with functions identical to DNA pol III are found in archaea and eukaryotes.

Experimental evidence indicates that most of the enzymes participating in DNA replication are part of a large protein complex called a **replisome**. There is one replisome at each replication fork. Replisomes have numerous components, including, in each replisome, two complete molecules of DNA pol III. One of these DNA pol III molecules carries out the 5'-to-3' synthesis of one daughter strand *continuously*, in the *same* direction in which the replication fork progresses. The second pol III in the replisome carries out synthesis of the other daughter strand. The continuously elongated daughter strand is called the **leading strand** (**Figure 7.18**). Notice that Figure 7.18 divides the replication bubble into four quadrants. The upper right and lower left quadrants contain leading strands.

The daughter strands in the upper left and lower right quadrants shown in Figure 7.18 have a 5'-to-3' direction of elongation that runs *opposite* to the direction of movement of the replication fork. These daughter strands are elongated *discontinuously*, in short segments, each of which is initiated by an RNA primer. The discontinuously synthesized daughter strand is called the **lagging strand**. Thus in Figure 7.18, the lower right and upper left quadrants of the replication bubble contain lagging strands (see also step ❺ of Figure 7.14).

Reiji Okazaki detected the synthesis of short fragments of DNA in the replication of the lagging strand. He observed that early in bacterial replication, newly synthesized DNA segments on one strand are 1000 to 2000 nucleotides long, while later in replication those newly synthesized segments have become much longer. Okazaki's discovery suggested that short segments of DNA are synthesized and then, as replication progresses, joined together. The short segments of newly replicated DNA are called **Okazaki fragments**, and they are the result of discontinuous synthesis of DNA on the lagging strand. Okazaki fragments in eukaryotes are much shorter than those in bacteria, 100 to 200 nucleotides in length. Similarly, archaeal Okazaki fragments are short.

RNA Primer Removal and Okazaki Fragment Ligation

To complete DNA replication, RNA primers must be removed and replaced with DNA, and Okazaki fragments must be joined together to form complete DNA strands. In *E. coli* these tasks are accomplished by the enzymes *DNA polymerase I* and *DNA ligase* that are each part of the replisome complex at each replication fork.

When DNA pol III on the lagging strand reaches an RNA primer, thus running out of template, it leaves a single-stranded gap between the last DNA nucleotide of the newly synthesized daughter strand and the first nucleotide of the RNA primer (**Figure 7.19**). The pol III, having very low affinity for these DNA–RNA single-stranded gaps, is then replaced by **DNA polymerase I (DNA pol I)**, which has high affinity for such gaps (Figure 7.19, ❶). The DNA pol I removes nucleotides of the RNA primer one by one and replaces them with DNA nucleotides, beginning with the 5' nucleotide of the RNA primer and progressing in the 3' direction until all the RNA nucleotides in the primer have been replaced by DNA nucleotides complementary to the template strand.

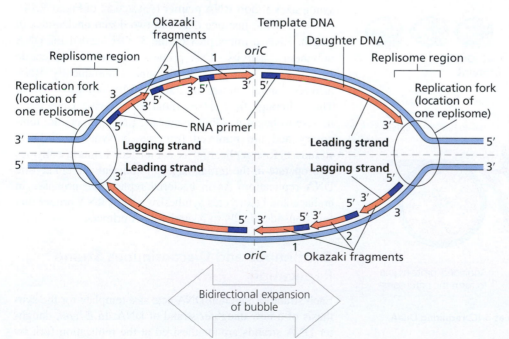

Figure 7.18   The replication bubble. Bidirectional expansion is driven by DNA synthesis at each replication fork. One replisome containing two DNA pol III enzymes operates at each fork to replicate both daughter strands.

Q Draw a second replication bubble to the right of the one illustrated. As these two replication bubbles expand toward one another, what kind of strand will each leading strand encounter when the bubbles make contact?

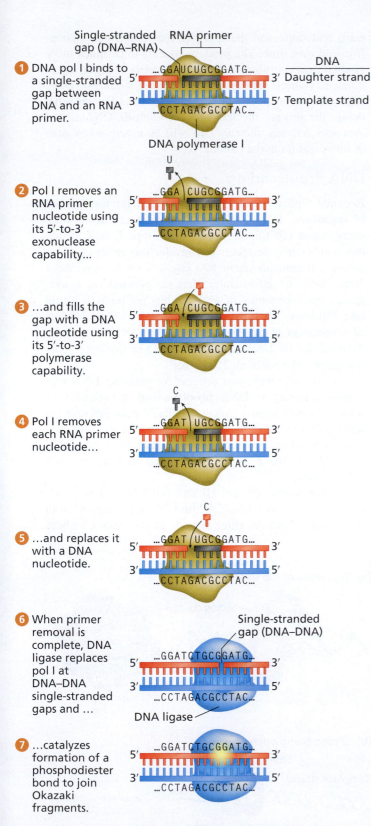

1 DNA pol I binds to a single-stranded gap between DNA and an RNA primer.

2 Pol I removes an RNA primer nucleotide using its 5'-to-3' exonuclease capability...

3 ...and fills the gap with a DNA nucleotide using its 5'-to-3' polymerase capability.

4 Pol I removes each RNA primer nucleotide...

5 ...and replaces it with a DNA nucleotide.

6 When primer removal is complete, DNA ligase replaces pol I at DNA–DNA single-stranded gaps and ...

7 ...catalyzes formation of a phosphodiester bond to join Okazaki fragments.

Figure 7.19 Removal and replacement of RNA primer nucleotides and ligation of Okazaki fragments in *E. coli*.

The pol I enzyme possesses two activities that accomplish the removal of RNA nucleotides and their replacement by DNA nucleotides. DNA pol I first uses its **5'-to-3' exonuclease activity** to remove the 5'-most nucleotide from the RNA primer (see step 6 in Figure 7.14). This creates one open space opposite the template, which is then filled with the correct DNA nucleotide by the **5'-to-3' polymerase activity** of DNA pol I. As DNA pol I removes each RNA primer nucleotide and replaces it with a DNA nucleotide, the pol I continually pushes the single-stranded gap in the 3' direction.

Once the entire RNA primer is replaced, a remaining single-stranded gap sits between two DNA nucleotides. At this point, **DNA ligase**, having exclusive and very high affinity for DNA–DNA single-stranded gaps, is attracted to the gap and there performs its single task of forming a phosphodiester bond between the two DNA nucleotides that joins two Okazaki fragments (see step 7 in Figure 7.14). Both pol I and DNA ligase are active on leading *and* lagging strands. The level of activity is greater on lagging strands, however, where every 1000 to 2000 nucleotides, they are needed to join Okazaki fragments during replication of *E. coli* DNA.

Overall, the pattern of DNA replication involving a leading strand and a lagging strand is similar in bacteria, eukaryotes, and archaea. For each domain, Table 7.3 lists three DNA polymerases that are principally responsible for carrying out the synthesis of RNA primers, DNA synthesis, and RNA primer removal and replacement.

Synthesis of Leading and Lagging Strands at the Replication Fork

As we have seen, the replisome components in *E. coli* include two DNA pol III enzymes, one of which synthesizes the leading strand and the other the lagging strand. As we describe momentarily, a similar organization exists in eukaryotic and archaeal DNA replication. Therefore, each replisome complex carries out replication of both the leading strand and the lagging strand. The replisome also includes pol I and ligase, as well as numerous other components that collectively carry out DNA replication.

The "processivity" of DNA polymerases on their own—that is, the ability of DNA polymerases to drive their own movement along template strands during replication—is comparatively low. This means that by themselves they are unable to provide the momentum required to both synthesize new DNA and progress along the template strand. To enhance the processivity of these polymerases, they are associated with an auxiliary protein complex known as a **sliding clamp**.

The sliding clamp, with its diameter of approximately 75Å, has a "doughnut hole" of about 35 Å that encircles double-stranded DNA (**Figure 7.20a**). Each sliding clamp locks onto a DNA template strand and affiliates with DNA pol III core enzyme, firmly anchoring the enzyme to the template to carry out the bulk of replication (**Figure 7.20b**).

Table 7.3	Properties of Selected Bacterial, Eukaryotic, and Archaeal DNA Polymerases	
Polymerase	**Functions**	
Bacterial polymerases		
DnaG	RNA primer synthesis	
I	RNA primer removal, proofreading, mutation repair	
III	DNA replication, proofreading	
Eukaryotic polymerases		
Primase/α	Primer synthesis and lagging strand synthesis	
β	Lagging strand synthesis, proofreading, DNA mutation repair	
ε	Leading strand synthesis, proofreading, DNA mutation repair	
Archaeal polymerases		
Primase	Primer synthesis	
PolB	DNA synthesis	
PolD	DNA synthesis	

The clamp is the key to the enzyme's high level of activity. When no more template nucleotides are available, the DNA pol III is dropped by the sliding clamp and replaced by DNA pol I, which as we have seen removes RNA primers and replaces them with DNA.

How does the replisome coordinate synthesis of the leading strand and the lagging strand? Molecular biologists thought they knew, until the first real-time observation of DNA replication was made in mid-2017. Models of DNA replication in bacteria since the 1960s have proposed that the replisome has two "arms" that each carry DNA pol III. The models depict the continuous 5′-to-3′ synthesis of the leading strand by pol III on one replisome arm as the replisome progresses behind the advancing replication fork while DNA pol III on the other arm of the replisome undertakes a "catch, synthesize, and release" process to synthesize new daughter DNA using the lagging strand template. In this model, the lagging strand template is grasped and rotated around so it is in position to allow the 5′-to-3′ synthesis of the lagging strand in the same direction as leading strand synthesis.

In mid-2017, for the first time, DNA replication was observed in real time in *E. coli* by Stephen Kowalczykowski and colleagues. The result was unexpected and not at all in agreement with the models of replication. Real-time observation showed that the expected coordination between synthesis of the leading strand and the lagging strand does not occur. Overall, the two strands are synthesized at about the same rate, but there are numerous

starts and stops, and the speed of replication varies about five-fold over time. The process appears to be much more random than coordinated; thus, the models of highly coordinated synthesis of leading and lagging strands of DNA appear to be incorrect, at least in bacteria. For the time being, the precise mechanism that controls DNA strand synthesis remains unclear. This will be a very active area of investigation in the coming years.

DNA Proofreading

Accurate replication of DNA is essential for the survival of organisms. DNA replication errors occur about once every billion (10^9) nucleotides in wild-type *E. coli*. To put this number into perspective, consider this textbook as an analogy. It contains about 800 pages, each holding about 5000 "bits" of information (letters, punctuation marks, spaces, etc.) for a total of 4×10^6 bits per book. It would take 250 books, each the size of this one, to equal 10^9 bits of information. If each bit were equal to a DNA nucleotide, the error rate for DNA replication would be like having *one* typographical error in all 250 books!

A critically important process for ensuring DNA replication accuracy is **DNA proofreading**, a capability of most DNA polymerases that momentarily stops and reverses replication to remove an incorrect nucleotide and replace it with a correct nucleotide. In *E. coli,* this proofreading ability resides in the **3′-to-5′ exonuclease activity** of DNA polymerases.

Polymerases like pol III and pol I have a structure resembling an open hand: A "thumb" and "fingers" hold the template and daughter strands in the "palm," where

(a) Two views of the sliding clamp

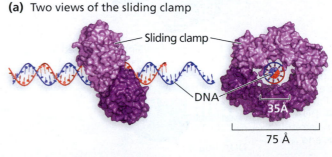

(b) Sliding clamp operation

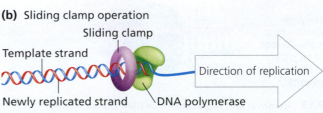

Figure 7.20 The DNA sliding clamp. (a) Two views of the sliding clamp, one showing the clamp on DNA in profile (left) and the other showing DNA through the "doughnut hole" of the sliding clamp (right). **(b)** The sliding clamp–DNA polymerase complex has high processivity during replication.

5′-to-3′ polymerase activity is centered (**Figure 7.21**). When a replication error occurs, the mismatched DNA bases of the template and daughter strands are unable to hydrogen bond properly. As a result, the 3′ OH end of the daughter strand becomes displaced, blocking the further addition of nucleotides and inducing rotation of the daughter strand into the 3′-to-5′ exonuclease site at the "heel" of the hand. Several nucleotides, including the mismatched one, are then removed from the 3′ end of the daughter strand, after which the daughter strand rotates back to the polymerase site in the palm and replication resumes. Like their counterparts in bacteria, the principal DNA replication polymerases in eukaryotes and archaea also have proofreading ability to help ensure the accuracy of DNA replication.

Genetic Analysis 7.2 checks your understanding and analysis of molecular events at the replication fork.

Supercoiling and Topoisomerases

During DNA replication, the molecule undergoes superhelical twisting, referred to as **supercoiling**. This is a form of twisting that goes beyond the double helical twists already present. Supercoiling occurs because the unwinding of portions of the helix to permit replication communicates torsional strain to other parts of the molecule (**Figure 7.22a**). It is like holding one side of a rubber band stationary while twisting the other side. Phospodiester bonds are under particular stress, but random breaks are prevented from occurring by a process that provides controlled relief of this stress. Circular chromosomes like those in many bacteria and archaea are particularly prone to supercoiling during DNA replication, as the figure shows. Linear chromosomes of eukaryotes manage this extra twisting more easily, but they also require controlled relief of torsional stress.

Enzymes known as **DNA topoisomerases** catalyze a controlled cleavage and rejoining of DNA to allow overwound DNA strands to unwind (**Figure 7.22b**). Relief of supercoiling is accomplished by different topoisomerases in different ways. Some topoisomerases break a phosphodiester bond in just one DNA strand, while others break both strands of DNA. Either mechanism allows the supercoiled strands to unwind superhelical twists. After unwinding is complete, broken phosphodiester bonds reform.

Replication at the Ends of Linear Chromosomes

Linear chromosomes, like those in the nuclei of your cells, have an altogether different problem presented by replication. Whereas the replication of circular chromosomes generates two complete copies of the original parental chromosome, linear chromosomes are unable to replicate fully and completely all the way to their ends. Instead, linear chromosome replication falls a little short of reaching the chromosome ends, and as a result, linear chromosomes get progressively shorter with each replication cycle.

The incomplete replication process occurs at the ends of chromosomes due to the presence of RNA primers very near the end of the lagging strand template. (**Figure 7.23**). A segment of DNA at the end of the lagging strand template is not replicated, shortening the chromosome with each replication cycle.

Although the loss of DNA with each replication cycle sounds potentially disastrous, the problem is solved by the

(a) DNA polymerase error

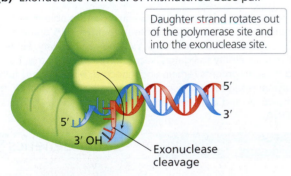

(b) Exonuclease removal of mismatched base pair

Daughter strand rotates out of the polymerase site and into the exonuclease site.

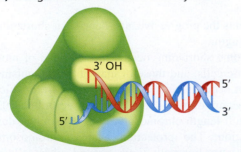

(c) Daughter strand resumes DNA synthesis

Figure 7.21   DNA polymerase proofreading activity.
(a) A replication error by polymerase. **(b)** Newly synthesized 3′ end of daughter strand shifts into exonuclease site, where nucleotides are removed. **(c)** The polymerase resumes 5′-to-3′ synthesis.

PROBLEM Two strains of *E. coli* have temperature-sensitive mutations that hamper their ability to complete DNA replication. At 25°C, both strains are able to complete replication, but neither is able to complete replication at 40°C. At 40°C, temperature-sensitive mutant 1 is able to synthesize DNA by DNA polymerase III activity, and it is able to remove RNA primers and replace them with DNA, but it accumulates many short segments of DNA (Okazaki fragments) that are not joined together. At 40°C, temperature-sensitive mutant 2 also synthesizes DNA by polymerase III activity, but it is unable to remove RNA primers and replace them with DNA. For each of these mutants, use the information provided here to identify the molecule that is most likely carrying the temperature-sensitive mutation. Identify which normal major events of DNA replication each mutant can complete at 40°C and which normal events are altered in each mutant.

> **BREAK IT DOWN:** Temperature-sensitive mutations are the result of proteins that have full function at a lower temperature but denature and lose function at higher temperatures (see Section 4.1)

Solution Strategies	Solution Steps
Evaluate	
1. Identify the topic this problem addresses and the nature of the required answer.	1. This problem addresses DNA replication and asks you to identify the function of particular proteins and enzymes that are active at different stages of replication.
2. Identify the critical information given in the problem.	2. Two *E. coli* strains with different temperature-sensitive mutations of DNA replication are described. Mutant strain 1 accumulates Okazaki fragments that cannot be joined together, and mutant strain 2 is unable to remove RNA primers.
Deduce	
3. Review the molecular events and principal molecules that are involved in RNA primer removal and RNA primer replacement. TIP: The function of principal proteins and enzymes in *E. coli* DNA replication is discussed in this section.	3. A review of Foundation Figure 7.14 and of Section 7.4 shows that in *E. coli*, DNA polymerase I is responsible for the removal of RNA primer nucleotides and their replacement with DNA nucleotides, and that DNA ligase joins Okazaki fragments together.
Solve	
4. Identify the molecule affected by mutation in mutant	4. Mutant 1 is most likely to have a defect in DNA ligase.
5. Identify the molecule affected by mutation in mutant 2.	5. Mutant 2 is most likely to have a defect in DNA polymerase I.
6. Identify which parts of DNA replication are completed at 40°C and which are affected by each mutation.	6. Mutant 1 is able to synthesize RNA primers by DnaG activity and is able to synthesize DNA with polymerase III activity. It is also able to remove RNA primers and replace the RNA nucleotides with DNA through polymerase I activity. However, mutant 1 is defective in its ability to ligate Okazaki fragments together by DNA ligase activity, and these fragments remain unconnected. Mutant 2 has fully functional DnaG and polymerase III to synthesize RNA primers and most DNA. It lacks active DNA pol I, however, and is therefore unable to remove RNA primers and replace them with DNA.

For more practice, see Problems 14, 15, and 18.   Visit the Study Area to access study tools.   **Mastering Genetics**

---

presence of hundreds to thousands of copies of repetitive DNA sequences called **telomeres** at the ends of linear chromosomes. Telomeres do not contain protein-coding genes. Instead, telomeres are made up of hundreds to thousands of end-to-end 6-bp repeats at the ends of vertebrate chromosomes and of longer repeats, up to about 12 bp each, in plants, yeast, and other eukaryotes. Total telomere length on each chromosome ranges from 2 to 20 kb at the birth of an organism, and decreases with age after that. Since telomere sequences are repetitive and contain no genetic information, a portion of a telomere can safely be lost in each replication cycle, without consequence to the organism. Gel-based and genome sequence analysis of telomeric DNA documents the progressive, age-dependent shortening of telomere length.

Chromosome shortening occurs in the nuclei of most of your somatic cells, and those of many other organisms, but it does not occur in cells of the germ line, from which sperm and eggs are derived. This feature of germ line cells ensures that full-length chromosomes are transmitted during reproduction. The protection against chromosome shortening in germ-line cells (and selected other cells in the body) is afforded by the DNA-synthesizing ability of the ribonucleoprotein **telomerase**, a complex consisting of several proteins and a molecule of RNA. The RNA in telomerase acts as a template for synthesizing a repetitive

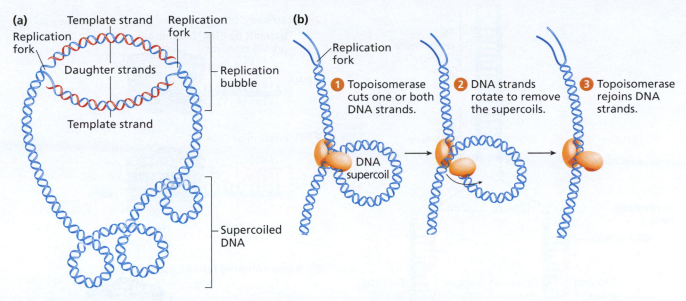

Figure 7.22   **DNA supercoiling in bacteria (a) and its cutting and release by topoisomerase (b).**

telomeric DNA sequence. Elizabeth Blackburn and Carol Greider discovered both telomeric repeat sequences and telomerase in 1987, in the ciliated protozoan *Tetrahymena*. Along with Jack Szostak, who described critical elements of the biochemistry of telomerase activity, they were awarded the 2009 Nobel Prize in Physiology or Medicine for their work. Telomerase is a reverse transcriptase enzyme, meaning that it transcribes DNA from an RNA template. It is encoded by the *TERT (telomerase reverse transcriptase)* gene.

Figure 7.24 depicts the repetitive telomeric sequence in *Tetrahymena* and illustrates the mechanism of telomerase synthesis of a telomere (see steps ❶ through ❺). The repetitive sequence 5′-TTGGGG-3′ is the characteristic telomeric repeat sequence of *Tetrahymena*. The template RNA in the *Tetrahymena* telomerase contains the repeat AACCCC that is used to elongate the telomere of one strand enough to allow new DNA replication to fill out the chromosome ends. All eukaryotes follow a similar scheme for telomere production, although the repetitive telomere sequence differs along species lines. Humans and other vertebrates, for example, have the telomeric repeat sequence 5′-TTAGGG-3′. Yeast, plants, and other eukaryotes have their own telomere sequences. At birth, the average human chromosome has about 2000 to 2500 TTAGGG repeats comprising the telomeres at each chromosome end. These repeats initially span 12 to 15 kb at each telomere.

In the decades since Blackburn, Greider, and Szostak identified telomere structure and the mechanism for their maintenance, the picture of telomeres has become more complex. In addition to repetitive DNA sequence, most eukaryotic telomeres are also characterized by the presence of a DNA sequence that forms a knotted fold known

as the **T loop**. The T loop protects the telomere from enzymatic degradation by joining with a protein complex known as **shelterin** (see Figure 7.24 step ❻). The combination of telomeric repeats and shelterin-protected T loops preserves telomeres for several dozen cycles of DNA replication. Inevitably, however, telomere length shortens, and when it becomes too short, it triggers apoptosis (programmed cell death).

Apoptosis induced by telomere shortening is associated with an observation in cell biology called the **Hayflick limit**, the apparent limit to the length of a cell's life span. Leonard Hayflick first described this limitation in 1965, pointing out that vertebrate cells live an average of 50 to 70 cycles before dying. The Hayflick limit appears to be explained by the progressive loss of telomere length as cells age.

Some research has suggested that preserving or lengthening telomers, perhaps by activating telomerase activity in somatic cells, may be an avenue to longer life spans. For example, some research in humans indicates that physical activity, which is associated with prolonged healthy living, may lengthen telomeres. Complicating this idea of generating telomerase activity to stabilize telomere length and potentially prolong life, however, is the finding that the activation of telomerase activity in somatic cells is a characteristic of cancerous cells in 80 to 90% of all cancers. The most likely functional role of telomerase activation in cancer development is the prevention of programmed cell death. The ability of cancer cells to evade normal cell death by preserving telomere length confers an element of immortality on cancer cells that is not possessed by normal somatic cells. We discuss this idea more fully in Application Chapter C: The Genetics of Cancer.

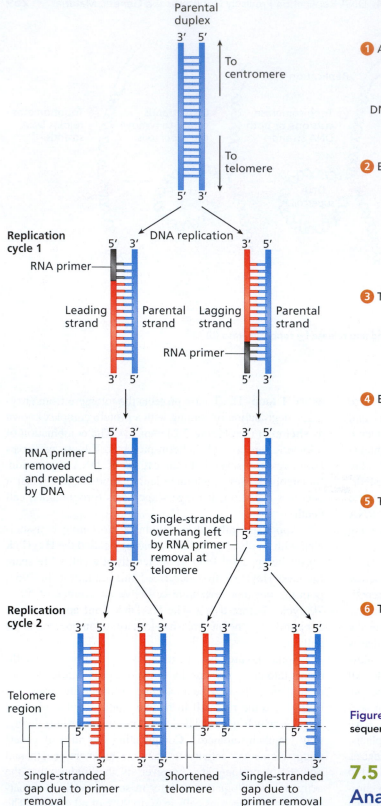

Figure 7.23 Loss of DNA at telomeres. Leading strands are synthesized to the ends of linear chromosomes, but lagging strands are shortened at each replication cycle, when the RNA primer sequence at the end of the template strand is removed but not replaced with DNA nucleotides.

🔍 **Looking at the results of replication cycle 2, and examining the DNA duplex at the right-hand side, would you call the red DNA strand a leading strand or a lagging strand?**

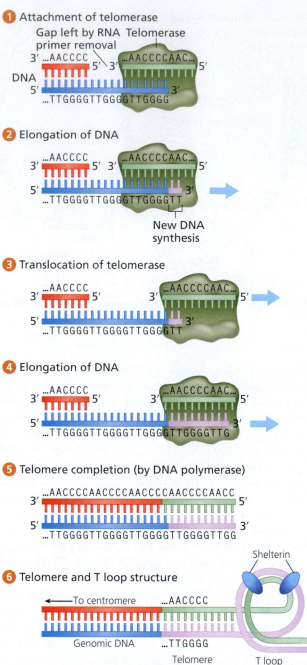

Figure 7.24 Telomerase synthesis of repeating telomeric sequence.

7.5 Methods of Molecular Genetic Analysis Make Use of DNA Replication Processes

Molecular biologists have used their understanding of the enzymes and processes of DNA replication to develop new laboratory methods for molecular genetic analysis. Two widely used methods that developed directly from this knowledge are the *polymerase chain reaction (PCR)* and a method for *dideoxynucleotide DNA sequencing* designed by Frederick Sanger. In this section, we look at both of these methods and at their use in deciphering DNA variation.

The Polymerase Chain Reaction

Developed in 1983 by Kary Mullis, the **polymerase chain reaction (PCR)** is an automated version of DNA replication that takes place in a test tube containing a total reaction volume of 20 to 50 microliters (one microliter is one-millionth of a liter). Despite this very small total reaction volume, a typical PCR reaction, beginning with just a few copies of a short, targeted DNA sequence, produces millions of copies of the sequence in a few hours. Reproduction of DNA through PCR has innumerable uses in modern biological research, including the evolutionary study of extinct species; the comparison of DNA among living species; forensic genetic applications such as paternity testing, crime scene analysis, and individual identification; and production of DNA segments for genome sequencing projects.

Polymerase chain reactions are in vitro DNA-replication reactions performed using (1) double-stranded DNA containing the target sequence that is to be copied, (2) a supply of the four DNA nucleotides, (3) a heat-stable DNA polymerase, and (4) two different single-stranded DNA primers (described in the list of steps below). These PCR components are mixed with a buffer solution, and then the automated reaction is run through 30 to 35 three-step "cycles." Each cycle doubles the number of copies of the targeted DNA sequence. The PCR process is generally identified as "amplification," and it is common to speak of "PCR amplification" in reference to the process and of "amplified DNA" as the product of the reaction.

PCR reactions are carried out in a device known as a *PCR thermal cycler*. Thermal cyclers are programmable, allowing the length and temperature of each cycle step to be adjusted to meet the needs of the experimenter. The thermal cycler takes just a few seconds to change temperature between steps.

Figure 7.25 illustrates the three steps of a PCR reaction. The steps and functions of each PCR cycle are as follows:

❶ *Denaturation.* The reaction mixture is heated to approximately 95°C, causing double-stranded DNA to *denature* into single strands as the hydrogen bonds between complementary strands break down. The step duration is usually 1 to 2 minutes.

❷ *Primer annealing.* The reaction temperature is reduced to between about 45°C and 68°C to allow *primer annealing*—the hybridization of the two short, single-stranded DNA primers to complementary sequences bracketing the target sequence. These primers have the same function as RNA primers in DNA replication. They are, as mentioned, short (12 to

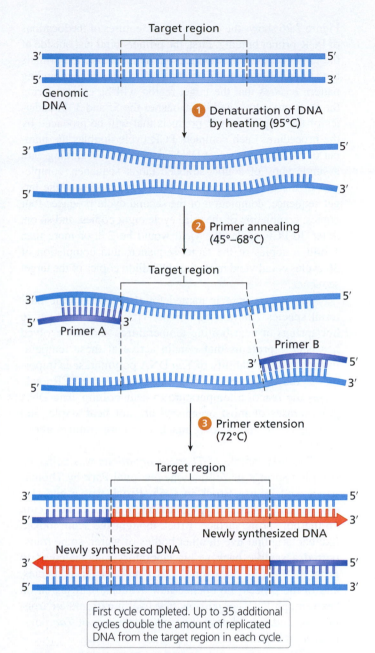

Figure 7.25 The three-step cycle of PCR. Amplification by PCR doubles the number of copies of the targeted DNA sequence each cycle.

24 nucleotides), and one primer binds to each of the denatured DNA strands. The step duration is usually 1 to 2 minutes.

❸ *Primer extension.* Raising the temperature of the reaction to 72°C allows *primer extension*, during which a specialized DNA polymerase known as *Taq* polymerase synthesizes DNA, beginning at the 3′ end of each primer. *Taq* polymerase, described in more detail below, synthesizes new DNA at the rate of about 1000 bp per minute. This step duration is usually 3 to 5 minutes.

Figure 7.26 shows the two important features of the locations of PCR-primer binding. First, the primers bind just outside of the target region for amplification, and, second, the primers bind to opposite complementary strands. This primer binding pattern ensures that the target region will be copied during the PCR procedure, and it establishes the 5′ and 3′ boundaries of the amplified PCR products that will be produced by the procedure. Each complete PCR cycle doubles the number of copies of the target DNA sequence, so beginning with a single copy of double-stranded target sequence, completion of the first PCR cycle produces two copies of the target sequence, completion of the second cycle produces four copies, completion of the third cycle eight copies, and so on. After 30 PCR cycles the yield would be 2^{30}, or more than 1 billion copies of the target sequence, and completion of 36 cycles could yield more than 68 billion copies of the target sequence.

Taq polymerase is named for the thermophilic bacterial species *Thermus aquaticus*. This bacterium lives in hot springs at near-boiling temperatures and has evolved heat-stable proteins that remain active at these temperatures. The heat stability of *Taq* DNA polymerase is important to the efficiency of PCR, since step 1 of a PCR cycle raises the reaction temperature to near boiling. The DNA polymerases of most organisms are not heat stable, and they denature and become inactive at temperatures above about 45°C.

The first sample of *Thermus aquaticus* was collected from hot springs in Yellowstone National Park by Thomas Brock and Louise Brock in 1965. Brock was a microbiologist, and his attention was drawn to some brown scum on the hot spring surface. Brock thought the scum looked like bacteria that live in other bodies of water, so he transported a sample back to his laboratory and managed to grow it. What he discovered was a new bacterial species, and in the process he opened new avenues of research on "extremophiles"—organisms that live in extreme environments—and helped pave the way for the use of *Taq* polymerase in PCR.

PCR has an enormous variety of applications, but it also has limitations, the most important of which are (1) the necessity of having some knowledge of the sequences needed for primers and (2) the difficulty of producing amplification products longer than 10 to 15 kb. In most cases, the length limitations on PCR restrict its use to the study of selected DNA segments or individual genes. The requirement for primer sequence information can be satisfied by informed guesses about the sequences likely to occur at primer binding sites or by using primers from one species to amplify similar sequences in another species. For example, a biologist wanting to study DNA-sequence similarity between species could use a pair of primers that amplify a *Drosophila* gene to examine the human genome for a related gene. There may be one or more base-pair mismatches between the *Drosophila* primers and the human DNA sequences they bind to, but the mismatches need not prevent primer annealing if the temperature of the PCR reaction is lowered during step 2 of the reaction. The lower temperature can increase the stability of hybridization of the primers and their target sequences enough to allow the former to prime the PCR amplification.

Separation of PCR Products

The PCR process selectively amplifies DNA fragments ranging in size from a few dozen base pairs to several thousand base pairs in length. The fragments generated are almost all of the same double-stranded target region. So highly concentrated are the results of PCR amplification that they can be analyzed directly using gel electrophoresis (see Chapter 1 for a discussion of this method).

Gel electrophoresis separates fragments of DNA by their sizes in base pairs. Recall from our discussion in Chapter 1 that DNA fragments containing fewer base pairs move more quickly in the electrical separation field than fragments with more base pairs. This means that smaller fragments, with higher electrophoretic mobility, migrate farther from the origin of migration than do fragments with more base pairs. The use of molecular-weight size markers in gel electrophoresis (DNA fragments containing known numbers of base pairs) allows researchers to determine the size of DNA fragments of unknown length by comparing their migration with that of the known size markers.

Figure 7.26a shows four hypothetical VNTR (variable number tandem repeat) alleles of a gene (V_1 to V_4) that consist of different numbers of repeats of the same short DNA sequence (see Section 5.5). Genetic markers of this type are commonly used in genetic studies, and they are especially common in forensic genetic analysis applications. We discuss the analysis of VNTR markers in forensic genetic settings in Application Chapter E: Forensic Genetics.

For an autosomal VNTR gene like the one illustrated in Figure 7.26a, the four alleles can form 10 different genotypes that each have their own distinctive set of one or two DNA fragment lengths (**Figure 7.26b**). Each homozygous genotype has a single band and each heterozygous genotype has two bands. The bands are identified by their repeat number.

The inheritance of the VNTR alleles follows a codominant pattern in which both alleles are detected in heterozygous genotypes. In the family represented in **Figure 7.26c**, the two parents have completely different heterozygous genotypes, and each parent transmits one allele to each child. As a consequence of the parents' completely different genotypes, each allele in each child can be traced to one of the parents, and each child has a heterozygous genotype. Notice that there are two DNA bands for each person in this family: VNTRs and other similar DNA genetic markers display codominant inheritance, and heterozygous individuals display DNA bands corresponding to each allele (see Section 4.1).

(a) Each allele produces a PCR fragment of a different length.

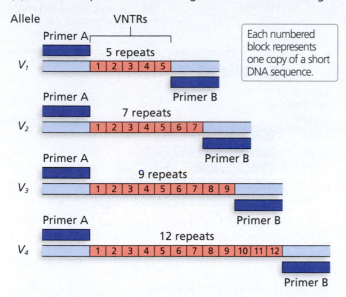

(b) VNTR band patterns

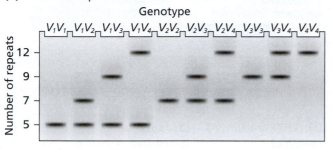

(c) Inheritance of VNTR variation

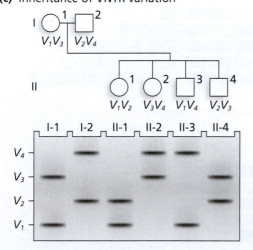

Figure 7.26 **Separation of variable number tandem repeat (VNTR) alleles after PCR amplification.** **(a)** Four VNTR alleles (V_1 to V_4) are characterized by different numbers of identical DNA repeat sequences. **(b)** Ten genotypes are possible for the VNTR gene, each having a unique pattern of PCR-fragment sizes. One band is seen for each homozygous genotype, and two bands for each heterozygous genotype. **(c)** Hereditary transmission of VNTR alleles follows a codominant pattern.

Dideoxynucleotide DNA Sequencing

The ultimate description of any DNA molecule is its sequence of bases. Depending on the purpose of the analysis or application, DNA sequence information may be sought for any-length sequence of DNA, from a small series of base pairs to a single chromosome to the genome as a whole. In addition, the phrase "genome sequence" can encompass all coding and regulatory sequences of genes along with all the other sequences in the DNA, including repetitive sequences, or it can be more limited. Most commonly, a "genome sequence" includes only those portions of the genome that are transcribed into RNA. We discuss approaches to creating and analyzing genomic sequence data in Chapter 16.

In addition to genetics research, DNA sequencing technology has found broad application in fields like agriculture, medicine, and evolutionary biology. And at the same time as its uses have broadened, laboratory and computer technologies have combined to make DNA sequencing faster and cheaper by orders of magnitude.

The first DNA sequencing protocols were developed in 1977, one by Allan Maxam and Walter Gilbert and another by Sanger. Of the two methods, Sanger's was more amenable to automation, and it is the basis for the high-throughput approach to genome sequencing that is the method of choice today. Therefore, before discussing the newest generations of automated DNA sequencing, let us begin with a look at Sanger's approach.

Sanger's DNA sequencing method is known as **dideoxynucleotide DNA sequencing** or **dideoxy DNA sequencing** or simply *Sanger sequencing*. Based on in vitro DNA replication reactions that closely resemble PCR, dideoxy sequencing, like PCR, uses DNA primers and DNA polymerase to replicate new DNA from a single-stranded template. In dideoxy sequencing reactions, the four standard deoxynucleotides (dNTP) of DNA are used in high concentrations, but to them is added a much smaller amount of a **dideoxynucleotide triphosphate (ddNTP).** Tens of thousands of identical DNA fragments are used in each sequencing reaction. The fragments are generated by cloning.

Dideoxynucleotides differ from deoxynucleotides in lacking two oxygen atoms (*dideoxy* means "two deoxygenated sites") rather than the usual one deoxygenated site. Recall that dNTPs are deoxygenated at the 2′ carbon and have a hydroxyl group (OH) at the 3′ carbon. In contrast, ddNTPs have hydrogen (H) atoms rather than hydroxyl groups at both the 2′ *and* 3′ carbons (**Figure 7.27a**). The absence of a hydroxyl group at the 3′ carbon in ddNTP prevents the ddNTP from forming a phosphodiester bond, so when a ddNTP is incorporated into a growing strand by DNA polymerase, the synthesis of the strand is terminated at that point (**Figure 7.27b**). Dideoxy sequencing therefore produces a large number of partial replication products, each terminated by incorporation of a ddNTP at a different site in the sequence.

(a)
Chemical structure

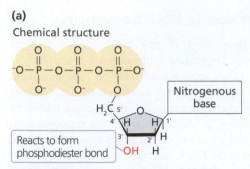

Deoxynucleotide triphosphate (dNTP)

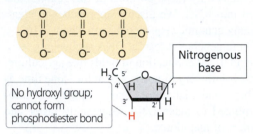

Dideoxynucleotide triphosphate (ddNTP)

(b)

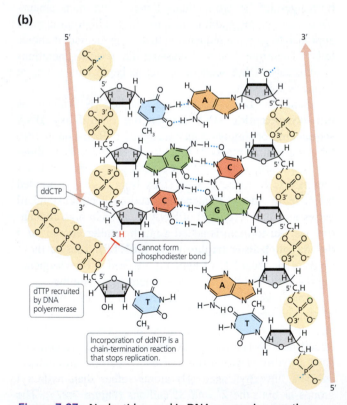

Figure 7.27 Nucleotides used in DNA sequencing reactions.
(a) Dideoxynucleotides (ddNTPs) are deoxygenated at both the 2′ and 3′ carbons and cannot form a phosphodiester bond for the further elongation of DNA. **(b)** The incorporation of a dideoxynucleotide of cytosine (ddCTP) terminates the replication reaction.

🔍 Circle the feature of the dideoxynucleotide in part (b) that prevents it from forming a phosphodiester bond.

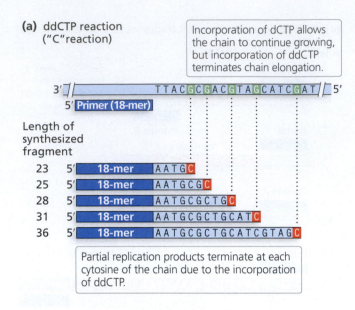

(a) ddCTP reaction ("C" reaction)

> Incorporation of dCTP allows the chain to continue growing, but incorporation of ddCTP terminates chain elongation.

3′ TTAC GCGACGTAGCATCGAT 5′
5′ Primer (18-mer)

Length of synthesized fragment

23	5′ 18-mer	AATG C
25	5′ 18-mer	AATGCG C
28	5′ 18-mer	AATGCGCTG C
31	5′ 18-mer	AATGCGCTGCAT C
36	5′ 18-mer	AATGCGCTGCATCGTAG C

> Partial replication products terminate at each cytosine of the chain due to the incorporation of ddCTP.

(b) ddGTP reaction ("G" reaction)

Length of synthesized fragment		Partial replication products
22	5′ 18-mer	AATG
24	5′ 18-mer	AATGCG
27	5′ 18-mer	AATGCGCTG
32	5′ 18-mer	AATGCGCTGCATCG
35	5′ 18-mer	AATGCGCTGCATCGTAG

(c) ddTTP reaction ("T" reaction)

Length of synthesized fragment		Partial replication products
21	5′ 18-mer	AAT
26	5′ 18-mer	AATGCGCT
30	5′ 18-mer	AATGCGCTGCAT
33	5′ 18-mer	AATGCGCTGCATCGT
38	5′ 18-mer	AATGCGCTGCATCGTAGCT

(d) ddATP reaction ("A" reaction)

Length of synthesized fragment		Partial replication products
19	5′ 18-mer	A
20	5′ 18-mer	AA
29	5′ 18-mer	AATGCGCTGCA
34	5′ 18-mer	AATGCGCTGCATCGTA
38	5′ 18-mer	AATGCGCTGCATCGTAGCTA

Figure 7.28 DNA sequencing reactions. (a) A target region of DNA is located by binding a single-stranded primer of 18 nucleotides (an "18-mer") that carries a 5′ label. Replication products terminated by ddCTP each have a different length. **(b)** Replication products terminated by ddGTP. **(c)** Termination products generated by ddTTP. **(d)** Termination products generated by ddATP.

Dideoxy DNA sequencing is carried out in four separate reaction mixtures—one for each of the four ddNTPs. Each reaction mixture contains the DNA strand to be sequenced, a single-stranded DNA primer, DNA polymerase, large amounts of each of the four standard nucleotides (dATP, dGTP, dCTP, and dTTP), and a small amount of *one* dideoxynucleotide, either that of adenine (ddATP), thymine (ddTTP), cytosine (ddCTP), or guanine (ddGTP).

Figure 7.28 shows that in each reaction mixture, DNA synthesis terminates at each site where a ddNTP is incorporated into the newly synthesized molecule. Figure 7.28a shows the DNA fragment being sequenced at the top, annealed to the 18-mer primer used to initiate DNA synthesis (18-mer means the primer is 18 nucleotides in length). It also shows that for the "C reaction mixture" (the mixture that includes ddCTP), each location at which a cytosine can be incorporated into the growing chain generates some DNA replication fragments that terminate at that location. Keep in mind that most of the cytosine in the C reaction mixture is the more highly concentrated dCTP, so it is most likely that this nucleotide will be incorporated into the growing chain. If so, replication continues. If, on the other hand, the less concentrated ddCTP is incorporated, as it will be in a small proportion of the replicating molecules, replication terminates. Figure 7.28a shows five different DNA fragment lengths

generated by ddCTP incorporation into C reaction mixture products.

The same process ensues in the three reaction mixtures containing, respectively, ddGTP, ddTTP, and ddATP (Figures 7.28b–d). Upon the completion of the four parallel sequencing reactions, there will be, for every nucleotide in the sequence, some partial replication DNA fragments terminating at that nucleotide.

Following completion of the ddNTP reactions, the contents of each reaction are loaded into separate lanes of a DNA electrophoresis gel, and the contents undergo separation by their length in base pairs (**Figure 7.29a**). Each DNA fragment in the gel can be radioactively labeled for visualization, allowing the sequence of the newly synthesized strand to be "read" off the gel. Knowing that the smallest DNA fragment migrates the farthest from the origin of migration, and knowing that newly synthesized DNA is elongated in the 5′-to-3′ direction and that the primer is located at the 5′ end of the sequenced strand, we can identify the consecutive nucleotides by the gel lane in which successively longer DNA fragments are located. Thus, the first incorporated nucleotide after the primer is A (i.e., ddATP is incorporated and terminates replication), followed by another A (ddATP incorporated), followed by T (ddTTP incorporated), and so on. Once the sequenced strand is determined, the complementary strand can be determined, using the knowledge that DNA strands are antiparallel and display complementary

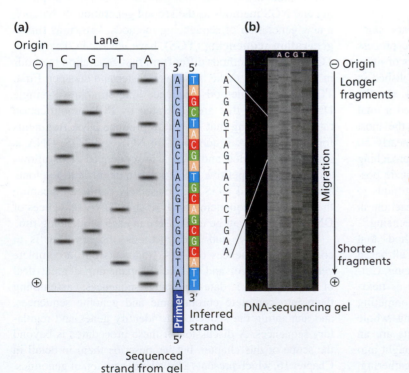

(a)

Sequenced strand from gel

(b)

DNA-sequencing gel

Figure 7.29 **Reading a dideoxy DNA sequencing gel. (a)** Replication of each fragment terminates with the addition of a ddNTP. Nucleotides of the newly synthesized "sequenced strand" are read off the gel. The 5′-to-3′ polarity of the sequenced strand corresponds to the smaller-to-larger fragment-length direction. The "inferred strand" is the complementary DNA strand, and it is antiparallel to the sequenced strand. **(b)** A photograph of a dideoxy sequencing gel with a segment of the sequence read.

Place 5′ and 3′ labels on the partial DNA sequence read from the DNA sequencing gel in part (b).

base pairing. An example of a dideoxy DNA sequencing gel is shown in **Figure 7.29b**, and a portion of the sequence is given.

Dideoxy sequencing is a slow and labor-intensive process that has been supplanted by high-throughput, automated DNA sequencing. When manual dideoxy DNA sequencing was used, it could generate 100 to 200 base pairs of a sequence per gel. A laboratory technician could hope to generate sequences for at most a few hundred base pairs in a day's work. Modern automated DNA sequencers, once they are loaded with DNA samples to be sequenced and with reaction ingredients, can run 24 hours a day, 365 days a year, and assemble genomic sequence at the rate of 10,000 to 20,000 bp per hour! **Genetic Analysis 7.3** tests your skills at interpreting dideoxy sequencing results.

New Generations of DNA Sequencing Technology

New generations of DNA sequencing technologies are continuing to be developed. These technologies sequence DNA fragments in parallel, meaning that hundreds of thousands to millions of DNA fragments are sequenced simultaneously. This brings the cost of DNA sequencing down so far that the goal of the "thousand dollar genome sequence"— that is, the availability of genome sequencing as an affordable component of everyday medicine—is within reach. It is likely that most readers of this book will have the opportunity to have their genomes sequenced.

Next-Generation Sequencing In the 40 years since Sanger introduced dideoxy DNA sequencing, the process has gotten both faster and cheaper by many orders of magnitude. The first human genome sequence, copublished in the scientific journals *Science* and *Nature* in 2001, was the result of nearly 15 years of work and represented a total investment of approximately $3 billion. Today, the most rapid automated DNA sequencers can produce nearly 50 human genome sequences a day for a cost is approaching $1000 per genome. These advances have been made possible by methods that sequence hundreds of thousands to millions of DNA fragments simultaneously in a reaction, in a process characterized as "massively parallel sequencing."

There are several different versions of methods that take a massively parallel approach, but they are all based on a similar elaboration of dideoxy DNA sequencing. Collectively, these advanced methods are identified as **next-generation sequencing**, or **NGS**. Enormous computing power and sophisticated ways of reconstructing whole genomes from the DNA sequences of fragments are an essential part of NGS. Advances in NGS have brought into being the field of bioinformatics to deal with the gathering,

management, and assembly of genome sequencing data generated by NGS.

NGS procedures begin with the fragmentation of genomic DNA. **Figure 7.30** illustrates this process as the first step of one version of NGS known as Illumina sequencing. In Illumina sequencing, the DNA is fragmented ❶, tagged with adaptor molecules attached to both ends of each strand ❷, and then denatured for analysis ❸. The adaptor molecules anchor the strand in a later step and may contain a PCR primer. The single-strand fragments are next placed in a flow cell and amplified to produce clusters of identical strands ❹ ❺. The mixture used for amplification contains DNA polymerase, the four dNTPs, and other necessary compounds. The dNTPs of A, T, G, and C are tagged with different fluorescent compounds that emit light in specific wavelengths when excited ❻. After each new nucleotide is incorporated into a growing strand, a laser light excites the fluorescent compound attached to the base, and a photoreceptor records the emission wavelength to identify the intensity ❼ ❽. Software records this information and converts it to identify the nucleotide as either A, T, C, or G ❾. This process repeats itself very rapidly as nucleotides are added to the strands. The result is a sequence for the fragments in each cluster. In this manner, next-generation sequencing identifies the sequence of a DNA strand "by synthesis" rather than "by chain termination" (the approach in dideoxy sequencing).

Third-Generation Sequencing Dideoxy DNA sequencing can be thought of as the first generation of DNA sequencing and NGS methods as the second generation. Inevitably, a new generation of sequencing methods, known as **third-generation sequencing (TGS)**, have now been developed. TGS and NGS methods differ from first generation methods in two ways that make them even faster and cheaper. First, TGS and NGS methods sequence long stretches of single DNA molecules that are generated by PCR amplification rather than cloning that is used to produce DNA fragments for dideoxy DNA sequencing. In NGS and TGS, DNA is first PCR amplified and then it is sequenced. This allows sequencing of repetitive DNA that can be difficult to clone, Second, TGS and NGS are "massively parallel," meaning that million of sequencing reads of short DNA sequences of DNA fragments can be undertaken in each sequencing run.

In both NGS and TGS methods, the key task is to compile the sequences of DNA fragments into a complete genomic sequence, and it requires managing a great deal of raw sequence data—aligning sequences, assembling them into complete chromosome and genome sequences, and annotating the sequences to identify genes and regulatory sequences. A discussion of these procedures is beyond the scope of this chapter, but we describe them in detail in Chapter 16, which presents a broader discussion of genomics.

PROBLEM From the dideoxy DNA sequencing gel shown here, deduce the sequence and strand polarities of the DNA duplex fragment.

> **BREAK IT DOWN:** Chain termination, caused by the incorporation of a dideoxynucleotide, produces the partially replicated DNA fragments detected in a DNA sequencing gel (p. 263).

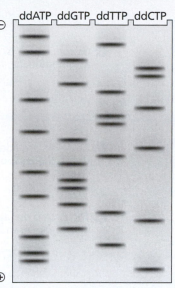

Solution Strategies	Solution Steps
Evaluate	
1. Identify the topic this problem addresses and the nature of the required answer.	1. This question concerns dideoxynucleotide DNA sequencing. The answer requires interpretation of a DNA sequencing gel to determine the double-stranded sequence of a fragment of DNA, including strand polarities.
2. Identify the critical information given in the problem.	2. A dideoxynucleotide DNA sequencing gel is shown.
Deduce	
3. Review the essential steps of dideoxy-nucleotide DNA sequencing.	3. DNA polymerase incorporates nucleotides in four parallel reactions. Each reaction mixture includes the four normal DNA nucleotides (dNTPs) and one labeled dideoxynucleotide (ddNTP). Incorporation of a dNTP allows continued strand synthesis, but incorporation of a ddNTP terminates synthesis.
4. Examine the gel and identify the "beginning" of DNA synthesis.	4. The 3′ end of the primer is used to initiate DNA synthesis. The first nucleotide incorporated during synthesis is cytosine, as determined by identifying the location of the smallest synthesized fragment: the "C" lane. The second and third nucleotides are both adenine. The first three nucleotides are therefore 5′-CAA-3′.

> **TIP:** DNA fragments toward the bottom of the gel (nearer the positive pole) are shorter than fragments higher up in the gel. The sequence of the synthesized strand shown in the gel is 5′ at the bottom and 3′ at the top.

Solve	
5. Write the rest of the sequence (along with the polarity) of the synthesized strand shown in the gel.	5. The synthesized strand is 5′-[primer]-CAATAGCTGAGGAGTCGATTCATGCCGATA-3′
6. Determine the sequence and polarity of the template strand used for DNA synthesis.	6. The template DNA strand is 3′-GTTATCGACTCCTCAGCTAAGTACGGCTAT-5′

For more practice, see Problems 28, 29, 30, and 34.   Visit the Study Area to access study tools.   **Mastering Genetics**

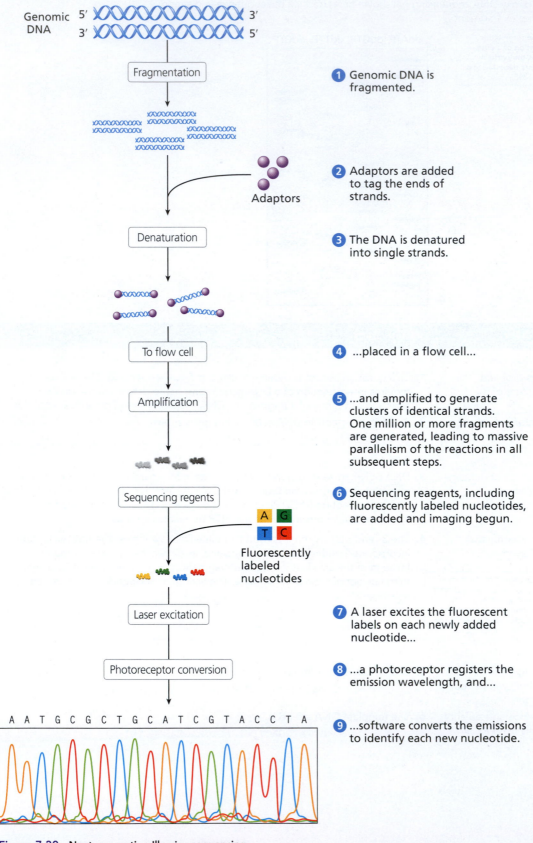

Genomic DNA 5′ 3′
            3′ 5′

Fragmentation

Adaptors

Denaturation

To flow cell

Amplification

Sequencing regents

A G
T C

Fluorescently
labeled
nucleotides

Laser excitation

Photoreceptor conversion

A A T G C G C T G C A T C G T A C C T A

① Genomic DNA is fragmented.

② Adaptors are added to tag the ends of strands.

③ The DNA is denatured into single strands.

④ ...placed in a flow cell...

⑤ ...and amplified to generate clusters of identical strands. One million or more fragments are generated, leading to massive parallelism of the reactions in all subsequent steps.

⑥ Sequencing reagents, including fluorescently labeled nucleotides, are added and imaging begun.

⑦ A laser excites the fluorescent labels on each newly added nucleotide...

⑧ ...a photoreceptor registers the emission wavelength, and...

⑨ ...software converts the emissions to identify each new nucleotide.

Figure 7.30   **Next-generation Illumina sequencing.**

CASE STUDY

DNA Helicase Gene Mutations and Human Progeroid Syndrome

At the latest count, the human genome contains 95 genes that each produce a different helicase enzyme. Most of these genes—64 of them—produce helicases that operate on RNA. The remaining 31 helicase genes produce DNA helicases. DNA helicases have a number of specific functions. Collectively, they are active in DNA replication, transcription, translation, recombination, damage repair, and other processes. Any process requiring the separation of two nucleic acid strands will involve helicase.

The helicase discussed in the body of this chapter belongs to a class of DNA helicases that are active in initiating DNA replication. In this Case Study, we discuss a different class of DNA helicase, one identified as the RECQ class, but some of them do take part in DNA replication and repair. Humans produce five RECQ helicases from five different autosomal genes. RECQ helicases are primarily active in meiotic crossing over and recombination. The designation "REC" for these helicases is short for "recombination." During meiotic recombination, RECQ helicases participate in the unwinding of DNA strands and work along with other proteins and enzymes to efficiently and accurately achieve reciprocal recombination of the type we discuss in Chapter 5. Rather than focus on the normal activities of RECQ helicases, however, we will now consider the mutations of three RECQ helicase genes that lead to three different hereditary conditions. In each case, mutation of a RECQ gene inherited in a recessive homozygous genotype is the cause of the condition.

HUMAN PROGEROID SYNDROME The three RECQ helicase gene mutations described in this Case Study each cause a specific form of premature aging. These diseases are among the eight hereditary conditions known collectively as *human progeroid syndrome* (Table 7.4). The term progeroid refers to premature aging, and although the specific symptoms of the eight progeroid conditions differ somewhat, there are some consistent general features that typify a progeroid condition. These common features are premature aging, short stature, and elevated risks for several conditions that are usually associated with advanced age, such as cancer; metabolic diseases, including diabetes type 2; osteoporosis (bone decalcification); and atherosclerosis (hardening of the arteries). In most progeroid conditions, life expectancy is much shorter than average, although the specific effect varies somewhat from case to case and the different conditions have different life expectancies.

Premature aging is not a sped-up version of normal aging. Instead, it involves an accumulation of gene and chromosome mutations that very early in the life of affected individuals cause the appearance of conditions normally associated with advanced age. In addition, specific physical abnormalities accompany each progeroid condition, making the appearance of individuals with a progeroid condition distinctive from that of an elderly person.

RECQ HELICASE–ASSOCIATED PROGEROID CONDITIONS The five human RECQ helicases are required for recombination and also function in the repair of damage

Table 7.4	Human Progeroid Conditions
Disorder	**Mutated Gene(s)**
RECQ helicase gene mutations	
Bloom syndrome (BS)	*BLM (RECQL2)*
Rothmund–Thomson syndrome (RTS)	*RECQL4*
Werner syndrome (WS)	*WRN (RECQL2)*
DNA repair-gene mutations	
Cockayne syndrome (two types)	*ERCC6* and *ERCC8*
Trichothiodystrophy (three types)	*ERCC2, ERCC3, GTF2H5* (three genes)
Xeroderma pigmentosum (seven types)	*XPA–XPG* (seven genes)
Lamin A (nuclear structure) mutation	
Hutchinson–Gilford progeria syndrome	*LMNA*
Unknown mutation	
Wiedemann–Rautenstrauch syndrome	Unknown

to DNA and in preventing genomic instability that would result in the accumulation of gene and chromosome mutations. Defects in these helicases lead to increased risks of chromosome and gene mutations associated with premature aging, elevated cancer risk, and other metabolic and physical abnormalities. In addition, individuals with RECQ-associated progeroid conditions display high sensitivity to mutagens, including ultraviolet light.

BLOOM SYNDROME Bloom syndrome (BS) is a very rare autosomal recessive condition, seen so infrequently that estimates of its incidence are not available. It is known that rates of BS are highest in Ashkenazi Jewish populations, where an incidence of about 1 in 50,000 is estimated. About one-third of the known cases of BS occur in individuals of Ashkenazi Jewish descent.

Individuals with BS have short stature; characteristic abnormal facial features; respiratory, digestive, and metabolic disturbances; sensitivity to light that causes a skin reaction; and a strongly elevated risk of cancer. The abnormalities associated with BS are present from infancy, and the average life span of a person with BS is about 30 years.

BS is caused by mutations of the *BLM* gene, also known as *RECQL3*. This DNA helicase plays a minor role in DNA replication, but it's primarily involved with recombination between homologous chromosomes and between the sister chromatids that make up individual chromosomes. Numerous *BLM* mutations have been described, and most appear to inactivate the activity of the helicase. Normally this helicase interacts with several other proteins to carry out and regulate specific steps of recombination. There is evidence that *BLM* mutations lead to defective homologous recombination, and also that *BLM* mutations lead to an excessive level of recombination between sister chromatids. Both these abnormalities contribute to chromosome defects that accumulate up to 100 times faster than average. The accumulated defects include the loss of chromosomal material, gene mutations, and chromosome instability. These gene and chromosome defects account for the elevated cancer risk associated with BS.

ROTHMUND–THOMSON SYNDROME Rothmund–Thomson syndrome (RTS) is a very rare autosomal recessive condition caused by mutation of the *RECQL4* gene. Only about 300 cases of RTS have been reported to date in the medical literature. Moreover, mutations of *RECQL4* have been identified in only about two-thirds of RTS patients, with no mutation of the gene detected in the other one-third of cases. Individuals with a *RECQL4* gene mutation experience difficulty initiating DNA replication and have errors in homologous recombination.

RTS symptoms first appear in infancy and include a skin rash that occurs in response to sun exposure. Abnormalities of bones and teeth are also present in infancy. Often, cataracts appear in childhood. RTS patients have short stature, gastrointestinal abnormalities, and an elevated risk of cancer, particularly the bone cancer osteosarcoma. Most of these abnormalities are manageable with intensive medical treatment, and unless cancer occurs, a life span approaching normal is possible.

WERNER SYNDROME Werner syndrome (WS) is a rare autosomal recessive condition that occurs in about 1 in 100,000 live births worldwide. Fewer than 2000 cases of WS are currently known in the world. WS is sometimes called an "adult onset progeria" because symptoms are not usually apparent until puberty. The usual growth spurt that occurs to most people during puberty does not occur in individuals with WS. This leads to short stature, and is followed by premature graying of the hair, hair loss, wrinkling and atrophy of the skin, loss of body fat, changes in facial shape, metabolic abnormalities, and a strongly elevated risk of cancer. Due to its onset around puberty, WS is usually diagnosed in the early 20s, and life expectancy is about 50 years, on average.

The *WRN* gene, also known as *RECQL2*, produces a DNA helicase that functions primarily during DNA replication and during DNA damage repair. As a DNA helicase, its function is localized to the nucleus, where it separates the strands of double-stranded DNA. More than 20 different mutations of *WRN* have been identified. These occur throughout the gene, and they have a range of effects on the production and function of the RECQL2 helicase protein. Some mutations completely block production of the helicase, whereas others severely reduce the level of function of the helicase. The RECQL2 helicase interacts with numerous other proteins as it carries out its normal activities, and these interactions are altered or prevented in WS. The consequent accumulation of gene and chromosome mutations and DNA damage leads to the disease symptoms.

SUMMARY   Mastering Genetics   For activities, animations, and review quizzes, go to the Study Area.

7.1 DNA Is the Hereditary Molecule of Life

- Griffith determined in 1928 that a molecular transformation factor was responsible for transformation of living R bacteria into an S form.

- In 1944, Avery, MacLeod, and McCarty's study of in vitro transformation caused by an S-cell extract identified DNA as the transformation factor and strongly suggested it is the hereditary material.

- Hershey and Chase determined in 1952 that bacteriophage T2 uses DNA, not protein, to reproduce within host *E. coli* cells.

7.2 The DNA Double Helix Consists of Two Complementary and Antiparallel Strands

- The DNA nucleotides consist of the five-carbon sugar deoxyribose, a phosphate group, and one of four nitrogen-containing nucleotide bases.

- The DNA nucleotide bases are the purines adenine and guanine, and the pyrimidines cytosine and thymine.

- Phosphodiester bonds form between 5′ phosphate and 3′ OH groups to join nucleotides into polynucleotide chains.

- Complementary base pairs consist of a purine and a pyrimidine. In DNA, A and T form two stable hydrogen bonds, whereas G and C form three stable hydrogen bonds.

- Complementary nucleic acid strands are antiparallel.

- The stacking of base pairs in DNA imparts helical twisting that creates major grooves and minor grooves in the duplex.

7.3 DNA Replication Is Semiconservative and Bidirectional

- Experimental evidence demonstrates that DNA replication is semiconservative, meaning each daughter molecule receives one parental strand and one newly synthesized strand that was produced using the parental strand as a template.

- Most DNA replication is bidirectional. A replication bubble with replication forks at each end expands as replication progresses.

- Bacterial genomes have a single replication origin, whereas eukaryotic genomes have many origins of replication.

- Eukaryotic replication origins initiate asynchronously during S phase.

- Eukaryotic DNA replication produces sister chromatids.

7.4 DNA Replication Precisely Duplicates the Genetic Material

▐ Bacterial, archaeal, and yeast DNA replication begins at specific locations that bind replication initiation proteins. Specific conserved sequences are found in bacteria, but other mechanisms direct replication initiation in eukaryotes.

▐ DNA replication begins with the synthesis of an RNA primer by primase, followed by synthesis of leading and lagging DNA strands by DNA polymerase operating in replisome complexes.

▐ To complete replication, RNA primers are removed by DNA polymerase, and DNA segments are joined by DNA ligase.

▐ DNA polymerases not only replicate DNA but also proof-read newly synthesized DNA for accuracy.

▐ Eukaryotic chromosomes have repetitive sequences called telomeres at their ends that shorten with each replication in somatic cell cycles.

▐ Telomerase is a ribonucleoprotein that synthesizes telomeric repeat sequences to maintain telomere length in germ-line and stem cells.

7.5 Methods of Molecular Genetic Analysis Make Use of DNA Replication Processes

▐ The polymerase chain reaction (PCR) is a method for producing large numbers of copies of target DNA sequences.

▐ Dideoxynucleotide DNA sequencing is a method for discovering the sequence of DNA fragments.

▐ Next-generation and third-generation DNA sequencing are much faster and far cheaper methods that have paved the way for large numbers of genome sequencing projects and personal human genome sequencing.

PREPARING FOR PROBLEM SOLVING

In addition to the list of problem-solving tips and suggestions given here, you can go to the Study Guide and Solutions Manual that accompanies this book for help at solving problems.

1. Be familiar with and able to describe the structure of DNA.

2. Know the four DNA nucleotide bases and be able to describe complementary base pairing and the antiparallel alignment of strands. If required by your instructor, know the structure of the DNA bases.

3. Be able to describe the evidence that identified DNA as the hereditary material.

4. Understand the overall process of DNA replication and be able to diagram the general structure of a replication bubble.

5. Be able to identify the major enzymatic activities during DNA replication.

6. Be prepared to use an understanding of DNA replication processes and biochemical activities to analyze and predict the results of experiments involving DNA replication.

7. Understand the polymerase chain reaction (PCR) process and results.

8. Be able to describe dideoxy DNA sequencing and to analyze DNA sequencing results.

PROBLEMS

Mastering Genetics Visit for instructor-assigned tutorials and problems.

Chapter Concepts

For answers to selected even-numbered problems, see Appendix: Answers.

1. What results from the experiments of Frederick Griffith provided the strongest support for his conclusion that a transformation factor is responsible for heredity?

2. Explain why Avery, MacLeod, and McCarty's in vitro transformation experiment showed that DNA, but not RNA or protein, is the hereditary molecule.

3. Hershey and Chase selected the bacteriophage T2 for their experiment assessing the role of DNA in heredity because T2 contains protein and DNA, but not RNA. Explain why T2 was a good choice for this experiment.

4. Explain how the Hershey and Chase experiment identified DNA as the hereditary molecule.

5. One strand of a fragment of duplex DNA has the sequence 5'-ATCGACCTGATC-3'.

   a. What is the sequence of the other strand in the duplex?

b. What is the name of the bond that joins one nucleotide to another in the DNA strand?

c. Is the bond in part (b) a covalent or a noncovalent bond?

d. Which chemical groups of nucleotides react to form the bond in part (b)?

e. What enzymes catalyze the reaction in part (d)?

f. Identify the bond that joins one strand of a DNA duplex to the other strand.

g. Is the bond in part (f) a covalent or a noncovalent bond?

h. What term is used to describe the pattern of base pairing between one DNA strand and its partner in a duplex?

i. What term is used to describe the polarity of two DNA strands in a duplex?

6. The principles of complementary base pairing and antiparallel polarity of nucleic acid strands in a duplex are universal for the formation of nucleic acid duplexes. What is the chemical basis for this universality?

7. For the following fragment of DNA, determine the number of hydrogen bonds and the number of phosphodiester bonds present:

$$5'-\text{ACGTAGAGTGCTC}-3'$$
$$3'-\text{TGCATCTCACGAG}-5'$$

8. Figure 1.6 presents simplified depictions of nucleotides containing deoxyribose, a nucleotide base, and a phosphate group. Use this simplified method of representation to illustrate the sequence $3'-\text{AGTCGAT}-5'$ and its complementary partner in a DNA duplex.

a. What kind of bond joins the C to the G within a single strand?

b. What kind of bonds join the C in one strand to the G in the complementary strand?

c. How many phosphodiester bonds are present in this DNA duplex?

d. How many hydrogen bonds are present in this DNA duplex?

9. Consider the sequence $3'-\text{ACGCTACGTC}-5'$.

a. What is the double-stranded sequence?

b. What is the total number of covalent bonds joining the nucleotides in each strand?

c. What is the total number of noncovalent bonds joining the nucleotides of the complementary strands?

10. DNA polymerase III is the main DNA-synthesizing enzyme in bacteria. Describe how it carries out its role of elongating a strand of DNA.

11. There is a problem completing the replication of linear chromosomes at their ends.

a. Describe the problem and identify why telomeres shorten in each replication cycle.

b. What is the function of telomerase, and how does it operate to synthesize telomeres?

12. Explain how RNA participates in DNA replication.

13. A sample of double-stranded DNA is found to contain 20% cytosine. Determine the percentage of the three other DNA nucleotides in the sample.

14. Bacterial DNA polymerase I and DNA polymerase III perform different functions during DNA replication.

a. Identify the principal functions of each molecule.

b. If mutation inactivated DNA polymerase I in a strain of *E. coli*, would the cell be able to replicate its DNA? If so, what kind of abnormalities would you expect to find in the cell?

c. If a strain of *E. coli* acquired a mutation that inactivated DNA polymerase III function, would the cell be able to replicate its DNA? Why or why not?

15. Diagram a replication fork in bacterial DNA and label the following structures or molecules.

a. DNA pol III
b. helicase
c. RNA primer
d. origin of replication
e. leading strand (label its polarity)
f. DNA pol I
g. topoisomerase
h. SSB protein
i. lagging strand (label its polarity)
j. primase
k. Okazaki fragment

16. Which of the following equations are true for the percentages of nucleotides in double-stranded DNA?

a. $(A+G)/(C+T) = 1.0$
b. $(A+T)/(G+C) = 1.0$
c. $(A)/(T) = (G)/(C)$
d. $(A)/(C) = (G)/(T)$
e. $(A)/(G) = (T)(C)$

17. Which of the following equalities is not true for double-stranded DNA?

a. $(G+T) = (A+C)$
b. $(G+C) = (A+T)$
c. $(G+A) = (C+T)$

18. List the order in which the following proteins and enzymes are active in *E. coli* DNA replication: DNA pol I, SSB, ligase, helicase, DNA pol III, and primase.

19. Two viral genomes are sequenced, and the following percentages of nucleotides are identified:

Genome 1: A = 28%, C = 22%, G = 28%, T = 22%
Genome 2: A = 22%, C = 28%, G = 28%, T = 22%

Are the DNA molecules in each genome single-stranded or double-stranded?

Application and Integration

For answers to selected even-numbered problems, see Appendix: Answers.

20. Matthew Meselson and Franklin Stahl demonstrated that DNA replication is semiconservative in bacteria. Briefly outline their experiment and its results for two DNA replication cycles, and identify how the alternative models of DNA replication were excluded by the data.

21. Raymond Rodriguez and colleagues demonstrated conclusively that DNA replication in *E. coli* is bidirectional. Explain why locating the origin of replication on one side of the circular chromosomes and the terminus of replication on the opposite side of the chromosome supported this conclusion.

22. Joel Huberman and Arthur Riggs used pulse labeling to examine the replication of DNA in mammalian cells. Briefly describe the Huberman–Riggs experiment, and identify how the results exclude a unidirectional model of DNA replication.

23. Why do the genomes of eukaryotes, such as *Drosophila*, need to have multiple origins of replication, whereas bacterial genomes, such as that of *E. coli,* have only a single origin?

24. Bloom syndrome (OMIM 210900) is an autosomal recessive disorder caused by mutation of a DNA helicase. Among the principal symptoms of the disease are chromosome instability and a propensity to develop cancer. Explain these symptoms on the basis of the helicase mutation.

25. How does rolling circle replication (see Section 6.2) differ from bidirectional replication?

26. Telomeres are found at the ends of eukaryotic chromosomes.
    a. What is the sequence composition of telomeres?
    b. How does telomerase assemble telomeres?
    c. What is the functional role of telomeres?
    d. Why is telomerase usually active in germ-line cells but not in somatic cells?

27. A family consisting of a mother (I-1), a father (I-2), and three children (II-1, II-2, and II-3) are genotyped by PCR for a region of an autosome containing repeats of a 10-bp sequence. The mother carries 16 repeats on one chromosome and 21 on the homologous chromosome. The father carries repeat numbers of 18 and 26.
    a. Following the layout of Figure 7.28c, which aligns members of a pedigree with their DNA fragments in a gel, draw a DNA gel containing the PCR fragments generated by amplification of DNA from the parents (I-1 and I-2). Label the size of each fragment.
    b. Identify all the possible genotypes of children of this couple by specifying PCR fragment lengths in each genotype.
    c. What genetic term best describes the pattern of inheritance of this DNA marker? Explain your choice.

28. In a dideoxy DNA sequencing experiment, four separate reactions are carried out to provide the replicated material for DNA sequencing gels. Reaction products are usually run in gel lanes labeled A, T, C, and G.
    a. Identify the nucleotides used in the dideoxy DNA sequencing reaction that produces molecules for the A lane of the sequencing gel.
    b. How does PCR play a role in dideoxy DNA sequencing?
    c. Why is incorporation of a dideoxynucleotide during DNA sequencing identified as a "replication-terminating" event?

29. The following dideoxy DNA sequencing gel is produced in a laboratory.

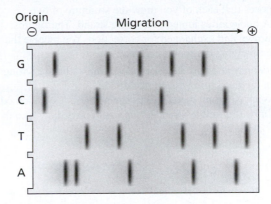

What is the double-stranded DNA sequence of this molecule? Label the polarity of each strand.

30. Using an illustration style and labeling similar to that in Problem 29, draw the electrophoresis gel containing dideoxy sequencing fragments for the DNA template strand 3'-AGACGATAGCAT-5'.

31. A PCR reaction begins with one double-stranded segment of DNA. How many double-stranded copies of DNA are present after the completion of 10 amplification cycles? After 20 cycles? After 30 cycles?

32. DNA replication in early *Drosophila* embryos occurs about every 5 minutes. The *Drosophila* genome contains approximately 1.8×10^8 base pairs. Eukaryotic DNA polymerases synthesize DNA at a rate of approximately 40 nucleotides per second. Approximately how many origins of replication are required for this rate of replication?

33. What would be the effects on DNA replication if mutation of DNA pol III caused it to lose each of the following activities:
    a. 5' to 3' polymerase activity
    b. 3' to 5' exonuclease activity

34. A sufficient amount of a small DNA fragment is available for dideoxy sequencing. The fragment to be sequenced contains 20 nucleotides following the site of primer binding:

5'-ATCGCTCGACAGTGACTAGC-[primer site]-3'

Dideoxy sequencing is carried out, and the products of the four sequencing reactions are separated by gel electrophoresis. Draw the bands you expect will appear on the gel from each of the sequencing reactions.

Collaboration and Discussion

For answers to selected even-numbered problems, see Appendix: Answers.

35. You are participating in a study group preparing for an upcoming genetics exam, and one member of the group proposes that each of you draw the structure of two DNA nucleotides joined in a single strand. The figures are drawn and exchanged for correction. You receive the accompanying diagram to correct:

    a. Identify and correct at least five things that are wrong in the depiction of each nucleotide.
    b. What is wrong with the way the nucleotides are joined?
    c. Draw this single-stranded segment correctly.

36. Suppose that future exploration of polar ice on Mars identifies a living microbe and that analysis indicates the organism carries double-stranded DNA as its genetic material. Suppose further that DNA replication analysis is performed by first growing the microbe in a growth medium containing the heavy isotope of nitrogen (^{15}N), that the organism is then transferred to a growth medium containing the light isotope of nitrogen (^{14}N), and that the nitrogen composition of the DNA is examined by CsCl ultracentrifugation and densitometry after the first, second, and third replication cycles in the ^{14}N-containing medium. The results of the experiment are illustrated here for each cycle. The control shows the positioning of the three possible DNA densities. Based on the results shown, what can you conclude about the mechanism of DNA replication in this organism? (Hint: See the description of the Meselson and Stahl experiment on pp. 245–247.)

37. The following diagram shows the parental strands of a DNA molecule undergoing replication. Draw the daughter strands present in the replication bubble, indicating

    a. the polarity of daughter strands
    b. the leading and lagging strands
    c. Okazaki fragments
    d. the locations of RNA primers

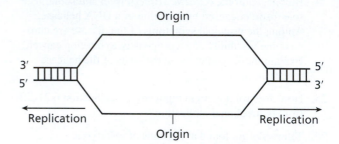

38. Go to the OMIM website (https://www.ncbi.nlm.nih .gov/omim) and type "dyskeratosis congenita autosomal dominant 1" (DKCA1) into the search bar. The result will include a clickable link to the disorder that has an OMIM number of 127550. Review the OMIM information you retrieve and notice that this disorder is caused by a mutation of a telomerase gene that results in abnormally rapid shortening of telomeres and the appearance of disease symptoms at progressively younger ages in successive generations of the affected families. Use this and other information on OMIM to assist with this problem.

    Go the reference number 15 at the bottom of the OMIM page for a link to a 2004 paper by Tom Vulliamy and colleagues that appeared in the journal *Nature Genetics*. Click on the "Full text" option and download a copy of the paper. Look at Table 1 of the paper on page 448. This table lists the lengths of telomeres measured in members of the families in this study. Telomeres shorten with age, and the telomere lengths in Table 1 are age-adjusted. The negative numbers for telomere lengths in the table indicate that telomeres are shorter than average for age, and the more negative the number, the shorter the telomere. Based on Table 1, discussion in the *Vulliamy et al. (2004)* paper, and information available on OMIM answer the following:

    a. How do telomere lengths in children compare with telomere lengths of their parents?
    b. Why are telomeres of people with DKCA1 shorter than average?

Molecular Biology of Transcription and RNA Processing

8

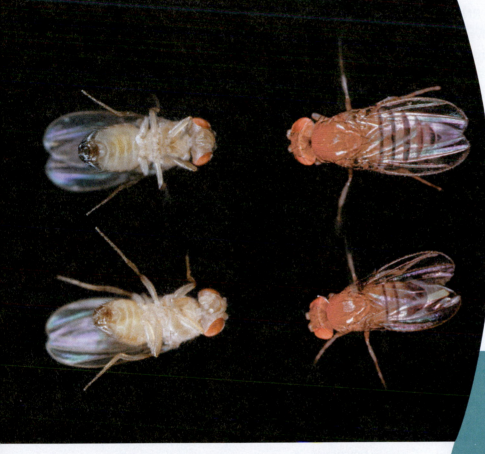

The molecular basis of sex determination in fruit flies (*Drosophila melanogaster*) involves variations in splicing of the precursor mRNA transcript of the *Tra* gene. One pattern of splicing helps direct female sex development, and an alternative splicing pattern helps direct male sex development.

At a critical juncture in a court proceeding, an attorney thinks two witnesses have given contradictory testimony. To verify this, the attorney asks the court clerk to read back the portions of the trial transcript containing the statements in question. This court transcript contains information that was first presented in verbal form and then precisely converted to a written form. Precision is essential, as the exact wording of each witness's testimony is critical to determining whether contradictory statements were made. An inaccurate or incomplete transcript would be of no value.

We can compare this situation to a process taking place at this very moment in millions of cells in your body, where

CHAPTER OUTLINE

8.1 RNA Transcripts Carry the Messages of Genes

8.2 Bacterial Transcription Is a Four-Stage Process

8.3 Eukaryotic Transcription Is More Diversified and Complex than Bacterial Transcription

8.4 Posttranscriptional Processing Modifies RNA Molecules

ESSENTIAL IDEAS

- Ribonucleic acid (RNA) molecules are transcribed from genes and are of several types. The most common types are messenger RNA (mRNA), transfer RNA (tRNA), and ribosomal RNA (rRNA), but other types have important functions as well.

- Bacterial transcription is a four-step process that begins with promoter recognition by RNA polymerase and ends with the completion of transcript synthesis.

- Eukaryotes and archaea have homologous transcription proteins and processes. Eukaryotes use different RNA polymerases to transcribe different kinds of RNA. Each type of polymerase initiates transcription at a different type of promoter.

- Eukaryotic RNAs undergo three processing steps after transcription. Alternative events during and after transcription allow different transcripts and proteins to be produced from the same DNA sequence.

information contained in the DNA sequence of your genes is being precisely transcribed into a different form. This genetic transcription takes genetic information originally contained in deoxyribonucleic acid and converts it into a new molecule called ribonucleic acid (RNA). As with the court transcript, the completeness and accuracy of an RNA transcript is essential to its success at conveying, in this case, the information originally provided by a gene.

Transcription, the process of transcribing information from DNA into RNA, is the first of the two genetic processes encompassed by the commonly used term "gene expression"—two processes that together generate proteins from the instructions in DNA. Transcription is the topic of this chapter. The second process is *translation*, and we cover that topic in Chapter 9. Figure 1.8 gives an overview of these two processes that, along with DNA replication, collectively form the central dogma of biology (DNA → RNA → protein).

More specifically, this chapter describes the mechanisms of transcription producing the three main forms of RNA: *messenger RNA (mRNA)*, *transfer RNA (tRNA)*, and *ribosomal RNA (rRNA)*. It also discusses the events in the nucleus of eukaryotic cells that modify the *precursor messenger RNA (pre-mRNA)* to yield the mature mRNA that subsequently undergoes translation to produce proteins. In our discussion, we compare and contrast the mechanisms of transcription in the three domains of life: Bacteria, Archaea, and Eukarya. Through these comparisons we will see that members of each domain share a number of features of transcription in common, as their common ancestry would suggest, but that their transcription processes also differ in certain ways.

The discovery of mRNA in particular raised numerous questions: How is a gene recognized by the transcription machinery? Where does transcription begin? Which strand of DNA is transcribed? Where does transcription end? How much transcript is made? How is RNA modified after transcription? We answer these questions and others by the chapter's end, but we begin with a discussion of RNA structure.

8.1 RNA Transcripts Carry the Messages of Genes

In the mid-1950s, with the structure of DNA in hand, molecular biology researchers turned their attention to identifying and describing the molecules and mechanisms responsible for conveying the genetic message of DNA. RNA was known to be chemically similar to DNA and present in abundance in all cells, but its diversity and biological roles remained to be discovered. Some roles were strongly suggested by cell structure. For example, in eukaryotic cells, DNA is located in the nucleus, whereas protein synthesis takes place in the cytoplasm, suggesting that DNA could not code directly for proteins but RNA perhaps could. Bacteria, however, lack a nucleus, so an open question was whether bacteria and eukaryotes used similar mechanisms and similar molecules to convey the genetic message for protein synthesis. The search was on to identify the types of RNA in cells and to identify the mechanisms by which the genetic message of DNA is conveyed for protein synthesis.

RNA Nucleotides and Structure

Both DNA and RNA are nucleic acids. They are composed of nucleotide building blocks that are joined together by phosphodiester bonds to form polynucleotide strands. One principal difference between their molecules is the stable single-stranded structure of RNA versus the double-stranded structure of DNA. A second difference is the frequently encountered folding of RNA molecules. Many RNA molecules adopt folded secondary structures by complementary base pairing of segments of the molecule as part of the process by which they become functional.

The RNA nucleotides, like those of DNA, are composed of a five-carbon sugar, a nucleotide base, and one or more phosphate groups. Each RNA nucleotide carries one of four possible nucleotide bases. But RNA nucleotides differ chemically from DNA nucleotides in two critical ways. The first difference concerns the identity of the RNA nucleotide bases. The purines adenine and guanine in RNA are identical to the purines in DNA. Likewise, the pyrimidine cytosine is identical in RNA and DNA. In RNA, however, the second pyrimidine is **uracil** (U) rather than the thymine carried by DNA. The four RNA **ribonucleotides** (A, U, G, C) are shown in **Figure 8.1**. The structure of uracil is similar to that of thymine, but notice, by comparing the structure of uracil in Figure 8.1 with that of thymine in Figure 7.5, that thymine has a methyl group (CH_3) at the 5 carbon of the pyrimidine ring, whereas uracil does not. In all other respects, uracil is similar to thymine, and when uracil undergoes base pairing, its complementary partner is adenine.

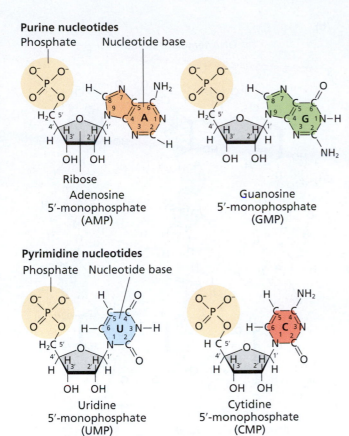

Purine nucleotides

Adenosine
5'-monophosphate
(AMP)

Guanosine
5'-monophosphate
(GMP)

Pyrimidine nucleotides

Uridine
5'-monophosphate
(UMP)

Cytidine
5'-monophosphate
(CMP)

Figure 8.1 **The four RNA ribonucleotides.** Shown in their mono-phosphate forms, each ribonucleotide consists of the sugar ribose, a phosphate group, and one of the RNA nucleotide bases adenine, guanine, cytosine, and uracil.

Ⓠ **Examine these four RNA nucleotides in comparison to the four DNA nucleotides illustrated in Figure 7.5 and identify one chemical difference and one nucleotide base difference between the nucleotides making up DNA and those making up RNA.**

The second chemical difference between RNA and DNA nucleotides is the presence of the sugar **ribose** in RNA rather than the deoxyribose occurring in DNA. The ribose gives RNA its name (ribonucleic acid). Compare the ribose molecules shown in Figure 8.1 with deoxyribose in Figure 7.5, and notice that ribose carries a hydroxyl group (OH) not found in deoxyribose at the 2' carbon of the ring. Except for this difference, ribose and deoxyribose are identical, having a nucleotide base attached to the 1' carbon and a hydroxyl group at the 3' carbon.

The similarity of the sugars of RNA and DNA leads to the formation in RNA of phosphodiester bonds between nucleotides of a strand and to a sugar-phosphate backbone that is identical to that of DNA. RNA-strand phosphodiester bond formation takes place by the same general mechanism as found in DNA (**Figure 8.2**). RNA is synthesized from a DNA template strand using the same purine–pyrimidine

complementary base pairing described for DNA, except that in RNA, adenine pairs with uracil rather than thymine. **RNA polymerase** enzymes catalyze the addition of each ribonucleotide to the 3' end of the nascent strand, forming a phosphodiester bond between the 5' carbon of one nucleotide and the 3' carbon of the adjacent nucleotide, eliminating two phosphates (the pyrophosphate group) from the incoming ribonucleotide triphosphate in the process, just as in DNA synthesis. Compare Figure 8.2 to Figure 7.6 to see the similarity of these nucleic acid synthesis processes.

Experimental Discovery of Messenger RNA

In their search for the RNA molecule responsible for transmitting the genetic information content of DNA to the site of protein production, researchers utilized many techniques. Among the methods used was the pulse–chase technique (see Section 7.3) to follow the trail of newly synthesized RNA in cells. Recall that the "pulse" step of this technique exposes cells to radioactive nucleotides that become incorporated into newly synthesized nucleic acids. After a short incubation period to incorporate the labeled nucleotides, a "chase" step replaces any remaining unincorporated radioactive nucleotides by introducing an excess of unlabeled nucleotides. An experimenter can then observe the changing location of labeled nucleic acid to determine the pattern of its movement and its ultimate destination and fate.

In 1957, microbiologist Elliot Volkin and geneticist Lazarus Astrachan used the pulse–chase method to study transcription in bacteria immediately following infection by a bacteriophage. Exposing newly infected bacteria to radioactive uracil, they observed rapid incorporation of the label, indicating a burst of transcriptional activity. In the chase phase of the experiment, when radioactive uracil was removed, Volkin and Astrachan found that the radioactivity quickly dissipated, indicating that the newly synthesized RNA broke down rapidly. They concluded that the synthesis of a type of RNA with a very short life span is responsible for the production of phage proteins that drive progression of the infection.

Similar pulse–chase experiments were soon conducted with eukaryotic cells. In these experiments, radioactivity was concentrated in the nucleus immediately after the pulse. This indicated that RNA was synthesized in the nucleus. Over a short period of time, however, radioactive RNA migrated to the cytoplasm, where translation takes place. The radioactivity dissipated after lingering in the cytoplasm for a period of time. These experiments led researchers to conclude that the RNA synthesized in the nucleus was likely to act as an intermediary carrying the genetic message of DNA to the cytoplasm for translation into proteins.

The discovery of mRNA was capped in 1961 when an experiment by the biologists Sydney Brenner, François,

(a)

(b)

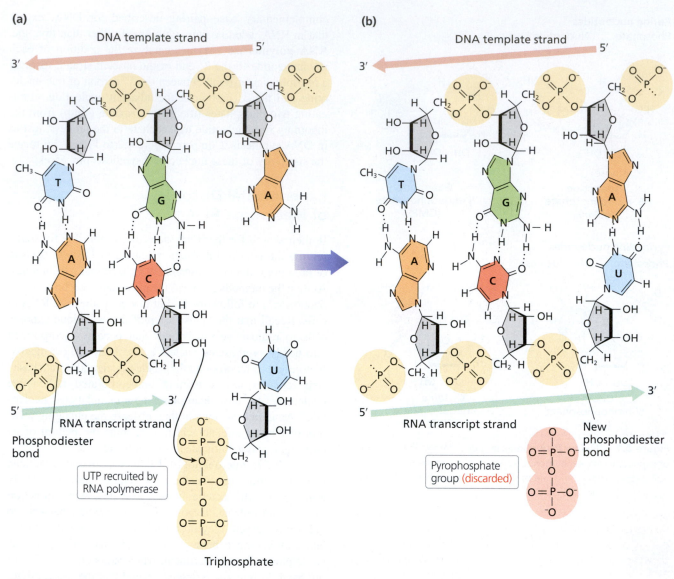

Figure 8.2 **RNA synthesis.** RNA polymerase catalyzes the formation of a phosphodiester bond to join a new RNA nucleotide to the 3′ end of a growing RNA strand. Two phosphate molecules are cleaved as a pyrophosphate group.

Jacob, and Matthew Meselson identified an unstable form of RNA that acted as the genetic messenger. Brenner and his colleagues knew from experimental evidence presented by George Palade in 1958 that ribosomes are composed of RNA and protein and function as the site of protein synthesis. They designed an experiment that used bacteriophage infection of bacterial cells to determine whether new phage protein synthesis that is part of a bacterial infection required newly constructed ribosomes or whether phage proteins could be produced using existing bacterial ribosomes. The experiment found that newly synthesized phage RNA associates with existing bacterial ribosomes to produce phage proteins and that newly formed ribosomes are not responsible for phage protein synthesis. The RNA that directed phage protein synthesis formed and degraded quickly, leading the experimenters to conclude that a phage "messenger" RNA with a short half-life is responsible for protein synthesis during infection.

Categories of RNA

In addition to *messenger RNA (mRNA)*, a wide variety of other RNAs are found in cells. These are RNA molecules that are not translated into proteins but perform their own particular functions. The two most prominent of them are *ribosomal RNA (rRNA)* and *transfer RNA (tRNA)*. We discuss ribosomal and transfer RNA to some degree in this chapter and describe their functions in the following chapter. The major and best understood forms of RNA are listed and briefly described in **Table 8.1**. RNAs that are listed there but are not discussed in this chapter will be described in more detail in later chapters.

Table 8.1	Major RNA Molecules

Type of RNA	Function
Messenger RNA (mRNA)	Used to encode the sequence of amino acids in a polypeptide. May be polycistronic (encoding two or more polypeptides) in bacteria and archaea. Encodes single polypeptides in nearly all eukaryotes (see Sections 8.2 and 8.4).
Ribosomal RNA (rRNA)	Along with numerous proteins, helps form the large and small ribosomal subunits that unite for translation of mRNA (see Sections 8.4 and 9.2).
Transfer RNA (tRNA)	Carries amino acids to ribosomes and binds there to mRNA by complementary base pairing to add the amino acids to the elongating polypeptide (see Sections 8.4 and 9.3).
Small nuclear RNA (snRNA)	Found in eukaryotic nuclei, where multiple snRNAs join with numerous proteins to form spliceosomes that remove introns from precursor mRNA (see Section 8.4).
MicroRNA (miRNA)	Eukaryotic regulatory RNAs that function by base pairing with certain mRNAs, altering their stability and efficiency of translation (see Section 13.3).
Small interfering RNA (siRNA)	Eukaryotic regulatory RNA made from long double-stranded molecules that are cut into shorter pieces used to regulate mRNA stability and translation (see Section 13.3).
Telomerase RNA	Located in the telomerase ribonucleoprotein complex, where it acts as a template to maintain and elongate telomere length of eukaryotic chromosomes (see Section 7.4).

All types of RNA are generated by the transcription of genes. Genes whose transcription yields **messenger RNA (mRNA)**, the short-lived intermediary form of RNA described by Brenner and his colleagues that conveys the genetic message of DNA to be translated, are protein-producing genes. The RNA transcripts of these genes direct protein synthesis by the process of translation that is described in the next chapter. Messenger RNA is the only form of RNA that undergoes translation. Transcription of mRNA and posttranscriptional processing of mRNA are principal areas of focus in this chapter.

Ribosomal RNA combines with numerous proteins to form the ribosome, the molecular machine responsible for translation. Specific segments of rRNA molecules interact with mRNA to initiate translation. **Transfer RNA** is the RNA that carries amino acids to the ribosomes for construction of proteins, and it is encoded in dozens of different forms in all genomes. Each tRNA is responsible for binding a particular amino acid that it carries to the ribosome. At the ribosome a group of nucleotides of a tRNA temporarily base pair with nucleotides of mRNA. The tRNA deposits its amino acid that is added to the protein chain being produced there.

Four types of RNA perform specialized functions in eukaryotic cells only. We discuss **telomerase RNA** in Section 7.4, where its role in providing a template for synthesis of the repeating DNA sequence composing telomeres is described. **Small nuclear RNA (snRNA)** of various types is found in the nucleus of eukaryotic cells, where it participates in mRNA processing and intron removal (Section 8.4). **Micro RNA (miRNA)** and **small interfering RNA (siRNA)** are recently recognized types of regulatory RNA that are particularly active in plant and animal cells. Micro RNAs and siRNAs have a widespread and important role in the posttranscriptional regulation of gene expression, controlling the stability or translatability of certain mRNAs. This component of regulated gene expression is described in Section 13.3.

8.2 Bacterial Transcription Is a Four-Stage Process

Transcription is the synthesis of a single-stranded RNA molecule by RNA polymerase. It is most clearly understood and described in bacteria, and *E. coli* is the model experimental organism from which the majority of our knowledge of bacterial transcription has been derived. In this section, we examine the four stages of transcription in bacteria: (1) promoter recognition and identification, (2) the initiation of transcript synthesis, (3) transcript elongation, and (4) transcription termination.

Like all RNA polymerases, bacterial RNA polymerase uses one strand of DNA, the **template strand**, to assemble the transcript by complementary and antiparallel base pairing of RNA nucleotides with DNA nucleotides of the template strand (see Figure 1.9 for a review). The **coding strand** of DNA, also known as the **nontemplate strand**, is complementary to the template strand. The gene—that is, the stretch of DNA regions that produces an RNA transcript—contains several segments with distinct functions (**Figure 8.3**). The **promoter** of the gene is immediately **upstream**—that is, within a few nucleotides of the 5′ start of transcription, which is identified as corresponding to the +1 nucleotide. The promoter is not transcribed. Instead, the promoter sequence is a transcription-regulating DNA sequence that controls the access of RNA polymerase to the gene. The **coding region** is the portion of the gene that is transcribed into mRNA and contains the information needed to

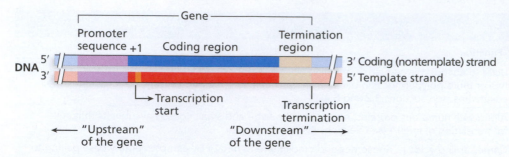

Figure 8.3   Gene structure and associated nomenclature.

🅠 If a consensus DNA sequence occurs upstream of the start of transcription, is it part of the coding sequence of a gene?

Bacterial RNA Polymerase

synthesize the protein product of the gene. The **termination region** is the portion of the gene that regulates the cessation of transcription. The termination region is located immediately **downstream**—that is, immediately 3′ to the coding segment of the gene.

Bacterial RNA Polymerase

A single type of *E. coli* RNA polymerase catalyzes transcription of all RNAs. The initial experimental evidence supporting this conclusion came from analysis of the effect of the antibiotic rifampicin on bacterial RNA synthesis. Rifampicin inhibits RNA synthesis by preventing RNA polymerase from catalyzing the formation of the first phosphodiester bond in the RNA chain. In rifampicin-sensitive (rif^S) bacterial strains, synthesis of all three major types of RNA (mRNA, tRNA, and rRNA) is inhibited in the presence of rifampicin. In contrast, rifampicin-resistant (rif^R) bacteria actively transcribe DNA into the three major RNAs when rifampicin is present. Molecular analysis identifies a single mutation of RNA polymerase in rif^R strains that allows it to remain catalytically active when exposed to rifampicin. Subsequent molecular studies have confirmed the presence of a single bacterial RNA polymerase.

Bacterial RNA polymerase is composed of a pentameric (five-polypeptide) **RNA polymerase core** that binds to a sixth polypeptide, called the **sigma subunit (σ)**, which induces a conformational change in the core enzyme that switches it to its active form. In its active form, the RNA polymerase is described as a **holoenzyme**, a term meaning an intact complex of multiple subunits, with full enzymatic capacity. **Figure 8.4** shows a common type of sigma subunit known as σ⁷⁰, but there are also other sigma subunits in *E. coli*.

The RNA polymerase core consists of two α subunits, designated αI and αII, two β subunits, and an ω (omega) subunit. The molecular weight of the five-subunit core RNA polymerase is approximately 390 kD (kiloDaltons), and with the sigma subunit added, the holoenzyme has a molecular weight of 430 kD. Each of these subunits is evolutionarily conserved in archaea and in eukaryotes.

By itself, the core RNA polymerase can transcribe DNA template-strand sequence into RNA sequence, but the core is unable to efficiently bind to a promoter or initiate RNA synthesis without a sigma subunit. The joining of the sigma subunit to the core enzyme to form a holoenzyme induces a conformational shift in the core segment that enables it to bind specifically to particular promoter consensus sequences.

Because this single RNA polymerase is responsible for all bacterial transcription, the bacterial RNA polymerase must recognize promoters for protein-coding genes as well as for genes that produce otherRNAs, such as tRNA and rRNA. But not all promoters of bacterial genes are identical. There is great diversity among bacterial promoter sequences, permitting certain genes to be expressed only under special circumstances. Bacteria manage the recognition of the promoters of these specialized genes by producing several different types of sigma subunits that can join the core polymerase. These so-called **alternative sigma subunits** alter the specificity of the holoenzymes for promoter regions by imparting distinct conformational changes to the core. These differences enable transcription of specific genes under the appropriate conditions, or at the correct time.

Bacterial Promoters

Promoters are double-stranded regulatory DNA sequences that bind transcription proteins such as RNA polymerase

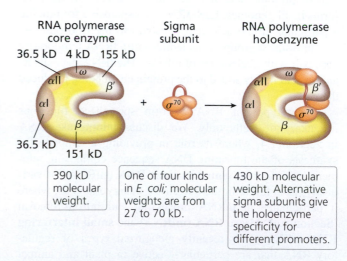

Figure 8.4   Bacterial RNA polymerase core plus a sigma (σ) subunit forms the fully active holoenzyme.

and direct the RNA polymerase to the nearby start of transcription. RNA polymerase is attracted to promoters by the presence of consensus sequences, short regions of DNA sequences that are highly similar, though not necessarily identical, to one another and are located in the same position relative to the start of transcription of different genes (see Section 7.4 for an introduction to consensus sequences).

Although promoters are double stranded, promoter consensus sequences are usually written in a single-stranded shorthand form that gives the 5′-to-3′ sequence of the coding (nontemplate) strand of DNA (Figure 8.5). The most commonly occurring bacterial promoter contains two consensus sequence regions that each play an important functional role in recognition by RNA polymerase and the subsequent initiation of transcription. These consensus sequences are located upstream from the +1 nucleotide (the start of transcription) in a region flanking the gene where the nucleotides are denoted by negative numbers and are not transcribed. At the −10 position of the *E. coli* promoter is the **Pribnow box sequence**, or the **−10 consensus sequence**, consisting of 6 bp having the consensus sequence 5′-TATAAT-3′. The Pribnow box is separated by about 25 bp from another 6-bp region, the **−35 consensus sequence**, identified by the nucleotides 5′-TTGACA-3′. The nucleotide sequences that occur upstream, downstream, and between these consensus sequences are highly variable and contain no other consensus sequences. Thus, in a functional sense, the −10 (Pribnow) and −35 consensus sequences are important because of their nucleotide content, their location relative to one another, and their location relative to the start of transcription. In contrast to the consensus sequences themselves, the nucleotides between −10 and −35 are important as spacers between the consensus elements, but their specific sequences are not critical. In the figure, untranslated mRNA at the 5′ end (5′ UTR) and at the 3′ end (3′

UTR) separate the 5′ mRNA end from the start codon and the stop codon from the rest of the mRNA, respectively.

Natural selection has operated to retain strong sequence similarity in consensus regions and to retain the position of the consensus regions relative to the start of transcription. The effectiveness of evolution in maintaining promoter consensus sequences is illustrated by comparison with the sequences between and around −10 and −35, which are not conserved and which exhibit considerable variation. In addition, the spacing between the sequences and their placement relative to the +1 nucleotide is stable. RNA polymerase is a large molecule that binds to −10 and −35 consensus sequences and occupies the space between and immediately around the sites. Crystal structure models show that the enzyme spans enough DNA to allow it to contact promoter consensus regions and reach the +1 nucleotide. Once bound at a promoter in this fashion, RNA polymerase can initiate transcription. Genetic Analysis 8.1 guides you through the identification of promoter consensus regions.

Transcription Initiation

RNA polymerase holoenzyme initiates transcription through a process involving two steps. In the first step, the holoenzyme makes an initial loose attachment to the double-stranded promoter sequence and then binds tightly to it to form the **closed promoter complex** (❶ in Foundation Figure 8.6). In the second step, the bound holoenzyme unwinds approximately 18 bp of DNA around the −10 consensus sequence to form the **open promoter complex** ❷. Following formation of the open promoter complex, the holoenzyme progresses downstream to initiate RNA synthesis at the +1 nucleotide on the template strand of DNA ❸.

Bacterial promoters often differ from the consensus sequence by one or more nucleotides, and some are different at several nucleotides. Since considerable DNA-sequence

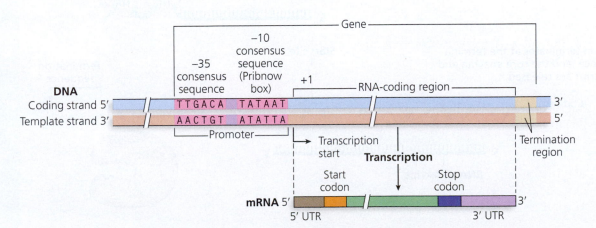

Figure 8.5 Bacterial promoter structure and consensus sequences. Two promoter consensus sequences—the Pribnow box at −10 and the −35 sequence—are essential promoter regulatory elements.

Bacterial Transcription

1 The RNA polymerase core enzyme and sigma subunit bind to −10 and −35 promoter consensus sequences.

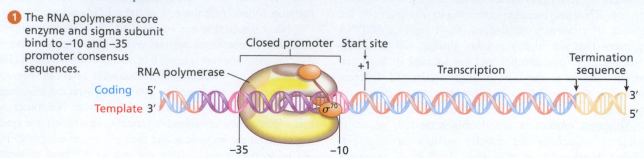

Closed promoter Start site +1 Transcription Termination sequence

RNA polymerase

Coding 5′
Template 3′
σ⁷⁰
−35 −10
3′
5′

2 DNA unwinds near the transcription start site to form the open promoter complex.

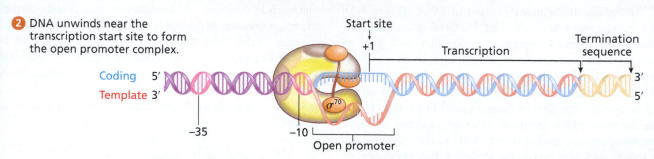

Start site +1 Transcription Termination sequence

Coding 5′
Template 3′
σ⁷⁰
−35 −10
Open promoter
3′
5′

3 RNA polymerase holoenzyme initiates transcription and begins RNA synthesis. The sigma subunit dissociates shortly after transcription initiation, and the core enzyme continues transcription.

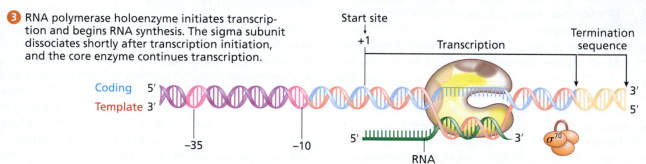

Start site +1 Transcription Termination sequence

Coding 5′
Template 3′
−35 −10
5′ RNA 3′
σ⁷⁰
3′
5′

4 The core enzyme synthesizes until it encounters the termination sequence. As RNA synthesis progresses, the DNA duplex unwinds to allow the template strand to direct RNA assembly. The duplex closes following synthesis.

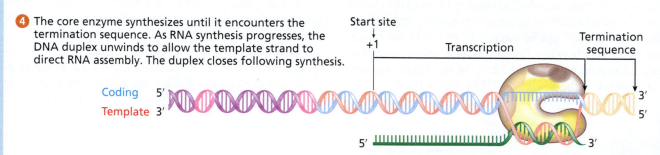

Start site +1 Transcription Termination sequence

Coding 5′
Template 3′
5′ 3′
3′
5′

5 Transcription terminates at the termination sequence, and the core enzyme and RNA transcript are released.

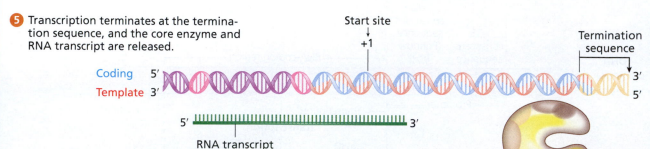

Start site +1 Termination sequence

Coding 5′
Template 3′
5′ RNA transcript 3′
3′
5′

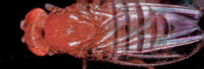

GENETIC ANALYSIS 8.1

PROBLEM DNA sequences in the promoter region of 10 *E. coli* genes are shown. Sequences at the −35 and −10 sites are boxed.

a. For these 10 genes, what are the −35 and −10 consensus sequences?

b. What would be the expected effects of a mutation in a promoter consensus region versus a mutation in the sequence between consensus regions?

> **BREAK IT DOWN:** Promoter consensus sequences are similar in different genes and bind transcriptionally active proteins (p. 281).

> **BREAK IT DOWN:** Research methods directed at detecting promoters and assessing their functionality are described in Research Technique 8.1 and Figure 8.12.

Gene	−35 region		−10 region	+1
A2	AATGC TTGACT CTGTAGCGGGAAGGCG-- TATAAT GCACACC- C CGC
bio	AAAAC GTGTTT TTTGTTGTTAATTCGGTG TAGACT TGT---AA ACCT
his	AGTTC TTGCTT TCTAACGTGAAAGTGGTT TAGGTT AAAAGAC- A TCA
lac	CAGGC TTTACA CTTTATGCTTCCGGCTCG TATGTT GTG-TGG- A ATT
lacI	GAATG GCGCAA AACTTTTCGCGGTATGG- CATGAT AGCGCCC- G GAA
leu	AAAAG TTGACA TCCGTTTTTGTATCCAG- TAACTC TAAAAGC- A TAT
recA	AACAC TTGATA CTGTATGAGCATACAG-- TATAAT TGCTTC-- A ACA
trp	AGCTG TTGACA ATTAATCATCGAACTAG- TTAACT AGTACGC- A AGT
tRNA	AACAC TTTACA GCGGGCCGTCATTTGA-- TATGAT GCGCCCC- G CTT
X1	TCCGC TTGTCT TCCTAGGCCGACTCCC-- TATAAT GCGCCTCC A TCG

Solution Strategies	Solution Steps
Evaluate	
1. Identify the topic this problem addresses and the nature of the required answer.	1. This question concerns bacterial promoters. The answer requires identification of consensus sequences for −35 and −10 regions of promoters and speculation about the consequences of promoter mutations.
2. Identify the critical information provided in the problem.	2. The problem provides promoter sequence information for 10 *E. coli* genes and identifies the segment of each promoter containing the −10 and −35 regions.
Deduce	
3. Examine the −10 and −35 sequences of these promoters, and look for common patterns.	3. The −10 and −35 sites are the location of RNA polymerase binding during transcription initiation. Count the numbers of A, T, C, and G in each position in the boxed regions.
TIP: A consensus sequence identifies the most common nucleotide at each position in a DNA segment.	
Solve	**Answer a**
4. Determine the consensus sequence at the −10 and −35 regions.	4. At the −10 site, and moving left to right (toward +1), the most common nucleotides in each position in the consensus region, and the number of times they occur in that position, are
TIP: Identify the most commonly occurring nucleotide in each position of each 6-nucleotide consensus region of these genes.	$$\begin{array}{cccccc} T & A & T & A & A & T \\ (9) & (9) & (6) & (5) & (5) & (9) \end{array}$$
	At the −35 site, also moving left to right (toward the +1), the most common nucleotides in each position, and the number of times they occur in that position, are
	$$\begin{array}{cccccc} T & T & G & A & C & A \\ (8) & (9) & (8) & (6) & (6) & (6) \end{array}$$
	Answer b
5. Compare and contrast the likely effects of consensus sequence mutations with those of mutations occurring between consensus regions.	5. Mutation in a consensus sequence is likely to alter the efficiency with which a protein binds to the promoter and to decrease the amount of gene transcription. In contrast, mutations between consensus sequences are unlikely to alter gene transcription because the sequences in these intervening regions do not bind tightly to RNA polymerase.

For more practice, see Problems 4, 7, and 16.

Visit the Study Area to access study tools. **Mastering Genetics**

variation occurs among promoters, it is reasonable to ask how RNA polymerase is able to recognize promoters and reliably initiate RNA synthesis. For an answer, we turn to the sigma subunits that confer promoter recognition and chain-initiation ability on RNA polymerase.

Four alternative sigma subunits identified in *E. coli* are named according to their molecular weight (**Table 8.2**). Each alternative sigma subunit leads to recognition of a different set of −10 and −35 consensus sequences by the holoenzyme. These different consensus sequence elements are found in promoters of different types of genes; thus, the sigma subunit that it becomes attached to determines the specific gene promoters a holoenzyme will recognize.

The sigma subunit σ^{70} is the most common in bacteria. It recognizes promoters of "housekeeping genes," the genes whose protein products are continuously needed by cells. Because of the constant need for their products, housekeeping genes are continuously expressed. Subunits σ^{54} and σ^{32} recognize, respectively, promoters of genes involved in nitrogen metabolism and genes expressed in response to environmental stress such as heat shock, and they are utilized when the action of these genes is required. The fourth sigma subunit, σ^{28}, recognizes promoters for genes required for bacterial chemotaxis (chemical sensing and motility).

The specificity of each type of sigma subunit for different promoter consensus sequences produces RNA polymerase holoenzymes that have different DNA-binding specificities. Microbial geneticists estimate that each *E. coli* cell contains about 3000 RNA polymerase holoenzymes at any given time and that each of the four kinds of sigma subunits is represented to a differing degree among them. Because sigma subunits readily attach and detach from core enzymes in response to changes in environmental conditions, the organism is able to change its transcription patterns to adjust to different conditions.

Transcription Elongation and Termination

Upon reaching the +1 nucleotide, the holoenzyme begins RNA synthesis by using the template strand to direct RNA assembly. The holoenzyme remains intact until the first 8 to 10 RNA nucleotides have been joined. At that point, the sigma subunit dissociates from the core enzyme, which continues its downstream progression (❸ in Foundation Figure 8.6). The sigma subunit itself remains intact and can associate with another core enzyme to transcribe another gene.

Downstream progression of the RNA polymerase core is accompanied by DNA unwinding ahead of the enzyme to maintain approximately 18 bp of unwound DNA ❹. As the RNA polymerase passes, progressing at a rate of approximately 40 nucleotides per second, the DNA double helix re-forms in its wake. When transcription of the gene is completed, the 5′ end of the RNA trails off the core enzyme ❺.

The end product of transcription is a single-stranded RNA that is complementary and antiparallel to the template DNA strand. The transcript has the same 5′-to-3′ polarity as the coding strand of DNA, the strand complementary to the template strand. The coding strand and the newly formed transcript also have identical nucleotide sequences, except for the presence of uracil in the transcript in place of thymine in the coding strand. For this reason, gene sequences are written in 5′-to-3′ orientation as single-stranded sequences based on the coding strand of DNA. This allows easy identification of the mRNA sequence of a gene by simply substituting U for T.

Gene transcription is not a one-time event, and shortly after one round of transcription is initiated, a second round begins with new RNA polymerase–promoter interaction. Following sigma subunit dissociation and core enzyme synthesis of 50 to 60 RNA nucleotides, a new holoenzyme can bind to the promoter and initiate a new round of transcription while the first core enzyme continues along the gene. In addition, if the transcript under construction is mRNA, the 5′ end is immediately available to begin translation (as we see in Section 9.2, this is only true of organisms that don't possess a nucleus). In contrast, transcripts of other RNAs, such as transfer and ribosomal RNA, must await the completion of transcription before undergoing the folding into secondary structures that readies them for cellular action.

Transcription Termination Mechanisms

Termination of transcription in bacterial cells is signaled by a DNA termination sequence that usually contains a repeating sequence producing distinctive 3′ RNA sequences. Termination sequences are downstream of the stop codon; thus,

Table 8.2	*Escherichia coli* RNA Polymerase Sigma Subunits			
Subunit	Molecular Weight (kD)	Consensus Sequence		Function
		−35	−10	
σ^{28}	28	TAAA	GCCGATAA	Flagellar synthesis and chemotaxis
σ^{32}	32	CTTGAA	CCCCATTA	Heat shock genes
σ^{54}	54	CTGGPyAPyPu[a]	TTGCA	Nitrogen metabolism
σ^{70}	70	TTGACA	TATAAT	Housekeeping genes

[a] Py = pyrimidine; Pu = purine.

they are transcribed after the coding region of the mRNA and so are not translated. Two transcription termination mechanisms occur in bacteria. The most common is **intrinsic termination**, a mechanism dependent only on the occurrence of specialized repeat sequences in DNA that induce the formation in RNA of a secondary structure leading to transcription termination. Less frequently, bacterial gene transcription terminates by **rho-dependent termination**, a mechanism characterized by a different terminator sequence and requiring the action of a specialized protein called the **rho protein**.

Intrinsic Termination   Most bacterial transcription termination occurs exclusively as a consequence of termination sequences encoded in DNA—that is, by intrinsic termination. Intrinsic termination sequences have two features. First, they are encoded by a DNA sequence containing an **inverted repeat**, a DNA sequence repeated in opposite directions but with the same 5′-to-3′ polarity. **Figure 8.7** shows the inverted repeats ("inverted repeat 1" and "inverted repeat 2") in a termination sequence, separated by a short spacer sequence that is not part of either repeat. The second feature of intrinsic termination sequences is a string of adenines on the template DNA strand that begins at the 5′ end of the inverted repeat 2 region ❶. Transcription of inverted repeats produces mRNA with complementary segments that are able to fold into a short double-stranded stem ending with a single-stranded loop ❷. This secondary structure is a **stem-loop structure**, also known as a **hairpin** ❸. A string of uracils complementary to the adenines on the template strand immediately follows the stem-loop structure at the 3′ end of the RNA.

The formation of a stem-loop structure followed immediately by a poly-U sequence near the 3′ end of RNA causes the RNA polymerase to slow down and destabilize. In addition, the 3′ U–A region of the RNA–DNA duplex contains the least stable of the complementary base pairs. The instability created by RNA polymerase slowing and the U–A base pairs induces RNA polymerase to release the transcript and separate from the DNA ❹. The behavior of RNA polymerase during intrinsic termination of transcription is like that of a bicycle rider at slow speed. Slow forward momentum creates instability and eventually the rider loses balance. In a similar way, RNA polymerase is destabilized as it slows while transcribing inverted repeat sequences, and it falls off DNA when the transcript is released where A–U base pairs form and then separate.

Rho-Dependent Termination   In contrast to the more common intrinsic termination, certain bacterial genes require the action of rho protein to bind to nascent mRNA and catalyze separation of mRNA from RNA polymerase to terminate transcription. Genes whose transcription is rho-dependent have termination sequences that are distinct from those in genes utilizing intrinsic termination. As the mRNA transcript grows, a segment of the gene known as the **rho utilization site** is transcribed. On mRNA this produces a segment of sequence known as the

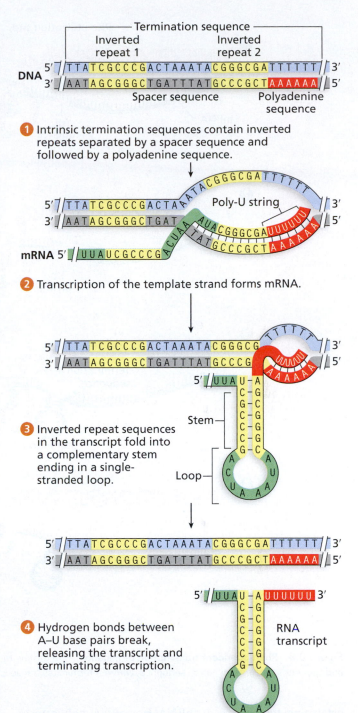

❶ Intrinsic termination sequences contain inverted repeats separated by a spacer sequence and followed by a polyadenine sequence.

❷ Transcription of the template strand forms mRNA.

❸ Inverted repeat sequences in the transcript fold into a complementary stem ending in a single-stranded loop.

❹ Hydrogen bonds between A–U base pairs break, releasing the transcript and terminating transcription.

Figure 8.7   Intrinsic termination. Inverted repeat DNA sequences alone initiate transcription termination.

rut site (**Figure 8.8 step ❶**). As RNA polymerase continues to elongate the mRNA in the 3′ direction, rho protein attaches to the rut site and quickly moves toward the RNA polymerase ❷. When RNA polymerase reaches and transcribes the termination sequence containing inverted repeat sequences, a stem-loop forms in the mRNA, causing the RNA polymerase to pause so that the rho protein catches up to it ❸. Rho protein then terminates transcription by

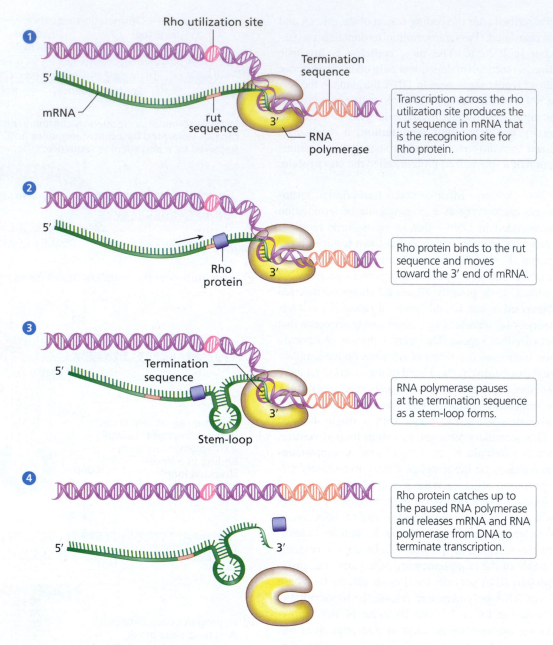

1. Rho utilization site

Transcription across the rho utilization site produces the rut sequence in mRNA that is the recognition site for Rho protein.

5′ mRNA — rut sequence — 3′ — RNA polymerase — Termination sequence

2. Rho protein binds to the rut sequence and moves toward the 3′ end of mRNA.

5′ — Rho protein — 3′

3. RNA polymerase pauses at the termination sequence as a stem-loop forms.

5′ — Termination sequence — Stem-loop — 3′

4. Rho protein catches up to the paused RNA polymerase and releases mRNA and RNA polymerase from DNA to terminate transcription.

5′ — 3′

Figure 8.8 Rho-dependent transcription termination. Rho protein binds to the rut sequence on mRNA and proceeds to the termination sequence, where it terminates transcription.

catalyzing the release of mRNA from RNA polymerase and causing RNA polymerase to drop off the DNA ❹.

8.3 Eukaryotic Transcription Is More Diversified and Complex than Bacterial Transcription

Bacteria use a single RNA polymerase core enzyme and several alternative sigma subunits to transcribe all genes. Eukaryotes, by contrast, each have three RNA polymerases that are specialized for the transcription of different genes.

The eukaryotic RNA polymerase responsible for the transcription of most polypeptide-producing genes differs from the bacterial RNA polymerase, but eukaryotic transcription progresses through the same four stages we described for bacteria: promoter recognition, transcription initiation, transcript elongation, and transcription termination. Several structural and functional factors make transcription more complex in eukaryotes.

First, eukaryotic promoters and consensus sequences are considerably more diverse than in *E. coli*, and, as indicated above, the three different RNA polymerases in eukaryotes recognize different promoters, transcribe different genes, and produce different RNAs. Second, the

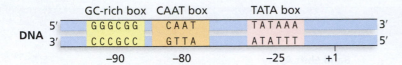

GC-rich box   CAAT box   TATA box

DNA	5′	GGGCGG	CAAT	TATAAA	3′
	3′	CCCGCC	GTTA	ATATTT	5′

−90   −80   −25   +1

Figure 8.9   Three common eukaryotic promoter consensus sequence elements. The TATA box and the CAAT box are common; the presence of the upstream GC-rich box is more variable.

molecular apparatus assembled at promoters to initiate and elongate transcription is more complex in eukaryotes. Third, eukaryotic genes contain introns and exons, requiring extensive posttranscriptional processing of mRNA. We describe this posttranscriptional processing in a later section. Finally, eukaryotic DNA is permanently associated with a large amount of protein to form a compound known as *chromatin*, the complex of DNA and proteins that makes up the eukaryotic chromosome and plays a central role in regulating eukaryotic transcription.

The three different RNA polymerases transcribing the major types of RNA coded by eukaryotic genomes are **RNA polymerase I (RNA pol I)**, which transcribes several ribosomal RNA genes; **RNA polymerase II (RNA pol II)**, which is primarily responsible for transcribing messenger RNAs that encode polypeptides, as well as for transcribing most small nuclear RNA genes; and **RNA polymerase III (RNA pol III)**, which transcribes all transfer RNA genes as well as one small nuclear RNA gene and one ribosomal RNA gene. RNA pol II and RNA pol III are also responsible for miRNA and siRNA synthesis.

Polymerase II Transcription of mRNA in Eukaryotes

RNA pol II transcribes eukaryotic polypeptide-coding genes into mRNA. The promoters for these genes are numerous and highly diverse, with different overall lengths and differences in the number and type of consensus sequences prominent among the sources of promoter variation. RNA polymerase II (RNA pol II) is a molecule composed of a dozen or more protein subunits, making it much more complex than the bacterial RNA polymerase, with its five subunits. In comparison, archaeal RNA polymerase has at least 11 or more subunits, making it more similar to RNA pol II than to bacterial RNA polymerase. Given the function of RNA pol II, it is reasonable to ask how RNA polymerases locate promoter DNA for different genes and how researchers determine which regions of a genome function as promoters.

Three lines of investigation help researchers to identify and characterize promoters of different polypeptide-coding genes: (1) promoters are identified by determining which DNA sequences are bound by proteins associated with RNA pol II during transcription, (2) putative promoter sequences from different genes are compared to evaluate their similarities, and (3) mutations that alter gene transcription are examined to identify how DNA base-pair changes affect transcription. **Research Technique 8.1** discusses the experimental identification and analysis of promoters.

The most common eukaryotic promoter consensus sequence, the *TATA box*, is shown in **Figure 8.9** as part of a set of three consensus segments that were the first eukaryotic promoter elements to be identified. A **TATA box**, also known as a **Goldberg–Hogness box**, is located approximately at position −25 relative to the beginning of the transcriptional start site. Consisting of 6 bp with the consensus sequence TATAAA, it is the most strongly conserved promoter element in eukaryotes. The figure shows two additional consensus sequence elements that are more variable in their frequency in promoters. A 4-bp consensus sequence identified as the **CAAT box** is most commonly located near −80 when it is present in the promoter. An upstream GC-rich region called the **GC-rich box**, with a consensus sequence GGGCGG located −90 or more upstream of the transcription start, has a frequency that is less than that of CAAT box sequences.

Comparison of eukaryotic promoters reveals a high degree of variability in the type, number, and location of consensus sequence elements (**Figure 8.10**). Some promoters contain all three of the consensus sequences identified above, others contain one or two of these consensus elements, some contain none at all, and many contain other types of consensus sequence elements altogether. For example, the thymidine kinase gene contains TATA, CAAT, and GC-rich boxes along with an octamer (OCT) sequence, called an OCT box. The histone *H2B* gene contains two OCT boxes in addition to a TATA box and a pair of CAAT boxes. All of these consensus sequence elements play important roles in the binding of *transcription factors*, a group of transcriptional proteins described below.

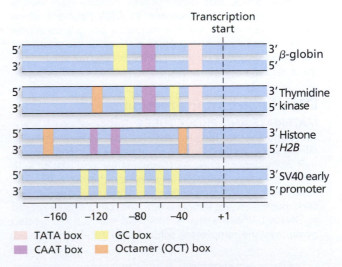

Figure 8.10   Selected examples of variability in eukaryotic promoters.

RESEARCH TECHNIQUE 8.1

Techniques for Finding Eukaryotic Promoters

PURPOSE The functional action of promoters in transcription depends on consensus DNA sequences that bind RNA polymerase and transcription factor proteins. To locate promoters, molecular biologists first scan DNA for potential promoter consensus sequences and then determine that the sequence binds transcriptionally active proteins. Fragments of DNA containing suspected promoter consensus sequence are examined by two experimental methods. The first, called *band shift assay*, verifies that the sequence of interest binds proteins. The second, called *DNA footprint protection assay*, identifies the exact location of the protein-binding sequence.

Band Shift Assay

MATERIALS AND PROCEDURES In this method, two identical samples of DNA fragments containing a suspected consensus sequence are analyzed. One DNA sample is a control to which no transcriptional proteins are added, and the other is the experimental DNA sample, with which transcriptional proteins are mixed. Both the control and the experimental DNA samples are subjected to gel electrophoresis that separates the fragments based on their size (molecular weight).

RESULTS In the band shift assay result, notice that the electrophoretic mobility of experimental DNA is slower than that of control DNA. This is the anticipated result if the experimental sample contains a consensus sequence that is bound by transcriptional proteins. The bound protein increases the molecular weight of the experimental sample and slows its migration relative to the same DNA without bound protein.

CONCLUSION The band shift assay results shown indicate different migration rates and therefore different molecular weights for the control and experimental DNA fragments. This is evidence that transcriptional proteins have bound to a sequence on the experimental DNA fragment, which would be consistent with the sequence being a consensus sequence and a potential promoter. However, the location of the bound sequence on the DNA fragment is not known from these results.

DNA Footprint Protection

MATERIALS AND PROCEDURES This experimental analysis begins with two identical samples of DNA fragments containing suspected consensus sequences as identified by band shift assay experiments. All fragments are end-labeled with ^{32}P to make their detection in gel electrophoresis easier. The experimental DNA sample is mixed with transcriptional proteins, but the control sample is not. Both samples are exposed to DNase I, which randomly cuts DNA that is not protected by protein. The samples are subjected to gel electrophoresis,

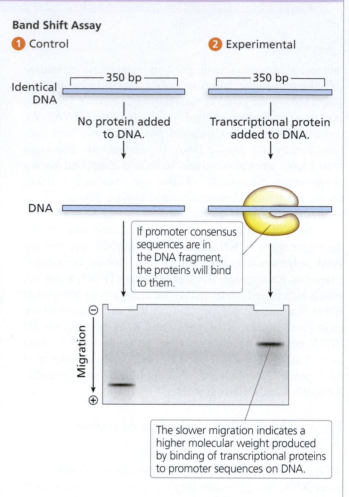

Band Shift Assay

1 Control   **2** Experimental

Identical DNA ├── 350 bp ──┤   ├── 350 bp ──┤

No protein added to DNA.   Transcriptional protein added to DNA.

DNA

If promoter consensus sequences are in the DNA fragment, the proteins will bind to them.

Migration

The slower migration indicates a higher molecular weight produced by binding of transcriptional proteins to promoter sequences on DNA.

and each end-labeled fragment produced is located by its radioactivity.

RESULTS In this DNA footprint protection assay, notice that the experimental DNA lane contains a gap in which no DNA fragments appear. The gap represents "footprint protection" for the portion of the fragment that is protected from DNase I digestion by bound transcriptional proteins. No such protection occurs for the control fragment, as there are no transcriptional proteins bound to any part of it.

CONCLUSION The gap created by footprint protection indicates that a DNA sequence on the experimental DNA fragment has been bound by transcriptional proteins, and the results provide information that can pinpoint where on the DNA fragment a protected DNA sequence is located. The final piece of evidence that a DNA fragment contains a promoter comes from mutational analysis that identifies functional changes caused by mutations of specific nucleotides of promoter consensus sequences. This analysis is described momentarily and is illustrated in **Figure 8.12**.

(continued)

RESEARCH TECHNIQUE 8.1 Continued

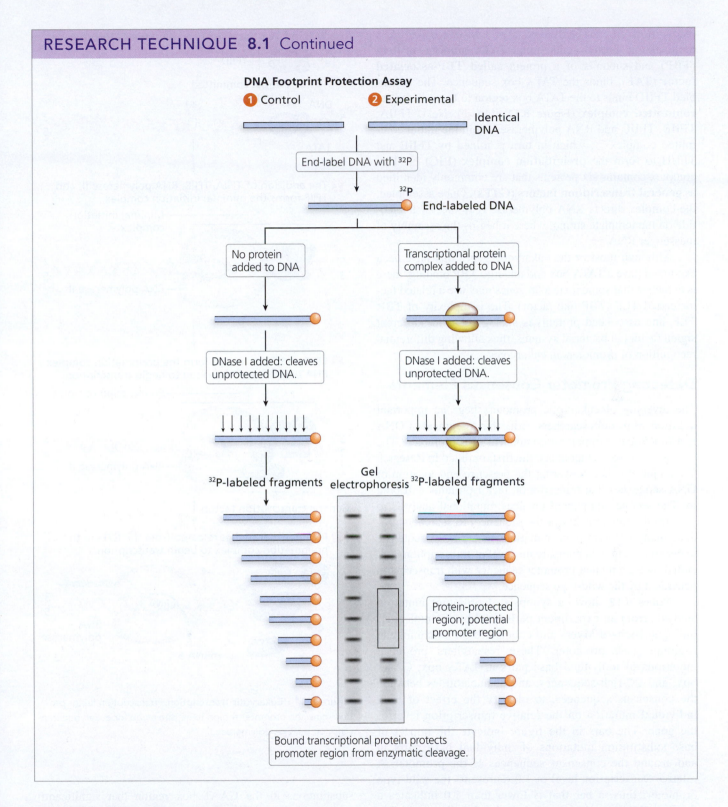

DNA Footprint Protection Assay

① Control   **②** Experimental

Identical DNA

End-label DNA with ³²P

³²P — End-labeled DNA

No protein added to DNA | Transcriptional protein complex added to DNA

DNase I added: cleaves unprotected DNA. | DNase I added: cleaves unprotected DNA.

³²P-labeled fragments   Gel electrophoresis   ³²P-labeled fragments

Protein-protected region; potential promoter region

Bound transcriptional protein protects promoter region from enzymatic cleavage.

Pol II Promoter Recognition

RNA polymerase II recognizes and binds to promoter consensus sequences in eukaryotes with the aid of proteins called **transcription factors (TF)**. The TF proteins bind to promoter regulatory sequences and influence transcription initiation by interacting, directly or indirectly, with RNA polymerase. Transcription factors that influence mRNA transcription, and therefore interact with RNA pol II, are given the designation TFII. Numerous individual TFII proteins are involved in this process. These proteins are assigned letter designations A, B, C, and so on.

In most eukaryotic promoters, the TATA box is the principal binding site for transcription factors during promoter recognition. At the TATA box, a protein called TFIID, a multisubunit protein containing **TATA-binding protein (TBP)** and subunits of a protein called **TBP-associated factor (TAF)**, binds the TATA box sequence. The assembled TFIID binds to the TATA box region to form the **initial committed complex** (**Figure 8.11 step ❶**). Next, TFIIA, TFIIB, TFIIF, and RNA polymerase II join the initial committed complex ❷, which in turn is joined by TFIIE and TFIIH to form the **preinitiation complex (PIC)** ❸. This complex contains six proteins that are commonly identified as **general transcription factors (GTFs)**. Once assembled, the complex directs RNA polymerase II to the +1 nucleotide on the template strand, where it begins the assembly of messenger RNA ❹.

Although most of the eukaryotic genes that have been examined have a TATA box and undergo TBP binding, there is evidence that some metazoan genes may use a related factor called TLF (*TBP-like factor*). The complexity of TBP, TLF, and associated proteins is analogous to the different sigma factors in bacterial systems, thus allowing differential recognition of promoters in eukaryotes.

Detecting Promoter Consensus Elements

The diversity of eukaryotic promoters begs an important question: How do researchers verify that a segment of DNA is a functionally important component of a promoter? The research has two components; the first, outlined in Research Technique 8.1, is discovering the presence and location of DNA sequences that transcription factor proteins will bind to. The second component involves mutational analysis to confirm the functionality of the sequence. Researchers produce many different point mutations in the DNA sequence under study and then compare the level of transcription generated by each mutant promoter sequence with transcription generated by the wild-type sequence.

Figure 8.12 shows a synopsis of promoter mutation analysis from an experiment performed by the molecular biologist Richard Myers and colleagues on a mammalian β-globin gene promoter. These researchers produced mutations of individual base pairs in TATA box, CAAT box, and GC-rich sequences, and of nucleotides between the consensus sequences, to identify the effect of each individual mutation on the relative transcription level of the gene. The bars in the figure indicate the impact of base substitution mutations of individual base pairs in and around the consensus sequences of the promoter. A relative transcription level of 1.0 represents the wild-type promoter; thus, a bar that is lower than 1.0 indicates a decrease in transcription level, and a bar that is higher than 1.0 indicates an increased level of transcription. The dots at nucleotide positions along the sequence indicate that no data are available since no mutation was made.

The researchers found that most base-pair mutations in the three consensus regions significantly decreased the transcription level of the gene, and they found two base

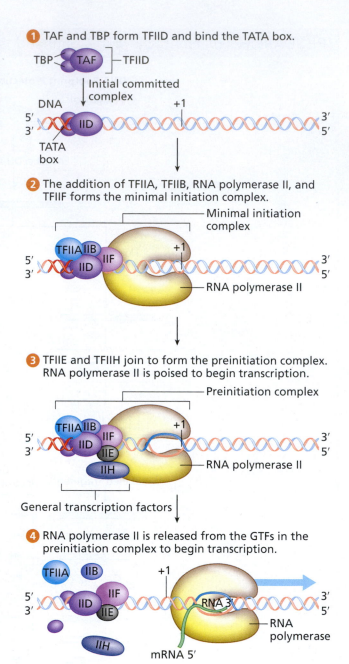

❶ TAF and TBP form TFIID and bind the TATA box.

❷ The addition of TFIIA, TFIIB, RNA polymerase II, and TFIIF forms the minimal initiation complex.

❸ TFIIE and TFIIH join to form the preinitiation complex. RNA polymerase II is poised to begin transcription.

General transcription factors

❹ RNA polymerase II is released from the GTFs in the preinitiation complex to begin transcription.

Figure 8.11 Eukaryotic transcription. Transcription factor proteins bind the promoter region to set the stage for eukaryotic transcription by RNA polymerase II.

substitutions in the CAAT box region that significantly increased transcription. In contrast, mutations outside the consensus regions had nonsignificant effects on transcription level. These results show the functional importance of specific DNA sequences in promoting transcription and confirm a functional role in transcription for TATA box, CAAT box, and GC-rich sequences. Notice that the sequences of these regulatory regions in this particular gene differ slightly from the consensus sequences shown in Figure 8.9. This is

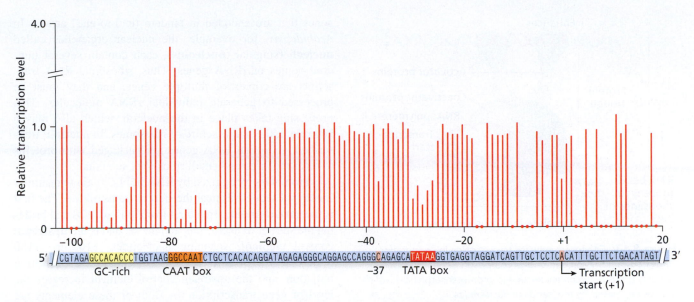

Figure 8.12 Mutation analysis of the β-globin gene promoter. The bars indicate that mutations in regions containing TATA box, CAAT box, and upstream GC-rich box sequences substantially reduce the relative transcription level. Orange dots indicate sites where no mutations were made and for which no data are available.

🔴 In this figure, the TATA box begins at −26 and ends at −30. In two or three sentences, describe the effect of mutations at positions −27 and −28 on relative transcription compared with mutations at −47 and −48. Explain the reason for the difference in mutation effect.

because the precise regulatory sequence of any gene may vary slightly from the consensus sequence.

Other Regulatory Sequences and Chromatin-Based Regulation of RNA Pol II Transcription

Often, promoters alone, while necessary, are not sufficient to initiate transcription of eukaryotic genes. In such cases, additional regulatory sequences, and additional transcription-activating proteins, are needed to drive transcription. This is particularly the case for multicellular eukaryotes that have many different types of cells with distinctive patterns of gene expression, including patterns that change as the organisms grow and develop. This type of transcriptional regulation is discussed in Section 13.2.

Enhancer sequences are one important group of DNA regulatory sequences that increase the level of transcription of specific genes. Enhancer sequences bind specific proteins that interact with the proteins bound at gene promoters, and together promoters and enhancers drive transcription of certain genes. In many situations, enhancers are located upstream of the genes they regulate; but enhancers can be located downstream as well. Some enhancers are relatively close to the genes they regulate, but others are thousands to tens of thousands of base pairs away from their target genes. Thus, important questions for molecular biologists are: What proteins are bound to enhancers, and how do enhancer sequences regulate transcription of

the gene given their different distances from the start of transcription?

One answer is that enhancers bind activator proteins and associated coactivator proteins to form a protein "bridge" that bends the DNA and links the transcription complex at the promoter to the activator–coactivator complex at the enhancer (**Figure 8.13**). The bend produced in the DNA may contain dozens to thousands of base pairs. The action of enhancers and the proteins they bind dramatically increases the efficiency of RNA pol II in initiating transcription, and as a result increases the level of transcription of genes regulated by enhancers.

At the other end of the transcription-regulating spectrum are **silencer sequences**, DNA elements that act to repress transcription of their target genes. Silencers bind proteins that bend DNA in such a way that genes become sequestered in the folded segment and thus are shielded from transcription activation by RNA pol II.

Overlying the operation of transcription-regulating DNA sequences and their interactions with DNA-binding proteins is the **chromatin** structure of eukaryotic DNA. "Chromatin," as mentioned earlier, is the name applied to the mixture of DNA and proteins that constitutes eukaryotic chromosomes, and its structure is both integral to the chromosome and dynamic. Specifically, chromatin can change to become more compact or less compact, either permitting or blocking RNA polymerase II and its transcription factor access to promoters and thus controlling the accessibility of regions of DNA to transcription. Different patterns of chromatin state occur in different types of cells; moreover, chromatin state for

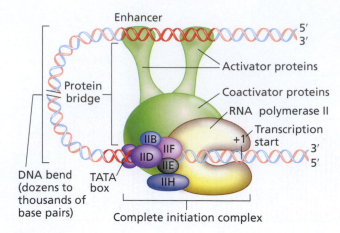

Figure 8.13 **Enhancers activate transcription in cooperation with promoters.** A protein bridge composed of transcriptional proteins forms between enhancer and promoter sequences, which may be separated by thousands of nucleotides.

a chromosome region can change during growth and development. This means that chromatin state can permit transcription of some genes in certain cell types or at certain times during development, but not in other cell types or at other times. The regulatory control of eukaryotic gene transcription exerted by changes in chromatin state is labeled an **epigenetic** process. These chromatin changes are identified as "chromatin modification" and as "chromatin remodeling," and are discussed in detail in Chapter 13. Epigenetic control of gene transcription is a prominent aspect of regulated gene expression in eukaryotes, and the chemical processes that control chromatin change are the subject of intensive research. Section 10.6 provides a further description of chromatin, and Section 13.2 delves into processes and consequences of epigenetic control of transcription.

In addition to the role of chromatin in transcription, the chromatin state of all chromosomes undergoes broad changes throughout the cell cycle. One category of chromatin known as **euchromatin** condenses chromosomes prior to cell division and decondenses them after cell division. Euchromatin constitutes the majority of the chromosomal material, and it is where most gene transcription takes place. The remaining chromatin is called **heterochromatin**, and while its level of condensation can change somewhat during the cell cycle, genes in heterochromatic regions of chromosomes exhibit a very low level of gene transcription.

RNA Polymerase I Promoters

The genes for rRNA are transcribed by RNA polymerase I, utilizing a transcription initiation mechanism similar to that used by RNA pol II. RNA polymerase I is the most specialized eukaryotic RNA polymerase, as it transcribes a limited number of genes. It is recruited to upstream promoter elements following the initial binding of transcription factors, and it transcribes ribosomal RNA genes.

In bacteria, rRNA genes are dispersed throughout the genome, but eukaryotic genomes contain clusters of rRNA

genes that are encoded in tandem (end-to-end) arrays. In *Arabidopsis*, for example, the nuclear organelles called **nucleoli** (singular, **nucleolus**), each contain several hundred copies of rRNA genes. Thus, ribosomal RNA transcripts are copies of multiple genes, and they must be processed to generate individual rRNA molecules. This processing takes place in the nucleoli, which also play a key role in the manufacture of ribosomes. In nucleoli, transcribed ribosomal RNA genes are packaged with proteins to form the large and small ribosomal subunits.

Promoters recognized by RNA pol I contain two similar functional sequences near the start of transcription. The first is the **core element**, stretching from -45 to $+20$ and bridging the start of transcription, and the second is the **upstream control element**, spanning nucleotides -100 to -150 (**Figure 8.14**). The core element is essential for transcription initiation, and the upstream control element increases the level of gene transcription ❶. Both of these elements are rich in guanine and cytosine; DNA sequence comparisons show that all upstream control elements have the same base pairs at approximately 85 percent of nucleotide positions, and the same is true of all core elements. Two upstream binding factor 1 (UBF1) proteins bind the upstream control element. Copies of a second protein, known as sigma-like factor 1 (SL1) protein, bind the core element ❷. The UBF1-SL1 complex recruits RNA pol I to the core element, to initiate transcription of rRNA genes ❸.

RNA Polymerase III Promoters

The remaining eukaryotic RNA polymerase, RNA polymerase III, is primarily responsible for transcription of tRNA genes. It also transcribes one rRNA and certain other RNA-encoding genes. The promoter structures for these genes differ significantly from the structure of promoters recognized by RNA pol I or RNA pol II. RNA pol III promoters most often have an **internal control region (ICR)** that is located within the transcribed region (**Figure 8.15**).

The ICRs most often contain two short DNA sequences, designated box A and box B in some genes and box A and box C in other genes ❶. The two box regions of the ICR are separated by about 25 base pairs. Reminiscent of the activity associated with transcription by RNA pol II, TFIII proteins bind to the two box regions prior to binding by RNA pol III ❷❸. Transcription begins near box A once RNA pol III is properly positioned ❹. RNA pol III promoters vary, and some have regulatory elements upstream of the start of transcription.

Archaeal Promoters and Transcription

Much less is known about promoters and transcription in archaeal species than in bacteria and eukaryotes. The information available to date, however, indicates that archaea have a single major RNA polymerase that transcribes mRNA, tRNA, and rRNA genes. The RNA polymerase of archaea is distinct from that of bacteria and represents a

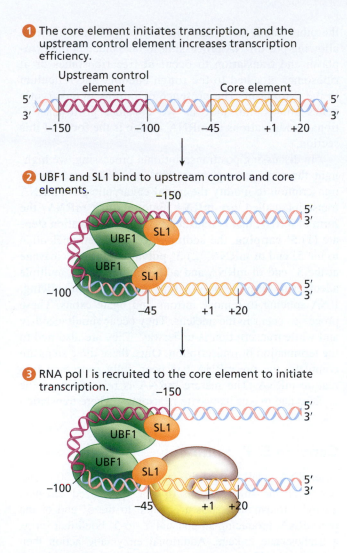

1. The core element initiates transcription, and the upstream control element increases transcription efficiency.

2. UBF1 and SL1 bind to upstream control and core elements.

3. RNA pol I is recruited to the core element to initiate transcription.

Figure 8.14 Promoter consensus sequences for transcription initiation by RNA polymerase I.

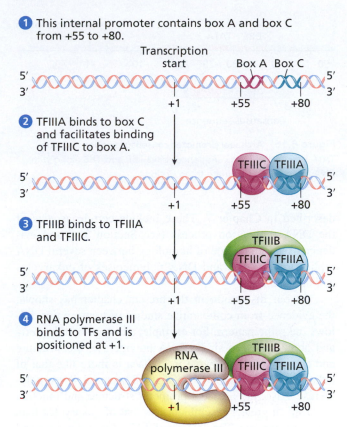

1. This internal promoter contains box A and box C from +55 to +80.

2. TFIIIA binds to box C and facilitates binding of TFIIIC to box A.

3. TFIIIB binds to TFIIIA and TFIIIC.

4. RNA polymerase III binds to TFs and is positioned at +1.

Figure 8.15 An internal promoter for transcription by RNA polymerase III.

The Evolutionary Implications of Comparative Transcription

Since the origin of life on Earth more than 4 billion years ago, the lineages of living organisms have branched off into three domains—Bacteria, Archaea, and Eukarya (see Figure 1.2). Among the many questions posed by the divergence of these domains are the questions of the degree of relationship between them and the order in which they diverged. At first glance, bacteria and archaea might seem to be most similar to one another, and eukaryotes would appear to be most different. Some of the superficial similarities between bacteria and archaea are that members of both groups are single-celled, their cells lack a nucleus, and most species of both domains have a single chromosome. Some comparisons of the biochemistry and DNA sequences of bacteria and archaea also reveal similarities.

At the same time, further inspection seems to suggest a closer relationship between archaea and eukaryotes than between bacteria and eukaryotes. The preponderance of evidence now indicates that eukaryotes are more closely related to archaea than to bacteria. Some of the striking similarities between eukaryotes and archaea were

simplified and ancestrally related version of the eukaryotic RNA polymerases and an overall transcription process that is most similar to that of RNA pol II.

Studies examining archaeal promoters and transcription initiation in the thermophilic archaeal species *Sulfolobus shibatae* have identified a TATA-binding protein (TBP, a subunit of TFIID) and transcription factor B (TFB), a homolog of eukaryotic TFIIB, as the only proteins required for interaction with RNA polymerase in the initiation of archaeal transcription (**Figure 8.16**). TBP binds to a TATA box in the archaeal promoter, and TFB binds a BRE box (TFB-recognition element) that is immediately upstream of the TATA box. With TBP and TFB bound to their promoter elements, RNA polymerase is directed approximately 25 base pairs downstream to the transcription start site in a process that appears to be quite similar to the start of transcription in eukaryotes.

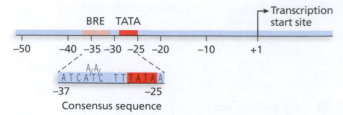

Figure 8.16 Archaeal promoter consensus sequences. The TATA box and BRE box sequences bind TBP and TFB along with RNA polymerase to initiate transcription.

described in Chapter 7. These include certain aspects of the DNA replication process (see Section 7.4) and evidence of a high degree of homology between several DNA replication proteins and DNA polymerases of eukaryotes and archaea.

As our discussion in the present chapter has shown, the evidence from comparative studies of transcription follows the same pattern. For example, although both bacteria and archaea have a single RNA polymerase, the structure and activity of the enzyme in archaea is more like that of eukaryotic RNA pol II than that of bacterial RNA polymerase. Also, the archaeal promoter structure and function has a much greater resemblance to that of eukaryotes than to that of bacteria. The sharing of TATA box sequences and the activity of TBP and other molecular components of transcription suggest a strong level of similarity between eukaryotes and archaea.

Overall, the current conclusion from comparative examination of bacterial, archaeal, and eukaryotic replication and transcription is that eukaryotes and archaea are more closely related to one another than either is to bacteria, supporting the pattern of divergence illustrated in Figure 1.2. In that figure, Eukarya and Archaea are seen to diverge from each other more recently than their lineage diverged from that of the Bacteria.

8.4 Posttranscriptional Processing Modifies RNA Molecules

Bacterial, archaeal, and eukaryotic RNA transcripts differ from one another in at least two important ways. First, eukaryotic transcripts are more stable than bacterial and archaeal transcripts. The half-life of a typical eukaryotic mRNA is measured in hours to days, whereas bacterial mRNAs have an average half-life measured in seconds to minutes. A second difference is the presence of introns in eukaryotic genes that are absent from most bacterial and archaeal genes. Keep in mind that in bacteria the lack of a nucleus leads to coupling of transcription and translation. Similarly, archaea lack a nucleus, leading to the possibility of synchrony between transcription and translation in those organisms. In eukaryotic cells, on the other hand, transcription takes place in the nucleus, allowing pre-mRNA processing to take place in the cytoplasm and translation to occur at free ribosomes or at ribosomes attached to the rough endoplasmic reticulum in the cytoplasm. The presence of introns in eukaryotic genes comes into play as we consider posttranscriptional modifications of mRNA, which is the focus of this section.

In discussing posttranscriptional processing, we highlight three processing steps that are coordinated during transcription to modify the initial eukaryotic gene mRNA transcript, called **pre-mRNA**, into **mature mRNA**, the form of mRNA that is translated. These modification steps are (1) **5′ capping**, the addition of a modified nucleotide to the 5′ end of mRNA; (2) **3′ polyadenylation**, cleavage at the 3′ end of mRNA and addition of a tail of multiple adenines to form the **poly-A tail**; and (3) **intron splicing**, RNA splicing to remove introns and ligate exons. These processes occur in the nucleus. They occur simultaneously and while transcription is underway. They are also tied to the termination of transcription. Once these three steps are complete, the pre-mRNA has been fully processed into mature mRNA. The mature mRNA is released from the nucleus and makes its way to ribosomes, where translation takes place.

Capping 5′ Pre-mRNA

After RNA pol II has synthesized the first 20 to 30 nucleotides of the mRNA transcript, a specialized enzyme, guanylyl transferase, adds a guanine to the 5′ end of the pre-mRNA, producing an unusual 5′-to-5′ bond that forms a triphosphate linkage. Additional enzymatic action then methylates (adds a methyl group to) the newly added guanine and may also methylate the next one or more nucleotides of the transcript. This addition of guanine to the transcript and the subsequent methylation is known as 5′ capping.

Guanylyl transferase initiates 5′ capping in three steps depicted in **Figure 8.17**. Before capping, the terminal 5′ nucleotide of mRNA contains three phosphate groups, labeled α, β, and γ in Figure 8.17. Guanylyl transferase first removes the γ phosphate, leaving two phosphates on the 5′ terminal nucleotide ❶. The guanine triphosphate containing the guanine that is to be added loses two phosphates (γ and β) to form a guanine monophosphate ❷. Then, guanylyl transferase joins the guanine monophosphate to the mRNA terminal nucleotide to form the 5′-to-5′ triphosphate linkage ❸. Methyl transferase enzyme then adds a methyl (CH_3) group to the 7-nitrogen of the new guanine, forming 7-methylguanosine (m^7G). Methyl transferase may also add methyl groups to 2′−OH of nearby nucleotides of mRNA.

The 5′ cap has several functions, including (1) protecting mRNA from rapid degradation, (2) facilitating mRNA transport across the nuclear membrane,

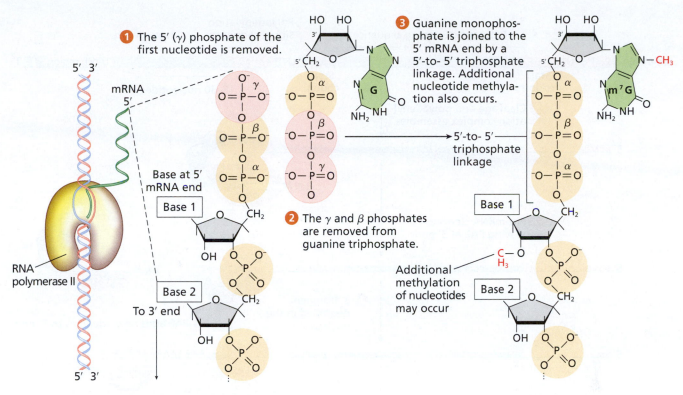

Figure 8.17 Capping the 5′ end of eukaryotic pre-mRNA.

❓ Circle the two features in the 5′ cap region that make it distinctively different from the 5′ end of an mRNA that does not have 5′ cap modifications.

(3) facilitating subsequent intron splicing, and (4) enhancing translation efficiency by orienting the ribosome on mRNA.

Polyadenylation of 3′ Pre-mRNA

Termination of transcription by RNA pol II is not fully understood, but it appears to be tied to the processing and polyadenylation of the 3′ end of pre-mRNA. It is clear that the 3′ end of eukaryotic mRNA is not generated by transcriptional terminating sequence as it is in bacteria. Rather, the 3′ end of the pre-mRNA is created by enzymatic action that removes a segment from the 3′ end of the transcript and replaces it with a string of adenine nucleotides, the poly-A tail. This step of pre-mRNA processing is thought to be associated with subsequent termination of transcription.

Figure 8.18 illustrates these steps. Polyadenylation begins with the binding of a factor called cleavage and polyadenylation specificity factor (CPSF) near a six-nucleotide mRNA sequence, AAUAAA, that is downstream of the stop codon and thus not part of the coding sequence of the gene. This six-nucleotide sequence is known as the **polyadenylation signal sequence**. The binding of cleavage-stimulating factor (CStF) to a uracil-rich sequence several dozen nucleotides downstream of the polyadenylation signal sequence quickly follows, and the binding of two other

cleavage factors, CFI and CFII, and polyadenylate polymerase (PAP) enlarges the complex ❶. The pre-mRNA is then cleaved 15 to 30 nucleotides downstream of the polyadenylation signal sequence ❷. The cleavage releases a transcript fragment bound by CFI, CFII, and CStF, which is later degraded ❸. Through the action of CPSF and PAP, the 3′ end of the cut pre-mRNA then undergoes the enzymatic addition of 20 to 200 adenine nucleotides that form the 3′ poly-A tail ❹. After addition of the first 10 adenines, molecules of poly-A-binding protein II (PABII) join the elongating poly-A tail and increase the rate of adenine addition ❺. The 3′ poly-A tail has several functions, including (1) facilitating transport of mature mRNA across the nuclear membrane, (2) protecting mRNA from degradation, and (3) enhancing translation by enabling ribosomal recognition of messenger RNA.

Certain eukaryotic mRNA transcripts do not undergo polyadenylation. The most prominent of these are transcripts of genes producing *histone proteins*, which are key components of chromatin (see Section 10.6). On these and other "tailless" mRNAs, the 3′ end contains a short stem-loop structure reminiscent of the ones seen in the intrinsic transcription termination mechanism of bacteria. There may be an evolutionary connection between bacterial transcription termination and stem-loop formation on "tailless" eukaryotic mRNAs.

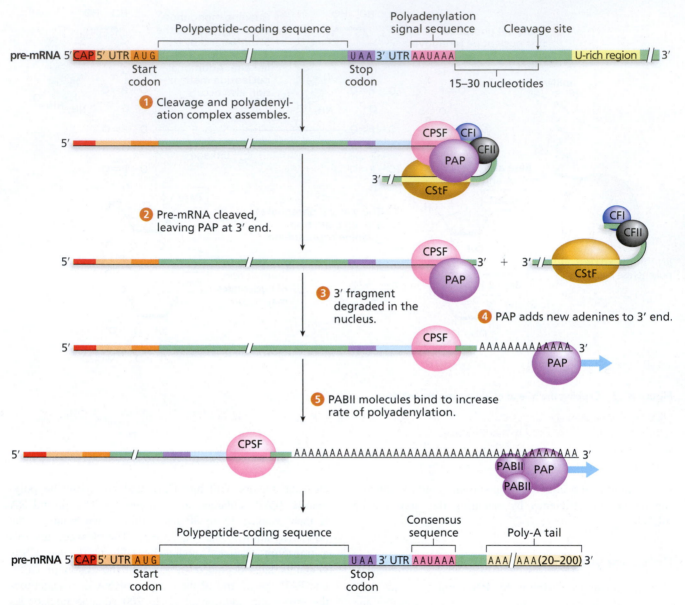

Figure 8.18 Polyadenylation of the 3′ end of eukaryotic pre-mRNA.

The Torpedo Model of Transcription Termination

The connection between polyadenylation and transcription termination lies in the activity of a specialized RNase (an RNA-destroying enzyme) that attacks and digests the residual RNA transcript that has remained attached to RNA pol II after 3′ transcript cleavage. Following polyadenylation and 3′ cleavage, the residual segment still attached to RNA pol II has no cap protecting its 5′ end. This end is attacked by the specialized RNase that rapidly digests the remaining transcript.

The RNase is thought of as a "torpedo" aimed at the residual mRNA attached to RNA pol II (**Figure 8.19**). Studies have shown that the torpedo RNase is a highly processive enzyme, meaning that it rapidly carries out its

enzymatic action. Once the RNase destroys the residual mRNA and catches up to RNA pol II, it triggers dissociation of the polymerase from template strand DNA to terminate transcription.

Introns

Most eukaryotic genes contain two kinds of segments. One kind, the exons, become part of mature mRNA and encode segments of proteins. The other kind, the introns, are intervening segments that separate exons. Introns are removed from pre-mRNA by processes that excise the introns and splice together the exons.

Introns are common in eukaryotic genes, are rare in bacterial genes, and are found occasionally in archaeal genes. There is also evidence of the presence of introns in a

Figure 8.19   The torpedo model of eukaryotic transcription termination. Eukaryotic transcription ❶ leads to torpedo RNase association with mRNA ❷, Enzymatic cleavage near the poly-A-signal sequence releases the mature mRNA. The torpedo RNase attacks the uncapped 5′ end of the residual mRNA ❸ and digests it ❹, leading RNA polymerase II to dissociate from the DNA and the torpedo RNase ❺.

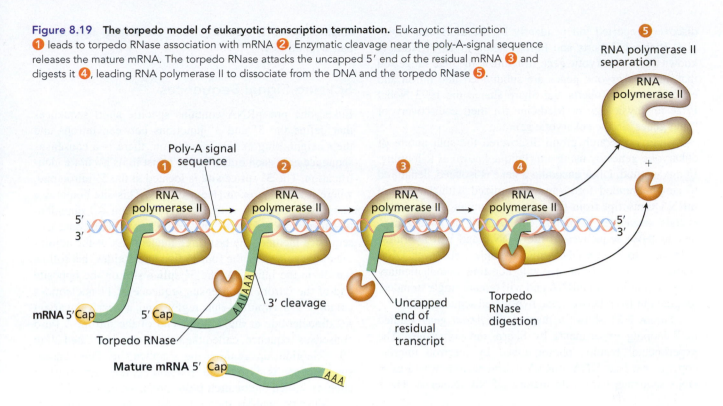

very small number of bacteriophage genes. The length and number of introns vary widely in eukaryotic genes. Among the members of the three domains of life there are four major types of introns (Table 8.3). In addition, there are several types of minor introns.

Most of our focus for the remainder of this chapter is on the most common type of intron—the type found in pre-mRNA transcripts. These introns are removed from pre-mRNA by a specialized enzymatic process involving the formation of a *spliceosome* complex that carries out excision and splicing. Two other types of introns known as group I and group II introns are removed by *self-splicing processes*, and a different enzymatic activity splices rRNA and tRNA gene transcripts. We discuss each of these processes below.

Pre-mRNA Splicing

Pre-mRNA intron removal requires exquisite precision to remove all intron nucleotides accurately without intruding on the exons, and without leaving behind additional nucleotides, so that the mRNA sequence encoded by the ligated (spliced) exons will completely and faithfully direct synthesis of the correct polypeptide. As an example of the need for

Table 8.3	Major Types of Introns	
Type of Intron	**Splicing Mechanism**	**Type of Organism/ Location**
Group I	Self-splicing	Eukaryotes, bacteria, bacteriophages
Group II	Self-splicing	Eukaryotic organelles, bacteria, archaea
Pre-mRNA	Spliceosome	Eukaryotic nuclear genes
rRNA and tRNA	Enzymatic	Eukaryotes, bacteria, archaea

precision in intron removal, consider the "precursor string" in Figure 8.20, made up of exon-like blocks of letters forming three-letter words interrupted by unintelligible intron-like blocks of letters. If editing removes the "introns" accurately, the "edited string" can be divided into three-letter words that form a "sentence." If an error in editing were to remove too many or too few letters, a nonsense sentence would result.

The finding that introns interrupt the genetically informative segments of eukaryotic genes was a stunning

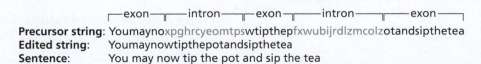

┌──exon──┬──intron──┬─exon─┬──────intron──────┬──────exon──────┐
Precursor string: Youmaynoxpghrcyeomtpswtipthepfxwubijrdlzmcolzotandsipthetea
Edited string: Youmaynowtipthepotandsipthetea
Sentence: You may now tip the pot and sip the tea

Figure 8.20 An analogy for intron removal and exon splicing.

discovery reported independently by the molecular biologists Richard Roberts and Phillip Sharp in 1977. Nothing known about eukaryotic gene structure at the time suggested that most eukaryotic genes are subdivided into intron and exon elements. Roberts and Sharp shared the 1993 Nobel Prize in Physiology or Medicine for their codiscovery of "split genes" in the eukaryotic genome.

Sharp's research group discovered the split nature of eukaryotic genes by using a technique known as R-looping. In this method, DNA encoding a gene is isolated, denatured to single-stranded form, and then mixed with the mature mRNA transcript from the gene. Regions of the gene that encode sequences in mature mRNA will be complementary to those sequences in the mRNA and will hybridize with them to form a DNA–mRNA duplex. However, DNA segments encoding introns will not find complementary sequences in mature mRNA and will remain single stranded, looping out from between the hybridized sequences.

Figure 8.21 shows a map of the *hexon* gene studied in R-looping experiments by Sharp and colleagues. The experimental results, photographed by electron microscopy, reveal four DNA–mRNA hybrid regions where exon DNA sequence pairs with mature mRNA sequence. Three

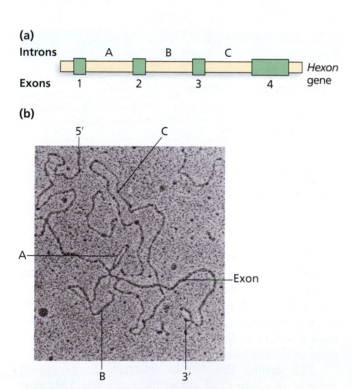

(a)

Introns

Exons

Hexon gene

(b)

Figure 8.21 R-loop experimental analysis. (a) The *hexon* gene contains four exons (1 to 4) and three introns (A to C). **(b)** Electron micrographs show hybridization of mature *hexon* gene mRNA with denatured *hexon* DNA. Exon regions of DNA hybridize with mature mRNA, but intron sequences do not hybridize and appear as single-stranded loops.

Q The electron micrograph in part (b) has a pointer indicating an "exon." Which specific exon does this pointer most likely indicate? Justify your answer.

single-stranded R-loop sequences are introns that do not pair with mRNA.

Splicing Signal Sequences

Eukaryotic pre-mRNA contains specific short sequences that define the 5′ and 3′ junctions between introns and their neighboring exons. In addition, there is a consensus sequence near each intron end to assist in its accurate identification. The **5′ splice site** is located at the 5′ intron end, where it abuts an exon (**Figure 8.22**). This site contains a consensus sequence with a nearly invariant GU dinucleotide forming the 5′-most end of the intron. The consensus sequence includes the last three nucleotides of the adjoining exon, as well as the four or five nucleotides that follow the GU in the intron. At the 3′ **splice site** on the opposite end of the intron, a consensus sequence of 11 nucleotides contains a pyrimidine-rich region and a nearly invariant AG dinucleotide at the 3′-most end of the intron. A third consensus sequence, called the branch site, is located 20 to 40 nucleotides upstream of the 3′ splice site. This consensus sequence is pyrimidine-rich and contains an invariant adenine, called the **branch point adenine**, near the 3′ end.

Mutation analysis shows that these consensus sequences are critical for accurate intron removal. Mutations altering nucleotides in any of the three consensus regions can produce abnormally spliced mature mRNA. The abnormal mRNAs—too short if exon sequence is mistakenly removed, too long if intron sequence is left behind, or altered in other ways that result in improper reading of mRNA sequence—produce proteins with incorrect sequences of amino acids (see Section 11.2).

Introns are removed from pre-mRNA by an snRNA–protein complex called the **spliceosome**. The spliceosome is something like a molecular workbench to which pre-mRNA is attached while spliceosome subunit components cut and splice it in a four-step process that, first, cleaves the 5′ splice site; second, forms a **lariat intron structure** that binds the 5′ intron end to the branch point adenine; third, cleaves the 3′ splice site; and finally, splices exons and releases the lariat intron to be degraded to its nucleotide components.

Figure 8.22 illustrates the steps of nuclear pre-mRNA splicing, beginning with the aggregation of five small nuclear ribonucleoproteins (snRNPs; pronounced "snurps") to form a spliceosome. The snRNPs are snRNA–protein subunits designated U1, U2, and U4 to U6. The spliceosome is a large complex made up of multiple snRNPs, but its composition is dynamic; it changes throughout the different stages of splicing when individual snRNPs come and go as particular reaction steps are carried out.

A Gene Expression Machine Couples Transcription and Pre-mRNA Processing

Each intron–exon junction is subjected to the same spliceosome reactions, raising the question of whether there is a particular order in which introns are removed

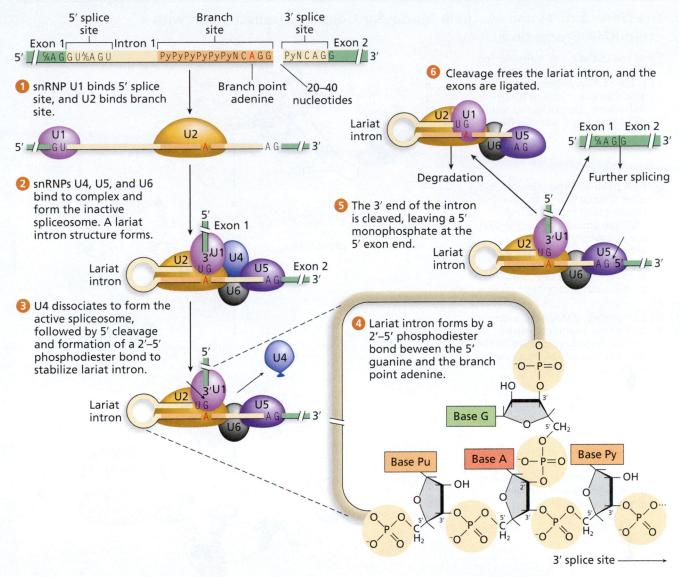

Figure 8.22 Intron removal from eukaryotic pre-mRNA by a spliceosome. The solidus between A and G in the 5' splice site (A/G) indicates that these two nucleotides are about equally frequent in this consensus sequence. In the 3' splice site, Py indicates either of the pyrimidines (C or U) and N indicates that any nucleotide can be present.

from pre-mRNA—or whether U1 and U2 search more or less randomly for 5' splice-site and branch-site consensus sequences, inducing spliceosome formation when they happen to encounter an intron. The answer is that introns appear to be removed one by one, but not necessarily in order along the pre-mRNA. A study of intron splicing of the mammalian *ovomucoid* gene demonstrates this feature of intron removal. The *ovomucoid* gene contains eight exons and seven introns. The pre-mRNA transcript is approximately 5.6 kb, and the mature mRNA is reduced to 1.1 kb. Analysis of *ovomucoid* pre-mRNAs at various stages of intron removal illustrates that each intron is removed separately, rather than all introns being removed at once, but the order of intron removal does not precisely match their 5'-to-3' order in pre-mRNA.

The three steps of pre-mRNA processing are tightly coupled. In comprehensive models developed over the past decade or so, the carboxyl terminal domain (CTD) of RNA polymerase II plays an important role in this coupling by functioning as an assembly platform and regulator of pre-mRNA processing machinery. The CTD is located at the site of emergence of mRNA from the polymerase and contains multiple heptad (seven-member) repeats of amino acids that can be phosphorylated. Binding of processing proteins to the CTD allows the mRNA to be modified as it is transcribed.

Current models propose that "gene expression machines" consisting of RNA polymerase II and an array of pre-mRNA–processing proteins are responsible for the coupling of transcription and pre-mRNA processing. **Foundation Figure 8.23** illustrates this gene expression

The Gene Expression Machine Model for Coupling Transcription with pre-mRNA Processing

1 At the initiation of transcription the carboxyl terminal domain (CTD) of RNA polymerase II affiliates with capping (CAP), polyadenylation (pA), and splicing (SF) factors, and torpedo RNase (RNase).

2 RNA pol II initiates transcription after dissociation of the general transcription factors (GTFs). Multiple amino acids in the CTD are phosphorylated. The pre-mRNA processing proteins on the CTD begin their work, starting with the CAP proteins carrying out 5' capping.

3 CAP protein dissociates, leaving part of the capping complex behind, including splicing factors (SF). The pre-mRNA continues to elongate.

4 Spliceosome complexes affiliate with pre-mRNA with the aid of SF proteins. Intron splicing takes place as RNA pol II continues elongation of mRNA.

5 Polyadenylation proteins identify the pA signal sequence and carry out polyadenylation. Transcription terminates. Splicing continues to completion. Torpedo RNase digests the residual mRNA.

6 Fully processed mature mRNA dissociates from RNA pol II, is released through nuclear pores, and is transported to cytoplasm for translation. RNA pol II dissociates from DNA.

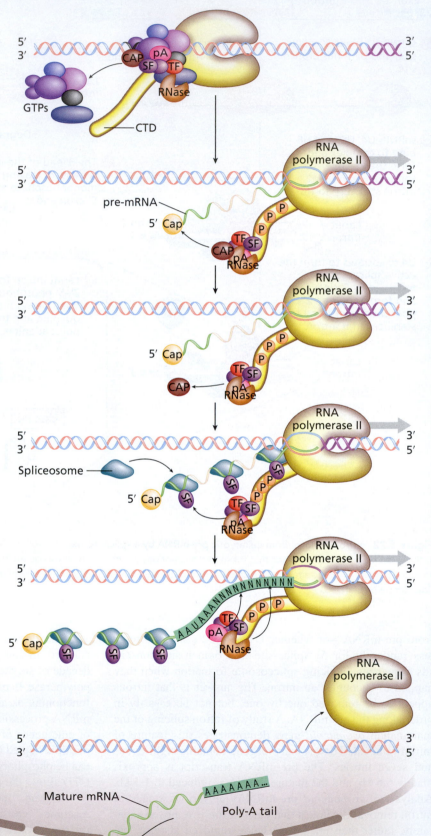

machine model. The CTD of RNA polymerase II associates with multiple proteins that carry out capping (CAP), intron splicing (SF), and polyadenylation (pA) so that the processes of transcription and pre-mRNA processing occur simultaneously. At the initiation of transcription, phosphorylation (P) along the CTD assists the binding of 5′-capping enzymes, which carry out their capping function and then dissociate. During transcription elongation, specific transcription elongation factors bind the CTD and facilitate splicing-factor binding. The CTD also contains the torpedo RNase responsible for digestion of the residual transcript left attached to RNA pol II by 3′ cleavage linked to polyadenylation. The torpedo RNase is loaded onto the transcript from the CTD to quickly trigger transcription termination (see Figure 8.19).

Alternative Patterns of RNA Transcription and Alternative RNA Splicing

Before the complete sequencing of the human genome in the early 2000s, estimates of the number of human genes varied, having been as high as 80,000 to 100,000 genes 20 years or so earlier. A principal reason for the size of these initial predictions was that human cells produce well over 100,000 distinct polypeptides. It came as something of a surprise, then, when gene annotation of the human genome revealed a total content of approximately 22,800 genes. The difference between the number of genes and the number of polypeptides is mirrored by similar findings in other eukaryotic genomes, especially those of mammals. It is common for large eukaryotic genomes to express more proteins than there are genes in the genomes. Three transcription-associated mechanisms can account for the ability of single DNA sequences to produce more than one polypeptide. First, a pre-mRNA can be spliced in alternative patterns in different types of cells. In other words, the same transcript might produce one mature mRNA (and a particular protein) in one type of cell and a different mature mRNA (and a different protein) in another type of cell, This process is called **alternative pre-mRNA splicing**. Second, **alternative promoters** can initiate transcription at distinct +1 start points in different cell types, and third, **alternative polyadenylation** uses different polyadenylation signal sequences in a gene to produce different mRNAs.

The products of the human *calcitonin/calcitonin gene-related peptide* (*CT/CGRP*) gene exemplify the process of alternative splicing and illustrate the production of several different proteins from the same sequence of DNA (**Figure 8.24**). The *CT/CGRP* gene produces the same pre-mRNA transcript in many cells, including thyroid cells and neuronal cells. The transcript contains six exons and five introns and includes two alternative polyadenylation sites, one in exon 4 and the other following exon 6. In thyroid cells, *CT/CGRP* pre-mRNA is spliced to form mature mRNA containing exons 1 through 4, using

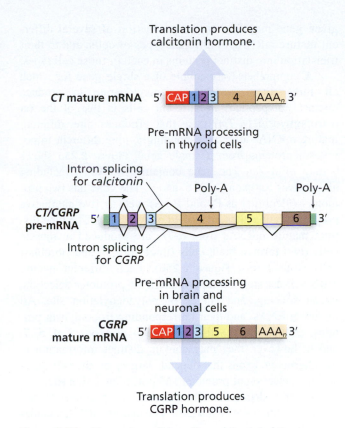

Figure 8.24 Alternative splicing. The *calcitonin/calcitonin gene-related peptide* (*CT/CGRP*) gene is transcribed into either calcitonin or CGRP.

🅠 Using the same labeling scheme shown for this pre-mRNA and mature mRNAs, draw two additional mature mRNAs that could be produced from this pre-mRNA.

the first poly-A site for polyadenylation. Translation produces calcitonin, a hormone that helps regulate calcium. In neuronal cells, the same pre-mRNA is spliced to form mature mRNA containing exons 1, 2, 3, 5, and 6. Polyadenylation takes place at the site that follows exon 6, since exon 4 is spliced out as though it were an intron. Translation in neuronal cells produces the hormone CGRP. Alternative splicing is common in mammals—approximately 70 percent of human genes are thought to undergo alternative splicing—but it is less common in other animals, and it is rare in plants.

The use of alternative promoters occurs when a gene contains more than one upstream sequence that can bind transcription factors and initiate transcription at different transcription start sites. Similarly, alternative polyadenylation is possible in those genes that contain more than one polyadenylation signal sequence that can activate 3′ pre-mRNA cleavage and polyadenylation. Alternative promoters and alternative polyadenylation are driven by the variable expression of transcriptional or polyadenylation proteins in a cell-type-specific manner, and the processes generate characteristic mature mRNAs and distinctive proteins in specific cells. The result is that transcription of a given gene may lead to the production of several different mature mRNAs in different types of cells, and to their translation into distinct proteins in each of those cell types.

A comprehensive example of a single gene for which all three alternative mechanisms operate to produce distinct polypeptides in different cells is that of the rat α-tropomyosin (α-*Tm*) gene that produces nine different mature mRNAs and, correspondingly, nine different tropomyosin proteins from a single gene. **Figure 8.25a** shows a map of α-*Tm*. The gene contains 14 exons, including alternatives for exons 1, 2, 6, and 9. The gene has two promoters (identified as P_1 and P_2) as well as five alternative polyadenylation sites (identified as A_1 to A_5). The nine distinct mature mRNAs from α-*Tm* are produced in muscle cells (two forms), brain cells (three forms), and fibroblast cells (four forms; **Figure 8.25b**). Each different mature mRNA illustrates a unique pattern of promoter selection, intron splicing, and choice of polyadenylation site. All mature mRNAs, and their corresponding tropomyosin proteins, contain the genetic information of exons 3, 4, 5, 7, and 8; however, they may contain distinct information in the alternative exons that depends largely on the cell-type–specific selection of promoter and polyadenylation site.

In striated muscle cells, for example, promoter P_1 and polyadenylation site A_2 are used. The mature mRNA includes the alternative exons 1a, 2b, 6b, 9a, and 9b. In contrast, tropomyosin in smooth muscle cells utilizes promoter P_1 and polyadenylation site A_5, and its mature mRNA contains exons 1a, 2a, 6b, and 9d. Brain cells produce three different tropomyosin proteins, each of which are translated from differentially spliced pre-mRNAs that also utilize different polyadenylation sites. In addition, two forms of the brain cell tropomyosin proteins are translated from mRNAs that utilize promoter P_2, and one from an mRNA utilizing P_1. Among the four different tropomyosin proteins produced in fibroblasts, the mRNAs all use polyadenylation site A_5, but they differ in selection of P_1 versus P_2, and alternative splicing occurs as well. **Genetic Analysis 8.2** guides you through analysis of the results of alternative mRNA processing.

Self-Splicing Introns

In addition to introns that are excised by spliceosomes, certain other RNAs can contain introns that self-catalyze their own removal. Two categories of self-excising introns, designated group I introns and group II introns, have been identified. The molecular biologist Thomas Cech and his colleagues discovered group I introns in 1981, when they observed that a 413-nucleotide precursor of an rRNA gene from the protozoan *Tetrahymena* could excise itself

(a) The rat α-tropomyosin gene

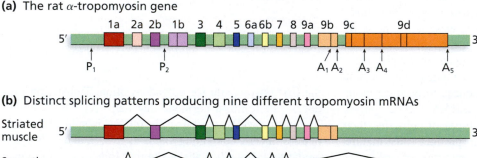

(b) Distinct splicing patterns producing nine different tropomyosin mRNAs

Striated muscle

Smooth muscle

TMBr-1, brain

TMBr-2, brain

TMBr-3, brain

TM-2, fibroblast

TM-3, fibroblast

TM-5a, fibroblast

TM-5b, fibroblast

Figure 8.25 Alternative pre-mRNA processing of the rat α-tropomyosin gene. Alternative splicing patterns are indicated by the bent lines connecting exons. Nine distinct mature mRNAs produced by different types of muscle, brain, and fibroblast cells each produce a different tropomyosin protein.

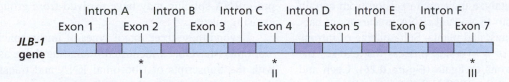

PROBLEM The *JLB-1* gene, expressed in several human organs, contains seven exons (1 to 7) and six introns (A to F). Three labeled oligonucleotide (i.e., small polynucleotide) probes (I to III), hybridizing to exons 2, 4, and 7, respectively, are indicated by asterisks below the gene map:

	Intron A	Intron B	Intron C	Intron D	Intron E	Intron F
	Exon 1	Exon 2	Exon 3	Exon 4	Exon 5	Exon 6	Exon 7

JLB-1 gene

I   II   III

Mature mRNA is isolated from three tissues expressing the *JLB-1* gene—blood, liver, and kidney—and examined by gel electrophoresis using the three oligonucleotide probes indicated above. The probes bind to complementary sequences in mRNA. Probe I and probe II bind to blood cell mRNA, but probe III does not. Probes II and III bind to liver cell mRNA, but probe I does not. And, probes I and III bind to kidney cell mRNA, but probe II does not. Use the information on these distinct probe-binding patterns to answer the following questions.

a. Thinking about pre-mRNA versus mature mRNA in these cells, explain the meaning of the different probe-hybridization patterns.

b. Identify the biological process or processes accounting for the observed patterns of probe hybridization.

> **BREAK IT DOWN:** Molecular probes bind only to their target sequences. A band appears in the gel only if the exon target of a probe is present in the mRNA (p. 17).

Solution Strategies	Solution Steps
Evaluate	
1. Identify the topic this problem addresses and the nature of the required answer.	1. This problem concerns the production of mature mRNAs from a single human gene expressed in different organs. The answer requires identification of the specific mechanisms responsible for the data obtained from each organ.
2. Identify the critical information provided in the problem.	2. The problem gives gene structure, the binding location of each of three molecular probes hybridizing the gene, and the results of three electrophoretic gel analyses of mature mRNA from different organs.
Deduce	
3. Identify the regions of *JLB-1* that are anticipated to be part of the pre-mRNA.	3. Pre-mRNA from this gene is anticipated to include all intron and exon sequences.
4. Identify the regions expected to be found in mature mRNA.	4. Some or all of the exon segments are expected in mature mRNA, along with modification at the 5′ mRNA end (capping) and the 3′ end (poly-A tailing).
Solve	Answer a
5. Interpret the hybridization pattern of molecular probes in each tissue.	5. Blood: Probes I and II hybridize, but probe III does not. This result indicates that exons 2 and 4 are present in the mature mRNA in blood, but exon 7 is not.
	Liver: Probe I fails to hybridize to mRNA from liver, indicating that exon 1 is missing from the liver mRNA. Probes II and III hybridize liver mRNA, indicating that exons 4 and 7 are included in the mature transcript.
TIP: Hybridization of a probe occurs when the probe finds its target sequence. The absence of hybridization indicates that the target sequence for a probe is not present.	Kidney: Probe II does not hybridize the kidney mRNA, indicating that exon 4 is missing from it. Probes I and III find hybridization targets, indicating that exons 2 and 7 are present in the transcript.
	Answer b
6. Interpret the hybridization patterns in each tissue and identify the process or processes that reasonably account for the observed patterns.	6. Blood: The absence of exon 7 is most likely due to either the use of an alternative polyadenylation site that generates 3′ cleavage of pre-mRNA ahead of exon 7 or to differential splicing that removes exon 7 from pre-mRNA during intron splicing.
TIP: Alternative promoters, alternative polyadenylation sites, and alternative splicing are three mechanisms that lead eukaryotic genomes to generate distinct proteins from the same gene.	Liver: The absence of exon 2 is most likely due either to use of an alternative promoter that initiates transcription at a point past exon 2 or to differential splicing of liver pre-mRNA.
	Kidney: The absence of exon 4 is most likely the result of differential splicing of pre-mRNA.

For more practice, see Problems 2, 3, and 8.

Visit the Study Area to access study tools.   **Mastering Genetics**

without the presence of any protein. Following up on this initial observation, Cech and others have shown that group I introns are large, self-splicing ribozymes (catalytically active RNAs) that catalyze their own excision from certain mRNAs and also from tRNA and rRNA precursors in bacteria, simple eukaryotes, and plants. Self-splicing of introns takes place by way of a two-step process that excises the intron and allows exons to ligate (**Figure 8.26**), Cech and Sidney Altman shared the 1989 Nobel Prize in Physiology or Medicine for their contributions to the discovery and description of the catalytic properties of RNA.

Group II introns, which are also self-splicing ribozymes, are found in transcripts of archaea and bacteria, and in the transcripts of genes in the eukaryotic organelles mitochondria and chloroplasts. Group II introns form highly complex secondary structures containing many

① Exon–intron base pairing. The G-binding site nucleotide attacks the UpA bond, bonding to the adenine and cleaving exon A.

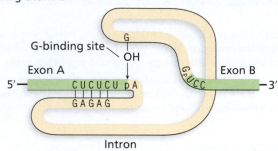

② The 3' end of exon A attacks the G$_p$U bond at the intron–exon junction.

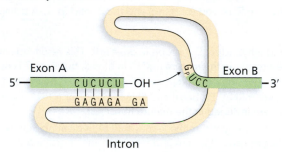

③ The intron is released, and exons ligate.

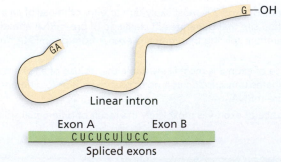

Figure 8.26 Self-splicing of group I introns.

stem-loop arrangements. Their self-excision takes place in a lariat-like manner utilizing a branch point nucleotide that in many cases is adenine. It is thought that nuclear pre-mRNA splicing may have evolved from group II self-excising introns.

Beyond these three major types of intron splicing, several others have been identified, including those associated with the transcripts of ribosomal RNA and transfer RNA that are processed to produce the nucleic acids that function in translation.

Ribosomal RNA Processing

In bacteria, archaea, and eukaryotes, rRNAs are transcribed as large precursor molecules that are cleaved into smaller RNA molecules by removal and discarding of spacer sequences intervening between the sequences of the different RNAs. The *E. coli* genome, for example, contains seven copies of an rRNA gene. Each gene copy is transcribed into a single 30S precursor RNA that is processed by the removal of intervening sequences to yield 5S, 16S, and 23S rRNAs, along with several tRNA molecules (**Figure 8.27a**; RNA molecules and subunits are described in Svedberg units, abbreviated S, which give an idea of their size). All seven gene copies produce the same three rRNAs, but each gene generates a different set of tRNAs. There is evidence that archaea use a similar process to produce some rRNA molecules.

Eukaryotic genomes have hundreds of rRNA genes clustered in regions of repeated genes on various chromosomes. Each gene produces a 45S precursor rRNA that contains an external transcription sequence (ETS) and two internal transcription sequences (ITS1 and ITS2) that are removed by processing. The transcript is processed in multiple steps to yield three rRNA molecules weighing 5.8S, 18S, and 28S (**Figure 8.27b**). Eukaryotic genomes differ somewhat in the steps that process the 45S pre-rRNA transcript. In general, however, the 45S transcript is cleaved to a 41S intermediate from which the 18S transcript is then removed, followed by cleavage that produces the 28S and 5.8S transcripts. The 5.8S and 28S products pair with one another and become part of the same ribosomal subunit. Eukaryotic rRNA processing takes place in the nucleolus, where ribosome assembly also occurs. After processing, the resulting rRNAs fold into complex secondary structures and are joined by proteins to form ribosomal subunits. Some chemical modifications of rRNA, particularly methylation of selected nucleotide bases, occur after completion of transcription.

Transfer RNA Processing

The production of tRNA, whether in bacteria, archaea, or eukaryotes, also requires posttranscriptional processing. Each type of tRNA has distinctive nucleotides and

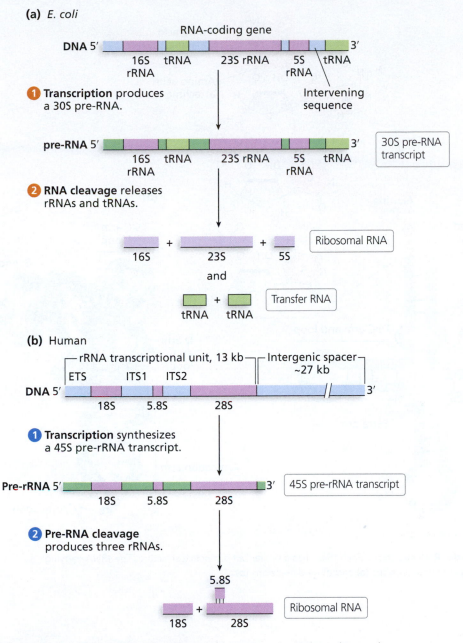

Figure 8.27 The processing of ribosomal and transfer RNA. (a) A large transcript is cleaved to produce rRNA and tRNA in *E. coli*. **(b)** Human rRNA genes are part of 40-kb repeating sequences that each produce three rRNAs.

a specific pattern of folding, but all tRNAs have similar structures and functions (**Figure 8.28**). Some bacterial transfer RNA molecules are produced simultaneously with rRNAs, as described above (see Figure 8.27a). Other tRNAs are transcribed as part of a large pre-tRNA transcript that is then cleaved to yield multiple tRNA molecules. In eukaryotes, tRNA genes occur in clusters on specific chromosomes. Each eukaryotic tRNA gene is individually transcribed by RNA polymerase III, and a single pre-tRNA is produced from each gene.

The number of different tRNAs produced depends on the type of organism. In bacteria, the exact number of

different tRNAs varies, but it is usually substantially *less than* 61, the number of codons found in mRNA. At a minimum, each species must have at least 20 different tRNAs, one for each amino acid, but most produce at least 30 to 40 different tRNAs. The low number of different tRNAs (compared with the number of codons) results from a phenomenon called *third-base wobble*, a relaxation of the "rules" of complementary base pairing at the third base of codons (see Section 9.4). Although third-base wobble plays a role in reducing the number of distinct tRNA genes needed in eukaryotic genomes, eukaryotes nevertheless produce a larger number of different tRNAs than bacteria do. Some

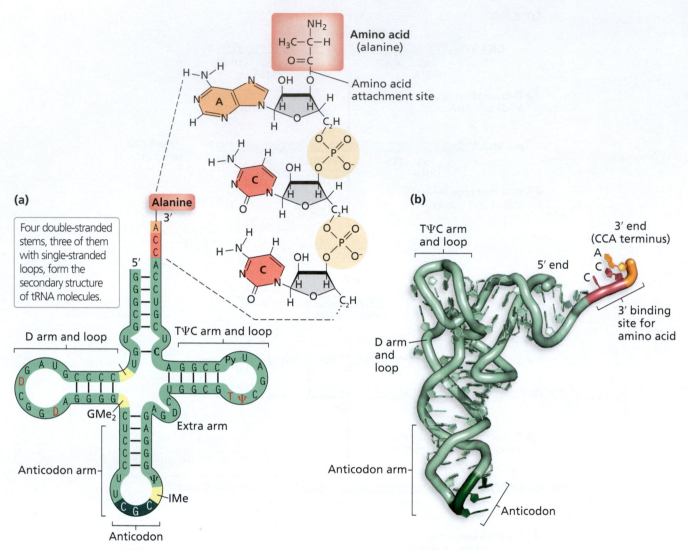

(a)

Four double-stranded stems, three of them with single-stranded loops, form the secondary structure of tRNA molecules.

D arm and loop

TΨC arm and loop

Extra arm

Anticodon arm

Anticodon

(b)

TΨC arm and loop

3' end (CCA terminus)

5' end

3' binding site for amino acid

D arm and loop

Anticodon arm

Anticodon

Amino acid (alanine)

Amino acid attachment site

Alanine

Figure 8.28 Transfer RNA structure. Each tRNA has a similar but distinctive structure. The tRNA carrying alanine is illustrated in two dimensions **(a)** and three dimensions **(b)**.

eukaryotic genomes contain a full complement of 61 different tRNA genes, one corresponding to each codon of the genetic code.

Bacterial tRNAs require processing before they are ready to assume their functional role of transporting amino acids to the ribosome. The precise processing events differ somewhat among tRNAs, but several features are common. First, many tRNAs are cleaved from large precursor tRNA transcripts to produce several individual tRNA molecules. Second, nucleotides are trimmed off the 5′ and 3′ ends of tRNA transcripts to prepare the mature molecule. Third, certain individual nucleotides in different tRNAs are chemically modified to produce a distinctive molecule. Fourth, tRNAs fold into a precise three-dimensional structure that includes

four double-stranded stems, three of which are capped by single-stranded loops; each stem and loop constitutes an "arm" of the tRNA molecule. Fifth, tRNAs undergo post-transcriptional addition of bases. The most common addition is three nucleotides, CCA, at the 3′ end of the molecule. This region is the binding site for the amino acid the tRNA molecule transports to the ribosome. Figure 8.28 shows tRNA^{Ala}, which carries alanine. The CCA terminus is indicated, along with chemically modified nucleotides in each arm that are characteristic of this tRNA. Both a two-dimensional and a three-dimensional representation are shown.

Eukaryotic and archaeal tRNAs undergo processing modifications similar to those of bacterial tRNAs. In addition, however, eukaryotic pre-tRNAs may contain small introns that are removed during processing. For example, an intron 14 nucleotides in length is removed from the precursor molecule by a specialized nuclease enzyme that cleaves the 5′ and 3′ splice sites of tRNA introns. The cleaved tRNA then folds into its functional form.

RNA Editing

A firmly established tenet in the central dogma of biology is the role of DNA as the repository and purveyor of genetic information. Notwithstanding the modifications made to precursor RNA transcripts after transcription, a fundamental principle of biology is that DNA dictates the sequence of mRNA nucleotides and controls the order of amino acids in proteins. And yet, in the mid-1980s, a phenomenon called **RNA editing** was uncovered that is responsible for post-transcriptional substitutions of some of the nucleotides of an mRNA.

The mRNAs from some nuclear genes in eukaryotes, some plant mitochondrial genes, and some mitochondrial genes of trypanosomes are edited by a specialized RNA called **guide RNA (gRNA)**. A portion of a guide RNA contains a sequence complementary to the region of mRNA that it edits. With the aid of a protein complex, a portion of guide RNA pairs with complementary nucleotides of pre-edited mRNA and acts as a template to direct the insertion (and occasionally the deletion) of uracil (**Figure 8.29**). Guide RNA releases edited mRNA after editing is complete. The protein translated from edited mRNA may differ from the protein produced from unedited transcript.

RNA editing is responsible for producing two different apolipoprotein B proteins from a single gene in human liver and intestinal cells. The same mRNA transcript is initially produced in both types of cells. In liver cells, the mRNA is used to produce an apolipoprotein B protein containing 4563 amino acids. RNA editing substitutes one nucleotide

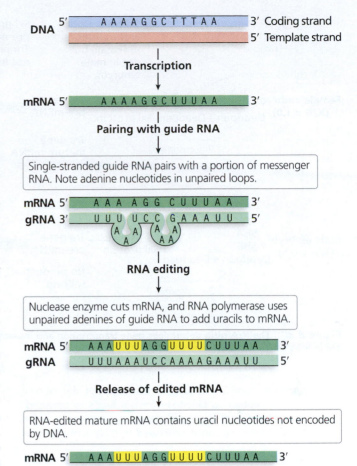

Figure 8.29   Guide RNA (gRNA) directs RNA editing.

of the mRNA in intestinal cells, and this produces a stop codon part way through the mRNA that stops translation early and results in an apolipoprotein B that is 2152 amino acids in length. These two proteins function differently in their respective cell types.

CASE STUDY

Sexy Splicing: Alternative mRNA Splicing and Sex Determination in Drosophila

What causes pre-mRNA to be edited in one way in one type of cell and in another way in a different type of cell? The answer has to do with differential gene expression in cells, leading to the presence or absence of specific proteins that determine which pattern of pre-mRNA splicing will take place in a given nucleus. A well-characterized example of the molecular basis of this kind of differential pre-mRNA splicing is provided by a part of the mechanism that determines female versus male sex in the fruit fly *Drosophila melanogaster.*

In Section 3.4 we described the X/autosome ratio (X/A ratio) that causes fruit fly embryos with one X chromosome to develop as males and those with two X chromosomes to develop as females. The molecular explanation of why this ratio causes *Drosophila* sex determination is much

deeper than simply the number of X chromosomes present and depends on a series of steps that begins with the transcription activation of the *sex-lethal* (*Sxl*) gene. The process includes alternative splicing of the pre-mRNA transcript of a second gene, the *transformer (Tra)* gene and to additional differential gene expression that directs sex development.

The X/A ratio in fly embryos initially influences the level of transcription and translation of two X-linked activator proteins called SisA and SisB compared with that of an autosomal gene producing a transcription repressor protein called Deadpan (**Figure 8.30**). Since the genes producing SisA and SisB are X-linked, early female embryos produce twice as much of each activator as do early male embryos, and the ratio of SisA + SisB to Deadpan differs between female

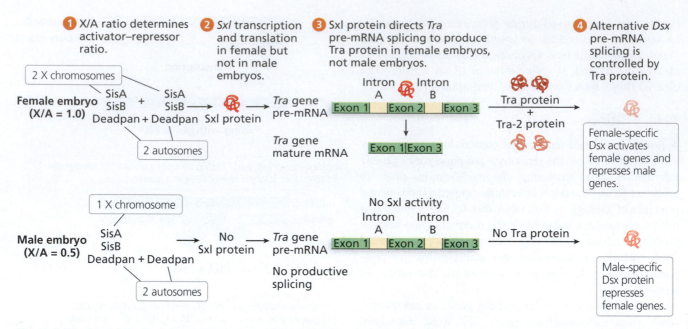

Figure 8.30 The X/A ratio determines gene transcription and transcript splicing pattern to determine sex in fruit flies.

and male embryos ❶. In early female embryos, the ratio of SisA + SisB protein to Deadpan protein leads to transcription of the *Sex lethal (Sxl)* gene and to the production of Sxl protein. *Sxl* transcription is repressed in male embryos and no Sxl protein is produced ❷.

Sxl protein is a pre-mRNA splicing regulator protein that operates on the pre-mRNA transcript of the *Transformer (Tra)* gene. In female embryos, *Tra* pre-mRNA is spliced to produce a functional Tra protein ❸. In male embryos, the absence of Sxl protein leads to alternative *Tra* pre-mRNA splicing that does not produce functional Tra protein. The Tra protein is also a splicing regulator; it operates on the

pre-mRNA of *Double sex (Dsx)* gene along with a second protein known as Tra-2 ❹. In female embryos, Tra protein and Tra-2 protein splice *Dsx* pre-mRNA in one alternative variant, which when translated produces female-specific Dsx protein. Female-specific Dsx activates transcription of female-specific genes and represses transcription of male-specific genes to produce female flies. Tra protein is absent in male embryos, and *Dsx* pre-mRNA is spliced in the other alternative variant. Dsx protein in male embryos represses female-specific genes and allows transcription of unrepressed male-specific genes, leading to male sex development.

SUMMARY   Mastering Genetics   For activities, animations, and review quizzes, go to the Study Area.

8.1 RNA Transcripts Carry the Messages of Genes

▌ RNA molecules are synthesized by RNA polymerases using as building blocks the RNA nucleotides A, G, C, and U to form single-stranded sequences complementary to DNA template strands.

▌ Messenger RNA is the transcript that undergoes translation to produce proteins. The many other forms of RNA are also transcribed, and may undergo modification, but are not translated.

8.2 Bacterial Transcription Is a Four-Stage Process

▌ Transcription has four stages: promoter recognition, chain initiation, chain elongation, and chain termination.

▌ A single RNA polymerase transcribes all bacterial genes. This polymerase is a holoenzyme composed of a

five-subunit core enzyme and a sigma subunit that aids the recognition of different forms of bacterial promoters.

▌ Bacterial promoters have two consensus sequence regions located upstream of the transcription start at approximately −10 and −35.

▌ The core enzyme of bacterial RNA polymerase carries out RNA synthesis following chain initiation by the holoenzyme.

▌ Transcription of most bacterial genes terminates by an intrinsic mechanism that depends only on DNA terminator sequences. Certain bacterial genes have a rho-dependent mechanism of transcription termination.

8.3 Eukaryotic Transcription Is More Diversified and Complex than Bacterial Transcription

▌ Eukaryotic cells contain three types of RNA polymerases that transcribe mRNA and the various other classes of RNA.

■ RNA polymerase II transcribes mRNA by interaction with numerous transcription factors that lead the enzyme to recognize promoters controlling transcription of polypeptide-coding genes.

■ Promoters recognized by RNA polymerase II have a TATA box and additional regulatory elements that bind transcription factors and RNA pol II during transcription initiation.

■ Tissue-specific and developmental modifications in transcription are regulated by enhancer and silencer sequences.

■ RNA polymerase I uses exclusive transcription factors to recognize upstream consensus sequences of ribosomal RNA genes. Ribosomal RNAs are processed in the nucleolus.

■ RNA polymerase III recognizes promoter consensus sequences that are upstream and downstream of the start of transcription for tRNA genes.

■ Archaeal transcription is a simplified version of eukaryotic transcription and has less in common with bacterial transcription.

■ Comparative studies of transcription reveal that the three domains of life share common transcriptional mechanisms that are attributable to their sharing of a common ancestor.

8.4 Posttranscriptional Processing Modifies RNA Molecules

■ 5′ capping of eukaryotic messenger RNA adds a methylated guanine through the action of guanylyl transferase shortly after transcription is initiated.

■ Polyadenylation at the 3′ end of eukaryotic messenger RNA is signaled by an AAUAAA sequence and is accomplished by a complex of enzymes.

■ RNA splicing is controlled by cellular proteins that identify introns and exons and form spliceosome complexes that remove introns and ligate exons.

■ Consensus sequences at the 5′ splice site, the 3′ splice site, and the branch point serve as guides during RNA splicing.

■ Alternative splicing is regulated by cell-type–specific variation of proteins that identify introns and exons.

■ Some RNA molecules have catalytic activity and are able to self-splice introns without the aid of proteins.

■ Ribosomal and transfer RNA molecules are generated by cleavage of large precursor molecules transcribed in bacterial, archaeal, and eukaryotic genomes.

■ RNA editing is a post-transcriptional altering of nucleotide sequence, causing the transcripts to differ from the corresponding template DNA sequence.

PREPARING FOR PROBLEM SOLVING

In addition to the list of problem-solving tips and suggestions given here, you can go to the Study Guide and Solutions Manual that accompanies this book for help at solving problems.

1. Understand the structure of bacterial and eukaryotic promoters; be familiar with the structure of genes and the relative positions of their landmarks (promoter, start of transcription, etc.); and be able to identify the template and nontemplate strands of a gene.

2. Be prepared to describe the mechanisms of bacterial and eukaryotic gene transcription initiation, including the complementary and 5′ and 3′ relationships between the nucleic acid strands.

3. Understand the two mechanisms of transcription termination in bacteria, and the connection between transcription termination of eukaryotic genes and posttranscriptional processing.

4. Be prepared to describe the posttranscriptional processing events that modify eukaryotic pre-mRNA.

5. Understand the experimental approaches that can identify promoters and their functional sequences.

6. Be prepared to interpret the results of experiments analyzing DNA binding of transcriptional proteins or the transcription of genes.

PROBLEMS

Mastering Genetics Visit for instructor-assigned tutorials and problems.

Chapter Concepts

For answers to selected even-numbered problems, see Appendix: Answers.

1. Based on discussion in this chapter,
   a. What is a gene?
   b. Why are genes for rRNA and tRNA considered to be genes even though they do not produce polypeptides?

2. In one to two sentences each, describe the three processes that commonly modify eukaryotic pre-mRNA.

3. Answer these questions concerning promoters.
   a. What role do promoters play in transcription?
   b. What is the common structure of a bacterial promoter with respect to consensus sequences?
   c. What consensus sequences are detected in the mammalian β-globin gene promoter?

d. Eukaryotic promoters are more variable than bacterial promoters. Explain why.

e. What is the meaning of the term *alternative promoter*? How does the use of alternative promoters affect transcription?

4. The diagram below shows a DNA duplex. The template strand is identified, as is the location of the +1 nucleotide.

```
     +1
5' ___|_____ 3' template strand

3' _____ 5' coding strand
```

a. Assume this region contains a gene transcribed in a bacterium. Identify the location of promoter consensus sequences and of the transcription termination sequence.

b. Assume this region contains a gene transcribed to form mRNA in a eukaryote. Identify the location of the most common promoter consensus sequences.

c. If this region is a eukaryotic gene transcribed by RNA polymerase III, where are the promoter consensus sequences located?

5. The following is a portion of an mRNA sequence:

$$3'-\text{AUCGUCAUGCAGA}-5'$$

a. During transcription, was the adenine at the left-hand side of the sequence the first or the last nucleotide used to build the portion of mRNA shown? Explain how you know.

b. Write out the sequence and polarity of the DNA duplex that encodes this mRNA segment. Label the template and coding DNA strands.

c. Identify the direction in which the promoter region for this gene will be located.

6. Compare and contrast the properties of DNA polymerase and RNA polymerase, listing at least three similarities and at least three differences between the molecules.

7. The DNA sequences shown below are from the promoter regions of six bacterial genes. In each case, the last nucleotide in the sequence (highlighted in blue) is the +1 nucleotide that initiates transcription.

a. Examine these sequences and identify the Pribnow box sequence at approximately −10 for each promoter.

b. Determine the consensus sequence for the Pribnow box from these sequences.

Gene 1   ...   TTCCGGCTCGTATGTTGTGTGG A ...

Gene 2   ...   CGTCATTTGATATGATGCGCCCC G ...

Gene 3   ...   CCACTGGCGGTGATACTGAGCAC A ...

Gene 4   ...   TTTATTGCAGCTTATAATGGTTAC A ...

Gene 5   ...   TGCTTCTGACTATAATAGACAGG G ...

Gene 6   ...   AAGTAAACACGGTACGATGTACCAC A ...

8. Bacterial and eukaryotic gene transcripts can differ—in the transcripts themselves, in whether the transcripts are modified before translation, and in how the transcripts are modified. For each of these three areas of contrast, describe what the differences are and why the differences exist.

9. Describe the two types of transcription termination found in bacterial genes. How does transcription termination differ for eukaryotic genes?

10. What is the role of enhancer sequences in transcription of eukaryotic genes? Speculate about why enhancers are not part of transcription of bacterial genes.

11. Describe the difference between introns and exons.

12. Draw a bacterial promoter and label its consensus sequences. How does this promoter differ from a eukaryotic promoter transcribed by RNA polymerase II? By RNA polymerase I? By RNA polymerase III?

13. For a eukaryotic gene whose transcription requires the activity of an enhancer sequence, explain how proteins bound at the enhancer interact with RNA pol II and transcription factors bound at the promoter.

14. Three genes identified in the diagram as *A*, *B*, and *C* are transcribed from a region of DNA. The 5'-to-3' transcription of genes *A* and *C* elongates mRNA in the right-to-left direction, and transcription of gene *B* elongates mRNA in the left-to-right direction. For each gene, identify the coding strand by designating it as an "upper strand" or "lower strand" in the diagram.

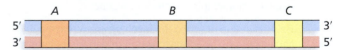

Application and Integration

For answers to selected even-numbered problems, see Appendix: Answers.

15. The eukaryotic gene *Gen-100* contains four introns labeled A to D. Imagine that *Gen-100* has been isolated and its DNA has been denatured and mixed with polyadenylated mRNA from the gene.

a. Illustrate the R-loop structure that would be seen with electron microscopy.

b. Label the introns.

c. Are intron regions single stranded or double stranded? Why?

16. The segment of the bacterial *TrpA* gene involved in intrinsic termination of transcription is the following:

$$3'-\text{TGGGTCGGGGCGGATTACTGCCCCGAAAAAAAAACTTG}-5'$$
$$5'-\text{ACCCAGCCCCGCCTAATGACGGGGCTTTTTTTTTGAAC}-3'$$

a. Draw the mRNA structure that forms during transcription of this segment of the *TrpA* gene.

b. Label the template and coding DNA strands.

c. Explain how a sequence of this type leads to intrinsic termination of transcription.

17. A 2-kb fragment of *E. coli* DNA contains the complete sequence of a gene for which transcription is terminated by the rho protein. The fragment contains the complete promoter sequence as well as the terminator region of

the gene. The cloned fragment is examined by band shift assay (see Research Technique 8.1). Each lane of a single electrophoresis gel contains the 2-kb cloned fragment under the following conditions:

Lane 1: 2-kb fragment alone
Lane 2: 2-kb fragment plus the core enzyme
Lane 3: 2-kb fragment plus the RNA polymerase holoenzyme
Lane 4: 2-kb fragment plus rho protein

a. Diagram the relative positions expected for the DNA fragments in this gel electrophoresis analysis.
b. Explain the relative positions of bands in lanes 1 and 3.
c. Explain the relative positions of bands in lanes 1 and 4.

18. A 3.5-kb segment of DNA containing the complete sequence of a mouse gene is available. The DNA segment contains the promoter sequence and extends beyond the polyadenylation site of the gene. The DNA is studied by band shift assay (see Research Technique 8.1), and the following gel bands are observed.

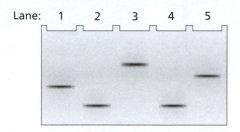

Match these conditions to a specific lane of the gel.

a. 3.5-kb fragment plus TFIIB and TFIID
b. 3.5-kb fragment plus TFIIB, TFIID, TFIIF, and RNA polymerase II
c. 3.5-kb fragment alone
d. 3.5-kb fragment plus RNA polymerase II
e. 3.5-kb fragment plus TFIIB

19. A 1.0-kb DNA fragment from the 5′ end of the mouse gene described in the previous problem is examined by DNA footprint protection analysis (see Research Technique 8.1). Two samples are end-labeled with ^{32}P, and

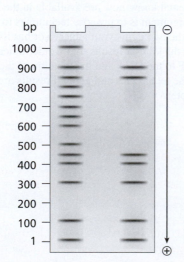

one of the two is mixed with TFIIB, TFIID, and RNA polymerase II. The DNA exposed to these proteins is run in the right-hand lane of the gel shown below and the control DNA is run in the left-hand. Both DNA samples are treated with DNase I before running the samples on the electrophoresis gel.

a. What length of DNA is bound by the transcriptional proteins? Explain how the gel results support this interpretation.
b. Draw a diagram of this DNA fragment bound by the transcriptional proteins, showing the approximate position of proteins along the fragment. Use the illustration style seen in Research Technique 8.1 as a model.
c. Explain the role of DNase I.

20. Wild-type *E. coli* grow best at 37°C but can grow efficiently up to 42°C. An *E. coli* strain has a mutation of the sigma subunit that results in an RNA polymerase holoenzyme that is stable and transcribes at wild-type levels at 37°C. The mutant holoenzyme is progressively destabilized as the temperature is raised, and it completely denatures and ceases to carry out transcription at 42°C. Relative to wild-type growth, characterize the ability of the mutant strain to carry out transcription at

a. 37°C
b. 40°C
c. 42°C
d. What term best characterizes the type of mutation exhibited by the mutant bacterial strain? (*Hint*: The term was used in Chapter 4 to describe the Himalayan allele of the mammalian *C* gene.)

21. A mutant strain of *Salmonella* bacteria carries a mutation of the rho protein that has full activity at 37°C but is completely inactivated when the mutant strain is grown at 40°C.

a. Speculate about the kind of differences you would expect to see if you compared a broad spectrum of mRNAs from the mutant strain grown at 37°C and the same spectrum of mRNAs from the strain when grown at 40°C.
b. Are all mRNAs affected by the rho protein mutation in the same way? Why or why not?

22. The human β-globin wild-type allele and a certain mutant allele are identical in sequence except for a single base-pair substitution that changes one nucleotide at the end of intron 2. The wild-type and mutant sequences of the affected portion of pre-mRNA are

	Intron 2	Exon 3
wild type	5′–CCUCCCACAG	CUCCUG–3′
mutant	5′–CCUCCCACUG	CUCCUG–3′

a. Speculate about the way in which this base substitution causes mutation of β-globin protein.
b. This is one example of how DNA sequence change occurring somewhere other than in an exon can produce mutation. List other kinds of DNA sequence changes occurring outside exons that can produce mutation. In each case, characterize the kind of change you would expect to see in mutant mRNA or mutant protein.

23. Microbiologists describe the processes of transcription and translation as "coupled" in bacteria. This term indicates that a bacterial mRNA can be undergoing transcription at the same moment it is also undergoing translation.

    a. How is coupling of transcription and translation possible in bacteria?
    b. Is coupling of transcription and translation possible in single-celled eukaryotes such as yeast? Why or why not?

24. A full-length eukaryotic gene is inserted into a bacterial chromosome. The gene contains a complete promoter sequence and a functional polyadenylation sequence, and it has wild-type nucleotides throughout the transcribed region. However, the gene fails to produce a functional protein.

    a. List at least three possible reasons why this eukaryotic gene is not expressed in bacteria.
    b. What changes would you recommend to permit expression of this eukaryotic gene in a bacterial cell?

25. The accompanying illustration shows a portion of a gene undergoing transcription. The template and coding strands for the gene are labeled, and a segment of DNA sequence is given. For this gene segment:

    a. Superimpose a drawing of RNA polymerase as it nears the end of transcription of the DNA sequence.
    b. Indicate the direction in which RNA polymerase moves as it transcribes this gene.
    c. Write the polarity and sequence of the RNA transcript from the DNA sequence given.
    d. Identify the direction in which the promoter for this gene is located.

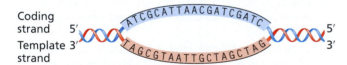

26. DNA footprint protection (described in Research Technique 8.1) is a method that determines whether proteins bind to a specific sample of DNA and thus protect part of the DNA from random enzymatic cleavage by DNase I. A 400-bp segment of cloned DNA is thought to contain a promoter. The cloned DNA is analyzed by DNA footprinting to help determine if it has the capacity to act as a promoter sequence. The accompanying gel has two lanes, each containing the cloned 400-bp DNA fragment treated with DNase I to randomly cleave unprotected DNA. Lane 1 is cloned DNA that was mixed with RNA polymerase II and several TFII transcription factors before exposure to

DNase I. Lane 2 contains cloned DNA that was exposed only to DNase I. RNA pol II and TFIIs were not mixed with that DNA before adding DNase I.

a. Explain why this gel provides evidence that the cloned DNA may act as a promoter sequence.
b. Approximately what length is the DNA region protected by RNA pol II and TFIIs?
c. What additional genetic experiments would you suggest to verify that this region of cloned DNA contains a functional promoter?

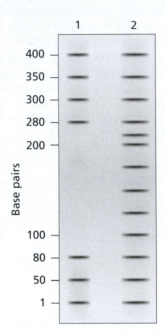

27. Suppose you have a 1-kb segment of cloned DNA that is suspected to contain a eukaryotic promoter including a TATA box, a CAAT box, and an upstream GC-rich sequence. The clone also contains a gene whose transcript is readily detectable. Your laboratory supervisor asks you to outline an experiment that will (1) determine if eukaryotic transcription factors (TF) bind to the fragment and, if so, (2) identify where on the fragment the transcription factors bind. All necessary reagents, equipment, and experimental know-how are available in the laboratory. Your assignment is to propose techniques to be used to address the two items your supervisor has listed and to describe the kind of results that would indicate binding of TF to the DNA and the location of the binding. (*Hint*: The techniques and general results are discussed in this chapter.)

Collaboration and Discussion

For answers to selected even-numbered problems, see Appendix: Answers.

28. Assume that a mutation affects the gene for each of the following eukaryotic RNA polymerases. Match each mutation with the possible effects from the list provided. More than one effect is possible for each mutation.

RNA Polymerase Mutation	Effect(s)
RNA pol I	_____
RNA pol II	_____
RNA pol III	_____
snRNA	_____

Possible Effects

a. Pre-mRNA does not have introns removed.
b. Some pre-mRNA is not synthesized.
c. Some rRNA is not synthesized.
d. Some tRNA is not synthesized.
e. Ribosomal RNA is not processed.

29. The DNA sequence below gives the first 12 base pairs of the transcribed region of a gene, and the template and nontemplate strands of DNA are identified. The transcription start is the thymine nucleotide at the end of the sequence given. Use the diagram to answer the list of questions. Make a copy of the diagram before you begin answering the questions, or have one group member diagram the answers for bacteria and another group member diagram the answers for eukaryotes.

Nontemplate strand _____ TTGCTACGGTCA _____

Template strand _____ AACGATGCCAGT _____

a. Write the polarity of the two DNA strands shown.
b. Give the mRNA transcript sequence and the polarity of the transcript.
c. Assuming the sequence shown is part of a bacterial gene, draw the approximate positions of the promoter sequence and the termination sequence.
d. Assuming the sequence shown is part of a bacterial gene, what consensus sequence(s) would you expect to identify in the promoter?
e. Write the anticipated bacterial consensus sequence(s) in the approximate position(s) on the diagram.
f. Assuming the sequence shown is part of a eukaryotic gene, what consensus sequence(s) would you expect to identify within about 100 base pairs of the start of transcription?
g. Write the anticipated eukaryotic consensus sequence(s) in the approximate position(s) on the diagram.

30. Genomic DNA from a mouse is isolated, fragmented, and denatured into single strands. It is then mixed with mRNA isolated from the cytoplasm of mouse cells. The image represents an electron micrograph result showing the hybridization of single-stranded DNA and mRNA.

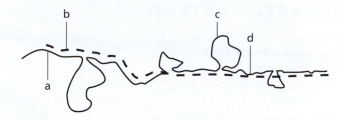

a. Which nucleic acid is indicated by the "a" pointer? Justify your answer.
b. Which nucleic acid is indicated by the "b" pointer? Justify your answer.
c. What term best identifies the nucleic acid region indicated by the "c" pointer?
d. What term best identifies the nucleic acid region indicated by the "d" pointer?
e. Based on this electron micrograph image, how many introns and exons are present in the mouse DNA fragment shown?

31. A portion of a human gene is isolated from the genome and sequenced. The corresponding segment of mRNA is isolated from the cytoplasm of human cells, and it is also sequenced. The nucleic acid strings shown here are from genomic coding strand DNA and the corresponding mRNA.

mRNA	5′ ACGCAUUACGUGGCUAGACAUUUAGC-CGAUCAGACUAGACAGCGCGCUAGCG-AUAGCGCUAAAGCUGACUCGCGAUCAGUCUC-GAGGGCACAUAGUCUA 3′
Genomic Coding Strand DNA	5′ ACGCATTACGTGGCTAGACATTTAGC-CGATCAGACTAGACAGCGCGCTAGCGAGTC-TACCTCAAGCCAUAATAGACAGTAGA-CATTGAAAGACATAGATAGACATAGAGA-CTTAGACATACGACCGGACATACCAAGAC-GAATACGAACACTATACAGCCUCAGTAGCGC-TAAAGCTGACTCGCGATCAGTCTCGAGGGCA-CATAGTCTA 3′

a. There is one intron in the DNA sequence shown. Locate the intron and underline the splice site sequences.
b. Does this intron contain normal splice site sequences?

9

The Molecular Biology of Translation

CHAPTER OUTLINE

9.1 Polypeptides Are Amino Acid Chains That Are Assembled at Ribosomes

9.2 Translation Occurs in Three Phases

9.3 Translation Is Fast and Efficient

9.4 The Genetic Code Translates Messenger RNA into Polypeptide

9.5 Experiments Deciphered the Genetic Code

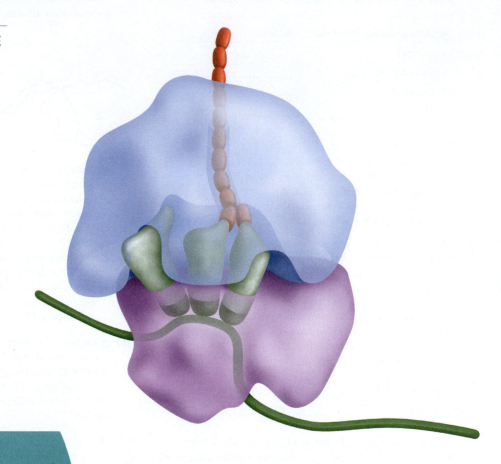

Ribosomes use codon sequences of messenger RNA to direct the assembly of polypeptides during translation. This rendering of a ribosome engaged in translation shows the large subunit (top), the small subunit (bottom), the path of mRNA through the small subunit, the spaces for E, P, and A sites into which tRNAs fit, and the egress of the polypeptide through the large subunit.

ESSENTIAL IDEAS

▪ Translation is the cellular process of polypeptide production carried out by ribosomes under the direction of mRNA.

▪ Ribosomes assemble on mRNA and initiate translation at the start codon.

▪ Transfer RNA molecules carry amino acids to ribosomes, which assemble polypeptides with the aid of ribosomal proteins.

▪ Polypeptide elongation and termination are similar in bacteria and eukaryotes.

▪ A virtually universal genetic code comprising 64 mRNA codons directs polypeptide assembly.

▪ Polypeptides undergo posttranslational folding and processing, and in eukaryotes are sorted into vesicles for transport to cellular destinations or for secretion.

Long before the discovery that DNA is the hereditary molecule, biologists had established the relationship between genes and proteins. In 1902, Archibald Garrod was the first to explicitly draw this connection when he proposed that the human hereditary disorder alkaptonuria was caused by an inherited defect in the enzyme homogentisic acid oxidase (see Section 4.3 and Figure 4.17b). As Garrod and other biologists expanded their exploration of the gene–protein connection, they found evidence that hereditary variation was closely tied to variations in proteins. Principal among the biologists who developed this connection were George Beadle and Edward Tatum, whose research established the "one gene—one enzyme" hypothesis (see Experimental Insight 4.1, pp. 125–126).

This chapter discusses translation, the mechanism by which the messenger RNA (mRNA) transcripts of genes are used to assemble amino acids into polypeptides (strings of amino acids) that form proteins. Translation is carried out by ribosomes that bring together mRNA transcripts and transfer RNA (tRNA) molecules carrying amino acids to facilitate the assembly of polypeptides. Polypeptides make up enzymes, structural proteins, transport proteins, signaling proteins, hormones, and other components that are assembled into cell structures or perform biological activities in or among cells.

The story of how polypeptides are produced by translation and of how scientists came to understand the process offers intriguing insight into the design of molecular genetic experiments. In this chapter, we describe some of these experiments and examine the molecular biology of translation. We also look at the homology of proteins that are active in translation in organisms from the three domains of life and describe how this and other features of translation are evidence of a single origin of life and of the evolutionary relationships between bacteria, archaea, and eukaryotes.

9.1 Polypeptides Are Amino Acid Chains That Are Assembled at Ribosomes

Twenty different amino acids are the basic building blocks of polypeptides. All amino acids have features in common and features that are distinct. The distinctive features impart specific characteristics that allow the amino acid to participate in certain chemical reactions or behave in a hydrophilic or hydrophobic manner. In part, the common features allow amino acids to be joined into polypeptides by covalent bond formation between adjacent amino acids in the chain.

Amino Acid Structure

The shared features of amino acids are a central carbon molecule known as the α-carbon, an amino (NH_3^+) group, and a carboxyl (COO^-) group (Figure 9.1). Each amino and carboxyl group is joined to the α-carbon. During polypeptide assembly, an enzyme in the ribosome catalyzes the formation of a **peptide bond** between the carboxyl group of one amino acid and the amino group of the next amino acid in the chain. Each amino acid added in this way becomes a new monomer in the growing polymer that is the elongating polypeptide. The term **polypeptide** signifies a string of amino acids that are joined by peptide bonds. Each *protein* has a unique sequence of amino acids, may be composed of one or more polypeptide chains, and generally has its own characteristic three-dimensional structure.

The distinctive portion of each amino acid is its side chain, known as an **R-group**, that is also joined to the α-carbon. The R-groups range in complexity from a single hydrogen atom to ringed structures that in themselves contain multiple carbon atoms. Each R-group imparts specific characteristics as shown in Table 9.1. Ten of the amino acids have nonpolar R-groups, meaning they have no charged atoms that can participate in formation of hydrogen bonds with other amino acids. Five other amino acids have polar R-groups that can carry partial charges and can participate in hydrogen bond formation with other amino acids. The five remaining amino acids have electrically charged R-groups: Three are basic and two are acidic. Electrically charged R-groups allow these amino acids to form ionic bonds and hydrogen bonds.

Polypeptide and Transcript Structure

Polypeptide assembly is orchestrated by ribosomes, which are ribonucleoprotein "machines" containing multiple molecules of ribosomal RNA (rRNA) and dozens of proteins.

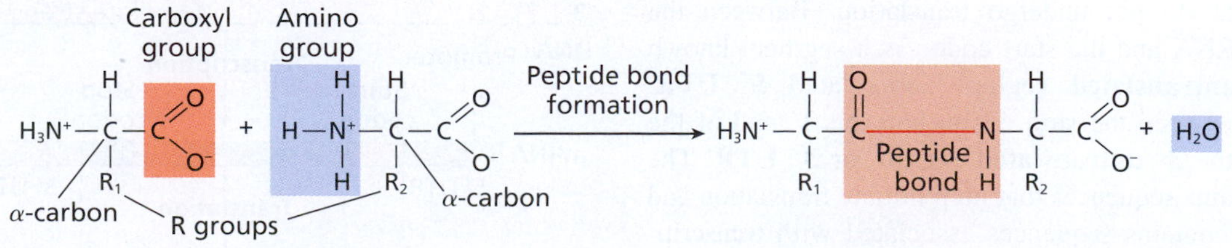

Figure 9.1 Amino acids and peptide bond formation. The carboxyl group (COO^-) of one amino acid reacts with the amino group (^+H_3N) of the adjacent amino acid to form a covalent peptide bond that links amino acids in a polypeptide chain. Amino acids contain a central carbon (the α-carbon) and an R-group, here identified as R1 and R2.

Table 9.1	Amino Acids Grouped by Their Side Chain Properties

Nonpolar side chains: Have no charged or electronegative atoms at pH 7.0 to form hydrogen bonds.

Alanine (Ala or A)	Methionine (Met or M)
Cysteine (Cys or C)	Phenylalanine (Phe or F)
Glycine (Gly or G)	Proline (Pro or P)
Isoleucine (Ile or I)	Tryptophan (Trp or W)
Leucine (Leu or L)	Valine (Val or V)

Polar side chains: Have partial charges at pH 7.0 and can form hydrogen bonds.

Asparagine (Asp or N)	Threonine (Thr or T)
Glutamine (Glu or Q)	Tyrosine (Tyr or Y)
Serine (Ser or S)	

Electrically charged side chains: At pH 7.0, can form hydrogen and ionic bonds.

Basic Side Chains	Acidic Side Chains
Arginine (Arg or R)	Aspartate (Asp or D)
Histidine (His or H)	Glutamate (Glu or E)
Lysine (Lys or K)	

Ribosomes of all organisms are composed of two subunits that assemble into a ribosome as translation begins. Ribosomes bind mRNA and provide an environment for complementary base pairing between mRNA codon sequences and the anticodon sequences of tRNA. (See Section 1.3 for a basic review of translation.) **Figure 9.2** encapsulates the essential elements of translation. Ribosomes translate mRNA in the $5' \rightarrow 3'$ direction, beginning with the start codon and ending with a stop codon. At each triplet codon, complementary base pairing between mRNA and tRNA determines which amino acid is added to the nascent (growing) polypeptide. The start codon and stop codon define the boundaries of the translated segment of mRNA. The resulting polypeptides have an N-terminal (amino-terminal) end corresponding to the 5' end of mRNA and a C-terminal (carboxyl-terminal) end that corresponds to the 3' end of mRNA (**Figure 9.3**).

Figure 9.3 identifies two segments of the mRNA transcript that do not undergo translation. Between the 5' end of mRNA and the start codon is a segment known as the **5' untranslated region**, abbreviated **5' UTR**. The region between the stop codon and the 3' end of the molecule is the **3' untranslated region**, or **3' UTR**. The 5' UTR contains sequences that help initiate translation and the 3' UTR contains sequences associated with transcription termination.

Polypeptides have four levels of organization (**Table 9.2**). The polypeptide **primary structure** is the sequence of amino acids contained in the polypeptide. The differences in the order of amino acids and in the lengths

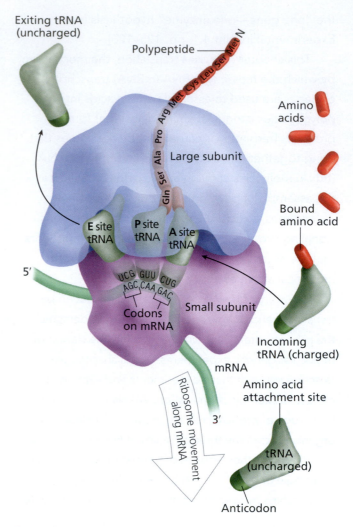

Figure 9.2   **Translation overview.**

of polypeptides (the number of amino acids they contain) are effectively limitless. There are billions of possible amino acid sequences. At the same time, the specific order of amino acids in any given polypeptide is critical to its proper folding and functioning.

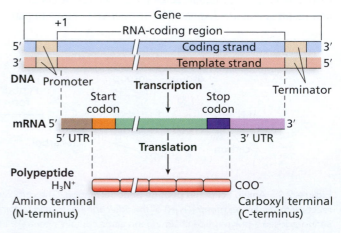

Figure 9.3   **Alignment of DNA, mRNA, and polypeptide.**

Table 9.2	Polypeptide Structure		
Level	**Description**	**Stabilized by**	**Example: Hemoglobin**
Primary	The sequence of amino acids in a polypeptide	Peptide bonds	Gly — Ser — Asp — Cys
Secondary	Formation of α-helices and β-pleated sheets in a polypeptide (thus, depends on primary structures)	Hydrogen bonding between groups along the peptide-bonded backbone	One α-helix
Tertiary	Overall three-dimensional shape of a polypeptide (includes contribution from secondary structures)	Bonds and other interactions between R-groups, or between R-groups and the peptide-bonded backbone	One of hemoglobin's subunits
Quaternary	Shape produced by combinations of polypeptides (each with its own tertiary structure)	Bonds and other interactions between R-groups, and between peptide backbones of different polypeptides	Hemoglobin consists of four polypeptide subunits

Polypeptide **secondary structure** consists of certain common configurations adopted by portions of polypeptides, owing primarily to hydrogen bonds and ionic interactions that form between amino acids. Hydrogen bond formation causes amino acids with polar R-groups to align with one another. This can result in local bending or twisting of the polypeptide into one of two possible structures: An **α-helix (alpha helix)** is a twisted coil of amino acids stabilized by hydrogen bonds between partially charged R-groups; a **β-pleated sheet (beta-pleated sheet)** is a roughly 130-degree bend created when hydrogen bonding between amino acids induces a segment of a polypeptide to fold.

A polypeptide's **tertiary structure** is the three-dimensional structure of the folded polypeptide as a whole. Polypeptides that are active are in their tertiary structure. Some polypeptides are capable of assuming two or more somewhat different tertiary structures. These may include an active structure and an inactive structure, or other combinations. A range of interactions involving the R-groups—hydrogen bonds, covalent bonds, ionic interactions, and hydrophobic interactions—produce the overall shape of the protein.

Primary, secondary, and tertiary structures of polypeptides are interdependent—the primary structure leads to certain secondary structure possibilities and these, in turn, lead to the formation of the one or more possible tertiary structures of a polypeptide. But some proteins in their active form consist of two or more polypeptides, and this level of organization is called the **quaternary structure**. Proteins that have two or more polypeptides (and therefore a quaternary structure) are often described as *multimers*. The individual polypeptides of a multimer may be identical or may be different. A protein composed of four identical polypeptides, for example, can be called a *homotetramer*, whereas a four-polypeptide protein that contains two or more different polypeptides can be identified as a *heterotetramer*. Table 9.2 summarizes these four levels of polypeptide structure for the red blood cell protein hemoglobin—a heterotetrameric protein that is responsible for carrying oxygen.

Ribosome Structures

The specific molecules composing bacterial, archaeal, and eukaryotic ribosomes differ, but the overall structures and functions of the ribosomes are similar, reflecting the fundamental nature of the translation process in all forms of life. In all three domains, ribosomes perform three essential tasks:

1. Bind messenger RNA and identify the start codon where translation begins.
2. Facilitate the complementary base pairing of mRNA codons and tRNA anticodons that determines amino acid order in the polypeptide.
3. Catalyze peptide bond formation between amino acids during polypeptide formation.

Differences in ribosomal composition between bacteria, archaea, and eukaryotes include the number and sequence of rRNA molecules and the number and type of ribosomal proteins. Although the archaeal and bacterial ribosomes are similar in size, and somewhat smaller than the eukaryotic ribosomes, most of the archaeal ribosomal proteins (and the tRNAs and protein factors involved in translation) display homology to their eukaryotic counterparts. In all three domains, ribosomes display key structural similarities, beginning with their each consisting of two main subunits, called the **large ribosomal subunit** and the **small ribosomal subunit**. By convention, subunit size is measured in Svedberg units (S), which describe the velocity of their sedimentation when subjected to a centrifugal force. Named in honor of Theodor Svedberg, a 1926 Nobel Laureate in Chemistry and inventor of the ultracentrifuge, higher S values indicate faster sedimentation rates and larger molecules. It should be noted that Svedberg units are not additive when ribosomal subunits are combined, because sedimentation is a composite property that is affected by multiple molecular factors, including size, shape, and hydration state.

The ribosomes of *E. coli* are the most thoroughly studied bacterial ribosomes and serve as a model for general ribosome structure (**Figure 9.4**). The small subunit of these bacterial ribosomes has a Svedberg value of 30S. It contains 21 proteins and a single 16S rRNA composed of 1541 nucleotides. The large subunit of this bacterial ribosome is a 50S particle composed of 32 proteins, a small 5S rRNA containing 120 nucleotides, and a large 23S rRNA containing 2904 nucleotides. When fully assembled, the intact *E. coli* ribosome has a Svedberg value of 70S.

Both the large and small subunits contribute to the formation of three regions that play important functional roles during translation: the **peptidyl site, or P site**, the **aminoacyl site, or A site**, and the **exit site, or E site**. The P site holds a tRNA to which the nascent polypeptide is attached. The A site binds a new tRNA molecule carrying the next amino acid to be added to the polypeptide. The E site provides an avenue of egress for tRNAs as they leave the ribosome after their amino acid has been added to the polypeptide chain. The small ribosomal subunit contains a channel to hold the mRNA. In addition, there is a channel in the large subunit through which the nascent polypeptide is extruded from the ribosome (see Figure 9.2).

Among eukaryotes, mammalian ribosomes are the most fully characterized. The small 40S ribosomal subunit contains 34 proteins and a single 18S rRNA composed of 1874 nucleotides. The large mammalian ribosomal subunit has a Svedberg value of 60S and contains 49 proteins, along with three molecules of rRNA. The rRNA molecules have values of 5S (120 nucleotides), 5.8S (160 nucleotides), and 28S (4718 nucleotides). The intact mammalian ribosome has a Svedberg value of 80S. Like the bacterial ribosome, the intact mammalian ribosome possesses a P site, an A site, an E site, and a channel for polypeptide egress.

The ribosomes of archaeal species have not been studied nearly as fully as those of bacteria and eukaryotes, but some information is available. The structure of the ribosomes of archaeal species reveals strong similarity to bacterial ribosomes. The large subunit of archaea contains a 23S and a 5S rRNA and 27 proteins. Analysis of the small

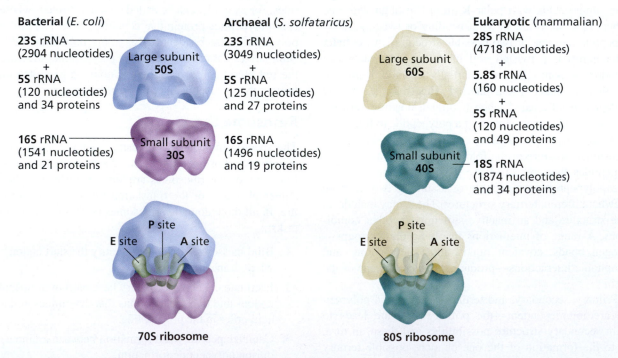

Bacterial (*E. coli*)

23S rRNA
(2904 nucleotides)
+
5S rRNA
(120 nucleotides)
and 34 proteins

Large subunit
50S

16S rRNA
(1541 nucleotides)
and 21 proteins

Small subunit
30S

E site   P site   A site

70S ribosome

Archaeal (*S. solfataricus*)

23S rRNA
(3049 nucleotides)
+
5S rRNA
(125 nucleotides)
and 27 proteins

16S rRNA
(1496 nucleotides)
and 19 proteins

Eukaryotic (mammalian)

28S rRNA
(4718 nucleotides)
+
5.8S rRNA
(160 nucleotides)
+
5S rRNA
(120 nucleotides)
and 49 proteins

Large subunit
60S

Small subunit
40S

18S rRNA
(1874 nucleotides)
and 34 proteins

E site   P site   A site

80S ribosome

Figure 9.4 Ribosomes of bacteria, archaea, and eukaryotes. The ribosomes of *E. coli* and of archaeal species (such as *Sulfolobus solfataricus*) are similar in rRNA and protein content, whereas mammalian ribosomes are somewhat different.

subunit structure revealed a 16S rRNA and 19 proteins. This is the basis for the conclusion that archaeal ribosomes have an overall size and structure similar to that of the 70S bacterial ribosome. As we discuss later, however, archaeal tRNAs and translation proteins are similar to those in eukaryotes.

The proteins contained in ribosomal subunits can be separated from one another by a specialized type of electrophoresis called two-dimensional gel electrophoresis. The 21 proteins that are part of the small ribosomal subunit in *E. coli* and the 32 proteins found in the large ribosomal subunit are efficiently separated by this method. **Research Technique 9.1** describes how two-dimensional gel electrophoresis is used to characterize the proteins found in *E. coli* ribosomal subunits.

A Three-Dimensional View of the Ribosome

Ribosomes are so small—a mere 25 nanometers (nm) in diameter—that almost 10,000 of them can fit in the same space as the period at the end of this sentence. No one has ever "seen" a ribosome with the naked eye, or even an optical microscope, but powerful molecular imaging techniques can resolve the three-dimensional configuration of ribosomes and ribosomal subunits, at levels of resolution that are measured in ångströms ($\mathring{A}$; $1\mathring{A} = 10^{-10}$ meters). Structural analyses based on these images have clarified how ribosomal subunits fit together, and have produced a detailed understanding of ribosomal interactions with mRNA and tRNA.

RESEARCH TECHNIQUE 9.1

Two-Dimensional Gel Electrophoresis and the Identification of Ribosomal Proteins

PURPOSE All ribosomes are composed of two subunits that are each a complex mixture of rRNA and, in most cases, dozens of proteins. One approach to determining the number of proteins contained in each ribosomal subunit uses a method of electrophoresis known as two-dimensional gel electrophoresis to separate the proteins, by their charge in the first dimension and then by their mass in the second dimension. Two-dimensional gel electrophoresis produces a distinctive "protein fingerprint" that displays each ribosomal protein in a different location in the two-dimensional gel.

MATERIALS AND PROCEDURES In preparation for the procedure, ribosomes are isolated from cells, the subunits are separated, and the subunits are treated to dissociate the proteins they contain. The mixture containing liberated ribosomal proteins is then separated in the first dimension by a version of gel electrophoresis known as isoelectric focusing, which separates proteins exclusively by their charge. Unlike conventional gel electrophoresis, which uses a buffered solution to maintain constant pH throughout the gel, isoelectric focusing gels contain a pH gradient. A protein's pH environment affects its charge, and for every protein there is a characteristic pH—called the isoelectric point—at which that protein has neutral charge and cannot move in an electrical field. In isoelectric focusing, proteins migrate through the pH gradient to their isoelectric point, where they stop.

Once isoelectric focusing is complete, a second protein separation is conducted, this time in the second (perpendicular) dimension and using SDS (sodium dodecyl sulfate) gel electrophoresis. SDS is a strong anionic detergent that denatures proteins by disrupting the interactions that keep them folded. Denatured proteins migrate through the gel at a rate determined by their mass, that is, by the number of amino acids they contain. In the SDS gel dimension of two-dimensional gel electrophoresis, each protein has a unique starting point

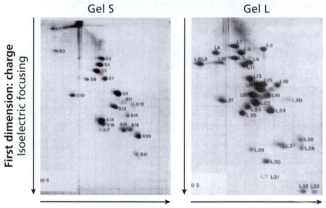

First dimension: charge Isoelectric focusing

Gel S   Gel L

Second dimension: mass SDS gel electrophoresis

corresponding to its isoelectric point. Proteins with large mass (more amino acids) migrate a short distance in the second dimension, whereas proteins with small mass (fewer amino acids) migrate a greater distance.

DESCRIPTION The pair of two-dimensional electrophoresis gels shown here, one containing proteins of the small subunit of the *E. coli* ribosome (gel S) and the other containing proteins of the large subunit (gel L), reveal protein spots (the protein fingerprint) corresponding to the final positions of the proteins that make up each ribosomal subunit. Each spot identifies the location of a unique protein that differs from the other proteins in the gel by a combination of charge and mass. The proteins in gel S are identified as S1 to S21, and in gel L as L1 to L34 (a few of the proteins are not visible or labeled in this gel).

CONCLUSION Two-dimensional gel electrophoresis identifies 21 proteins in the small subunit of the *E. coli* ribosome and 32 proteins in the large ribosomal subunit. Each protein obtained by two-dimensional electrophoresis can be subjected to additional biochemical examination to specifically identify the protein and investigate its role in translation.

More specifically, structural analysis of ribosomes and other molecular complexes in cells is made possible by a technique known as cryo-electron microscopy (cryo-EM), pioneered by Robert Glaeser in the 1970s and perfected by Jacques Dubochet in the 1980s. Cryo-EM uses liquid nitrogen or liquid ethane, with temperatures nearly as low as −200°C, to instantaneously freeze macromolecules and thus preserve them in their native state. A frozen macromolecule is then placed on a microcaliper and scanned from various angles by electron beams that collect data analyzed by specialized software to create a three-dimensional picture of molecular structure. Cryo-EM creates exquisitely precise three-dimensional images of ribosome structure—much like CAT-scan imaging of the human body—revealing atomic-level details of ribosome structure (**Figure 9.5**). These images have identified the location and dimensions of the E, A, and P sites, for example, and have clarified the mechanical activities of ribosomes during translation. This work was recognized with the 2009 Nobel Prize in Chemistry awarded to Ada Yonath, Thomas Steitz, and Venki Ramakrishnan.

9.2 Translation Occurs in Three Phases

Translation occurs in three phases: initiation, elongation, and termination. The three phases are generally similar in bacteria, archaea, and eukaryotes, and yet they differ in several ways, particularly during translation initiation, where distinct mechanisms are used to identify the start codon in mRNA.

Translation Initiation

Translation initiation in all organisms begins when the small ribosomal subunit binds near the 5′ end of mRNA and identifies the start codon sequence. In the next stage, the **initiator tRNA**, the tRNA carrying the first amino acid of the polypeptide, binds to the mRNA start codon. In the final stage of initiation, the large subunit joins the small subunit to form an intact ribosome, and translation begins. During these stages, *initiation factor proteins* help control ribosome formation and binding of the initiator tRNA, and guanosine triphosphate (GTP) provides energy. The tRNAs used during translation each carry a specific amino acid and are identified as **charged tRNAs**. In contrast, a tRNA without an amino acid is **uncharged**. Specialized enzymes discussed in a later section are responsible for recognizing different tRNAs and charging each one with the correct amino acid.

Starting translation at the authentic (correct) start codon is essential for translation of the correct polypeptide. Errant translation starting at the wrong codon, or even at the wrong nucleotide of the start codon, may produce an abnormal polypeptide and result in a nonfunctional protein. Thus, critical questions for biologists studying translation initiation were these: How does the ribosome locate the authentic start codon? And if more than one AUG (start codon) sequence occurs near the 5′ end of the mRNA, how is the authentic start codon identified? Bacteria and eukaryotes use different mechanisms to identify the authentic start codon.

Bacterial Translation Initiation In *E. coli*, six critical molecular components come together to initiate the translation process: (1) mRNA, (2) the small ribosomal

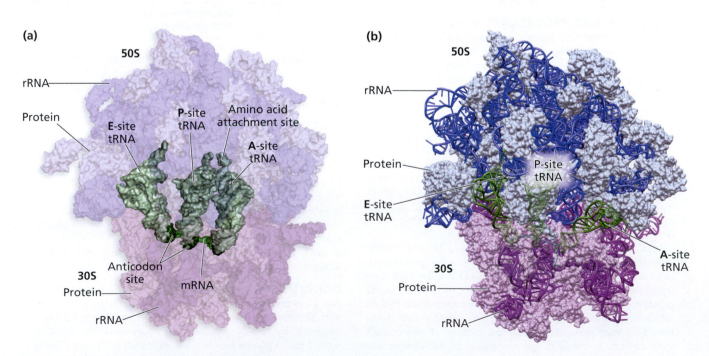

Figure 9.5   **Ribosome structure and tRNA-binding sites interpreted from cryo-EM–generated data.**

subunit, (3) the large ribosomal subunit, (4) the initiator tRNA, and (5) three essential initiation factor proteins. The sixth component, GTP (guanosine triphosphate) provides energy for this and other steps of translation through the cleavage of individual phosphate molecules.

For most of translation initiation in bacteria, the 30S ribosomal subunit is affiliated with an **initiation factor (IF)** protein called IF3, which facilitates binding between the mRNA and the 30S subunit. IF3 also prevents the 30S subunit from binding to the 50S subunit (**Figure 9.6**).

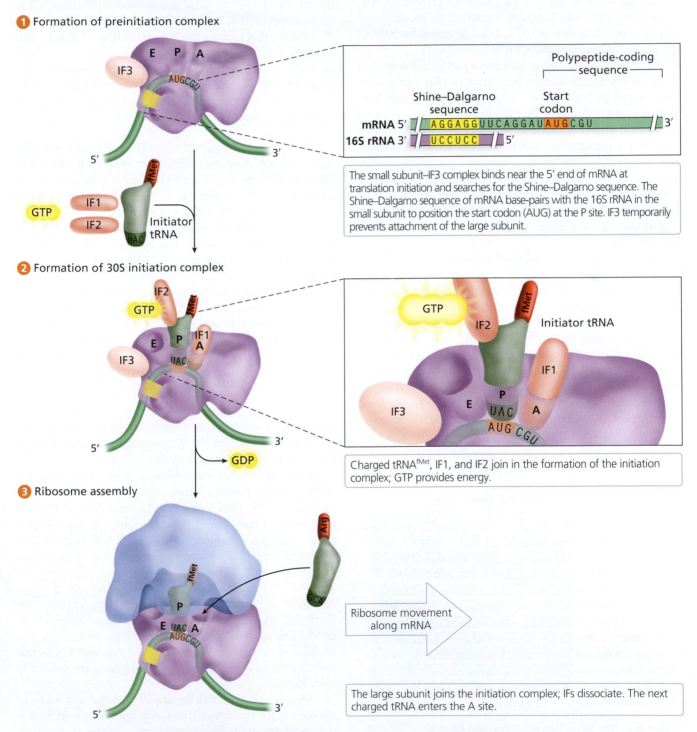

1 Formation of preinitiation complex

The small subunit–IF3 complex binds near the 5′ end of mRNA at translation initiation and searches for the Shine–Dalgarno sequence. The Shine–Dalgarno sequence of mRNA base-pairs with the 16S rRNA in the small subunit to position the start codon (AUG) at the P site. IF3 temporarily prevents attachment of the large subunit.

2 Formation of 30S initiation complex

Charged tRNA^fMet, IF1, and IF2 join in the formation of the initiation complex; GTP provides energy.

3 Ribosome assembly

Ribosome movement along mRNA

The large subunit joins the initiation complex; IFs dissociate. The next charged tRNA enters the A site.

Figure 9.6 Initiation of bacterial translation. The Shine–Dalgarno sequence orients the mRNA on the small subunit.

Q In a sentence or two describe the mechanism that places the start codon of a bacterial mRNA in position to begin translation.

The small subunit—IF3 complex binds near the 5′ end of mRNA, searching for the AUG sequence that serves as the start codon. The **preinitiation complex** forms when the authentic start codon sequence is identified by base pairing that occurs between the 16S rRNA in the 30S ribosome and a short mRNA sequence located a few nucleotides upstream of the start codon in the 5′ UTR of mRNA (Figure 9.6, **❶**). John Shine and Lynn Dalgarno identified the location and sequence of this region in 1974, and it is named the **Shine–Dalgarno sequence** in recognition of their work.

The Shine–Dalgarno sequence is a purine-rich sequence of about six nucleotides located three to nine nucleotides upstream of the start codon. A complementary pyrimidine-rich segment containing the sequence UCCUCC is found near the 3′ end of 16S rRNA, and it pairs with the Shine–Dalgarno sequence to position the mRNA on the 30S subunit (see Figure 9.6). The Shine–Dalgarno sequence is another example of a consensus sequence. As with the consensus sequences we describe for promoters (see Section 8.2), the precise nucleotide sequence and exact position of the Shine–Dalgarno sequence vary slightly from one mRNA to another (**Figure 9.7**).

In the next step of translation initiation (Figure 9.6, **❷**), the initiator tRNA binds to the start codon at what will be part of the P site after ribosome assembly. The amino acid on the initiator tRNA is a modified methionine called **N-formylmethionine (fMet)**; thus, the charged initiator tRNA is abbreviated **tRNA^fMet**. This tRNA has a 3′-UAC-5′ anticodon sequence that is a complementary mate to the start codon sequence. An initiation factor (IF) protein designated IF2 and a molecule of GTP are bound at the P site to facilitate binding of tRNA^fMet. Initiation factor 1 (IF1) also joins the complex to forestall attachment of the 50S subunit. At this point, the **30S initiation complex**, consisting of mRNA

bound to the 30S subunit, tRNA^fMet located at the start codon, three initiation factors, and a molecule of GTP, has been formed.

In the final step of initiation (Figure 9.6, **❸**), the 50S subunit joins the 30S subunit to form the intact ribosome. The energy for the union of the two subunits is derived from hydrolysis of GTP to GDP (guanosine diphosphate). The dissociation of IF1, IF2, and IF3 accompanies the joining of subunits that creates the **70S initiation complex**. This complex is a fully active ribosome with a P site, an A site, an E site, and a channel for exit of the polypeptide. The first tRNA (tRNA^fMet) is already paired with mRNA at the P site, and the open A site contains the second codon and is awaiting the next charged tRNA.

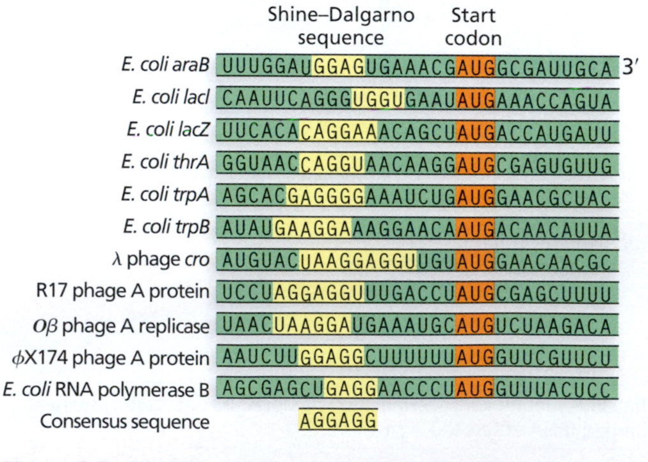

Eukaryotic Translation Initiation The eukaryotic 40S ribosomal subunit complexes with three **eukaryotic initiation factor (eIF)** proteins (eIF1, eIF1A, and eIF3) to form the preinitiation complex (**Figure 9.8, ❶**). In step **❷**, the preinitiation complex joins with the initiator tRNA and eIF5.

The **initiation complex** is formed by binding of the mRNA. This initiates the process called **scanning** (Figure 9.8, **❸**), in which the small ribosomal subunit moves along the 5′ UTR in search of the start codon. About 90% of eukaryotic mRNAs use the first AUG encountered by the initiation complex as the start codon, but the remaining 10% use the second or, in some cases, the third AUG as the start codon. The initiation complex is able to accurately locate the authentic start codon because the codon is embedded in a consensus sequence that reads

$$5′-ACC\mathbf{AUG}G-3′$$

(the start codon itself is shown in bold). This consensus sequence is called the **Kozak sequence** after Marilyn Kozak, who discovered it in 1978.

Locating the start codon leads to recruitment of the 60S subunit to the complex, using energy derived from GTP hydrolysis. This final step **❹** in the formation of the 80S ribosome is accompanied by dissociation of the eIF proteins. In the 80S ribosome, the initiator tRNA^Met is located at the P site; the A site is vacant, awaiting arrival of the second tRNA (**Genetic Analysis 9.1**).

Archaeal Translation Initiation and Its Implications for Evolution Archaeal ribosome subunits are composed of rRNAs that are more similar in size to those of bacteria than to those of eukaryotes. However, the ribosomal RNAs that make up the central structure of the subunits are distinct in each domain.

Despite the similarity in size of archaeal and bacterial ribosomes, the process of translation initiation in archaea is decidedly eukaryote-like. One example of this similarity is the archaeal use of methionine as the common first amino acid of polypeptide chains. This is like eukaryotes and unlike bacteria, which use N-formyl-methionine. A second aspect of archaeal translation initiation concerns the presence of

	Shine–Dalgarno sequence	Start codon
E. coli araB	UUUGGAUGGAGUGAAACG**AUG**GCGAUUGCA 3′	
E. coli lacI	CAAUUCAGGGUGGUGAAU**AUG**AAACCAGUA	
E. coli lacZ	UUCACA**CAGGAA**ACAGCUAUG**ACC**AUGAUU	
E. coli thrA	GGUAACC**AGGU**AACAAGG**AUG**CGAGUGUUG	
E. coli trpA	AGCACG**AGGGG**AAAUCUG**AUG**GAACGCUAC	
E. coli trpB	AUAUG**AAGGA**AAGGAACA**AUG**ACAACAUUA	
λ phage cro	AUGUACU**AAGGAGGU**UGU**AUG**GAACAACGC	
R17 phage A protein	UCCU**AGGAGGU**UUGACCU**AUG**CGAGCUUUU	
Oβ phage A replicase	UAACU**AAGGA**UGAAAUGC**AUG**UCUAAGACA	
φX174 phage A protein	AAUCUU**GGAGG**CUUUUUU**AUG**GUUCGUUCU	
E. coli RNA polymerase B	AGCGAGCUGAGG**AACCCU**AUG**GUUUACUCC	
Consensus sequence	**AGGAGG**	

Figure 9.7 The Shine–Dalgarno consensus binding sequence. The AUG start codon (orange) is near the Shine–Dalgarno sequence (gold), which binds to the 3′ end of 16S rRNA.

❓ Name two features of a Shine–Dalgarno sequence that are essential to its ability to function in translation initiation.

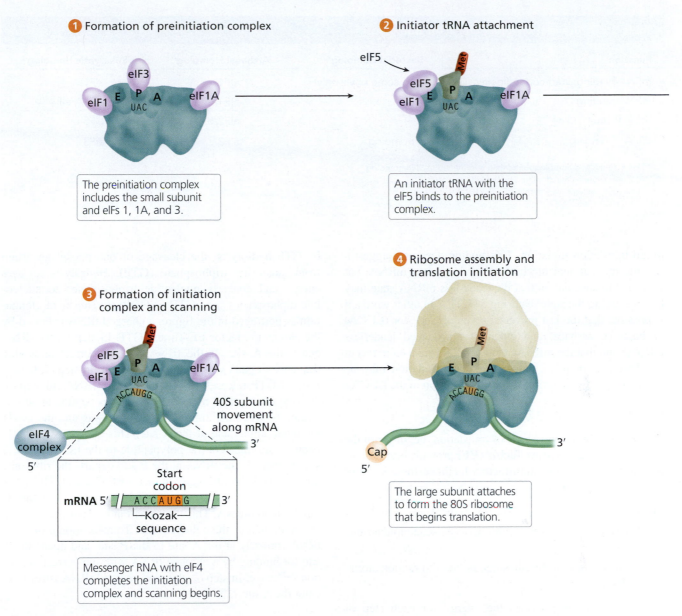

1 Formation of preinitiation complex

The preinitiation complex includes the small subunit and eIFs 1, 1A, and 3.

2 Initiator tRNA attachment

An initiator tRNA with the eIF5 binds to the preinitiation complex.

3 Formation of initiation complex and scanning

40S subunit movement along mRNA

Start codon

mRNA 5′ ACCAUGG 3′
Kozak sequence

Messenger RNA with eIF4 completes the initiation complex and scanning begins.

4 Ribosome assembly and translation initiation

The large subunit attaches to form the 80S ribosome that begins translation.

Figure 9.8 **Initiation of eukaryotic translation.** The Kozak sequence orients the mRNA on the small subunit and places the authentic start codon in position to begin translation.

Q In a sentence or two describe the mechanism that places the authentic start codon of a eukaryotic mRNA in position to begin translation.

Shine–Dalgarno sequences. These are relatively common in the mRNAs of some archaeal species but not in others.

More significantly, the homology seen between transcription factor initiation proteins of archaea and eukaryotes is strong, whereas the homology between those of archaea and bacteria is less so (**Table 9.3**). Recall from our discussion in Section 1.4 that amino acid or nucleic acid sequences that are homologous have a common ancestral origin. Proteins that have greater degrees of homology have more recent common ancestral history than do proteins with lower levels of homology. Based on the protein homology information in Table 9.3, it appears that translation initiation in archaea is more complex than in bacteria and that known

archaeal initiation factor proteins (**aIFs**) are homologous in structure and function to eIFs.

The archaea have multiple mechanisms of mRNA–ribosome interaction at translation initiation. This is most apparent at 5′ mRNA ends, many of which—some studies say more than 50% in certain archaeal species—appear not to have a 5′ UTR. Those mRNAs lacking a 5′ UTR are said to be "leaderless" mRNAs and are apparently missing all or most of the translation-initiating segments, including the Shine–Dalgarno sequence in some cases. The mechanism through which leaderless mRNA translation is initiated is not yet known. Archaeal species producing mRNAs with 5′ UTRs typically have Shine–Dalgarno sequences

Table 9.3 Translation Initiation Factor Homologs

Function	Bacterial Homolog[a]	Archaeal Homolog[b]	Eukaryotic Homolog[c]
mRNA binding; start codon fidelity	IF3 (in some phyla only)	aIF1	eIF1
mRNA binding	IF1	aIF1a	eIF1A/eIF4
tRNA P-site binding	IF2	aIF2/5	eIF5
tRNA^{Met} binding	No homolog	aIF3	eIF3

[a] The absence of a homologous protein is identified as "No homolog."
[b] Archaeal proteins are identified by the letter a.
[c] Eukaryotic proteins are identified by the letter e.

to aid translation initiation. This finding does not suggest a specific translational mechanism for leaderless mRNA, but it has led to speculation that the leaderless mRNA state may be ancestral to the state featuring 5′ UTRs. In other words, it is possible that the last universal common ancestor (LUCA) of bacteria, archaea, and eukaryotes produced leaderless mRNAs and that the mRNAs with 5′ UTRs are a more recent development. In this context, archaeal translation may be something of a relic reminiscent of translation in the LUCA.

Polypeptide Elongation

Elongation, the second phase of translation, begins with the recruitment of **elongation factor (EF)** proteins into the initiation complex. Elongation factors facilitate three steps of polypeptide synthesis:

1. Recruitment of charged tRNAs to the A site
2. Formation of a peptide bond between sequential amino acids
3. Translocation of the ribosome in the 3′ direction along mRNA

GTP cleavage provides the energy for each step of elongation in bacteria, archaea, and eukaryotes. Moreover, the steps in the elongation process are the same in all three types of organisms: Although the elongation factors differ, the ribosomal P, A, and E sites of all three organisms serve nearly identical functions. The rates of elongation seem also to be similar; bacteria add about 20 new amino acids per second to a nascent polypeptide chain, and eukaryotes elongate the polypeptide at a rate of 15 amino acids per second. The elongation rate in archaea has not been established. Lastly, numerous studies indicate high fidelity of translation in all organisms. An error rate of approximately one amino acid in each 10,000 added to polypeptides is estimated for bacteria.

Polypeptide Elongation in Bacteria The steps depicted in **Foundation Figure 9.9**, while specifically describing translation in bacteria, give a generally accurate picture of how different elongation factor proteins (EFs) and other ribosomal proteins carry out elongation in all organisms. As noted above, the energy required for these steps is generated

by GTP hydrolysis, the cleavage of one phosphate group from guanosine triphosphate (GTP). Hydrolysis releases energy and converts nucleotide triphosphates to nucleotide diphosphates (i.e., GTP → GDP). In step ❶ of elongation as portrayed in the figure, a charged tRNA is bound by the elongation factor EF-Tu and GTP. In step ❷, the tRNA enters the A site. If the tRNA has the correct anticodon sequence, it pairs with the mRNA codon. In step ❸, hydrolysis of GTP releases EF-Tu–GDP from tRNA. In step ❹, the enzyme peptidyl transferase catalyzes peptide bond formation between the amino acid at the P site and the newly recruited amino acid at the A site. This elongates the polypeptide and transfers the polypeptide to the tRNA at the A site. In step ❺, the tRNA at the P site departs the ribosome through the E site. Elongation factor EF-G uses GTP hydrolysis to translocate the ribosome by moving it in the 3′ direction on mRNA. This translocation is exactly one codon in length, that is, three nucleotides. Translocation moves the tRNA formerly at the A site to the P site, and opens the A site for binding by a charged tRNA with the correct anticodon sequence. In step ❻, the next charged tRNA is ready to enter the A site.

Elongation of Eukaryotic and Archaeal Polypeptides Evolution has acted to strongly conserve the basic biochemistry of polypeptide elongation in all three domains of life. The elongation factors that carry out polypeptide elongation in eukaryotes and archaea are shown in **Table 9.4**. All organisms use two elongation factors to carry out polypeptide elongation, and the illustration of polypeptide elongation in Figure 9.9 is an equally accurate

Table 9.4 Translation Elongation Factor Homologs

Function	Bacterial Homolog	Archaeal Homolog	Eukaryotic Homolog
Adjusts tRNA in A site	EF-Tu	aEF-1	eEF-1
Promotes translocation	EF-G	aEF-2	eEF-2

Bacterial Translation Elongation

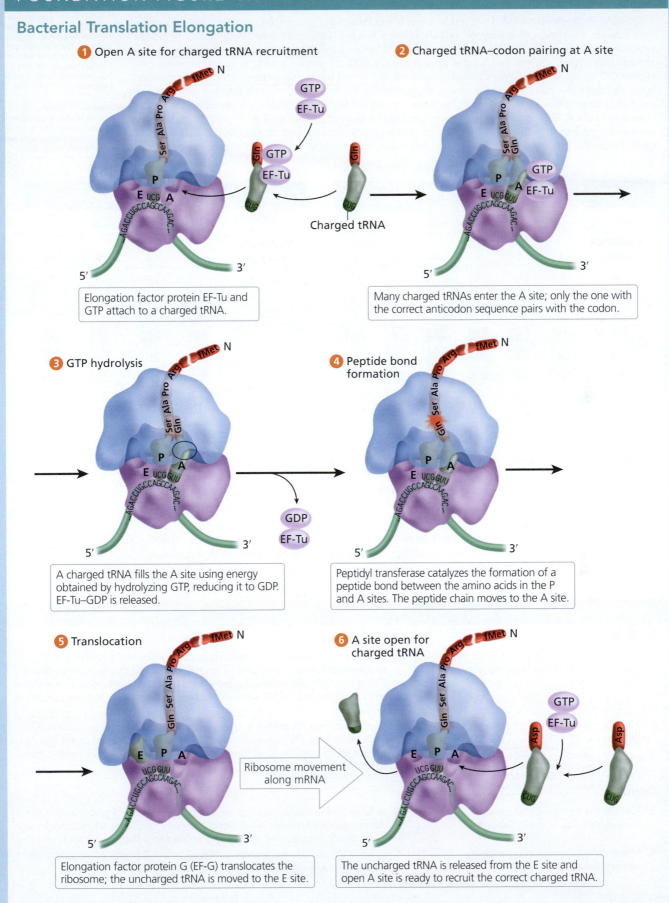

1 Open A site for charged tRNA recruitment

Elongation factor protein EF-Tu and GTP attach to a charged tRNA.

2 Charged tRNA–codon pairing at A site

Many charged tRNAs enter the A site; only the one with the correct anticodon sequence pairs with the codon.

3 GTP hydrolysis

A charged tRNA fills the A site using energy obtained by hydrolyzing GTP, reducing it to GDP. EF-Tu–GDP is released.

4 Peptide bond formation

Peptidyl transferase catalyzes the formation of a peptide bond between the amino acids in the P and A sites. The peptide chain moves to the A site.

5 Translocation

Elongation factor protein G (EF-G) translocates the ribosome; the uncharged tRNA is moved to the E site.

6 A site open for charged tRNA

The uncharged tRNA is released from the E site and open A site is ready to recruit the correct charged tRNA.

Ribosome movement along mRNA

PROBLEM In an investigation designed to identify the consensus sequence containing the AUG codon that initiates translation of eukaryotic mRNA, Marilyn Kozak (1986) compared the amounts of protein produced from 10 mutant mRNA molecules having different single-base substitutions flanking the AUG. Protein production was gauged by the optical density (OD) of protein bands in electrophoretic gels. Higher OD values indicated more protein produced. In the two tables shown here, AUG, the start codon, is highlighted (dark blue) and its adenine (A) is labeled the +1 nucleotide of the translated region. Kozak examined six single-base mutants at nucleotides −3 and +4 (light blue). These are identified by number (1 to 6) in **Table A**. She also examined four single-base mutants of positions −2 and −1 (light blue). These are numbered 7 to 10 in **Table B**. The OD for protein production by each mutant was measured and is given below the mutant in the table. Use the OD values to determine answers to the problem questions.

> **BREAK IT DOWN:** The Kozak consensus sequence, 5′–ACCAUGG–3′, includes the AUG start codon sequence and several surrounding mRNA nucleotides and is critical to ribosome recognition of the authentic start codon (p. 322).

> **BREAK IT DOWN:** Efficient translation of mRNA produces more protein and is indicated by higher OD values for mutants possessing that capability (p. 322).

Table A	Six Position −3 and +4 Mutants					
Nucleotide Position	**Mutant Number**					
	1	**2**	**3**	**4**	**5**	**6**
−3	G	A	U	C	G	A
−2	C	C	C	C	C	C
−1	C	C	C	C	C	C
+1	A	A	A	A	A	A
+2	U	U	U	U	U	U
+3	G	G	G	G	G	G
+4	U	U	G	G	G	G
OD	0.7	2.6	0.9	0.9	3.1	5.0

Table B	Four Position −2 and −1 Mutants			
Nucleotide Position	**Mutant Number**			
	7	**8**	**9**	**10**
−3	A	A	A	A
−2	C	G	G	C
−1	A	A	G	G
+1	A	A	A	A
+2	U	U	U	U
+3	G	G	G	G
OD	3.3	1.8	1.9	2.0

a. Looking just at the nucleotides in positions −3 and +4 for the six mutants in Table A, decide which nucleotides give the highest level of protein production.

b. Describe the impact of each nucleotide (A, T, C, and G) in the −3 position.

c. Looking just at nucleotides at positions −2 and −1 for the four mutants in Table B, decide which nucleotides give the highest level of protein production.

d. Why did Kozak use only A in the −3 position to test the effects of nucleotides at positions −2 and −1?

e. Putting together data from both Table A and Table B, give the sequence of the mRNA region from −3 to +4 that produces the highest level of translation.

Solution Strategies	Solution Steps

Evaluate

1. Identify the topic this problem addresses and the nature of the required answer.

2. Identify the critical information given in the problem.

> **TIP:** Notice that AUG is the start codon sequence in all mutants tested. As a consequence, differences in OD result from differences among the surrounding nucleotides.

Deduce

3. Identify the constant and variable nucleotides displayed in Table A.

4. Identify the constant and variable nucleotides shown in Table B.

1. This problem involves examination and interpretation of the effects that sequence differences surrounding the mRNA start codon have on translation. The answer requires comparing the effects of base substitutions on translation and identifying the mRNA sequence corresponding to the highest translation level.

2. Two tables provide mRNA sequence for different sequence variants. For each variant, an OD value describes the approximate level of protein produced by translation of the sequence. Higher OD values correspond to more protein production.

3. In Table A, the nucleotide C is constant at positions −1 and −2, and the start codon nucleotides A, U, and G occupy positions +1, +2, and +3, respectively. Nucleotide variability is limited to positions −3 and +4.

4. In Table B, only the nucleotide at the −1 and −2 positions vary; all other nucleotides are constant.

Solve

5. Specify the nucleotides in the −3 and +4 positions (Table A) that give the highest OD.

6. Assess how each nucleotide in the −3 position affects OD.

7. Evaluate how nucleotide differences at the −1 and −2 positions (Table B) affect OD.

8. Explain the decision to base Table B evaluations only on sequences with A in the −3 position.

> TIP: Compare OD values and nucleotide differences from both tables to determine the most efficient consensus sequence.

9. Identify the start codon consensus sequence that results in the highest level of translation.

Answer a

5. In Table A, the presence of A in position −3 and G in position +4 produces the highest OD value. At the +4 position, G produces two high OD values and two low ODs, and T produces one high and one low OD.

Answer b

6. At position −3, A produces the highest and the third-highest OD values; G produces the second-highest and the lowest OD; T and C produce the same low OD value.

Answer c

7. In Table B, a C in position −2 and an A in position −1 produce the highest OD. Considering only the variable position −2, C produces higher OD values than does G.

Answer d

8. Adenine is selected as the nucleotide in position −3 for Table B evaluations based on the high average OD value reported for this nucleotide in the −3 position in Table A in comparison with other nucleotides. The average OD for A in the −3 position in Table A is $\frac{(5.0 + 2.6)}{2} = 3.8$ versus the next-highest average of $\frac{(3.1 + 0.7)}{2} = 1.9$ for G in the −3 position.

Answer e

9. Data from the two tables combined identify the sequence ACC**AUG**G (start codon in bold) as the most efficient consensus sequence for the start codon. For the nucleotide positions immediately surrounding the start codon, A is most efficient at −3, C is more efficient than G at −2, C is more efficient than A or G at −1, and G is more efficient than U at +4.

For more practice, see Problems 34, 35, and 36.   Visit the Study Area to access study tools.   **Mastering Genetics**

---

portrayal of the process in eukaryotes and archaea. Based on sequence comparisons, the archaeal and eukaryotic elongation factor homologs are more alike than are archaeal and bacterial EFs.

Translation Termination

The elongation cycle continues until one of the three stop codons, UAG, UGA, or UAA, enters the A site of the ribosome. There are no tRNAs with anticodons complementary to stop codons, so the entry of a stop codon into the A site is a translation-terminating event. All organisms use **release factors (RF)** to bind a stop codon in the A site (**Figure 9.10** ❶). The catalytic activity of RFs releases the polypeptide bound to tRNA at the P site ❷. Polypeptide release causes ejection of the RF from the P site and leads to the separation of the ribosomal subunits ❸.

In bacteria, two release factors, RF1 and RF2, recognize stop codons. RF1 recognizes UAG and UAA, and RF2 recognizes UAA and UGA. A third bacterial release factor, RF3, is active in recycling RF1. Eukaryotic and archaeal translation are terminated by the action of a single release factor, identified as eRF1 in eukaryotes and aRF1 in archaea, that recognizes all three stop codons in organisms of both of these domains. Eukaryotes have a second RF that,

like RF3 of bacteria, participates in recycling eRF1. The currently available information on sequence and function of RFs suggests that archaea and eukaryotes have RFs that are more like one another than either is like bacterial RFs (**Table 9.5**).

9.3 Translation Is Fast and Efficient

With mRNA transcripts of hundreds to thousands of genes in cells, translation is an active and ongoing process that must efficiently initiate, elongate, and terminate polypeptide synthesis. In recent decades, research has uncovered several aspects of the translation machinery that help explain the speed, accuracy, and efficiency of polypeptide production.

The Translational Complex

Cell biologists estimate that each bacterial cell contains about 20,000 ribosomes, collectively constituting nearly one-quarter of the mass of the cell. The number of ribosomes per eukaryotic cell is variable, but it too is in the tens of thousands. Given these numbers, it is not surprising that translation is almost never a matter of a solitary ribosome

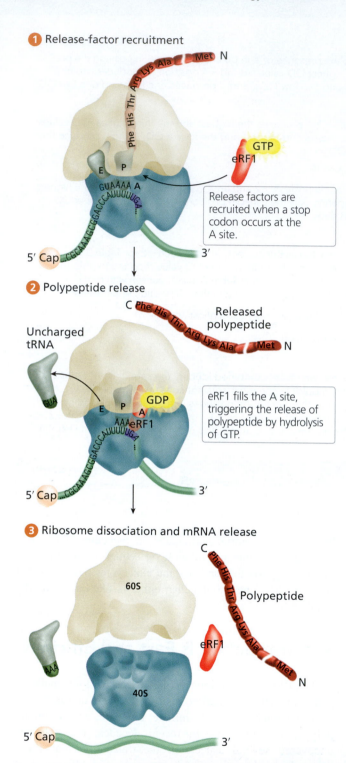

1 Release-factor recruitment

Release factors are recruited when a stop codon occurs at the A site.

2 Polypeptide release

Uncharged tRNA

Released polypeptide

eRF1 fills the A site, triggering the release of polypeptide by hydrolysis of GTP.

3 Ribosome dissociation and mRNA release

60S

eRF1

Polypeptide

40S

5′ Cap   3′

Figure 9.10   Termination of translation by release factor (eRF) proteins in eukaryotes. A similar process terminates bacterial and archaeal translation.

In a sentence or two describe the mechanism that terminates translation in bacteria and eukaryotes.

translating a single mRNA. Rather, electron micrographs reveal structures called **polyribosomes**, busy translational complexes containing multiple ribosomes that are each actively translating the same mRNA (**Figure 9.11**). Each

Table 9.5	Translation Termination Factor Homologs		
Function	Bacterial Homolog	Archaeal Homolog	Eukaryotic Homolog
Stop codon recognition	RF1 and RF2	aRF1	eRF1
Recycling RF1 and eRF1	RF3	No homolog	eRF3
Ribosome recycling	RRF	No homolog	No homolog

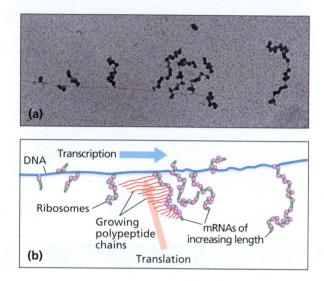

Figure 9.11   Polyribosomes in bacteria. (a) Electron micrograph of polyribosomes shows that as mRNAs are being transcribed from DNA, multiple ribosomes are bound to each mRNA, to translate it and to produce polypeptides. **(b)** Artist rendition of the polyribosome electron micrograph. Transcription moves left to right, so the mRNA length increases toward the right. Translation is shown on one mRNA. It begins at the bottom (the 5′ mRNA end) and progresses in the 3′ direction toward the top.

ribosome in the polyribosome structure independently synthesizes a polypeptide, markedly increasing the efficiency of utilization of an mRNA.

In bacteria, the absence of a nucleus and of pre-mRNA processing leads to the "coupling" of transcription and translation seen in Figure 9.11. This means that multiple ribosomes can be engaged in translation of the 5′ region of mRNAs whose 3′ end is still being synthesized by RNA polymerase. In Figure 9.11, transcription occurs along DNA in the left-hand to right-hand direction. Translation of the mRNA transcripts begins before transcription is complete and stops when the mRNA degrades. The average half-life of bacterial mRNA is a few minutes, but many polypeptides can be translated in that time span.

By contrast, transcription and translation in eukaryotes are uncoupled. Transcription takes place in the nucleus, where pre-mRNA is processed to form mature mRNA. Translation occurs in the cytoplasm after release of mature mRNA.

However, once in the cytoplasm, each individual eukaryotic mRNA is translated by multiple ribosomes simultaneously. The half-life of an average mature mRNA is several hours, and many polypeptides can be produced in that time span.

Translation of Polycistronic mRNA

Each polypeptide-producing gene in eukaryotes produces monocistronic mRNA, meaning mRNA that contains the transcript of a single gene. According to the scanning model described earlier for translation in eukaryotes, each eukaryotic mRNA contains a single authentic start codon and a nucleotide sequence that codes only one kind of polypeptide chain. In contrast, groups of bacterial and archaeal genes often share a single promoter, and the resulting mRNA transcript contains information that synthesizes several different polypeptides. These **polycistronic mRNAs** are produced as part of operon systems that regulate the transcription of sets of bacterial genes functioning in the same metabolic pathway (a form of regulation we discuss in Section 12.2). The term "cistron" is equivalent to "gene"; thus, a polycistronic mRNA contains the transcripts of two or more genes.

To repeat, polycistronic mRNAs consist of multiple polypeptide-producing segments, so when a polycistronic mRNA is translated, two or more polypeptides are produced. Each of the polypeptides encoded by a polycistonic mRNA has its own start codon and stop codon. In the case of bacteria, and in all but the leaderless mRNAs in archaea, most, but not all, translation-initiating regions contain a Shine–Dalgarno sequence. Intercistronic spacer sequences separate the cistrons of polycistronic mRNA, and they are not translated (**Figure 9.12**).

Bacterial intercistronic spacers are variable in length: Some are just a few nucleotides long, although most are 30 to 40 nucleotides long. If the intercistronic spacer is a few nucleotides in length, it is short enough to be spanned by a ribosome. In such systems, the ribosome remains intact after completing synthesis of one polypeptide, and it goes on to translate the other genes encoded in the polycistronic mRNA. On the other hand, when the intercistronic spacer is longer, the initial ribosome dissociates and new translation initiation must occur to translate the next polypeptide encoded by the polycistronic mRNA.

9.4 The Genetic Code Translates Messenger RNA into Polypeptide

In chemical terms, nucleic acids and amino acids are very different compounds, and there is no *direct* mechanism by which mRNA could synthesize a polypeptide. Nevertheless, the nucleotide sequences of mRNA do provide a means by which the amino acid sequences of polypeptides can be specified. This vehicle is the "genetic code," the name used to describe the correspondence between nucleotide triplets in mRNA and individual amino acids.

The conversion of an mRNA sequence into a polypeptide depends on interactions between mRNA and the transfer RNAs (tRNAs) that carry amino acids to the ribosome. At ribosomes, complementary base pairing binds consecutive sets of three mRNA nucleotides—the codons—to the three nucleotide bases of the correct tRNA anticodons. Once the correct tRNA is bound by a codon, it transfers its amino acid to the end of a growing polypeptide chain. Transfer RNA molecules facilitate the translation of genetic information from one chemical language (nucleic acid) to another (amino acid). That is, tRNA is an adaptor molecule that interprets and then acts on the information carried in mRNA.

Our review of translation and the genetic code in Section 1.3 depicts a triplet genetic code containing 64 different codons, more than enough to encode the 20 common amino acids used to construct polypeptides (**Figure 9.13**; see also the genetic code inside the front cover). The greater number of codons than amino acids leads to *redundancy* in the genetic code, as evidenced by the observation that single amino acids are specified by from one to as many as six different codons. Codons that specify the same amino acid are called **synonymous codons**.

To an extent, this redundancy has a specific pattern. Notice, for example, that the two synonymous codons for histidine (His) and the two synonymous codons for glutamine (Gln) all share the same first two bases in the same order: C and A. What distinguishes one codon pair from the other is that both His codons have a pyrimidine at the third position, whereas the two Gln codons have a purine in the third position. As you look at Figure 9.13, you will

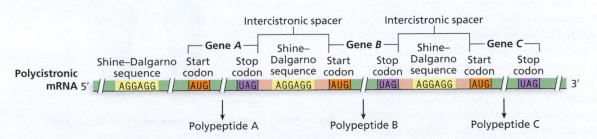

Figure 9.12 Polycistronic mRNA. A polycistronic mRNA is a transcript of multiple genes. A separate polypeptide is produced from each gene.

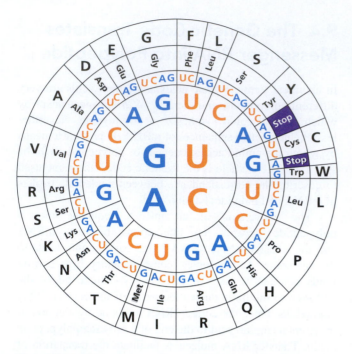

Figure 9.13   The genetic code. To read this circular table of the genetic code, start with the inner ring, which contains the nucleotide in the first position (5′ nucleotide) of a codon. The second-position nucleotide is in the second ring from the center, and the third-position nucleotide is in the third ring. Three-letter and one-letter abbreviations for the corresponding amino acids occupy the outermost rings. See also the genetic code inside the front cover.

🅠 Translate the mRNA sequence 5′ CCAUCAGGC 3′. Write an mRNA sequence that will encode the amino acid string Cys-Phe-Asn. What are the full names of these three amino acids?

see many examples of synonymous codons in which the first two nucleotides of the codons are the same. In the third position, synonymous codons will have either of the two purines or either of the two pyrimidines.

The Genetic Code Displays Third-Base Wobble

The triplet genetic code is a biological example of Ockham's razor, the principle that the simplest hypothesis is the most likely to be correct: During the late 1950s, arithmetic logic led many researchers to conclude that the genetic code was most likely triplet. This simple solution to the question of how amino acid sequences could be coded by nucleic acid sequences posited that a doublet genetic code (two nucleotides per codon) could produce just 16 (4^2) combinations of codons, which is not enough different combinations to specify 20 amino acids. On the other hand, a quadruplet genetic code would generate 4^4, or 256, different combinations of codons—far too many for the needs of genomes. In contrast, a triplet genetic code, yielding 4^3, or 64, different codons, provides enough variety to encode 20 amino acids with some, but not excessive, redundancy. Among the 64 codons, 61

specify amino acids, and the remaining 3 are the stop codons that terminate translation. Only two amino acids, methionine (Met)—with the codon AUG—and tryptophan (Trp)—with the codon UGG—are encoded by single codons. The other 18 amino acids are specified by two to six codons.

Each transfer RNA molecule carries a particular amino acid to the ribosome, where complementary base pairing between each mRNA codon sequence and the corresponding anticodon sequence of a correct tRNA takes place. This complementary base pairing requires antiparallel alignment of the mRNA and tRNA strands. Recall that Figure 8.28 illustrates a two-dimensional and a three-dimensional view of a tRNA molecule. The tRNA in Figure 8.28 has the anticodon sequence 3′-CGC-5′. This corresponds to the mRNA codon sequence 5′-GCG-3′, which specifies alanine (Ala). To visualize the codon–anticodon base-pairing arrangement, consider the codon sequence for aspartic acid (Asp), 5′-GAC-3′. Base-pairing rules predict that the tRNA anticodon sequence is 3′-CUG-5′ (**Figure 9.14**). Asp is also specified by a synonymous codon, 5′-GAU-3′, that pairs with tRNA carrying the anticodon sequence 3′-CUA-5′. Transfer RNA molecules with different anticodon sequences that carry the same amino acid are called **isoaccepting tRNAs**.

Does the presence of synonymous codons and isoaccepting tRNAs mean that a genome must provide 61 different tRNA genes and transcribe a tRNA molecule to match each codon? The answer is no. In fact, most genomes have 30 to 50 different tRNA genes. As an example, the *E. coli* genome encodes 47 different tRNAs that are collectively able to recognize all 61 codon sequences specifying an amino acid.

How does a genome that encodes fewer than 61 different tRNA molecules recognize all 61 functional codons? The answer lies in relaxation of the strict complementary base-pairing rules at the third base of the codon. The mechanics of translation provide for flexibility in the pairing of the third base, the 3′-most nucleotide, of the codon. **Third-base wobble** is the name given to the mechanism that relaxes the requirement for complementary base pairing between the third base of a codon and the corresponding nucleotide of its anticodon.

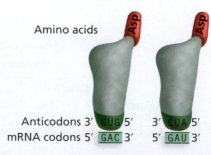

Figure 9.14   Complementary base pairing of codons and anticodons. Isoaccepting aspartic acid (Asp) tRNAs illustrate complementary antiparallel base pairing of codon and anticodon sequences.

Francis Crick devised the wobble hypothesis in 1966, proposing the possibility of nonstandard base pairing between the third-position nucleotides of the codon and anticodon. For example, **Figure 9.15** shows third-base wobble for two pairs of the six codons of serine (Ser) and the three codons of isoleucine (Ile). Stated differently, two tRNAs with distinct anticodon sequences are enough to recognize the four Ser codons; and a single tRNA recognizes all three Ile codons.

Third-base wobble occurs through flexible base pairing between the wobble nucleotide—that is, the 3′ nucleotide of a codon—and the 5′ nucleotide of an anticodon. At this position, base pairing between the nucleotides of the codon and anticodon need not be complementary. They must, however, be a purine and a pyrimidine (with one exception explained momentarily). Third-base wobble pairings are summarized in **Table 9.6**. The nucleotides at the wobble position in different anticodons include all the RNA nucleotides and also the modified nucleotide **inosine (I)**. Inosine is structurally similar to G but lacks the amino group attached to guanine's 2 carbon. As a result, inosine base-pairs with either purines or pyrimidines.

The patterns of third-base wobble are tied directly to the patterns of genetic code redundancy. Specifically, synonymous codons that share the first two nucleotides of the codons and differ only by having alternative purines or pyrimidines in the third position are subject to third-base wobble. Different organisms take greater or lesser advantage of wobble and have evolved different numbers of different tRNA genes. Theoretical calculations find that a minimum of 31 tRNA anticodon sequences are required to recognize the 61 mRNA codon sequences, but as far as is known, all organisms encode more than the minimum required number of tRNAs.

The (Almost) Universal Genetic Code

In astonishing testimony to the conclusion that life on Earth had a single origin, and to the power of natural selection to, in this case, maintain virtually complete uniformity over hundreds of millions of years, every living organism uses the same genetic code to synthesize polypeptides. In all living things, from bacteria to humans, the hereditary script carried by a given sequence of mRNA is translated by a similar mechanism and produces the same polypeptide. The universality of the genetic code has led to technologies in which bacterial systems are used to express biologically important plant or animal protein products.

As with most general rules, however, there are a few exceptions to the universality of the genetic code; thus, biologists characterize the genetic code as *almost* universal. The 10 known exceptions to the universal genetic code are summarized in **Table 9.7**. Most are found in mitochondria, but three exceptions occur in the translation of genetic information encoded in nuclear DNA.

Familiarize yourself with Figure 9.13 and the genetic code information inside the front cover by using them to decipher the mutations shown in **Genetic Analysis 9.2**.

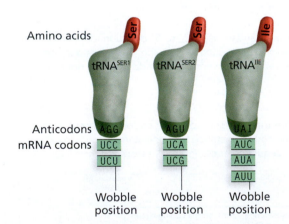

Figure 9.15 Third-base wobble. Relaxation of complementary base pairing at the third position of a codon can reduce the number of different tRNAs required during translation. In this example, wobble base pairing allows two serine (Ser) tRNAs (left) to recognize two different codons each. Wobble permits a single isoleucine (Ile) tRNA to recognize all three isoleucine codons.

Table 9.6	Third-Base Wobble Pairing between Codon and Anticodon Nucleotides
3′ Nucleotide of Codon	**5′ Nucleotide of Anticodon**
A or G	U
G	C
U	A
U or C	G
U, C, or A	I

Table 9.7	Genomes Using Modifications of the Universal Genetic Code		
Codon	**Universal Code**	**Unusual Code**	**Genome**
AGA, AGG	Arg	Stop	Mitochondria in plants, animals, and yeast
AUA, AUU	Ile	Met	Mitochondria in plants, animals, and yeast
UGA	Stop	Trp	Mitochondria in plants, animals, and yeast, and in *Mycoplasma* species
CUN[a]	Leu	Thr	Mitochondria in yeast
UAA, UAG	Stop	Gln	Green algae, protozoa
UGA	Stop	Cys	Protozoa

[a]N = any third-position nucleotide.

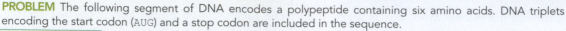

PROBLEM The following segment of DNA encodes a polypeptide containing six amino acids. DNA triplets encoding the start codon (AUG) and a stop codon are included in the sequence.

> **BREAK IT DOWN:** The DNA coding strand differs from mRNA by the presence of T in DNA in place of the U in RNA (p. 276).

```
5'-... CCCAGCCTAGCCTTTGCAAGAGGCCATATCGAC ...-3'
3'-... GGGTCGGATCGGAAACGTTCTCCGGTATAGCTG ...-5'
```

a. Write the sequence and polarity of the mRNA encoded by this gene.

b. Determine the amino acid sequence of the polypeptide, and identify the N- and C-terminal ends of the polypeptide.

> **BREAK IT DOWN:** The genetic code (see inside the front cover or Figure 9.13) is used for translation (p. 316).

c. If a base-substitution mutation changes the first transcribed G of the template strand to an A, how will this alter the polypeptide?

> **BREAK IT DOWN:** A base substitution on the template DNA strand would lead to a corresponding change on the coding strand so as to complement the nucleotide that is new on the template strand (p. 241).

Solution Strategies	Solution steps

Evaluate

1. Identify the topic this problem addresses and the nature of the required answer.

1. This problem concerns the identification of DNA coding and template strands; the transcription of DNA to mRNA and translation of mRNA into a polypeptide; and an evaluation of a mutation of the DNA sequence. The answer requires identification of the DNA strands, identification of start and stop codons, and determination of the amino acid sequence of wild-type and mutant polypeptides.

2. Identify the critical information given in the problem.

2. DNA sequence that includes a start (AUG) codon and a stop codon is given.

Deduce

3. Identify the start codon by inspecting both DNA strands for 5'-ATG-3' sequences that potentially encode start (AUG) codons.

> **TIP:** The AUG start codon is the most common codon for translation initiation corresponds to the DNA triplet 5'-ATG-3' on the coding strand.

3. Scanning both DNA strands in their 3'-to-5' direction identifies a single 5'-ATG-3' sequence. The sequence is on the lower strand in the diagram beginning with the seventh nucleotide from the right.

Survey the putative template strand identified in the previous step and determine if DNA triplets 5'-TAG-3', 5'-TGA-3', and 5'-TAA-3' corresponding to possible stop codons occur as the seventh codon of an mRNA sequence.

> **TIP:** The stop codons UAG, UGA, and UAA correspond to DNA triplets on the coding strand.

4. Since just one DNA triplet encoding a start codon is present, a scan of the strand at the correct distance from the start codon finds a 5'-TAG-3' triplet sequence encoding a UAG stop codon:

```
3'-GGGTCG GAT CGGAAACGTTCTCCG GTA TAGCTC-5'
```

> **TIP:** Substituting U for T on the coding strand produces mRNA sequence. Alternatively, arranging RNA nucleotides complementary to the template strand and assigning antiparallel polarity produces mRNA.

Solve

5. Identify the mRNA sequence encoding the six amino acids of the polypeptide.

> **TIP:** The mRNA sequence can be determined from either the coding strand or the template strand of DNA.

Answer a

5. The mRNA sequence is

```
5'-AUG GCC UCU UGC AAA GGC UAG-3'
```

Answer b

6. List the amino acid sequence of the polypeptide.

6. The polypeptide sequence is

```
N-Met-Ala-Ser-Cys-Lys-Gly-C
```

Answer c

7. Identify the effect of the G → A base substitution on the polypeptide.

7. Substituting the first transcribed G → A on the template strand alters the second codon of mRNA by changing GCC → GUC and substitutes valine (Val) for alanine (Ala) in the second position of the polypeptide sequence.

For more practice, see Problems 7, 12, and, 30.

Visit the Study Area to access study tools. **Mastering Genetics**

Charging tRNA Molecules

Transfer RNA molecules are transcribed from tRNA genes. Recall that the three-dimensional structure of tRNAs features a CCA terminus at the 3′ end of tRNA molecules as the site of attachment of an amino acid (see Figure 8.28). Each tRNA carries only one of the 20 amino acids, and correct charging of each tRNA is crucial for the integrity of the genetic code.

The charging of tRNAs is catalyzed by enzymes called **aminoacyl-tRNA synthetases,** or more simply, **tRNA synthetases.** There are 20 different tRNA synthetases, one for each of the amino acids. To charge an uncharged tRNA, a tRNA synthetase catalyzes a reaction that forms a bond between the carboxyl group of the amino acid and the 3′ hydroxyl group of adenine in the CCA terminus. Experimental analysis reveals that the recognition of isoaccepting tRNAs by tRNA synthetase is a complex process that involves contact with multiple nucleotides of the target tRNA (**Figure 9.16**). When tRNA is in contact with tRNA synthetase, the tRNA acceptor stem fits into an active site of tRNA synthetase. The active site contains the amino acid that will be added to the tRNA acceptor stem, as well as ATP that provides energy for amino acid attachment. Mutational analysis reveals the sequence sensitivity of tRNA synthetases. These studies show that mutations in any of the four arms of tRNA or in the anticodon sequence itself can render a tRNA unrecognizable to its tRNA synthetase.

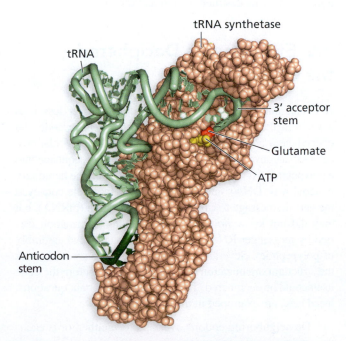

Figure 9.16   Interaction of aminoacyl-tRNA synthetase with tRNA. Aminoacyl-tRNA synthetase contacts multiple points on tRNA to identify the proper tRNA to charge with an amino acid (glutamate, in this example). Amino acid attachment occurs in a cleft of the synthetase that accommodates ATP, the amino acid, and the 3′ acceptor stem of tRNA.

Protein Folding and Posttranslational Polypeptide Processing

Translation produces polypeptides, but the production of functional proteins is not complete until the polypeptides are folded into their functional tertiary or quaternary structures. Recall from Section 9.1 that these steps involve the formation of hydrogen and covalent bonds. They may also involve specific chemical modifications of amino acids in polypeptides. In addition, other categories of posttranslational events provide further modifications and sort the proteins for transport to their destinations.

The removal of one or more amino acids from a polypeptide is a common form of **posttranslational polypeptide processing.** Earlier in the chapter, we identified AUG as the usual start codon and noted that it encodes the modified amino acid fMet in bacterial cells and methionine in eukaryotes. Yet fMet is never found in functional bacterial proteins, and amino acids other than methionine are frequently the first amino acid of polypeptides in eukaryotes. The absence of fMet from functional bacterial proteins is the result of posttranslational cleavage of fMet from each bacterial polypeptide (**Figure 9.17a**).

Even more extensive posttranslational processing occurs at the N-terminal end of eukaryotic polypeptides. As noted, methionine is rarely the first amino acid of eukaryotic polypeptides, but this is usually because of the removal of a larger piece of the N-terminal end of the polypeptide, in segments known as **leader regions.** These are segments of up to several amino acids in length that are removed as part of the transmembrane passage or vesicle transportation of polypeptides. Eukaryotic polypeptides frequently pass or are transported out of cells, and the removal of leader regions is part of that process.

In addition to cleavage of N-terminal amino acids, other amino acid residues can be chemically modified. One of the most common modifications of individual amino acids is performed by enzymes known as kinases that carry out phosphorylation of proteins by adding a phosphate group to individual amino acids (**Figure 9.17b**). This is an important regulatory process that can switch a protein from an inactive to an active form, or vice versa. Other enzymes may add methyl groups, hydroxyl groups, or acetyl groups to individual amino acids of polypeptides. The addition of carbohydrate side chains to polypeptides to form a glycoprotein is another important kind of posttranslational modification.

Posttranslational processing may also include the cleavage of a polypeptide into multiple segments that each form functional proteins or that aggregate after elimination of one or more segments to form a functional protein. Production of the hormone insulin, which facilitates transport of glucose into cells, includes two posttranslational modification steps that remove segments of the original polypeptide (**Figure 9.17c**). The polypeptide product translated from the insulin gene is called preproinsulin. It is an inactive protein that contains a leader segment, called the pre–amino acid segment, at the N-terminal end and a

(a) Cleavage of N-terminal amino acids

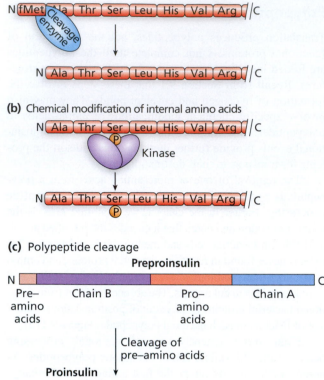

(b) Chemical modification of internal amino acids

(c) Polypeptide cleavage

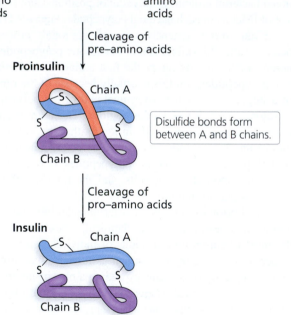

Disulfide bonds form
between A and B chains.

Figure 9.17   Examples of posttranslational processing.

connecting segment, called the pro–amino acid segment, that separates the A-chain segment and the B-chain segment, the two functional pieces of the polypeptide. In posttranslational processing of preproinsulin, the pre–amino acids of the signal sequence are removed, after the polypeptide is transported through the cell membrane, to form proinsulin. Next, three disulfide bonds form within and between the A-chain and B-chain segments, followed by polypeptide cleavage that removes the pro–amino acid segment. What results is a functional insulin molecule consisting of 20 amino acids in the A-chain segment and 31 amino acids in the B-chain segment.

The Signal Hypothesis

Like the passengers in a busy airline terminal, the proteins produced in a cell have different destinations, to which they travel with the aid of a "ticket" that tells the cell where to transport them. The destination is often an organelle or the cell membrane; in certain cases, the polypeptide is destined for transport out of the cell. The ticket that communicates the destination of a polypeptide is a **signal sequence** of 15 to 20 or so amino acids at the N-terminal end. The signal sequence is a specialized leader region that helps dictate the mode of transit and the final destination of polypeptides.

First articulated in the early 1970s by Günter Blobel, the **signal hypothesis** proposes that the first 15 to 20 amino acids of many polypeptides contain an "address label" in the form of a signal sequence that designates the protein's destination in the cell. Blobel posited that the signal sequence directs proteins to the endoplasmic reticulum (ER). From there, they are transported to the Golgi apparatus, where they are sorted and secreted to their cellular or extracellular destinations (**Figure 9.18**).

Blobel's signal hypothesis is now a widely accepted model for the identification of the cellular destinations of proteins. In fact, follow-up research has identified the mechanism by which proteins are processed and packaged for export from a cell. While proteins destined to remain in a cell are typically translated at "free" ribosomes (ribosomes that float freely in the cytoplasm), large numbers of ribosomes are attached to the rough endoplasmic reticulum (rough ER) and translate proteins destined for intercellular transport.

9.5 Experiments Deciphered the Genetic Code

A remarkable set of experiments performed over less than 4 years in the early 1960s deciphered the genetic code and opened the way for biologists to understand the molecular processes that convert a messenger RNA nucleotide sequence into a polypeptide. At the time, biologists knew *what* the hereditary material was (DNA), and they knew *what* molecule conveyed the genetic message to ribosomes for translation (mRNA), but they did not know *how* the protein-coding information carried by messenger RNA was deciphered during the assembly of polypeptides. Several questions had to be answered about the structural organization of the genetic code before the code itself could be deciphered. The three most important questions, listed here, are examined in the sections below:

1. Do neighboring codons overlap one another, or is each codon a separate sequence?

2. How many nucleotides make up a messenger RNA codon?

3. Is the polypeptide-coding information of messenger RNA continuous, or is coding information interrupted by gaps?

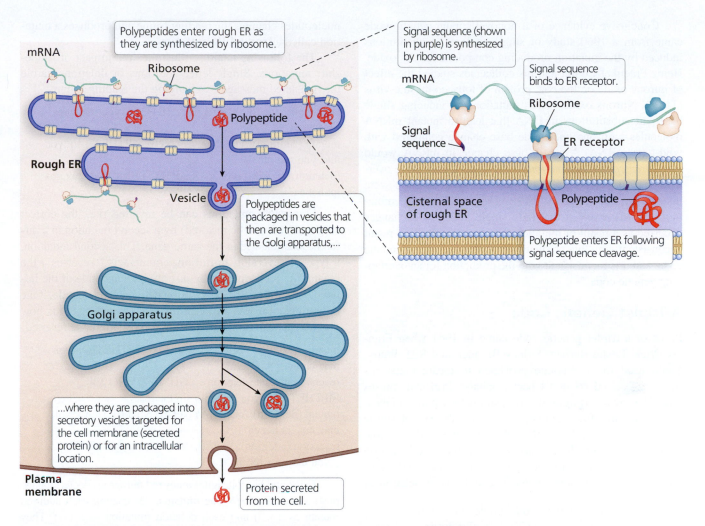

Figure 9.18   Translation at endoplasmic reticulum–bound ribosomes and the signal hypothesis. Translated polypeptides enter the cisternal space through ER receptors to which ribosomes are attached. The cleavage of signal sequences facilitates packaging and transmembrane transport of polypeptides in vesicles.

No Overlap in the Genetic Code

Consider the partial messenger RNA sequence:

...ACUAAG...

In reasoning employed before the genetic code was known (but surmising that a triplet code was most likely), researchers figured that if the genetic code was triplet and nonoverlapping, this sequence could contain at most two complete codons, each specifying an amino acid:

codon	1	2
	...ACU	AAG...
amino acid	1	2

In an overlapping triplet genetic code, on the other hand, these six nucleotides could spell out four complete codons and two partial codons. The sequence would in this case fully encode four amino acids and contribute to the coding of two others:

...ACUAAG...

amino acid	1	ACU
	2	CUA
	3	UAA
	4	AAG
	5	AG...
	6	G...

In 1957, based on his analysis of the available information on amino acid sequences of proteins, Sidney Brenner became convinced that an overlapping triplet genetic code was impossible because it was too restrictive. Brenner identified the amino acid following each lysine in a large number of proteins and found 17 different amino acids in that position. He reasoned that if the overlapping genetic code model were true, only four neighboring amino acids would have been possible. He concluded that an overlapping genetic code restricted evolutionary flexibility and was unsupported by biochemical observations.

Conclusive evidence of a nonoverlapping genetic code came from a 1960 study of single-nucleotide substitutions induced by the mutation-producing compound nitrous oxide. Heinz Fraenkel-Conrat and his colleagues studied the effect of nitrous oxide on the coat protein of tobacco mosaic virus (TMV). Nitrous oxide causes mutations by inducing single base-pair substitutions in DNA that lead to mutant mRNA molecules with one nucleotide base change compared with wild-type mRNA. A single base change in mRNA would alter *three consecutive codons* if the genetic code were overlapping, but just a *single codon* if the genetic code were nonoverlapping (**Figure 9.19**). Fraenkel-Conrat's mutation analysis revealed that only single amino acid changes occurred as a result of mutation by nitrous oxide. This result is consistent with that predicted for a nonoverlapping genetic code, and it is inconsistent with the prediction for an overlapping genetic code.

A Triplet Genetic Code

Proof of a triplet genetic code came in 1961 when Francis Crick, Leslie Barnett, Sidney Brenner, and R. J. Watts-Tobin used the compound proflavin to create mutations in a gene called *rII* in T4 bacteriophage. Proflavin causes mutations by inserting or deleting single base pairs in DNA. Such deletions, for example, lead to the absence of single nucleotides from mRNA, thus changing the reading frame of the mRNA. **Reading frame** refers to the specific codon sequence determined by the point at which the grouping of nucleotides into triplets begins. The addition or deletion of

nucleotides changes the reading frame and produces a mutation called a **frameshift mutation**.

The following analogy illustrates the impact of frameshift mutations. Single-letter additions or deletions garble the translated message by changing the reading frame:

wild-type: YOUMAYNOWSIPTHETEA ("you may now sip the tea")
mutant (addition): YOUMA C YNOWSIPTHETEA ("you mac yno wsi pth ete a")
(deletion): YOUMAYNO | | SIPTHETEA ("you may nos ipt het ea")

Frameshift mutations can be reverted (i.e., the correct reading frame can be restored) by a second mutation in a different location within the same gene. This second mutation, a type of **reversion mutation,** counteracts ("reverses") the reading frame disruption by inserting a nucleotide, if the initial mutation was a deletion, or by deleting a nucleotide, if the initial mutation was an insertion. For example, here is how the two frameshift mutations shown above might be reverted:

mutant (addition): YOUMA C YNOWSIPTHETEA (you mac yno wsi pth ete a)
reversion mutant (deletion): YOUMA C YNO | | SIPTHETEA ("you mac yno sip the tea")
mutant (deletion): YOUMAYNO | | SIPTHETEA ("you may nos ipt het ea")
reversion (addition): YOUMAYNO | | SIP R THE TEA ("you may nos ipr the tea")

Crick and his colleagues analyzed numerous bacteriophage proflavin-induced *rII*-gene mutants, designating each addition mutant as a (+) and each deletion mutation as a (−). They *guessed* that the first *rII*-gene mutant they examined, a mutation designated FC 0, resulted from insertion ("FC" stands for Francis Crick). Designating FC 0 as a (+) mutation turned out to be a correct guess. Based on their assumptions that (1) the genetic code is a nonoverlapping triplet and (2) FC 0 is an insertion, or (+), mutation, the data reported by Crick and colleagues supported the notion of a triplet genetic code by showing that the presence of one or two (+) or one or two (−) mutations disrupts the reading frame but that the reading frame is restored by the presence of *three* (+) mutations or *three* (−) mutations.

(a) An overlapping genetic code would change three consecutive codons with each base mutation.

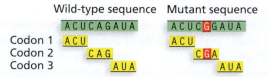

	Wild-type sequence	Mutant sequence
	A C U C A G A U A	A C U C G G A U A
Codon 1	A C U	A C U
Codon 2	C U C	C U C
Codon 3	U C A	U C G
Codon 4	C A G	C G G
Codon 5	A G A	G G A
Codon 6	G A U	G A U
Codon 7	A U A	A U A
Codon 8	U A...	U A...

(b) A nonoverlapping genetic code would change one codon with each base mutation.

	Wild-type sequence	Mutant sequence
	A C U C A G A U A	A C U C G G A U A
Codon 1	A C U	A C U
Codon 2	C A G	C G A
Codon 3	A U A	A U A

Figure 9.19 Predictions for the results of mutation of an overlapping and a nonoverlapping genetic code. (a) Wild-type and mutant DNA sequences for an overlapping genetic code. A base-pair substitution mutation is predicted to change three consecutive codons, and therefore three consecutive amino acids. **(b)** Wild-type and mutant DNA for a nonoverlapping genetic code. A base-pair substitution mutation is predicted to change only one amino acid.

No Gaps in the Genetic Code

In their 1961 research, Crick and colleagues also suggested that the genetic code is read as a continuous string of mRNA nucleotides uninterrupted by any kind of gap, space, or pause. If a gap or spacer were present between mRNA codons, the mRNA transcript might be represented as follows (*x* indicates the gap between codons):

YOUxMAYxNOWxSIPxTHExTEAx ("you may now sip the tea")

If the genetic code were structured in some such way, with each codon set off from its neighbors, insertion or deletion of a nucleotide would not cause the kind of frameshift mutation that Crick and colleagues had observed. Instead, insertion or deletion of nucleotides could be expected to alter the affected codon but not the identity of adjoining codons. For example, consider the following insertion mutation, where the separation between codons confines the alteration to a single word:

YOUx,MA T Yx,NOWx,SIPx,THEx,TEAx, ("you ma t y now sip the tea")

Deciphering the Genetic Code

Once it had been established that the genetic code consists of triplets, researchers sprang to the task of establishing which triplets are associated with each amino acid in the process of translation. Marshall Nirenberg and Johann Heinrich Matthaei performed a simple experiment in 1961 that laid the groundwork for later experiments in deciphering the genetic code. Their experimental design was straightforward: Construct synthetic strings of repeating nucleotides, and use an in vitro translation system to translate the sequence into a polypeptide. For example, Nirenberg and Matthaei synthesized an artificial mRNA containing only uracils, known as a poly(U). They devised an in vitro translation system composed of the known cellular components of bacterial translation—ribosomes, charged transfer RNA molecules, and essential translational proteins. Regardless of where translation might begin along the poly(U) mRNA, the only possible codon it contained was UUU. The researchers were therefore hoping to determine which amino acid corresponds to the UUU codon.

Twenty separate in vitro translations of poly(U) mRNA were carried out, each time using a pool of 19 unlabeled amino acids and one amino acid labeled with radioactive carbon (^{14}C). To determine which amino acid is encoded by poly(U) mRNA, Nirenberg and Matthaei used a different radioactive amino acid in each translation. They detected production of a highly radioactive polypeptide after conducting translation in a system containing radioactively labeled phenylalanine (**Figure 9.20**). The radioactive polypeptide was poly-phenylalanine (poly-Phe). Since the only possible triplet codon in the mRNA was UUU, Nirenberg and Matthaei reasoned that 5'-UUU-3' codes for phenylalanine. They went on to construct poly(A), poly(C), and poly(G) synthetic mRNAs and identified 5'-AAA-3' as a codon for lysine (Lys), 5'-CCC-3' as a proline (Pro) codon, and 5'-GGG-3' as a codon for glycine (Gly) (**Table 9.8**).

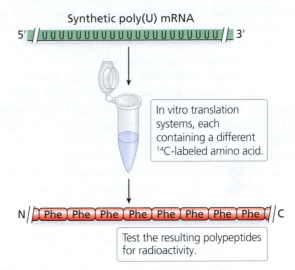

Figure 9.20 Use of synthetic mRNAs to determine genetic code possibilities. Synthetic poly(U) mRNA, forming only UUU codons, is translated in vitro in a series of experiments, each using a different ^{14}C-labeled amino acid—in this example, phenylalanine. A polypeptide consisting of phenylalanine (Phe) is formed.

Table 9.8	Examples of Polypeptide Production from Synthetic mRNAs		
Synthetic mRNA	**mRNA Sequence**	**Polypeptides Synthesized**	**Observation**
Repeating nucleotides	Poly-U UUUU...	Phe-Phe-Phe...	Polypeptides have one amino acid.
	Poly-C CCCC...	Pro-Pro-Pro...	
Repeating dinucleotides	Poly-UC UCUC...	Ser-Leu-Ser-Leu...	Polypeptides have two alternating amino acids.
	Poly-AG AGAG...	Arg-Glu-Arg-Glu...	
Repeating trinucleotides	Poly-UUC UUCUUCUUC...	Phe-Phe...; and Ser-Ser...; and Leu-Leu...	Three polypeptides have one amino acid each.
	Poly-AAG AAGAAGAAG...	Lys-Lys...; and Arg-Arg...; and Glu-Glu...	
Repeating tetranucleotides	Poly-UAUC UAUCUAUC...	Tyr-Leu-Ser-Ile-Tyr-Leu-Ser-Ile...	Some polypeptides have four repeating amino acids. Others identify stop codons.
	Poly-GUAA GUAAGUAA...	None (UAA is a stop codon)	

Note: Data adapted from Khorana (1967).

Har Gobind Khorana extended the experimental strategy of Nirenberg and Matthaei by developing methods for synthesizing mRNA molecules that contained di-, tri-, and tetranucleotide repeats. His construction of repeat-sequence mRNAs allowed him to define many additional codons. For example, Khorana used the dinucleotide repeat UC to form a synthetic mRNA with the sequence

$$5'-\text{UCUCUCUCUCUCUCUCUC}-3'$$

This mRNA can be translated in either a reading frame that begins with uracil or a reading frame that begins with cytosine. In both cases, the reading frame produces alternating UCU–CUC codons. Khorana identified the amino acids of the resulting polypeptide and found it contained alternating serine (Ser) and leucine (Leu), but he could not tell which codon corresponded to which amino acid.

When Khorana used mRNA containing trinucleotide repeats, most of these mRNAs produced three different polypeptides that each consisted of only one kind of amino acid. For example, the reading frame for poly-UUC can begin with either of the uracils or with cytosine. Messenger RNA is read as consecutive UUC codons if the first uracil initiates the reading frame, as UCU if the second uracil begins the reading frame, or as CUU if cytosine is at the start of the reading frame. Although the different reading frames each produced a polypeptide containing one amino acid, Khorana was again unsure which codon specified which amino acid.

Nirenberg and Philip Leder contributed the final piece of the genetic code puzzle in 1964, when they devised an experiment to resolve the ambiguities of codon identity remaining from Khorana's experiments. They synthesized many different mini-mRNAs that were each just three nucleotides in length (**Figure 9.21**). The tiny mRNAs were added in separate experiments (using one type of mini-mRNA per experiment) to in vitro translation systems containing ribosomes and also containing 19 unlabeled amino acids and 1 ^{14}C-labeled amino acid that were each attached to the correct tRNA. The mRNA formed a complex with the ribosome and, by codon-anticodon base pairing, with the tRNA carrying the amino acid that corresponded to the codon in the mRNA. Each in vitro mixture was then poured through a filter that captured the large ribosome–mRNA–tRNA complexes but permitted unbound tRNAs to pass through. The filter was subsequently tested to determine if the mRNA had bound a ^{14}C-labeled tRNA. Nirenberg and Leder tested all 64 possible codons and were able to identify codon–amino acid correspondences for the entire genetic code. In addition, they identified the nucleotide composition of the three stop codons, UAA, UAG, and UGA. Try solving Genetic Analysis 9.3 to further test your skill at interpreting the genetic code.

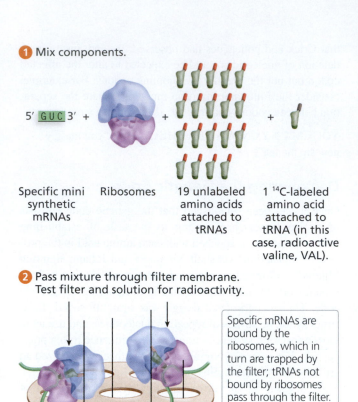

❶ Mix components.

5' GUC 3' +

Specific mini synthetic mRNAs

Ribosomes

19 unlabeled amino acids attached to tRNAs

1 ^{14}C-labeled amino acid attached to tRNA (in this case, radioactive valine, VAL).

❷ Pass mixture through filter membrane. Test filter and solution for radioactivity.

Specific mRNAs are bound by the ribosomes, which in turn are trapped by the filter; tRNAs not bound by ribosomes pass through the filter.

Filter membrane

GUC mRNA binds the tRNA carrying the radioactively labeled amino acid valine. Radioactivity is in the filter.

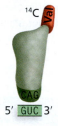

^{14}C Val

CAG

5' GUC 3'

Figure 9.21 Deciphering the genetic code with synthetic mini-mRNAs. A synthetic mini-mRNA GUC is attached to a ribosome and exposed to 19 tRNAs carrying 19 unlabeled amino acids and a ^{14}C-labeled valine (Val) ❶. The ^{14}C-labeled valine tRNA hybridizes to the GUC mini-mRNA within the ribosome ❷. The mRNA–ribosome–tRNA complex is caught by the filter membrane, where radioactivity is detected. The unbound tRNAs wash through the membrane.

? If the same experiment were performed using a 5'-GUC-3' mRNA and radioactively labeled Ser instead of Val, would the radioactivity be found in the filter or would it pass through the filter? Why?

PROBLEM A portion of an mRNA encoding C-terminal amino acids and the stop codon of a wild-type polypeptide is

5'-...CAACUGCCUGACCCACACUUAUCACUAAGUAGCCUAGCAGUCUGA...-3'

BREAK IT DOWN: The mRNA sequence is complementary to the DNA template strand and differs from the DNA coding strand only by having uracil instead of thymine (p. 276).

The wild-type amino acid sequence encoded by this portion of mRNA contains the amino acid Asn encoded by the codon 5'-AAC-3' along with several additional amino acids as shown.

N...Asn-Cys-Leu-Thr-His-Thr-Tyr-His-C

The C-terminal ends of three independently obtained mutant proteins produced by this gene are as follows.

Mutant 1:   N...Asn-Cys-Leu-Thr-His-Thr-C
Mutant 2:   N...Asn-Cys-Leu-Thr-His-Thr-Tyr-His-Lys-C
Mutant 3:   N...Asn-Cys-Leu-Thr-His-Thr-Tyr-His-Tyr-Ser-Ser-Leu-Ala-Val-C

Identify the mutational events that produce each of the mutant proteins.

BREAK IT DOWN: Mutations occur at the level of DNA. Comparison of each mutant DNA and amino acid sequences with the wild-type sequence will reveal how the DNA sequence is changed (p. 241).

Solution Strategies	Solution Steps

Evaluate

1. Identify the topic this problem addresses and the nature of the required answer.

2. Identify the critical information given in the problem.

1. This problem concerns examination of mRNA and comparison of a wild-type protein sequence to sequences of three mutant proteins to determine the alteration producing each mutant. The answers require the identification of specific mRNA sequence changes leading to each mutant protein.

2. In this problem the C-terminal end of a wild-type protein and the mRNA sequence that encodes it are given. Also given are the C-terminal sequences of three mutant proteins encoded by mutant mRNA sequences derived by alteration of the wild-type sequence.

Deduce

3. Use the genetic code to identify the codons corresponding to the wild-type amino acids and to identify the stop codon.

4. Compare each mutant polypeptide to the wild type and determine which codon contains the mutation.

TIP: Any of three stop codons (UAG, UGA, or UAA) terminates translation immediately after the codon specifying the amino acid at the C terminus of a polypeptide.

3. Two codons, AAC and AAU, encode asparagine (Asn). If we skip the 5'-most nucleotide of the mRNA sequence and begin reading at the A in the second position, the first codon is AAC followed by UGC-CUG-ACC-CAC-ACU-UAU-CAC-UAA. These codons encode the wild-type amino acids, and UAA is the stop codon.

4. Mutant 1—The polypeptide sequence is truncated two amino acids short of the normal stop codon. The Tyr codon (UAU) appears to have changed to a stop codon.

   Mutant 2—The wild-type sequence is extended by the addition of lysine (Lys), indicating that mutation changed the stop codon to a codon specifying Lys and is now followed immediately by a new stop codon.

   Mutant 3—The wild-type sequence is extended by six amino acids. This suggests another mutation affected the stop codon.

Solve

5. Identify the mutation and its consequence for translation in Mutant 1.

6. Identify the mutation and its consequence in Mutant 2.

7. Identify the mutation and its consequence in Mutant 3.

TIP: Examine the wild-type nucleotide sequence at the place where mutation is expected to have occurred, and identify ways in which base substitution, insertion, or deletion could have had the observed effect on the amino acid sequence.

5. Two different base substitutions altering the tyrosine (Tyr) codon UAU to a stop codon could cause Mutant 1. The wild-type UAU codon was most likely altered by base substitution to form either a UAA or a UAG stop codon.

6. Lysine (Lys), which was added to the mutant polypeptide, is encoded by AAA or AAG. Deletion of the U from the wild-type stop codon would produce an AAG codon followed by UAG, a stop codon.

7. Tyrosine, specified by codons UAU and UAC, is found in place of the normal stop codon. This is followed by a serine codon (UCN or AGU/C), rather than the GUA (Val) that follows the "in-frame" stop codon in the wild type. A base-pair insertion that adds a U or a C into the third position of the normal UAA stop codon forms a UAU or a UAC tyrosine (Tyr) codon. The altered reading frame from that point would then read AGU (Ser), followed by AGC (Ser), CUA (Leu), GCA (Ala), GUC (Val), and UGA (stop).

For more practice, see Problems 5, 11, 16, and 32.   Visit the Study Area to access study tools.   **Mastering Genetics**

CASE STUDY

Antibiotics and Translation Interference

We have all taken antibiotics at various times during our lives to counteract a painful or persistent microbial infection. As a result of the efficiency of these compounds, we have experienced rapid relief of symptoms and elimination of the infection. These beneficial effects are accomplished by selective cell death or through blocking cell proliferation. Specifically, the antibiotic either kills microorganisms without harming our own cells in the process or it acts to prevent further microbial cell growth. What is the biochemical basis of antibiotic action? How do antibiotic compounds specifically target microbial cells for destruction?

PROTEIN SYNTHESIS INHIBITION BY ANTIBIOTIC COMPOUNDS You will probably not be surprised to learn that different antibiotics target different aspects of microbe biology. But you may be surprised to learn that many different antibiotics target microbial translation as their mode of action (**Table 9.9**). Familiar antibiotics such as tetracycline, streptomycin, and chloramphenicol target different stages of microbial translation, as

Table 9.9	Antibiotic Inhibitors of Protein Synthesis
Antibiotic	**Inhibitory Action**
Chloramphenicol	Blocks polypeptide formation by inhibiting peptidyl transferase in the 70S ribosome (antibacterial action)
Erythromycin	Blocks translation by binding to 50S subunit and inhibiting polypeptide release (antibacterial action)
Streptomycin	Inhibits translation initiation and causes misreading of mRNA by binding to the 30S subunit (antibacterial action)
Tetracycline	Binds to the 30S subunit and inhibits binding of charged tRNAs (antibacterial action)
Cycloheximide	Blocks polypeptide formation by inhibiting peptidyl transferase activity in the 80S ribosome (antieukaryote action)
Puromycin	Causes premature termination of translation by acting as an analog of charged tRNA (antibacterial and antieukaryote action)

do less familiar antibiotics such as erythromycin, puromycin, and cycloheximide. Each antibiotic contains a different active compound that takes advantage of unique features of bacterial translation to disrupt the production of bacterial proteins while not interfering with the translation of proteins in our cells.

TRANSLATION DISRUPTION BY AMINOGLYCOSIDES *Streptomycin* is one of several antibiotics in a class of biochemical compounds called *aminoglycosides*. Streptomycin inhibits bacterial translation by interfering with binding of N-formylmethionine tRNA to the ribosome, thus preventing the initiation of translation. Streptomycin can also cause misreading of mRNA during translation by generating mispairing between codons and anticodons. For example, the codon UUU normally specifies phenylalanine, but streptomycin induces pairing between a UUU codon and the tRNA carrying isoleucine, whose codon is AUU. This error leads to amino acid changes in proteins and potentially to defective protein activity. Other aminoglycosides, such as neomycin, kanamycin, and gentamicin, also cause mispairing between codons and anticodons and can generate defective proteins. *Erythromycin* also impairs bacterial translation, but it does so in a very different way. It binds to the 50S (large) subunit in the tunnel from which the newly synthesized polypeptide emerges. The effect of its binding is to block the polypeptide from passing out of the ribosome. This causes the ribosome to stall on mRNA, bringing translation to a halt. Table 9.9 provides details about these and other actions of antibacterial agents.

TRANSLATION BLOCKAGE BY ANTIFUNGAL COMPOUNDS Single-celled eukaryotic microorganisms, such as fungi, can also cause human infections. To fight these infections, antibiotics such as *puromycin* and cycloheximide, which target translational activities of fungal cells, are used. Puromycin has a three-dimensional structure similar to that of the 3′ end of a charged tRNA. It stops translation of bacterial and eukaryotic mRNAs by binding at the ribosomal A site and acting as an analog of charged tRNA. When puromycin is bound at the A site, its amino group forms a peptide bond with the carboxyl group of the P-site amino acid. However, puromycin does not contain a carboxyl group. This difference prevents formation of any additional peptide bonds and puts an end to translation. *Cycloheximide* exclusively blocks fungal translation by binding to the 60S subunit and inhibiting peptidyl transferase activity, much like chloramphenicol does to bacterial peptidyl transferase (see Table 9.9).

SUMMARY   Mastering Genetics   For activities, animations, and review quizzes, go to the Study Area.

9.1 Polypeptides Are Amino Acid Chains That Are Assembled at Ribosomes

- Polypeptides contain 20 kinds of amino acids that carry side chains, giving them specific properties.
- Translation takes place at the ribosome, where mRNA codons are coupled to transfer RNA anticodons by complementary base pairing.

- Polypeptides have four structural levels: the amino acid order (primary), intrachain folding (secondary), three-dimensional functional folding (tertiary), and multimeric protein structure (quaternary).
- Polypeptides have an N-terminal (amino) end and a C-terminal (carboxyl) end.
- Ribosomes are composed of two subunits that each consist of ribosomal RNA and numerous proteins.

- Ribosomes have three functional sites of action: the P site, where the polypeptide is held; the A site, where tRNA molecules bind to add their amino acid to the end of the polypeptide; and the E site, which provides an exit point for uncharged tRNAs.

9.2 Translation Occurs in Three Phases

- Bacterial translation is initiated with the binding of the Shine–Dalgarno sequence on the 5′ mRNA end to a complementary sequence of nucleotides on the 3′ end of the 16S rRNA in the small ribosomal subunit. The nearby start codon is the site where translation commences.

- In eukaryotic mRNA, the 5′ cap is the binding site for eukaryotic initiation factors that cause the small ribosomal subunit to begin scanning in search of the start codon, which is part of the Kozak sequence.

- Archaea carry multiple translation-initiation factors that are homologous to eukaryotic initiation factors, but archaea also produce a high proportion of leaderless mRNAs that have an unknown translation-initiation mechanism.

- During polypeptide synthesis, charged tRNAs enter the A site, and peptidyl transferase catalyzes peptide bond formation, transferring the polypeptide from the A-site tRNA to the P-site tRNA. Elongation factor proteins translocate the ribosome, shifting the tRNA–polypeptide complex from the A site to the P site and opening the A site for the next charged tRNA.

- Translation terminates when a stop codon enters the A site. Release factor proteins, rather than tRNA, bind to stop codons. Release factors cause release of the polypeptide and lead to the dissociation of the ribosome from mRNA.

9.3 Translation Is Fast and Efficient

- An mRNA undergoes simultaneous translation by several ribosomes that attach to it sequentially to form a polyribosome.

- Usually, a ribosome will dissociate from mRNA upon encountering a stop codon, but the small size of some

intercistronic spacers in bacterial polycistronic mRNAs permits a ribosome to translate two or more polypeptides consecutively from the mRNA before dissociating.

- The evolutionary evidence derived from homologies among translationally active proteins of members of the three domains of life suggests that archaea are more closely related to eukaryotes than they are to bacteria.

9.4 The Genetic Code Translates Messenger RNA into Polypeptide

- Each mRNA codon is composed of three consecutive nucleotides. Of the 64 codons contained in the genetic code, 61 specify amino acids and 3 are stop codons.

- The genetic code is redundant, meaning that most amino acids are specified by more than one codon. Redundancy of the genetic code is made possible by third-base wobble that relaxes the strict complementary base-pairing requirements at the third base of the codon.

- The genetic code is essentially universal among living organisms. The few exceptions to the genetic code are found mainly in mitochondria.

- Properly charged tRNAs play the central role in converting mRNA sequence into polypeptide sequence.

- Specialized enzymes called aminoacyl-tRNA synthetases catalyze the addition of a specific amino acid to each tRNA.

- Proteins in eukaryotic cells are sorted to their cellular destinations by signal sequences at their N-terminal ends. Signal sequences are removed from polypeptides in the ER, where they are sorted for their cellular destinations.

9.5 Experiments Deciphered the Genetic Code

- In vitro experimental analysis demonstrates that the genetic code is triplet and does not contain gaps or overlaps.

- The genetic code was deciphered by analysis of in vitro translation of synthetic messenger RNA.

PREPARING FOR PROBLEM SOLVING

In addition to the list of problem-solving tips and suggestions given here, you can go to the Study Guide and Solutions Manual that accompanies this book for help at solving problems.

1. Know the general structure of genes and the relationships between a gene, its mRNA transcript, and the polypeptide translated from the mRNA. Be able to describe the relative positions of the transcription start, transcription termination, 5′ UTR, 3′ UTR, start codon, and stop codon, and be able to assign polarity to strands of nucleic acids and to identify the N-terminal and C-terminal ends of polypeptides.

2. Be familiar with the genetic code and be able to use it to deduce the primary structure of a polypeptide from an mRNA sequence.

3. Be familiar with amino acid structure and with the four levels of polypeptide structure.

4. Be able to use an amino acid sequence to determine the corresponding mRNA and DNA sequences.

5. Know the general structure of ribosomes and the steps and processes that initiate translation.

6. Be able to describe the steps of polypeptide elongation and the processes that produce polypeptides.

7. Know the similarities and the differences between bacterial and eukaryotic translation.

8. Be prepared to describe mechanisms of posttranslational polypeptide processing.

9. Be familiar with the experimental evidence that deciphered the genetic code.

Chapter Concepts

For answers to selected even-numbered problems, see Appendix: Answers.

1. Some proteins are composed of two or more polypeptides. Suppose the DNA template strand sequence 3'-TACGTAGGCTAACGGAGTAAGCTAACT-5' produces a polypeptide that joins in pairs to form a functional protein.
   a. What is the amino acid sequence of the polypeptide produced from this sequence?
   b. What term is used to identify a functional protein like this one formed when two identical polypeptides join together?

2. In the experiments that deciphered the genetic code, many different synthetic mRNA sequences were tested.
   a. Describe how the codon for phenylalanine was identified.
   b. What was the result of studies of synthetic mRNAs composed exclusively of cytosine?
   c. What result was obtained for synthetic mRNAs containing AG repeats, that is, AGAGAGAG...?
   d. Predict the results of experiments examining GCUA repeats.

3. Several lines of experimental evidence pointed to a triplet genetic code. Identify three pieces of information that supported the triplet hypothesis of genetic code structure.

4. Outline the events that occur during initiation of translation in *E. coli*.

5. A portion of a DNA template strand has the base sequence 5'-...ACGCGATGCGTGATGTATAGAGCT...-3'
   a. Identify the sequence and polarity of the mRNA transcribed from this fragmentary template strand sequence.
   b. Assume the mRNA is written in the correct reading frame. Determine the amino acid sequence encoded by this fragment. Identify the N- and C-terminal directions of the polypeptide.
   c. Which is the third amino acid added to the polypeptide chain?

6. Describe three features of tRNA molecules that lead to their correct charging by tRNA synthetase enzymes.

7. Identify the amino acid carried by tRNAs with the following anticodon sequences.
   a. 5'-UAG-3'
   b. 5'-AAA-3'
   c. 5'-CUC-3'
   d. 5'-AUG-3'
   e. 5'-GAU-3'

8. For each of the anticodon sequences given in the previous problem, identify the other codon sequence to which it could potentially pair using third base wobble.

9. What is the role of codons UAA, UGA, and UAG in translation? What events occur when one of these codons appears at the A site of the ribosome?

10. Compare and contrast the composition and structure of bacterial and eukaryotic ribosomes, identifying at least three features that are the same and three features that are unique to each type of ribosome.

11. Consider translation of the following mRNA sequence:
    5'-...AUGCAGAUCCAUGCCUAUUGA...-3'
    a. Diagram translation at the moment the fourth amino acid is added to the polypeptide chain. Show the ribosome; label its A, P, and E sites; show its direction of movement; and indicate the position and anticodon triplet sequence of tRNAs that are currently interacting with mRNA codons.
    b. What is the anticodon triplet sequence of the next tRNA to interact with mRNA?
    c. What events occur to permit the next tRNA to interact with mRNA?

12. The diagram of a eukaryotic ribosome shown below contains several errors.

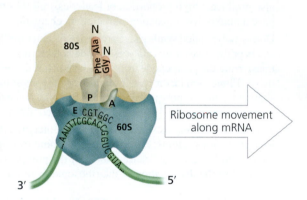

    a. Examine the diagram carefully, and identify each error.
    b. Redraw the diagram, and correct each error using the mRNA sequence shown.

13. Third-base wobble allows some tRNAs to recognize more than one mRNA codon. Based on this chapter's discussion of wobble, what is the *minimal* number of tRNA molecules necessary to recognize the following amino acids?
    a. leucine
    b. arginine
    c. isoleucine
    d. lysine

14. The genetic code contains 61 codons to specify the 20 common amino acids. Many organisms carry fewer than 61 different tRNA genes in their genomes. These genomes take advantage of isoaccepting tRNAs and the rules governing third-base wobble to encode fewer than 61 tRNA genes. Use these rules to calculate the *minimal* number of tRNA genes required to specify all 20 of the common amino acids.

15. The three major forms of RNA (mRNA, tRNA, and rRNA) interact during translation.
    a. Describe the role each form of RNA performs during translation.
    b. Which of the three types of RNA might you expect to be the least stable? Why?
    c. Which form of RNA is least stable in eukaryotes? Why is this form least stable?

d. Compared to the average stability of mRNA in *E. coli*, is mRNA in a typical human cell more stable or less stable? Why?

16. The accompanying figure contains sufficient information to fill in every row. Use the information provided to complete the figure.

DNA

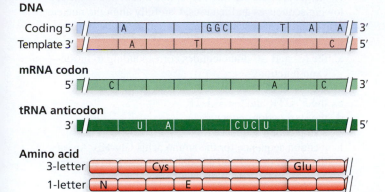

mRNA codon

tRNA anticodon

Amino acid

17. The line below represents a mature eukaryotic mRNA. The accompanying list contains many sequences or structures that are part of eukaryotic mRNA. A few of the items in the list, however, are not found in eukaryotic mRNA. As accurately as you can, show the location, on the line, of the sequences or structures that belong in eukaryotic mRNA; then, separately, list the items that are not part of eukaryotic mRNA.

5' _____ 3'

a. stop codon
b. poly-A tail
c. intron
d. 3' UTR
e. promoter
f. start codon
g. AAUAAA
h. 5' UTR
i. 5' cap
j. termination sequence

18. After completing Problem 17, carefully draw a line below the mRNA to represent its polypeptide product in accurate alignment with the mRNA. Label the N-terminal and C-terminal ends of the polypeptide. Carefully draw two lines above and parallel to the mRNA, and label them "coding strand" and "template strand." Locate the DNA promoter sequence. Identify the locations of the +1 nucleotide and of a transcription termination sequence.

19. Define and describe the differences in the primary, secondary and tertiary structures of a protein.

20. Describe the roles and relationships between
    a. tRNA synthetases and tRNA molecules.
    b. tRNA anticodon sequences and mRNA codon sequences.

Application and Integration

For answers to selected even-numbered problems, see Appendix: Answers.

21. In an experiment to decipher the genetic code, a poly-AC mRNA (ACACACAC...) is synthesized. What pattern of amino acids would appear if this sequence were to be translated by a mechanism that reads the genetic code as
    a. a doublet without overlaps?
    b. a doublet with overlaps?
    c. a triplet without overlaps?
    d. a triplet with overlaps?
    e. a quadruplet without overlaps?
    f. a quadruplet with overlaps?

22. Identify and describe the steps that lead to the secretion of proteins from eukaryotic cells.

23. The amino acid sequence of a portion of a polypeptide is
    N...Cys-Pro-Ala-Met-Gly-His-Lys...C
    a. What is the mRNA sequence encoding this polypeptide fragment? Use N to represent any nucleotide, Pu to represent a purine, and Py to represent a pyrimidine. Label the 5' and 3' ends of the mRNA.
    b. Give the DNA template and coding strand sequences corresponding to the mRNA. Use the N, Pu, and Py symbols as placeholders.

24. Har Gobind Khorana and his colleagues performed numerous experiments translating synthetic mRNAs. In one experiment, an mRNA molecule with a repeating UG dinucleotide sequence was assembled and translated.
    a. Write the sequence of this mRNA and give its polarity.

b. What is the sequence of the resulting polypeptide?
c. How did the polypeptide composition help confirm the triplet nature of the genetic code?
d. If the genetic code were a doublet code instead of a triplet code, how would the result of this experiment be different?
e. If the genetic code was overlapping rather than nonoverlapping, how would the result of this experiment be different?

25. An experiment by Khorana and his colleagues translated a synthetic mRNA containing repeats of the trinucleotide UUG.
    a. How many reading frames are possible in this mRNA?
    b. What is the result obtained from each reading frame?
    c. How does the result of this experiment help confirm the triplet nature of the genetic code?

26. The human β-globin polypeptide contains 146 amino acids. How many mRNA nucleotides are required to encode this polypeptide?

27. The mature mRNA transcribed from the human β-globin gene is considerably longer than the sequence needed to encode the 146–amino acid polypeptide. Give the names of three sequences located on the mature β-globin mRNA but not translated.

28. Figure 9.7 contains several examples of the Shine–Dalgarno sequence. Using the seven Shine–Dalgarno

sequences from *E. coli*, determine the consensus sequence and describe its location relative to the start codon.

29. Figure 9.17 shows three posttranslational steps required to produce the sugar-regulating hormone insulin from the starting polypeptide product preproinsulin.

    a. A research scientist is interested in producing human insulin in the bacterial species *E. coli*. Will the genetic code allow the production of human proteins from bacterial cells? Explain why or why not.

    b. Explain why it is not feasible to insert the entire human insulin gene into *E. coli* and anticipate the production of insulin.

    c. Recombinant human insulin (made by inserting human DNA encoding insulin into *E. coli*) is one of the most widely used recombinant pharmaceutical products in the world. What segments of the human insulin gene are used to create recombinant bacteria that produce human insulin?

30. A DNA sequence encoding a five–amino acid polypeptide is given below.

    ...ACGGCAAGATCCCACCCTAATCAGACCGTACCATTCACCTCCT...
    ...TGCCGTTCTAGGGTGGGATTAGTCTGGCATGGTAAGTGGAGGA...

    a. Locate the sequence encoding the five amino acids of the polypeptide, and identify the template and coding strands of DNA.

    b. Give the sequence and polarity of the mRNA encoding the polypeptide.

    c. Give the polypeptide sequence, and identify the N-terminus and C-terminus.

    d. Assuming the sequence above is a bacterial gene, identify the region encoding the Shine–Dalgarno sequence.

    e. What is the function of the Shine–Dalgarno sequence?

31. A portion of the coding strand of DNA for a gene has the sequence

    5'-...GGAGAGAATGAATCT...-3'

    a. Write out the template DNA strand sequence and polarity as well as the mRNA sequence and polarity for this gene segment.

    b. Assuming the mRNA is in the correct reading frame, write the amino acid sequence of the polypeptide using three-letter abbreviations and, separately, the amino acid sequence using one-letter abbreviations.

32. A eukaryotic mRNA has the following sequence. The 5' cap is indicated in italics (*CAP*), and the 3' poly(A) tail is indicated by italicized adenines.

    5'-*CAP*CCAAGCGUUACAUGUAUGGAGAGAAUGAAACUGAGGCUUG
    CCACGUUUGUUAAGCACCUAUGCUACCG*AAAAAAAAAAAAAAAAA
    AAAAAAA*-3'

    a. Locate the start codon and stop codon in this sequence.

    b. Determine the amino acid sequence of the polypeptide produced from this mRNA. Write the sequence using the three-letter and one-letter abbreviations for amino acids.

33. Diagram a eukaryotic gene containing three exons and two introns, the pre-mRNA and mature mRNA transcript of the gene, and a partial polypeptide that contains the following sequences and features. Carefully align the nucleic acids, and locate each sequence or feature on the appropriate molecule.

    a. the AG and GU dinucleotides corresponding to intron–exon junctions

    b. the +1 nucleotide

    c. the 5' UTR and the 3' UTR

    d. the start codon sequence

    e. a stop codon sequence

    f. a codon sequence for the amino acids Gly-His-Arg at the end of exon 1 and a codon sequence for the amino acids Leu-Trp-Ala at the beginning of exon 2

34. Table C contains DNA-sequence information compiled by Marilyn Kozak (1987). The data consist of the percentage of A, C, G, and T at each position among the 12 nucleotides preceding the start codon in 699 genes from various vertebrate species and at the first nucleotide after the start codon. (The start codon occupies positions +1 to +3, and the first nucleotide immediately after the start codon occupies position +4.) Use the data to determine the consensus sequence for the 13 nucleotides (−12 to −1 and +4) surrounding the start codon in vertebrate genes.

35. Table D lists α-globin and β-globin gene sequences for the 11 or 12 nucleotides preceding the start codon and the first nucleotide following the start codon (see Problem 34). The data are for 16 vertebrate globin genes reported by Kozak (1987). The sequences are written from −12 to +4 with the start codon sequence in capital letters. Use the data in this table to

    a. Determine the consensus sequence for the 16 selected α-globin and β-globin genes.

    b. Compare the consensus sequence for these globin genes to the consensus sequence derived from the larger study of 699 vertebrate genes in Problem 34.

36. The six nucleotides preceding the start codon and the first nucleotide after the start codon in eukaryotes exhibit strong sequence conservation as determined by the percentages of nucleotides in the −6 to −1 positions and the +4 position (see Problem 34). Use the data given in the table for Problem 35 to determine the seven nucleotides that most commonly surround the start in vertebrates.

Table C													
Position	−12	−11	−10	−9	−8	−7	−6	−5	−4	−3	−2	−1	[start] +4
Percent A	23	26	25	23	19	23	17	18	25	61	27	15	[AUG] 23
Percent C	35	35	35	26	39	37	19	39	53	2	49	55	[AUG] 16
Percent G	23	21	22	33	23	20	44	23	15	36	13	21	[AUG] 46
Percent T	19	18	18	18	19	20	20	20	7	1	11	9	[AUG] 15

Table D		

	Gene Sequence				**Gene Sequence**	
	−12	**start +4**			**−12**	**start +4**
α-Globin Family				**β-Globin Family**		
Human adult	agagaacccaccATGg			Human fetal	agtccagacgccATGg	
Human embryonic	caccctgccgccATGt			Human embryonic	aggcctggcatcATGg	
Baboon	ccagcgcgggcATGg			Rabbit adult	aaaccagacagaATGg	
Mouse adult	caggaagaaaccATGg			Rabbit embryonic	agaccagacatcATGg	
Rabbit adult	gaaggaaccaccATGg			Chicken adult	ccaaccgccgccATGg	
Goat embryonic	tcagctgccaccATGt			Chicken embryonic	cccgctgccaccATGg	
Duck adult	ggagctgcaaccATGg			*Xenopus* adult	tcaactttggccATGg	
Chicken embryonic	ctctcctgcacaATGg			*Xenopus* larval	tctacagccaccATGg	

37. In terms of the polycistronic composition of mRNAs and the presence or absence of Shine–Dalgarno sequences, compare and contrast bacterial, archaeal, and eukaryotic mRNAs.

38. Organisms of all three domains of life usually use the mRNA codon AUG as the start codon.

a. Do organisms of the three domains use the same amino acid as the initial amino acid in translation? Identify similarities and differences.

b. Despite AUG being the most common start codon sequence, very few proteins have methionine as the first amino acid. Why is this the case?

Collaboration and Discussion

For answers to selected even-numbered problems, see Appendix: Answers.

39. Answer the following questions about the accompanying diagram.
    a. Is the DNA nearest **A** the template strand or the coding strand?
    b. Which end of the DNA is closest to **A**?
    c. What structure is closest to **B**?
    d. What is the name of the molecule closest to **C**?
    e. Which end of the molecule is closest to **C**?
    f. What structure is closest to **D**? Be specific.
    g. What structure is closest to **E**? Be specific.
    h. What name is given to the object looking like a string of beads that is closest to **F**?
    i. Indicate where fMet is located in the string to the right of **G**.
    j. Which end of the polypeptide is closest to **G**?
    k. What process(es) are illustrated in the diagram?
    l. Does the diagram depict molecular activity in a bacterium or a eukaryote? Explain the reasoning for your answer.

a. 3'−UAC−5'
b. 3'−CCU−5'
c. 3'−AUG−5'

41. Base-substitution mutations often change the amino acid specified by a codon. For each of the amino acid changes listed, determine which ones can result from a one–base-pair substitution. For those that can result from a one–base-pair substitution, give the possible wild-type and mutant codons, listing multiple possibilities if there is more than one option. (Use either Figure 9.13 or the genetic code inside the front cover to help solve this problem).

Wild-type	Mutant
a. Ser	Ala
b. Cys	Ser
c. Pro	Glu
d. Lys	Stop
e. Met	His
f. Met	Ile

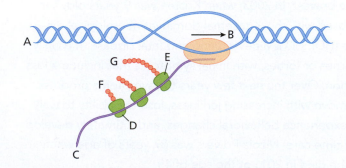

40. For each of the following tRNA anticodon sequences, give the sequence of the corresponding codon sequence, the amino acid carried by the tRNA, and the corresponding DNA coding strand sequence and polarity.

42. For the sequences given in the following list, indicate whether DNA replication, transcription, pre-mRNA processing, or translation will be most immediately affected by deletion of the sequence. As precisely as you can, specify what step of the process is directly affected by the deletion.
    a. start codon
    b. TATA box
    c. 5' splice site
    d. *ori* sequence
    e. −10 consensus sequence
    f. Shine–Dalgarno sequence
    g. 5' cap
    h. termination sequence

Human Genetic Screening

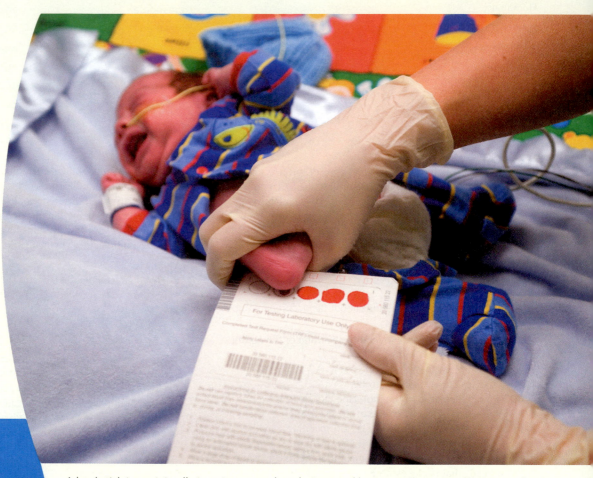

A heel stick is a minimally invasive procedure, being used here to collect a small amount of blood from a newborn infant. The blood is used to screen for disorders on the Recommended Uniform Screening Panel (RUSP) list of human hereditary diseases, as discussed in this chapter.

Kristen Powers is not the most famous graduate of Stanford University, but she is one of the bravest. In 2003, when Kristen was 9 years old, her mother Nicola was diagnosed with the autosomal dominant neurological disorder Huntington disease (HD). HD is a devastating and fatal disease. It usually strikes people in their thirties or forties, with initial symptoms that include a loss of balance and coordination. Over the next few years the symptoms progress. People with the disease move with increasing jerkiness, lose the ability to walk and perform daily tasks, experience behavioral changes, and ultimately develop dementia and require full-time care. Nicola Powers was 37 years of age when she was diagnosed, and she died in 2011 at the age of 45.

Nicola had not known that HD ran in her family. She had lost touch with her biological father after her parents' divorce and did not find out he had HD until after her own diagnosis. By then, Kristen and her younger brother Nate had been born, and they each had a 50% chance of having the disease.

The gene that is mutated in HD is on chromosome 4. Called *huntingtin*, it was cloned in the early 1990s, and the mutation was identified. A few years later, a genetic test for the mutant allele was developed. Kristen, like all those who live with the possibility of having inherited this fatal disease, had the option of undergoing genetic testing to determine whether or not she inherited the mutation.

The choices surrounding testing for HD are extraordinarily difficult and, whatever the outcome, life-changing. A negative test result means that the mutation is not detected and the person will not develop HD. On the other hand, a positive test result means that the mutation is present, and its presence seals the fate of the carrier; the person tested knows that he or she will develop symptoms. Whether in 1 year, 5 years, 10 years, or 30 years, they will inevitably appear and progress. Certain medications are currently available that may help slow the disease, but there is as yet no cure for HD.

What would you do if you were in Kristen's position? Would you want to know whether or not you inherited a fatal genetic disease? How would having that information affect your life choices, your plans, and your family? Kristen faced all these questions and many others as an adolescent watching her mother's condition worsen, but she decided in her early teenage years that she wanted to be tested. At about the same time she decided she wanted to make a documentary film about her choice, her test results, and the aftermath of testing.

North Carolina, where Kristen lived, is like all states in requiring a person to be at least 18 years old before being tested for HD. From the time of her decision until she turned 18, however, Kristen raised funds and began making her documentary, which she titled *Twitch*. Prior to undergoing genetic testing, she met with behavioral counselors, genetic counselors, and medical professionals at the University of North Carolina to help prepare her for the test and the test results. She also talked extensively with her family. Her father, stepmother, and brother were supportive of her choice but apprehensive. They realized, among other things, that whatever Kristen's genetic fate might be, it would have no impact on the genetic fate of her brother Nate.

Shortly after she turned 18, Kristen decided she was ready. Having no plans to keep her results a secret, she arranged to have a film crew at the genetic counseling session when her results were presented. Her hardest decision, she said, was whether or not to have her father in the room. She had never seen him cry, and although she knew she could take the news of a positive result, she wasn't sure she wanted to get a positive result and then watch her father cry.

In May 2012, about 2 weeks after her DNA was collected for the test, Kristen, who was already packing to move west to attend Stanford University in the fall, returned to the University of North Carolina with her father, stepmother, and brother. The first thing her genetic counselor said when she stepped into the room was, "Kristen, I have some good news for you."

Kristen does not carry the HD gene mutation. Neither does her brother Nate, who also decided to be tested when he turned 18. That means neither of them will get the disease and neither of them will pass the disease to their children.

The odds worked out for Kristen and for Nate, but that's not always the case. Kristen graduated from Stanford University in 2016, and she finished *Twitch*. The documentary is about HD, her mother's disease progression, Kristen's decision making regarding testing, the consequences of her test result, and the stigma and trauma of HD. See it, if you can. It carries an important message we should all hear. You can go to http://www.twitchdocumentary.com to read Kristen's story and gain access to *Twitch*.

Genetic testing of the kind Kristen underwent for the HD mutation is called **presymptomatic genetic testing**. As in Kristen's case, the goal is to determine whether or not a person carries a mutation that will cause disease in the future. This kind of genetic testing is only one of several we describe in this Application Chapter, and there are just a few genetic diseases for which it can be done. A more common kind of genetic testing that we describe here is **carrier genetic testing**, also called **genetic carrier screening**, used to determine if a person is a heterozygous carrier of a recessive allele that can cause disease in a homozygous recessive genotype. Another, nearly ubiquitous form of genetic testing is **newborn genetic screening**, which you probably underwent when you were born. As described in Application Chapter A, it is mandated in all 50 U.S. states and in many other countries around the world. It is really a set of three dozen or more tests that screen newborn infants for rare genetic diseases that can be treated if they are identified at birth. **Prenatal genetic testing**, a fourth category of genetic testing, is done to identify inherited diseases, detect chromosome abnormalities, and identify skeletal or developmental abnormalities. A fifth category, **preimplantation genetic screening**, is performed under very specific and limited circumstances. It is used to check for hereditary diseases in fertilized embryos generated by in vitro fertilization. Finally, the most recent entrant in the genetic testing arena is **direct-to-consumer genetic testing**. This category is made up of different tests offered by for-profit companies that either duplicate genetic carrier testing available in a medical setting or provide information about the inheritance of genetic markers that are associated with, but do not cause, certain hereditary conditions. One kind of genetic testing we don't discuss here, but do discuss in Application Chapter C: The Genetics of Cancer, is genetic testing for mutations that increase a person's chances of developing cancer.

B.1 Presymptomatic Diagnosis of Huntington's Disease

Kristen Powers's case highlights the significance of presymptomatic genetic testing for individuals who may have inherited a disease like HD. The ability to extract predictive power from inherited genetic variation is attributable to decades of advances in gene mapping and genetic analysis, and increasingly, to genome sequencing. One broad goal of physicians

and human biologists is to provide personal genomic information to everyone, enabling each of us to make more informed decisions about the most effective ways to prevent and manage certain diseases. It is likely that within the lifetime of the typical college student reading this book, human genetic science will reach a point at which one's personal genome will routinely be a part of one's medical record.

What human genetics and human medicine can do now, however, is make use of numerous available forms of molecular genetic analysis for the detection of mutations causing certain diseases. In this section, we examine the use of PCR and DNA sequencing analysis (see Section 7.5 for discussions of these methods) in presymptomatic identification of the gene mutation causing Huntington disease (OMIM 143100). The gene, abbreviated *HD*, encodes the huntingtin protein that is expressed in brain cells and in other cells of the body. The normal function of wild-type huntingtin is not known, but it interacts with dozens of other proteins. In mutant form, huntingtin appears to aggregate with itself and other proteins, hastening the death of neurons in the brain that lead to the progressive loss of motor control—the unintentional and uncontrollable movement known as chorea—that is characteristic of the disease.

Trinucleotide Repeat Expansion

Huntington disease is one of several human diseases that are caused by a type of mutation known as trinucleotide repeat expansions. We discuss this category of mutation in Section 11.2. The *HD* gene normally has a variable number of CAG repeats in the DNA sequence of the gene. Up to 34 end-to-end repeats of the CAG DNA triplet can be part of an *HD* allele with wild-type function. This repeating string encodes glutamine amino acids as part of the huntingtin protein. Variation in CAG repeat number is due to the fact that repeating DNA sequences are hotspots of mutation. Replication errors can lead to increases or to decreases in the number of CAG repeats. If the length of the repetitive CAG sequence is increased beyond 34 repeats, the unstable huntingtin protein they produce functions abnormally and can result in Huntington disease.

Detecting the Number of Repeats

Initially, DNA sequencing methods were used for identifying the CAG triplet repeat expansions of mutant *HD* genes. **Figure B.1** shows dideoxy DNA sequencing analysis of the

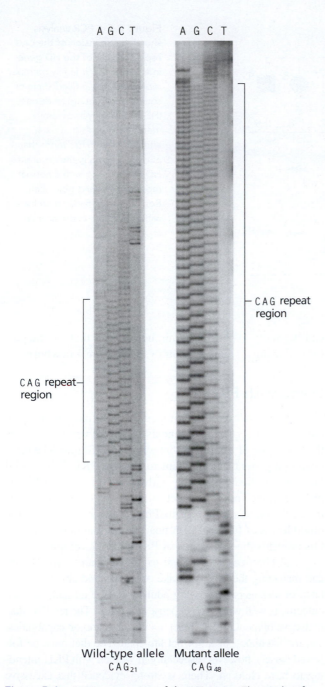

Figure B.1   **DNA sequencing of the *HD* gene.** The results of DNA sequencing show a wild-type *HD* allele with 21 CAG repeats and a mutant *HD* allele with 48 CAG repeats. The mutant allele causes Huntington disease (HD).

CAG repeat segment of the *HD* gene for a wild-type allele with 21 CAG repeats and for a mutant allele with 48 CAG repeats.

The polymerase chain reaction provides an improved way of visualizing the CAG triplet repeat expansion and of following the transmission of alleles in the families of people with HD. Employing primers that bind on opposite sides of the CAG repeat region, researchers amplify fragments of DNA by PCR and separate them by gel electrophoresis. The binding sites of the PCR primers are identical for all alleles, but

differences are seen in the lengths of amplified PCR products because of different numbers of CAG repeats between the primer-binding sites. Amplified DNA fragments containing the primers are shorter if they are generated from wild-type DNA sequences than from mutant alleles, because wild-type alleles have a smaller number of repeats than do mutant alleles. In the Huntington disease family shown in **Figure B.2**, each person with HD is heterozygous and carries one wild-type allele with fewer than 35 repeats of the CAG sequence and one expanded allele with more than 35 repeats. In contrast, family members shown here who do not have HD carry two alleles that each contain fewer than 35 CAG repeats.

B.2 Newborn Genetic Screening

You likely did not know that virtually all infants born in the United States or in one of many other countries within the past two decades have undergone genetic screening in their first days of life for three dozen or more hereditary diseases. You were likely one of these infants, and your parents may not have even been aware (and may not now know) that you were tested. The fact that you would be tested was disclosed to them, but in the rush of activity around your birth, they may not have noticed the testing taking place. No results would have been reported to them unless there was a positive finding that required follow-up or additional testing. Newborn genetic screening represents what many hope is just the beginning of a comprehensive approach to understanding and managing human health, wellness, and disease in the genomics era. New molecular tools will continue to improve our understanding of human genetics and will lead to new and more effective treatments for hereditary conditions. You can read more about newborn genetic screening in the context of genetic counseling in Application Chapter A: Human Hereditary Disease and Genetic Counseling.

Phenylketonuria and the First Newborn Genetic Test

The first human genetic disease for which newborn screening was approved for widespread use was phenylketonuria (PKU). PKU is an autosomal recessive condition caused by the absence of an enzyme called phenylalanine hydroxylase (PAH) that converts the amino acid phenylalanine (Phe) into another amino acid, tyrosine (Tyr). Phe is ingested as protein in the diet, and PKU is one of several genetic conditions that result from mutations in the complex biochemical pathway extending from Phe ingestion (see Section 4.3 and Figure 4.17b). In PKU, there is an excessive buildup of Phe and of a normally rare by-product called phenylpyruvic acid (PPA). The combination of these two compounds is toxic to developing cells of the nervous system. Infants with PKU are healthy at birth (in the absence of other problems) and develop normally for a few months. But starting at about 6 months of age, development begins to slow; then it stops,

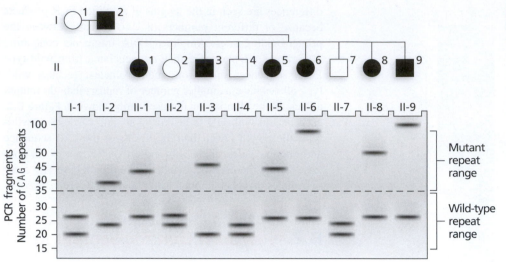

Figure B.2 PCR analysis showing expansion of the CAG repeat region of the *HD* gene in a family. Each family member represented by a filled circle or square has Huntington disease (HD). PCR analysis of family members reveals that each affected person has more than 35 CAG repeats in their mutant *HD* allele, along with a normal repeat-range wild-type allele. Both alleles of family members without HD are in the normal repeat range.

and soon the infant is experiencing permanent mental and developmental impairment. Prior to the availability of treatment, PKU was the cause of thousands of cases of profound mental incapacity annually around the world.

Fortunately, discovery of the abnormality in Phe metabolism led directly to creation of a disease management protocol able to prevent the development of PKU symptoms. Understanding of the abnormality also led Robert Guthrie to develop a newborn test for PKU. The **Guthrie test**, as it was known, was a simple, inexpensive procedure that accurately identified newborn infants with PKU, using just a few drops of their blood obtained from a "heel stick" (see the chapter opener photo). A heel stick is done using a small sterile lance to puncture the skin on the heel of the foot (where very few nerve endings are located), drawing a small amount of blood. Heel sticks are performed in the first few hours after birth, and they are the principal way material is collected for newborn genetic screening.

The original Guthrie test involved an examination of bacterial growth on a Petri dish. A positive Guthrie test, indicating possible PKU, was identified by bacterial growth in the presence of a few drops of the infant's blood along with a compound that normally inhibits bacterial growth. The excessive level of Phe in an affected infant's blood allowed abnormal bacterial growth to occur.

Today, the newborn test for PKU is done using mass spectrometry (MS). MS is an analytical chemistry technique that ionizes a test substance and then measures the abundance of specific gas ions that are released. MS is particularly useful for identifying the composition of proteins, nucleic acids, and other organic chemical compounds. An MS analysis of a newborn infant's blood sample can identify scores of proteins in the blood, as well as the concentrations of other compounds, including amino acids such as Phe. MS can complete numerous chemical analyses of heel stick blood in a matter of minutes. This substantially cuts the time and expense required by the Guthrie test,

and it greatly expands the number of tests that can be performed using a small amount of blood from a newborn.

Living with PKU

A positive result for PKU immediately initiates an array of other tests to verify the diagnosis, followed within hours by the beginning of treatment that will last a lifetime. The principal component of treatment to prevent PKU is a special low-protein diet, beginning with an infant formula that is phenylalanine-free. This diet, along with regular monitoring of the child's blood for its Phe concentration, keeps the blood levels of Phe and PPA near the normal ranges. Doing this prevents the symptoms of PKU from developing.

The Phe-free diet is more expensive than a typical diet, and managing the dietary intake of infants and children—and later, of teenagers and young adults—can be difficult; but the outcome is well worth the expense and effort. The result is normal development, fully intact mental and motor capabilities, and the likelihood of a normal life span. The diet must be followed closely, however; especially in women with PKU intending to have children. There is strong evidence that excessive levels of Phe in their blood circulation are a risk factor for birth defects in their children. Moreover, there is evidence of significant declines in mental capacity in people with PKU when their blood Phe levels have been persistently high for an extended period of time.

There are also a number of dietary traps to be avoided by those with PKU. One of the most common dietary pitfalls is the artificial sweetener known as aspartame, an ingredient of NutraSweet and many other "sugar-free" products (**Figure B.3**). This compound is manufactured by linking together two amino acids, aspartic acid and phenylalanine. On ingestion, the aspartame is broken down and Phe is released. Occasional exposures to the artificial sweetener are not serious, but persistent intake can lead

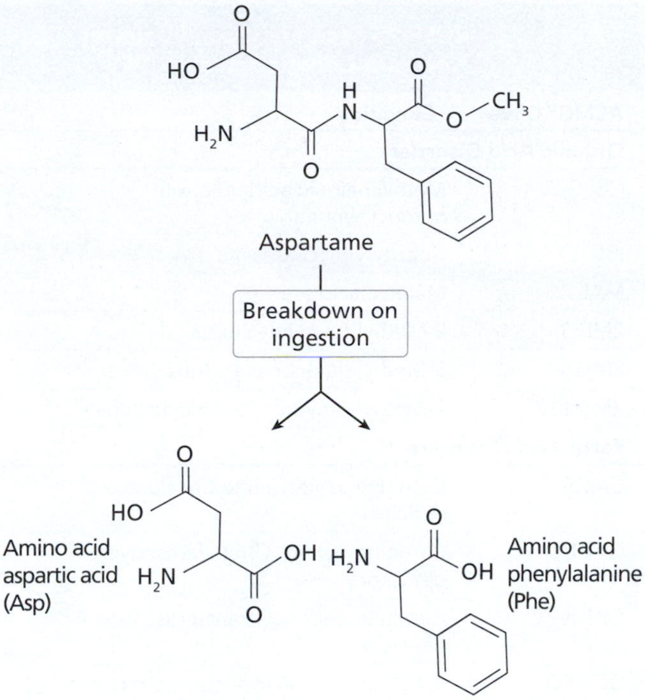

Aspartame

Breakdown on ingestion

Amino acid aspartic acid (Asp)

Amino acid phenylalanine (Phe)

Figure B.3   Aspartame. This artificial sweetener aspartame (found in sugar substitutes like NutraSweet) is composed of two amino acids—aspartic acid (Asp) and phenylalanine (Phe). After consumption, the breakdown of the sweetener releases both amino acids. Phe is the compound to be avoided by people with phenylketonuria; thus aspartame poses a danger to these individuals.

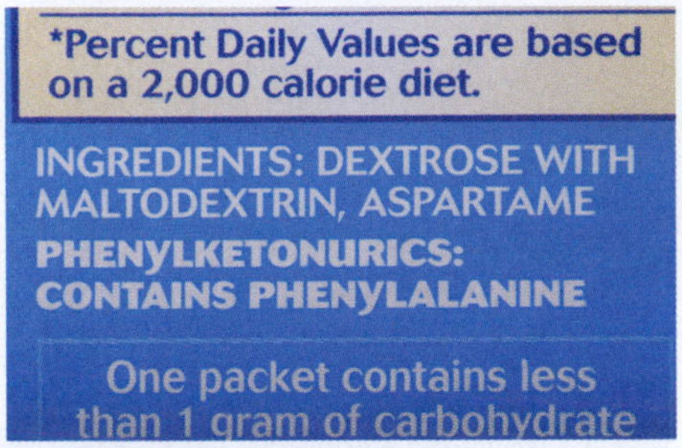

Figure B.4   An aspartame warning label. The danger of Phe to people with phenylketonuria has prompted the U.S. Food and Drug Administration and similar agencies in other countries to require warning labels on all products containing aspartame.

to serious complications of the disease. For this reason, all food and beverage products containing this artificial sweetener carry a warning label to phenylketonurics (**Figure B.4**).

Years ago those with PKU were doomed to suffer from severe mental impairment and numerous other problems that led to short lives of complete dependency. Today, newborn detection of PKU and a specialized diet means that people with the condition can avoid these impairments and are just as likely as anyone else to be honors students. It is estimated that worldwide since the 1960s, more than 50,000 babies born with PKU have gone on to develop normal cognitive ability thanks to newborn genetic testing and the special diet. Two organizations, the National PKU Alliance (npkua. org) and National PKU News (pkunews.org), provide support and information for people with phenylketonuria, their families, and their friends.

The Recommended Uniform Screening Panel

Apart from the success of the Guthrie test and the Phe-free diet that prevents PKU, advances in newborn genetic screening occurred slowly at first. By 1999, just five disorders

could be screened in newborn infants, and states were slow to mandate the available tests. But in that year, the U.S. Department of Health and Human Services (HHS) set up advisory panels to search out additional testable and treatable genetic diseases and to make recommendations to the secretary of HHS for newborn genetic testing. In 2003, the HHS secretary's Advisory Committee on Heritable Disorders in Newborns and Children established a list of genetic diseases recommended for such testing: the **Recommended Uniform Screening Panel (RUSP)**. As a consequence, by 2007, all U.S. states provided newborn genetic screening for 25 disorders. As of November 2016, the American College of Medical Genetics lists 34 "core" hereditary conditions on the RUSP list (**Table B.1**). These are recommended for screening by all states, and nearly all states test for all of these core conditions. There are an additional 25 "secondary" conditions for states to consider for inclusion on their test list (**Table B.2**).

There are two principal criteria for placement of a genetic disease on these RUSP lists. First, the disease must be reliably detected in newborn infants, and second, the disease must either be preventable or its symptoms and prognosis must be substantially improved with treatment. Many of the disorders currently on these lists are metabolic disorders of organic acid, fatty acid, or amino acid production or breakdown. They are caused by the absence or severely reduced action of single proteins. Like PKU (in Table B.1) or argininemia (ARG; in Table B.2 and described in Application Chapter A), these conditions are often treated with dietary restrictions and drug therapy. Hemoglobin disorders are generally treated with drug therapy and blood transfusions. Endocrine and other disorders are commonly treated by drug therapy, dietary restrictions, or other interventions.

Most of the diseases on the RUSP list are rare, occurring in just a few of every 25,000 to 100,000 infants born. Yet despite their individual rarity, their combined frequency is high enough that newborn genetic screening is estimated to save or improve the lives of approximately 12,000

Table B.1	RUSP 34 Core Conditions for Newborn Genetic Screening[a]
ACMG[b] Code	**Condition**
Organic Acid Disorders	
CblA, CblB	Methylmalonic acidemia (cobalamin disorders)
GA1	Glutaric acidemia type 1
HMG	3-Hydroxyl-3-methylglutaric aciduria
IVA	Isovaleric acidemia
MCD	Holocarboxylase synthase deficiency
MUT	Methylmalonic acidemia (methylmalonyl-CoA mutase)
PROP	Propionic acidemia
βKT	β-Ketothiolase deficiency
3-MCC	3-Methylcrotonyl-CoA carboxylase deficiency
Fatty Acid Disorders	
CUD	Carnitine uptake defect
LCHAD	Long-chain L-3-hydroxylacyl-CoA dehydrogenase deficiency
MCAD	Medium-chain acyl-CoA dehydrogenase deficiency
TFP	Trifunctional protein deficiency
VLCAD	Very long-chain acyl-CoA dehydrogenase deficiency
Amino Acid Disorders	
ASA	Argininosuccinic aciduria
CIT	Citrullinemia type 1
HCY	Homocystinuria
MSUD	Maple sugar urine disease
PKU	Phenylketonuria
TYR 1	Tyrosinemia type 1
Endocrine Disorders	
CAH	Congenital adrenal hyperplasia
CH	Primary congenital hyperthyroidism
Hemoglobin Disorders	
Hb SC	Hemoglobin SC disease
Hb SS	Hemoglobin SS disease (sickle cell disease)
Hb SβTh	Hemoglobin S, beta-thalassemia disease
Other Disorders	
BIOT	Biotinidase deficiency
CCHD	Critical congenital heart disease
CF	Cystic fibrosis
GALT	Galactosemia
GSD II	Glycogen storage disease type II
HEAR	Hearing loss
MPS 1	Mucopolysaccharidosis type 1
SCID	Severe combined immunodeficiency
X-ALD	X-linked adrenoleukodystrophy

[a] As of November 2016.
[b] American College of Medical Genetics and Genomics.

Table B.2	RUSP 25 Secondary Conditions for Newborn Genetic Screening[a]
ACMG[b] Code	**Condition**
Organic Acid Disorder	
Cbl C, D	Methylmalonic acidemia with homocystinuria
IBG	Isobutyrylglycinuria
MAL	Malonic aciduria
2MBG	2-Methylbutyrylglycinuria
3MGA	3-Methylglutaconic aciduria
2M3HBA	2-Methyl-3-hydroxybutyric aciduria
Fatty Acid Disorders	
CACT	Carnitine acylcarnitine translocase deficiency
CPT IA	Carnitine palmitoyltransferase type 1 deficiency
CPT II	Carnitine palmitoyltransferase type II deficiency
DE RED	2,4-Dienoyl-CoA reductase deficiency
GA2	Glutaric acidemia type II
MCAT	Medium-chain ketoacyl-CoA thiolase deficiency
M/SCHAD	Medium/short-chain L-3-hydroxylacyl-CoA reductase deficiency
SCAD	Short-chain acyl-CoA dehydrogenase deficiency
Amino Acid Disorders	
ARG	Argininemia
BIOPT (BS)	Biopterin defect in cofactor biosynthesis
BIOPT (REG)	Biopterin defect in cofactor regeneration
CIT II	Citrullinemia type II
H-PHE	Benign hyperphenylalaninemia
MET	Hypermethioninemia
TYR II	Tyrosinemia type II
TYR III	Tyrosinemia type III
Hemoglobin Disorders	
Var Hb	Various hemoglobinopathies
Other Disorders	
GALE	Galactoepimerase deficiency
GALK	Galactokinase deficiency T-cell related lymphocyte deficiencies

[a] As of November 2016.
[b] American College of Medical Genetics and Genomics.

infants every year in the United States. Even if detected early, a disease may not be fully preventable, and many of these diseases require costly treatment that may be lifelong. Those costs, however, are far lower than the cost of providing lifelong care to a patient with full-blown disease symptoms. Furthermore, the emotional and other benefits for families may be incalculable. One recent study of the costs, benefits, and impact of newborn genetic screening was conducted in the state of Washington for the 10-year period from 2004, when the state first mandated screening, through 2014. The study found that during this period there was a 20% decrease in infant mortality and a 14% decrease in serious developmental disabilities, and that the cost savings was many times the cost of carrying out the screening program.

You can learn more about the conditions on the RUSP list in your state, and about other hereditary and childhood diseases, at two websites: the HHS-sponsored website http://www.babysfirsttest.org/newborn-screening/states provides details on the RUSP, and the National Institutes of Health-sponsored website for the Eunice Kennedy Shriver Institute for Child Health and Human Development (http://www.nichd.nih.gov) offers details on the effects of RUSP diseases on infants and children.

B.3 Genetic Testing to Identify Carriers

Genetic carrier screening is used to determine the genotypes of adults for the purpose of identifying those who are heterozygous for mutations that cause serious or fatal diseases in children with homozygous recessive genotypes. This type of genetic testing has been in use for three decades and examines either blood proteins or DNA, depending on the genetic condition of interest.

Testing Blood Proteins

The first and most frequently used adult carrier genetic screens examine blood proteins of individuals from populations known to have elevated frequencies of certain mutant alleles and therefore higher numbers of heterozygous carriers. In these carrier genetic screening tests, the heterozygous genotype could be determined by detection of both the wild-type protein product and the mutant protein product in a blood sample. Figure 1.13 shows an example of detection of the heterozygous genotype in a carrier of the recessive allele for sickle cell disease (SCD; OMIM 141900). SCD is one of the conditions examined in carrier screening. It is particularly prevalent among people of African and Mediterranean ancestry. Carrier genetic testing for Tay–Sachs disease (OMIM 272800) and Gaucher disease Type I (OMIM 230800) have been frequent subjects of testing in populations of Ashkenazi Jewish ancestry since the 1990s. The purpose of identifying heterozygotes is so that male and female partners who are both heterozygous for a serious condition will know of their one in four chance of having a child with the condition and can make informed decisions about the pregnancy and care of the newborn infant.

DNA-Based Carrier Screening and Diagnostic Verification

In the past two decades, the direct testing of DNA has become possible. DNA genetic testing allows the direct detection of mutant DNA sequences producing mutant, disease-causing alleles. The purpose of DNA-based genetic testing is twofold. One use is to identify carrier status for conditions that do not have signature protein variation in the blood. The other use is to verify clinical diagnoses by determining that a person suspected of having a particular hereditary condition is homozygous for variant alleles causing the condition. DNA-based genetic testing is often capable of identifying more different disease-causing alleles than is possible with genetic tests of blood-protein variants. Dozens of different hereditary diseases and conditions are detected and diagnosed by the direct examination of DNA.

For example, DNA genetic testing for cystic fibrosis (OMIM 219700), which occurs predominantly in people of Caucasian ancestry, not only can detect the most common disease-causing allele (that produces serious cases of cystic fibrosis and accounts for almost 50 percent of the cystic fibrosis alleles in the population) but also can identify dozens of other mutant alleles of the same gene. Any genotype that contains two mutant copies of the gene will result in cystic fibrosis in a child. Homozygosity for the most common mutant allele produces a severe form of the disease, but either homozygosity for another of the mutations or so-called *compound heterozygosity*, the presence of two different mutant alleles in a genotype, can lead to milder, but still serious, forms of cystic fibrosis. The same is true for many of the diseases detected by DNA analysis. In a clinical setting, this information can have an important impact on patient care and case management. With a disease like cystic fibrosis, cases that are potentially more serious may be more responsive to certain types of care than less serious cases are.

Carrier Screening Criteria

Whether carrier genetic screening is performed by assessment of blood proteins or by DNA testing, there are two different screening strategies that can be followed. The first strategy is a population-based or community-based screening effort. In these instances, members of certain populations in which a particular hereditary disease is prevalent are recruited to participate in carrier testing programs. Carrier testing programs for Tay–Sachs disease and Gaucher disease in Ashkenazi Jewish populations are examples. The participants in these programs are all free of the disease and they might or might not have family members with the disease. The purpose of the genetic screening is to identify individuals who are heterozygous carriers of the disease so that they can use this information for decisions such as family planning. Prospective parents who each know their genotypes will have solid genetic information to use for these purposes.

Alternatively, a woman who is a member of a population in which a certain disease is prevalent but who does not know her genotype can take the second approach to carrier screening. If, for example, a woman in a population in which cystic fibrosis is prevalent intends to have a child, she can have her genotype identified. If she is homozygous for the dominant allele, she has no chance of having a child with cystic fibrosis, and testing goes no further. If, on the other hand, she is a heterozygous carrier of a mutation producing cystic fibrosis, her partner can be tested to determine his genotype. If he is homozygous for the dominant allele, then there is no chance the child will have cystic fibrosis. If he is also a heterozygous carrier, however, then the couple can seek additional medical and genetic services to minimize the chance that a child of theirs could have cystic fibrosis.

Pharmacogenetic Screening

A special category of carrier testing is the developing area of **pharmacogenetic screening** that can be important in guiding drug treatment of disease, as it can predict individual responsiveness or reaction to certain medications. Inherited genetic variation has been shown to influence the effectiveness of, or to increase the likelihood of adverse reactions to, about one dozen commonly used drugs. Among the dozen or so well-documented examples of a genotype–drug influence is the use of the blood thinner warfarin that is often given to help prevent blood clots in heart patients. Proper dosages of warfarin are critical for management of blood-clotting risk. The *CYP2C9* gene (*cytochrome P*) produces an enzyme that metabolizes warfarin. More than 30 alleles of the gene have been identified. Most genotypes metabolize warfarin at the wild-type rate, but individuals who are homozygous for either the *CYP2C9*2* or the *CYP2C9*3* allele, and also those who have a heterozygous genotype involving the two alleles (i.e., *CYP2C9*2/CYP2C9*3*), metabolize warfarin at a significantly lower rate than wild type, and they require a lower drug dose to prevent overdosing.

B.4 Prenatal Genetic Testing

Prenatal genetic testing is the longest-standing category of genetic evaluations, predating the other genetic screening approaches we have described. These analytical and diagnostic methods are used to examine fetuses beginning a few weeks after conception and in some cases until near the term of a pregnancy. Several different methods are used for prenatal genetic screening. Some are invasive, meaning that they involve a small risk of fetal injury or loss, whereas others are noninvasive and carry no risk to the fetus. The various methods are used for different purposes and to identify different kinds of hereditary conditions,

some that cause severe disability to a fetus and some that are fatal.

The abnormalities screened in prenatal genetic testing fall into three categories (Table B.3). The first is chromosomal abnormalities: an extra or a missing chromosome, extra or missing chromosome segments, or structural abnormalities of chromosomes. The most common criteria for recommending prenatal screening of chromosomes are maternal age over 35, a previous child born with a chromosome abnormality, or the presence of a chromosome abnormality in one parent. The second category of conditions examined by prenatal genetic screening is developmental or growth conditions. These include neural tube (spinal cord and brain) abnormalities, bone or skeletal abnormalities, such as osteogenesis imperfecta (brittle bone disease), and stature-dwarfing conditions. A history of any of these conditions in a family or in a prior pregnancy is a common criterion for recommending this screening. The final category of prenatal genetic screening conditions is hereditary disease. Several genetic diseases tested prenatally also appear on the RUSP list for newborn genetic testing. Once again, a family history or a previous child with the condition are common reasons a physician might recommend prenatal screening.

Invasive Screening Using Amniocentesis or Chorionic Villus Sampling

Amniocentesis uses a needle to penetrate the uterus and placenta of a pregnant woman to withdraw 10 to 20 mL (2–3 tablespoons) of amniotic fluid. This fluid contains fetal cells that can be cultured and used for genetic testing

Table B.3	Examples of Conditions Detected by Prenatal Genetic Screening Methods
Type of Condition	**Detection Methods**
Chromosome conditions such as . . .	
Trisomies of 21, 18, or 13	Primarily by amniocentesis or CVS following MSS
Sex chromosome abnormalities	
Structural abnormalities	
Skeletal or developmental conditions such as . . .	
Neural tube defects	Primarily by ultrasound, some are detected by prenatal analysis of DNA following amniocentesis or CVS
Cleft lip and palate	
Osteogenesis imperfecta	
Genetic conditions such as . . .	
Tay–Sachs disease	Detected by preimplantation screening, prenatal biochemical or DNA analysis following amniocentesis or CVS, heterozygous carrier screening, some detected by newborn genetic screening
Cystic fibrosis	
Sickle cell disease	
PKU	

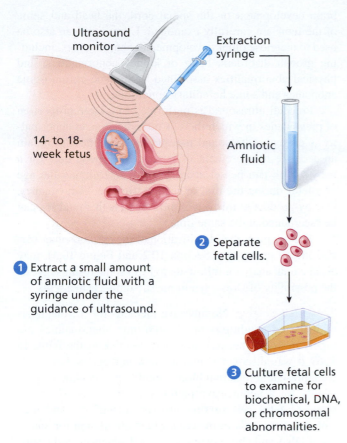

① Extract a small amount of amniotic fluid with a syringe under the guidance of ultrasound.

② Separate fetal cells.

③ Culture fetal cells to examine for biochemical, DNA, or chromosomal abnormalities.

Figure B.5 Amniocentesis. Amniotic fluid contains fetal cells that can be isolated and cultured. The cultured cells can be used for biochemical tests, DNA analysis, or chromosome examination.

or chromosome examination (**Figure B.5**). Amniocentesis is usually an out-patient procedure performed using a local anesthetic and is usually performed between the 14th and 18th week of pregnancy. It carries about a one in 400 risk of fetal loss (spontaneous abortion) or other fetal injury.

Chorionic villus sampling (CVS) uses a small tube passed transvaginally into the uterus to suction off a sample of tissue from the chorion on the outside of the placenta (**Figure B.6**). The chorion is the part of the placenta that is composed of fetal cells. Cells collected by CVS can be cultured and examined for chromosome analysis and genetic testing. CVS can be performed as early as the 10th week of pregnancy, but it appears to carry a slightly higher risk than amniocentesis.

Both amniocentesis and CVS yield fetal cells that can be used for biochemical analysis, DNA analysis, or chromosome analysis. Biochemical tests examine proteins and enzymes to ascertain abnormalities of function or abnormalities of protein levels that indicate genetic disease. DNA analysis examines selected genes, looking for inherited variation producing genetic disease. To examine chromosomes, cells must first be cultured. The cells are then ruptured, and after that the nuclei are deposited and ruptured on microscope slides, allowing the chromosomes to spill out for microscopic examination. A digital photograph is taken of the chromosomes, and the image is rearranged to align the homologous pairs. This manipulated image, called a *karyotype*, allows accurate counting of chromosomes and assessment of their individual structures.

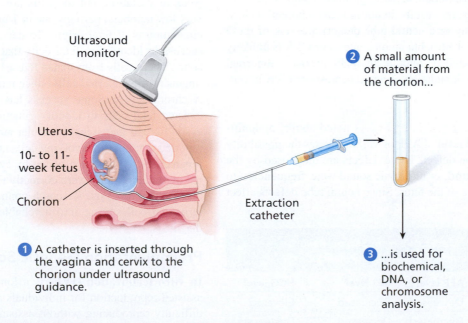

② A small amount of material from the chorion...

① A catheter is inserted through the vagina and cervix to the chorion under ultrasound guidance.

③ ...is used for biochemical, DNA, or chromosome analysis.

Figure B.6 Chorionic villus sampling (CVS). Cells obtained by CVS can be used directly in biochemical tests, DNA analysis, or chromosome examination.

Noninvasive Prenatal Testing

One of the most common reasons a physician might recommend amniocentesis or CVS in a pregnancy has to do with the risk of the numerical chromosome condition called trisomy 21, or Down syndrome. In this condition, the fetus carries three copies of chromosome 21 rather than the normal two copies. The term *trisomy* means "three chromosomes." Maternal age over 35 is strongly linked to an elevated risk of trisomy 21, as we discuss in Section 10.2. Before a recommendation for amniocentesis or CVS is made, however, a noninvasive prenatal test called *maternal serum screening* is usually performed.

Maternal Serum Screening

Maternal serum screening (MSS), also called triple screening, measures the levels of three proteins in a pregnant woman's blood circulation between the 15th and 20th week of gestation. MSS requires nothing more than drawing a small amount of blood from a vein. The three proteins are alpha fetoprotein (AFP), a form of the hormone estriol (uE3), and human chorionic gonadotropin (HCG). The levels of these three proteins are associated with elevated risks of two chromosome trisomy conditions, as **Table B.4** indicates. A significantly elevated level of AFP by itself is an indicator of a possible neural tube defect.

It is important to recognize that MSS, which is used routinely in many obstetric practices, is a *screening test*, not a *diagnostic test*. In other words, MSS results can indicate the increased likelihood of a chromosome trisomy or a neural tube defect, but they do not mean a condition is present. Protein levels detected in MSS are simply associated with these conditions. Should an MSS produce results in the normal ranges (i.e., the results do not indicate a potential chromosome trisomy or a neural tube defect), the risk of these conditions is not zero, but amniocentesis or CVS is unlikely to be recommended. Should an MSS produce abnormal results, a recommendation of amniocentesis or CVS is very likely as a follow up.

Prenatal Ultrasound Imaging As noted above, a significantly elevated level of AFP in MSS indicates the possibility of a neural tube defect. These defects are diagnosed by the use of **ultrasound**, or ultrasonic sound wave frequencies, to produce images of the fetus. Since neural tube defects affect brain development or the spinal cord, the head and spine of the fetus are carefully examined. Ultrasound can also be used to diagnose other developmental abnormalities, including growth disorders, heart or kidney abnormalities, and physical abnormalities associated with some chromosome anomalies and some hereditary conditions.

Prenatal ultrasound is performed in a large proportion of pregnancies in which there is no indication an abnormality is present. Ultrasound may be used routinely to obtain an accurate measurement of fetal age. The due date for a baby's birth can be set accurately by determining the age of a fetus during the first or second trimester of pregnancy. One by-product of this use of ultrasound is that fetal sex can be ascertained at the same time.

Karyotyping, the identification of the chromosomes carried in cell nuclei (see Section 10.2 and Figure 10.4), may also be indicated as a follow-up to MSS if the result suggests the possibility of Down syndrome (trisomy 21) in a fetus.

Fetal Cell Sorting Noninvasive methods for the diagnosis of inherited conditions or chromosome abnormalities are highly desirable because they pose no risk to the fetus. In 1969 it was discovered that a small number of fetal cells were present in maternal blood circulation, opening the possibility for a noninvasive pathway to diagnosis. The technique of **fetal cell sorting** involves identifying and then isolating fetal cells in maternal blood circulation for analysis of DNA and chromosomes. Several advances in the sorting and analysis of fetal cells have been made, but moving from research to reliable application as a clinical technique remains elusive.

Fetal cells, and some fetal DNA from ruptured fetal cells, are present in maternal circulation as early as the 8th week of gestation, but the cells are fragile and present in very low numbers; perhaps one in 1 billion cells in maternal circulation is of fetal origin. To date, there has been some success in identifying fetal cells that contain a Y chromosome. These cells from males fetuses are the easiest to distinguish from maternal cells, since female cells contain only X chromosomes. Some success has also been seen using isolated fetal cells to identify genetic disorders, including cystic fibrosis and spinal muscular atrophy. Studies in 2012 reported that in tests involving cells taken from a number of pregnancies, all fetuses affected by cystic fibrosis or by spinal muscular atrophy were correctly identified using molecular genetic analysis. Research continues in an attempt to turn fetal cell sorting into a reliable method for prenatal diagnosis.

Preimplantation Genetic Screening

In vitro fertilization (IVF) is a long-standing method of assisted reproduction for individuals and couples who have difficulty reproducing without assistance, or choose not to do so. In this method, ovulation is induced in a woman with the aid of hormone injections. A large number of eggs are then removed from the surface of the ovaries. The number

Table B.4	Maternal Serum Screen Results Indicating an Abnormality		
Condition	AFP level	uE3 level	HCG level
Trisomy 21	Decreased	Decreased	Elevated
Trisomy 18	Decreased	Decreased	Decreased
Neural tube defect	Elevated	Not applicable to this condition	

collected depends on the age and fertility of the egg donor. These eggs can either be frozen for later use or used immediately for fertilization by sperm. Following fertilization in a laboratory dish, embryos go through a small number of cell divisions over 3 to 5 days, and they are then ready for implantation into the uterus.

The success rate of IVF for a fertilized embryo varies with the age of the woman into whom the fertilized embryos are implanted, but for all ages it is less than 50%. Women under age 35 have about a 40% success rate. Those who are 35 to 37 have about a 35% success rate. The success rate is about 25% for ages 38 to 40, and it drops to about 15% for women over 40. As a consequence of these low rates, it is common for a woman to have to undergo two or more IVF implantation treatments to attain a successful pregnancy.

IVF was first successfully used to assist human reproduction in 1978. In that year, in England, Louise Brown became the first human IVF baby. IVF was introduced into the United States in 1981 and since that time has resulted in more than one million babies being born. IVF is expensive and not usually covered by medical insurance. Depending on the methods used and on other circumstances, the cost for each IVF cycle is about $12,000–$17,000.

There are numerous reasons for opting for IVF, but one of them is the risk of a genetic disease. The most common situations are those in which either both prospective parents are heterozygous carriers of an autosomal recessive condition or a prospective mother is a carrier of an X-linked recessive condition. In either case, couples may choose IVF in combination with preimplantation genetic screening (PGS) as a way of minimizing the risk of having a child with the condition.

PGS begins with IVF. After in vitro fertilization, embryos are normally allowed to rest for several cycles of mitotic division prior to implantation. Once they reach the 8-cell or the 16-cell stage, one cell can be removed from the embryo without risk of harm. DNA is taken from this single cell, and the segment targeted for genetic analysis is amplified by PCR (polymerase chain reaction). Any embryo that tests positive for the genetic condition will not be used for implantation, whereas those that test negative are known to be free from the condition and will be implanted. To date, thousands of healthy babies have been born subsequent to PGS.

B.5 Direct-to-Consumer Genetic Testing

There is no doubt that the genomics era has provided new opportunities to gain insight on the impact of genomic variation. In addition to the discoveries that human biologists and medical professionals have made through the recent technical advances in genomics, for-profit companies have now developed commercial applications that provide several kinds of personal genetic information directly to individual customers.

Direct-to-consumer genetic analysis is a new and growing wave in personal genetic testing. The Palo Alto, California-based company 23andMe is one of the more readily recognized for-profit companies involved in the direct-to-consumer genetics market. 23andMe, and companies like it, offer several kinds of personal genetic information and testing. One testing component is carrier genetic testing for more than 40 recessive conditions. These are the same tests included in our discussion in Section B.3, with results identifying carriers of recessive genetic conditions. A second genetic-testing component identifies inherited variants influencing drug response. We described this interaction above under "Pharmacogenetic Testing." Direct-to-consumer genetic testing can also identify the likely presence of certain physical traits in people based on the alleles in their genome. For example, individual differences in caffeine metabolism, an aversion to cilantro (coriander), the presence of freckling, lactose intolerance, male pattern baldness, and red or blond hair color can be identified as likely to be present based on the inheritance of specific genetic variants. Personal genetic testing for ancestry relationships and evidence of individual geographic origins can also be provided. We discuss the details of these genetic analyses in Application Chapter E: Forensic Genetics.

The most recent application of personal genetic testing, however, is perhaps one of the most far-reaching. In April 2017 the U.S. Food and Drug Administration (FDA) and 23andMe announced the approval of genetic testing to identify individuals' risks of developing 10 medical conditions that are influenced, but are not exclusively caused, by genetics. Each of the 10 conditions covered by the agreement is more likely to occur in individuals who carry specific single nucleotide polymorphism (SNP) variants or alleles of certain genes. These SNP variants or markers are not equivalent to recessive or dominant mutant alleles that cause a condition. Instead, these markers are *associated with* the occurrence of a condition. In the context of inherited traits, the presence of an **association** means that people who inherit a particular SNP variant or marker are significantly more likely to develop a specific hereditary condition than those who do not inherit the SNP variant or marker. Stated another way, the presence of a SNP variant or marker is often necessary for a genetic condition to develop, but it is not sufficient. Some additional nongenetic event or set of events are required for the genetic condition to manifest itself. This means that heredity can make individuals susceptible to developing the condition, but other factors must also have their effect for the condition to develop.

Table B.5 identifies the 10 genetic conditions covered by the FDA-23andMe agreement. It also identifies the gene affected and the specific SNP variants or markers that are

Table B.5	Ten Conditions Associated with Inherited Variation[a]		
Condition	**Complications**	**Gene**	**Variant(s) or Marker(s)**
Alpha-1 antitrypsin deficiency	Lung and liver disease	SERPINA1	PI*Z, PI*S
Alzheimer disease (late onset)	Memory and cognitive symptoms	APOE	rs7412, rs429358
Celiac disease (gluten sensitivity)	Digestive symptoms	HLA	DQ2, DQ8
Factor XI deficiency	Blood-clotting disorder	F11	IVS14+1 G>A, F283L, E117X
Gaucher disease	Organ and tissue damage	GBA	V394L, N370S, 84GG
G6PD deficiency	Red blood cell damage	G6PD	VAL68MET, ASN126ASP
Hereditary hemochromatosis	Iron overload	HFE	H63D, S65C, C282Y
Hereditary thrombophilia	Blood-clotting disorder	F2, F5	Prothrombin G20210A, Factor V Leiden
Parkinson disease	Neurological symptoms	LRRK2, GBA	G2019S, N370S
Primary dystonia (early onset)	Muscle control problems	DYT1	deltaE320

[a] Ten conditions approved by the U.S. FDA for risk association screening by 23andMe.

associated with development of the condition. Some of the SNP variants associated with a condition are identified by their specific sequence location in the human genome. This genomic-sequence-location address is called the **rs** or **rsid number**, "rsid" being an abbreviation for the *r*eference *S*NP *ID* cluster that identifies the genomic location of a SNP or identifies the allele associated with the condition.

The association between the identified SNP or allelic marker and each of these conditions is strong. In each case, the presence of specific alleles or SNPs identifies the inheritance of alleles that increase the likelihood of developing a condition. An example is the condition alpha-1 antitrypsin deficiency (AATD), a degenerative lung and liver condition that most frequently results in chronic obstructive pulmonary disease (COPD), a severe breathing difficulty. The alpha-1 antitrypsin protein (AATP) is produced by the *SERPINA1* gene, and its occurrence is the result of inheriting specific variant alleles producing a protease inhibitor (PI) protein. The most common form of the PI protein, known as PI*M, protects sensitive lung and other tissues from the protein-destroying (protease) activity of the protein trypsin. AATP is produced when either of two variant forms of the protein called PI*Z and PI*S are present. Both of these variant proteins are defective in protease inhibition. Individuals with genotypes encoding a variant protease inhibitor protein, that is, *PI*Z/PI*Z*, *PI*Z/PI*S*, or *PI*S/PI*S*, are at increased risk of developing COPD, especially when they are also smokers or are exposed to high levels of particulate matter in the air and other airborne pollutants over a long period of time.

The genetic test offered by 23andMe identifies individual genotypes for this gene, and this identification is the basis for assigning the risk of AATD. Importantly, genotyping for this condition and the other nine conditions does not diagnose the presence or absence of the diseases. The presence of a given genotype can only indicate the presence of a significant elevation of risk of an associated condition. In the case of AATP genotyping, having one or two alleles encoding PI*Z or PI*S significantly increases an individual's likelihood of developing COPD, but it does not necessarily mean that a person will develop the condition.

One might ask, what is the value of having such a genetic test if it identifies increased risk but does not identify the actual presence of a condition? The answer is that knowing you have a genotype associated with an increased risk of disease can be an important element in personal decision making. In this instance, knowing the increased risk of AATD and the likelihood of COPD can motivate the person to undergo regular pulmonary screening for breathing difficulties and for early signs of disease. It can also influence personal decisions such as whether to smoke or whether to work in an environment with a high level of exposure to airborne pollutants.

One pivotal but as yet unresolved issue to consider when providing genetic information that is associated with but is not diagnostic of disease is the question of whether to also provide individuals with the information and support they need to make informed decisions. Test results can identify those individuals who are at high genetic risk for a condition, but the accessing of support and additional information from a genetic counselor or other medical professional is likely to be left up to the individuals themselves. These needs may be long-term or life-long. Among the conditions listed in Table B.5 are Parkinson disease and late onset Alzheimer disease, conditions that might never develop or might not manifest symptoms for several decades after genetic testing. A significant public health issue arising from direct-to-consumer genetic testing concerns how genetic counseling and medical monitoring for the conditions will be accessed, paid for, and managed. Direct-to-consumer genetic testing will likely never achieve the level of follow-up genetic counseling as genetic testing conducted under the auspices of a medical practice, so it is incumbent on consumers to think carefully about their personal needs in regard to obtaining, understanding, and managing the genetic information they seek and about the source from which that genetic information is obtained.

B.6 Opportunities and Choices

The kinds of genetic testing described in this chapter offer us an unprecedented view of ourselves that was unavailable to previous generations. Today, we have the chance to know if we carry a mutant allele that might combine with another mutant allele to produce a serious or fatal disorder. We can screen our pregnancies for possible chromosome, developmental, or genetic problems. Newborn infants and their families can be spared the worst ravages of certain hereditary conditions, and we can even use genetics to look into our futures to foresee the onset of certain diseases. At the same time, with the exception of newborn genetic screening mandated by state laws, the various testing and screening approaches described are options, not requirements.

With opportunities come risks, and with the possibility of obtaining information, certain choices must be faced and certain decisions must be made—the choice of whether or not to obtain information through available genetic testing and the decision about what to do once the information is in hand. There is no universally right or wrong decision, nor is there one right decision for every situation. Whether for decision making today, using currently available knowledge and technology, or for decision making in the future, when additional information and choices are available, what is most important is the access to accurate information and the freedom to make the individual choices that are right for each person and each new situation. The roles of genetic counseling and related support services, as described in Application Chapter A: Human Hereditary Disease and Genetic Counseling are and will continue to be integral parts of these information-gathering, information-delivery, and decision-making processes.

PROBLEMS

Mastering Genetics   Visit for instructor-assigned tutorials and problems.

For answers to selected even-numbered problems, see Appendix: Answers.

1. Answer the following questions for autosomal conditions such as PKU.
   a. If both parents are heterozygous carriers of a mutant allele, what is the chance that their first child will be homozygous recessive for the mutation?
   b. Parents who are each heterozygous carriers for a recessive mutant allele have a child who *does not* have the condition. What is the chance this child is a heterozygous carrier of the condition?
   c. If the first child of parents who are both heterozygous carriers of a recessive mutant allele is homozygous recessive, what is the chance the second child of the couple will be homozygous recessive? What is the chance the second child will be a heterozygous carrier of the recessive mutation?

2. Homocystinuria is a rare autosomal recessive condition on the RUSP list of conditions screened by newborn genetic testing. The condition results from a mutation that blocks the degradation of the amino acid methionine. The absence of a critical enzyme causes the buildup of the compound homocysteine, which is one of the intermediate compounds in the methionine breakdown pathway. Homocystinuria causes mental impairment, heart problems, seizures, eye abnormalities, and a number of other symptoms that shorten life if not treated. The condition is treated by a specialized diet that is low in methionine and by the ingestion of several supplements.
   a. Why do you think eating a low-methionine diet is critical to controlling homocystinuria?
   b. The low-methionine diet must be maintained throughout life to manage homocystinuria. Why do you think this is the case?

3. Log on to the National Institute for Child Health and Disease (http://www.nichd.nih.gov), locate the search box at the top right corner of the homepage, and enter "RUSP" to search for information on the Required Uniform Screening Panel. From the options that appear, select "Brief History of Newborn Screening" and locate the discussion listing the criteria for adding a disease to the RUSP list. What are the criteria for listing a disease on the RUSP list?

4. What are community-based genetic screening programs? What is the intent of such screening programs? Why are members of specific communities or populations offered the chance to participate in such programs?

5. Describe the gene and protein defects in phenylketonuria (PKU). How are these defects connected to disease symptoms?

6. A couple and some of their relatives are screened for Gaucher disease in a community-based screening program. The woman is homozygous for the dominant allele, represented by *G*. The woman's father, sister, and paternal grandmother are heterozygous carriers of the mutant allele, represented by *g*. Her paternal grandfather, her mother, and both of her mother's parents are homozygous for the dominant allele. The man is heterozygous and he has a brother with Gaucher disease. The man's parents and grandparents have not been tested, but it is known that none of them has Gaucher disease.
   a. Draw a pedigree of this family, including the woman, the man, their siblings, parents, and grandparents.
   b. On the pedigree, write the genotypes (*GG, Gg,* or *gg*) for each person who has been tested or for whom you

can deduce a genotype. If a genotype cannot be determined completely, list the alleles you know or deduce must be present.

c. Explain why you are able to assign genotypes to the man's parents despite their not being tested.

7. Diseases and conditions on the RUSP list are tested on every newborn infant, and if the baby has one of the conditions, the parents are immediately informed. What kind of information and counseling should be provided to the parents along with the diagnosis?

8. Do you think it is important that participation in community-based genetic screening be entirely voluntary? Why or why not?

9. If a man and a woman are each heterozygous carriers of a mutation causing a disease on the RUSP list, what do you think are the three or four most important factors they should consider in their decision making about having children?

10. Suppose a man and a woman are each heterozygous carriers of a mutation causing a fatal hereditary disease not on the RUSP list. Prenatal genetic testing can identify the genotype of a fetus with regard to this disease and can identify fetuses with the disease. What do you think are the three or four most important factors this couple should consider in their decision making about having children?

11. The most common reason a physician might recommend that a woman have maternal serum screening and a karyotype analysis is concern that her fetus may have Down syndrome. Log on to the OMIM website at www.ncbi .nlm.nih.gov/omim and look up Down syndrome (OMIM 190685).

a. List the main symptoms of Down syndrome.
b. Look at the "Mapping" and "Molecular Genetics" sections and describe what is meant by the Down syndrome critical region (DSCR).
c. Summarize what is known about the location and genes found within the DSCR.
d. How might those genes lead to the main symptoms of Down syndrome?

12. If you were to look up Gaucher disease on the OMIM website, you would see that there are three major types, designated Type I (OMIM 230800), Type II (OMIM 230900), and Type III (OMIM 231000). All three types are mutations of the gene for acid-β-glucosidase, encoded on chromosome 1. Different mutations of this gene produce the three types of Gaucher disease that differ somewhat in their symptoms and disease severity.

a. For each mutation, speculate about whether the acid-β-glucosidase enzyme is merely reduced in function or whether its production is eliminated, and explain why.
b. Thinking about the production or function of the acid-β-glucosidase enzyme, why do you suppose different mutations of this gene produce differences in symptoms and disease severity?

13. Imagine yourself in the same position as Kristen Powers, faced with the decision of whether or not to undergo a genetic test that will discover if you have inherited Huntington's disease. List five life decisions or choices that you think are likely to be affected by the results of the genetic test. Do you think you would make the same choice to test that Kristen made? Why or why not?

14. Select one of the hereditary conditions from either the RUSP core conditions list or the RUSP list of secondary conditions and do some online research to find the following information:

a. The frequency of the condition in newborn infants (note any populations in which the condition is more frequent).
b. The defect that characterizes the condition.
c. The symptoms and consequences of the condition if it is not treated.
d. The recommended treatment for those with the condition.
e. The duration of treatment.
f. The anticipated outcome if treatment is applied.

Eukaryotic Chromosome Abnormalities and Molecular Organization

10

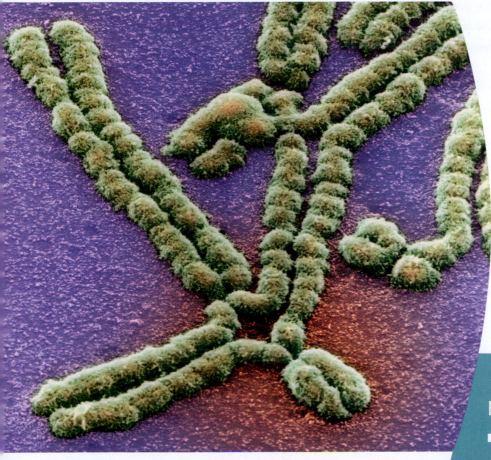

CHAPTER OUTLINE

10.1 Chromosome Number and Shape Vary among Organisms

10.2 Nondisjunction Leads to Changes in Chromosome Number

10.3 Changes in Euploid Content Lead to Polyploidy

10.4 Chromosome Breakage Causes Mutation by Loss, Gain, and Rearrangement of Chromosomes

10.5 Chromosome Breakage Leads to Inversion and Translocation of Chromosomes

10.6 Eukaryotic Chromosomes Are Organized into Chromatin

ESSENTIAL IDEAS

▪ The unique chromosome content of each genome can be visualized and analyzed by microscopic and molecular methods to yield information about normal chromosomes and to compare between species.

▪ Nondisjunction causes changes in the number of chromosomes and may result in gametes containing the wrong chromosome number.

▪ Changes in the number of sets of chromosomes alter phenotypes and can confer evolutionary advantages.

▪ Chromosome breakage can change chromosome structure and may lead to loss or duplication of genes.

▪ Chromosome breakage can lead to chromosome inversions and translocations.

▪ Large amounts of protein affiliate with eukaryotic chromosomes to form a complex called chromatin that condenses chromosomes during cell division and plays an important role in regulating gene transcription.

Chromosome translocations are mutations that rearrange chromosome structure. This electron micrograph shows two pairs of homologous chromosomes that have exchanged segments and must form a tetravalent structure involving the four chromosomes to synapse their homologous regions during prophase

The genome of a species is the totality of hereditary information carried in the DNA of the species. This information is contained in chromosomes. Bacterial and archaeal species generally carry all of their genomic information in a single chromosome. Some bacterial species have their genomes divided into two or more chromosomes, but all bacterial and archaeal species have only a single copy of each gene. As a consequence, these species are haploid, and the number of chromosomes they possess is represented by the variable *n*.

Eukaryotic genomes differ substantially from those of bacteria and archaea by having at least two copies of each gene. All animal species and many plant species are diploids, having two gene copies in their genome. Their cell nuclei carry the characteristic diploid number of chromosomes for the species—a number described as 2*n*. Numerous plant species have more than two copies of each gene and therefore more than a diploid number of chromosomes. These species are *polyploid* and may have up to 12*n* or more as their chromosome number.

Chromosomes are composed of a single, long DNA molecule. The chromosomes of bacteria and archaea are associated with small amounts of protein that help compact the chromosome in cells. In contrast, eukaryotic chromosomes contain as much protein as they do DNA. The protein and DNA are combined in a complex called *chromatin*, and this complex is critical for accomplishing four essential functions. First, the chromatin helps compact chromosomes so they fit efficiently into the eukaryotic nucleus. Second, chromatin helps stabilize DNA and protects it from damage. Third, chromatin promotes chromosome condensation and decondensation that are required for cell division. Finally, chromatin is a major factor in regulating DNA replication and gene transcription.

We begin this chapter with a discussion of natural variation in chromosome number and structure among eukaryotic species. After that we look at several kinds of abnormalities of chromosome number and structure. We then return to normal chromosomes to describe the basic organization of chromatin. The latter discussion sets the stage for a more detailed examination in Section 13.2 of the role of chromatin and chromatin modification in the regulation of eukaryotic gene transcription.

10.1 Chromosome Number and Shape Vary among Organisms

The content of a genome, the number of chromosomes contained in a nucleus, and the relative size and shape of each chromosome are species-specific characteristics. Chromosome number varies widely among species, though closely related species tend to have similar numbers. Similarly, chromosome shapes vary, with three or four general

chromosome shapes being found in most species. Each pair of chromosomes in a diploid genome is distinctive in the size, shape, and genetic content of the homologs, and these differences can be visualized by molecular and microscopic methods. The use of these methods enables researchers to identify individual chromosomes of genomes. It is important to note that even though chromosome numbers, sizes, and shapes are species-specific, none of these parameters is directly associated with the complexity of the organism (Table 10.1).

Chromosomes in Nuclei

Early observers of chromosomes in the nucleus, including Edmund Beecher Wilson, Walter Sutton, and Theodore Boveri, hypothesized that chromosomes contained the genetic material and noticed that their movement and separation during meiosis, and their union at fertilization mirrored the separation and transmission of genes. Biologists now know that these early investigators were correct, and contemporary biologists have learned a great deal about structure of chromosomes and their behavior during the cell cycle.

Chromosome behavior during interphase has been of particular interest, since chromosomes are highly decondensed and difficult to visualize during this period. Cell biologists Thomas Cremer and Christoph Cremer have used specialized methods to determine that interphase chromosomes are partitioned into their own chromosome territories (Figure 10.1). A **chromosome territory** is a small region of the nucleus that is the domain of a single chromosome. It is not bounded by any sort of membrane, nor is it demarcated in any distinctive manner. Chromosomes do not occupy

Table 10.1	Chromosome Number in Selected Animal Species
Species	**Diploid Chromosome Number (2*n*)**
Carp (*Cyprinus carpio*)	104
Cat (*Felis catus*)	38
Chicken (*Gallus domesticus*)	78
Chimpanzee (*Pan troglodytes*)	48
Cow (*Bos taurus*)	60
Dog (*Canis familiaris*)	78
Frog (*Rana pipiens*)	26
Fruit fly (*Drosophila melanogaster*)	8
Horse (*Equus caballus*)	64
Human (*Homo sapiens*)	46
Mouse (*Mus musculus*)	40
Rat (*Rattus norvegicus*)	42
Rhesus monkey (*Macaca mulatta*)	42

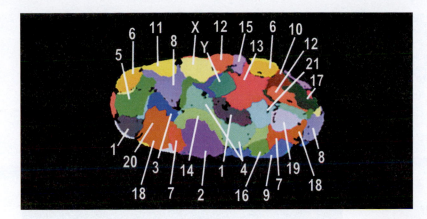

Figure 10.1 **Interphase chromosome territories.** Different fluorescent dyes are used to label each pair of interphase chromosomes in a human cell nucleus. Each chromosome inhabits a defined territory.

exactly the same territory in each nucleus (the nucleus does not have reserved seating for each chromosome), but once situated, a chromosome does not stray from its territory until the initiation of M phase of the cell cycle. Chromosomes are dynamically active within their territories during interphase and can be seen to move, twist, and turn during transcription and DNA replication. The chromosomes appear to be anchored by their centromeres and may assume positions that allow a characteristic pattern of gene transcription during interphase.

Adjacent chromosome territories are separated by an **interchromosomal domain** that contains no chromatin. These domains are channels for the movement of proteins, enzymes, and RNA molecules within the nucleus and among chromosome territories. The distribution of chromosome territories places the largest and most gene-rich chromosomes toward the center of the nucleus, whereas the territories of smaller chromosomes containing fewer genes are located toward the outer edges of the nucleus.

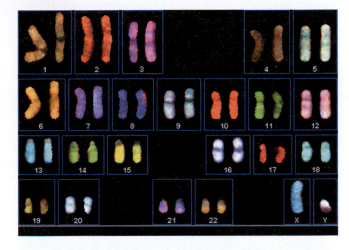

Figure 10.2 **A human karyotype.** With the use of 24 distinct fluorescent labels, this normal human male karyotype displays a different color pattern for each chromosome. Autosomal pairs are numbered 1 to 22, and the X and Y chromosomes are labeled.

Chromosome Visualization

Great variation in the characteristic number of chromosomes in animal species is evident in Table 10.1. These characteristic numbers of chromosomes can be counted in each nucleus once chromosomes condense in preparation for cell division. Chromosome condensation begins in early prophase and reaches its maximum at metaphase. With the aid of specialized molecular and microscopic techniques, chromosomes can be individually visualized and identified beginning in about mid-prophase through metaphase. Micrographs of the chromosomes of a cell can then be digitally reorganized in an image that places each chromosome next to its homologous mate and lines up the pairs in descending order of size. An organized image of the chromosomes from a nucleus is called a **karyotype**.

Figure 10.2 shows a typical human karyotype. The autosomal chromosomes in it are numbered 1 through 22 and arrayed in descending order of total length. The X and Y chromosomes are identified individually. The chromosomes in this karyotype were stained with special compounds called fluorophores. These are compounds that emit

fluorescent light when excited by ultraviolet or visible light during microscopy. The fluorescent emissions were collected by a photoreceptor and converted by software into the colors shown. Different compounds were used to label the different chromosomes, resulting in a characteristic color for each pair.

Total chromosome size allows the ordering of chromosomes in a karyotype, but the shape of the chromosomes is important as well. Chromosomes are divided by their centromere into segments known as **chromosome arms** that are almost always of unequal lengths. One chromosome arm, called the **short arm**, also known as the **p arm**, is shorter than the other arm that is known as the **long arm**, or the **q arm** (**Figure 10.3**). The position of the centromere determines the relative lengths of the short and long arms, leading to descriptive terms for the shapes of metaphase chromosomes. A **metacentric chromosome** has a more or less centrally located centromere and chromosome arms of similar lengths. **Submetacentric chromosomes** have a centromere nearer one end, producing one arm that is distinctly shorter than the other. The centromere of

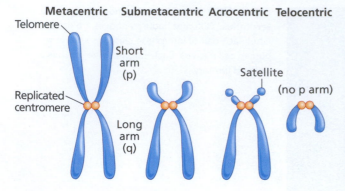

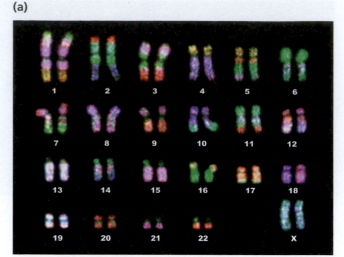

(a)

Figure 10.3 Chromosome shape. The position of the centromere and the ratio of the lengths of the long arm (q arm) and short arm (p arm) at metaphase determine chromosome shape.

🅠 Look at chromosome 1 in Figure 10.2. Is this chromosome metacentric, submetacentric, or acrocentric? Explain the rationale for your answer.

acrocentric chromosomes is nearly at the end of the chromosome. The "short arm" of acrocentric chromosomes is often composed of highly repetitive DNA. These repetitive regions are known as "satellites" in part because secondary chromosome constrictions appear to partially pinch off the repetitive segment of the short arm. **Telocentric chromosomes** have a terminal centromere and no short arm.

The contemporary approach to examining chromosome number, structure, and genetic content uses in situ methods to label specific segments of chromosomes or individual genes. Chromosomal in situ methods are those in which the chromosomes remain in the nucleus during staining and microscopy, as was the case for the preparation of the karyotype in Figure 10.2. The method known as **fluorescent in situ hybridization (FISH)** can use many different fluorophore labels to identify individual chromosomes or segments of chromosomes (**Figure 10.4a**) or it can use gene-specific fluorophores to locate individual genes (**Figure 10.4b**). In combination with the fluorescent labels, FISH uses molecular probes to recognize the chromosome sequences of interest. See the discussion in Section 1.4 and Figure 1.14 for a review of molecular probes. Like all molecular probes targeting DNA sequences, FISH probes consist of DNA that will seek out and bind to a complementary sequence. The attachment of a fluorophore label to a probe allows the visualization of the binding location or locations of the probe. Different fluorophores emitting light in a different part of the visible spectrum can be used in an experiment to allow different chromosomes or different sequences to be identified.

Chromosome Banding

Chromosome condensation, beginning, as mentioned, in early prophase, is driven by chromatin compaction. This means that as chromosomes condense, the proteins that have all along been affiliated with the chromosomes act to

(b)

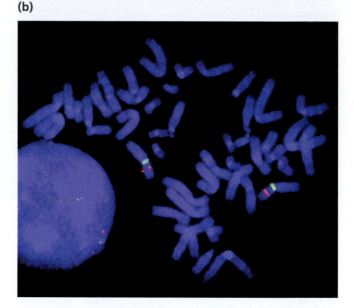

Figure 10.4 Fluorescent in situ hybridization (FISH). (a) Multiple probes and fluorescent compounds make each chromosome distinctive. **(b)** Two FISH probes hybridizing with target sequences on a human chromosome are detected by production of differently colored fluorophore emissions.

compact the DNA by forming ever more condensed loops of genetic material that reaches maximum compaction at the end of metaphase. At this point, chromosomes are in their most condensed state. Using nonfluorescent chromosome staining methods and microscopy, cytogeneticists can finely resolve each chromosome to reveal characteristic patterns of light and dark **chromosome banding** that are produced along the length of condensed chromosomes. These methods have been used for several decades, and they are the foundation both of chromosome nomenclature and of our understanding of different levels of chromatin compaction.

During the late 1960s and early 1970s, the first chromosome banding techniques were developed by experimentation with human and other mammalian chromosomes.

Generating karyotypes and obtaining chromosome banding patterns is a multistep process that begins with the growing of cells in culture. Cultures of growing cells are treated with chemicals that stop the cell cycle in metaphase, when chromosomes are most condensed. Individual cells from the arrested cell culture are then dropped onto a microscope slide. This bursts the cells and ruptures the nuclear membrane, allowing the chromosomes contained in a nucleus to spill out to form a "chromosome spread." After some additional treatment, any one of several different dyes or stains can be used on the chromosomes to reveal regional differences in chromatin compaction that produce a series of alternating chromosome bands. Banded chromosomes can be examined using microscopy, and the banded chromosome spreads are often photographed for karyotyping.

An international symposium in Paris, France, was convened in 1971 to agree on the standard banding pattern for each human chromosome as well as on a standardized nomenclature for identifying chromosome banding patterns based on karyotypes of metaphase chromosomes. This nomenclature remains in use today to ensure accuracy in identifying each chromosome and in describing any chromosome variants or abnormalities. The standardized banding is based on the highly reproducible patterns of some 300 or so lightly and darkly stained bands in chromosome-specific patterns seen on human chromosomes. The banding method is known as **G (Giemsa) banding**, and it is named after the staining compound called Giemsa stain that is used to generate the chromosome bands.

The standardized G-banding nomenclature uses letters and numbers to identify the major and minor band regions of each chromosome. The numbering begins at each chromosome centromere and progresses outward along each arm toward the telomere (**Figure 10.5**). Major regions are subdivided to permit a designation for each light- and dark-band region of a chromosome. Each band is given a designation that specifies the chromosome number, chromosome arm, and band location. An example is 5q2.3.1, which is the dark band on the long arm of chromosome 5 indicated in Figure 10.5.

Chromosome banding by G banding and other techniques was at one time limited to chromosomes in metaphase. Recently, however, advanced techniques have allowed cytogeneticists to stain chromosomes earlier in the cell cycle. Chromosome banding in prometaphase chromosome spreads produces as many as 2000 chromosome bands. Like the bands seen in metaphase chromosomes, these bands are highly reproducible, and chromosome-specific banding patterns for this phase of the cell cycle are now standardized.

Heterochromatin and Euchromatin

Each human chromosome band contains between 1 million and 10 million base pairs of DNA, enough to include multiple genes. The patterns and variations observed in chromosome banding are dependent on the various degrees

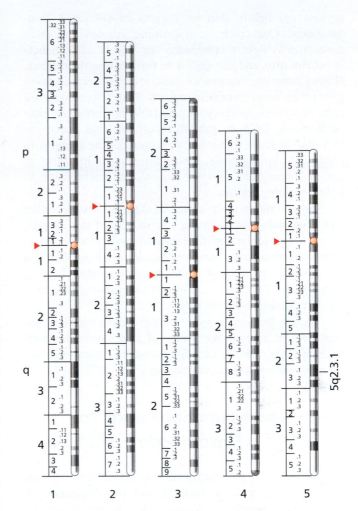

Figure 10.5 Standardized human chromosome banding patterns. Human chromosomes 1 to 5 in late prophase. Heterochromatic regions are shown as gray and black bands, euchromatic regions as white bands. Centromeres are indicated by the colored dots on each chromosome.

⊙ Locate chromosome band 3q2.3. Is it heterochromatic, euchromatic, or a mixture of the two?

of chromatin condensation. Originally, chromatin condensation was thought to reflect consistent but relatively unimportant regional variation in chromosomes, but there is now clear evidence that chromatin state is directly related to gene transcription. This means that chromosome banding patterns are associated with the distribution of expressed genes.

In general, the chromosome regions populated by actively transcribed genes are relatively less condensed than chromosome regions with few transcribed genes, which are more heavily compacted. Regions of lesser chromatin compaction are identified as **euchromatin,** or as **euchromatic regions**. Most expressed genes are located in euchromatic regions, where condensation is variable during the cell cycle. Euchromatic chromosome regions are lightly staining regions of G-banded chromosomes. Conversely, chromosome regions in which chromatin is tightly condensed are said to contain **heterochromatin** and are called **heterochromatic regions**. Heterochromatic regions contain many fewer expressed genes than do euchromatic regions. With fewer expressed gene sequences, heterochromatic DNA is more likely than euchromatic DNA to contain repetitive DNA sequences that may be located in multiple regions of the genome. In G-banded chromosomes, heterochromatin is identified as darkly staining chromosome regions and euchromatin as lightly staining regions.

We will return to the theme of chromatin condensation and gene transcription in the last section of this chapter, where we describe the fundamental molecular organization of chromatin and discuss a mutation in *Drosophila* that demonstrates the role of chromatin condensation in gene transcription. Chromatin and its role in regulating gene transcription is also discussed in Section 13.2.

Genetic Analysis 10.1 gives you practice with these concepts as you interpret the results of a hypothetical experiment involving the use of FISH probes that have unknown sequence targets within chromosomes.

10.2 Nondisjunction Leads to Changes in Chromosome Number

In Section 3.2, we discussed the connection between Mendel's two laws of heredity and the disjunction of homologous chromosomes and sister chromatids during meiosis. In the discussion that now follows, we focus on **nondisjunction**, the failure of chromosomes and sister chromatids to properly disjoin during cell division. As we describe, nondisjunction is the cause of abnormalities of chromosome number in cells.

The changes in chromosome number we describe in this section exert their effects primarily by addition or removal of one or more chromosomes of the normal complement in a nucleus. Such changes are mutations that add or remove large numbers of genes. In animal species, but less so in plant species, these abnormalities almost always alter the phenotype, and can have an effect on the development and reduce fertility and viability of the affected organism.

Chromosome Nondisjunction

With a few unusual exceptions, the number of chromosomes is the same for males and females of a species, and the number of chromosomes in nuclei of normal cells is a multiple of the haploid number (n), the number in a single set of chromosomes. In nearly all animal species, the total chromosome number is $2n$ (diploid), but in plants, $3n$ (triploid) or higher multiples of n are relatively common. Chromosome numbers that are a multiple of the haploid number are identified as **euploid**. In contrast, the addition or removal

of a chromosome alters the euploid number and generates a chromosome count known as **aneuploidy** (i.e., "not euploid"). Chromosome nondisjunction is the cause of aneuploidy.

Nondisjunction in germ-line cells produces aneuploid gametes—reproductive cells that have one or more extra or missing chromosomes. These errors lead to the production of aneuploidy of fertilized eggs. Meiotic nondisjunction can occur in either meiosis I or II and most often affects just a single homologous pair or a single pair of sister chromatids in a gametocyte (gametocytes are the cells that undergo meiosis to produce gametes). Meiosis I nondisjunction is the failure of homologous chromosomes to separate. It results in both homologs moving to a single pole. One of the gametocytes produced in meiosis I contains both chromosomes, and the other contains neither chromosome (**Figure 10.6**). These gametocytes, contain aneuploid chromosome numbers of $n + 1$ and $n - 1$ (assuming only one chromosome pair is affected). Meiosis II usually proceeds normally even when meiosis I is aberrant, and its completion sends the sister chromatids to different gametes. If nondisjunction occurs in meiosis I, each of the four resulting gametes are aneuploid—either $n + 1$ or $n - 1$. The union of an aneuploid gamete with a normal haploid gamete at fertilization results in a fertilized egg with an aneuploid number of chromosomes that will be either **trisomic** ($2n - 1$), having three of one of the chromosomes rather than a homologous pair, or **monosomic** ($2n - 1$) having just a single copy of one of the chromosomes rather than a homologous pair.

Nondisjunction occurring in meiosis II typically follows a normal meiosis I that produced normal secondary gametocytes, both containing the haploid (n) number of chromosomes (**Figure 10.7**). Since these gametocytes are separate cells, they independently divide during meiosis II; thus, if nondisjunction occurs, only one of the secondary gametocytes will be affected. Among the four resulting gametes, two are normal because a normal disjunction took place during each meiotic division. The other two gametes are aneuploid: one contains $n + 1$ chromosomes and the other $n - 1$ chromosomes. Trisomic or monosomic fertilized eggs are produced when one of these aneuploid gametes unites with a normal gamete at fertilization.

Gene Dosage Alteration

In 1913, at about the same time Calvin Bridges was demonstrating the chromosome theory of heredity by examining nondisjunction in fruit flies (see Section 3.3), Albert Francis Blakeslee and John Belling reported the phenotypic consequences of aneuploidy in the diploid ($2n = 24$) jimson weed (*Datura stramonium*), in which 12 chromosome pairs are identified as A to L. Blakeslee and Belling identified 12 phenotypically distinct lines of trisomic *Datura*, one for each of the chromosome pairs (**Figure 10.8**). Their results documented that aneuploidy causes phenotypic consequences. Over ensuing decades, this observation was expanded and it was found that aneuploidy profoundly

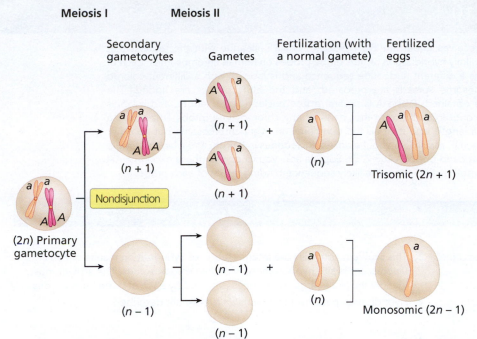

Meiosis I   Meiosis II

Secondary gametocytes   Gametes   Fertilization (with a normal gamete)   Fertilized eggs

Nondisjunction

(n + 1)

(n + 1)

(n + 1)

(n − 1)

(n − 1)

(n − 1)

(2n) Primary gametocyte

(n)

(n)

Trisomic (2n + 1)

Monosomic (2n − 1)

Figure 10.6   Meiosis I nondisjunction. Homologous chromosomes fail to disjoin in meiosis I, and all resulting gametes are aneuploid. Fertilization by a normal haploid gamete produces fertilized eggs that are trisomic (2n + 1) or monosomic (2n − 1).

affects the phenotype and development of nearly all animal species. The effects on the phenotype of plants were also further documented.

The phenotypic and developmental abnormalities associated with aneuploidy result from changes in **gene dosage**, the number of copies of a gene in the genome. Aneuploidy changes the dosage of *all the genes* on the affected

chromosome. In a diploid organism, where two copies of a gene, on a homologous pair of chromosomes, generate 100% of gene dosage, a monosomic mutant has just one gene copy and just 50% of normal gene dosage for each gene on the chromosome. In contrast, a trisomic mutant has three copies and 150% of normal gene dosage for each of the genes on the chromosome.

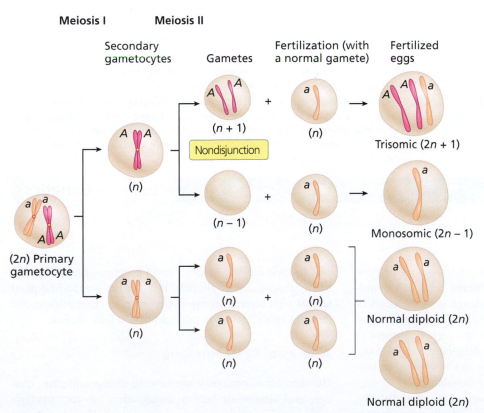

Meiosis I   Meiosis II

Secondary gametocytes   Gametes   Fertilization (with a normal gamete)   Fertilized eggs

Nondisjunction

(n + 1)

(n − 1)

(n)

(n)

(n)

(n)

(n)

(n)

(2n) Primary gametocyte

(n)

(n)

Trisomic (2n + 1)

Monosomic (2n − 1)

Normal diploid (2n)

Normal diploid (2n)

Figure 10.7   Meiosis II nondisjunction. Sister chromatid disjunction fails in meiosis II. Normal fertilization of the resulting gametes generates trisomy, monosomy, or normal diploidy at fertilization.

367

PROBLEM Suppose Dr. O. Sophila receives three new FISH probes from a colleague with the request that Dr. Sophila's laboratory determine the likely hybridization targets of the probes on human chromosomes. Each of the three FISH-probe designs contains a different nucleotide sequence and is labeled with a different-colored fluorophore. Chromosome spreads are prepared, and the FISH probes are added. The following results are obtained: Probe A is several dozen nucleotides in length, and it labels each chromosome centromere but no other parts of any chromosome; probe B is about a dozen nucleotides in length, and it labels the telomeres on every chromosome but no other parts of any chromosome; probe C is about a dozen nucleotides in length, and it labels a single spot on each copy of chromosome 4 at band position 4q3.2. Dr. Sophila asks you to ponder these experimental results and to help his colleague by hypothesizing about the likely sequence-binding target of each probe.

BREAK IT DOWN: Review the discussion of FISH on p. 364.

Solution Strategies	Solution Steps
Evaluate	
1. Identify the topic of this problem and the nature of the required answer.	1. This problem concerns the interpretation of hybridization results of FISH (fluorescent in situ hybridization) in human chromosomes. The answer must identify the likely target sequences detected by each of three FISH probes.
2. Identify the critical information given in the problem.	2. Hybridization patterns for three FISH probes are described.
Deduce	
3. Review your knowledge of the different portions of chromosomes to which these probes hybridize. [See discussions in Section 3.1 (centromeres) and Section 7.4 (telomeres).]	3. Centromeres contain specialized DNA sequences that are bound by microtubules during cell division. Telomeres are located at chromosome ends and are composed of hundreds of copies of short, repetitive DNA sequences.
TIP: FISH probes hybridize by complementary base pairing. Probes longer than about 20 base pairs may hybridize even if there are a few mismatches.	
4. Recall the makeup of eukaryotic chromosomes in terms of their content of protein-coding genes and other types of DNA sequences.	4. Eukaryotic DNA contains most of the expressed genes. Heterochromatic DNA contains few expressed genes and is more likely than eukaryotic regions to contain repetitive sequences.
Solve	
5. Provide an interpretation of the DNA sequence targeted by probe A.	5. By hybridizing exclusively to centromeric regions, probe A is likely to be targeting these specialized DNA sequences.
6. Provide an interpretation of the DNA sequence targeted by probe B.	6. Hybridization exclusively to telomeres indicates that probe B is targeting the short repetitive DNA sequences of telomeres.
7. Provide an interpretation of the DNA sequence targeted by probe C.	7. Probe C hybridizes to a single location on homologous copies of chromosome 4 that is most likely to be a protein-coding gene. The band 4q3.2 is a euchromatic region of the chromosome, where many expressed genes are located. The identity of the gene cannot be determined, however, without additional information.

For more practice, see Problems 11 and 28.　　Visit the Study Area to access study tools. **Mastering Genetics**

Changes in gene dosage lead to an imbalance of gene products from the affected chromosome relative to unaffected chromosomes, and this imbalance is at the heart of alterations of normal development and the production of abnormal phenotypes. Most animals are highly sensitive to changes in gene dosage, and their developmental biology, especially within the nervous system, does not proceed normally in the presence of gene dosage imbalance.

In contrast to animals, that are profoundly, often lethally, affected when aneuploidy occurs, gene dosage changes are more easily tolerated in many species of plants, owing in part to their having developmental programs that differ distinctly from those of animals. It is not unusual to find plant strains with more than two copies of each chromosome. We describe this situation in more detail in a later section.

Aneuploidy in Humans

Humans are enormously sensitive to changes in gene dosage, and almost all human aneuploidies are incompatible with life. Theoretically, there are potentially 24 different kinds of trisomy in humans—one for each autosome, and

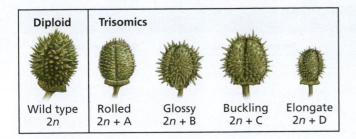

Diploid	Trisomics			
Wild type 2*n*	Rolled 2*n* + A	Glossy 2*n* + B	Buckling 2*n* + C	Elongate 2*n* + D

Figure 10.8 The appearance of the seed head in wild-type diploid and in four trisomic lines of jimson weed (*Datura stramonium*).

one each for the X and Y chromosomes—and an equal number of potential monosomies. Yet only autosomal trisomies of chromosomes 13, 18, and 21, and no autosomal monosomies, are seen with any measurable frequency in newborn human infants. Multiple forms of sex-chromosome trisomy are detected with some frequency at birth, however, as is one type of sex-chromosome monosomy (Table 10.2). A wide variety of other chromosome abnormalities occur in newborn infants as well. Each of the aneuploidy conditions identified in Table 10.2, along with the other chromosome abnormalities that occur, result in significant phenotypic abnormalities.

Human biologists know that other trisomies and monosomies, not just the ones listed in the table, also occur at conception, but the resulting zygotes almost never survive to be born alive. The explanation for this outcome is that the abnormalities of development that are produced are so severe that either implantation in the uterine wall does not occur, or early zygotic mitotic division is so disrupted that the zygote dies, or fetal development comes to a halt and the fetus spontaneously aborts.

The best available data on human reproduction and the rate of aneuploidy comes from studies that monitor women for hormone changes associated with conception and the earliest stages of pregnancy. These studies make two surprising observations. First, in the first trimester of pregnancy, about half of all human conceptions spontaneously abort, and second, more than half of the spontaneously terminated human pregnancies carry abnormalities of chromosome number or chromosome structure. These observations point to a surprisingly high (15–25%) frequency of meiotic nondisjunction in humans. Other errors producing gametes with abnormal chromosomes add to this level of chromosome error in meiosis.

To ascertain the biological basis for the high rate of meiotic nondisjunction in humans, trisomy 21 (Down syndrome)—the most common autosomal trisomy at birth—has been the focus of intense study. Epidemiologic studies conducted over several decades have linked the risk of a child having trisomy 21 to the age of the mother at conception. Table 10.3 illustrates the connection between maternal age and the risk of trisomy 21.

One theory explaining this association has to do with the fact that meiosis begins in the ovaries of female fetuses.

Table 10.2	Human Aneuploidies and Frequencies at Birth		
Aneuploidy	Syndrome	Frequency at Birth	Syndrome Characteristics
Autosomal Aneuploidy			
Trisomy 13	Patau syndrome	1 in 15,000	Mental retardation and developmental delay, possible deafness, major organ abnormalities, early death
Trisomy 18	Edward syndrome	1 in 8000	Mental retardation and developmental delay, skull and facial abnormalities, early death
Sex-Chromosome Aneuploidy			
Trisomy 21	Down syndrome	1 in 1500	Mental retardation and developmental delay, characteristic facial abnormalities, short stature, variable life span
47, XXY	Klinefelter syndrome (males)	1 in 1000	Variable secondary sexual characteristics, infertility, frequent breast swelling; no impact on mental capacity
47, XYY	Jacob syndrome (males)	1 in 1000	Tall stature common; possible reduction but not loss of fertility; no impact on mental capacity
47, XXX	Triple X syndrome (females)	1 in 1000	Tall stature common; possible reduction of fertility; menstrual irregularity; no impact on mental capacity
45, XO	Turner syndrome (females)	1 in 5000	No secondary sexual characteristics; infertility, short stature; webbed neck common; no impact on mental capacity

Table 10.3	Risk of Down Syndrome (Trisomy 21) by Maternal Age[a]		
Maternal Age Range	**Total Live Births Studied**	**Trisomy 21 Births**	**Rate per 1000 Births**
15–19	30,272	18	0.49
20–24	117,593	87	0.73
25–29	108,746	96	0.90
30–34	49,487	72	1.56
35–39	19,522	73	4.19
40–44	4880	73	18.02
45–49	304	19	55.02

[a] Data adapted from E. B. Hook and A. Lindsjo, Down syndrome in live births by single year maternal age interval in a Swedish study: Comparison with results from a New York State study. *Am. J. Hum. Genet.* 30 (1978): 19–27.

In the 500,000 or so follicles in each of the two fetal ovaries, meiosis reaches the point of homologous chromosome synapsis in prophase I and then arrests. At puberty, or at any point over a woman's span of reproductive fertility, monthly hormone cycling reinitiates meiosis in a few follicles. Meiosis I (homologous chromosome separation) leads to an egg that is released into the fallopian tube. If the egg is fertilized by a sperm cell, meiosis II is stimulated to occur, the two parental haploid nuclei fuse, and fertilization is complete. If maternal age at conception is functionally linked to the risk of trisomy 21, then researchers should find that nondisjunction errors in maternal meiosis I are more often the cause than are errors in maternal meiosis II. In fact, molecular genetic analysis of the chromosomes in infants with trisomy 21 has indeed determined that more than 90% of cases of trisomy 21 are attributable to a maternal nondisjunction, and that the majority of nondisjunction events are errors in meiosis I. Predominantly, infants with trisomy 21 have two identical copies of a maternal chromosome 21 and one copy of a paternal chromosome 21. This circumstance arises through maternal meiosis I nondisjunction.

Molecular and genomic analyses have also determined that a small number of genes on chromosome 21 are responsible for mental and developmental delays and heart abnormalities, which are the principal symptoms of trisomy 21. The critical portion of chromosome 21 for trisomy 21 is the *Down syndrome critical region* (DSCR). Its discovery came from the study of individuals with the symptoms of Down syndrome who have two complete copies of chromosome 21 and an additional fragment of a third copy of the chromosome. Only when the additional fragment contains DSCR are the symptoms of trisomy 21 present.

Research in mice has pointed to a potential explanation for the role of DSCR in generating the symptoms of Down syndrome. Among a handful of candidate genes located in the DSCR, one gene, *DYRK*, has a homolog that produces dosage-sensitive learning defects. Mice with an extra copy of the *DYRK* homolog have a reduction in brain size. *DSCAM* is a second gene whose increased dosage is linked to Down syndrome. This gene also has homologs in mouse and *Drosophila*, where its protein product participates in the formation of the heart and components of the developing nervous system.

A different kind of change in gene dosage is seen in humans with Turner syndrome, a monosomy of the X chromosome in which there is one X chromosome but no second sex chromosome (see Table 10.2). Despite the occurrence of random X-inactivation in human female embryos that leads to one expressed X chromosome and one inactive X chromosome in each nucleus, two sex chromosomes are necessary for normal early development. In female embryos that are XO (Turner syndrome), the single copy of the gene *SHOX*, located in pseudoautosomal region 2 on the short arm of the X chromosome (and in males also on the Y chromosome; Section 3.2), is insufficient to direct certain aspects of normal development. The haploinsufficiency of *SHOX* appears to play a central role in producing Turner syndrome.

Genetic Analysis 10.2 guides you through an analysis of chromosome 21 nondisjunction.

Mosaicism

Our discussion of random X-inactivation of mammalian females in Chapter 3 identified the phenomenon as an example of naturally occurring mosaicism, in which different cells of the organism contain differently functioning X chromosomes (see Section 3.6). Mosaicism is the condition of being composed of two or more cell types having different genetic or chromosomal makeup. In addition to the random X-inactivation process, mosaicism can also develop as a consequence of mitotic nondisjunction early in embryogenesis. Mosaicism derived in this way is one of the many kinds of chromosome abnormalities that occur in newborn infants. For example, 25–30% of cases of Turner syndrome, the X-chromosome monosomy (XO), occur in females exhibiting mosaicism in which some cells are 45, XO and others are 46, XX. Some individuals with mosaic Turner syndrome carry 47, XXX cells as well. This kind of mosaicism is usually derived from mitotic nondisjunction in a 46, XX zygote (**Figure 10.9**).

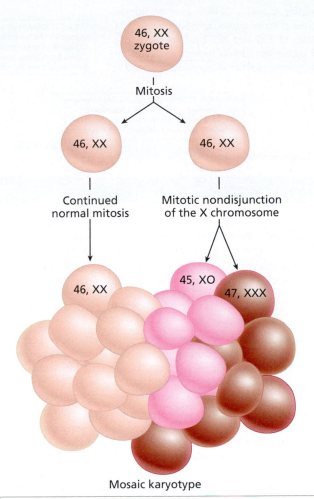

46, XX zygote

|
Mitosis

46, XX   46, XX

| |

Continued   Mitotic nondisjunction
normal mitosis   of the X chromosome

46, XX   45, XO
                 47, XXX

Mosaic karyotype

Turner syndrome mosaic females contain 46, XX and 45, XO cells, and they may also have cells with 47, XXX.

Figure 10.9 Chromosome mosaicism. Mosaicism usually begins with a normal diploid zygote. Mitotic nondisjunction produces one or more aneuploid cell lines that persist and are found in the newborn.

Uniparental Disomy

A rare abnormality of chromosome content called **uniparental disomy** has been identified in humans. Uniparental disomy occurs when both copies of a homologous chromosome pair originate from a single parent. It was first identified in connection with two chromosomal conditions, Angelman syndrome (OMIM 105830) and Prader–Willi syndrome (OMIM 176270), that are usually the result of a partial deletion of the 15q11.12 portion of chromosome 15 but can also be caused by uniparental disomy of that chromosome.

Uniparental disomy has two mechanisms of origin. The rarer mechanism requires nondisjunction of the same chromosome in both sperm and egg, with the result that a fertilization occurs in which one gamete contributes two copies of the chromosome and the other does not contribute a copy of the chromosome. The second mechanism is more common. It involves nondisjunction in one parent that results in an

aneuploid gamete contributing two copies of a chromosome and the other parent contributing a normal gamete with a single copy of the chromosome. In the case of either Angelman syndrome or Prader–Willi syndrome, the chromosome involved is chromosome 15. Union of the gametes described above—with two copies and one copy, respectively, of chromosome 15—results in trisomy 15 in the fertilized egg. This is a condition that is invariably incompatible with survival. By a process known as **trisomy rescue**, however, some fertilized eggs that are initially trisomic can survive and lead to the formation of a zygote that can survive. In trisomy rescue, one of the extra copies of the chromosome is ejected in one of the first mitotic divisions following fertilization. Which of the three chromosomes is ejected is apparently random. Thus, one result of trisomy rescue can be a cell with one chromosome from each parent. Zygotes with this result have normal chromosome content. Alternatively, trisomy rescue could result in a zygote that retains two copies of the chromosome from the same parent, and this is uniparental disomy.

10.3 Changes in Euploid Content Lead to Polyploidy

Polyploidy is the presence of three or more sets of chromosomes in the nucleus of an organism. Polyploidy is common, particularly in plant species, and can result either from the duplication of full sets of chromosomes or from the combining of chromosome sets from different species. Many types of polyploidy are possible—triploids ($3n$), tetraploids ($4n$), pentaploids ($5n$), hexaploids ($6n$), octaploids ($8n$), and so on. Polyploids whose karyotype is comprised of chromosomes derived from a single species are designated **autopolyploids** (*auto* = "self"), and polyploids with chromosome sets from two or more species are called **allopolyploids** (*allo* = "different"). Terms such as *autotetraploid* ($4n$ chromosomes that all derive from a single species) and *allohexaploid* ($6n$ with chromosomes from two or more species) are used to describe a polyploid organism's genomic content.

Causes of Autopolyploidy and Allopolyploidy

Two mechanisms are most commonly the cause of polyploidy. The first mechanism derives from meiotic nondisjunction. In these cases, one or both gametes have an extra set of chromosomes that are contributed at fertilization. For example, nondisjunction during oogenesis can produce an egg that is $2n$. When fertilized by pollen that is n, the resulting plant will be triploid ($3n$). Similarly, both egg and pollen could be $2n$, resulting in a plant that is $4n$. The second mechanism is mitotic nondisjunction that results in a doubling of chromosome number. For example, a $2n$ cell experiencing mitotic nondisjunction can become $4n$. These two mechanisms can also combine to increase polyploidy. For example, the autotriploid plant that results from the union of a $2n$ egg

PROBLEM Suppose polymerase chain reaction (PCR) is used to amplify (clone) a DNA marker on human chromosome 21 from a mother, a father, and their child who was born with trisomy 21 (Down syndrome). The mother has marker alleles of 310 and 380 bp. The father has marker alleles of 290 and 340 bp. What PCR bands would you expect to detect on an electrophoresis gel for their child with Down syndrome if nondisjunction occurred in

> **BREAK IT DOWN:** PCR generates large numbers of copies of specific target sequences of DNA. See Section 7.5 for PCR details (p. 261).

> **BREAK IT DOWN:** Trisomy 21 is caused by the inheritance of three copies of chromosome 21—two copies from one parent and the third copy from the other parent.

a. maternal meiosis I   b. maternal meiosis II
c. paternal meiosis I   d. paternal meiosis II

> **BREAK IT DOWN:** Autosomal DNA markers are inherited as autosomal codominant alleles. The four parental marker alleles are different, so you can expect to see two alleles from one parent and the third allele from the other parent.

Solution Strategies	Solution Steps
Evaluate	
1. Identify the topic of this problem and the nature of the required answer.	1. This problem deals with chromosome nondisjunction and requires a prediction of PCR results expected for different nondisjunction events.
2. Identify the critical information given in the problem.	2. The four alleles inherited on parental copies of chromosome 21 are given. These four alleles are of different lengths, making it possible to identify each chromosome uniquely.
Deduce	
3. Review the abnormal chromosome combinations that result from nondisjunction in meiosis I and meiosis II. TIP: See Figures 10.6 and 10.7, p. 367.	3. Meiosis I nondisjunction is the failure of homologous chromosomes to disjoin. An abnormal secondary gametocyte contains homologous copies of the chromosome that are different from one another. Meiosis II nondisjunction is the failure of sister chromatids to disjoin. An abnormal secondary gamete contains identical copies of the chromosome.
4. Identify the alleles that would be present on the two copies of chromosome 21 produced by maternal meiotic I nondisjunction and by paternal meiotic I nondisjunction.	4. The marker alleles present if meiosis I nondisjunction occurs will include the two alleles from one parent's homologous copies of chromosome 21. These are 310 and 380 for maternal meiosis I nondisjunction and 290 and 340 for paternal meiosis I nondisjunction.
5. Identify the alleles that would be present on the two copies of chromosome 21 produced by maternal meiosis II nondisjunction and by paternal meiosis II nondisjunction.	5. The marker alleles present if meiosis II nondisjunction occurs will include two identical markers from one parent. These are either both 310 or both 380 for maternal meiosis II nondisjunction, or both 290 or both 340 for paternal meiosis II nondisjunction.
Solve	Answer a
6. List the alleles expected if trisomy 21 is produced by maternal meiosis I nondisjunction.	6. The gel for the trisomy 21 child's DNA will have three bands, since all three chromosomes carry different PCR alleles. In the case of maternal meiosis I nondisjunction, two bands will be maternal and one will be paternal. The gel band patterns are either 310, 380, 290 or 310, 380, 340.
	Answer b
7. List the alleles expected if trisomy 21 is produced by maternal meiosis II nondisjunction.	7. The gel will have two PCR bands—one representing the two identical maternal alleles and the other representing the one paternal allele. There are four possible gel band patterns for the child with trisomy 21: (1) 310, 290; (2) 310, 340; (3) 380, 290; or (4) 380, 340.
	Answer c
8. List the alleles expected if trisomy 21 is produced by paternal meiosis I nondisjunction.	8. The gel will have PCR bands for both of the paternal chromosomes and one of the maternal chromosomes. There are two possible patterns for these three PCR gel bands: (1) 290, 340, 310; or (2) 290, 340, 380.
	Answer d
9. List the alleles expected if trisomy 21 is produced by paternal meiosis II nondisjunction.	9. The gel will have two PCR bands—one representing the two identical paternal alleles and the other representing the one maternal allele. There are four possible gel band patterns for the child: (1) 290, 310; (2) 290, 380; (3) 340, 310; or (4) 340, 380.

For more practice, see Problem 25.

Visit the Study Area to access study tools. **Mastering Genetics**

and an n pollen could become $6n$ (autohexaploid) by a doubling of the chromosomes through mitotic nondisjunction. In all of the examples described here, all the chromosomes present in the polyploid cell originate from the same species; thus, these are examples of autopolyploidy.

The strawberries you eat each summer are autooctaploids ($8n$) and have had chromosome sets duplicated by the processes outlined here. Strawberries have a haploid number of $n = 7$ and a diploid number of $2n = 14$, thus the commercial octaploid varieties contain $8n = 56$ chromosomes. Octaploid strawberries are prized for their bright red color, sweet taste, and juicy texture. In these traits, as we describe below, strawberries reveal some of the reasons why agricultural products are so often polyploids. Octaploid strawberries are larger (and much better tasting) than their diploid counterparts (**Figure 10.10**).

In contrast to autopolyploids, the multiple sets of chromosomes in allopolyploids originate in different species. The union of a haploid gamete from species 1 (n_1) and a haploid gamete from species 2 (n_2) produces a hybrid organism that may have either an even number or an odd number of chromosomes, depending on the haploid number that is normal for each species. The chromosomes of the two contributing species are not homologous and may have difficulty pairing in meiosis. However, mitotic duplication of chromosomes doubles the total chromosome number and generates homologous pairs of chromosomes.

An example of these events is the emergence of a new species of salt grass, *Spartina anglica*, along the English coastline in the late 1800s. *S. anglica* is a naturally occurring allopolyploid possessing 122 chromosomes. It arose through the interspecific hybridization of native salt grass, *Spartina*

maritima ($2n = 60$), with a non-native salt grass, *Spartina alterniflora* ($2n = 62$; **Figure 10.11**). Haploid gametes from the two parental species fused to produce an interspecific hybrid with 61 chromosomes. Chromosome nondisjunction that doubled the chromosome number to 122 generated fertility in the hybrid and stabilized its genome. With an even number of chromosomes, balanced gametes were able to form. This established the new species that grew vigorously and spread its range along the English coast.

Consequences of Polyploidy

Polyploids of plant species frequently occur naturally and are also produced by human manipulation. When produced for commercial purposes, plant polyploidy has three main consequences. First, fruit and flower size are increased. The nuclei and cells of polyploid strains are larger than those of

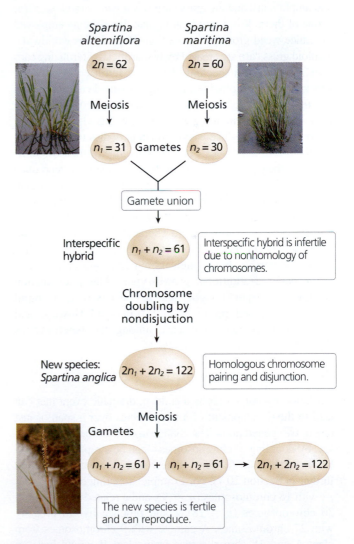

Figure 10.11   The production of a new allopolyploid species. Two salt grass species, *Spartina maritima* ($2n = 60$) and *Spartina alterniflora* ($2n = 62$) produced an interspecific hybrid ($2n = 61$) that subsequently doubled its chromosome number by nondisjunction to produce the new salt grass species *Spartina anglica*, an allotetraploid ($4n = 122$).

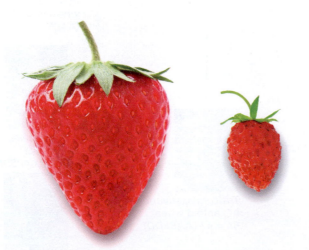

Figure 10.10   Polyploidy increases fruit size. The most common strains of commercial strawberries are octaploid ($8n$) and bear larger fruits than do diploid ($2n$) strawberry strains.

🔵 In Chapter 1, Experimental Insight 1.1 (pp. 10–11) describes a kitchen experiment in which you can isolate DNA and says that strawberries are a good source of DNA. Why do you think that is the case?

diploid strains, and many familiar fruit and vegetable varieties benefit from this effect. Apples ($3n = 51$), bananas ($3n = 33$), strawberries ($8n = 56$), peanuts ($4n = 40$), and potatoes ($4n = 48$) are just a few examples.

Increased fruit and flower size in polyploid plants comes at the cost of fertility—the second consequence. The problem is particularly acute for odd-numbered polyploids ($3n$, $5n$, etc.), in which the odd number of chromosomes cannot be evenly divided at the first meiotic division. The result is an unequal distribution of chromosomes that makes almost all of the resulting gametes nonviable. In some cases, this reproductive disadvantage can be turned into commercial advantage: Certain "seedless" fruits and vegetables in the produce aisle of your local grocery store are odd-numbered polyploids.

The grass carp furnishes an animal example of the commercial benefits of infertility. While most animals do not tolerate polyploidy, there are some exceptions among certain fishes and amphibians, and the grass carp (*Ctenopharyngodon idella*) is one of them. It is a weed-eating fish that is being employed to reduce weed growth in more than 50 countries worldwide. Triploid grass carp are created by first artificially fertilizing carp eggs and then heat-shocking the newly fertilized eggs. Heat-shock causes the diploid fertilized eggs to divide unevenly, producing a triploid cell that goes on to develop into a fish that is fully viable. The triploid grass carp eat weeds vigorously and, in doing so, help reduce weed growth in bodies of water without the use of herbicides. As a consequence of their triploidy, however, the carp are infertile, so they are unable to reproduce and don't invade the habitats into which they are introduced. The triploid grass carp must be restocked periodically if its continued presence is desired to control weed growth.

Polyploids exhibit a third characteristic of commercial importance—an increase in heterozygosity relative to diploids that comes about when inbred lines are crossed and is the basis of additional growth vigor. This phenomenon is known as **hybrid vigor**, and it consists of more rapid growth, increased production of fruits and flowers, and improved resistance to disease among the heterozygous (hybrid) progeny of inbred lines.

Polyploidy and Evolution

Evolution by polyploidy is a sudden, dramatic event that can lead to the development of a new species over a span of just one or two generations. The change in chromosome number—say, by doubling of chromosomes—can be a reproductive isolation mechanism (a form of new-species creation explored further in Section 20.7). For example, a mating between plant A, with 18 chromosomes ($n = 9$), and a related plant B, with 36 chromosomes ($n = 18$), could produce hybrid progeny with 27 chromosomes. A gamete with 9 chromosomes from plant A and 18 chromosomes from plant B would have an odd-numbered ploidy, which dramatically reduces fertility. Viable progeny are produced by self-fertilization of the hybrid.

Numerous examples of speciation (the creation of new species) by polyploidization have been documented in plants, but perhaps no common plant species embody the

evolutionary impact of polyploidy more dramatically than *Triticum aestivum*, common bread wheat, and *Triticum spelta*, spelt wheat (**Figure 10.12**). Both of these species are allohexaploids. Their development came about through the

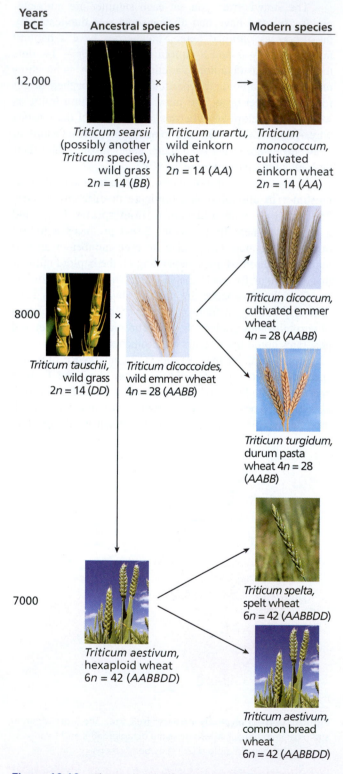

Figure 10.12 The evolution of modern wheat (*Triticum aestivum*), spelt wheat (*T. spelta*), durum pasta wheat (*T. turgidum*), and other modern species from crosses of ancestral species.

union of diploid genomes of three ancestral species in two hybridization events. This evolutionary history of modern wheat begins about 12,000 years ago with the hybridization of two diploid species that contain 14 chromosomes each. Einkorn wheat, *T. monococcum*, is a cultivated variety of wheat that can still be found around the world and is the modern form of wild einkorn wheat, *T. urartu*. Represented by the chromosome designation *AA*, *T. urartu* hybridized with a wild grass species, either *T. searsii* or *T. tripsacoides*, each with chromosomes represented as *BB*, to form an allotetraploid variety called emmer wheat, *T. dicoccoides*. Emmer wheat has 28 chromosomes and a chromosome formula *AABB* and was being cultivated approximately 8000 years ago when it underwent a second hybridization event with another wild diploid grass species, *T. tauschii* (chromosome formula *DD*), to form *T. aestivum* and *T. spelta* (both *AABBDD*), the modern allohexaploid species, which each have 42 chromosomes.

10.4 Chromosome Breakage Causes Mutation by Loss, Gain, and Rearrangement of Chromosomes

In animals, as mentioned earlier, the proper balance of gene dosage is critical for normal growth and development. For this reason, mutations that result in the loss or gain of whole chromosomes or chromosome segments have the potential to produce severe abnormalities. In this section, we examine changes to chromosome structure that occur by chromosome breakage and other events that lead to the loss or gain of chromosomal segments by the partial duplication or the partial deletion of a chromosome.

Partial Chromosome Deletion

When a chromosome breaks, both strands of DNA are severed at a location called a **chromosome break point**. The ends at the breakpoint of a broken chromosome retain their chromatin structure, and they can adhere to one another, to other truncated chromosome ends, or to the ends of intact chromosomes. Chromosome breakage can result in partial chromosome deletion by the loss of a portion of a chromosome. The size of the deletion and the specific genes deleted are significant factors in the degree of ensuing phenotypic abnormality. Larger chromosome deletions are detected by microscopy through the observation of altered chromosome banding patterns. In these larger deletions, many genes are affected, and the likelihood of substantial phenotypic consequences is very high.

A chromosome break that detaches all or part of one arm of a chromosome leads to a **terminal deletion** (**Figure 10.13a**). The chromosome fragment broken off in terminal deletion contains one of the chromosome ends, or *termini*, consisting of a telomere and additional genetic material.

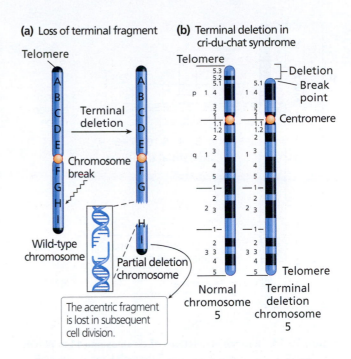

(a) Loss of terminal fragment

(b) Terminal deletion in cri-du-chat syndrome

Figure 10.13 **Chromosome terminal deletion.** **(a)** A double-stranded DNA break at a chromosome break point in region H leads to terminal deletion of the acentric fragment. **(b)** Terminal deletion of chromosome 5 in cri-du-chat syndrome.

Any part of a broken chromosome that the breakage leaves **acentric,** meaning without a centromere, can be lost during cell division. Without a centromere, the acentric fragment lacks a kinetochore and therefore is unable to attach spindle fibers and cannot migrate to a pole of the cell during division.

Organisms carrying one wild-type chromosome and a homolog with a terminal deletion are called **partial deletion heterozygotes**. A human condition known as cri-du-chat syndrome (OMIM 123450) is an example of a chromosome syndrome caused by terminal deletion, in this case the loss of 5p15.2–5p15.3 (**Figure 10.13b**). The syndrome is named for the distinctive cat-cry sound emitted by infants with the condition.

In contrast to a terminal deletion, which results from a single break at one end of a chromosome, an **interstitial deletion** is the loss of an internal segment of a chromosome that results from two chromosome breaks followed by a joining of the ends from either side of the lost segment. Interstitial deletions can be seen in many organisms, including humans. WAGR syndrome (OMIM 194072) and a closely related condition, WAGRO (OMIM 612469), both result from an interstitial deletion in humans affecting chromosome bands 11p1.3 and the adjoining band, 11p2. Studies of chromosome 11 structural abnormalities in patients with WAGR syndrome and WAGRO syndrome reveal partial chromosome deletions of various sizes, with the smallest common deletion region at 11p1.3 to 11p2 (**Figure 10.14**). The initials WAGR stand for *W*ilms tumor (a type of hereditary kidney cancer), *a*niridia (the absence of the iris in the eye), *g*enitourinary abnormalities, and mental *r*etardation. WAGRO has the same four developmental abnormalities as

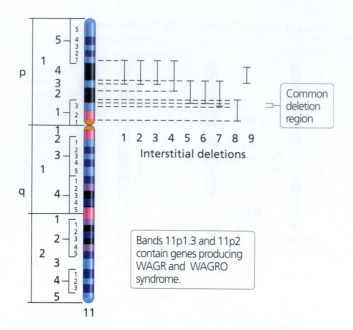

Figure 10.14 **Interstitial deletions of chromosome 11 in WAGR and WAGRO syndromes.** Deletions 5 through 8 result in WAGR, but deletions 1 through 4 and 9 do not. The smallest common deletion region affects bands 11p1.3 and 11p2.

WAGR, with the addition of obesity. Patients with the largest deletions have all five conditions, whereas patients with smaller deletions may have just one or two of the disorders.

WAGR syndrome and WAGRO syndrome result from gene dosage imbalance as a consequence of partial chromosome deletion. Researchers have identified two critical gene deletions in WAGR syndrome and an additional critical gene deletion in WAGRO syndrome. The gene *PAX6* produces a DNA-binding protein that is a transcription-regulating protein in development of the eye. The loss of this gene produces aniridia. The gene *WT1* produces a transcription-regulating protein that is essential for genitourinary development, and its loss is also tied to Wilms tumor and to mental disability. The third critical gene deleted in WAGRO syndrome is *BDNF*, which produces a protein expressed in the brain to protect striatal neurons from damage and destruction. When this gene is deleted, it produces obesity. Other mutant alleles of *BDNF* are associated with anorexia, bulimia, memory impairment, and obsessive-compulsive disorder. *BDNF* may play a role in the mental impairment that is part of WAGR syndrome.

Unequal Crossover

The process of reciprocal recombination (crossing over) achieves the recombination of alleles on homologous chromosomes without causing a gain or loss of chromosomal material that would result in mutation (see Sections 5.2 and 12.6). Occasionally, however, crossing over between homologs is inaccurate, resulting in chromosome mutations that are due to **unequal crossover.** These mutations result in the

partial duplication and **partial deletion** of chromosome segments on the resulting recombinant chromosomes. An organism carrying one homolog with duplicated material is a **partial duplication heterozygote**, whereas one with material deleted from one chromosome is a partial deletion heterozygote. Both states change the dosage of genes carried on the duplicated or deleted chromosome segments, and phenotypic abnormalities due to dosage effects can occur.

Unequal crossover is rare and occurs most commonly when repetitive regions of homologous chromosomes misalign. The human condition known as Williams–Beuren syndrome (WBS; OMIM 194050) is frequently found in partial deletion heterozygotes for a segment of chromosome 7. In wild-type chromosome 7, this region contains duplicate copies of the gene *PMS*, designated *PMS$_A$* and *PMS$_B$*, that are located near one another and have 17 genes located in between (**Figure 10.15a**). Misalignment of the homologous chromosomes results in mispairing of *PMS$_A$* on one chromosome with *PMS$_B$* on the homologous chromosome. A copy

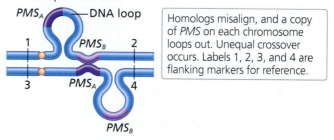

(a) Normal chromosome 7 structure

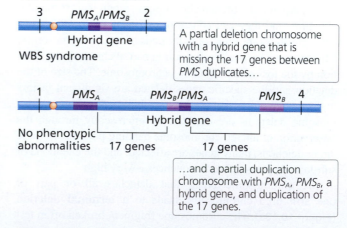

(b) Homologous chromosome misalignment and unequal crossover

(c) Deletion and duplication recombinant chromosomes
The recombinants are...

Figure 10.15 **Unequal crossover in creation of Williams–Beuren syndrome.**

of *PMS* on each chromosome is looped out from each homolog during misalignment (**Figure 10.15b**). Unequal crossing over between the misaligned chromosomes results in one recombinant chromosome that has a partial deletion chromosome 7 that results in WBS. This chromosome contains a nonfunctional hybrid PMS_A–PMS_B gene and is missing intact PMS_A and PMS_B genes as well as the 17 genes normally found between PMS_A and PMS_B (**Figure 10.15c**). The partial duplication chromosome (containing the PMS_A and PMS_B genes, a hybrid PMS_A–PMS_B gene, and duplicated copies of the 17 intervening genes) does not cause readily identifiable phenotypic abnormalities.

Detecting Duplication and Deletion

Large deletions or duplications of chromosome segments can be detected by microscopic examination that reveals altered chromosome banding patterns resulting from the structural change to the chromosome. Such deletions and duplications are generally quite large. In human chromosomes, duplications and deletions of about 100,000 to 200,000 base pairs are at the lower limit of chromosome banding visualization. **Microdeletions** and **microduplications** are considerably smaller and are generally not easily detected by chromosome banding analysis. Instead, molecular techniques such as FISH (fluorescent in situ hybridization; Section 10.1) can be used to detect the absence or duplication of a particular gene or chromosome sequence (**Figure 10.16**).

(a) Wild-type chromosome

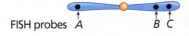

FISH probes *A*   *B* *C*

(b) Microinterstitial deletion

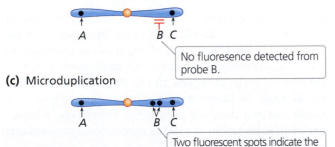

A   *B* *C*

No fluoresence detected from probe B.

(c) Microduplication

A   *B* *C*

Two fluorescent spots indicate the target of probe B is duplicated.

Figure 10.16 Detection of chromosome microdeletion and microduplication by FISH. (a) Three FISH probes identify genes *A*, *B*, and *C*. **(b)** Microdeletion of a chromosome segment containing *B* prevents probe hybridization. **(c)** Microduplication results in hybridization of probe *B* to duplicated genes.

⊙ Refer back to Figure 10.14. If a fluorescent label for chromosome band 11p2 was used to stain different copies of the chromosome, each having one of the nine partial deletions shown, which partial deletion chromosomes would be labeled by fluorescence and which would not?

Irrespective of the mechanism that may have created a partial chromosome duplication or deletion, prophase I homologous chromosome synapsis during meiosis produces a telltale signature of their existence. Homologous pairs that are mismatched because one contains a large duplication or deletion will form an **unpaired loop** in synapsis (**Figure 10.17**). Along most of the length of the homologous pair, normal synaptic pairing occurs. But in regions of structural difference, the extra material present on one chromosome bulges out to allow synaptic pairing on either side. The material in the loop is normal genetic material if one chromosome carries a deletion, and it is duplicated genetic material if one homolog carries a duplication.

Deletion Mapping

Pseudodominance is a genetic phenomenon that occurs when a normally recessive allele is "unmasked" and expressed in the phenotype because the dominant allele on the homologous chromosome has been deleted. Pseudodominance is used to map genes in deleted chromosome regions by a method known as **deletion mapping**.

We discussed a version of deletion mapping in Section 6.5 in connection with Benzer's fine-structure analysis of the genes involved in bacterial lysis by bacteriophage. In that analysis, Benzer mapped mutations by ascertaining whether it was possible to form a wild-type lysis recombinant between a lysis-deficient phage with a point mutation (a revertible mutation) and one with a deletion mutation (a nonrevertible mutation). In studies using deletion mutation analysis in diploid organisms, the unmasking of a recessive allele (the observation of pseudodominance) is central to gene mapping. **Figure 10.18** shows deletion mapping using pseudodominance to map the *Notch* gene (*n*) in *Drosophila*. The *Notch* gene resides on the X chromosome, and its location is revealed by the detection of pseudodominance in female fruit flies that are heterozygous for partial X-chromosome deletions. Pseudodominance appears when the portion containing the dominant allele has been deleted from one X chromosome, allowing the recessive allele that still resides on the other, intact X chromosome to be

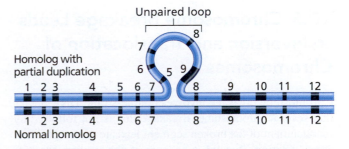

Unpaired loop

Homolog with partial duplication

Normal homolog

Figure 10.17 An unpaired loop at synapsis. The partial duplication heterozygote shown here has duplicated genetic material of bands 5 through 9. The extra material forms an unpaired loop at synapsis to allow homologous regions to align correctly.

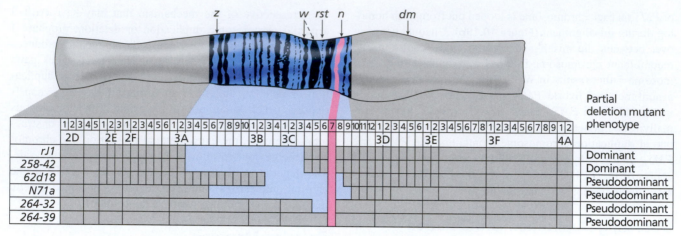

Figure 10.18   Deletion mapping of the *Drosophila Notch* (*n*) gene. The open blue sections of the grid without bisecting lines show the extent of each partial deletion of the *Drosophila* X chromosome for six partial deletion mutants. The retention of the dominant character or the emergence of notch by pseudodominance is indicated in the right-hand column. The smallest X-chromosome segment missing from all pseudodominant mutants is region 3C7, indicating this as the location of the gene.

expressed. In the figure, the gray segments in the grid represent chromosome segments remaining on the partial deletion X chromosomes of six different mutants. The colored portions of the grid identify segments that have been deleted from that chromosome in each mutant. The first two partial deletions (rJ1 and 258-42) do not lead to pseudodominance (in other words, the dominant wild-type phenotype is observed), indicating that the regions deleted do not contain the *Notch* gene. The next two partial deletions, 62d18 and N71a, do result in pseudodominance (in other words, the recessive phenotype is observed), indicating that the *Notch* gene locus containing the dominant allele is in the region 3C4 to 3C8. To home in on the location of *Notch*, progressively smaller partial deletions are used to identify the smallest deletion segment common to all deletions resulting in pseudodominance. In this instance the smallest partial deletion common to genomes expressing pseudodominance for *Notch* is region 3C-7, which is missing from mutant 264-39. This is where the gene resides. Genetic Analysis 10.3 guides you through analysis of deletion mapping.

10.5 Chromosome Breakage Leads to Inversion and Translocation of Chromosomes

Chromosome breakage involves double-strand DNA breaks that sever a chromosome. Breakage that is not followed by reattachment of the broken segment leads to partial chromosome deletion—but what happens if the broken chromosome reassembles with the broken segment reattached in the *wrong orientation* or if the broken segment reattaches to a *nonhomologous* chromosome? The answers are that reattachment in the wrong orientation produces a **chromosome**

inversion, whereas attachment to a nonhomologous chromosome results in **chromosome translocation**. We discuss two types of chromosome inversion events and two types of chromosome translocation in this section. A repeating theme that emerges is that as long as no critical genes or regulatory regions are mutated by chromosome breakage, and as long as dosage-sensitive genes are retained in their proper balance, individuals that have a chromosome inversion or a chromosome translocation might not experience any phenotypic abnormalities. However, complications during meiosis may affect the efficiency of chromosome segregation, and fertility may be affected in those individuals.

Chromosome Inversion

Chromosome inversions occur as a result of chromosome breaks followed by reattachment of the free segment in the reverse orientation. Two kinds of chromosome inversion are observed, depending on whether the centromere is part of the inverted segment (**Figure 10.19**). **Paracentric inversion** results from the inversion of a chromosome segment on a single arm and *does not* involve the centromere, whereas **pericentric inversion** reorients a chromosome segment that *includes* the centromere.

Inversion most commonly affects just one member of a homologous pair of chromosomes, and individuals who have one inverted chromosome and a homologous chromosome without the inversion are designated as **inversion heterozygotes**. The definition might be more specific—for instance, *paracentric inversion heterozygote* or *pericentric inversion heterozygote*—if the type of inversion is known.

Chromosome inversion causes a difference in linear order of genes on homologous chromosomes by a 180-degree reorientation of the inverted segment. Again, if the chromosome breakage event leading to the inversion

PROBLEM In *Drosophila*, the X-linked recessive mutant traits singed bristle, lozenge eye, and cut wing are encoded at linked genes. Five strains of *Drosophila* produced by the cross of pure-breeding wild-type and pure-breeding mutant flies (*SLC/SLC* × *slc/slc*) are expected to have the trihybrid genotype *SLC/slc* and express the wild-type phenotypes. Females of each strain exhibit pseudodominance for one or more of the traits, however, due to partial deletion of the X chromosome.

> **BREAK IT DOWN:** Pseudodominance can emerge in heterozygous organisms when the dominant allele on one copy of a chromosome pair is deleted, leaving only the recessive allele on the unaltered chromosome (p. 377).

Comparative X-chromosome maps showing the extent of deletions in each pseudodominant strain (indicated by dashed lines) are given here along with the pseudodominant phenotypes found in each strain. Use this information to locate each gene as accurately as possible along the X chromosome.

> **BREAK IT DOWN:** Gene mapping by pseudodominance seeks to identify the smallest region of chromosome that might contain a particular gene (p. 378).

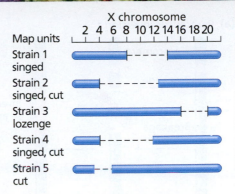

Solution Strategies	Solution Steps
Evaluate	
1. Identify the topic this problem addresses and the nature of the required answer.	1. This problem addresses deletion mapping using pseudodominance to locate the position of each gene. The answer requires construction of a map of gene locations.
2. Identify the critical information given in the problem.	2. The deletion regions on chromosomes and the corresponding pseudodominant phenotypes are given.
Deduce	
3. Review the meaning of pseudodominance and the connection between chromosome deletion and pseudodominance.	3. Pseudodominance is the appearance of a recessive trait in a presumed heterozygous organism due to deletion of a chromosome segment carrying the dominant allele. In deletion mapping using pseudodominance, the location of a gene maps to the smallest common deletion region shared by all organisms expressing the pseudodominant trait.
Solve	
4. Interpret the meaning of the pseudodominant phenotype in strain 1. TIP: Compare deletion mutants that share pseudodominance phenotypes to see where their deletions overlap.	4. Strain 1 is missing chromosome material from the 8th to the 14th map unit. The appearance of the pseudodominant phenotype singed indicates that the *singed* gene maps to this interval.
5. Compare strain 2 with strain 1, and interpret the meaning of the new pseudodominant phenotype cut.	5. Strain 2 has a deletion from map units 4 to 13 that includes both *singed* and *cut*. This narrows the location of *singed* to the interval between 8 and 13 map units. The *cut* location is between the 4th and 8th map unit, based on its appearance with the deletion of this interval.
6. Assess pseudodominance of strain 3.	6. Co-occurrence of the deletion between map units 16 and 20 and the appearance of the pseudodominant lozenge phenotype maps the *lozenge* gene to this location.
7. Assess strains 4 and 5, and refine the locations of the genes further where possible. TIP: Again, compare deletion mutants that share pseudodominance phenotypes to see where their deletions overlap.	7. Strain 4 contains a deletion between map units 4 and 12, confining the location of *singed* to the interval between 8 and 12. This strain provides no additional information about the location of *cut*. The deletion between map units 3 and 6 in strain 5 includes *cut* and refines its location to between map units 4 and 6.
8. Identify gene locations based on the deletion-mapping analysis.	8. Based on the data for pseudodominance in these five strains, *cut* resides in the interval between units 4 and 6, *singed* lies between 8 and 12, and *lozenge* is between 16 and 20.

For more practice, see Problems 8, 22, and 24.

Visit the Study Area to access study tools. **Mastering Genetics**

(a) Paracentric inversion

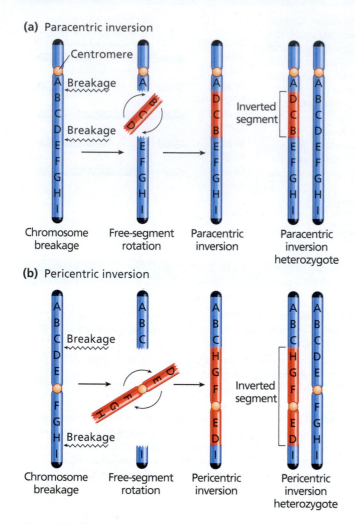

Chromosome breakage — Free-segment rotation — Paracentric inversion — Paracentric inversion heterozygote

(b) Pericentric inversion

Chromosome breakage — Free-segment rotation — Pericentric inversion — Pericentric inversion heterozygote

Figure 10.19 Paracentric and pericentric chromosome inversion. The letters represent regions of chromosomes, not single genes.

does not mutate any critical genes or regulatory DNA sequences, there may be no phenotypic consequence to the inversion heterozygote. Nevertheless, the difference in gene order between the homologs leads to a need for some chromosomal gymnastics during prophase I when homologous chromosomes synapse. To bring the homologs of an inversion heterozygote into synaptic alignment, the formation of an unusual **inversion loop** is required. Such inversion loops form readily, as chromosomes are flexible enough to form the required structures without breakage.

Figure 10.20 illustrates the formation of an inversion loop in a paracentric heterozygote and also demonstrates the generation of partial chromosome duplication and partial chromosome deletion as a result of certain crossover events that may occur between the homologs. Specifically, crossing over *inside* the region of the inversion loop results in duplications and

Figure 10.20 The consequences of crossover in the inversion loop in paracentric inversion heterozygotes.

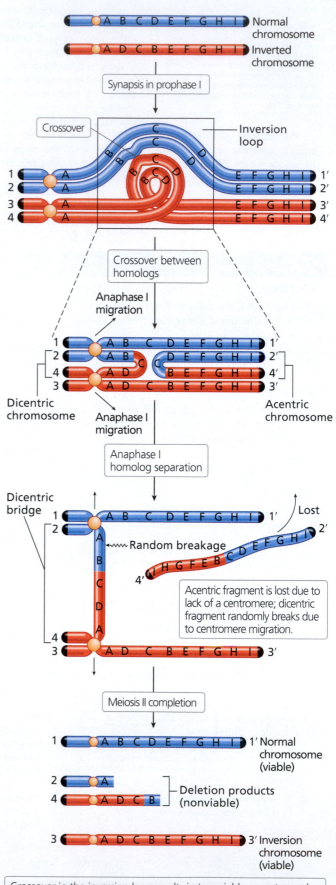

Crossover in the inversion loop results in two viable gametes and two nonviable gametes.

deletions among the recombinant chromosomes. By contrast, crossing over taking place *outside* the inversion loop region proceeds in the normal, reciprocal manner and none of the recombinant chromosomes gains or loses any genetic material.

The crossover examined in Figure 10.20 occurs within the inversion loop, between chromosome regions B and C. After crossover occurs, one normal-order chromosome (1 • ABCDEFGHI 1′) and one inverted-order chromosome (3 • ADCBEFGHI 3′) are unchanged by recombination (the dot represents the centromere). The recombinant chromosomes, however, are abnormal: One is a **dicentric chromosome** with two centromeres (2 • ABCDA • 4), and the other is an acentric fragment that has no centromere 2′ IHGFEDCBEFGHI 4′). At anaphase I, when centromeres on homologous chromosomes normally migrate toward opposite poles, a **dicentric bridge** forms as the dicentric chromosome is pulled toward both poles of the cell. Eventually the bridge snaps under the tension, at a random break point. Both products of the break have a centromere, but both are also missing genetic material. In contrast, the acentric fragment, lacking a centromere, has no mechanism by which to migrate to a pole of the cell and will be lost during meiosis. The completion of meiosis of this paracentric inversion heterozygote results in two viable gametes, one with the normal-order chromosome (1 • ABCDEFGHI 1′) and one with the inverted-order chromosome (3 • ADCBEFGHI 3′), and two nonviable gametes with partial deletion chromosomes.

Crossover in the inversion loop in a pericentric inversion heterozygote also yields two viable gametes and two nonviable gametes (**Figure 10.21**). One viable gamete contains the normal-order chromosome (1 ABCDE • FGHI 1′) and one contains the inversion-order chromosome (3 ABCHGF • EDI 3′). Each of the two nonviable gametes has a combination of deletions and duplications (2 ABCDE • FGHCBA 4 and 4′ IDE • FGHI 2′).

Three observations about recombination in inversion heterozygotes have important genetic implications:

1. **The probability of crossover within the inversion loop is linked to the size of the inversion loop.** Small inversions produce small inversion loops that have a low frequency of crossover. On the other hand, larger inversions produce loops that span more of the chromosome and correlate with a higher probability of crossover.

2. **Inversion suppresses the production of recombinant chromosomes.** The viable gametes produced by inversion heterozygotes contain either the normal-order chromosome or the inversion-order chromosome, but no recombinant chromosomes are viable, due to duplications and deletions of chromosome segments. The absence of recombinant chromosomes in progeny is identified as **crossover suppression**. In reality, crossovers do occur between homologous chromosomes carried by inversion heterozygotes, but because the recombinant chromosomes contain

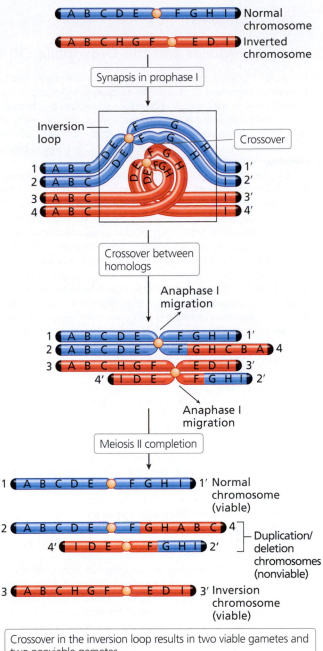

Crossover in the inversion loop results in two viable gametes and two nonviable gametes.

Figure 10.21 **The consequences of crossover in the inversion loop in pericentric inversion heterozygotes.**

Q If two chromosome homologs each contain the same inversions, would they form an inversion loop? Why or why not?

duplications and deletions, there is little possibility of viability for any progeny formed from the gametes that contain them. Geneticists have taken advantage of crossover suppression in research by marking crossover-suppressed chromosomes with dominant alleles that aid in the interpretation of genetic crosses. **Experimental Insight 10.1** describes research by Hermann Muller, who used the so-called ClB ("See-el-bee")

EXPERIMENTAL INSIGHT 10.1

Hermann Muller and the *Drosophila* ClB Chromosome Method

Hermann Muller, a student of Thomas Hunt Morgan, made numerous important contributions to genetics. Among these were his discoveries that X-rays induce mutations by chromosome breakage and his development of a genetic method to identify recessive lethal X-ray–induced mutations of the X chromosome in *Drosophila* called the ClB ("see-el-bee") method.

To identify X-ray-induced recessive lethal mutations, Muller first created an X chromosome called the ClB chromosome, where "C" stands for *crossover suppression*, "l" for presence of a recessive *lethal* mutation, and "B" for a dominant mutation producing an abnormal *bar*-shaped eye. Crossover suppression is a result of the presence of multiple inversions on the chromosome that prevent the production of viable recombinant chromosomes by crossing over between the ClB and wild-type X chromosomes in females. Bar eye is a dominant mutant phenotype that alters the shape of the eye. It permanently marks the ClB chromosome since it cannot be reshuffled by recombination. In other words, a bar-shaped eye will be observed in all surviving flies that inherit the ClB chromosome. Potentially lethal recessive mutations [*m*(?)] are generated on X chromosomes of wild-type males by X-ray exposure.

Muller began his search for lethal X-ray–induced mutations by exposing wild-type male fruit flies to X-rays with the intent of inducing mutations in germ-line cells (see the figure). In Cross I, X-ray–exposed males were crossed to a bar-eyed female (ClB/+). Male progeny of Cross I that are hemizygous for ClB (ClB/Y) die as a result of the lethal mutation (*l*) on the X chromosome, whereas wild-type males (+/Y) survive. Female progeny of the cross either are wild type [+ / *m*(?)] or they have bar-shaped eyes and carry a copy of the ClB chromosome (ClB/+).

In Cross II, Muller mated bar-eyed female progeny from Cross I to wild-type males from Cross I. Cross II has two possible outcomes depending on whether or not a recessive lethal mutation was induced by X-irradiation. If X-ray exposure *did not* induce a lethal mutation on the X chromosome, then Muller expected a 2:1 ratio of females to males (Cross II progeny alternative A). In this outcome, all females survive. About half have bar eye and half are carriers of the potential mutant *m*(?). Males inheriting the ClB chromosome are hemizygous for the recessive lethal mutation on the ClB chromosome and they die. Males inheriting the *m*(?) X chromosome [*m*(?)/Y] will survive. The phenotype of these surviving males will be wild type if there is no mutation on the X chromosome or mutant if a nonlethal mutation on the X chromosome was produced by X-irradiation.

On the other hand, if X-irradiation induced a recessive lethal mutation, no males are predicted from Cross II (Cross II progeny alternative B) since all males inherit a recessive lethal X-linked mutation. Males inheriting the ClB chromosome would die, but so would males inheriting the *m*(?) X chromosome carrying the X-ray–induced lethal mutation. In this outcome, only female progeny are produced. Female progeny in this category of Cross II progeny that do not have bar eye are heterozygous carriers of the recessive lethal

(continued)

Cross I: ♀ ClB/+ × ♂ Wild type (X-ray exposed)

X-Rays → *m*(?)

+   ClB
Bar eye

Females
ClB   *m*(?) and +   *m*(?)
Bar eye   Wild type

Males
+   and   ClB
Wild type   Dies

Cross II: ♀ ClB/*m*(?) × ♂ Wild type

ClB   *m*(?)   +

Cross II progeny possibility 1

If no lethal mutation is induced by X-irradiation, a 2:1 ratio of ♀ : ♂ is expected.

Females
ClB   + and *m*(?)   +
Bar eye   Wild type

Males
m(?)   and   ClB
Wild type or mutant   Dies

Cross II progeny possibility 2

Alternatively, if lethal mutation is induced, hemizygous *m*(?)/Y males die and only female progeny are produced.

Females
ClB   + and *m*(?)   +
Bar eye   Wild type (mutation carrier)

Males
m(?)   and   ClB
Dies   Dies

Additional study and possible characterization of the induced lethal mutation

mutation. They can be used in additional studies to characterize the nature of the lethal mutation.

Identifying X-ray–induced recessive lethal mutations using the ClB method is highly accurate: It requires only a determination of whether or not males are produced by Cross II. Nonlethal X-ray induced mutations can also be identified, by examining the males produced by Cross II.

Muller used the ClB method to demonstrate that X-ray exposure induces mutations at a rate more than 150 times greater than the spontaneous mutation rate in *Drosophila*. His work led to the characterization of many of these mutations and to the identification of the linear relationship between the level of X-ray exposure and the frequency of induced lethal mutations.

---

chromosome to identify and later investigate lethal X-linked mutations induced in *Drosophila* by X-ray exposure.

3. **Fertility may be altered if an inversion heterozygote carries a very large inversion.** When an inversion spans all or nearly all the length of a chromosome, any crossover that occurs will produce two viable and two nonviable gametes. This means that approximately half the gametes will be lost in the specific case of an inversion heterozygote who carries a very large inversion. No such loss of fertility is expected for organisms with small inversions.

Chromosome Translocation

Chromosome translocation takes place when chromosome breakage is followed by the reattachment of a broken segment to a *nonhomologous* chromosome. Once again, if no critical genes are severed or have their regulatory regions disrupted by the breakage or translocation events, **translocation heterozygotes**, with one normal chromosome and one altered chromosome in each affected homologous pair, may display no outward phenotype effects. Even if no phenotypic abnormalities are detected, however, certain translocation heterozygotes can experience semisterility as a result of abnormalities of chromosome segregation, as described below.

Three principal types of translocation are observed. **Unbalanced translocation** arises from a chromosome break and subsequent reattachment of the fragment to a nonhomologous chromosome in a one-way event; that is, a piece of one chromosome is translocated to a nonhomologous chromosome and there is no reciprocal event (**Figure 10.22a**). **Reciprocal balanced translocation** is produced when breaks occur on two nonhomologous chromosomes and the resulting fragments switch places when they are reattached (**Figure 10.22b**). **Robertsonian translocation**, also known as **chromosome fusion**, involves the fusion of two nonhomologous chromosomes. Chromosome fusion is accompanied by loss of one of the centromeres and by the loss of a chromosome short (p) arm (**Figure 10.22c**). The chromosomes involved in Robertsonian translocation are usually acrocentric or telocentric chromosomes. These have little or no genetic information in the short arm, thus the organism does not suffer

harm by the chromosome fusion event. Were chromosome fusion to lead to the loss of critical genes, the organism would not survive. One consequence of Robertsonian translocation is the reduction of chromosome number.

Patterns of Reciprocal Balanced Translocation In reciprocal balanced translocation, one member of each homologous pair is altered by translocation, and none of the four chromosomes has a fully homologous partner. Instead, the translocated chromosome segments homologous to the normal member of each pair are dispersed on two other chromosomes. The absence of complete homology between chromosome pairs requires formation of an unusual tetravalent synaptic structure, a cross-like configuration made up of the four chromosomes related by the translocation, to enable homologous regions to synapse during metaphase I, as shown in **Figure 10.23**. The chromosomes in the figure are labeled I, II, III, and IV so that we may more easily follow their progress in meiosis and meiotic outcomes.

Two main patterns of chromosome segregation emerge from the tetravalent structures found in translocation heterozygotes. *Alternate segregation* and *adjacent-1 segregation* each occur in approximately 50% of meiotic divisions, although the actual proportions vary somewhat among different species. At anaphase I in **alternate segregation**, chromosomes I and IV move to one cell pole and chromosomes II and III move to the opposite pole. At the completion of meiosis, all gametes are viable because each contains a complete set of genetic information for the two chromosomes. Fertilization of a gamete containing chromosomes I and IV will produce a normal zygote, whereas fertilization of a gamete containing chromosomes II and III will produce a zygote with reciprocal balanced translocation heterozygosity, like the parent chromosomes at the top of the figure.

In anaphase I of **adjacent-1 segregation**, chromosomes I and III are moved to one cell pole and chromosomes II and IV go to the opposite pole. None of the gametes formed by this pattern of segregation is viable because of duplications and deletions of genetic information. Gametes containing chromosomes I and III have a duplication of the F and G regions, along with deletion of the R and S regions. Conversely, gametes containing chromosomes II and IV have a duplication of the R and S regions and a deletion of regions F and G.

(a) Unbalanced translocation

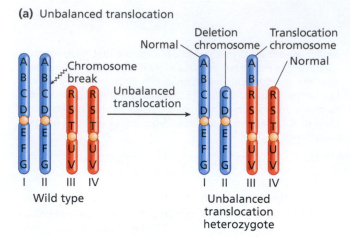

(b) Reciprocal balanced translocation

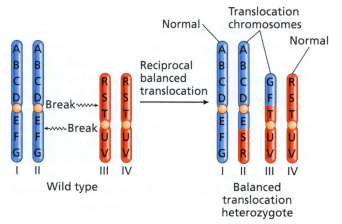

(c) Robertsonian translocation (chromosome fusion)

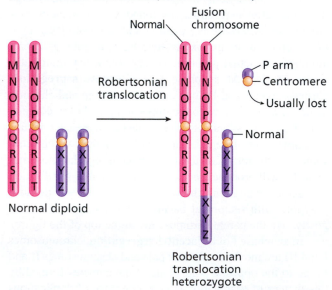

Figure 10.22 **Unbalanced, reciprocal balanced, and Robertsonian chromosome translocations.**

🔍 Refer back to Figure 10.2 and suppose that a male has a Robertsonian translocation involving chromosomes 18 and 22. State two ways in which the karyotype of the person with the translocation would look different from the normal karyotype shown in the figure.

Occasionally, an unusual pattern of segregation known as adjacent-2 segregation takes place. It is rare because it requires that chromosomes I and II, which have homologous centromeres, move to the same pole of the cell at anaphase I. Correspondingly, chromosomes III and IV, which also have homologous centromeres, also move to the same cell pole (opposite chromosomes I and II). This is atypical of the usual pattern at anaphase I, in which homologous chromosomes (that carry homologous centromeres) are separated in the reduction division. None of the gametes or progeny resulting from adjacent-2 segregation is viable.

In summary, cell biologists conclude that in balanced translocation heterozygotes, only alternate segregation produces viable gametes and viable progeny. This pattern accounts for just one-half of all meiotic events in these individuals; thus, the semisterility of translocation heterozygotes is due to reduction by about one-half in the number of viable gametes that can be produced.

Patterns Of Robertsonian Translocation In organisms with a Robertsonian translocation, also known as chromosome fusion, two nonhomologous chromosomes fuse to form a single, larger chromosome, resulting in a reduction in chromosome number. If two pairs of chromosomes fuse by Robertsonian translocation (meaning each chromosome of pair "A" fuses to a different chromosome of pair "B"), the number of chromosomes in a genome is reduced to $2n - 2$. This is a frequently observed mechanism by which chromosome number diverges in related organisms.

Evolution of just this kind is happening to the mice on Madeira, a tiny island off the western coast of Portugal: They are in the process of differentiating into two species! Madeira, about 20 miles long and 8 miles wide, has steep volcanic mountains running down the middle that form a barrier to easy mouse migration. The common house mouse (*Mus musculus*) was introduced to Madeira by sailors in the 1400s. Today, Madeira has two distinct populations of mice, one on either side of the central mountain range.

In addition to the mountain range separating these two populations, each has also undergone multiple chromosome fusions that have reduced their diploid number. The usual chromosome number for *Mus musculus* is 20 pairs ($2n = 40$). On Madeira, however, one population has $2n = 22$, and the other has $2n = 24$. Because each population has a different chromosome number, interpopulation hybrids are sterile. Such hybrids carry 23 chromosomes (11 from one parent and 12 from the other) and therefore cannot form viable gametes. This is an example of reproductive isolation that can lead to speciation based on differences in chromosome structure and chromosome number. The Case Study at the end of the chapter returns to this theme in discussing the evolution of human chromosome composition and number.

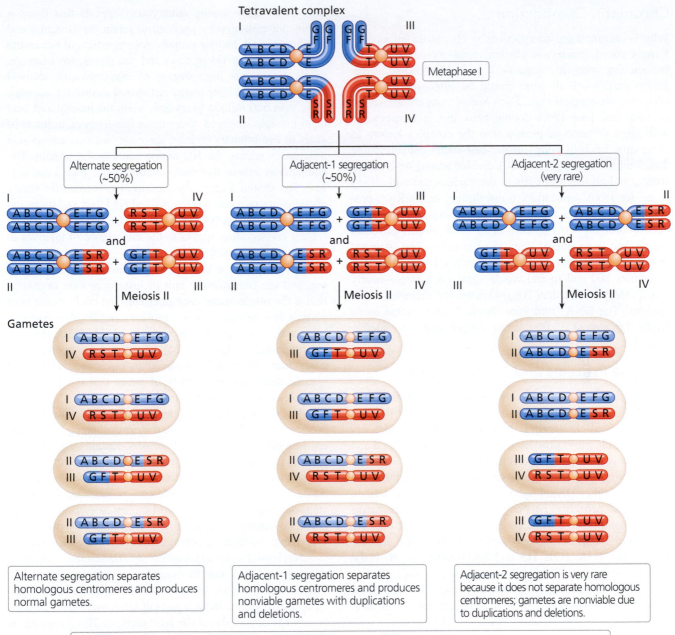

Figure 10.23 The tetravalent synaptic structure and alternate and adjacent chromosome segregation in reciprocal balanced translocation heterozygotes.

10.6 Eukaryotic Chromosomes Are Organized into Chromatin

We return now to the subject of chromosome structure and the chromatin organization of eukaryotic chromosomes. This molecular organization is essential to the normal function and distribution of chromosomes in cell division, and it plays a pivotal role in the regulation of gene expression that typifies all kinds of eukaryotic cells. In this section we describe the typical chromatin organization of chromosomes and its impact on chromosomes throughout the cell cycle. At the end of this section we introduce the concept of the influence of chromatin compaction on gene expression by examining a mutant phenotype in fruit flies. In Section 13.2 we take up further discussion of the regulation of gene expression in eukaryotes, exploring the normal and essential role chromatin plays in these processes.

Chromatin Compaction

Why is chromosome compaction by chromatin important? Simply stated, eukaryotic chromosomes would not fit into the nucleus without compaction, and chromosome segregation during cell division would be impossible without chromosome condensation. Each one of your chromosomes contains one long DNA double helix that is incorporated with large amounts of protein into the complex known as chromatin. Each of your somatic cell nuclei contains more than 6 billion base pairs of DNA divided among 46 chromosomes, and all that DNA fits in the nucleus and still allows space for DNA replication, transcription, and mRNA processing, thanks to a remarkable feat of biomolecular engineering brought about by chromatin. If all 46 chromosomes were taken from one of your somatic cell nuclei, stripped of their proteins, and unwound to a relaxed state, the DNA molecules laid end to end would span 1.8 meters—nearly 6 feet. This is more than 260,000 times the diameter of the nucleus! The DNA from your shortest chromosome alone would be almost 15,000 times longer than the nuclear diameter.

Histone Proteins and Nucleosomes

By weight, each eukaryotic chromosome is approximately half DNA and half proteins, and about one-half of the protein content of chromatin is **histone protein**. The histones are five small, basic proteins that are positively charged and bind tightly to negatively charged DNA. Equally abundant in the chromatin, but more diverse, is an array of hundreds of types of other DNA-binding proteins named, by default, **nonhistone proteins**. This large array of proteins performs a variety of tasks in the nucleus, not all of which are defined.

The five types of histone proteins in chromatin are designated **H1**, **H2A**, **H2B**, **H3**, and **H4** (Table 10.4). H1 is the largest and most variable histone protein, containing 215 to 244 amino acids, depending on the species. The other four histones are considerably smaller and more uniform in size, containing between 102 and 129 amino acids.

Among eukaryotes, there is very strong evolutionary conservation of the amino acid sequences of histone proteins. This consistency among eukaryotes suggests that there is significant evolutionary pressure to retain the structure and function of each histone protein. A comparison of the amino acid sequences of H4 in cows and pea plants, for example, demonstrates this high degree of evolutionarily retained identity. Cows and pea plants last shared a common ancestor more than 500 million years ago, when the animal and land plant lineages diverged. Over those hundreds of millions of years of evolutionary change, there are just two amino acid differences among the 102 amino acids in the protein. The comparison tells us that since the time when plants and animals last shared a common ancestor, extraordinarily strong evolutionary pressure has maintained H4 DNA and its amino acid sequence identity in organisms. This example of evolutionary conservation speaks to the importance of histones in eukaryotic chromosome organization.

Histones are the principal agents in chromatin packaging, and the fundamental unit of histone protein organization is the **nucleosome core particle**. The nucleosome core particle is a heterooctameric protein complex that contains two molecules each of four histones—H2A, H2B, H3, and H4 (Foundation Figure 10.24). These proteins are continuously transcribed and translated in eukaryotic cells, and histone genes are one family of genes that are present in multiple copies in eukaryotic genomes.

Nucleosome core particles self-assemble. The histone proteins first self-assemble into dimers containing two different histones each: H2A–H2B dimers contain one molecule each of histone 2A and histone 2B, and H3–H4 dimers contain one molecule each of histone 3 and histone 4. Current evidence indicates that nucleosome core particles are formed in steps that begin with two H3–H4 dimers assembling to form a histone tetramer. The tetramer is then joined by two H2A–H2B dimers to form the octameric nucleosome core particle.

Nucleosome core particles are flat-ended structures approximately 11 nm in diameter by 5.7 nm thick (see Figure 10.24a). Each nucleosome core particle is wrapped by approximately 146 base pairs of DNA that twist one-and-two-thirds times around the core particle. This wrapping is the first level of DNA condensation, and it condenses the DNA approximately sevenfold.

Table 10.4	Histone Protein Characteristics			
Histone[a]	Ratio of Basic/Acidic Amino Acids	Molecular Weight (D)	Number of Amino Acids	Location
H1	5.4	23,000	224	Linker DNA
H2A	1.4	13,960	129	Nucleosome
H2B	1.7	13,774	125	Nucleosome
H3	1.8	15,273	135	Nucleosome
H4	2.5	11,236	102	Nucleosome

[a] Histone proteins from calf thymus gland.

Condensing the Nuclear Material
The hierarchy of chromatin organization and chromosome condensation.

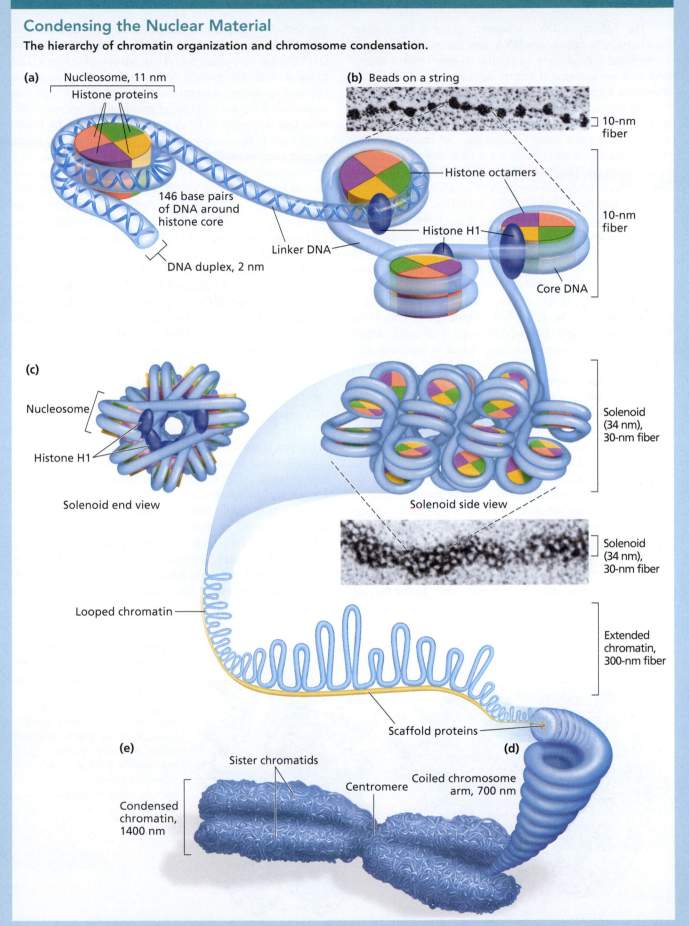

(a) Nucleosome, 11 nm
Histone proteins
146 base pairs of DNA around histone core
Linker DNA
DNA duplex, 2 nm

(b) Beads on a string
10-nm fiber
Histone octamers
10-nm fiber
Histone H1
Core DNA

(c)
Nucleosome
Histone H1
Solenoid end view

Solenoid (34 nm), 30-nm fiber
Solenoid side view
Solenoid (34 nm), 30-nm fiber

Looped chromatin
Extended chromatin, 300-nm fiber

Scaffold proteins

(e)
Sister chromatids
Condensed chromatin, 1400 nm
Centromere
(d) Coiled chromosome arm, 700 nm

The 146 bp of DNA wrapped around a nucleosome core particle is called **core DNA**, and the combination of a nucleosome core particle wrapped with core DNA is identified as a **nucleosome**. Electron micrographs of chromatin fibers in a highly decondensed state show a regular series of circular structures strung together by connecting filaments (see Figure 10.24b). This form of chromatin is identified as the "beads on a string" morphology of chromatin. The "beads" are nucleosomes that are a little more than 11 nm in diameter, and the "string" is called **linker DNA**. Linker DNA is the DNA between regions of core DNA.

The length of linker DNA segments varies among organisms, although in each species it is a consistent length and thus nucleosomes occur at regular intervals. In the yeast *Saccharomyces cerevisiae*, linker DNA is 13 to 18 bp in length. Linker DNA is about 35 bp long in the fruit fly *Drosophila*. In humans and other mammals, linker DNA spans about 40 to 50 bp; in sea urchins, linker DNA is very long—approximately 110 bp. If the 146 bp in length of core DNA is added to the length of linker DNA, the nucleosome repeat distance of the beads-on-a-string structure is approximately 160 to 260 bp. This beads-on-a-string form of chromatin is identified as the **10-nm fiber**, since the diameter of nucleosomes is approximately 10 nm.

This nucleosome-based model of chromatin was proposed by Roger Kornberg in 1974. Kornberg based his model on biochemical observations that chromatin contains a ratio of one molecule of each of the four core histone proteins (H2, H2A, H3, and H4) to each 100 base pairs and one molecule of the histone H1 to each 200 base pairs.

Structural protein–imaging (described momentarily) supported Kornberg's model, but the molecular proof of the model's validity came from research by Markus Noll, who treated eukaryotic chromatin with different concentrations of the enzyme DNase I to cut DNA where it is not protected by bound proteins. Recall from Research Technique 8.1

(pp. 288–289) and discussion in Section 8.3 in connection with DNA footprint-protection analysis that DNase I cuts DNA that has no protein bound to it but is unable to cut DNA in regions bound by protein. Noll's most important result was obtained by mixing mammalian chromatin with a high concentration of DNase I and using gel electrophoresis to determine that the length of DNA fragments produced by DNase I digestion measured approximately 200 bp in length. This is precisely the length Kornberg predicted, as it is the sum of the approximately 145 bp of DNA wrapping a nucleosome core particle and the 55 bp of linked DNA between nucleosomes.

Kornberg's model was also supported by structural protein studies, X-ray diffraction imaging, and cryogenic electron microscopy (cryo-EM). The latter has produced detailed images of nucleosome structure and revealed the likely points of interaction between the octameric nucleosome core particle and core DNA. Timothy Richmond and his colleagues have described the crystal structure of the nucleosome using cryo-EM at 2.8-Å resolution (**Figure 10.25**). Richmond's analysis indicates that there are 1.65 turns of core DNA around each nucleosome core particle. The analysis identifies additional molecular interactions between the N-terminal (amino terminal) tails of histone proteins and core and linker DNA. These interactions are critically important to the types of chromatin structure present in different regions of eukaryotic chromosomes.

The 10-nm fiber is an unnatural state for chromatin. To achieve it, chromatin must be chemically treated and held in conditions that are not found in cells. Under in vitro conditions, chromatin forms the **30-nm fiber**, although it is not certain this structure forms in vivo (see Figure 10.24c). Electron micrographs and molecular modeling help us visualize how the 30-nm fiber is assembled. It is produced by coalescence of the 10-nm fiber into a cylindrical filament of coiled nucleosomes that is hollow in the middle. Due to its coiled structure and open middle, the 30-nm fiber is often also called the **solenoid structure** (like the coil of wire in

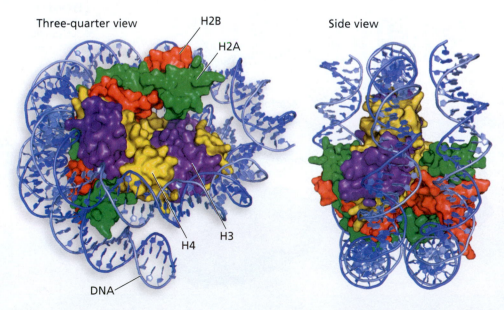

Three-quarter view   H2B   H2A   Side view

H4   H3

DNA

Figure 10.25 Nucleosome structure. A computer-generated rendering of the X-ray crystal structure of the nucleosome imaged at 2.8-Å resolution by cryo-electron microscopy shows the eight histone protein molecules in the color-coded nucleosome core particle. DNA wraps one and two-thirds turns around the core particle, a span of approximately 146 bp.

the starter of a car). Each turn of the solenoid structure contains six to eight nucleosomes. The diameter of the solenoid is approximately 34 nm. Research examining in vivo chromatin structures will soon be able to determine occur in cells or only in vitro.

The histone protein H1 plays a key role in stabilizing the solenoid structure. The long N-terminal and C-terminal ends of the H1 protein attach to adjacent nucleosome core particles. H1 protein pulls the nucleosomes into an orderly solenoid array and lines the inside of the structure. Experimental analysis shows that chromatin from which H1 has been removed can form 10-nm fibers but not 30-nm fibers. Chromatin exists in a 30-nm-fiber state or a more condensed state during interphase.

Higher Order Chromatin Organization and Chromosome Structure

Beyond the 30-nm stage, chromatin compaction and the presence of nonhistone proteins are integral to the structure of chromosomes and the process of chromosome condensation that initiates with the onset of prophase in the M phase of the cell cycle. Nonhistone proteins perform multiple roles in influencing chromosome structure and in facilitating M phase chromosome condensation. Interphase chromosome structure results from the formation of looped domains of chromatin similar to supercoiled bacterial DNA (see Figure 10.24d). The loops are variable in size, containing from tens to hundreds of kilobase pairs and consisting of 30-nm–fiber DNA looped on a category of nonhistone proteins that are the foundation of chromosome shape. The diameter of looped chromatin is approximately 300 nm, so looped chromatin is called the **300-nm fiber**. With continued condensation, the chromatin loops form the sister chromatids. In metaphase, chromosome condensation reaches its zenith, resulting in chromosomes that are easily visualized by microscopy (see Figure 10.24e).

The **chromosome scaffold** is a filamentous framework made up of a large number of distinct nonhistone **scaffold proteins**. The chromosome scaffold gives a chromosome its shape. The scaffold is in some ways like the steel infrastructure that provides the shape, strength, and support for a building. In the case of chromosomes, the chromatin is "hung" on the scaffold. **Figure 10.26a** shows a fully condensed chromosome at metaphase, and **Figure 10.26b** shows the protein scaffold of a metaphase chromosome after being stripped of DNA. The shape of the chromosome scaffold is clearly reminiscent of the metaphase chromosome structure, consisting of sister chromatids joined at the centromere, which is visible as a constriction near the midpoint of the scaffold. The stringy gray material surrounding the scaffold is the DNA of the chromosome.

Chromatin loops containing 20,000 to 100,000 bp of DNA are anchored to the chromosome scaffold by other nonhistone proteins at sites called **matrix attachment regions (MARs)**. Contemporary models of chromatin organization predict that the chromatin loops progressively consolidate and are further compressed by nonhistone proteins. Ultimately, the compaction of chromatin achieved by metaphase is approximately a 250-fold compaction of the 300-nm fiber, which, as shown in Foundation Figure 10.24, already represents significant compaction.

Nucleosome Disassembly, Synthesis, and Reassembly during Replication

Our current discussion of histones as a basic organizing element of chromatin and our discussion of DNA replication in Chapter 7 invites a question about the chromatin organization of newly synthesized DNA. Specifically, when the amount of DNA doubles during S phase, do the number of nucleosomes also double to organize the newly synthesized DNA? If so, how are the new nucleosomes constructed? It would be of interest to know whether old nucleosomes are recycled during replication or whether the new nucleosomes are composed entirely of newly produced proteins.

Experimental research has answered these questions. The evidence collected by numerous investigators finds that

Figure 10.26   The chromosome scaffold of a metaphase chromosome. (a) A metaphase chromosome. **(b)** Stripped of chromatin, the chromosome scaffold is composed of nonhistone proteins that form an infrastructure that anchors DNA loops and gives the chromosome its shape.

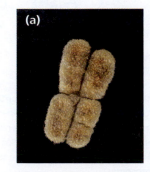

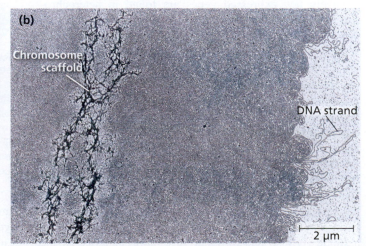

the assembly of nucleosome core particles in connection with replication is driven by the partial denaturing of old nucleosome octamers. These are partially broken down into dimers and tetramers that are then randomly joined with other dimers and tetramers—some old and some new—to form the nucleosome core particles that organize newly synthesized DNA.

The current models propose that as the replication fork passes, nucleosomes break down into H3–H4 tetramers (each tetramer contains two molecules of H3 and two molecules of H4) and H2A–H2B dimers (one molecule of each histone in a dimer). The H3–H4 tetramers reattach at random to one of the sister chromatid products of replication. Meanwhile, H2A–H2B dimers dissociate from the chromosome, and they may disassemble into individual histone molecules. Quickly, however, disassembled H2A and H2B histones reform into dimers or are joined by newly synthesized H2A and H2B histones to form dimers. New H3 and H4 molecules are also synthesized, and they form tetramers that attach to H2A–H2B dimers and to sister chromatids. H2A–H2B dimers also join H3–H4 tetramers already attached to sister chromatids. Enough new synthesis of all four histone proteins takes place to double the number of nucleosomes. All combinations of old and new histone components aggregate in assembling new nucleosomes after DNA replication, as Figure 10.27 illustrates.

Collectively, these activities provide the histone octamers needed to organize newly synthesized DNA.

This feature has important implications for maintaining the heterochromatic and euchromatic regions described in Section 10.1 and for maintaining the transcription-regulating capacity of chromatin in cells.

Position Effect Variegation: Effect of Chromatin State on Transcription

Our final discussion concerns the first experimental evidence indicating the critical role chromatin state plays in the transcription of genes in eukaryotes. Most expressed genes are located in euchromatic regions of chromosomes, where DNA is not as tightly affiliated with histones. In contrast, relatively few expressed genes are found in heterochromatic regions, where histones and other proteins tightly bind DNA. The experimental evidence that first suggested a direct link between gene transcription and the level of DNA compaction by chromatin came from research into a phenomenon called **position effect variegation (PEV)**.

Position effect variegation was discovered in connection with a red and white variegated eye color seen in certain *Drosophila* mutants. Recall that the wild-type X-linked allele w^+ produces red eye color in the fruit flies. In the 1920s and 1930s, Hermann Muller created mutations in fruit flies using X-rays. In one experiment, he irradiated flies with wild-type red eye color and generated flies with mutant variegated eye color. He noticed that the pattern of variegation differed from fly to fly and that the two eyes of a single fly also had different variegation patterns. At the

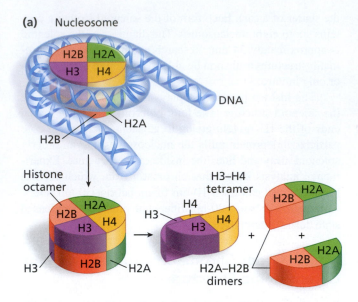

(a) Nucleosome

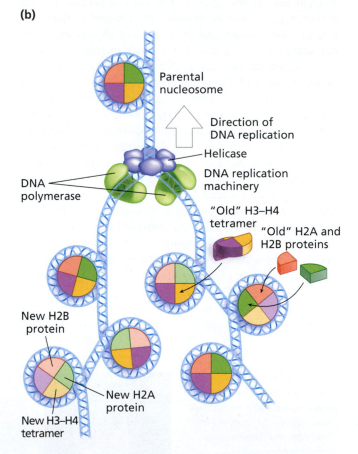

(b)

Figure 10.27 Nucleosome inheritance after DNA replication. Following the passage of the replication fork, "old" H3–H4 tetramers are randomly assigned to daughter strands, and newly synthesized H3–H4 tetramers inhabit strands not bound by old tetramers. Old and new H2A–H2B dimers join the tetramers to form complete nucleosomes.

time Muller studied this trait, the production of the white eye color was known to be caused by a mutation, but the variability of variegation pattern was puzzling.

Looking at the chromosomes of mutant flies with variegated eye color, Muller discovered that the X chromosome had undergone an inversion. Exposure to X-rays had broken the X chromosome, and the broken ends reattached to form a paracentric inversion. Muller examined the banding patterns in the inverted X chromosome and noticed that variegated flies had a particular kind of paracentric inversion. Their inversions had moved the *w* gene from its normal location near the telomere of the X chromosome to a new location very near the chromosome centromere (**Figure 10.28**).

The chromosome region immediately surrounding the centromere is a heterochromatic region that in *Drosophila* and most eukaryotes contains very few expressed genes. During S phase there is a temporary dissociation of nucleosomes as DNA replicates. The reassociation of nucleosomes after DNA replication leads to the reformation of heterochromatin around the region of the centromere, but the distance to which the reformed heterochromatin extends can vary from chromosome to chromosome. This variability is permissible because the centromeric region normally contains few if any expressed genes. Specifically, on some X chromosomes the centromeric heterochromatin spreads a greater distance outward from the centromere than on other X chromosomes. A greater extent of heterochromatin spread leads to more DNA sequence being included in the heterochromatic region.

Muller was not able to provide a molecular explanation for variegation, but research in the decades since Muller made his observations about eye color variegation have provided an explanation for both the patches of red and white eye color and the variability of the variegation pattern. The X- chromosome-to-X-chromosome variability of centromeric heterochromatin spread following DNA replication

has a very specific consequence for the expression of the w^+ alleles that are close to the centromere as a result of paracentric inversion. As Figure 10.28b indicates, if centromeric heterochromatin spread is limited (top image) and does not reach the new position of w^+, the allele is expressed in the cell. All cells descending from this initial cell grow in a cluster in the eye, and the cells in such a cluster will have red pigment and form red patches in the variegated eye. If, on the other hand, centromeric heterochromatin spread is more extensive, and the relocated w^+ allele is covered by reformed heterochromatin (bottom image), the allele is not expressed in the cell. All cells descending from this one also grow in a cluster in the eye, and they have no pigment (i.e., they are white). This is the source of white patches in the variegated eye. Because the spread of centromeric heterochromatin can vary from chromosome to chromosome, and the development of patches of eye tissue is also variable from eye to eye, there is a great deal of observed variation in the patterns of eye color variegation.

Since the time when Muller first described position effect variegation and the time when its molecular basis was identified, geneticists and cell biologists have come to understand that chromatin structure and the degree of chromatin compaction are critical components of gene expression in eukaryotic genomes. Research on PEV and on chromatin state have led to two central conclusions: (1) Gene expression can be controlled by the state of the chromatin in which a gene is located, and (2) gene expression or gene silencing can be dictated by chromatin structure that is transmissible from one cell generation to the next. We discuss these and other topics related to the modification of eukaryotic gene expression in Section 13.3.

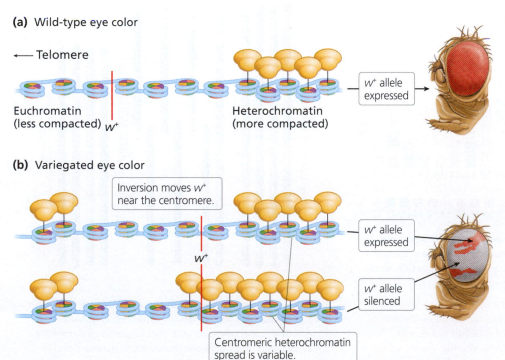

(a) Wild-type eye color

⟵ Telomere

Euchromatin (less compacted) w^+

Heterochromatin (more compacted)

w^+ allele expressed

(b) Variegated eye color

Inversion moves w^+ near the centromere.

w^+

w^+ allele expressed

w^+ allele silenced

Centromeric heterochromatin spread is variable.

Figure 10.28   Position effect variegation of eye color in *Drosophila*. (a) The w^+ allele is expressed in wild-type X chromosomes. Markers indicate the heterochromatin compaction region. **(b)** It is also expressed in inverted X chromosomes as long as the centromeric heterochromatin does not spread to cover the gene. If the spread of centromeric heterochromatin covers the new gene location in inverted X chromosomes, w^+ is silenced.

CASE STUDY

Human Chromosome Evolution

Researchers can trace the evolution of human chromosomes by comparing chromosome structure and genetic composition of humans with those of other species that share an ancestor with us. We describe two such comparative approaches here: One approach compares syntenic clusters of genes (genes grouped on the same chromosome) in related species which identify how species diversification has affected the distribution of those genes among chromosomes. The second approach compares banding patterns of chromosomes in closely related species to reconstruct the chromosome-level events that have produced the contemporary chromosomes of the species.

In **Figure 10.29**, syntenic clusters of genes on 20 chromosomes (19 autosomes and the X chromosome) in the mouse genome are colored to show their correspondence to the sequences making up the 23 chromosomes (22 autosomes and the X chromosome) in humans. Published in 2002 by a large research group known as the Mouse Genome Sequencing Consortium, this study compares 342 syntenic chromosome segments. The average size of the syntenic segments is a little less than 10 million base pairs. Syntenic groups of genes found in the human genome are dispersed among several chromosomes in the mouse genome. Interestingly, human chromosomes 17 and 20 each correspond entirely to a portion of mouse chromosomes 11 and 2, respectively. In both cases, the human chromosome corresponds to a long cluster of contiguous syntenic groups in the identified mouse chromosome. Comparison of X chromosomes of human and mouse reveal very strong sequence and genetic similarity.

This comparison leads to two salient evolutionary conclusions. First, mouse and human share similar syntenic

clusters because their common ancestor carried these clusters. Human and mouse chromosomes have diverged from those of their common ancestor by numerous rearrangements, including chromosome translocation, chromosome fusion, and chromosome inversion, that have changed many attributes of chromosome structure, but they also retain large segments of genes and sequences as syntenic clusters. Second, for X-linked genes specifically, the strong syntenic relationship has been maintained by natural selection driven by the requirements of embryonic development and the necessity to maintain a balance in dosage of X-linked genes by random X-inactivation.

Figure 10.30 illustrates the banding patterns of chromosomes 1, 2, and 3 of human (H), chimpanzee (C), gorilla (G), and orangutan (O). These four closely related primate species last shared a common ancestor between 30 and 35 million years ago. In each of the three chromosomes, strong similarity of banding patterns directly reflects the strong genetic similarity between the species. Structural and numerical differences between the chromosomes allow reconstruction of the evolutionary events that shaped the contemporary chromosomes of each species. By comparing the human chromosome with each of the others, we can reconstruct some of that evolutionary history as follows.

- Chromosome 1 is very similar in the four primate species, with the exception of a pericentric inversion and the addition of a small segment near the centromere of the human chromosome (1q1.2 to 1q2.1).

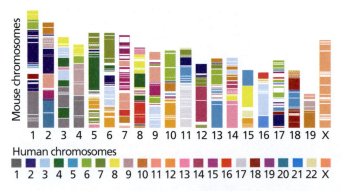

Figure 10.29 Evolutionary conservation of chromosome synteny between mouse and human chromosomes. Each of 23 human chromosomes is uniquely colored and its segments superimposed on 20 mouse chromosomes.

Q The genetic composition of the mouse and that of the human X chromosome look very similar based on this image. Thinking back to the discussion of X-linked genes and X-inactivation in Section 3.6, explain why this makes sense in evolutionary terms.

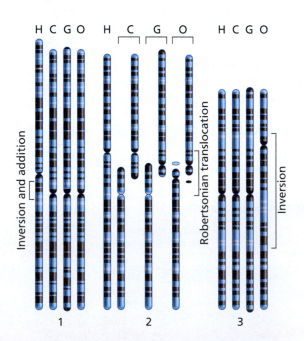

Figure 10.30 Human and great ape chromosome evolution. Chromosomes 1, 2, and 3 of human (H), chimpanzee (C), gorilla (G), and orangutan (O) are compared to determine the events leading to different chromosome numbers and structures.

- Chromosome 2 holds the explanation for the difference in diploid number between humans (2n = 46) and our close relatives (2n = 48). The reduction in human diploid number is the result of a Robertsonian translocation fusing two small acrocentric chromosomes that belong to separate chromosome pairs in chimp, gorilla, and orangutan.

- Chromosome 3 shows strong similarity of banding pattern in the four species with the exception of the orangutan chromosome, which has undergone a pericentric inversion that changed the relative arm lengths and altered the position of the centromere in comparison with the other primate chromosomes.

SUMMARY   Mastering Genetics   For activities, animations, and review quizzes, go to the Study Area.

10.1 Chromosome Number and Shape Vary among Organisms

- Chromosomes are categorized by shape on the basis of the centromere position and the ratio of long-arm (q arm) length to short-arm (p arm) length.

- Specialized molecular probes are used for in situ hybridization to locate specific genes or chromosome-specific DNA sequences. These probes often utilize fluorescent labels for detection.

- During interphase, each chromosome inhabits a territory of its own in the nucleus.

- Each chromosome has a distinctive banding pattern created by applying stains or dyes to solutions of condensed chromosomes from a single nucleus that are spread on microscope slides.

- Heterochromatic DNA forms darkly staining bands that contain relatively few expressed genes.

- Euchromatic DNA forms lightly staining bands that contain the majority of expressed genes.

10.2 Nondisjunction Leads to Changes in Chromosome Number

- In euploid nuclei, the number of chromosomes is equal to a multiple of the haploid number (n), whereas aneuploid nuclei have additional or missing chromosomes.

- Chromosome nondisjunction is the failure of homologous chromosomes or sister chromatids to separate and is a common cause of aneuploid gametes.

- Aneuploidy alters the phenotype of an organism by changing the balance of gene dosage of critical genes.

- Human aneuploidy manifests as trisomy of certain autosomes and as trisomy or monosomy of sex chromosomes.

- Chromosomal mosaics are organisms containing cells with two or more genetic or chromosomal constitutions.

- Uniparental disomy occurs when both homologous copies of a chromosome originate in a single parent.

10.3 Changes in Euploid Content Lead to Polyploidy

- Polyploids carry three or more haploid sets of chromosomes.

- Allopolyploids carry chromosome sets from different species, whereas autopolyploids have multiple chromosome sets from a single species.

- Polyploidy is common in plant species, causing increases in fruit and flower size that alter fertility and producing hybrid vigor.

10.4 Chromosome Breakage Causes Mutation by Loss, Gain, and Rearrangement of Chromosomes

- Chromosome breakage can result in terminal deletion or in interstitial deletion and may alter chromosome banding patterns.

- Heterozygosity for partial deletion or partial duplication produces phenotypic abnormalities through disturbances of gene dosage balance.

- Homologous chromosome synapsis involving a partial deletion or partial duplication chromosome produces a characteristic unpaired loop.

- Microdeletions and microduplications too small to be seen by banding changes are detected by molecular methods.

- The detection of pseudodominance provides important positional indicators for deletion mapping of genes.

10.5 Chromosome Breakage Leads to Inversion and Translocation of Chromosomes

- Chromosome breakage can lead to inversion or translocation of chromosome segments.

- Chromosome inversion heterozygotes have one chromosome with the normal order but have an inversion in the homolog. Homologs in these organisms form an inversion loop at synapsis.

- Paracentric inversions have two break points on one arm only, and the inversion does not include the centromeric region. Pericentric inversions have break points on each arm, and the centromeric region is included in the inverted region.

- Chromosome inversion is a crossover-suppression mechanism.

- A tetravalent synaptic structure containing chromosomes involved in reciprocal translocation leads to two main patterns of chromosome segregation in meiosis.

- The reduction in the number of viable gametes produced by reciprocal balanced translocation heterozygotes results in semisterility.

- Robertsonian translocation occurs by the fusion of nonhomologous chromosomes.

10.6 Eukaryotic Chromosomes Are Organized into Chromatin

▉ Eukaryotic nuclei contain multiple chromosomes, and they are highly compacted.

▉ Eukaryotic chromosomes are composed of chromatin—a mixture of DNA, histone proteins, and nonhistone proteins.

▉ Eight histone protein molecules form nucleosomes around which 146 bp of DNA wraps to form the 10-nm fiber.

▉ The 10-nm fiber condenses to form the 30-nm fiber.

▉ Nonhistone proteins form the chromosome scaffold that gives structure to chromatids and aids in additional chromosome compaction during prophase of the cell cycle.

▉ Chromatin loops form with the aid of the proteins that comprise the chromosome scaffold.

▉ Studies of position effect variegation (PEV) have determined that the structure of chromatin surrounding a gene directly influences transcription.

PREPARING FOR PROBLEM SOLVING

In addition to the list of problem-solving tips and suggestions given here, you can go to the Study Guide and Solutions Manual that accompanies this book for help at solving problems.

1. Be familiar with general chromosome nomenclature, including the system used to describe chromosome banding.

2. Be prepared to describe the basis for chromosome banding and the molecular components and general structure of chromatin.

3. Understand the role of chromatin in chromosome condensation and the general role chromatin structure plays in gene transcription.

4. Be familiar with experimental approaches to analysis of chromosomes, including G banding, karyotype analysis, DNase I analysis, and the interpretation of PEV (position effect variegation).

5. Understand the errors in meiosis that lead to abnormalities in chromosome number and the role chromosome breakage plays in generating structural abnormalities of chromosomes.

6. Understand the mechanisms and origins of polyploidy and its consequences for the phenotype of organisms.

7. Be prepared to describe and predict the effects of abnormalities of chromosome number and structure on the phenotype of organisms.

PROBLEMS

Mastering Genetics   Visit for instructor-assigned tutorials and problems.

Chapter Concepts

For answers to selected even-numbered problems, see Appendix: Answers.

1. Give descriptions for the following terms:
   a. histone proteins
   b. nucleosome core particle
   c. scaffold proteins
   d. G bands
   e. euchromatin
   f. heterochromatin
   g. nucleosome
   h. chromosome territory

2. The human genome contains 2.9×10^9 base pairs. Approximately how many nucleosomes are required to organize the 10-nm–fiber structure of the human genome? Show the calculation you use to determine the answer.

3. In eukaryotic DNA,
   a. where are you most likely to find histone protein H4?
   b. where are you most likely to find histone protein H1?
   c. along a 6000-bp segment of DNA, approximately how many molecules of each kind of histone protein do you expect to find? Explain your answer.
   d. how does the role of H1 differ from the role of H3 in chromatin formation?

4. Describe the importance of light and dark G bands that appear along chromosomes.

5. Human late prophase karyotypes have about 2000 visible G bands. The human genome contains approximately 22,000 genes. Consider the region 5p1.5 through the end of the short arm of chromosome 5 that is identified on the late prophase chromosome in Figure 10.5, and assume the entire region is deleted. Approximately how many genes will be lost as a result of the deletion?

6. Consider synapsis in prophase I of meiosis for two plant species that each carry 36 chromosomes. Species A is diploid and species B is triploid. What characteristics of homologous chromosome synapsis can be used to distinguish these two species?

7. From the following list, identify the types of chromosome changes you expect to show phenotypic consequences.
   a. pericentric inversion
   b. interstitial deletion
   c. duplication
   d. terminal deletion

e. trisomy
f. reciprocal balanced translocation
g. paracentric inversion
h. monosomy
i. polyploidy

8. If the haploid number for a plant species is 4, how many chromosomes are found in a member of the species that has one of the following characteristics? Explain your reasoning in each case.

a. diploidy
b. pentaploidy
c. octaploidy
d. trisomy
e. triploidy
f. monosomy
g. tetraploidy
h. hexaploidy

9. Mating between a male donkey ($2n = 62$) and a female horse ($2n = 64$) produces sterile mules. Recently, however, a very rare event occurred—a female mule gave birth to an offspring by mating with a horse.

a. Determine how many chromosomes are in the mule karyotype, and explain why mules are generally sterile.
b. How many chromosomes does the mule–horse offspring carry?
c. Why is it very unlikely that the offspring will have fully horse-like genetic characteristics?

10. A researcher interested in studying a human gene on chromosome 21 and another gene on the X chromosome uses FISH probes to locate each gene. The chromosome 21 probe produces green fluorescent color, and the X chromosome probe produces red fluorescent color.

a. If the subject studied is female, how many green and red spots will be detected? Explain your answer.
b. If the subject studied is male, how many green and red spots will be detected? Explain your answer.

11. In what way does position effect variegation (PEV) of *Drosophila* eye color indicate that chromatin state can affect gene transcription?

Application And Integration

For answers to selected even-numbered problems, see Appendix: Answers.

12. A pair of homologous chromosomes in *Drosophila* has the following content (single letters represent genes):

Chromosome 1   RNMDHBGKWU

Chromosome 2   RNMDHBDHBGKWU

a. What term best describes this situation?
b. Diagram the pairing of these homologous chromosomes in prophase I.
c. What term best describes the unusual structure that forms during pairing of these chromosomes?
d. How does the pairing diagrammed in part (b) differ from the pairing of chromosomes in an inversion heterozygote?

13. An animal heterozygous for a reciprocal balanced translocation has the following chromosomes:

MN • OPQRST
MN • OPQRjkl
cdef • ghijkl
cdef • ghiST

a. Diagram the pairing of these chromosomes in prophase I.
b. Identify the gametes produced by alternate segregation. Which if any of these gametes are viable?
c. Identify the gametes produced by adjacent-1 segregation. Which if any of these gametes are viable?
d. Identify the gametes produced by adjacent-2 segregation. Which if any of these gametes are viable?
e. Among the three segregation patterns, which is least likely to occur? Why?

14. Dr. Ara B. Dopsis has an idea he thinks will be a boon to agriculture. He wants to create the "pomato," a hybrid between a tomato (*Lycopersicon esculentum*) that has 12 chromosomes and a potato (*Solanum tuberosum*) that has 48 chromosomes. Dr. Dopsis is hoping his new pomato will have tuber growth like a potato and the fruit production of a tomato. He joins a haploid gamete from each species to form a hybrid and then induces doubling of chromosome number.

a. How many chromosomes will the hybrid have before chromosome doubling?
b. Will this hybrid be infertile?
c. How many chromosomes will the polyploid have after chromosome doubling?
d. Can Dr. Dopsis be sure the polyploid will have the characteristics he wants? Why or why not?

15. A normal chromosome and its homolog carrying a paracentric inversion are shown here. The dot (•) represents the centromere.

Normal   ABC • DEFGHIJK
Inversion   abc • djihgfek

a. Diagram the alignment of chromosomes during prophase I.
b. Assume a crossover takes place in the region between F and G. Identify the gametes that are formed following this crossover, and indicate which if any gametes are viable.
c. Assume a crossover takes place in the region between A and B. Identify the gametes that are formed by this crossover event, and indicate which if any gametes are viable.

16. The accompanying chromosome diagram represents a eukaryotic chromosome prepared with Giemsa stain. Indicate the heterochromatic and euchromatic regions of the chromosome, and label the chromosome's centromeric and telomeric regions.

Centromere

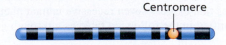

a. What term best describes the shape of this chromosome?

b. Do you expect the centromeric region to contain heterochromatin? Why or why not?

c. Why are expressed genes not found in the telomeric region of chromosomes?

d. Are you more likely to find the DNA sequence encoding the digestive enzyme amylase in a heterochromatic, euchromatic, centromeric, or telomeric region? Explain your reasoning.

17. Histone protein H4 isolated from pea plants and cow thymus glands contains 102 amino acids in both cases. A total of 100 of the amino acids are identical between the two species. Give an evolutionary explanation for this strong amino acid sequence identity based on what you know about the functions of histones and nucleosomes.

18. A survey of organisms living deep in the ocean reveals two new species whose DNA is isolated for analysis. DNA samples from both species are treated to remove nonhistone proteins. Each DNA sample is then treated with DNase I that cuts DNA not protected by histone proteins but is unable to cut DNA bound by histone proteins. Following DNase I treatment, DNA samples are subjected to gel electrophoresis, and the gels are stained to visualize all DNA bands in the gel. The staining patterns of DNA bands from each species are shown in the figure. The number of base pairs in small DNA fragments is shown at the left of the gel. Interpret the gel results in terms of chromatin organization and the spacing of nucleosomes in the chromatin of each species.

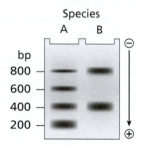

19. In humans that are XX/XO mosaics, the phenotype is highly variable, ranging from females who have classic Turner syndrome symptoms to females who are essentially normal. Likewise, XY/XO mosaics have phenotypes that range from Turner syndrome females to essentially normal males. How can the wide range of phenotypes be explained for these sex-chromosome mosaics?

20. A plant breeder would like to develop a seedless variety of cucumber from two existing lines. Line A is a tetraploid line, and line B is a diploid line. Describe the breeding strategy that will produce a seedless line, and support your strategy by describing the results of crosses.

21. In *Drosophila*, seven partial deletions (1 to 7) shown as gaps in the following diagram have been mapped on a chromosome. This region of the chromosome contains genes that express seven recessive mutant phenotypes, identified in the following table as *a* through *g*. A researcher wants to determine the location and order of genes on the chromosome, so he sets up a series of crosses in which flies homozygous for a mutant allele are crossed with flies that are homozygous for a partial deletion. The progeny are scored to determine whether they have the mutant phenotype ("m" in the table) or the wild-type phenotype ("+" in the table). Use the partial deletion map and the table of progeny phenotypes to determine the order of genes on the chromosome.

Chromosome

Deletion			
1			
2			
3			
4			
5			
6			
7			

	Mutation						
Deletion	a	b	c	d	e	f	g
1	+	m	+	m	+	+	+
2	m	+	+	+	+	m	+
3	m	+	+	+	+	+	m
4	m	+	+	m	+	m	m
5	+	m	+	m	m	+	+
6	m	m	m	m	+	m	m
7	m	+	+	+	+	+	+

22. Two experimental varieties of strawberry are produced by crossing a hexaploid line that contains 48 chromosomes and a tetraploid line that contains 32 chromosomes. Experimental variety 1 contains 40 chromosomes, and experimental variety 2 contains 56 chromosomes.

a. Do you expect both experimental lines to be fertile? Why or why not?

b. How many chromosomes from the hexaploid line are contributed to experimental variety 1? To experimental variety 2?

c. How many chromosomes from the tetraploid lines are contributed to experimental variety 1? To experimental variety 2?

23. In the tomato, *Solanum esculentum*, tall (*D*−) is dominant to dwarf (*dd*) plant height, smooth fruit (*P*−) is dominant to peach fruit (*pp*), and round fruit shape (*O*−) is dominant to oblate fruit shape (*oo*). These three genes are linked on chromosome 1 of tomato in the order *dwarf–peach–oblate*. There are 12 map units between *dwarf* and *peach* and 17 map units between *peach* and *oblate*. A trihybrid plant (*DPO/dpo*) is testcrossed to a plant that is homozygous recessive at the three loci (*dpo/dpo*). The accompanying table shows the progeny plants. Identify the mechanism responsible for

the resulting data that do not agree with the established genetic map.

Progeny Phenotype	Number
Tall, smooth, round	473
Dwarf, peach, oblate	476
Tall, smooth, oblate	12
Dwarf, peach, round	8
Tall, peach, oblate	17
Dwarf, smooth, round	13
Tall, peach, round	0
Dwarf, smooth, oblate	1
	1000

24. A boy with Down syndrome (trisomy 21) has 46 chromosomes. His parents and his two older sisters have a normal phenotype, but each has 45 chromosomes.

   a. Explain how this is possible.
   b. How many chromosomes do you expect to see in karyotypes of the parents?
   c. What term best describes this kind of chromosome abnormality?
   d. What is the probability the next child of this couple will have a normal phenotype and have 46 chromosomes? Explain your answer.

25. Experimental evidence demonstrates that the nucleosomes present in a cell after the completion of S phase are composed of some "old" histone dimers and some newly synthesized histone dimers. Describe the general design for an experiment that uses a protein label such as ^{35}S to show that nucleosomes are often a mixture of old and new histone dimers following DNA replication.

26. DNase I cuts DNA that is not protected by bound proteins but is unable to cut DNA that is complexed with proteins. Human DNA is isolated, stripped of its nonhistone proteins, and mixed with DNase I. Samples are removed after 30 minutes, 1 hour, and 4 hours and run separately in gel electrophoresis. The resulting gel is stained to make all DNA fragments in it visible, and the results are shown in the figure. DNA fragment sizes in base pairs (bp) are estimated by the scale to the left of the gel.

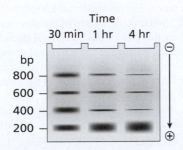

a. Examine the gel results and speculate why longer DNase I treatment produces different results.

b. Draw a conclusion about the organization of chromatin in the human genome from this gel.

27. Genomic DNA from the nematode worm *Caenorhabditis elegans* is organized by nucleosomes in the manner typical of eukaryotic genomes, with 145 bp encircling each nucleosome and approximately 55 bp in linker DNA. When *C. elegans* chromatin is carefully isolated, stripped of nonhistone proteins, and placed in an appropriate buffer, the chromatin decondenses to the 10-nm fiber structure. Suppose researchers mix a sample of 10-nm–fiber chromatin with a large amount of the enzyme DNase I that randomly cleaves DNA in regions not protected by bound protein. Next, they remove the nucleosomes, separate the DNA fragments by gel electrophoresis, and stain all the DNA fragments in the gel.

   a. Approximately what range of DNA fragment sizes do you expect to see in the stained electrophoresis gel? How many bands will be visible on the gel?
   b. Explain the origin of DNA fragments seen in the gel.
   c. How do the expected results support the 10-nm–fiber model of chromatin?

28. A small population of deer living on an isolated island are separated for many generations from a mainland deer population. The populations retain the same number of chromosomes and but hybrids are infertile. One chromosome (shown here) has a different banding pattern in the island population than in the mainland population.

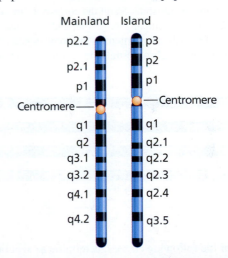

a. Describe how the banding pattern of the island population chromosome most likely evolved from the mainland chromosome. What term or terms describe the difference between these chromosomes?
b. Draw the synapsis of these homologs during prophase I in hybrids produced from the cross of mainland with island deer.
c. In a mainland–island hybrid deer, recombination takes place in band q1 of the homologous chromosomes. Draw the gametes that result from this event.
d. Suppose that 40% of all meioses in mainland–island hybrids involve recombination somewhere in the chromosome region between q2.1 and p2. What proportion of the gametes of hybrid deer are viable? What is the cause of the decreased proportion of viable gametes in hybrids relative to the parental populations?

Collaboration And Discussion

For answers to selected even-numbered problems, see Appendix: Answers.

29. A eukaryote with a diploid number of $2n = 6$ carries the chromosomes shown below and labeled (a) to (f).

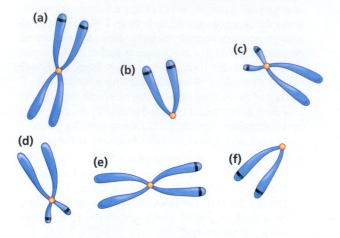

   a. Carefully examine and redraw these chromosomes in any valid metaphase I alignment. Draw and label the metaphase plate, and label each chromosome by its assigned letter.
   b. Explain how you determined the correct alignment of homologous chromosomes on opposite sides of the metaphase plate.

30. Human chromosome 5 and the corresponding chromosomes from chimpanzee, gorilla, and orangutan are shown here. Describe any structural differences you see in the other primate chromosomes in relation to the human chromosome.

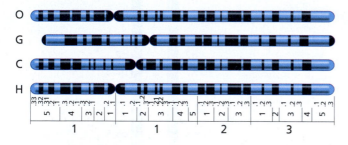

31. For the following crosses, determine as accurately as possible the genotypes of each parent, the parent in whom nondisjunction occurs, and whether nondisjunction takes place in the first or second meiotic division. Both color blindness and hemophilia, a blood-clotting disorder, are X-linked recessive traits. In each case, assume the parents have normal karyotypes (see Table 10.2).

   a. A man and a woman who each have wild-type phenotypes have a son with Klinefelter syndrome (XXY) who has hemophilia.
   b. A man who is color blind and a woman who is wild type have a son with Jacob syndrome (XYY) who has hemophilia.
   c. A color-blind man and a woman who is wild type have a daughter with Turner syndrome (XO) who has normal color vision and blood clotting.

   d. A man who is color blind and has hemophilia and a woman who is wild type have a daughter with triple X syndrome (XXX) who has hemophilia and normal color vision.

32. A healthy couple with a history of three previous spontaneous abortions has just had a child with cri-du-chat syndrome, a disorder caused by a terminal deletion of chromosome 5. Their physician orders karyotype analysis of both parents and of the child. The karyotype results for chromosomes 5 and 12 are shown here.

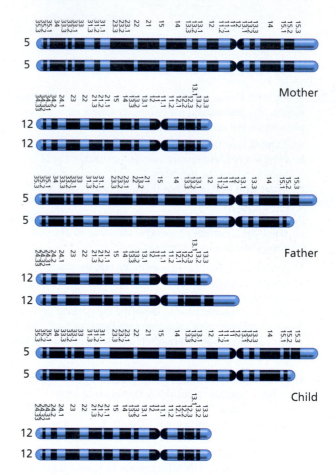

   a. Are the chromosomes in the child consistent with those expected in a case of cri-du-chat syndrome? Explain your reasoning.
   b. Which parent has an abnormal karyotype? How can you tell? What is the nature of the abnormality?
   c. Why does this parent have a normal phenotype?
   d. Diagram the pairing of the abnormal chromosomes.
   e. What segregation pattern occurred to produce the gamete involved in fertilization of the child with cri-du-chat syndrome?
   f. What is the approximate probability that the next child of this couple will have cri-du-chat syndrome?
   g. Do the karyotypes of the parents help explain the occurrence of the three previous spontaneous abortions? Explain.

Gene Mutation, DNA Repair, and Homologous Recombination

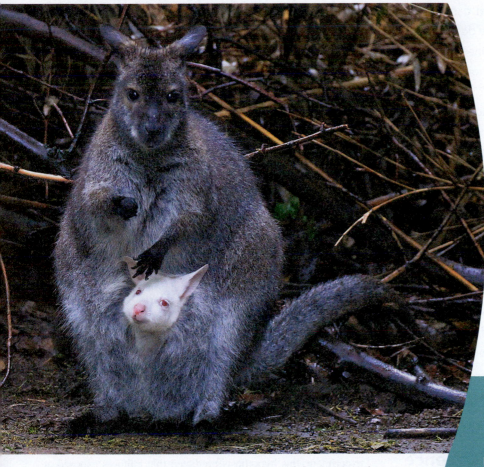

The baby kangaroo peeking out of its mother's pouch has autosomal recessive albinism, a condition that occurs in about 1 in 20,000 births due to spontaneous mutation.

CHAPTER OUTLINE

11.1 Mutations Are Rare and Random and Alter DNA Sequence

11.2 Gene Mutations May Arise from Spontaneous Events

11.3 Mutations May Be Caused by Chemicals or Ionizing Radiation

11.4 Repair Systems Correct Some DNA Damage

11.5 Proteins Control Translesion DNA Synthesis and the Repair of Double-Strand Breaks

11.6 DNA Double-Strand Breaks Initiate Homologous Recombination

11.7 Transposable Genetic Elements Move throughout the Genome

ESSENTIAL IDEAS

▪ Gene mutations are rare and random.

▪ Mutations change DNA sequence and can alter polypeptide composition and protein function. Mutations can also cause phenotypic variation.

▪ Spontaneous nucleotide changes can lead to mutation.

▪ Chemical mutagens and radiation can damage DNA and produce mutations.

▪ DNA repair systems can directly repair DNA damage or can remove and replace damaged segments.

▪ Specialized enzymes can bypass a blockage of DNA replication caused by unrepaired damage.

▪ Controlled DNA double-strand breaks initiate homologous recombination and also recombination between homologous chromosomes in meiosis.

▪ Transposable genetic elements move throughout the genome and may mutate genes and alter genomes.

Mutation can be defined most simply as a heritable change in DNA sequence, a definition that covers an enormous range of changes. Mutation is indispensable in two ways. First, from an evolutionary perspective, mutations generate new hereditary variety. These new variants can influence the evolution of a species through the action of any of the four evolutionary processes described in Section 1.4. For example, mutations that cause phenotypic changes can be subject to natural selection. A few of these changes will have a positive effect on the fitness of organisms, and natural selection will favor their perpetuation in populations. Many, however, will have a negative consequence for the organism, and selection will operate to reduce the frequency of the mutant allele or eliminate it entirely from the population.

The second way in which mutations are indispensable has to do with their role in genetic analysis. Whether for studying the phenotypic effects of variant alleles on organisms, the processes that damage DNA, the molecular biology of DNA damage detection and repair, the structure and function of genes, or the patterns of hereditary transmission, mutation analysis is at the heart of genetics.

In this chapter, we focus on mutation at the level of the individual gene—that is, gene mutation. We first discuss the nature of gene mutation and then describe spontaneous changes to DNA nucleotide base structure and the occasional DNA replication errors that can generate gene mutations. We also examine the DNA-damaging actions of chemical and physical agents and the role this damage plays in producing gene mutation, after which we describe DNA damage repair mechanisms and the connection between mechanisms of DNA double-strand break repair and homologous recombination. We end the chapter with a discussion of the role of transposition in generating mutations.

11.1 Mutations Are Rare and Random and Alter DNA Sequence

Gene mutations are random and their occurrence is rare. The **mutation rate** is measured in two primary ways: at the phenotypic level, by counting the number of mutations affecting a phenotype; and at the molecular level, by determining the frequency of mutations per base pair. By either measure, average mutation rates are very low. Owing to the mechanisms of DNA replication that are shared by bacteria, archaea, and eukaryotes, there is a remarkable similarity between mutation rates at the DNA level—on the order of about 10^{-9} per replicated base pair in all organisms. Mutation rates at the phenotypic level are more frequent and more variable among organisms; 10^{-6} to 10^{-8} per gene are typical.

Certain genes in specific genomes have elevated mutation rates. These genes are identified as being **mutation hotspots**. There are multiple reasons why a gene might be a hotspot, but large gene size is a frequent cause. For example, the human X-linked *dystrophin (DYS)* gene, whose mutation causes Duchenne muscular dystrophy, and the autosomal gene *NF1*, whose mutation causes autosomal dominant neurofibromatosis, each have a mutation rate of about 10^{-4}.

These high mutation rates are due to the large size of those genes. *DYS* is the largest gene in the human genome, spanning almost 2.5 million base pairs, and *NF1* is well over 1 million base pairs in length.

Proof of the Random Mutation Hypothesis

Despite some difference in average mutation rates per gene (10^{-6} to 10^{-7} for most genes in most organisms), mutations occur at random in genomes. The random nature of mutations was first experimentally demonstrated by Salvador Luria and Max Delbrück in 1943 in an experiment called the **fluctuation test**. This experiment tested the nature of bacterial mutations that produced resistance to bacteriophage infection and thus protected the bacterium *Escherichia coli* (*E. coli*) from lysis.

At the time there were two competing hypotheses to explain the occurrence of mutations. One, the **random mutation hypothesis** (which turned out to be the correct hypothesis) predicted that mutations occur at random. With respect to cultures of bacteria and their bacteriophage resistance, the random mutation hypothesis predicted that different cultures would develop resistance mutations at different times. When a bacteriophage-resistant mutation occurs early in the history of a bacterial culture, large numbers of resistant bacteria will be present when the culture is tested. Other cultures may develop a resistance mutation later in their history and will have fewer resistant bacteria when tested. Under the random mutation hypothesis, a comparison of the number of resistant bacteria in several different cultures will reveal a great deal of fluctuation, or variation, in the number, hence the name of the experiment (**Figure 11.1a**). The alternative hypothesis, known as the **adaptive mutation hypothesis**, proposed that environmental change triggers mutation. For the bacterial culture experiment, this hypothesis predicted that cultures exposed at the same time to a trigger (bacteriophage exposure, in this case) would respond the same way. This means that the number of bacteriophage-resistant bacteria in each culture should be about equal, with little variation (**Figure 11.1b**).

Luria and Delbrück began with a single large culture of bacteria that had never been exposed to bacteriophage. They split the large culture into about two dozen smaller cultures and allowed them to grow for multiple generations, still free from bacteriophage exposure. After several generations of growth, samples from each culture were plated on growth plates containing bacteriophage, and the number of phage-resistant bacterial colonies was counted on each. The results revealed a great deal of fluctuation in the number of phage-resistant bacteria in different cultures, closely mirroring the predictions of the random mutation hypothesis.

In genetics, the term "random mutation" means that mutations occur by chance, with each base pair having an equal probability of mutating. Mutations do not occur with any predetermined purpose, and they occur independently of whether they will prove to be favorable or detrimental or to have no impact on the fitness of an organism.

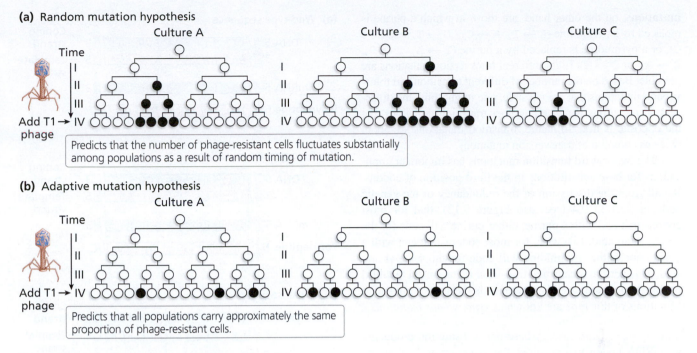

(a) Random mutation hypothesis

Figure 11.1 **The fluctuation test of Luria and Delbrück.**

Germ-Line and Somatic Mutations

Gene mutation can occur in any cell at any time. Mutations that occur in germ-line cells, such as those giving rise to sperm and egg, can be passed from one generation to the next. These are identified as **germ-line mutations**. The seven traits studied by Mendel and the various human autosomal and X-linked conditions described in this book are examples of inherited variation originating with germ-line mutations. All of the body's cells that are not in the germ line are somatic cells, and mutations in these cells are called **somatic mutations**. Somatic mutations can be passed to subsequent generations of cells in a cell lineage through mitotic cell division, but only the direct descendants of the original mutated cell carry the gene mutation.

Point Mutations

The most common kinds of gene mutations are those that substitute, add, or delete one or more DNA base pairs. These kinds of mutations are confined to a specific base pair or location in a gene and are called **point mutations**. There are point mutations of several types, each having characteristic consequences. They can occur anywhere in the genome. Those that occur in the coding sequence of a gene can lead to changes in the amino acid composition of the protein product of the gene. In contrast, those occurring in a regulatory sequence of a gene can alter the amount of wild-type protein product produced by the gene. When base-pair substitution mutations occur in the coding sequence of a gene, they are further categorized at the molecular level by the manner in which they alter the informational content of the gene: They may be synonymous mutations (also known as silent mutations), missense

mutations, or nonsense mutations. Table 11.1 and the following discussions summarize the types of point mutations.

Base-Pair Substitution Mutations

The replacement of one nucleotide base pair by another is a common type of point mutation. These mutations, called **base-pair substitution mutations**, are of two types. **Transition mutations** are those in which one purine replaces the other ($A \rightarrow G$; $G \rightarrow A$) or one pyrimidine replaces the other ($C \rightarrow T$; $T \rightarrow C$). The four different transition mutations shown in the previous sentence are all that are possible. **Transversion**

Table 11.1	Point Mutations
Type	**Consequence**
Coding-Sequence Mutations	
Synonymous	No amino acid sequence change.
Missense	Changes one amino acid.
Nonsense	Creates stop codon and terminates translation.
Frameshift	Wrong sequence of amino acids.
Regulatory Mutations	
Promoter	Changes timing or amount of transcription.
Polyadenylation	Alters sequence of mRNA.
Splice site	Improperly retains an intron or excludes an exon.
DNA replication mutation, e.g., triplet-repeat expansion	Increases (or less often, decreases) number of short repeats of DNA.

mutations, on the other hand, are those in which a purine is replaced by a pyrimidine (A → T, A → C, G → T, and G → C), or a pyrimidine is replaced by a purine (T → A, T → G, C → A, or C → G). Eight different transversion mutations are possible. Based on the number of different transition and transversion mutations that are possible, one might think that transversion mutations would outnumber transition mutations, but the opposite is true. In nature, transition mutations are about twice as common as transversion mutations.

The bias toward transition mutations has important implications for base substitutions in the third position of codons. Recall from the discussion of the redundancy of the genetic code in Section 9.4 (see also Figure 9.13), that for most codons that end with a purine, either purine will code for the same amino acid. Likewise, for most codons that end with a pyrimidine, either pyrimidine will code for the same amino acid. This pattern means that transition mutations in the third positions of codons are likely to encode the same amino acid. Mutations of this type are known as *synonymous mutations*.

Synonymous Mutation A base-pair substitution producing an mRNA codon that specifies the same amino acid as the wild-type mRNA is known as a **synonymous mutation** (also known as a *silent mutation*). **Figures 11.2a** and **11.2b** illustrate a synonymous mutation in which an A–T to G–C transition mutation changes the wild-type leucine codon (5′–UUA–3′) to a mutant codon (5′–UUG–3′) that also encodes leucine.

Missense Mutation A base-pair substitution that results in an amino acid change to the protein is a **missense mutation**. **Figure 11.2c** shows a T–A to A–T transversion mutation that alters the wild-type 5′–UGG–3′ codon to 5′–AGG–3′, changing the amino acid from tryptophan to arginine. Protein function may be altered by a missense mutation. The specific consequence of the protein change (i.e., whether it results in complete or only partial loss of protein function) depends on what kind of amino acid change takes place and where in the polypeptide chain the change occurs. The tall versus short stature of pea plants (stem length) studied by Mendel is caused by a missense mutation. See **Experimental Insight 11.1** for a discussion.

Nonsense Mutation A base-pair substitution that creates a stop codon in place of a codon specifying an amino acid is a **nonsense mutation**. The G–C to A–T base-pair substitution shown in **Figure 11.2d** that changes the UGG (Trp) codon to a UGA (stop) codon is an example of a nonsense mutation.

Frameshift Mutations

Insertion or deletion of one or more base pairs in the coding sequence of a gene leads to addition or deletion of mRNA nucleotides. This can alter the reading frame of the codon sequence, beginning at the point of mutation. The result would be a **frameshift mutation**, in which the mutant polypeptide contains an altered amino acid sequence from the point of mutation to the end of the polypeptide (**Figure 11.3**).

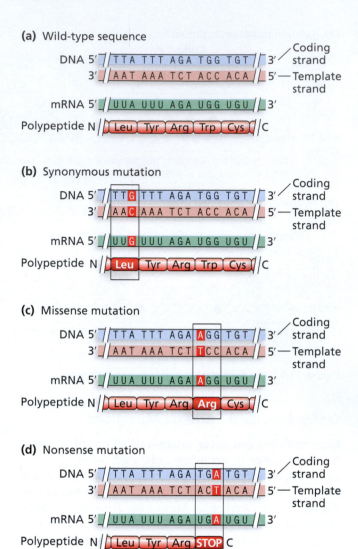

Figure 11.2 **The consequences of base-pair substitutions.**

In addition to producing the wrong amino acids in a portion of the polypeptide, frameshift mutations commonly generate premature stop codons that result in a truncated polypeptide. For these reasons, frameshift mutations usually result in the complete loss of protein function and thus produce null alleles. The yellow versus green seed pod trait studied by Mendel is caused by an insertion of six base pairs of DNA. Since the insertion is a multiple of three nucleotides, it adds two codons to the mutant allele mRNA without changing the reading frame. Thus, this particular mutant is not the result of a frameshift mutation. Nevertheless, the insertion of DNA base pairs is a common mechanism producing frameshift mutations. (See the discussion of Mendel's pod-color mutation in Experimental Insight 11.1 for details.).

Regulatory Mutations

Some point mutations have the effect of reducing or increasing the amount of wild-type gene transcript and the amount of wild-type polypeptide without affecting the transcript

(a) Wild-type sequence

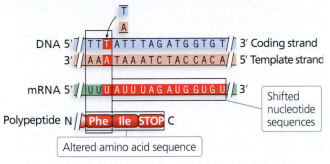

(b) Frameshift mutation: Insertion of single base pair

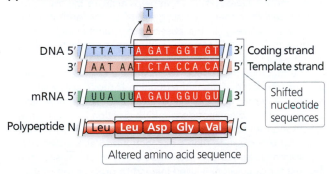

(c) Frameshift mutation: Deletion of single base pair

Figure 11.3 Frameshift mutation.

and polypeptide sequences. These mutations, classified as **regulatory mutations**, occur in noncoding regions of genes, such as promoters, introns, and regions coding 5′-UTR and 3′-UTR segments of mRNA. None of these regions directly encodes amino acids, but mutations in these regions can lead to the production of abnormal or abnormal amounts of mRNAs that, in turn, produce mutant phenotypes. Three types of regulatory mutations are commonly recognized: promoter mutations, splicing mutations, and cryptic splice sites.

Promoter Mutations Promoter consensus sequences, such as those recognized by RNA polymerase II and its associated transcription factors in eukaryotes, direct the efficient initiation of transcription. Mutations that alter consensus sequence nucleotides and interfere with efficient transcription initiation are **promoter mutations**. The human β-globin gene offers multiple examples of promoter mutations, with various consequences for transcription. **Figure 11.4a** lists mutations at six positions of the human β-globin gene promoter that each result in a moderate reduction in the amount

of β-globin gene transcript and in a reduced amount of β-globin protein. Each of the six promoter mutations shown here reduces transcription, but none eliminates transcription entirely. Some promoter mutations of other genes result in the complete elimination of transcription.

Splicing Mutations On the DNA coding strand, the dinucleotide GT occurs invariably at the 5′ splice site of introns to demarcate the boundary between the 5′ end of the intron and the 3′ end of the adjacent exon (the GT of coding strand DNA corresponds to the GU dinucleotide of mRNA; see Figure 8.22). In the human β-globin gene, an AG dinucleotide occurs at the 3′ end of exon 1. Each of these dinucleotides is part of the consensus sequence at which the spliceosome forms. Mutations of either of these dinucleotide sequences or of nearby nucleotides in the consensus sequence within the intron can result in splicing errors in the removal of intron sequences from pre-mRNA.

(a) Mutations in promoter

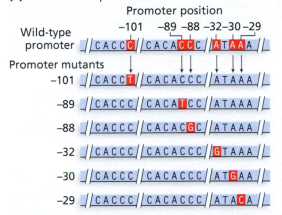

(b) Mutations in intron 1

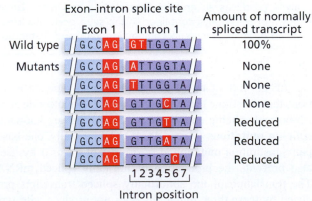

Figure 11.4 Regulatory mutations of the human β-globin gene. (a) These base-pair substitution mutations in the promoter reduce transcription of the gene. **(b)** These base-pair substitutions in intron 1 reduce or eliminate normal pre-mRNA splicing.

🔵 Section 8.4 describes the 5′ splice site consensus sequence as being encoded by a GT sequence in eukaryotic mRNA (GU in mRNA) followed by a few additional nucleotides. How does the information on mutations shown in part (b) support the idea that there is a consensus sequence at this splice site?

EXPERIMENTAL INSIGHT 11.1

Mendel's Mutations

Table 2.8 on page 57 and the accompanying text briefly describe the wild-type and mutant alleles of the four genes studied by Mendel that have been identified to date. For three of the genes, described in this Experimental Insight, the inherited phenotype differences result from point mutations of various types. Variation of the fourth gene is described in the Case Study at the end of this chapter.

STEM LENGTH: A MISSENSE MUTATION

The *Le* gene variation was identified in 1997 by research groups led by Diane Lester and David Martin, who determined that the wild-type dominant allele of this gene (*Le*) produces an enzyme active in the biosynthetic pathway that produces the growth hormone gibberellin 3β-hydroxylase. The effect of the dominant allele is to generate the wild-type level of growth hormone production, which, in turn, produces the long stems that characterize tall pea plants. The recessive mutant allele (*le*) is unable to produce the enzyme, and this reduces the biosynthesis of the growth hormone to about 5% of the wild-type level. The result is poor stem growth and short plants.

The *le* allele is the result of a missense mutation that changes an alanine to a threonine in the polypeptide product of the gene. This missense change is brought about by a G–C to A–T transition mutation in the *le* allele's DNA sequence. It is an example of a missense mutation that inactivates the function of the allele's protein product. In this case, the consequence of the mutation is the significant reduction of the synthesis of a growth hormone.

POD COLOR: AN INSERTION MUTATION

The 2007 studies of the *Sgr* ("stay green") gene by research groups led by Ian Armstead and Sylvain Aubry identified the molecular basis for the dominant wild-type yellow seed pod and the recessive mutant green seed pod. The wild-type allele produces an enzyme that participates in the breakdown of chlorophyll contained in the seed pod. This breakdown normally occurs in conjunction with pod maturation, and it results in mature seed pods that are yellow. The mutant allele produces a very poorly functioning enzyme, largely disabling a critical step of chlorophyll breakdown. Consequently, chlorophyll is retained in mature pods, making them green.

The mutant allele contains a 6-bp insertion that changes the enzyme product by adding two additional codons to mRNA and two amino acids to the protein. This insertion of 6 bp, being a multiple of three nucleotides, as found in a codon, does not change the reading frame. Thus, in the mutant protein, the amino acid sequence is normal except for the presence of the two additional amino acids. Since the mutant protein is largely normal, it is able to retain partial function, albeit significantly reduced in comparison with the wild type.

FLOWER COLOR: AN mRNA-SPLICING MUTATION

Purple flower color is dominant in pea plants, and it results from the production of the pigment anthocyanin. The recessive mutant phenotype is white flower color, and in these plants there is no anthocyanin production. A research group led by Roger Hellens identified the *bHLH* gene as the source of the white flower mutation in pea plants. This gene produces a transcription factor protein that helps activate the transcription of several genes, including some in the anthocyanin-production pathway. In the absence of a functioning protein product from the *bHLH* gene, anthocyanin production does not take place.

The mutation in the recessive allele is a G–C to A–T base-pair substitution that alters the guanine at the 5' splice site of one of the introns of the allele. Recall that 5' splice sites have an invariant GU dinucleotide in mRNA (Section 8.4). The base substitution identified by Hellens changes the 5' sequence to an AU dinucleotide that is not recognized as a splice site. An alternative splice site (known as a cryptic splice site; see the text for discussion) is used instead to process the mutant mRNA transcript. The aberrant splicing elongates the mature mRNA by eight nucleotides. This addition of mRNA nucleotides results in a frameshift during translation, and the protein product is nonfunctional.

In intron 1 of the β-globin gene, two separate mutations that substitute the guanine of the GT dinucleotide abolish normal splicing entirely in mutations that are known as **splicing mutations** (**Figure 11.4b**). Additionally, one base-pair substitution mutation at position 5 of intron 1 by itself also prevents the production of normally spliced mRNA. The translation of the abnormally spliced transcripts produced by these three mutations does not produce wild-type β-globin protein. Other base-pair substitution mutations in intron 1 result in production of a mixture of normally and abnormally spliced transcript and produce some wild-type β-globin protein, but in reduced amounts.

One of Mendel's traits, the purple versus white flower phenotype, is caused by a splicing mutation. See the discussion of Mendel's flower color mutation in Experimental Insight 11.1 for details concerning this pre-mRNA–splicing mutation.

Cryptic Splice Sites Certain base-pair substitution mutations produce new splice sites that replace or compete with authentic splice sites during pre-mRNA processing. These newly formed splice sites are known as **cryptic splice sites**. Intron 1 of the human β-globin gene is 130 nucleotides in length. A base-pair substitution mutation that changes G to A at position 110 of intron 1 creates an AG dinucleotide that is a cryptic splice site (**Figure 11.5**). The cryptic splice site is spliced in about 90% of the intron 1 3' splicing events. This aberrant splicing leaves 19 additional nucleotides in the mature mRNA; these nucleotides have been removed in the other 10% of mature transcripts, which are spliced at the authentic 3' splice site for intron 1.

Polyadenylation Mutations Processing of the 3' end of eukaryotic mRNAs is initiated by the presence of a 5'–AAU–AAA–3' polyadenylation signal sequence (see Section 8.4),

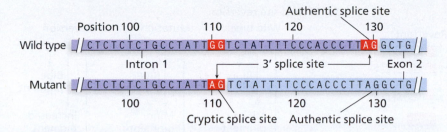

Figure 11.5 Cryptic splicing. Base-pair substitution of G–C to A–T at position 110 of intron 1 of the human β-globin gene creates a cryptic 3′ splice site.

and mutation of this sequence can block proper 3′ processing of mRNA. One example of this mutation is found in a rare variant of the human α-globin gene in which the DNA coding strand sequence is mutated from 5′-AATAAA-3′ to 5′-AATAAG-3′. The A–T to G–C base substitution blocks recognition of the polyadenylation signal sequence, generates abnormal mRNA, and leads to a severe reduction in the amount of functional α-globin protein.

Forward Mutation and Reversion

Forward mutation, often identified simply as "mutation," converts a wild-type allele to a mutant allele. In contrast, mutations identified as **reverse mutation** or, more commonly, as **reversion**, convert a mutation to a wild-type or near wild-type state. The mechanisms of base-pair substitution described earlier are examples of processes that create mutation. Reversions can be caused by similar mechanisms.

In one type of reversion, called a **true reversion**, the DNA sequence reverts to encoding its original message owing to a second mutation at the same site or within the same codon (**Figure 11.6a**). Alternatively, reversion can occur by a second mutation elsewhere in the gene. This is an **intragenic reversion**. An example is given in **Figure 11.6b**. Here the initial mutation was caused by deletion of two base pairs, and the intragenic reversion is a compensatory insertion of two base pairs near the site of the initial mutation, restoring the allele to a near wild-type form.

Figure 11.6c illustrates an example of a **second-site reversion**, produced by mutation in a different gene. In this case, the original mutation inactivates gene *A* and results in the loss of function of the major pigment-transporting protein in a flower. A minor pigment-transporting gene, *B*, remains active, transporting a small amount of blue pigment from gene *C*. The initial mutation produces a light-blue flower. The second-site reversion is a mutation of gene *B* that increases gene transcription and thus increases production of the pigment-transporting protein. The mutation of gene *B* compensates for the mutation of gene *A* and restores the wild-type dark-blue flower phenotype. Second-site mutations are also known as **suppressor mutations** because the second mutation, by restoring wild-type appearance, can be said to "suppress" the mutant phenotype generated by the first mutation.

In **Genetic Analysis 11.1**, you can practice identifying types of mutations by the alterations they produce in polypeptides.

11.2 Gene Mutations May Arise from Spontaneous Events

Spontaneous mutations are naturally occurring mutations that arise occasionally through errors during DNA replication or, much more often, through spontaneous changes in the chemical structure of nucleotide bases.

Spontaneous DNA Replication Errors

DNA replication has extraordinarily high fidelity. Replication errors resulting in base-pair mismatches between a template strand and a newly synthesized strand of DNA occur at an approximate rate of 1×10^{-9} in wild-type *E. coli*, and a similar accuracy rate is found in eukaryotic DNA replication. The overall efficiency of the replication process is attributable to the accuracy of DNA polymerases, to the "proofreading" capabilities of DNA polymerases, and to the efficiency of DNA base-pair mismatch repair systems that operate in all organisms during and immediately after replication (and discussed in Section 11.4).

Insertions and Deletions of Nucleotide Repeats One category of spontaneous mutation seen occasionally consists of mutations that alter the number of DNA repeats and that occur by a process called **strand slippage**. In the mid-1960s, George Streisinger and his colleagues described the first known example of strand slippage, which generated frameshift mutations caused by adding to the number of nucleotide repeats in a gene of the bacteriophage T4. Streisinger proposed that strand slippage occurs when the DNA polymerase of the replisome temporarily dissociates from the template strand as it moves across a region of repeating DNA sequence (**Figure 11.7**). He suggested that while synthesis of the new DNA strand is proceeding, a portion of newly replicated DNA can form a temporary double-stranded hairpin structure induced by the complementary base pairing of nucleotides in the loop. Slippage of the daughter strand on the template strand or pausing or slippage of DNA polymerase is apparently responsible for formation of these loops. The resumption of replication leads to rereplication of a portion of the repeat region, increasing the length of the repeat region in the daughter strand. Changes in the number of DNA sequence repeats of a VNTR allele (see Figure 7.27) or of other alleles with repeating DNA sequence come about by this mechanism.

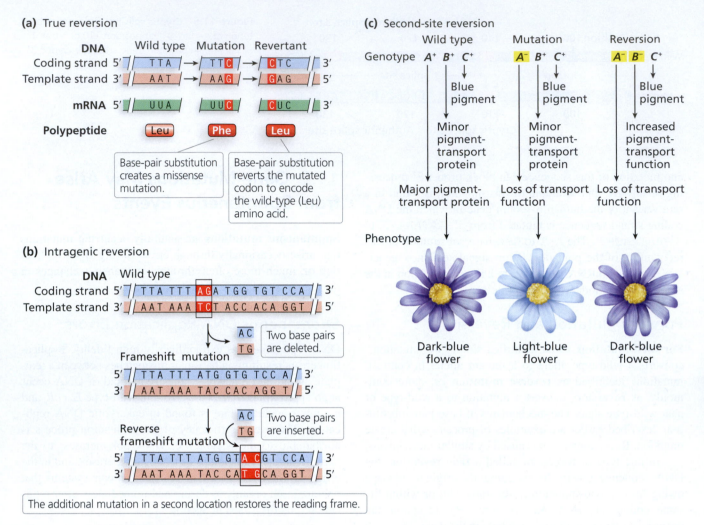

Figure 11.6   Reversion mutations. (a) This true reversion restores the wild-type amino acid sequence to the polypeptide. **(b)** This intragenic reversion reverts a frameshift mutation caused by a 2-bp deletion by insertion of 2 bp at a nearby site in the gene. **(c)** Second-site reversion restores a nearly wild-type phenotype through a compensatory mutation of a second gene.

🔘 Using the genetic code (Figure 9.13), make a base substitution mutation in a DNA triplet so as to produce a nonsense mutation, and then make a reversion mutation in the triplet so as to produce the original amino acid but with a different codon than the wild-type sequence.

Strand slippage mutations were first identified in the mid-1980s when an unusual X chromosome disorder called fragile X syndrome (OMIM 309550) was shown to be caused by increases in the number of DNA sequence repeats in a gene known as *FMR1*. Since then, a number of strand slippage mutations have been identified as the causes of several hereditary diseases in humans and other organisms. The human diseases are classified as **trinucleotide repeat expansion disorders** (Table 11.2). The wild-type alleles of the genes in question normally contain a variable number of DNA trinucleotide repeats. On rare occasions, these gene regions undergo mutations through strand slippage that cause the number of trinucleotide repeats to increase. For each of these disorders, expansion of the number of trinucleotide repeats beyond the wild-type range results in a hereditary disorder. Most often

the mutations block the production of wild-type mRNA and reduce or eliminate the production of wild-type protein.

Mispaired Nucleotides   The accuracy of DNA replication is due in large measure to complementary base pairing, A with T and G with C. We saw in Section 9.4, however, that third-base wobble during translation offers occasional exceptions to complementary base-pair rules. Similar noncomplementary base pairing occasionally occurs during DNA replication. These so-called **non–Watson-and-Crick base pairs** can include the mispairing of guanine with thymine or the mispairing of cytosine with adenine. Both sets of mispaired nucleotides form two hydrogen bonds.

The mispairing of a nucleotide in a newly synthesized DNA strand is identified as an **incorporated error**.

PROBLEM In a mutant analysis, a goal is often to identify the type of mutation that has occurred. In this problem, a fragment of a polypeptide with the wild-type amino acid sequence is given:

Met–His–Ala–Trp–Asn–Gly–Glu–His–Arg

The amino acid sequences of three mutants are shown below. For each mutant, identify the type of mutation that has occurred and specify how the mRNA sequence has been changed.

Mutation 1: Met–His–Ala–Trp–Lys–Gly–Glu–His–Arg
Mutation 2: Met–His–Ala
Mutation 3: Met–Met–Leu–Gly–Met–Ala–Glu–His–Arg

> **BREAK IT DOWN:** Use the wild-type amino acid sequence to determine the mRNA sequence, including all possible synonymous codons, as the starting point for mutant analysis. (Use the genetic code, p. 330; see also inside the front cover)

> **BREAK IT DOWN:** Identification of the mutations requires deducing each mutant mRNA sequence and comparing it to the wild-type mRNA sequence. (pp. 401–402)

Solution Strategies	Solution Steps
Evaluate	
1. Identify the topic this problem addresses and the nature of the required answer.	1. This problem concerns mutations affecting the amino acid sequence of a gene. The type of change causing each mutation must be identified, and the effect of the mutation on mRNA must be described.
2. Identify the critical information given in the problem.	2. The wild-type amino acid sequence and the corresponding portions of the mutant polypeptides are given.
Deduce	
③ Determine the sequence of the wild-type mRNA.	③ The sequence of the wild-type mRNA is 5′–AUG CAU/C GCN UGG AAU/C GGN GAA/G CAU/CA/CGN–3′

> **TIP:** Use N if the position could be occupied by any nucleotide, A/G for the alternative purines, and U/C for alternative pyrimidines.

> **TIP:** Use the genetic code in Figure 9.13 or in Table B inside the front cover.

Solution Strategies	Solution Steps
Solve	
4. Compare each mutant sequence with the wild-type polypeptide, and identify the probable types of mutations.	4. Mutant 1: This is a missense mutation in which the mutant polypeptide has one amino acid changed from Asn to Lys. Mutant 2: This is a nonsense mutation in which a Trp codon is changed to a stop codon. Mutant 3: This mutant contains alterations of five consecutive amino acids, beginning with the second amino acid (His to Met). The wild-type sequence is restored beginning with the seventh amino acid (Glu). This mutant results from two frameshift mutations. The first alters the reading frame, and the second restores it.
5. Determine the mRNA change producing the missense mutant.	5. The wild-type (Asn) codon is AAU/C, and the mutant (Lys) codon is AAA/G. This change results from either a transition or a transversion mutation.
6. Determine the mRNA change producing the nonsense mutant.	6. The wild-type Trp (UGG) codon is changed to a stop codon. The change is either UGG to UGA or UGG to UAG. In either case, this is a transition mutation.
7. Determine the mRNA change producing the frameshift mutant.	7. The appearance of Met in position 2 means the second codon of the frameshift mutant is AUG. This change requires deletion of the first C of the wild-type sequence and means that U, not C, is present as the sixth nucleotide of the wild type. Beginning with Glu, the wild-type amino acid sequence is restored. This requires insertion of G immediately after the Ala codon.

For more practice, see Problems 4, 11, 22, and 32.   Visit the Study Area to access study tools.   **Mastering Genetics**

Figure 11.8 provides an example in which DNA replication cycle 1 produces a wild-type DNA duplex (with an A–T base pair highlighted in the box) and a second DNA duplex with a G–T base pair (highlighted) as an incorporated error. This means there is an abnormality in DNA that might be repaired or might lead to a mutation. DNA replication cycle 2 is where the mispairing of nucleotides is converted into a mutation (the sequence change that will be transmitted through replication) in an event known as a **replicated error**. Here an A–T to G–C base-pair substitution takes place. The figure shows the thymine-containing strand producing a wild-type DNA duplex with an A–T base pair, and

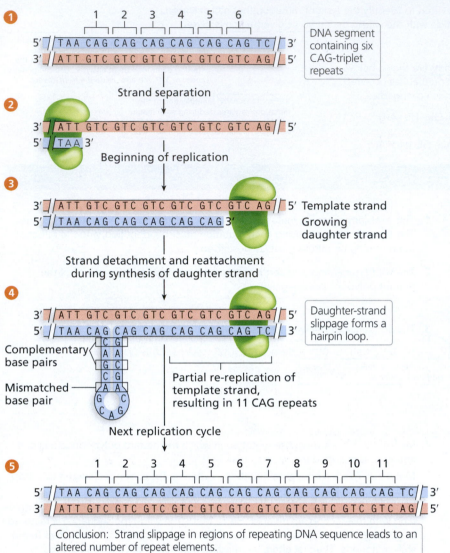

Figure 11.7   Strand slippage during DNA replication.

①

1   2   3   4   5   6

5′ ⫽TAA CAG CAG CAG CAG CAG CAG TC⫽ 3′
3′ ⫽ATT GTC GTC GTC GTC GTC GTC AG⫽ 5′

DNA segment containing six CAG-triplet repeats

Strand separation

②

3′ ⫽ATT GTC GTC GTC GTC GTC GTC AG⫽ 5′
5′ ⫽TAA 3′

Beginning of replication

③

3′ ⫽ATT GTC GTC GTC GTC GTC GTC AG⫽ 5′   Template strand
5′ ⫽TAA CAG CAG CAG CAG CAG 3′   Growing daughter strand

Strand detachment and reattachment during synthesis of daughter strand

④

3′ ⫽ATT GTC GTC GTC GTC GTC GTC AG⫽ 5′
5′ ⫽TAA CAG CAG CAG CAG CAG CAG TC⫽ 3′

Daughter-strand slippage forms a hairpin loop.

Complementary base pairs
C G
A A
G C
C G
Mismatched base pair
A A
G   C
C A G

Partial re-replication of template strand, resulting in 11 CAG repeats

Next replication cycle

⑤

1   2   3   4   5   6   7   8   9   10 11

5′ ⫽TAA CAG CAG CAG CAG CAG CAG CAG CAG CAG CAG CAG TC⫽ 3′
3′ ⫽ATT GTC GTC GTC GTC GTC GTC GTC GTC GTC GTC GTC AG⫽ 5′

Conclusion: Strand slippage in regions of repeating DNA sequence leads to an altered number of repeat elements.

the guanine-containing strand producing a duplex with a base substitution (G–C base pair) mutation. Both the wild type and the mutant contain complementary base pairs, so there is no possibility of detection by DNA repair systems.

DNA replication frequently plays an important role in permanently establishing incorporated errors and other kinds of DNA damage as mutations. Several examples are seen in this and the following section.

Table 11.2   Human Trinucleotide Repeat Disorders

Disease	OMIM Number	Repeat Sequence	Repeat Range		Principal Disease Phenotype
			Normal	Disease	
Fragile X syndrome	309550	CGG	6–50	200–2000	Mental retardation
Friedreich ataxia	229300	GAA	6–29	200–900	Loss of coordination
Huntington disease	143100	CAG	10–34	40–200	Uncontrolled movement
Jacobsen syndrome	147791	CGG	11	100–1000	Growth retardation
Myotonic dystrophy (type I)	160900	CTG	5–37	80–1000	Muscle weakness
Spinal and bulbar muscular atrophy	313200	CAG	14–32	40–55	Muscle wasting
Spinocerebellar ataxia (multiple forms)	271245	CAG	4–44	45–140	Loss of coordination

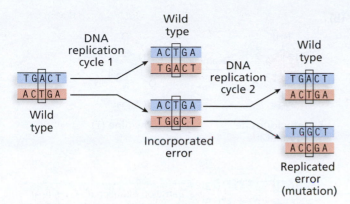

Figure 11.8   Incorporated errors and mutations. DNA base mispairing generates an incorporated error that if not repaired will generate a replicated error (a mutation) by DNA replication.

Spontaneous Nucleotide Base Changes

DNA nucleotide bases are organic chemical structures that can sustain damage or can spontaneously undergo structural alteration. These alterations embody damage to the duplex, but DNA replication may need to occur before they are preserved as mutations in the DNA sequence.

Two types of spontaneous damage to individual nucleotides are associated with subsequent mutation. **Depurination** is the loss of one of the purines, adenine or guanine, from a nucleotide by breakage of the covalent

bond at the 1′ carbon of deoxyribose that links the sugar to the nucleotide base (**Figure 11.9**). This forms a DNA lesion known as an **apurinic (AP) site** that lacks a purine nucleotide base. The missing nucleotide base can be replaced by DNA repair processes, but if it is not repaired the base will be missing during the next round of DNA replication. Lacking a template nucleotide base, the newly synthesized strand incorporates a nucleotide (most often an adenine) opposite the AP site. If the incorporated nucleotide is incorrect, a base substitution mutation will result following DNA replication.

Living cells lose thousands of purines a day, making depurination one of the most frequent spontaneous chemical changes affecting DNA. Most AP sites are replaced by the correct purine before the next DNA replication cycle, but depurination is a common cause of base-pair substitution mutations. Pyrimidine nucleotide bases are also lost but at a much lower rate than purines.

The second spontaneous nucleotide change leading to mutation is **deamination**, the loss of an amino (NH_2) group from a nucleotide base. Each of the DNA nucleotide bases contains an amino group, but deamination of cytosine is the event most often associated with mutation. When cytosine is deaminated, the amino group is replaced by an oxygen atom, forming the nucleotide base uracil (**Figure 11.10a**). DNA mismatch repair readily recognizes uracil as an RNA nucleotide base and removes it from DNA. The excised uracil is replaced by cytosine, and wild-type sequence is restored.

(a) Depurination

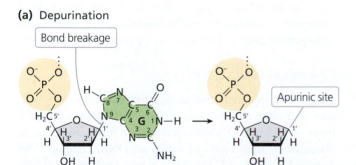

Figure 11.9   Depuration. (a) Breakage of the 1′ carbon bond releases a purine base. **(b)** Loss of a guanine from one strand of DNA creates an AP site. DNA replication adds adenine opposite the AP site. **(c)** The second cycle of DNA replication leads to a G–C to T–A mutation.

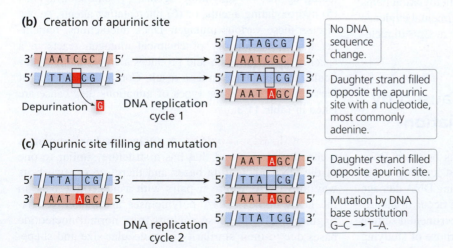

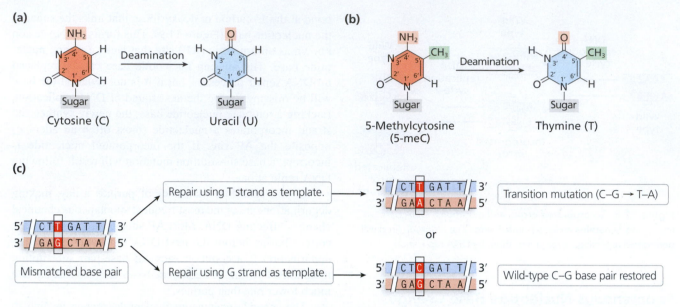

Figure 11.10 **Deamination.** **(a)** Unmethylated cytosine is deaminated to form uracil. **(b)** Deamination of 5-methylcytosine forms thymine that is mismatched to guanine. **(c)** Mismatch repair can create a C – G to T–A transition mutation or can remove the thymine to restore wild-type sequence.

A different scenario occurs, however, when deamination takes place on a cytosine that has been methylated. A methylated cytosine has the hydrogen atom at the number 5 carbon replaced with a CH_3 (methyl) group. Deamination of 5-methylcytosine (5meC) creates thymine and generates a base-pair mismatch between the newly formed thymine on one strand and the previously complementary guanine on the other strand (**Figure 11.10b**). If DNA base-pair mismatch repair does not correct the mismatch, the next round of DNA replication will include a C–G to T–A base-pair substitution (**Figure 11.10c**).

Deamination of 5-methylcytosine is associated with hotspots of mutation. Cytosines that are side by side with guanines in a DNA strand are identified as CpG dinucleotides; the *p* signifies the single phosphate group between the nucleotides, and the C is upstream of the G. Cytosines of CpG dinucleotides are frequent targets for methylation, particularly in mammalian promoters, where methylation helps regulate transcription (Section 13.2). Experimental evidence shows that base-pair substitution mutations at CpG dinucleotides are common in mammals.

11.3 Mutations May Be Caused by Chemicals or Ionizing Radiation

Mutations can be produced by interactions between DNA and chemical agents or between DNA and ionizing radiation. The agents generating mutation-inducing DNA damage are called **mutagens**. These mutations can occur in nature, but frequently mutagens are used in an experimental setting to generate **induced mutations** for the purpose of studying

the types of damage done to DNA by mutagen exposure, the mutational process itself, or the organism's repair responses to DNA damage. This section looks at some of the specific ways chemical mutagens and ionizing radiation interact with DNA to create particular mutations. Some mutagens are exotic or rare, but others are routinely present in the everyday life of an organism. For this reason, the study of mutagenesis through the production of induced mutations is an important form of biological and public health research.

Chemical Mutagens

Chemical compounds that induce mutations do so by specific and characteristic interactions with DNA nucleotide bases or with the DNA molecule. As a result, they can be classified by their mode of action on DNA, creating DNA damage by acting as (1) nucleotide base analogs, (2) deaminating agents, (3) alkylating agents, (4) oxidizing agents, (5) hydroxylating agents, or (6) intercalating agents. As we discuss these various mutagen–DNA interactions, remember that each category of chemical mutagen reacts in a specific way with DNA and produces a consistent and particular kind of mutation as a result. Compounds in each of these categories and the types of mutations they cause are listed in **Table 11.3**.

Nucleotide Base Analogs A **nucleotide base analog** is a chemical compound that has a structure similar to one of the DNA nucleotide bases and therefore can work its way into DNA, where it pairs with a nucleotide base in the DNA duplex. DNA polymerases are unable to distinguish nucleotide base analogs from normal nucleotide bases due to their similarity in molecular size and shape.

Table 11.3	Examples of Mutagenic Agents and Their Consequences	
Mutagen	**Type of Agent**	**Mutagenic Event**
2-Aminopurine	Nucleotide base analog	Transition mutation
5-Bromodeoxyuridine	Nucleotide base analog	Transition mutation
Ethyl methanesulfonate	Alkylating agent	Transition mutation
Hydroxylamine	Hydroxylating agent	Transition mutation
Nitrous oxide	Deaminating agent	Transition mutation
Oxygen radicals	Oxidizing agent	Transversion mutation
Acridine orange	Intercalating agent	Frameshift mutation
Proflavin	Intercalating agent	Frameshift mutation

Consequently, base analogs are incorporated into DNA strands during replication. For example, the compound 5-bromodeoxyuridine (BU) is a derivative of uracil and is very similar to thymine in size and shape. In its common form, called the keto form, BU is an analog of thymine and base pairs with adenine (**Figure 11.11a**). BU also has a rare form, called the enol form, that it assumes by undergoing a change in molecular configuration. In its enol form, BU base-pairs with guanine (**Figure 11.11b**). Two different base-substitution pathways can result from the incorporation of BU into DNA. A transition mutation from an A–T base pair to a G–C base pair occurs when the keto form of BU initially mispairs with adenine (**Figure 11.11c**). If BU switches to its enol form before the next DNA replication cycle, it mispairs with guanine, and in the following replication cycle the G-containing strand incorporates a cytosine in the daughter strand, completing the A–T to G–C transition mutation. **Figure 11.11d** depicts the second base-substitution pathway for BU incorporation. This pathway produces a G–C to A–T transition mutation. In this pathway, the rare enol form of BU initially mispairs with guanine. If BU switches to its more common keto form before the next DNA replication cycle, it directs the incorporation of adenine into the daughter strand, and then this daughter strand directs the incorporation of thymine into its daughter strand in the following replication cycle.

Deaminating Agents Nitrous acid (HNO_2) is a deaminating agent, meaning an agent that removes an amino group (NH_2) from a nucleotide base with a mutagenic effect. One example is how nitrous acid deaminates adenine. The product of this deamination is the modified nucleotide hypoxanthine that can mispair with cytosine and lead to an A–T to G–C base-pair substitution mutation (**Figure 11.12a**).

Alkylating Agents Alkylating agents add bulky side groups such as methyl (CH_3) and ethyl (CH_3–CH_2) groups to nucleotide bases. Ethyl methanesulfonate (EMS) is a powerful alkylating agent that adds an ethyl group to

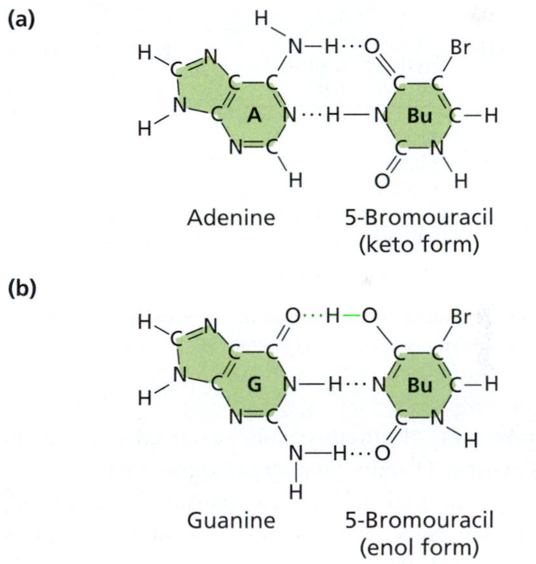

(a)

Adenine   5-Bromouracil (keto form)

(b)

Guanine   5-Bromouracil (enol form)

(c)

Wild-type	Bu incorporation	Base mispair in replication cycle 1	Mutation in replication cycle 2
A	A	G	G
..	..	...	...
T	Bu (keto)	Bu (enol)	C

(d)

Wild-type	Bu incorporation	Base mispair in replication cycle 1	Mutation in replication cycle 2
G	G	A	A
...	...	..	..
C	Bu (enol)	Bu (keto)	T

Figure 11.11 Mutation by incorporation of the nucleotide base analog 5-bromouridine (BU).

Ⓠ **Does a mutation exist before or after DNA replication cycle 1? Why?**

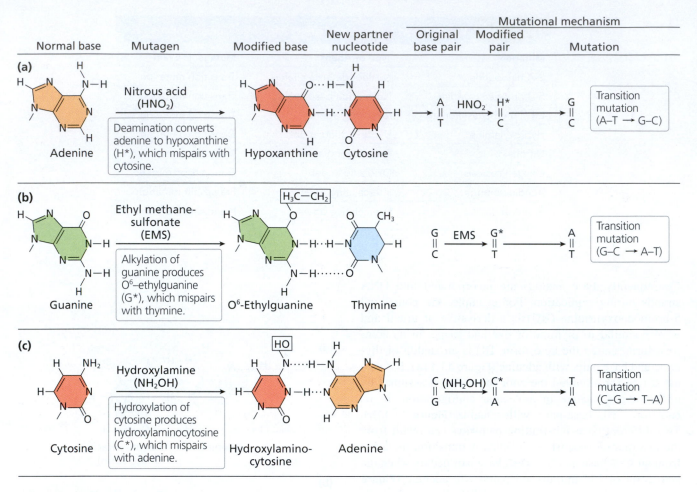

Figure 11.12 Examples of the action of chemical mutagens. In (a), H* is hypoxanthine. In (b) and (c), the asterisks (*) denote modified nucleotides.

thymine, producing 4-ethylthymine, or an ethyl group to guanine, creating O^6-ethylguanine (**Figure 11.12b**). This interferes with normal DNA base pairing by distorting the DNA double helix. EMS induces transition mutations through its action on guanine.

Hydroxylating Agents Hydroxylation is the addition of a hydroxyl (OH) group to a recipient compound by a donor called a hydroxylating agent. Hydroxylamine is a hydroxylating agent that adds a hydroxyl group to cytosine by displacing an H_2, thus creating hydroxylaminocytosine (**Figure 11.12c**). Hydroxylaminocytosine often pairs with guanine but frequently mispairs with adenine, leading to transition mutations.

DNA Intercalating Agents Certain small molecular compounds called **DNA intercalating agents** can squeeze their way between DNA base pairs. DNA-intercalating compounds, such as proflavin, benzo(a)pyrene (a component of cigarette smoke), and aflatoxin (a toxin found in mold-contaminated peanuts), can find their way between base pairs and distort the duplex (**Figure 11.13**). Intercalating agents generate helical distortions that lead to DNA

strand nicking (the breakage of a phosophdiester bond on one DNA strand) that is not efficiently repaired. In the next DNA replication cycle, the nicked strands can gain or lose one or more nucleotides. As a result, intercalating agents cause frameshift mutations.

Radiation-Induced DNA Damage

Hermann Muller was the first to describe the mutagenic power of X-rays, but now we know that all forms of energy above the visible spectrum—ultraviolet (UV) radiation, X-irradiation, gamma rays, and cosmic rays—are mutagenic. In low doses, X-ray irradiation causes mutations by inducing chromosome breaks; at higher doses, however, X-rays are energetic enough to kill fruit flies outright.

Minimizing human X-ray exposure is a prominent public health and medical focus, but the mutagenic radiation source of greater concern is the UV radiation that is a component of sunlight. This is the mutagen to which we and other organisms are most often exposed. Like chemical mutagens, the mutagenicity of UV radiation derives from specific lesions it creates in DNA. UV irradiation alters DNA nucleotides by inciting the formation of additional

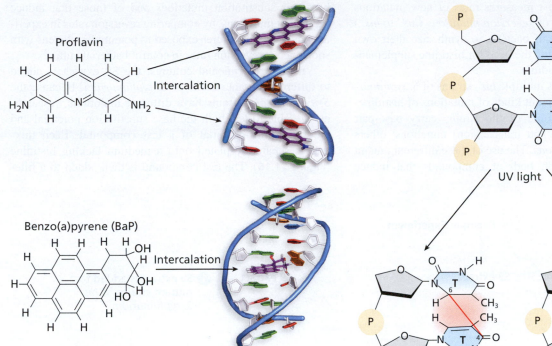

Figure 11.13 **DNA intercalating agents.** Proflavin and benzo(a)pyrene intercalate into the double helix and distort its shape, generating strand nicking that can produce frameshift mutations.

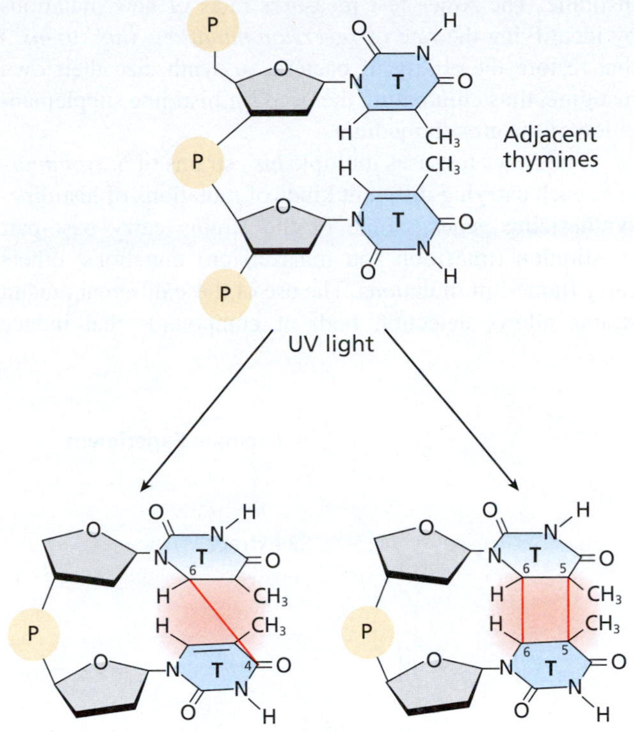

Figure 11.14 **UV photoproducts.** UV irradiation forms photoproducts from adjacent pyrimidines, distorting the double helix and potentially blocking replication.

bonds that create aberrant structures called **photoproducts**. These photoproducts most often form between two adjacent pyrimidine nucleotide bases in a DNA strand. Two adjacent thymines are the most frequent locations for the creation of UV photoproducts that contain one or two additional covalent bonds (**Figure 11.14**). One common photoproduct called a **thymine dimer** contains two additional covalent bonds that join the 5 and 6 carbons of adjacent thymines. Another, called a **6-4 photoproduct**, also joins adjacent thymines, in this case by formation of a bond between the 6 carbon of one thymine and the 4 carbon of the other thymine.

Organisms that experience regular UV exposure—and they range from bacteria to humans—have DNA repair systems that identify and correct most pyrimidine dimers. But a few pyrimidine dimers may escape repair; and when they do, DNA replication can be disrupted. These disruptions lead to mutations, and they are a primary cause of the strong association between excessive UV exposure and skin cancer. Some of the specific DNA repair mechanisms that repair UV-induced photoproducts are discussed in the following section.

The Ames Test

In our day-to-day lives, we encounter scores of naturally occurring and synthetic chemicals and compounds—in the food we eat, the air we breathe, the cars we drive, and even the books we read. Each year new chemical compounds are introduced as part of various commercial and industrial processes. How do we determine which of these chemicals can

increase the mutation frequencies of genes and therefore pose a hazard to our health? Occasionally, the mutagenic or carcinogenic potential of a compound is so great that evidence of its danger is relatively easy to identify. Much more often, however, the mutagenicity of a compound is more subtle, and careful analysis of experimental data is required to ascertain it.

For nearly 40 years, thousands of natural and synthetic compounds have been assayed for mutagenic potential by a simple biological test developed by Bruce Ames. This procedure, called the **Ames test**, exposes bacteria to experimental compounds in the presence of a mixture of purified enzymes produced by the mammalian liver. In animals, ingested chemicals are routed to the liver, where they are broken down by detoxifying enzymes. Using a critical subset of detoxifying liver enzymes called the S9 extract, the Ames test mimics the biological defense processes that take place in the liver of animals exposed to chemical compounds. During enzymatic breakdown in the liver, numerous intermediate products can be produced, some of which may be mutagenic, even if the original compound was not. The purpose of the Ames test is to detect whether the original compound or any of its normal breakdown products is mutagenic.

The Ames test most commonly uses strains of the bacterium *Salmonella typhimurium* that carry mutations affecting their ability to synthesize the amino acid histidine. These bacteria are designated *his⁻* to indicate that their mutation prevents histidine synthesis. They will not grow unless they are provided with a medium that is supplemented with histidine. The Ames test measures rates of new mutations by identifying the rate of *reversion mutations* (*his⁻* to *his⁺*) that restore the ability of bacteria to synthesize their own histidine, thus eliminating the need for histidine supplementation of the growth medium.

The Ames test uses multiple *his⁻* strains of *S. typhimurium*, each carrying different kinds of mutations of histidine-synthesizing genes. Some of the strains carry base-pair substitution (transition and transversion) mutations; others carry frameshift mutations. The use of these different mutant strains allows detection both of compounds that induce

base-pair substitution mutations and of those that induce frameshift mutations, by comparing reversion rates in experimental bacterial cultures exposed to potential mutagens with spontaneous reversion rates in control bacterial cultures.

In the experimental cultures, the S9 extract is added to different mutant strains of *S. typhimurium*. Because the *S. typhimurium* strains have different mutations, researchers are able to test both the base substitution potential and the frameshift potential of a test compound. Each mixture is separately plated onto a medium lacking histidine (**Figure 11.15**). The test compound is then added to a filter

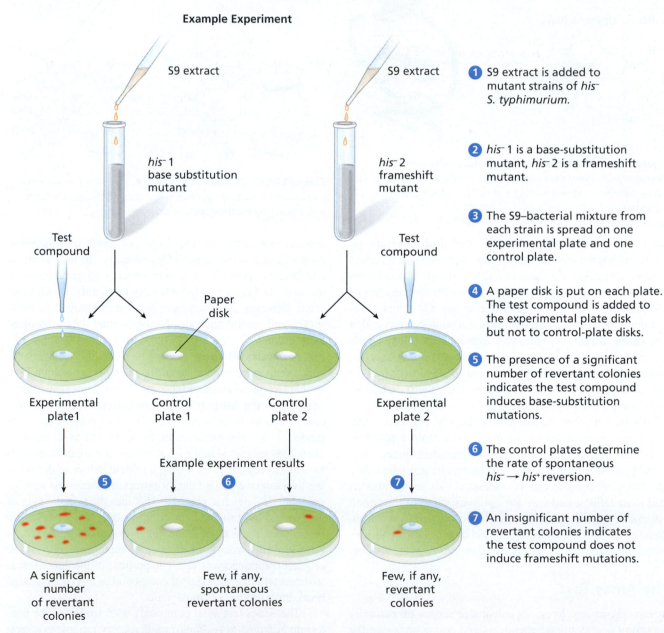

Figure 11.15 The Ames test for potential mutagenicity of chemical compounds.

On the culture plate containing the Ames test of a powerful chemical mutagen, there will often be an empty zone, with no revertants growing, immediately surrounding the paper disk. Farther away from the disk, however, revertants will grow. Why does this zone of no growing revertants occur?

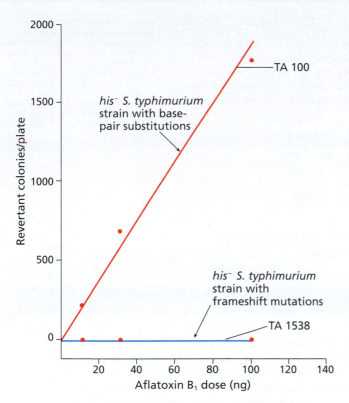

Figure 11.16 **Mutagenicity of aflatoxin B$_1$ determined by the Ames test.** Aflatoxin B$_1$ induces a high rate of reversions in *his$^-$* bacteria with base-pair substitution mutations (strain TA 100), but not in frameshift mutants (strain TA 1538).

paper disk in the center of each test plate, and the plates are incubated. On the corresponding control plates, bacteria are exposed to S9 but not to the test compound.

The test compound in the paper filter diffuses outward into the growth medium. It is more concentrated near the filter and less concentrated away from the filter. Thus, bacteria closer to the filter are exposed to a higher concentration of the test compound than those that are more distant from the filter. Often, the gradient of the test compound concentration leads to the finding of more revertant colonies near the filter than farther away from the filter.

The results of an Ames test are interpreted by counting the number of growing colonies on each plate and comparing the numbers with one another and with the control plates. The number of growing colonies on the control plates allows the determination of the spontaneous rates of reversion from *his$^-$* to *his$^+$*. The numbers of growing colonies on the experimental plates are compared with the control plate results to determine if there is a statistically significant increase in the number of revertant colonies on an experimental plate. If there is, the test compound or one of the breakdown products formed by the activity of S9 enzymes is likely mutagenic.

In **Figure 11.16**, the effect of the very powerful mutagen known as aflatoxin B$_1$ is shown. The Ames test reversion results show a linear dose-response curve (i.e., the number of revertants is proportionate to the dosage of aflatoxin B$_1$), revealing the strong mutagenic potential of aflatoxin B$_1$. Aflatoxin B$_1$

is produced by the fungus *Aspergillus* that grows on nuts and maize (corn). This powerful mutagen induces large numbers of base-pair substitution reversion mutations in the *his$^-$* strain designated TA 100 that contains a base-pair substitution and is highly sensitive to aflatoxin B$_1$. At all doses tested, the reversion rate for aflatoxin B$_1$ in base-pair substitution *his$^-$* strains is elevated above that of the *his$^-$* strain TA 1538, which contains a frameshift mutation. This result indicates that aflatoxin B$_1$ actively induces reversion of base-pair substitution mutants but not of frameshift mutants. **Genetic Analysis 11.2** guides you through an analysis of an Ames test of potential mutagens.

11.4 Repair Systems Correct Some DNA Damage

It is clear that the structural and informational integrity of DNA is under continuous assault from spontaneous chemical change and from various chemical and physical mutagens. Despite this ongoing challenge, organisms preserve the fidelity of their DNA by repairing most lesions that occur and leaving very few mutations—most of which are deleterious—to accrue. Too great an accumulation of mutations may doom an organism and ultimately affect survival of the species; on the other hand, too small a pool of mutations will limit the range of genetic variability and may hamper the species' ability to evolve.

Organisms must therefore strike a balance between the accumulation of mutations and the repair of DNA damage before mutations accrue. The multiple repair mechanisms that have evolved for this purpose are often partially redundant with regard to the lesions they identify and repair. In broad terms, these damage repair processes fall into two categories: (1) those that directly repair DNA damage and restore it to its wild-type state; and (2) those that allow the organism to circumvent problems such as blocked DNA replication, which can occur when damage is not repaired but which leave the DNA damage in place.

Direct Repair of DNA Damage

We have already encountered one way to repair DNA lesions and to reverse DNA damage before it causes mutation. This mechanism is proofreading by DNA polymerase (see Chapter 7), which identifies DNA base-pair mismatches during DNA replication, removes a segment of DNA containing the erroneous nucleotide, and resynthesizes the excised sequence. In this section, four additional repair systems are described that also carry out direct repair of DNA damage (**Table 11.4**).

Photoreactive Repair UV radiation is the most common mutagen that most organisms encounter on a daily basis. UV exposure induces the formation of photoproducts that can inhibit DNA replication as well as lead to mutation. One common way organisms identify and repair UV-induced

PROBLEM Three potentially hazardous compounds, A, B, and C, are assayed by the Ames test. Two strains of *his⁻* bacteria (1 and 2) are used. Auxotrophy in strain 1 is caused by a frameshift mutation and in strain 2 by the substitution of one base pair, resulting in a nonsense mutation. Each strain is treated with the different compounds. An S9 fraction (supernatant of solubilized rat liver enzymes) was added to each mixture of auxotrophic bacteria plus one of the compounds.

After treatment, the cells were plated on minimal medium. Control plates contain each of the two strains treated with S9 alone, without A, B, or C present. The accompanying table shows the number of prototrophic colonies observed on the plates:

BREAK IT DOWN: The Ames test examines the potential mutagenicity of compounds or their breakdown products by exposing bacteria and determining the rate of reversion from mutant to wild-type phenotype (pp. 413–414).

BREAK IT DOWN: Growth of a bacterial colony on a minimal medium plate indicates it is wild type (see Research Technique 6.1, pp. 189–190).

Compound Tested	Strain 1	Strain 2
A	904	6
B	5	4
C	3	680
Control (no compound)	6	3

a. Assess the growth results for each compound and determine whether it is mutagenic.
b. Determine the type of mutation most likely induced by any mutagens.

BREAK IT DOWN: See the Ames test sample data in Figure 11.16 (p. 415).

Solution Strategies	Solution Steps
Evaluate	
1. Identify the topic this problem addresses and the nature of the required answer.	1. This problem concerns interpretation of the results of an Ames test of three compounds. The answer must identify which if any of the compounds are mutagenic and describe the nature of that mutagenicity.
2. Identify the critical information given in the problem.	2. The number of revertant colonies is given for each compound. A control result is also given. The cause of auxotrophy in each mutant strain is identified.
Deduce	
3. Describe the meaning of growth results on the control plate.	3. The control plates have had no test compound added. The growing colonies on these plates are spontaneous revertants from each of the auxotrophic tester strains.
4. Deduce the meaning of growth results on each of the experimental plates.	4. Compound A produces many revertants in strain 1 but no reversion over spontaneous levels in strain 2. Compound C generates many revertants in strain 2 but does not produce revertants at a rate greater than the control in strain 1. Compound B does not increase the reversion rate above the spontaneous level in either strain.
Solve	Answer a
5. Identify the mutagenic compounds and justify your answer.	5. Compounds A and C are mutagenic, but compound B is not. The large numbers of revertant colonies on the strain 1 test of compound A and the number of revertants on the strain 2 test of compound C identify these compounds as mutagens. Compound B does not show an increased rate of reversion relative to the background numbers on the control plates.
	Answer b
6. Describe the nature of mutagenicity for each compound.	6. Compound A causes frameshift mutations by inducing a high rate of reversion of *his⁻* strain 1 auxotrophs. Compound C causes a high rate of reversions of strain 2 auxotrophs by inducing base-pair substitution reversions.

TIP: Base-pair substitution mutagens generally revert base-pair substitution auxotrophs, and frameshift mutagens revert frameshift auxotrophs.

Table 11.4	Common Systems for Direct DNA Repair
Photoreactive repair	Repair of UV-induced photoproducts catalyzed by photolyase activated by visible light
Base excision repair (BER)	Removal of an incorrect or damaged DNA base and repair by synthesis of a new strand segment (nick translation)
Nucleotide excision repair (NER)	Removal of a strand segment containing DNA damage and replacement by new DNA synthesis
Mismatch repair	Removal of a DNA base-pair mismatch by excision of a segment of the newly synthesized strand followed by resynthesis of the excised segment

DNA damage is through **photoreactive repair**. This direct DNA repair mechanism is found in bacteria, single-celled eukaryotes, plants, and some animals (e.g., *Drosophila*) but not in humans. Photoreactive repair utilizes the enzyme photolyase to bind to a UV-induced photo product. Once bound, photolyase uses visible light to direct energy into breaking the bonds that produce the photoproduct. In *E. coli*, photolyase is the product of the *phr* (photoreactive repair) gene. Mutations of this gene result in a substantial increase in UV-induced mutations in bacteria. Photolyase mutations in other organisms similarly result in increases in the mutation rate.

Base Excision Repair Damage to a DNA base or the presence of an incorrect base can initiate the direct DNA-repair process known as **base excision repair (BER)**. This process first identifies and removes the damaged DNA base. It then breaks one strand of DNA near the excised base and utilizes the single-stranded break as the site from which to initiate synthesis of a short DNA segment that replaces several nucleotides, including the damaged base. **Figure 11.17**

illustrates an example of BER that is initiated by the recognition and removal of a uracil that is mispaired with a guanine. The uracil was derived from the deamination of 5-methylcytosine, as described in the previous section. The enzyme DNA *N*-glycosylase removes the uracil, creating an AP (apyrimidinic) site. The enzyme AP endonuclease then cuts the sugar-phosphate backbone at the 5′ side of the AP site. This single-stranded break is called a "nick." In a process called **nick translation**, DNA polymerases recognize the nick and initiate the removal and replacement of DNA nucleotides, including the AP site. Nick translation is essentially identical to the process that removes and replaces the RNA primer during DNA 1 replication. After replacing several nucleotides, DNA ligase seals the sugar-phosphate backbone, and repair is complete. Different DNA polymerases undertake BER in bacteria and eukaryotes, and the precise mechanisms of repair vary somewhat, but the overall process of BER is the same in all organisms.

Nucleotide Excision Repair A third process for directly repairing DNA damage is **nucleotide excision repair (NER)**. It is a very common repair process found in virtually all bacterial and eukaryotic species, including humans. NER is frequently used to repair UV-induced damage to DNA. For this reason it is also known as **ultraviolet (UV) repair** (**Figure 11.18**). In UV-damage repair, NER is carried out by the protein products of four UV repair genes called *uvrA*, *uvrB*, *uvrC*, and *uvrD*. Two molecules of UVR A protein and one molecule of UVR B protein bind on one strand of DNA opposite the site of the photoproduct. The two molecules of UVR A dissociate from the strand, and a molecule of UVR C joins UVR B to form a UVR BC complex. Each UVR C cleaves a bond about four or five nucleotides to the 3′ side or the 5′ side of the photoproduct. The single-stranded fragment of approximately 12 nucleotides containing the photoproduct is released with the help of UVR D, which is a DNA helicase. A DNA polymerase binds to the exposed 3′ OH end created by the removal of a strand segment and synthesizes a replacement for the lost segment, using the complementary strands as a template. When synthesis is complete, DNA ligase binds to the gap to reseal the sugar-phosphate backbone. This

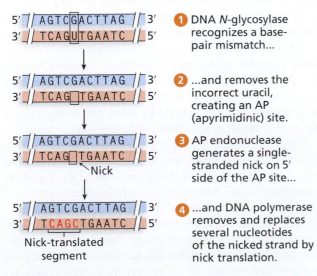

① DNA *N*-glycosylase recognizes a base-pair mismatch...

② ...and removes the incorrect uracil, creating an AP (apyrimidinic) site.

③ AP endonuclease generates a single-stranded nick on 5′ side of the AP site...

④ ...and DNA polymerase removes and replaces several nucleotides of the nicked strand by nick translation.

Figure 11.17 **Base excision repair.** DNA *N*-glycosylase and AP (apurinic) endonuclease remove mismatched and damaged nucleotides from DNA.

UV-damaged DNA

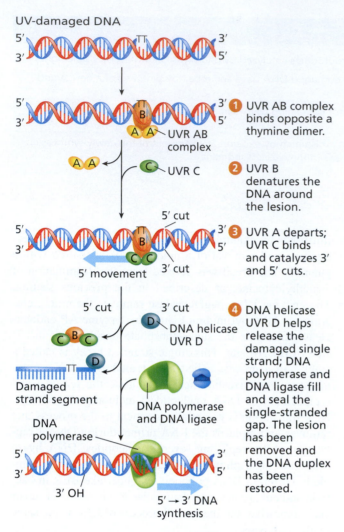

1 UVR AB complex binds opposite a thymine dimer.

2 UVR B denatures the DNA around the lesion.

3 UVR A departs; UVR C binds and catalyzes 3' and 5' cuts.

4 DNA helicase UVR D helps release the damaged single strand; DNA polymerase and DNA ligase fill and seal the single-stranded gap. The lesion has been removed and the DNA duplex has been restored.

Figure 11.18 **An example of nucleotide excision repair.** UVR proteins remove UV-induced damage from DNA strands.

🅠 **What would be the likely short-term and long-term consequences of a mutation that inactivated the production of UVR A protein?**

process removes the lesion and restores the DNA duplex to its wild-type sequence and structure.

The human hereditary cancer-prone condition xeroderma pigmentosum (XP; various OMIM numbers) is caused by mutation of any of seven different genes involved in human NER. The Case Study in Chapter 4 (pp.136–137) describes genetic complementation results that led to the identification of five of the human NER genes (the data reveal five complementation groups, each corresponding to a different NER gene). Two additional NER genes were discovered in other studies. Individuals with XP have extreme UV sensitivity and develop UV-induced precancerous and cancerous lesions through UV exposure. The UV sensitivity is so great that most XP individuals must avoid almost all sun exposure to limit their cancer risk, and in extreme cases they must even avoid exposure to fluorescent lights, which emit a low level of UV irradiation.

Mismatch Repair The final example of direct repair of DNA damage is that of DNA base-pair **mismatch repair**. The proofreading that accompanies DNA replication is an efficient system that helps keep the mutation rate low (see Section 7.4). Still, some mismatched nucleotide base pairs escape proofreading. These can be detected and repaired by mismatch repair. Mismatch repair has been most extensively studied in *E. coli*, but similar processes that include the action of homologous genes in eukaryotes, including humans, have also been examined.

When faced with a base-pair mismatch, repair enzymes must correctly identify the nucleotide to be replaced, and this requires distinguishing between the original DNA strand, with the correct nucleotide, and the new DNA strand with the mismatched nucleotide. The identification is accomplished by the sensitivity of mismatch repair enzymes to the methylation (the addition of CH_3 groups) of specific nucleotides in the original DNA strand. In *E. coli*, methylation is a common feature of DNA, and prior to replication, DNA parental strands are fully methylated. However, the daughter DNA duplexes produced by replication are only hemimethylated—that is, fully methylated on just the parental strand. A period of time must pass before the newly synthesized strands are fully methylated, and it is in this window of time that the methyl-sensitive components of mismatch repair operate.

Three *E. coli* genes, *MutS*, *MutL*, and *MutH*, produce proteins—MutS, MutL, and MutH, respectively—that recognize and bind to DNA containing base-pair mismatches as follows. MutH searches out hemimethylated sequences and has as its most common target the sequence 5'-GATC-3'. This sequence forms a palindrome (i.e., the same sequence reading 5' to 3' on both DNA strands). MutS locates and binds to the site of a base-pair mismatch and then forms a complex with MutL. The complex binds in turn to MutH (**Figure 11.19**). MutH breaks a phosphodiester bond on the 5' side of the guanine of a GATC sequence on the unmethylated daughter strand, and exonuclease enzymes remove from that strand a segment of DNA that extends beyond the mismatched base pair. This leaves a gap in the newly synthesized strand, and it is filled by DNA polymerase, using the original strand as a template to fill the gap.

After mismatch repair was described in *E. coli*, a similar repair mechanism was identified in yeast and other eukaryotes. Homologs of *MutS* and *MutL* are found in eukaryotes, but no homolog of *MutH* has been identified. Although the operation of mismatch repair in eukaryotes is not well understood, defects in the system are known to be associated with cancer development. Strong evidence indicates that a rare type of human hereditary cancer known as hereditary nonpolyposis colorectal cancer (HNPCC) is caused by mutations of *hMLH1* or *hMLH2*, the human homologs of *MutS* and *MutL*. As is the case with mutations

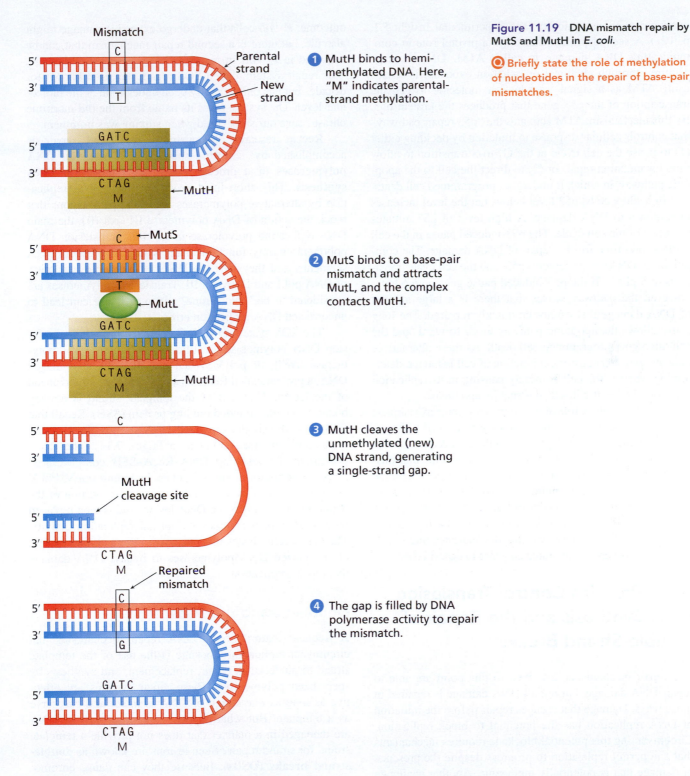

Mismatch

5′
3′

C
T

Parental strand

New strand

GATC

CTAG
M

MutH

C — MutS

5′
3′

T

MutL

GATC

5′
3′

CTAG
M

MutH

C

5′
3′

MutH cleavage site

5′
3′

CTAG
M

Repaired mismatch

C
G

5′
3′

GATC

5′
3′

CTAG
M

Figure 11.19 DNA mismatch repair by MutS and MutH in *E. coli*.

Q Briefly state the role of methylation of nucleotides in the repair of base-pair mismatches.

① MutH binds to hemi-methylated DNA. Here, "M" indicates parental-strand methylation.

② MutS binds to a base-pair mismatch and attracts MutL, and the complex contacts MutH.

③ MutH cleaves the unmethylated (new) DNA strand, generating a single-strand gap.

④ The gap is filled by DNA polymerase activity to repair the mismatch.

of genes involved in NER, mutations of the base-pair mismatch repair process appear to lead to the accumulation of mutations and to the development of cancer.

DNA Damage-Signaling Systems

The biochemical mechanisms that recognize DNA damage and mount a damage-repair response are crucial to the health and survival of an organism. They consist of tightly regulated genetic processes involving numerous genes and proteins. In humans and other mammals, a certain multiprotein complex acts as a genomic sentry to identify damage. This damage-response process is active throughout the cell cycle and is especially important in regulating the G_1-to-S transition, preventing the cell cycle from progressing to S phase until the cell has adequately repaired any mutations.

One important protein in this process is BRCA1, the product of the first gene implicated in familial breast and ovarian cancer susceptibility (see Experimental Insight 5.1, p. 171). A second protein that plays a pivotal role in communicating DNA damage is called ATM. DNA damage acquired through chemical or radiation exposure is sensed using ATM as a signal transduction molecule to activate transcription of the *p53* gene that produces the protein p53. By this mechanism, ATM activates the "p53 repair pathway" that controls cellular response to mutation by deciding either (1) to pause the cell cycle at the G_1-to-S transition to allow time for mutation repair or (2) to direct the cell to the apoptotic pathway, in which it undergoes programmed cell death.

In healthy cells, p53 level is low, but the level increases in response to DNA damage. A high level of p53 initiates G_1 arrest of the cell cycle. The p53-induced pause in the cell cycle allows time for the repair of DNA damage. The completion of DNA repair depletes p53, and the cell cycle transitions to S phase. If the p53-induced pause goes on too long, however, the pathway senses that there is a large amount of DNA damage that cannot be quickly repaired. The long pause allows the apoptotic pathway to go forward, and the cell undergoes programmed cell death. As these alternatives indicate, *p53* sits at a critical junction of cell behavior, determining whether the cell is merely pausing in its replication cycle or whether it will self-destruct by apoptosis.

Given the critical role of p53, it may not come as a surprise that mutation of the *p53* gene is strongly associated with cancer development. We take up details of the connection between mutations of *p53*, the occurrence of cancer, and the transmission of *p53* mutation in the human familial cancer syndrome known as Li–Fraumeni syndrome (OMIM 151623) in Application Chapter C: The Genetics of Cancer. Mutation of *p53* is also implicated, more broadly, in other cancers. Information accumulated over the past two decades indicates that *p53* is one of the most commonly mutated genes in cancer cells.

11.5 Proteins Control Translesion DNA Synthesis and the Repair of Double-Strand Breaks

The repair mechanisms described to this point are able to repair DNA damage, but not all DNA damage is repaired in those ways. Damage that escapes repair before the initiation of DNA replication has the potential to block replication. Circumventing this potential blockage requires mechanisms that can permit replication to progress despite the presence of damage that is potentially mutagenic. Another challenge to organisms is the occasional breakage of one or both DNA strands, which can also block DNA replication and may lead to cell death if it is not successfully overcome.

Translesion DNA Synthesis

In response to widespread DNA damage, molecular activities in the cell may direct the cell to initiate apoptosis. The activity of the p53 protein in eukaryotic cells can lead to this

outcome. *E. coli* cells that undergo extensive damage might also die, but there is a second repair mechanism that can be activated in *E. coli* in response to massive DNA damage. This repair system, called SOS repair, has been known for decades but has only recently been understood at the molecular level. The system takes its name from the old maritime phrase "save our ship," used when sinking was imminent.

Recent research demonstrates that SOS repair is accomplished by activating specialized **translesion DNA polymerases** in a process known as **translesion DNA synthesis**. This short-lived process allows DNA replication by alternative polymerases able to bypass lesions that block the action of DNA polymerase III (pol III), the main DNA-replicating polymerase in *E. coli*. Translesion DNA polymerases only function in the synthesis of short DNA segments, and they lack the DNA proofreading capability of DNA pol I and DNA pol III. Translesion polymerases are considered to be "error-prone," since their use can lead to uncorrected DNA replication errors.

The SOS system in *E. coli* operates through a translesion DNA polymerase identified as polymerase V ("polymerase five"), or pol V. When pol III stalls at damaged DNA, a protein called RecA coats the template strand ahead of the lesion. This part of the template strand is already bound by single-stranded binding protein (SSB). Recall that SSB coats the single, separated DNA strands ahead of the replication fork (see Foundation Figure 7.14). The RecA protein in the resulting DNA–RecA–SSB complex activates transcription of several genes, including pol V. Pol V displaces polymerase III, synthesizes a short portion of the daughter strand across the DNA lesion, and is then replaced by pol III, which resumes its normal replication activity. The evidence indicates that eukaryotes use a similar system of specialized DNA polymerases to bypass DNA damage that blocks replication.

Double-Strand Break Repair

A frequent feature of the DNA repair mechanisms that circumvent replication blockage is the use of the template strand to guide DNA repair, replacement, and synthesis by specialized polymerases. These repair systems are effective as long as one strand of DNA is intact and can serve as a template. But what happens if *both strands* of DNA are damaged in a manner that does not provide a template strand for strand repair? Such lesions are known as **double-strand breaks (DSBs)**. Because they can cause chromosome instability and incomplete replication of the genome, double-strand breaks are potentially lethal to cells and elevate the risk of cancer and the chance of chromosome structural mutations.

To protect organisms from the unpleasant consequences of double-strand breaks, two mechanisms have evolved to carry out **double-strand break repair**. The first is an error-prone repair process known as *nonhomologous end joining* that repairs double-strand breaks occurring before

DNA replication. The second is an error-free process called *synthesis-dependent strand annealing* that repairs double-strand breaks occurring after the completion of DNA replication.

Nonhomologous End Joining

Nonhomologous end joining (NHEJ) is a four-step process for repairing double-strand breaks that inevitably leads to mutation (**Figure 11.20**). In this process, double-strand breaks are recognized by a protein complex containing the proteins PK$_{CS}$, Ku70, and Ku80. This complex attaches to each of the broken ends of the DNA duplex. The complex then trims back (resects) the free ends of each broken strand. Resection leaves blunt ends on each side of the break. Lastly, the blunt ends are ligated by a specialized DNA ligase.

Completion of NHEJ produces an intact DNA duplex and allows replication across the repaired region in the upcoming replication cycle, but the repair is often imperfect because resection removes nucleotides that cannot be replaced. For this reason, NHEJ is error prone.

Synthesis-Dependent Strand Annealing

In eukaryotes, once DNA replication is complete, each chromosome is composed of two identical sister chromatids. Double-stranded breaks at this stage can be repaired by exploiting the intact sister chromatid to repair the damaged chromatid in an error-free repair process known as **synthesis-dependent strand annealing (SDSA)**.

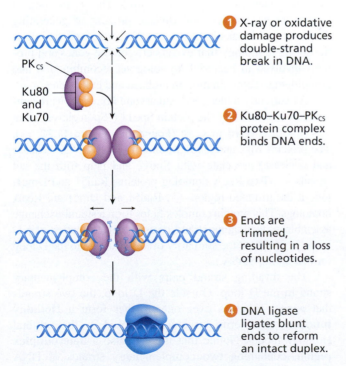

❶ X-ray or oxidative damage produces double-strand break in DNA.

❷ Ku80–Ku70–PK$_{CS}$ protein complex binds DNA ends.

❸ Ends are trimmed, resulting in a loss of nucleotides.

❹ DNA ligase ligates blunt ends to reform an intact duplex.

Figure 11.20 Nonhomologous end joining (NHEJ). NHEJ is an error-prone system that rejoins DNA strands following a double-stranded break.

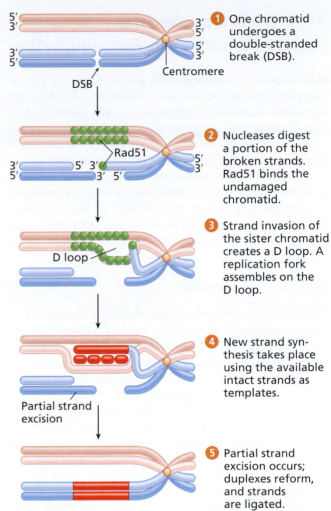

❶ One chromatid undergoes a double-stranded break (DSB).

❷ Nucleases digest a portion of the broken strands. Rad51 binds the undamaged chromatid.

❸ Strand invasion of the sister chromatid creates a D loop. A replication fork assembles on the D loop.

❹ New strand synthesis takes place using the available intact strands as templates.

❺ Partial strand excision occurs; duplexes reform, and strands are ligated.

Figure 11.21 Synthesis-dependent strand annealing (SDSA).

Figure 11.21 shows a double-stranded break. Notice that one chromatid has two broken DNA strands but that the sister chromatid is undamaged. SDSA begins with trimming of one of the broken strands. This is followed by attachment of the protein Rad51. Rad51 binds to the strands and facilitates the invasion of the intact chromatid by the resected end of a strand from the sister chromatid. This **strand invasion** process displaces one strand of the intact duplex and creates a **displacement (D) loop**. DNA replication within the D loop synthesizes new DNA strands from intact template strands. The sister chromatids are reformed by dissociation and annealing of the nascent strands to repair the breaks. By accomplishing the removal of DNA in the immediate vicinity of a double-stranded break and the replacement of the excised DNA with a duplex identical to that in the sister chromatid, SDSA carries out error-free repair of double-stranded breaks. This mechanism for repairing double-strand breaks is closely related to the molecular mechanism that generates homologous recombination during meiosis.

11.6 DNA Double-Strand Breaks Initiate Homologous Recombination

Homologous recombination is the exchange of genetic material between homologous molecules of DNA. All organisms undertake homologous recombination. In bacteria, homologous recombination occurs during events such as conjugation and as a consequence of the repair of double-strand breaks. Archaea undertake homologous recombination under circumstances similar to those in bacteria. In eukaryotes, recombination between homologous chromosomes is essential in prophase I of meiosis, where it is initiated by controlled double-strand DNA breaks in a process that is reminiscent of synthesis-dependent strand annealing.

The Holliday Model

The first viable molecular model of meiotic recombination was proposed by Robin Holliday in 1964 and was based on the study of homologous recombination in *E. coli*. Known as the **Holliday model**, it offered a plausible scheme for meiotic recombination by hypothesizing that spontaneously generated single-stranded breaks in one chromatid led to invasion of a homologous molecule. Holliday's scheme for breaking and rejoining DNA strands suggested that some encounters between homologous chromosomes would produce crossovers whereas others would not.

The original Holliday model ultimately proved to be too simplistic and has been superseded by more accurate models of meiotic recombination. The more recent models rely on some of the features of the Holliday model but incorporate new knowledge and steps. Perhaps the most important features distinguishing the current model of meiotic recombination from the original Holliday model are, first, that meiotic recombination is now known to be initiated by *double-stranded DNA breaks* and, second, that the double-stranded breaks initiating meiotic recombination are generated in a programmed manner by the activity of a specialized enzyme.

The Bacterial RecBCD Pathway

Homologous recombination in all organisms shares many features in terms of the mechanical processes involved as well as the homologies of proteins that are active in recombination. The first, and still the most detailed, molecular description of homologous recombination comes from research on *E. coli*. This homologous recombination model describes the action of several proteins that are critical to initiating and completing homologous recombination.

Known as the **RecBCD pathway**, the system of homologous recombination in bacteria relies on the occurrence of DNA double-strand breaks to initiate the process. Double-strand DNA breaks attract the protein RecA (described above as part of the SOS system in *E. coli*). Bacterial RecA

is a homolog of the eukaryotic and archaeal protein Rad51, which performs a similar function in those organisms (recall its role in synthesis-dependent strand annealing, above). The multiprotein complex known as RecBCD then attaches to the region of a bacterial chromosome to which RecA is bound, and this complex promotes single-strand invasion and the formation of D loops. The process is highly similar in appearance to the strand invasion and D-loop formation we saw in SDSA. RecBCD activity is followed by binding of RuvAB and RuvC proteins. The Ruv complex completes homologous recombination between the bacterial DNA molecules.

The Double-Stranded Break Model of Homologous Recombination

The bacterial RecBCD pathway of homologous recombination was the starting point for the study of meiotic recombination in eukaryotes, where numerous protein homologies have since been identified. The outline of the current model of meiotic recombination was proposed in 1983 by Jack Szostak, Terry Orr-Weaver, Rodney Rothstein, and Franklin Stahl. Their model was the first to predict that the creation of double-stranded breaks controlled by the activity of a specific protein was the foundation of meiotic recombination. The accumulated experimental evidence has confirmed this view, and the research has added major new details to the original proposal by Szostak and his colleagues.

Among these new findings is the determination that the double-strand breaks that precede meiotic recombination are under precise protein control. This is in contrast to a more generalized and diverse process of generating double-strand breaks in bacterial DNA. A second finding is the strong homology that exists between the genes and proteins involved in bacterial homologous recombination and homologous recombination in archaea and eukaryotes.

As currently understood, eukaryotic homologous recombination is initiated by the protein Spo11 ("Spoh eleven") that was first discovered in yeast (**Foundation Figure 11.22** ❶). The proteins Mrx and Exo1 (homologs of RecBCD helicase and nuclease) associate with Spo11 and help trim the cut strands ❷. Two RecA homolog proteins, Rad51 and Dmc1, join at the trimmed region ❸. Rad51 and Dmc1 are RecA homologs. This protein complex helps form a strand-exchange assemblage, facilitating strand invasion and formation of a D loop ❹, ❺. (Note the similarity of this structure to the D loop formed during SDSA.)

The invading strand pairs with the complementary strand in the D loop. Outside the D loop, the two strands that appear to cross over one another form a **Holliday junction**, an interim structure proposed in the original Holliday model. Notice that there is also a **heteroduplex region**, containing two complementary strands of DNA that originated in different homologs. Also identified as **heteroduplex DNA**, these regions are a molecular signature of homologous recombination. Because the two strands

Molecular model of homologous recombination in meiosis.

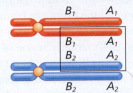

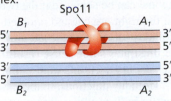 Meiotic recombination diagrammed between these nonsister chromatids of homologous chromosomes

1 Spo11 creates double-strand break in one DNA duplex.

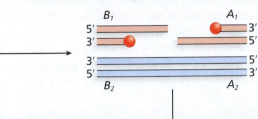

2 Enzymatic digestion 5′ → 3′ by Mrx and Exo creates single-stranded segments.

4 The strand-exchange filaments promote strand invasion.

3 Dmc1 and Rad51c assemble strand-exchange nucleoprotein filaments.

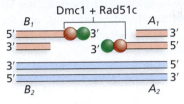

5 Strand invasion creates one D loop and the first heteroduplex region. Rad52, Rad59, and other proteins participate.

6 Strand extension by DNA polymerase displaces D loop DNA and pairs with complementary single-stranded DNA to form the second heteroduplex region.

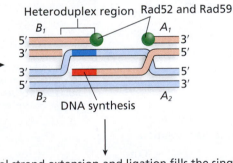

8 Double Holliday junctions form after the nick is sealed; chromatids contain offset heteroduplexes.

7 DNA pol strand extension and ligation fills the single-stranded gap in the strand paired with D loop DNA.

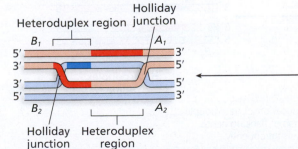

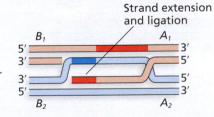

of the heteroduplex DNA originate in different homologs, there may be mismatched base pairs between them. In other words, if heterozygosity is present in the DNA sequences forming a heteroduplex region, one or more base pairs will be mismatched in the heteroduplex DNA.

Extension of the invading strand and DNA synthesis within the broken strand are guided by intact template strands ⑥ and are assisted by additional proteins, including Rad52 and Rad59, that are RecBCD homologs ⑦. At this point, a second heteroduplex region has formed. The 3′ end of the invading strand next connects with the 5′ end of a strand segment that was initially part of the invading strand ⑧, to form a second Holliday junction. Now the nonsister chromatids of the recombining chromosomes are interconnected to one another by the presence of **double Holliday junctions** (**DHJs**): The recombining chromosomes contain DHJs and two heteroduplex regions.

The DHJs appearing in step ⑧ of Foundation Figure 11.22 are present during prophase I of meiosis. For meiosis to proceed, the homologous chromosomes must be disentangled. This involves cutting and rejoining the DNA strands in at least one of the Holliday junctions, and the pattern of cutting and rejoining is what leads to genetic recombination between the homologs.

The resolution of Holliday junctions generates genetic recombination. **Figure 11.23a** shows the double Holliday junction structure present at the end of the events in Foundation Figure 11.22. Through **opposite sense resolution**—that is, the cutting and rejoining of the DNA strands in one of the Holliday junctions (the one on the left is illustrated here) and cutting and rejoining of the two strands outside the second Holliday junction—genetic recombination is achieved, leaving heteroduplex DNA in both recombinant chromosomes. One recombinant chromosome is B_1A_2 and the other is B_2A_1. The same outcome can be achieved if the two Holliday junction strands at the right are cut and rejoined and the strands outside the Holliday junction on the left are cut and rejoined. **Figure 11.23b** illustrates **same sense resolution**, the resolution that comes about by cutting and rejoining of the DNA strands in *both* Holliday junctions. In this case, heteroduplex DNA is present in both resulting chromosomes, but genetic recombination *does not* take place. Opposite sense resolution is more common than same sense resolution; thus, homologous recombination in meiosis is likely to lead to the production of recombinant chromosomes. There is evidence that some homologous recombination events do not produce recombinant chromosomes, however; and same sense resolution explains this outcome.

(a) Opposite sense resolution

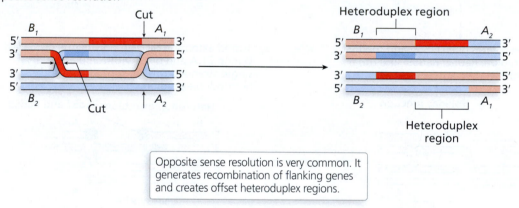

Opposite sense resolution is very common. It generates recombination of flanking genes and creates offset heteroduplex regions.

(b) Same sense resolution

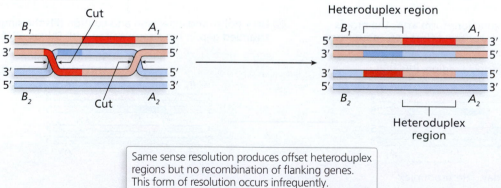

Same sense resolution produces offset heteroduplex regions but no recombination of flanking genes. This form of resolution occurs infrequently.

Figure 11.23 Resolution of the double Holliday junctions of homologous chromosomes. (a) Opposite sense resolution generates genetic recombinants. (b) Same sense resolution does not produce genetic recombination.

11.7 Transposable Genetic Elements Move throughout the Genome

Transposable genetic elements are DNA sequences of various lengths and sequence composition that have evolved the ability to move within the genome by an enzyme-driven process known as **transposition**. Transposition has two principal effects on genomes. First, transposition can be a mutational event—one that has a biological basis as opposed to a chemical or physical (irradiation) cause. Second, transposition can increase genome size through duplication of the transposable genetic elements.

The movement of transposable genetic elements throughout the genome occurs in two ways. One is through the excision of a transposable element from its initial location and its insertion in a new location. This process is potentially mutagenic, but it does not contribute to a meaningful increase in genome size. The second mechanism of transposition is a duplication mechanism that generates a copy of the transposable element for insertion in a new location. As a result, the genome is left with both the original copy of the element and the new copy as well. This process can be mutagenic and can also lead to an increase in genome size, particularly when large numbers of copies of the transposable element are present.

The Characteristics and Classification of Transposable Elements

Transposable elements have been found in all organisms. They exist in a wide array of types that vary from the simplest, encoding only the information required for transposition of the element, to much more complex structures that encode numerous functions beyond transposition. Antibiotic resistance is an example of the additional functions that can be included.

Despite these differences, transposable elements have two distinctive sequence features that make them recognizable in genomes and leave a "molecular signature" of their presence: (1) The transposable element itself contains **terminal inverted repeats** on both its ends, and (2) the inserted transposable element is bracketed by **flanking direct repeats**. **Figure 11.24** illustrates a transposable

genetic element from *E. coli* that has 5-bp flanking direct repeats on either side of the element and two 6-bp terminal inverted repeats surrounding the central region that contains the DNA sequence of the transposable element.

Terminal inverted repeats are part of the sequence of a transposable element, but flanking direct sequences are not. The transposition process generates these flanking sequences, as shown in **Figure 11.25**. Staggered cuts of both strands of a DNA sequence targeted for insertion leave short single-stranded ends where the cut occurred. The DNA target sequence can potentially be any sequence in the genome. The enzyme **transposase**, produced by the transposable element, is the enzyme that generates the staggered cuts of the target sequence. Figure 11.25 shows that transposition of the genetic element into the target sequence leaves short single-stranded gaps. These are filled by DNA synthesis, completing the insertion of the transposable genetic element. The insertion event illustrated here generates the same 5-bp flanking direct repeats as are next to the transposable element shown in Figure 11.24 (which also has the same 6-bp terminal inverted repeats).

Transposable elements fall into two categories. **DNA transposons** (also called Class II transposable elements) transpose as DNA sequences. Their transposition produces flanking direct repeats at the site of insertion. At a minimum, all DNA transposons carry the transposase gene that produces the transposase enzyme required for the movement of the transposon, but many DNA transposons also carry other genes.

The second category of transposable elements are **retrotransposons** (also called Class I transposable elements), which transpose through an RNA intermediate. Retrotransposons are composed of DNA, but they are transcribed into RNA before transposition, and the RNA transcript is then copied back into DNA by the specialized enzyme reverse transcriptase. The reverse-transcribed DNA is then inserted into a new location, where flanking direct repeats are formed. Some, but not all, retrotransposons carry the reverse transcriptase gene, an enzyme that copies single-stranded RNA into DNA. Retrotransposons carrying the reverse transcriptase gene can initiate their own transposition, whereas those lacking the gene must utilize reverse transcriptase synthesized by another retrotransposon.

DNA transposons follow one of two modes of insertion. **Replicative transposition** can be thought of as a "copy-and-paste" process, whereby the original copy of the transposable element remains in place and a new copy is transposed to another location. Alternatively, some DNA transposons undergo **nonreplicative transposition**; this can be thought of as a "cut-and-paste" mechanism. In this process, the original copy of the transposon is excised, and it is then reinserted into a new location. As indicated above, both modes of transposition can cause mutations, but whereas replicative transposition increases the transposable element copy number and potentially increases genome size, nonreplicative transposition does not. Retrotransposons are also a frequent source of increases in genome size in eukaryotic genomes.

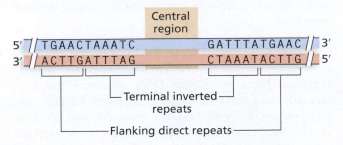

Figure 11.24 The general structure of DNA transposons.

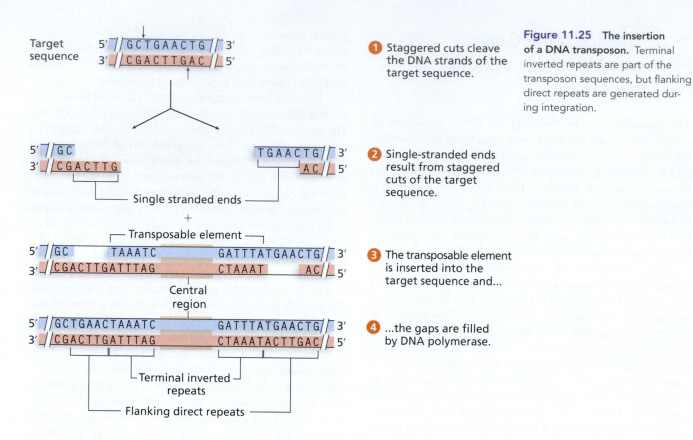

Figure 11.25 **The insertion of a DNA transposon.** Terminal inverted repeats are part of the transposon sequences, but flanking direct repeats are generated during integration.

1. Staggered cuts cleave the DNA strands of the target sequence.

2. Single-stranded ends result from staggered cuts of the target sequence.

3. The transposable element is inserted into the target sequence and...

4. ...the gaps are filled by DNA polymerase.

The Mutagenic Effect of Transposition

Transposable elements create mutations by their insertion into wild-type alleles. The insertion of new DNA into a functional gene is the equivalent of inserting a random string of letters into a sentence. Just like the sentence is rendered unintelligible and therefore nonfunctional by a random insertion, so is the wild-type allele rendered unable to produce a wild-type gene product and thus nonfunctional by the random insertion of a transposon. This mutational process is known as **insertional inactivation**.

Numerous examples of insertional inactivation mutations by transposition are known in bacteria, plants, and animals, including humans. A number of human hereditary conditions are caused by transposition. The blood clotting disorder hemophilia A (OMIM 300841) is caused by absence of activity of the blood clotting protein factor VIII ("factor eight"). The *F8* gene is X-linked, and one of the many mutations of the gene is the result of the insertion of a transposable element. A second example is Coffin–Lowry syndrome (OMIM 303600). This X-linked condition produces skeletal malformations, growth retardation, hearing deficits, and mental impairment. Among numerous mutations of the *RPS6KA3* gene that controls Coffin–Lowry syndrome is one involving the insertion of a transposable element that inactivates the gene. But the original example of mutation by insertional inactivation was the round versus wrinkled pea phenotype examined

by Mendel. Research led by Cathie Martin in the early 1990s identified the gene Mendel examined and described its mutation by the insertion of a transposable element. The Case Study at the end of this chapter describes how transposition alters the DNA, mRNA, and protein from the mutant allele.

Transposable Elements in Bacterial Genomes

Bacterial genomes, as well as plasmids and viruses, contain three types of transposable elements: (1) simple transposons known as **insertion sequences (ISs)**, containing sequences encoding terminal inverted repeats surrounding a gene (sometimes two genes) encoding transposase, (2) *composite transposons*, designated Tn in bacteria, that contain a transposase gene, two flanking IS elements, and one or more additional genes and, (3) *noncomposite transposons*, similar to composite transposons but lacking insertion sequences.

Insertion Sequences Numerous IS elements are found in bacterial, archaeal, and viral genomes and also in plasmids. These are simple DNA sequences that contain only the genetic information necessary for their own transposition. Ranging between about 800 and 2000 bp, IS elements insert by either replicative or nonreplicative transposition. All IS elements have terminal inverted repeats surrounding the transposase gene, and a few have one additional gene. The smallest of the IS elements, designated *IS1*, is typical of many IS elements. Totaling 768 bp in length, *IS1* contains the transposase gene surrounded by two 23-bp terminal inverted repeats and two 9-bp flanking direct repeats.

Composite Transposons Bacterial **composite transposons** (Tn) are considerably larger than IS elements, and they can contain multiple genes in addition to their transposase gene. The additional genes in Tn elements are variable and are contained in a central region that is flanked by the two IS elements. The genes in the central region confer characteristics such as antibiotic resistance and resistance to the toxic consequences of heavy metal exposure. These transposable elements can thus carry genes that may confer a growth advantage in certain environments.

Tn10 has a structure typical of most composite transposons (**Figure 11.26**). It contains two copies of the *IS10* element, each with its terminal inverted repeats. These are designated *IS10R* on the right (R) side and *IS10L* on the left (L) side, and they flank the central region. Each of the IS elements is about 1300 bp in length, and the *Tn10* central region is about 6600 bp in length. It contains a *Tet^R* gene for resistance to the antibiotic tetracycline. The total length of *Tn10* is about 9300 bp. The *Tn10* transposon readily inserts into plasmid DNA, allowing rapid dissemination of tetracycline resistance among bacterial strains that carry the plasmid.

Noncomposite Transposons Bacteria can also carry a third type of DNA transposon, known as a **noncomposite transposon**. These transposons do not contain insertion sequences but do carry additional genes. They transpose in the same manner as composite transposons. The noncomposite transposon *Tn3*, for example, carries two 38-bp inverted repeats flanking a 4957-bp central region that encodes three enzymes: transposase and resolvase, both of which are required for transposition, and β-lactamase, which provides resistance to the antibiotic ampicillin.

Genetic Analysis 11.3 guides you through an assessment of potential terminal inverted repeat sequences of IS elements.

Transposable Elements in Eukaryotic Genomes

Transposable genetic elements are plentiful and highly varied in eukaryotic genomes. These elements fall into two groups. The first are similar to bacterial transposable elements. These are generally short sequences that carry inverted repeats. Examples of these bacterial-like transposable elements, described in this section, include *Ac* and *Ds* elements in maize and *P* elements in *Drosophila*. The second category of eukaryotic transposable elements are the retrotransposons, which transpose through an RNA intermediate. Examples of these elements, also discussed in this section, are human *Alu* sequences and *Ty* and *copia* elements of yeast and *Drosophila*, respectively.

Eukaryotic genome sequence analysis finds that substantial proportions of many genomes are composed of transposable DNA. For example, nearly half of the human genome—well more than 1 billion base pairs—is composed of transposable DNA. Much of this DNA is repetitive in sequence, indicating that up to tens to hundreds of thousands of copies of various transposable elements are present. Many eukaryotic genomes exhibit a similar profile, evidence that transposition has been a major factor in eukaryotic genome evolution. It is equally evident that transposition continues to play an active role in the evolution of genomes and in mutation.

The Discovery of *Ds* and *Ac* Elements in Maize

Transposable genetic elements were discovered in eukaryotes. Barbara McClintock discovered transposition in a series of studies of a mutant phenotype of kernel color in maize (*Zea mays*) that she conducted in the 1930s. When McClintock proposed her model of transposition it was not well received. The overwhelming prevailing notion at the time was that except for the rare occurrence of gene mutations, genomes were stable, and the idea that pieces of the genome could jump from place to place seemed untenable. Resistance to McClintock's ideas barely wavered for more than two decades before it began to crumble in the face of the discovery of transposable genetic elements in bacteria.

McClintock had been studying the *C* gene for maize. The dominant wild-type allele *C* produces purple kernels, and a mutant c_1 allele produces yellow kernels. One gene that is closely linked to *C* produces plump (*Sh*) or shrunken (*sh*) kernels, and a second closely linked gene produces shiny (*Wx*) or waxy (*wx*) kernels (**Figure 11.27a**). In experiments with several trihybrid strains of maize with the genotype *C Sh Wx/c_1 sh wx*, McClintock found a

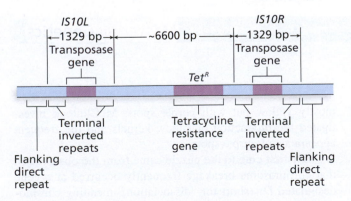

Figure 11.26 Structure of a composite transposon, *Tn10*.

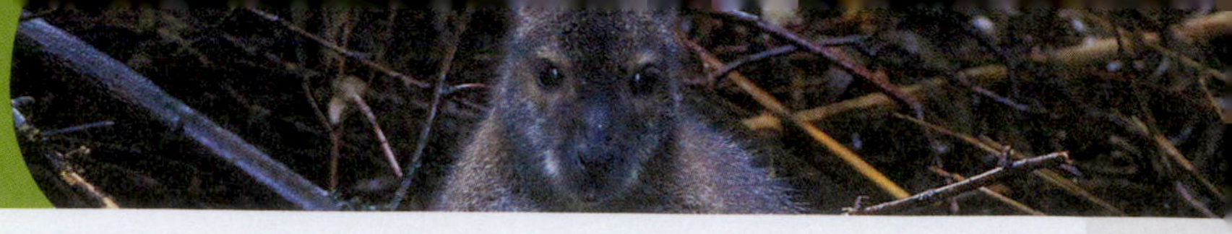

PROBLEM Each pair of DNA sequences shown below occur on the same strand of DNA and are separated by a large number of nucleotides. Which of these sequences might be found flanking an insertion sequence? Explain your answer, and identify the relevant parts of your selected sequences.

a. 5'-TTAGCAC...CAGGATT-3'

b. 5'-GGCCAAT...ATTGGCC-3'

c. 5'-CCGACCGTA...CCGACCGTA-3'

d. 5'-AGTATACCGC...GCGGTATGGC-3'

> **BREAK IT DOWN:** Terminal inverted repeat sequences are characteristically found at the ends of insertion sequences (p. 425).

Solution Strategies	Solution Steps
Evaluate	
1. Identify the topic this problem addresses and the nature of the required answer.	1. This problem requires you to recognize DNA sequences that might flank a bacterial insertion sequence. You must identify one or more of the given choices as candidate flanking sequences, explain your answer, and identify the relevant portions of the sequences.
2. Identify the critical information given in the problem.	2. We are given four single-stranded segments of DNA, each identifying the sequences sitting on opposite sides of potential insertion sequences.
Deduce	

3. Determine the double-stranded sequences for each of the single-stranded sequences listed.	3. The double-stranded sequences are
	
	a. 5'-TTAGCAC...CAGGATT-3'
	   3'-AATCGTG...GTCCTAA-5'
	
	b. 5'-GGCCAAT...ATTGGCC-3'
	   3'-CCGGTTA...TAACCGG-5'
	
	c. 5'-CCGACCGTA...CCGACCGTA-3'
	   3'-GGCTGGCAT...GGCTGGCAT-5'
	
	d. 5'-AGTATACCGC...GCGGTATGGC-3'
	   3'-TCATATGGCG...CGCCATACCG-5'

4. Review what you know about the sequences flanking insertion elements.	4. The sequences flanking insertion elements are inverted repeat sequences.
Solve	
5. Identify any sequence that might be found flanking an insertion sequence.	5. Sequences b and d in step 3 are the ones most likely to be found flanking insertion sequences. The inverted repeat sequences in double-stranded DNA are highlighted. 5'-**GGCCAAT**...**ATTGGCC**-3' 3'-**CCGGTTA**...**TAACCGG**-5' 5'-**AGTATAC**CGC...GCG**GTATGGC**-3' 3'-**TCATATG**GCG...CGC**CATACCG**-5'

For more practice, see Problems 12 and 19.
Visit the Study Area to access study tools. **Mastering** Genetics

---

few unusual kernels that were mostly purple but had yellow (colorless) sectors that varied among different kernels. Invariably, however, the purple regions were plump and shiny, but the yellow sectors were shrunken and waxy. At the same time, the kernel color mutation appeared to be unstable. Specifically, the appearance of the mutant yellow kernel phenotype often changed to an appearance that was mostly yellow but with purple spots. McClintock investigated the production of yellow kernels and the frequent appearance of purple spots.

Her first clue to the puzzle came from the observation that chromosome breakage frequently occurred at a gene designated *Ds* (short for "dissociation," meaning chromosome breakage), but only when another gene called *Ac* (for

(a) Trihybrid, wild-type phenotype

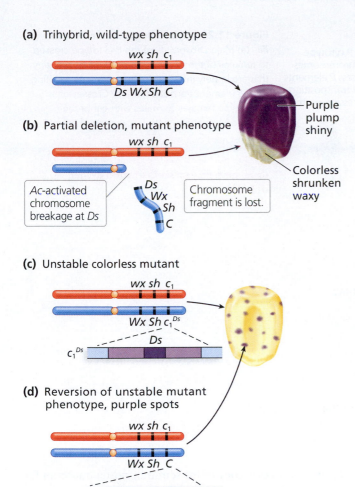

(b) Partial deletion, mutant phenotype

Ac-activated chromosome breakage at *Ds*

Chromosome fragment is lost.

Purple plump shiny

Colorless shrunken waxy

(c) Unstable colorless mutant

(d) Reversion of unstable mutant phenotype, purple spots

Ac-activated excision of *Ds*

Figure 11.27 **Production of colorless sectors and reversion of the unstable colorless mutation in maize by the transposable genetic elements Ds and Ac.**

"activator," meaning it activated chromosome breakage) was present. *Ac* elements contain a transposase gene that is used to activate transposition. The *Ds* elements appeared to move around the maize genome, and they appeared to be the cause of the unstable kernel color mutation. She called *Ds* a "control element," meaning that it controlled the expression of other genes. *Ds* elements do not contain a transposase gene and require an *Ac* element to activate their transposition.

McClintock's examination of maize chromosomes and kernel color revealed that when the trihybrid ($C\ Sh\ Wx/c_1\ sh\ wx$) had both chromosomes intact and complete, kernels were purple. Chromosome breakage and loss of the $C\ Sh\ Wx$ chromosome segment produced a yellow sector that was also shrunken and waxy (**Figure 11.27b**). The *Ac*-activated transposition of *Ds* into the *C* gene inactivated the expression of *C*, and kernels were yellow (**Figure 11.27c**). Lastly, she discovered that purple spotting of otherwise yellow kernels came about

when a *Ds* element inserted into a *C* gene was excised by *Ac* action. This process took place cell by cell, resulting in purple spotting in those segments of a kernel that were derived from a cell in which *Ds* was excised (**Figure 11.27d**). Kernel segments in which *Ds* remained in *C* were yellow.

Drosophila P Elements

The genome of *Drosophila melanogaster* carries several different types of transposable elements, but the most prominent of these is a DNA transposon called a **P element**. These DNA transposons were not part of the genome of *D. melanogaster* collected from the wild before about 1960. Today, however, all *D. melanogaster* collected in the wild carry *P* elements in their genome, suggesting that *P* elements were introduced into *D. melanogaster* about 1960, perhaps by cross-species transfer from a distantly related species. Since their introduction to the genome, *P* elements have quickly proliferated. The *Drosophila* life cycle can produce 20 to 25 generations per year; thus, *P* elements have been evolving for about 1000 generations or so in *D. melanogaster* since first being introduced into the genome.

The *P* elements exist in multiple forms. Full-length *P* elements encode transposase and are capable of autonomous transposition. These *P* elements are approximately 2900 bp in length, and they have a central region containing a gene for transposase that is encoded in four exons and three introns flanked by 31-bp inverted repeats. Transcription and translation of the transposase gene in full-length *P* elements produces an 87-kD transposase enzyme that activates *P* element transposition in germline cells. Several types of nonfunctional *P* elements are also found in the *D. melanogaster* genome, none producing functional transposase and all being shorter than 2900 bp.

The *P* elements were discovered in *D. melanogaster* by Margaret Kidwell in 1985, when she identified **hybrid dysgenesis**, a phenomenon in which sterility occurs in the F_1 progeny of a cross between laboratory-bred female flies and males derived from natural populations (**Figure 11.28**). In these crosses, the female laboratory fly has the so-called M cytotype (*M* is for "maternal"), and the wild-type male fly has the P ("paternal") cytotype. The P-cytotype male has three to four dozen *P* elements scattered throughout its genome. In contrast, the M-cytotype female has no *P* elements. The progeny of this cross between laboratory (female, M cytotype) and wild flies (male, P cytotype) are hybrids that have a normal external appearance, but they are dysgenic—in other words they are biologically deficient. The term *hybrid dysgenesis* refers to the combination of sterility, a high mutation rate, and a propensity for chromosomal aberrations and nondisjunction present in these flies. Importantly, the mutations found in dysgenic flies are unstable, reverting to wild-type or mutating again at a high rate. Curiously, the reciprocal

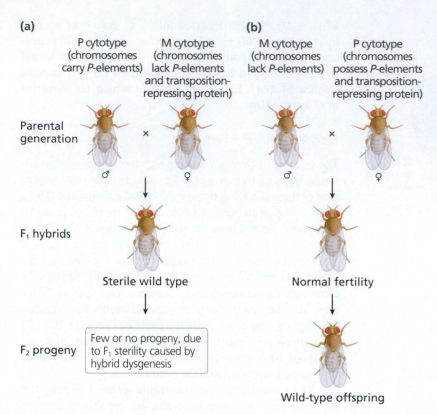

(a)

P cytotype (chromosomes carry *P*-elements) × M cytotype (chromosomes lack *P*-elements and transposition-repressing protein)

(b)

M cytotype (chromosomes lack *P*-elements) × P cytotype (chromosomes possess *P*-elements and transposition-repressing protein)

Parental generation

♂   ♀   ♂   ♀

F₁ hybrids

Sterile wild type   Normal fertility

F₂ progeny

Few or no progeny, due to F₁ sterility caused by hybrid dysgenesis

Wild-type offspring

Figure 11.28 Hybrid dysgenesis in *Drosophila*. (a) Male *Drosophila* of the P cytotype crossed to females of the M cytotype produce F₁ progeny that are largely infertile due to mutations resulting from *P* element transposition. **(b)** Crosses of P-cytotype females to males with either the P or the M cytotype yield F₁ progeny of normal fertility.

Q Do sperm carry cytoplasmic material? How does this help explain the hybrid dysgenesis illustrated in part (a)?

cross—a P-cytotype female (this genome contains *P* elements) crossed to an M-cytotype male (this genome is *P* element-free) results in normal flies that show no evidence of hybrid dysgenesis.

The key to the action of *P* elements appears to be that the transposase genes are silenced by a suppressor protein in P-cytotype strains. This inhibits their transposition and potential for causing mutations. In matings of P-cytotype males and M-cytotype females, sperm from P-cytotype males contains virtually no cytoplasmic material. The chromosomes carry *P*-elements, but as there is no cytoplasmic material, sperm do not possess the transposition repressor protein. The eggs of M-cytotype females contain abundant cytoplasmic material but carry no transposition repressor protein because the chromosomes in the M cytotype are free of *P* elements. At fertilization, sperm add *P* element–laden chromosomes into an egg lacking transposition-repressing protein. Extensive transposition takes place, creating multiple mutations by insertion of *P* elements into functional genes or by inducing chromosome breaks that result in hybrid dysgenesis.

Retrotransposons

Retrotransposons are the most common transposable elements in eukaryotic genomes. They are related to RNA-containing retroviruses that reverse transcribe their genetic information into DNA to parasitize host cells, but retrotransposons do not infect cells, instead they transpose throughout the genome. Retrotransposons use reverse transcriptase to

synthesize a DNA copy of the retrotransposon transcript for insertion into new genome locations.

Fully functional retroviruses that infect cells encode at least three genes, called *gag*, *env*, and *pol*. *Gag* and *env* encode proteins that form the retroviral particle. New retroviral particles are produced within infected cells and perpetuate the infection by invading new cells. The *pol* gene encodes the enzyme *reverse transcriptase* that directs the synthesis of double-stranded DNA from single-stranded RNA.

Figure 11.29 illustrates the structures of three eukaryotic retrotransposons that transpose within eukaryotic genomes. Two constant features of retrotransposons are seen. First, all retrotransposons encode reverse transcriptase (*pol*) to catalyze transposition, and some contain *gag*, but none contains *env*. Second, the gene or genes carried by retrotransposons are flanked by **long terminal repeats (LTRs)** that may be up to several hundred base pairs in length.

LINE, SINE, and *Alu* Elements of Humans As mentioned above, more than 45% of the human genome is composed of transposable DNA. Among the functional transposable genetic elements in the human genome, LINE (long interspersed nuclear elements) and SINE (short interspersed nuclear elements) families of elements stand out because of their relative abundance and their ability to cause spontaneous human gene mutations. LINEs are up to several thousand base pairs in length and have an average length of about 900 bp. SINEs are much shorter and have their sequences truncated at one end of the element, most likely because the reverse

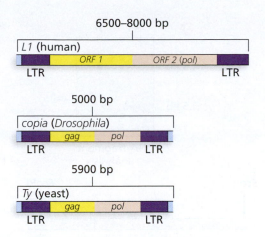

Figure 11.29 Eukaryotic retroviral structures.

transcription process used for their transfer terminates before the entire sequence has transposed.

Almost 1 million copies of LINE sequences are found in the human genome. Collectively, these sequences constitute a little more than 20% of the total genome sequence. Human *L1* elements are the most common members of the LINE family of elements in the human genome, which contains approximately 600,000 copies of *L1* alone, constituting more than 17% of the total genome. The *L1* elements vary in length from about 6500 to 8000 bp. Full-length *L1* elements encode a protein with nuclease and reverse transcriptase function and may also encode a second RNA-binding protein, but shortening of the element affects its ability to transpose. Full-length *L1* elements actively transpose in the human genome and produce mutations. The transposable element referred to earlier in the chapter as the cause of the X-linked blood-clotting disorder hemophilia A is an *L1* element.

SINE elements, too, are common, composing a little more than 10% of human genome sequence. The most common human SINE element is called an *Alu* element. *Alu* elements vary in length from 100 to 300 bp and are each flanked

by direct repeats of 7 to 20 bp. They are so named because each element can be cleaved into two segments by the restriction endonuclease *Alu*I ("Al-LOO-one") that recognizes the 4-bp restriction enzyme target sequence 5′-AGCT-3′.

The human genome contains more than 1 million *Alu* elements, and they actively generate mutations. The mutational mechanisms identified are alterations of gene expression by *Alu* insertion into regulatory DNA sequences such as promoters, *Alu* insertions into exons that alter the reading frame (frameshift mutations), disruption of normal mRNA splicing following *Alu* insertion into introns, and unequal crossover events between homologous chromosomes involving *Alu* elements. Overall, *Alu* elements are estimated to transpose in about 1 in 200 people and to be directly responsible for about 0.3% of all human hereditary disease, much of it due to new mutations.

***Ty* Elements of Yeast** Many different forms of *Ty* retrotransposons of yeast are found, all sharing the common features of retrotransposons. In *Ty* elements, the central element is approximately 6 kb, flanked by LTRs that are each about 330 bp in length. Both LTRs contain promoters that direct the transcription of different genes in the central region. Approximately 50 to 100 copies of *Ty* elements are present in the typical *Saccharomyces cerevisiae* genome. The *Ty* elements cause mutation in yeast genes by insertion.

Copia* Elements of *Drosophila Multiple forms of the retrotransposon *copia* are found in the *Drosophila* genome. *Copia* elements have a central element of 5 to 8.5 kb that contains *pol* and *gag* genes and is flanked by LTRs of 250 to 600 bp each. The word *copia* comes from the Latin for "abundance," and befitting this designation, more than 5% of the *Drosophila* genome is composed of *copia* retrotransposons. This abundance leads to many mutations throughout the genome that are usually the result of insertion of *copia* into a wild-type gene.

CASE STUDY

Mendel's Peas Are Shaped by Transposition

Gregor Mendel left good descriptions, data, and analyses of the crosses he used for establishing the law of segregation and the law of independent assortment, but he did not leave any seeds to give geneticists direct access to the genes themselves. Experimental Insight 11.1 identifies three of the genes studied by Mendel that have now been identified and analyzed. Details of the discovery in 1990 of a fourth gene are described here. It is the gene responsible for the round and wrinkled seed shapes described by Mendel, now known as *SBE1*, the starch-branching enzyme 1 gene.

The gene was identified and shown to be responsible for the seed shape variation Mendel reported by a laboratory group led by Cathie Martin (Bhattacharyya et al., 1990). In their paper, the group reports DNA, mRNA, and protein evidence

that the recessive mutant allele, *r*, is altered by the insertion of approximately 800 bp of DNA. The insertion is of transposable DNA, and its effect is insertional inactivation of the ability to produce a starch-branching enzyme that is the normal gene product. The researchers also provide a physiological explanation for the appearance of wrinkled seed shape.

PROTEIN ANALYSIS Prior to the start of this study, considerable evidence already suggested that seed shape variation was due to differences in starch synthesis. Among candidate enzymes known to be important in starch synthesis was SBE1. The researchers used *RR* (pure-breeding round) plants as a source of SBE1 to raise an antibody for use as a probe for the enzyme. They then used protein gel electrophoresis and protein analysis to test for reactivity between the anti-SBE1 antibody and proteins extracted from *RR* and *rr* (pure-breeding wrinkled) plants. The antibody detected the enzyme in *RR* plant protein gels but not in *rr* plant protein gels ❶. This indicates that *RR* plants produce SBE1 but that *rr* plants do not.

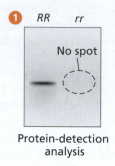

Protein-detection
analysis

MESSENGER RNA ANALYSIS The researchers next tested mRNA from the *SBE1* gene for evidence of the basis of the mutation. Testing mRNA from *RR* and *rr*, the researchers detected a 3300-nucleotide mRNA derived from *RR* plants and a 4100-nucleotide mRNA from *rr* plants. They found as well that the larger transcript from *rr* plants was about tenfold less abundant than the smaller transcript from *RR* plants ❷. These results indicate that the transcript of *SBE1* in *rr* plants is longer than in *RR* plants and that it is produced at just a fraction of the percentage present in *RR* plants.

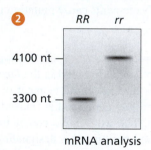

mRNA analysis

DNA ANALYSIS DNA encoding the *SBE1* gene was isolated from *RR* and *rr* plants and was fragmented for analysis by DNA gel electrophoresis. This analysis revealed a DNA fragment approximately 3.5 kb in length from *RR* plants and a corresponding DNA fragment of about 4.3 kb from *rr* plants ❸. One possible explanation for this result is the insertion of approximately 800 bp of DNA into the *r* allele. Subsequent analysis revealed that an 800-bp insertion of transposable DNA into the *R* allele was the mutational event that generated the *r* allele ❹. This event caused insertional inactivation of the *r* allele of *SBE1*.

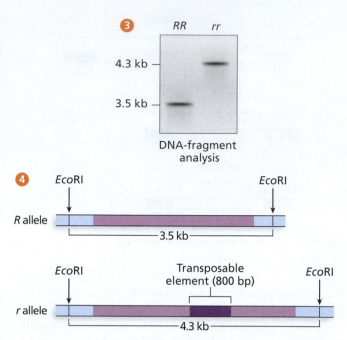

DNA-fragment
analysis

WRINKLED SEED DEVELOPMENT The physiological explanation of wrinkled seed development is tied to the loss of function of SBE1. In mature round peas, almost half of the dry weight is starch. About 35% of the starch is in a simple linear form known as amylose. The remainder is in complexly branched forms, most commonly a form known as amylopectin. Free molecules of sucrose make up about 5% of the dry weight. Amylose is actively converted to amylopectin by SBE1 in round seeds. In wrinkled seeds, only about 30% of starch is amylopectin, and about 70% is amylose. Amylose readily loses molecules of free glucose, and the sugar accounts for more than 10% of the dry weight of wrinkled seeds.

During early seed development, SBE1 is active in immature seeds that will become round, but it is inactive due to mutation in immature seeds that will become wrinkled. In seeds that will be wrinkled, the high percentage of free sucrose causes cells to import large amounts of water to dilute the excess sugar. The extra water results in larger cells and larger immature seeds that stretch the seed membrane. As all pea seeds mature, they dehydrate to the same level, and this is when wrinkling appears in *rr* seeds. The overstretched membranes of those seeds collapse, much like an overinflated balloon that has lost air, causing the seeds to look wrinkled. Membranes of *RR* and *Rr* seeds have not been stretched by extra water importation. They are resilient, and the seeds appear round.

SUMMARY **Mastering Genetics** For activities, animations, and review quizzes, go to the Study Area.

11.1 Mutations Are Rare and Random and Alter DNA Sequence

▪ Mutations occur at random in genomes.

▪ Mutation frequencies are low in all organisms.

▪ Mutational hotspots are genes or regions where mutations occur much more often than average.

▪ Base-pair substitution mutations can be either transitions or transversions.

▪ Base-pair substitutions can change one amino acid of a polypeptide, can create a new stop codon, or can leave the polypeptide unchanged.

- Frameshift mutations result from the insertion or deletion of one or more base pairs that shift the mRNA reading frame during translation.
- Regulatory mutations alter gene transcription or pre-mRNA splicing.
- Forward mutation alters a wild-type allele to mutant form, and reversion changes a mutant back to wild-type or near wild-type form.

11.2 Gene Mutations May Arise from Spontaneous Events

- DNA replication errors can substitute base pairs, and strand slippage can modify the number of repeats of a DNA sequence.
- Different kinds of spontaneous changes in nucleotide structure can result in mutation of DNA sequence by base-pair mismatching.

11.3 Mutations May Be Caused by Chemicals or Ionizing Radiation

- Mutagenic chemicals interact in characteristic reactions with DNA nucleotides and generate specific mutations.
- Chemical compounds may create mutations by acting as nucleotide base analogs, adding or removing side groups from nucleotides, or intercalating into DNA.
- Energy in the ultraviolet range and higher (shorter in wavelength) is mutagenic. Ultraviolet radiation induces the formation of photoproducts that lead to base-pair substitution mutations.
- The Ames test identifies mutagenic chemical compounds by testing for increased reversion rates in auxotrophic bacteria exposed to a test compound in the presence of detoxifying enzymes from the eukaryotic liver.

11.4 Repair Systems Correct Some DNA Damage

- Direct repair of DNA lesions removes damaged nucleotides and prevents mutation.
- Mismatched DNA nucleotides, photoproducts induced by UV radiation, and modified nucleotide side chains are removed by direct repair.
- Nucleotide excision repair and UV repair remove segments of DNA single strands containing damaged nucleotides and direct new synthesis to fill the resulting single-stranded gap.
- Genetically controlled systems monitor the genome and regulate DNA repair.

11.5 Proteins Control Translesion DNA Synthesis and the Repair of Double-Strand Breaks

- SOS repair, controlled by the RecA protein, is a specialized process activated during replication in bacteria in response to widespread DNA damage.
- Translesion DNA synthesis uses translesion DNA polymerases to complete replication when damage is present.
- Nonhomologous end joining repairs double-strand DNA breaks occurring before DNA replication.
- Synthesis-dependent strand annealing repairs double-strand breaks occurring after the completion of replication.

11.6 DNA Double-Strand Breaks Initiate Homologous Recombination

- Homologous recombination is controlled by the RecBCD pathway in bacteria. In eukaryotes, meiotic recombination is initiated through the activity of Spo11 that regulates the production of double-strand breaks.
- In meiotic recombination, strand invasion and new DNA synthesis form heteroduplex DNA in both homologous chromosomes.
- Heteroduplex DNA contains base-pair mismatches if DNA sequences are heterozygous.
- DNA strands forming double Holliday junctions are cut and rejoined to different homologs before their separation in meiosis.
- Resolution of double Holliday junctions generates heteroduplex DNA and can produce recombinant or nonrecombinant chromosomes.

11.7 Transposable Genetic Elements Move throughout the Genome

- Transposable genetic elements, found in all genomes, are DNA sequences that can move about the genome by either a "cut-and-paste" or a "copy-and-paste" process.
- DNA transposons encode transposase and perhaps other genes and transpose as DNA sequences.
- Retrotransposons encode reverse transcriptase and perhaps other genes and transpose through an RNA intermediate.
- Transposase is the enzyme responsible for transposition, and it is encoded by many transposable genetic elements.
- Transposition can produce mutations through insertional inactivation that modifies gene expression or by contributing to unequal crossing over between homologous chromosomes.
- Transposable elements can contribute to great expansion of genome size.

PREPARING FOR PROBLEM SOLVING

In addition to the list of problem-solving tips and suggestions given here, you can go to the Study Guide and Solutions Manual that accompanies this book for help at solving problems.

1. Understand how to analyze and predict the effects of mutations on DNA, mRNA, and proteins.

2. Understand how the phenotypic effects of mutations are described and analyzed.

3. Be prepared to describe the molecular mechanisms that generate mutations.

4. Know the processes that ensure the accuracy of DNA replication.

5. Understand the molecular basis of homologous recombination.

PROBLEMS

Mastering Genetics Visit for instructor-assigned tutorials and problems.

Chapter Concepts

For answers to selected even-numbered problems, see Appendix: Answers.

1. Identify two general ways chemical mutagens can alter DNA. Give examples of these two mechanisms.

2. Nitrous acid and 5-bromodeoxyuridine (BU) alter DNA by different mechanisms. What type of mutation does each compound produce?

3. What is the difference between a transition mutation and a transversion mutation?

4. What are the differences between a synonymous mutation, a missense mutation, and a nonsense mutation?

5. UV irradiation causes damage to bacterial DNA. What kind of damage is frequently caused and how does photolyase repair the damage?

6. Ultraviolet (UV) radiation is mutagenic.
   a. What kind of DNA lesion does UV energy cause?
   b. How do UV-induced DNA lesions lead to mutation?
   c. Identify and describe two DNA repair mechanisms that remove UV-induced DNA lesions.

7. Researchers interested in studying mutation and mutation repair often induce mutations with various agents. What kinds of gene mutations are induced by
   a. chemical mutagens? Give two examples.
   b. radiation energy? Give two examples.

8. The effect of base-pair substitution mutations on protein function varies widely from no detectable effect to the complete loss of protein function (null allele). Why do the functional consequences of base-pair substitution vary so widely?

9. Describe the purpose of the Ames test. How are *his⁻* bacteria used in the Ames test? What mutational event is identified using *his⁻* bacteria?

10. In numerous population studies of spontaneous mutation, two observations are made consistently: (1) most mutations are recessive, and (2) forward mutation is more frequent than reversion. What do you think are the likely explanations for these two observations?

11. Two different mutations are identified in a haploid strain of yeast. The first prevents the synthesis of adenine by a nonsense mutation of the *ade-1* gene. In this mutation, a base-pair substitution changes a tryptophan codon (UGG) to a stop codon (UGA). The second affects one of several duplicate tRNA genes. This base-pair substitution mutation changes the anticodon sequence of a tRNA^{Trp} from

    $$3'-ACC-5' \text{ to } 3'-ACU-5'$$

   a. Do you consider the first mutation to be a forward mutation or a reversion? Why?
   b. Do you consider the second mutation to be a forward mutation or a reversion? Why?
   c. Assuming there are no other mutations in the genome, will this double-mutant yeast strain be able to grow on minimal medium? If growth will occur, characterize the nature of growth relative to wild type.

12. What is the phenotypic effect of inserting a *Ds* element into the maize *C* gene? How do *Ds* and *Ac* produce maize kernels that are mostly yellow with purple spots?

13. Answer the following questions concerning the accuracy of DNA polymerase during replication.
   a. What general mechanism do DNA polymerases use to check the accuracy of DNA replication and identify errors during replication?
   b. If a DNA replication error is detected by DNA polymerase, how is it corrected?
   c. If a replication error escapes detection and correction, what kind of abnormality is most likely to exist at the site of replication error?
   d. Identify two mechanisms that can correct the kind of abnormality resulting from the circumstances identified in part (c).
   e. If the kind of abnormality identified in part (c) is not corrected before the next DNA replication cycle, what kind of mutation occurs?
   f. DNA mismatch repair can accurately distinguish between the template strand and the newly replicated strand of a DNA duplex. What characteristic of DNA strands is used to make this distinction?

14. Several types of mutation are identified and described in the chapter. These include (1) promoter mutation, (2) splice site mutation, (3) missense mutation, (4) frameshift mutation, and 5) nonsense mutation. Match the following mutation descriptions with the type(s) of mutations listed above. More than one mutation type might match a description.

   a. A mutation that changes several amino acids in a protein and results in a protein that is shorter than the wild-type product.

   b. A mutation that produces about 5% of the wild-type amount of an mRNA.

   c. A mutation that produces a mutant protein that differs from the wild-type protein at one amino acid position.

   d. A mutation that produces a protein that is shorter than the wild-type protein but does not have any amino acid changes in the portion produced.

   e. A null mutation that does not produce any functional protein product.

15. A 1-mL sample of the bacterium *E. coli* is exposed to ultraviolet light. The sample is used to inoculate a 500-mL flask of complete medium that allows growth of all bacterial cells. The 500-mL culture is grown on the benchtop, and two equal-size samples are removed and plated on identical complete-medium growth plates. Plate 1 is immediately wrapped in a dark cloth, but plate 2 is not covered. Both plates are left at room temperature for 36 hours and then examined. Plate 2 is seen to contain many more growing colonies than plate 1. Thinking about DNA repair processes, how do you explain this observation?

16. A strain of *E. coli* is identified as having a null mutation of the *RecA* gene. What biological property do you expect to be absent in the mutant strain? What is the molecular basis for the missing property?

17. Describe the difference between DNA transposons and retrotransposons.

18. How are flanking direct repeat sequences created by transposition?

19. Using the adenine–thymine base pair in this DNA sequence

$$...GCTC...$$

$$...CGAG...$$

   a. Give the sequence after a transition mutation.
   b. Give the sequence after a transversion mutation.

20. The partial amino acid sequence of a wild-type protein is

   ... Arg–Met–Tyr–Thr–Leu–Cys–Ser ...

The same portion of the protein from a mutant has the sequence

   ... Arg–Met–Leu–Tyr–Ala–Leu–Phe ...

   a. Identify the type of mutation.
   b. Give the sequence of the wild-type DNA template strand. Use $^A/_G$ if the nucleotide could be either

purine, $^T/_C$ if it could be either pyrimidine, N if any nucleotide could occur at a site, or the alternative nucleotides if a purine and a pyrimidine are possible.

21. The two DNA and polypeptide sequences shown are for alleles at a hypothetical locus that produce different polypeptides, both five amino acids long. In each case, the lower DNA strand is the template strand:

allele A_1	5'... ATGCATGTAAGTGCATGA ... 3'
	3'... TACGTACATTCACGTACT ... 5'
A_1 polypeptide	N–Met–His–Val–Ser–Ala–C
allele A_2	5'... ATGCAAGTAAGTGCATGA ... 3'
	3'... TACGTTCATTCACGTACT ... 5'
A_2 polypeptide	N–Met–Gln–Val–Ser–Ala–C

Based on DNA and polypeptide sequences alone, is there any way to determine which allele is dominant and which is recessive? Why or why not?

22. Many human genes are known to have homologs in the mouse genome. One approach to investigating human hereditary disease is to produce mutations of the mouse homologs of human genes by methods that can precisely target specific nucleotides for mutation.

   a. Numerous studies of mutations of the mouse homologs of human genes have yielded valuable information about how gene mutations influence the human disease process. In general terms, describe how and why creating mutations of the mouse homologs can give information about human hereditary disease processes.

   b. Despite the homologies that exist between human and mouse genes, some attempts to study human hereditary disease processes by inducing mutations in mouse genes indicate there is little to be learned about human disease in this way. In general terms, describe how and why the study of mouse gene mutations might fail to produce useful information about human disease processes.

23. The fluctuation test performed by Luria and Delbrück is consistent with the random mutation hypothesis. Briefly describe their experiment and identify how the results match the prediction of the random mutation hypothesis. What would have to be different about the experimental results for them to agree with the prediction of the adaptive mutation hypothesis?

24. In this chapter, three features of genes or of DNA sequence that contribute to the occurrence of mutational hotspots were described. Identify those three features and briefly describe why they are associated with mutational hotspots.

25. Briefly compare the production of DNA double-strand breaks in bacteria versus the double-strand breaks that precede homologous recombination.

26. During mismatch repair, why is it necessary to distinguish between the template strand and the newly made daughter strand? Describe how this is accomplished.

Application and Integration

For answers to selected even-numbered problems, see Appendix: Answers.

27. Following the spill of a mixture of chemicals into a small pond, bacteria from the pond are tested and show an unusually high rate of mutation. A number of mutant cultures are grown from mutant colonies and treated with known mutagens to study the rate of reversion. Most of the mutant cultures show a significantly higher reversion rate when exposed to base analogs such as proflavin and 2-aminopurine. What does this suggest about the nature of the chemicals in the spill?

28. In an Ames test using *his⁻ Salmonella* bacteria a researcher determines that adding a test compound plus the S9 extract produces a large number of *his⁺* revertants, but mixing the *his⁻* strain plus the test compound without adding S9 does not produce an elevated number of *his⁺* revertants.

    a. What is the reason for the different experimental results described?
    b. Is the test compound still considered to be a potential mutagen? Explain why or why not.

29. A wild-type culture of haploid yeast is exposed to ethyl methanesulfonate (EMS). Yeast cells are plated on a complete medium, and 6 colonies (colonies numbered 1 to 6) are transferred to a new complete medium plate for further study. Four replica plates are made from the complete medium plate to plates containing minimal medium or minimal medium plus one amino acid (replica plates numbered 1 to 4) with the following results:

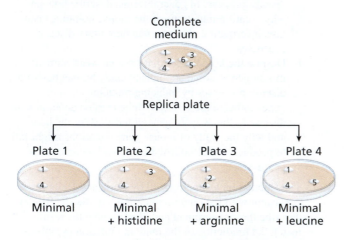

a. Identify the colonies that are prototrophic (wild type). What growth information leads to your answer?
b. Identify the colonies that are auxotrophic (mutant). What growth information leads to your answer?
c. Identify any colonies that are *his⁻*, *arg⁻*, *leu⁻*.
d. For colonies 1, 3, and 5, write "+" for the wild-type synthesis and " − " for the mutant synthesis of histidine and leucine.
e. Are there any colonies for which genotype information cannot be determined? If so, which colony or colonies?

30. A fragment of a wild-type polypeptide is sequenced for seven amino acids. The same polypeptide region is sequenced in four mutants.

Wild-type polypeptide	N . . . Thr–His–Ser–Gly–Leu–Lys–Ala . . . C
Mutant 1	N . . . Thr–His–Ser–Val–Leu–Lys–Ala . . . C
Mutant 2	N . . . Thr–His–Ser–C
Mutant 3	N . . . Thr–Thr–Leu–Asp–C
Mutant 4	N . . . Thr–Gln–Leu–Trp–Ile–Glu–Gly . . .

a. Use the available information to characterize each mutant.
b. Determine the wild-type mRNA sequence.
c. Identify the mutation that produces each mutant polypeptide.

31. Experiments by Charles Yanofsky in the 1950s and 1960s helped characterize the nature of tryptophan synthesis in *E. coli*. In one of Yanofsky's experiments, he identified glycine (Gly) as the wild-type amino acid in position 211 of tryptophan synthetase, the product of the *trpA* gene. He identified two independent missense mutants with defective tryptophan synthetase at these positions that resulted from base-pair substitutions. One mutant encoded arginine (Arg) and another encoded glutamic acid (Glu). At position 235, wild-type tryptophan synthetase contains serine (Ser), but a base-pair substitution mutant encodes leucine (Leu). At position 243, the wild-type polypeptide contains glutamine, and a base-pair substitution mutant encodes a stop codon. Identify the most likely wild-type codons for positions 211, 235, and 243. Justify your answer in each case.

32. Alkaptonuria is a human autosomal recessive disorder caused by mutation of the *HAO* gene that encodes the enzyme homogentisic acid oxidase. A map of the *HAO* gene region reveals four *Bam*HI restriction sites (B1 to B4) in the wild-type allele and three *Bam*HI restriction sites in the mutant allele. *Bam*HI utilizes the restriction sequence 5′-GGATCC-3′. The *Bam*HI restriction sequence identified as B3 is altered to 5′-GGAACC-3′ in the mutant allele. The mutation results in a Ser-to-Thr missense mutation. Restriction maps of the two alleles are shown below, and the binding sites of two molecular probes (probe A and probe B) are identified.

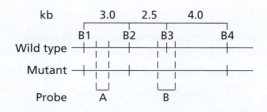

DNA samples taken from a mother (M), father (F), and two children (C1 and C2) are analyzed by Southern blotting of *Bam*HI-digested DNA. The gel electrophoresis results are illustrated.

a. Using *A* to represent the wild-type allele and *a* for the mutant allele, identify the genotype of each family member. Identify any family member who is alkaptonuric.

b. In a separate figure, draw the gel electrophoresis bandpatterns for all the genotypes that could be found in children of this couple.

c. Explain how the DNA sequence change results in a Ser-to-Thr missense mutation.

33. In an experiment employing the methods of the Ames test, two *his*⁻ strains of *Salmonella* are used. Strain A contains a base substitution mutation, and Strain B contains a frameshift mutation. Four plates are prepared to test the mutagenicity of the compound ethyl methanesulfonate (EMS). Plate 1 is a control plate with Strain A and S9 extract but no EMS. Plate 2 is also a control plate and contains Strain B and S9 extract but no EMS. Plate 3 contains Strain A along with S9 extract and EMS, and Plate 4 contains Strain B, S9 extract, and EMS.

a. Characterize the expected distribution of colony growth on the four plates. Defend your growth prediction for each plate.

b. What event is being detected by growth of a colony on any of the four plates?

c. Why is the S9 extract added to each of the plates?

d. Suppose the compound being tested was proflavin instead of EMS. Would this change the Ames test results? Explain why or why not.

34. Using your knowledge of DNA repair pathways, choose the pathway that would be used to repair the following types of DNA damage. Explain your reasoning.

a. a change in DNA sequence caused by a mistake made by DNA polymerase during replication

b. heavily damaged bacterial DNA

c. a thymine dimer induced as a result of UV exposure

d. a double-strand break that occurs just after replication in an actively dividing cell

e. a double-stranded break that occurs during G_1 and prevents completion of DNA replication

f. a cytosine that has been deaminated to uracil

35. Ataxia telangiectasia (OMIM 208900) is a human inherited disorder characterized by poor coordination (ataxia), red marks on the face (telangiectasia), increased sensitivity to X-rays and other radiation, and an increased susceptibility to cancer. Recent studies have shown that this disorder occurs as a result of mutation of the *ATM* gene. Propose a mechanism for how a mutation in the *ATM* gene leads to the characteristics associated with the disorder. Be sure to relate the symptoms of this disorder to functions of the ATM protein. Further, explain why DNA repair mechanisms cannot correct this problem.

36. A geneticist searching for mutations uses the restriction endonucleases *Sma*I and *Pvu*II to search for mutations that eliminate restriction sites. *Sma*I will not cleave DNA with CpG methylation. It cleaves DNA at the restriction digestion sequence

$$\downarrow$$
5'-CCC GGG-3'
3'-GGG CCC-5'
$$\uparrow$$

*Pvu*II is not sensitive to CpG methylation. It cleaves DNA at the restriction sequence

$$\downarrow$$
5'-CAG CTG-3'
3'-GTC GAC-5'
$$\uparrow$$

a. What common feature do *Sma*I and *Pvu*II share that would be useful to a researcher searching for mutations that disrupt restriction digestion?

b. What process is the researcher intending to detect with the use of these restriction enzymes?

c. Explain why CpG dinucleotides are hotspots of mutation.

Collaboration and Discussion

For answers to selected even-numbered problems, see Appendix: Answers.

37. In a mouse-breeding experiment a new mutation called Dumbo is identified. A mouse with the Dumbo mutation has very large ears. It is produced by two parental mice with normal ear size. Based on this information, can you tell whether the Dumbo mutation is a regulatory mutation or a mutation of a protein coding gene? Why or why not?

38. Considering the Dumbo mutation in Problem 37, what kinds of additional evidence would help you determine whether Dumbo is a mutation of a regulatory sequence or of a protein coding gene?

39. Thinking back to the discussion of gain-of-function and loss-of-function mutations in Section 4.1, and putting those concepts together with the discussion of base substitution mutations in this chapter, explain why gain-of-function mutations are often dominant and why loss-of-function mutations are often recessive. Give an example of a type of gain-of-function mutation that is dominant and of a loss-of-function mutation that is recessive.

40. Common baker's yeast (*Saccharomyces cerevisiae*) is normally grown at 37°C, but it will grow actively at temperatures down to approximately 25°C. A haploid culture of wild-type yeast is mutagenized with EMS. Cells from the mutagenized culture are spread on a complete-medium plate and grown at 25°C. Six colonies (1 to 6) are selected from the original complete-medium plate and transferred to two fresh complete-medium plates. The new complete plates (shown) are grown at 25°C and 37°C. Four replica plates are made onto minimal medium or minimal plus adenine from the 25°C complete-medium plate. The new plates are grown at either 25°C or 37°C and the growth results are shown.

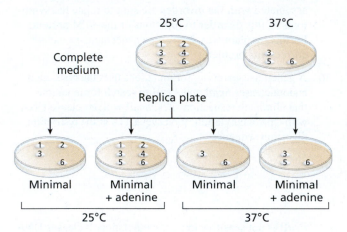

a. Which colonies are prototrophic and which are auxotrophic? What growth information is used to make these determinations?
b. Classify the nature of the mutations in colonies 1, 2, and 5.
c. What can you say about colony 4?

41. The two gels illustrated contain dideoxynucleotide DNA-sequencing information for a wild-type segment and mutant segment of DNA corresponding to the N-terminal end of a protein. The start codon and the next five codons are sequenced.

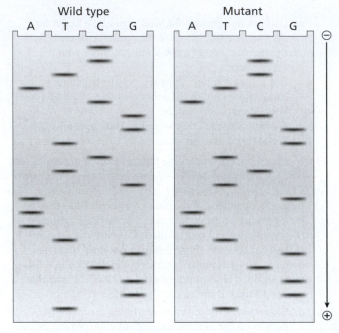

a. Write the DNA sequence of both alleles, including strand polarity.
b. Identify the template and nontemplate strands of DNA.
c. Write out the mRNA sequences encoded by each template strand, and underline the start codons.
d. Determine the amino acid sequences translated from these mRNAs.
e. What is the cause of the mutation?

Regulation of Gene Expression in Bacteria and Bacteriophage

CHAPTER OUTLINE

12.1 Transcriptional Control of Gene Expression Requires DNA–Protein Interaction

12.2 The *lac* Operon Is an Inducible Operon System under Negative and Positive Control

12.3 Mutational Analysis Deciphers Genetic Regulation of the *lac* Operon

12.4 Transcription from the Tryptophan Operon Is Repressible and Attenuated

12.5 Bacteria Regulate the Transcription of Stress Response Genes and Also Translation

12.6 Riboswitches Regulate Bacterial Transcription, Translation, and mRNA Stability

12.7 Antiterminators and Repressors Control Lambda Phage Infection of *E. coli*

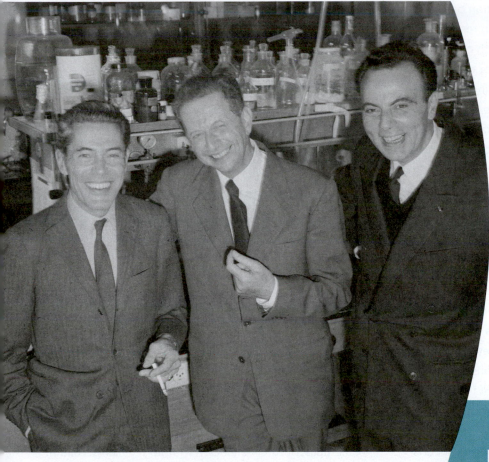

Jacques Monod (left), André Lwoff (middle), and François Jacob (right) on October 14, 1965, following the announcement of the awarding of the Nobel Prize in Physiology or Medicine for their work describing the lactose (*lac*) operon in *E. coli*.

Take a moment to think about the ever-changing environment endured by the billions of *Escherichia coli* (*E. coli*) that populate your intestinal tract. These bacteria are accustomed to a diverse and constantly shifting set of environmental factors and nutritional conditions, as well as to competition from the many other bacterial species in your gut. In all these rapidly changing environmental conditions, bacterial survival depends on the cell's ability to deal with whatever conditions prevail at the moment. Although certain bacteria engage in *quorum sensing*, a mechanism causing certain genes to be coordinated among the individuals within a dense population of bacteria, each individual bacterial cell is largely self-reliant when it comes to producing the proteins necessary to carry out

ESSENTIAL IDEAS

- Gene expression in bacteria is controlled primarily through transcriptional regulation, often by regulating groups of genes known as operons.
- Transcription of lactose (*lac*) operon genes is induced by lactose and is repressed in the absence of lactose.
- Transcription of the repressible tryptophan (*trp*) operon adjusts to the level of available tryptophan.
- Specialized regulatory processes control transcriptional response to environmental stress and regulate translation.
- Bacteria can regulate transcription, translation, and the stability of mRNA with mRNA sequences and RNA-binding regulatory proteins.
- Bacteriophage use transcriptional regulation to express the genes responsible for infecting their hosts.
- Competition between regulatory proteins determines the course of bacteriophage lambda infection in bacteria.

439

metabolism and to generate the compounds it needs to stay alive and to reproduce.

What is the best strategy for the survival of *E. coli* in a rapidly changing environment? Should the organism transcribe and translate all its genes at all times, or should gene transcription and translation be regulated in a closely monitored manner that can respond in a matter of minutes to changes in growth conditions as they arise? Answering these kinds of questions was critically important to understanding how evolution has shaped the processes of gene expression in organisms. On one hand, if bacteria transcribed and translated all their genes at all times, they could be instantly ready for almost any environmental shift that might occur. On the other hand, continuously expressing all genes would be terribly costly in metabolic terms and entail a great deal of unnecessary transcription and translation. Unregulated gene expression could also result in antagonistic interactions between proteins operating in different metabolic systems. Biologists in the 1950s and 1960s hypothesized that energetic and metabolic expenditures associated with regulated gene expression would be evolutionarily favored over the high cost of continuous gene expression. But to demonstrate the validity of that hypothesis, examples of regulated gene expression had to be identified and studied.

The first research describing the gene actions and molecular mechanism for regulated gene expression was by Francois Jacob, Jacques Monod, André Lwoff, and others, who showed how the lactose (*lac*) operon system in *E. coli* was transcriptionally regulated in response to the presence or absence of the milk sugar lactose. This research was a milestone in biology that introduced a new way of thinking about the expression of genes. It opened the door to research on mechanisms that regulate gene expression—research that is just as active today as it has ever been.

In this chapter, the regulatory systems we discuss are principally found in *E. coli*, the most widely used model bacterium. We begin with a general introduction to regulated gene expression and introduce the concept that the interaction between DNA-binding regulatory proteins and regulatory DNA sequences regulates transcription. Next we explore the organization, function, and regulation of the *E. coli* lactose (*lac*) operon system, whose gene transcription is induced (turned on) by the presence of the sugar lactose in the growth medium. This topic is followed by a discussion of mutational analysis and the molecular explanation for the transcriptional control of *lac* operon genes. We then turn our attention to the genetic structure and molecular control of transcription of the tryptophan (*trp*) operon that contains the genes needed to synthesize the amino acid tryptophan. After moving on to discussions of posttranscriptional regulation of bacterial genes and of a mechanism that uses regulatory mRNA sequences to control gene expression, we examine the regulatory process that controls infection of bacterial cells by bacteriophage λ (lambda).

12.1 Transcriptional Control of Gene Expression Requires DNA–Protein Interaction

Certain bacterial genes—specifically, those whose products are needed continuously to perform routine tasks—undergo **constitutive transcription,** a term identifying the genes as being transcribed continuously with no regulatory control. In contrast, the need for agile and calibrated responses to changing environmental conditions has resulted in the evolution of mechanisms for the **regulated transcription** of many bacterial genes.

Regulation of the transcription of bacterial genes is the predominant mode by which bacteria regulate responses to the environment, and it takes place at two levels. At both levels, control results from interactions between DNA-binding proteins and specific regulatory sequences of DNA. The first level of control regulates the *initiation of transcription*, determining whether a particular gene or group of genes is transcribed at all. The second transcriptional control level determines the *amount of transcription*, regulating either the duration of transcription or the amount of mRNA transcript produced from the gene.

Additionally, posttranscriptional regulatory mechanisms are important, controlling mRNA stability, the level of translation of mRNA, or the activity of proteins and enzymes. Table 12.1 provides an overview of bacterial regulatory mechanisms that are described in this chapter.

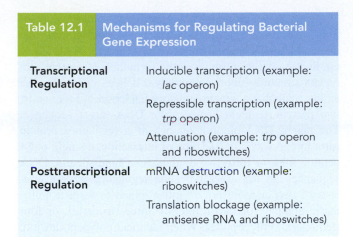

Table 12.1	Mechanisms for Regulating Bacterial Gene Expression
Transcriptional Regulation	Inducible transcription (example: *lac* operon)
	Repressible transcription (example: *trp* operon)
	Attenuation (example: *trp* operon and riboswitches)
Posttranscriptional Regulation	mRNA destruction (example: riboswitches)
	Translation blockage (example: antisense RNA and riboswitches)

Negative and Positive Control of Transcription

Mechanisms of transcriptional control are described as negative or positive. **Negative control** of transcription involves the binding of a *repressor protein* to a regulatory DNA sequence, with the consequence of *preventing* transcription of a gene or a cluster of genes. On the other hand, **positive control** of transcription involves the binding of an *activator protein* to regulatory DNA, with the result of *initiating* gene transcription.

Repressor proteins are a broad category of regulatory proteins that exert negative control of transcription. In their active form, repressor proteins bind to regulatory DNA sequences, including those called **operators**, as we describe below, under "Regulatory DNA-Binding Proteins," for the lactose operon. Repressor protein binding blocks transcription initiation by RNA polymerase. The repressor protein acts by occupying the space on regulatory DNA where the polymerase would otherwise bind or by preventing formation of the open promoter complex necessary for transcription initiation. Repressor proteins can be activated or inactivated by interactions with other compounds.

Repressor proteins commonly contain two active sites through which their functional role is performed. The **DNA-binding domain** is responsible for locating and binding operator DNA sequence or other target regulatory sequences. The **allosteric domain** binds a molecule or protein and, in so doing, causes a change in the conformation of the DNA-binding site. The property belonging to some enzymes of changing conformation at the active site as a result of binding a substance at a different site is known as **allostery**.

Allosteric domains operate in two modes. Certain repressor proteins undergo inactivation of their DNA-binding domain because of allosteric changes brought about by an **inducer** compound binding to the allosteric site (**Figure 12.1a**). If the inducer is removed from the allosteric site, the repressor's conformation is switched, the

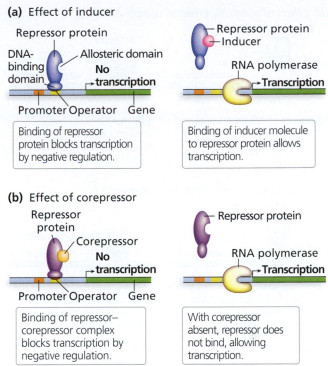

(a) Effect of inducer

Binding of repressor protein blocks transcription by negative regulation.

Binding of inducer molecule to repressor protein allows transcription.

(b) Effect of corepressor

Binding of repressor–corepressor complex blocks transcription by negative regulation.

With corepressor absent, repressor does not bind, allowing transcription.

Figure 12.1 Mechanisms of negative control of transcription.

Briefly describe the role an inducer substance plays in allostery.

DNA-binding site is reactivated, and the protein can repress transcription. On the other hand, some repressor proteins require binding of a **corepressor** molecule at the allosteric site to activate the DNA-binding site (**Figure 12.1b**). In this case, transcriptional repression is reversed when the corepressor is removed from the allosteric site.

Positive control of transcription is accomplished by **activator proteins** that bind to regulatory DNA sequences called **activator binding sites**. Activator protein binding facilitates RNA polymerase binding at promoters and helps initiate transcription. Activator proteins have a DNA-binding domain that binds the activator binding site of DNA. In one mode of action for activator proteins, the DNA-binding domain remains inactive until the allosteric domain of the protein is bound by an **allosteric effector compound**. The induced allosteric change leads to the formation of a functional DNA-binding domain, allowing the activator protein to bind to DNA (**Figure 12.2a**). Alternatively, certain activator proteins have a functional DNA-binding domain that is converted to an inactive conformation by binding of an **inhibitor** compound in the allosteric binding domain (**Figure 12.2b**).

Regulatory DNA-Binding Proteins

Most DNA-binding proteins that exert regulatory control bind DNA at specific sequences to accomplish their regulatory activity. These interactions occur by association of the amino acid side chains of the proteins with the specific

(a) Effect of allosteric effector compound

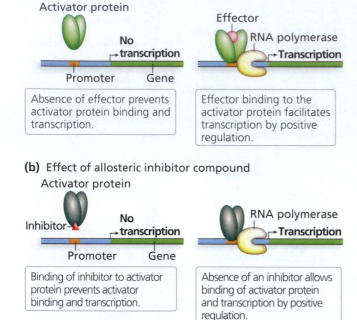

Absence of effector prevents activator protein binding and transcription.

Effector binding to the activator protein facilitates transcription by positive regulation.

(b) Effect of allosteric inhibitor compound

Binding of inhibitor to activator protein prevents activator binding and transcription.

Absence of an inhibitor allows binding of activator protein and transcription by positive regulation.

Figure 12.2 **Mechanisms of positive control of transcription.**

Ⓠ Briefly describe the difference between negative control of transcription and positive control of transcription.

nucleotide bases and the sugar-phosphate backbone of DNA. The proteins make their contact with specific base pairs located in the major groove and the minor groove of the DNA helix using the unique patterns of hydrogen, nitrogen, and oxygen atoms that characterize each base pair.

To achieve protein–DNA specificity in these interactions, the protein must simultaneously contact multiple nucleotides. A common motif in the structures of DNA-binding regulatory proteins is the formation of protein secondary structures, most commonly α helices, containing the amino acids that contact regulatory nucleotides. Frequently, two protein segments contact the DNA target sequence. The paired DNA-binding regions of a regulatory protein form in two ways. In one type of interaction, a single polypeptide folds to form two domains that bind specific DNA sequences. In the other type, the regulatory protein consists of two or more polypeptides joined to form a multimeric complex of two (dimeric), three (trimeric), or four (tetrameric) polypeptides. When identical polypeptides join together, the prefix *homo-* is used. A "homodimer" contains two identical polypeptides in the functional protein. When different polypeptides join together, the complex is identified by the prefix *hetero-*, as in "heterodimer."

Extensive studies of transcription-regulating proteins in bacteria have identified the characteristic structural features of DNA-binding regulatory proteins and the DNA sequence they bind. Bacterial regulatory DNA sequences frequently contain inverted repeats or direct repeats. Each polypeptide of a homodimeric regulatory protein, or each of the binding regions of a folded polypeptide, interacts with one of the inverted repeat segments. By far the most common structural motif seen in these proteins in bacteria is the **helix-turn-helix (HTH) motif** (**Figure 12.3**). In the HTH motif, two α-helical regions in each of two polypeptides in a homodimer interact with inverted repeat regulatory sequences in DNA. In each of the polypeptides, one

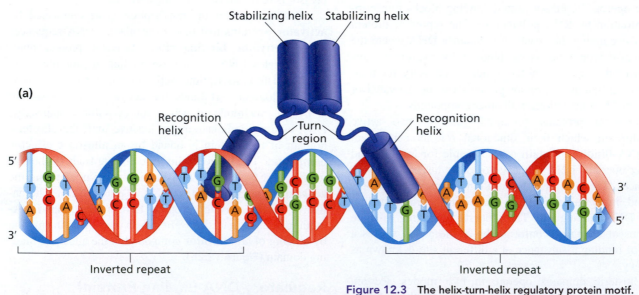

Figure 12.3 **The helix-turn-helix regulatory protein motif.**
(a) DNA-binding proteins forming an HTH motif are usually dimeric. Two subunits of an HTH dimer are shown as pairs of helices joined by a "turn" connecting them. The recognition helices bind DNA that often is composed of inverted repeat sequence in the major or minor grooves. The stabilizing helices interact with one another to help hold the complex together. **(b)** Inverted repeat sequences are often targets of DNA-binding regulatory domains of proteins such as HTH proteins.

of the two α-helical regions is the recognition helix that fits into the major groove of DNA and binds the inverted repeat sequences. The second helix of each polypeptide is the stabilizing helix. It lies across the major groove and contacts the sugar-phosphate backbone, ensuring a strong DNA–protein interaction and properly orienting the recognition helix to sit in the major groove. The recognition helix and the stabilizing helix of each polypeptide are connected by a short amino acid string identified as the "turn," hence the name of the helix-turn-helix motif. Many different DNA-binding regulatory proteins with the HTH motif have been identified in bacteria as we discuss in later sections of this chapter.

12.2 The *lac* Operon Is an Inducible Operon System under Negative and Positive Control

One conclusion evolutionary biologists have reached in comparing the genomes of different forms of life is that evolution has operated to restrict the total size of bacterial genomes compared with most others and to limit the percentage of repetitive (noncoding) DNA in them to less than 15 percent on average. These limitations are imposed by various factors, including the dependence of bacteria on their abilities to reproduce rapidly and respond quickly to environmental changes. Possession of a relatively small genome and small percentage of noncoding DNA speeds the DNA replication process and shortens the time required to replicate the genome during cell division. The need for rapid responsiveness to environmental change and for restricted genome size dictates another evolutionary adaptation in bacteria: the clustering and coordinated transcriptional regulation of genes involved in the same metabolic processes.

Clusters of genes undergoing coordinated transcriptional regulation by a shared regulatory region are called **operons**. Operons are common in bacterial genomes, and the genes that are part of a given operon almost always participate in the same metabolic or biosynthesis pathway. Besides having a single promoter shared by the operon genes, operons contain additional regulatory DNA sequences that interact with promoters to exert transcriptional control.

In this discussion, we focus on the **lactose (*lac*) operon** of *E. coli*. This operon is responsible for the production of three polypeptides that permit *E. coli* to utilize the sugar lactose as a carbon source for growth and metabolic energy. In this section, we explain how the *lac* operon works, describe the circumstances under which its genes are transcribed, and identify the regulatory mechanisms that control operon gene transcription. In the following section, we turn our attention to mutational and molecular analyses of the *lac* operon to understand the function of operon genes and to explore the molecular interactions that regulate operon gene transcription.

Lactose Metabolism

The monosaccharide sugar glucose is the preferred energy source of *E. coli*, just as it is for your cells. Glucose is metabolized by the biochemical pathway called glycolysis, a sequence of biochemical reactions that oxidizes glucose, and closely related compounds, to produce pyruvate and ATP (adenosine triphosphate), the compound used universally by cells to store and produce energy. This pathway occurs in virtually all cells as part of fermentation and cellular respiration. Glycolysis is the principal energy-producing reaction in your cells and those of *E. coli*. But like humans and other organisms, *E. coli* is capable of metabolizing sugars such as galactose, lactose, and fructose as well. Glucose is the preferred sugar because it can be directly metabolized in glycolysis. The alternative sugars require separate metabolism to first produce glucose or a glucose derivative that can then be processed by glycolysis. Thus, *E. coli* will consume all available glucose before a genetic switch is flipped that changes the metabolic pathway to one that uses an alternative sugar.

The genetic switch to lactose utilization requires that lactose be present in the cell, but the lactose is not used by the cell until after glucose has been depleted. The *lac* operon, whose genes and regulatory sequences control lactose utilization in *E. coli*, is an **inducible operon** system, meaning that under the specific circumstances of lactose presence in the growth medium and glucose absence, transcription of the operon genes is activated, or induced. The inducible nature of the *lac* operon and other inducible operons also means that expression of operon genes is limited to the circumstance of the *inducer compound* being available. Other nutritional requirements may have to be met as well for transcription induction to occur.

Lactose is a disaccharide consisting of two monosaccharides, glucose and galactose, that are joined by a covalent β-galactoside linkage (**Figure 12.4**). Bacteria that have a *lac*⁺ phenotype ("lack plus") are able to grow on a medium containing lactose as the only sugar. *lac*⁺ strains accomplish this growth by producing a gated channel at the cell membrane that allows lactose to enter the cell. The channel is formed by the enzyme permease. On entering the cell ❶, lactose is processed by the enzyme β-galactosidase that processes lactose in two ways. The principal activity of β-galactosidase is to break the β-galactoside linkage to release glucose and galactose ❷. Glucose produced by lactose breakdown can immediately enter glycolysis. The molecule of galactose can be further processed to produce glucose. In addition to producing glucose and galactose, β-galactosidase also converts some lactose to an isomer called **allolactose** ❸. Allolactose plays a critical role in regulating the transcription of *lac* operon genes by acting as the inducer compound. Allolactose that is not used for induction can be cleaved by β-galactosidase ❹. Bacteria that are unable to grow on a lactose-containing medium are identified as having a *lac*⁻ phenotype ("lack minus"). These strains are either unable to import lactose to the cell, unable to break it down once it is in the cell, or both.

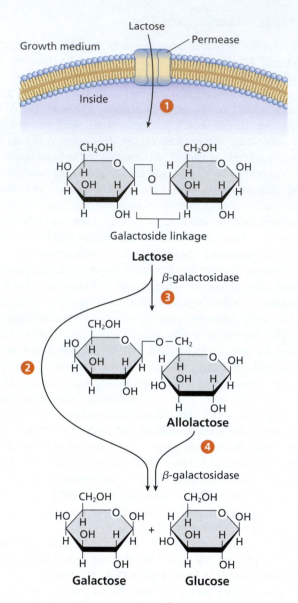

Figure 12.4 Lactose metabolism. ❶ Lactose enters the *E. coli* cell from the growth medium with the aid of permease. ❷ Most of the lactose has its galactoside linkage cleaved by β-galactosidase to yield galactose and glucose. ❸ β-galactosidase converts some lactose to its isomeric form, allolactose that acts as the inducer. ❹ Excess allolactose is cleaved by β-galactosidase.

lac Operon Structure

The *lac* operon consists of a multipart regulatory region and a structural gene region containing three genes (**Figure 12.5a**). The regulatory region contains three protein-binding regulatory sequences. One is the promoter that binds RNA polymerase, another is the operator (*lacO*) sequence that binds the Lac repressor protein, and the third is the **CAP binding site**. These three regions partially overlap and are immediately upstream of the start of transcription of *lac* operon genes.

The three structural genes of the *lac* operon are identified as ***lacZ***, a gene encoding the enzyme β-galactosidase; ***lacY***,

which encodes the enzyme permease; and ***lacA***, which encodes transacetylase. These three genes are transcribed as a **polycistronic mRNA**, an mRNA molecule that is the transcript of all the genes in the operon. Each gene transcript that is part of a polycistronic mRNA contains a start and a stop codon sequence. The translation of a polycistronic mRNA generates a distinct polypeptide for each gene.

The β-galactosidase produced by the *lacZ* gene is responsible for cleaving the β-galactoside linkage of lactose to release molecules of glucose and galactose. As mentioned above, the enzyme also converts a small amount of lactose into allolactose, which has a chemical structure very similar to that of lactose. The permease enzyme encoded by *lacY* functions at the cell membrane to facilitate the entry of lactose into the cell. Transacetylase, the product of *lacA*, is not essential for lactose utilization, although in bacteria it protects against potentially damaging by-products of lactose metabolism. Our discussion focuses only on transcription of *lacZ* and *lacY*, and on the action of β-galactosidase and permease, since transacetylase is not essential for lactose utilization.

Adjacent to, but not part of the *lac* operon, is the regulatory gene, *lacI* ("lack eye"), that produces the Lac repressor protein. The *lacI* gene has its own promoter that is not regulated and drives constitutive transcription. The Lac repressor protein is a homotetramer that has two functional domains. The first is a DNA-binding domain that binds the operator regions, and the second is an allosteric domain that binds the inducer substance allolactose.

Figure 12.5b shows the DNA sequence composition of the *lac* operon promoter (*lacP*) and the *lac* operator (*lacO*), which are directly adjacent and together only span about 80 base pairs. Owing to the slight overlap mentioned above, the operator sequence includes the +1 nucleotide that starts transcription. The *lac* promoter contains the −10 and −35 consensus sequence sites that are critical for RNA polymerase binding (see Section 8.2). Notice that the CAP binding site is near the −35 and −10 regions of the promoter. We discuss this relationship in the next subsection.

lac Operon Function

The *lac* operon is transcriptionally silent when no lactose is available and when glucose is available to the cell (**Figure 12.6a**). In the absence of production of β-galactosidase, there is no allolactose in the cell and the constitutively produced Lac repressor protein binds to *lacO*, using its DNA-binding domain. By its presence at the operator, Lac repressor blocks RNA polymerase from binding to *lacP* and prevents transcription initiation. This transcriptional regulatory interaction is an example of negative control of transcription that is achieved through the binding of repressor protein to the transcription-regulating operator sequence.

In contrast, the availability of lactose in the growth medium and the unavailability of glucose lead to the induction of transcription of the *lac* operon structural genes (**Figure 12.6b**). On this basis, the *lac* operon is identified as

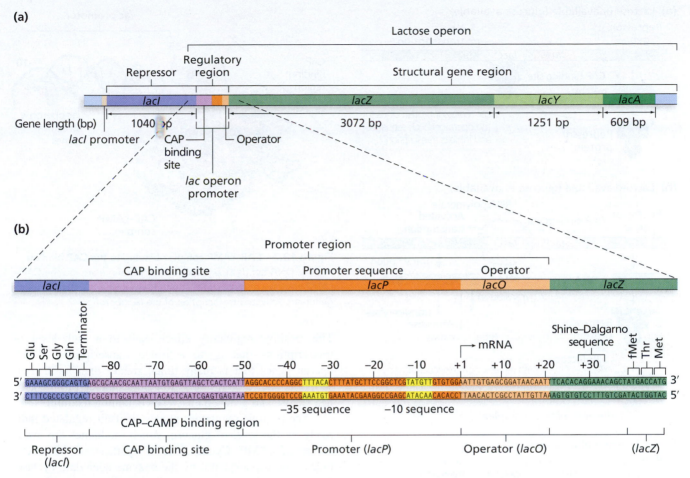

Figure 12.5 **The lactose (lac) operon of E. coli.** **(a)** The repressor protein (lacI) is encoded by a 1040-bp segment under separate transcriptional regulation. The transcription regulatory region consists of a CAP binding site, a promoter consensus sequence region, and an operator sequence. The three structural genes of the *lac* operon encode the enzymes β-galactosidase (lacZ), permease (lacY), and transacetylase (lacA). **(b)** The DNA sequence of the regulatory region of the *lac* operon, including the −10 and −35 consensus sequences, the operator, and the CAP binding site.

◉ Describe the position of the *lac* operator with respect to the positions of the *lac* promoter and the +1 nucleotide.

an inducible operon. With synthesis of β-galactosidase, the production of allolactose occurs. By binding to the allosteric domain of the repressor protein, allolactose forms the **inducer–repressor complex**. The formation of this complex induces an allosteric change that alters the conformation of the DNA-binding domain of the repressor protein to a form that does not recognize or bind the operator. An essential part of the induction of transcription is the binding of the CAP–cAMP complex to the CAP binding site, which facilitates achievement of the highest level of transcription. The polycistronic mRNA is synthesized, and translation produces β-galactosidase, permease, and transacetylase.

When both glucose and lactose are available, *E. coli* utilize glucose. The presence of lactose, however, generates a small amount of allolactose that carries out its normal inducer function by binding to repressor protein. The inducer–repressor interaction opens the promoter region, and RNA polymerase binds.

By itself, however, RNA polymerase is very ineffective at accomplishing transcription of the *lac* operon genes. This is due to the absence of binding of the CAP–cAMP complex at the CAP binding site (more on this in a moment). RNA polymerase by itself is only able to manage **basal transcription** (**Figure 12.6c**)—transcription that produces only a small number of polycistronic mRNAs and leads to the translation of a few molecules of β-galactosidase, permease, and transacetylase per cell.

Basal transcription driven solely by RNA polymerase that gains access to the *lac* promoter through the inducer–repressor complex mechanism is insufficient to generate enough copies of the polycistronic mRNA to drive active lactose metabolism. A second regulatory process featuring positive control of transcription is required to fully activate *lac* operon gene transcription. Positive control of *lac* operon transcription lies in a DNA–protein interaction that occurs at the **CAP–cAMP binding region** of the *lac* operon

(a) Lactose unavailable (glucose available)

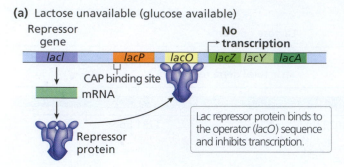

(b) Lactose available (glucose unavailable)

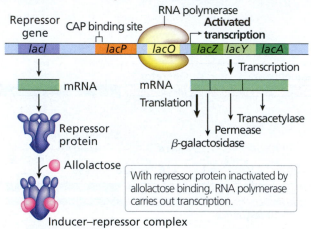

(c) Lactose and glucose available

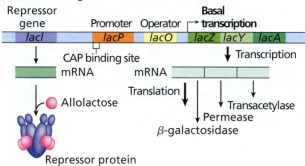

Figure 12.6 *lac* operon transcription regulation. **(a)** When glucose is available and lactose is unavailable, *lac* operon genes are not transcribed. **(b)** Lactose availability in the absence of glucose induces activated transcription of operon genes by binding of the CAP–cAMP complex at the CAP site (see the text for a description). **(c)** The presence of both glucose and lactose leads to basal transcription of the operon.

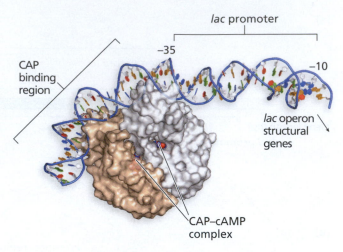

Figure 12.7 **CAP–cAMP complex binding to the CAP binding region.** DNA bends at an approximate 90° angle around the CAP–cAMP complex and facilitates strong RNA polymerase binding that generates activated transcription of the *lac* operon.

This positive regulatory effect leads to a high level of transcription—that is, to activated transcription—of *lac* operon genes that is many times greater than basal transcription. Activated transcription allows the cell to metabolize lactose and grow on a lactose-containing medium.

The positive regulatory process is itself regulated indirectly by the level of glucose, which modulates the availability of cAMP. Cyclic AMP is synthesized from ATP (adenosine triphosphate) by the enzyme adenylate cyclase. During glycolysis, the availability of adenylate cyclase is limited and cAMP synthesis is reduced. Thus, when glucose is available, cAMP is very low in concentration, almost no CAP–cAMP can form, and *lac* operon gene transcription is highly inefficient. This effect of glucose in blocking *lac* operon gene transcription, even when lactose is present, is known as **catabolite repression**, during which the presence of the preferred catabolite (glucose) represses the transcription of genes for an alternative catabolite (lactose).

With your budding understanding of *lac* operon gene transcription, perhaps the following question—a kind of chicken-and-egg conundrum—has occurred to you. Lactose must enter the cell so that allolactose can be produced to act as an inducer. Lactose cannot enter the cell without the aid of permease that helps bring lactose into the cell. But because the *lacY* gene that produces permease is part of the *lac* operon, and transcription is not induced until lactose is present inside the cell, how does lactose enter the cell in the first place? It does so in two ways. One stems from the reversibility of the interaction between the repressor protein and the *lac* operator. In the presence of glucose and the absence of lactose, the repressor protein is almost always bound to the operator sequence. Occasionally and spontaneously, however, the repressor protein loses contact with the operator sequence. While short-lived, this spontaneous release is just enough to allow momentary transcription of the operon and

promoter. This site is located at approximately –60 of *lacP* (see Figures 12.5b and 12.6c). The CAP binding site contains the sequence that attracts the **CAP–cAMP complex**, a small molecular complex composed of a protein known as the catabolite activator protein (CAP) and the nucleotide cyclic adenosine monophosphate (cAMP). Binding of the CAP–cAMP complex to its binding site causes DNA to bend around the complex, and it increases the ability of RNA polymerase to transcribe *lac* operon genes (**Figure 12.7**).

production of a few molecules of β-galactosidase and permease. This small amount of permease and β-galactosidase, amounting to no more than a few molecules per cell, is sufficient to bring a small number of lactose molecules across the cell membrane and to generate allolactose. This trickle of lactose quickly induces more transcription, launching a transcriptional cascade that soon causes the cell to switch its metabolism to lactose utilization.

The second way also involves the production of a tiny amount of permease and β-galactosidase—in this case, through basal transcription that takes place when both glucose and lactose are available to a cell. Basal transcription becomes fully activated transcription when glucose is exhausted and only lactose is available to a cell.

12.3 Mutational Analysis Deciphers Genetic Regulation of the *lac* Operon

The identification and description of the *lac* operon began with a series of publications in the early 1960s by François Jacob, Jacques Monod, André Lwoff, and several other colleagues. Their genetic analysis of numerous *lac* operon mutants led to the identification of each gene and regulatory region, and to the functional description of the operon as provided in the previous section. Jacob, Monod, and Lwoff were awarded the Nobel Prize in Physiology or Medicine in 1965 for this work (see the chapter opener photo). Their work also laid the foundation for a description of *lac* operon

transcription regulation at the DNA sequence level. We discuss several of their analyses of *lac* operon mutants and elements of the molecular analysis of *lac* operon transcriptional regulation in this section. As you read this discussion, refer to Tables 12.2 and 12.3 for a list of *lac* operon genes and regulatory sequences, as well as example genotypes and phenotypes associated with mutations we discuss. You can also refer to Research Technique 6.1, which discusses the determination of the genotype of a bacterial strain based on its pattern of growth and no growth in various media.

Analysis of Structural Gene Mutations

The genetic analysis of the *lac* operon by Jacob, Monod, and colleagues was made possible by the study of operon mutations. Several dozen lac^- mutants were generated by treatment of *E. coli* with mutagens. The mutants were first subjected to genetic complementation experiments to determine whether the lac^- phenotypes of different mutants resulted from mutation of the same gene or from mutations of different genes. Investigations showed that lac^- mutants formed two complementation groups, indicating that two genes are responsible for the lac^- phenotype. The two complementation groups are today known to correspond to *lacZ* (β-galactosidase) and *lacY* (permease).

The complementation analysis was carried out using partial diploid bacterial strains that were produced by conjugation between F′ (*lac*) and F⁻ bacteria (see Section 6.3). Recall that exconjugants produced by F′ × F⁺ conjugation have two copies of a portion of the genome and are thus partially diploid. In the case of *lac* operon partial diploids, one copy of the *lac* operon information resides on the recipient

Table 12.2	*lac* Operon Genes and Regulatory Sequences		
Gene/Sequence	**Product/Sequence Type**	**Function**	**Important Mutants**
Protein-Producing Genes			
lacI	Repressor protein	Contains two binding sites, one for the operator and one for allolactose, the inducer.	I^-: Unable to bind to operator. I^S: So-called super repressor. Unable to bind the inducer (allolactose), blocking all transcription.
lacZ	β-galactosidase	Cleaves lactose into two monosaccharides (glucose and galactose).	Z^-: No functional β-galactosidase.
lacY	Permease	Facilitates lactose transport across the cell membrane.	Y^-: No functional permease.
lacA	Transacetylase	Protects against harmful by-products of lactose metabolism.	A^-: No transacetylase.
Regulatory Sequences			
lacO	Operator	Binds repressor protein to block transcription of operon genes.	O^C: Fails to bind repressor protein, resulting in continuous (constitutive) transcription.
lacP	Promoter	Binds RNA polymerase.	P^-: Fails to bind RNA polymerase or does so weakly.

Table 12.3 Synthesis of β-Galactosidase and Permease by Haploids and Partial Diploids with Structural Gene Mutations

Genotype	β-Galactosidase[a]		Permease[a]		Description
	Lactose	No Lactose	Lactose	No Lactose	
1. $I^+ P^+ O^+ Z^+ Y^+$	+	−	+	−	Wild-type (lac^+)
2. $I^+ P^+ O^+ Z^- Y^+$	−		+	−	No functional β-galactosidase (lac^-)
3. $I^+ P^+ O^+ Z^+ Y^-$	+	−	−	−	No functional permease (lac^-)
4. $I^+ P^+ O^+ Z^+ Y^-/I^+ P^+ O^+ Z^- Y^+$	+	−	+	−	Wild-type response by complementation (lac^+).

[a]Symbols + and − indicate production and no production, respectively, of functional enzymes.

bacterial chromosome, and the second copy of the operon is acquired on the F′ plasmid. The genotype of partial diploids is written with the F′ segment on the left and the recipient chromosome on the right. The homologous chromosomes are separated by a slash (/). For example, the genotype of a partial diploid demonstrating complementation of *lac* gene mutations can be written as follows:

$$F' \ I^+ \ P^+ \ O^+ \ Z^+ \ Y^- \ / \ I^+ \ P^+ \ O^+ \ Z^- \ Y^+$$

Analyzed as haploid genotypes, each portion of the partial diploid genotype above would produce the *lac⁻* pheno-type. The F′ haploid lacks the ability to produce perme-ase (*lacY⁻*), and the bacterial haploid is unable to produce β-galactosidase (*lacZ⁻*). Genetic complementation occurs in this partial diploid, however, and the resulting pheno-type is *lac⁺* (see Table 12.3). The molecular basis of genetic complementation in this case is that the F′ portion of the partial diploid provides β-galactosidase by its *lacZ⁺* gene, and the recipient portion of the partial diploid provides per-mease by its *lacY⁺* gene. Based on the analysis of structural gene mutations, Jacob, Monod, and colleagues concluded that there are two protein-producing genes required for *lac⁺* growth behavior and that *lacZ* and *lacY* wild-type alleles are usually dominant to mutant alleles. Recombination mapping analysis revealed close genetic linkage of the three struc-tural genes of the *lac* operon, but the order of these struc-tural genes (*lacZ–lacY–lacA*) was ultimately determined by mutational analysis.

Another type of structural gene mutation that proved useful for understanding the process of translation of the *lac* polycistronic mRNA was base substitution nonsense mutations that generate stop codons in inappropriate loca-tions. If one of these mutations, known as **polar mutations**, occurs early in the *lacZ* portion of the polycistronic mRNA, it has the curious effect of significantly reducing or pre-venting translation of the other gene sequences in the tran-script. How could this be? The answer is that there is just one Shine–Dalgarno sequence in the *lac* operon mRNA. It occurs upstream of the start codon for the *lacZ* gene (see Figure 12.5). Normally, individual ribosomes identify the Shine–Dalgarno sequence and translate the entire length

of the *lac* operon polycistronic mRNA, producing three polypeptides. The presence of the polar (nonsense) muta-tion in the *lacZ* gene stops translation by the ribosome. As there is no other Shine–Dalgarno sequence in the tran-script, the ribosome is unable to translate the *lacY* or *lacA* sequences. Thus, when a polar mutation occurs in the *lacZ* gene, no permease is produced, even if the strain is *lacY⁺*.

lac Operon Regulatory Mutations

Mutations of regulatory components of the *lac* operon alter the inducible response of the operon to the presence of lac-tose and allolactose in the cell. Certain mutations of the *lac* operon lead to **constitutive mutants**, which are unre-sponsive to the presence or absence of lactose in the growth medium. These mutants continuously transcribe the operon genes, rather than transcribing the genes in an inducible manner. Other regulatory mutations block all response to lactose and render the cell *lac⁻*. Eventually, genetic mapping of constitutive mutations identified two distinct sites of con-stitutive mutations of the *lac* operon: *lacO* and *lacI*. Consti-tutive mutations of *lacO* render the operator DNA sequence unrecognizable to the wild-type DNA-binding portion of the repressor protein. On the other hand, constitutive muta-tions of *lacI* result in production of a repressor protein with a mutated DNA-binding region that is unable to recognize and bind wild-type operator sequence. Both mutations pre-vent negative regulation of *lac* operon transcription.

It was the initial discovery of the existence of two sites of *lac* operon constitutive mutations that suggested to Jacob and Monod that a negative regulatory system with two com-ponents exercises transcriptional control of the structural genes. They postulated that one constitutive mutation site is the gene producing a regulatory protein and the second is the target DNA-binding site for the regulatory protein.

Operator Mutations The genetic evidence indicating that the operator is the DNA sequence binding the repres-sor protein comes from the finding that *lac* operator (*lacO*) mutations are exclusively **cis-acting**; that is, they influence the transcription of genes only *on the same chromosome*.

(a) I^+ (wild type)

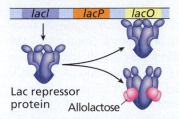

Lac repressor protein   Allolactose

Repressor binds operator when the inducer is absent and forms an inducer–repressor complex when inducer is present.

(b) O^c (operator constitutive mutation)

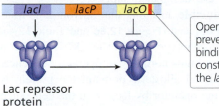

Lac repressor protein

Operator-site mutation prevents repressor protein binding and leads to constitutive synthesis of the *lac* operon.

(c) I^- (repressor mutation)

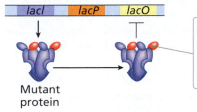

Mutant protein

Repressor protein mutation prevents repressor binding to the operator and produces constitutive synthesis of the *lac* operon.

(d) I^s (super-repressor mutation)

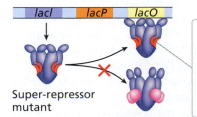

Super-repressor mutant

Repressor protein mutation blocks binding to the inducer, preventing formation of the inducer–repressor complex. Mutant repressor protein binds to the operator, preventing transcription.

Figure 12.8 Regulatory mutations of lacI and *lacO*. (a) Wild-type *lacI* and *lacO*. **(b)** Operator-constitutive (*lacO^C*) mutation. **(c)** *lacI^-* (operator-binding domain) mutation. **(d)** *lacI^S* (super-repressor) mutation of the allosteric binding domain.

⊙ **In which of the mutants shown in (b), (c), and (d) is the allosteric domain wild type, and in which is it mutated?**

In the wild-type organism, $lacI^+$ produces repressor protein that has an allosteric (allolactose) binding domain and a functional operator binding domain. Repressor protein uses its operator binding domain to bind the regulatory sequence and block transcription (**Figure 12.8a**). Bacteria with operator mutations are constitutive for transcription of *lac* operon genes and have the genotype $I^+ P^+ O^C Z^+ Y^+$ (**Figure 12.8b** and **Table 12.4**). The O^C allele designation signifies an "operator-constitutive mutation." In O^C mutants, the nucleotide sequence of the operator region is altered and is no longer recognized by wild-type repressor protein. In the absence of repressor protein bound to the operator sequence, constitutive transcription of the operon genes takes place and β-galactosidase and permease are produced continuously.

The crucial experiments revealing the cis-acting nature of *lacO* were performed with partial diploids. First it was shown that creation of partial diploids by conjugation of a constitutive lac^+ strain ($I^+ P^+ O^C Z^+ Y^+$) with a lac^- strain producing defective β-galactosidase ($I^+ P^+ O^+ Z^- Y^+$) does not alter the constitutive transcription of β-galactosidase. Note that $lacO^C$ in the partial diploid appears dominant to $lacO^+$. Dominance on the part of $lacO^C$ arises because transcription of the wild-type $lacZ^+$ allele is exclusively controlled by the $lacO^C$ mutation, since these two alleles are on the same chromosome. The wild-type operator has no effect on the $lacZ^+$ allele because operator DNA is a cis-acting element, not a trans-acting element.

In a second experiment, the *lacZ* alleles were on different chromosomes (Z^+ was with O^+ and Z^- was with O^C), and the partial diploid genotype F' $I^+ P^+ O^C Z^- Y^+$/$I^+ P^+ O^+ Z^+ Y^-$ was produced using two lac^- strains. In this case, the F' strain is constitutive for permease production but does not produce functional β-galactosidase due to a *lacZ* mutation. The bacterial recipient strain produces β-galactosidase by the wild-type inducible mechanism, but it does not produce functional permease, due to mutation of *lacY*. The partial diploid produces permease constitutively, but β-galactosidase is produced only when transcription is induced by lactose. This result could occur only if the operator is a cis-acting element. In this case, because the operator allele in cis to Z^+ is wild type, β-galactosidase production

Table 12.4	Synthesis of β-Galactosidase and Permease by Haploids and Partial Diploids with Regulatory Mutations				
Genotype	**β-Galactosidase**		**Permease**		**Description**
	Lactose	No Lactose	Lactose	No Lactose	
$I^- P^+ O^+ Z^+ Y^+$	+	+	+	+	Constitutive transcription due to *lacI^-* mutation.
$I^+ P^+ O^C Z^+ Y^+$	+	+	+	+	Constitutive transcription due to *lacO^C* mutation.
$I^S P^+ O^+ Z^+ Y^+$	−	−	−	−	Transcription is not inducible, due to *lacI^S* mutation.
$I^+ P^- O^+ Z^+ Y^+$	−	−	−	−	No effective transcription, due to *lacP^-* mutation.

falls under the inducible control of the wild-type operator sequence. Notice that in this partial diploid, the wild-type operator appears to be dominant to the O^C mutant.

The apparent difference in the dominance relationship of O^+ and O^C alleles is understandable if the *lac* operator is a cis-acting element that only controls the transcription of genes on the same DNA molecule. Taken together, the two experiments reveal the *lac* operator to be **cis-dominant**, meaning that the only genes the operator is able to influence are genes located downstream on the same gene. For the *lac* operon, the "dominant" operator allele can differ, depending on the alleles for the structural genes carried on each chromosome. If both wild-type structural genes are in cis to *lacO^C*, the mutant operator is dominant because it constitutively transcribes both genes. This is the case in the first experiment. On the other hand, if wild-type structural genes are on different chromosomes, as in the second experiment, then the *lacO^+* allele is dominant because it exerts inducible transcriptional control on one of the two genes required for lactose metabolism.

Constitutive Repressor Protein Mutations Experimental evidence supporting the hypothesis that the repressor gene produces a regulatory protein comes from the analysis of mutants that constitutively transcribe *lac* operon genes where the mutant allele is recessive to the wild-type allele.

To see the dominance relationship of these alleles, let's first consider a haploid cell with the *lac* operon genotype $I^- P^+ O^+ Z^+ Y^+$. This cell constitutively transcribes and produces both β-galactosidase and permease (**Figure 12.8c**). Similarly, a haploid strain with the genotype $I^- P^+ O^+ Z^+ Y^-$ produces β-galactosidase constitutively, but no permease is produced, and bacteria with the genotype $I^- P^+ O^+ Z^- Y^+$ constitutively produce permease but do not produce β-galactosidase.

In contrast, a partial diploid with the genotype F′ $I^+ P^+ O^+ Z^- Y^+/I^- P^+ O^+ Z^+ Y^-$ expresses both enzymes in their normal inducible manner. The I^+ allele can be on either the F′ plasmid or the recipient chromosome and have the same effect, inevitably resulting in the dominance of I^+ over I^-. This outcome indicates that *lacI* produces a regulatory protein that is **trans-acting**—capable of influencing the expression of genes on other chromosomes. In this context, *trans* refers to a protein capable of diffusing through the cell and binding to a cis-acting target sequence.

The molecular explanation of the trans-acting ability of the *lac* repressor protein is that a *lacI^-* mutant alters the DNA-binding domain of the protein, rendering it incapable of binding the operator sequence. In the absence of negative control, transcription is constitutive. In partial diploids that are I^+/I^-, however, repressor protein with a functional DNA-binding domain is present in the cell and responds normally to the addition or removal of lactose from the cell.

Super-Repressor Protein Mutations A second set of repressor protein mutations produces a different consequence

for *lac* operon transcription. These mutants produce mutant repressor protein with an altered allosteric domain. The mutant proteins are unable to bind allolactose and are unresponsive to lactose addition or removal from cells. The DNA-binding domain is unaffected by the allosteric domain mutation, but as a result of the nonfunctional allosteric domain, mutant repressor proteins cannot release the operator even in the presence of allolactose.

Haploids and partial diploids with mutations of the allosteric domain of the repressor protein are identified as I^S mutants and are designated super-repressors. These mutants are **noninducible**, meaning that operon gene transcription cannot be induced (**Figure 12.8d** and Table 12.4). Haploids with the genotype $I^S P^+ O^+ Z^+ Y^+$ produce a repressor protein that binds normally to operator sequence, but lacking a functional allosteric domain, the protein is not removed from the operator by lactose in the cell. Such mutants are *lac^-* and cannot be induced to metabolize lactose. Cultures of partial diploid bacteria with the genotype F′ $I^S P^+ O^+ Z^+ Y^+/I^+ P^+ O^+ Z^+ Y^+$ may initially have some inducible responsiveness to lactose, but this ability is lost as mutant repressor protein binds to operator sequences. This partial diploid reveals the dominance of I^S over I^+.

Promoter Mutations Mutations of promoter consensus sequences significantly reduce transcription or may eliminate it entirely (see Figure 8.12). To know the specific effect of a promoter mutation usually requires direct testing of transcription in the mutant organism. Promoters, like operators, are cis-acting regulatory sequences, and most mutations of *lacP* significantly reduce, and may entirely eliminate, transcription of *lacZ* and *lacY* genes, which are located in cis. This reduces β-galactosidase and permease production to such a low point that haploid bacteria with the genotype $I^+ P^- O^+ Z^+ Y^+$ are *lac^-*.

Table 12.5 summarizes the conditions for *lac* operon gene transcription given the presence or absence of glucose and lactose. Active transcription of operon genes takes place only when glucose is depleted from the cell and lactose is present. Under these conditions, the following events occur:

1. Cyclic AMP level rises as a result of the availability of adenylcyclase.

2. CAP–cAMP complex forms and binds to the CAP site of the *lac* promoter, thus activating transcription.

3. Allolactose is produced by a side reaction of the metabolism of lactose by β-galactosidase.

4. Repressor protein conformation is modified by interaction with allolactose, causing the protein to release from the operator, thus allowing operon gene transcription.

Basal transcription occurs when both glucose and lactose are present, due to the presence of allolactose to bind repressor protein. When lactose is absent, no inducer–repressor complex can form, and no transcription takes

Table 12.5	Transcription Conditions for the *lac* Operon					
Glucose	**Lactose**	**cAMP**	**Allolactose**	***lac* Operon Transcription**	**Explanation**	
Present	Absent	Absent	Absent	None	Glucose is present to provide energy. There is no allolactose to bind repressor. There is no CAP–cAMP complex to bind CAP site.	
Present	Present	Absent	Present	Basal	Glucose is present to provide energy; absence of cAMP prevents positive transcription regulation, but allolactose is present and acts as an inducer to allow a small amount of transcription.	
Absent	Absent	Present	Absent	None	CAP–cAMP forms, but no allolactose is present to block repressor binding at operator.	
Absent	Present	Present	Present	High	Inducer and CAP–cAMP are available to induce and positively regulate transcription.	

place. To test your understanding of the *lac* operon, see **Genetic Analysis 12.1**, which guides you through analysis of some *lac* operon mutants.

Molecular Analysis of the *lac* Operon

In the 50 years since Jacob, Monod, and colleagues described their genetic analysis of the *lac* operon, molecular analysis and genome sequence analysis have identified the DNA sequences of its components (see Figure 12.5b). This and other accumulated molecular information weaves a virtually complete picture of *lac* operon transcription regulation, revealing it to be somewhat more complex than, but wholly consistent with, the description presented above.

Experimental Insight 12.1 discusses two important sets of experimental molecular evidence derived from DNA footprint protection analyses that pertain to transcriptional regulation of the *lac* operon. The first showed that the repressor protein binding location at the *lac* operator overlaps with the promoter binding location of RNA polymerase. This observation supports the hypothesis that repressor protein binding blocks RNA polymerase binding and transcription initiation and, conversely, that when the repressor protein is not bound to the operator, RNA polymerase can access and initiate transcription at the promoter. The second set of results identifies three segments of operator DNA sequence. These operator segments, designated O_1, O_2, and O_3, interact with the repressor protein, and the nature of the interactions suggests a mechanism by which repressor protein binding can block RNA polymerase access to the promoter.

Additional molecular analysis reveals that the repressor protein is a homotetrameric HTH protein formed by the union of four identical 360–amino acid polypeptides (**Figure 12.9**). The four polypeptides are joined together

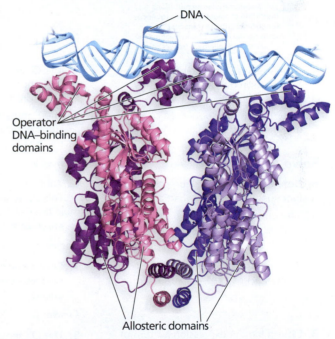

Figure 12.9   The homotetrameric structure of the *lac* repressor protein. Operator binding and allosteric domains are formed on opposite sides of the protein.

at their C-terminal ends and are arranged as two identical bundles. One end of each bundle forms an operator DNA–binding domain (identified as the "recognition helix" in Figure 12.3), and the other end forms the regulatory domain (identified as the "stabilizing domain" in Figure 12.3. The regulatory domain also contains an allosteric domain where allolactose can bind. The three operator DNA segments that are the targets of repressor protein binding share a conserved 21-bp inverted repeat sequence. In each sequence, a central G–C base pair is at the midpoint of a twofold axis

PROBLEM Evaluate the following *lac* operon partial diploids. Indicate whether the production of functional β-galactosidase from *lacZ* and of permease from *lacY* is "inducible," "constitutive," or "noninducible" for each partial diploid.

a. $I^- P^+ O^+ Z^+ Y^+/I^+ P^+ O^+ Z^- Y^-$

b. $I^+ P^+ O^C Z^+ Y^-/I^+ P^+ O^+ Z^- Y^+$

c. $I^+ P^+ O^C Z^- Y^+/I^S P^+ O^+ Z^+ Y^+$

> **BREAK IT DOWN:** Partial diploids have two copies of each *lac* operon gene and regulatory sequence. Success evaluating the *lac* operon depends on knowing the function of each operon component. Study Table 12.4 thoroughly (p. 449).

> **BREAK IT DOWN:** The transcription of *lac* genes is inducible if it is responsive to lactose presence and absence, constitutive if it is always on regardless of lactose availability, or noninducible if it cannot be activated (pp. 451–453).

Solution Strategies	Solution Steps
Evaluate	
1. Identify the topic this problem addresses and the nature of the required answer.	1. This problem concerns an analysis of patterns of transcriptional regulation and the production of functional β-galactosidase and permease by *lac* operon genotypes. The answer requires a determination of whether the enzymes are produced inducibly, constitutively, or not at all.
2. Identify the critical information given in the problem.	2. The *lac* operon genotypes of three partial diploids are given.
Deduce	
3. Describe the consequences of any mutations in genotype *a*.	3. The I^- mutation produces a repressor protein that is unable to bind operator sequence. The Z^- mutation will not produce functional β-galactosidase, and the Y^- mutation will not produce functional permease.
TIP: Assess regulatory mutations first; then consider the consequences for structural gene transcription in each partial diploid by evaluating the effect of each allele on transcription.	PITFALL: You must understand the wild-type function of each operon component before evaluating genotypes. Do not attempt to memorize patterns of "+" and "−" for operon components in hopes of determining *lac*+ or *lac*− phenotypes.
4. Describe the consequences of any mutations in genotype *b*.	4. The O^C mutation alters the operator sequence and prevents binding and transcriptional repression by repressor protein. The Z^- and Y^- mutations block production of functional β-galactosidase and permease.
5. Describe the consequences of any mutations in genotype *c*.	5. The I^S mutation produces a super-repressor protein that has an altered allosteric domain and will not interact with allolactose. The O^C and Z^- alter function as described above.
Solve	Answer a
6. Determine the expression pattern of functional enzymes for partial diploid *a*.	6. Wild-type repressor protein is trans-active and binds the wild-type operator. This cis-acting operator blocks transcription of Z^+ and Y^+ when lactose is not in the cell, but permits transcription when lactose is present. Therefore, both enzymes are produced inducibly.
	Answer b
7. Determine the expression pattern of functional enzymes for partial diploid *b*.	7. O^C is cis-active on Z^+, resulting in constitutive transcription. Y^+ is under the cis-active transcriptional control of O^+. Therefore, β-galactosidase is produced constitutively, and permease is produced inducibly.
	Answer c
8. Determine the expression pattern of functional enzymes for partial diploid *c*.	8. The O^C sequence is not recognized by either the wild-type repressor or the super-repressor. Both repressors have wild-type DNA-binding sequences. Cis-active O^C constitutively transcribes Y^+. The super-repressor binds O^+, and its cis activity renders Z^+ and Y^+ noninducible. Therefore, β-galactosidase is noninducible, and permease production is constitutive.

EXPERIMENTAL INSIGHT 12.1

Regulatory Proteins Binding to *lac* Operon Regulatory Sequences

DNase I footprint protection analysis of the kind described in Research Technique 8.1 has been used to precisely identify the binding location of Lac repressor protein relative to the location of RNA polymerase binding in the regulatory region of the *lac* operon. Identical control and experimental DNA fragments containing regulatory sequences are end-labeled with ^{32}P. The experimental fragments are then exposed to DNA-binding proteins, but the control fragments are not. All fragments are then exposed to DNase I that randomly digests those segments not protected by bound proteins. The resulting DNase I–digested DNA fragments are separated by gel electrophoresis to reveal the "footprint" of protein protection.

The figure here shows the results of footprint analysis of a 123-bp segment of the *lac* operon regulatory region from position +39 to 84. Control DNA in the first lane **①** is not protein-protected. The gel shows that the promoter regions protected by **②** RNA polymerase and **③** Lac repressor protein partially overlap one another. The relative positions of these protein-protected regions are consistent with the model that repressor protein binding can interfere with RNA polymerase binding.

Separate DNase I footprint analysis of the *lac* operator region detects three segments of DNA sequence that are protected by Lac repressor protein: O_1, O_2, O_3. Lane a of

the gel shown is control DNA not bound by protein, and is therefore unprotected DNA. The experimental analysis identifies one protected segment, designated O_1, as the principal operator sequence. The two other regions of protein-protected operator DNA sequence are designated O_2 and O_3. Lanes b through g of the DNA footprint-protection gel are protected by repressor protein at changing concentrations that are lowest in lane b and highest in lane f. The photo shows the footprint gaps corresponding to these operator elements.

Lanes of the gel also identify two regions, designated C_1 and C_2, that are protected from DNase I digestion by the CAP–cAMP complex. These segments contain the consensus sequences for the CAP binding site that partially overlaps operator regions O_1 and O_3. The relative positions of these protein-binding sites indicate two kinds of interactions between proteins binding the *lac* promoter and operator. First, when CAP–cAMP is bound to the CAP binding site, RNA polymerase gains enhanced access to the promoter, establishing conditions for efficient transcription of *lac* operon genes. Second, the overlap of the CAP binding region with O_1 suggests that when repressor protein is bound to DNA, the CAP–cAMP complex is unable to bind, thus preventing positive regulation of transcription.

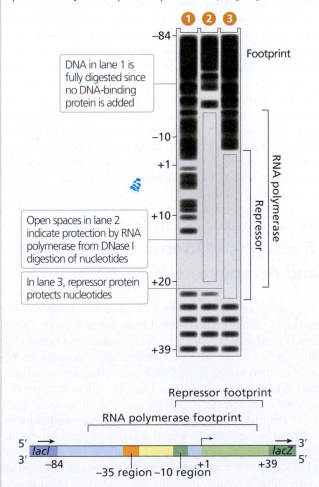

DNase I footprint protection analysis of the *lacP* and *lacO* regions and model.

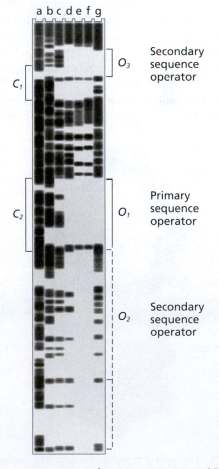

Lac repressor protein footprint protection and DNA binding.

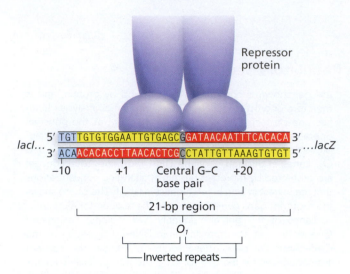

Figure 12.10 **The *lacO* region O_1 containing an inverted repeat sequence.** The central G–C base pair is the pivot point of this region of twofold nucleotide symmetry of an inverted repeat sequence.

Q Offer an explanation of why the two halves of the Lac repressor protein bind to an inverted repeat sequence.

of symmetry (**Figure 12.10**). On either side of the central G–C base pair are inverted repeat sequences of 10 bp each that are the specific binding location for polypeptides in each half of the repressor protein. Nevertheless, their interaction with the protein is such that O_1 must be bound before binding to O_3 can occur. Mitchell Lewis and his colleagues examined the crystal structure of DNA-bound repressor protein in a 1996 study and determined that the tetrameric repressor protein binds to O_1 and O_3 and induces **DNA loop** formation that draws the O_1 and O_3 regions closer together (**Figure 12.11**). This DNA loop structure contains part of the

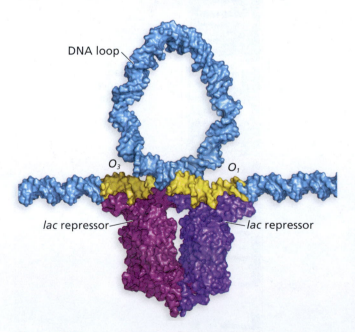

Figure 12.11 **Lac repressor protein binding.** The crystal structural model of Lac repressor binding at *lacO*.

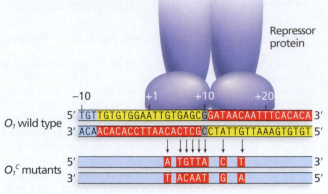

Figure 12.12 **Constitutive operator (O^C) mutations.** Eight different base-substitution mutations in *lacO* region O_1 that each produce operator-constitutive mutations. Each mutation disrupts the twofold symmetry of the operator inverted repeat sequences and prevents Lac repressor protein binding.

lac promoter and prevents transcription by blocking access of RNA polymerase.

Parallel experiments examining mutated operator DNA sequences reveal how constitutive operator mutations are caused by alterations of the DNA sequence in region O_1. **Figure 12.12** shows several base-pair substitutions that cause constitutive operator (O^C) mutations. Each of these changes disrupts the twofold symmetry of O_1, masking the sequence from recognition by repressor protein. Since O_1 is the primary binding target of the repressor protein and must be bound before binding to O_3 can occur, O_1 mutation also disrupts binding to O_3. The inability of repressor protein to bind to mutant operator sequence means that the transcription-repressing DNA loop cannot form. This in turn leaves the promoter available for binding by RNA polymerase and opens the door to continuous transcription and constitutive expression of the *lac* operon genes.

12.4 Transcription from the Tryptophan Operon Is Repressible and Attenuated

The *lac* operon is an example of an inducible operon that produces proteins responsible for the breakdown of a sugar that is an alternative energy source to glucose. Operons like *lac* that are involved in catabolism of alternative energy sources are typically inducible, because they are called upon only when glucose is depleted and the alternative sugar is available. In contrast, operons involved in anabolic pathways (pathways that synthesize compounds needed by the cell) can be regulated by negative feedback mechanisms that operate through activity of the end product of the pathway to block operon gene transcription. Operons of this kind are **repressible operons**, meaning that transcription of operon genes can be repressed by a negative feedback mechanism.

In addition to the negative feedback mechanism, certain repressible operons have a second regulatory capability known as **attenuation** that has the ability to fine-tune transcription to match the moment-to-moment requirements of the cell, achieving a more-or-less steady state of compound availability. The difference between attenuation and inducibility can be clarified by an analogy. Inducible operons, such as *lac*, are akin to light switches that provide illumination in one setting ("on") and no illumination in the alternative setting ("off"). Inducible operons are turned on and off by molecular switches controlled by DNA-binding proteins. Attenuation, on the other hand, works more like a dimmer switch that allows illumination to be incrementally adjusted up or down. For several amino acid operons, the regulation of gene expression has evolved to maintain steady amino acid levels in cells. In such systems, feedback inhibition turns off operon gene transcription when the amino acid is readily available, and attenuation fine-tunes the amino acid level to maintain a steady-state concentration.

Feedback Inhibition of Tryptophan Synthesis

The tryptophan (*trp*) operon ("trip operon") in the *E. coli* genome contains five structural genes that share a regulatory region containing a promoter (*trpP*), an operator (*trpO*), and a **leader region** (*trpL*) that contains the **attenuator region** (**Figure 12.13**). The regulatory region spans 312 base pairs, and the five structural genes span approximately 6800 base

pairs. The five structural genes transcribed in the operon are, in order, *trpE*, *trpD*, *trpC*, *trpB*, and *trpA*. Together, the protein products of these genes are responsible for synthesis of the amino acid tryptophan. Outside the operon, a sixth gene, *trpR*, encodes the repressor protein that is not activated until it pairs with tryptophan.

Transcription of *trp* operon genes is regulated by a feedback inhibition system that responds to free tryptophan in the cell. In this system, tryptophan acts as a corepressor by binding to and activating the Trp repressor protein that is not active without its bound corepressor. Feedback inhibition is the principal mechanism turning on and turning off *trp* operon gene transcription (**Figure 12.14**). In the absence of tryptophan, the inactive repressor is unable to bind *trpO*, and operon gene transcription takes place. When tryptophan is present, however, it binds the repressor to activate it, and the repressor–corepressor complex binds the operator to block transcription. This is an efficient mechanism that shuts down transcription of genes whose expression is not needed at the moment. Such systems have evolved because they save metabolic energy that would otherwise be wasted transcribing unneeded mRNA and later recycling the unused transcript.

Based on this description, and knowing about the feedback inhibition of gene transcription, one might expect that *trpR⁻* bacteria that are mutant for the repressor protein would show constitutive transcription of operon genes regardless of whether tryptophan is present. Surprisingly, however, this is not the case. In wild-type bacteria (*trpR⁺*),

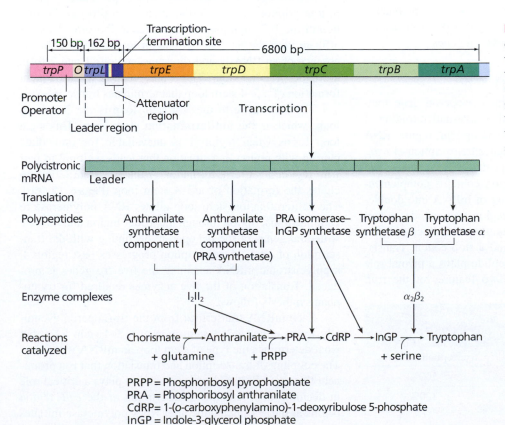

Figure 12.13 **The tryptophan (*trp*) operon.** Transcription is initiated from the promoter *trpP* and progresses through the tryptophan leader (*trpL*) region to transcribe the five operon genes (*trpE* to *trpA*) into a polycistronic mRNA. The protein products of the operon genes catalyze successive steps of tryptophan synthesis.

PRPP = Phosphoribosyl pyrophosphate
PRA = Phosphoribosyl anthranilate
CdRP = 1-(*o*-carboxyphenylamino)-1-deoxyribulose 5-phosphate
InGP = Indole-3-glycerol phosphate

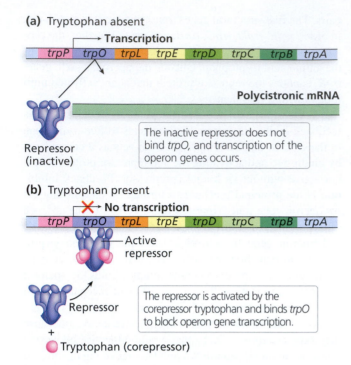

Figure 12.14 *Trp* operon transcription regulation by the repressor, with tryptophan absent (a) and with tryptophan present (b).

tryptophan synthesis is very low when tryptophan is present in the cell, but whereas tryptophan synthesis by $trpR^-$ strains is higher under the same conditions, it is not at 100% capacity (**Table 12.6**). Both $trpR^+$ and $trpR^-$ strains synthesize tryptophan at 100% of capacity when tryptophan is absent. This suggests that a second regulatory mechanism is also affecting transcription of *trp* operon genes.

Attenuation of the *trp* Operon

The second mechanism regulating *trp* operon gene transcription is attenuation, controlled by alternative folding of the mRNA synthesized from the 162-bp *trpL* region. RNA polymerase binds to *trpP* and initiates transcription of *trpL*. The *trpL* region contains four repeat DNA sequences, and the mRNA transcript of this region contains complementary repeats that lead to the folding of mRNA into double-stranded regions. The *trp* leader region also encodes a start codon, a short polypeptide of 14 amino acids (including the methionine of the start codon), and a stop codon. Translation of this 14–amino acid polypeptide plays a pivotal role in attenuation (**Figure 12.15a**). Two features of the *trpL*

Table 12.6	Percentage of Full Tryptophan Expression for $trpR^+$ and $trpR^-$ Strains	
	Tryptophan Present	**Tryptophan Absent**
$trpR^+$	8%	100%
$trpR^-$	33%	100%

region are critical to its attenuation function. First, the four repeat sequences, designated 1, 2, 3, and 4, can form different stem-loop structures (**Figure 12.15b–d**). (Stem-loop structures are discussed in Section 8.2 in connection with intrinsic transcription termination in bacteria; see Figure 8.7.) Second, among the codons for the 14 amino acids encoded by *trpL* mRNA, there are two back-to-back tryptophan codons (UGG) that function to sense the availability of tryptophan and are essential for attenuation.

The formation of stem loops of *trpL* mRNA is directly tied to the continuation or termination of transcription of the five *trp* operon genes. In the *trpL* region mRNA, region 1 is complementary to region 2, region 2 is complementary to region 3, and region 3 is complementary to region 4. Two of these stem-loop structures, the *3–4 stem loop* and the *2–3 stem loop*, are central to attenuation. The third type of stem loop, the *1–2 stem loop*, plays a minor role in attenuation.

The **3–4 stem loop** of mRNA, which is the **termination stem loop**, signals transcription termination. This is identified as the transcription termination site in Figure 12.15. Formation of the 3–4 stem loop halts RNA polymerase progress along the DNA, terminating transcription in the leader region before it reaches the structural genes of the operon (**Figure 12.16a**). Notice that region 4 is followed immediately by a poly-uracil sequence (a poly-U tail). This configuration—an mRNA stem loop followed by a uracil string—is the same as one described in connection with intrinsic termination of transcription in bacteria (see Figure 8.7). Formation of a 3–4 stem loop may be accompanied by formation of a 1–2 stem loop, which can induce a pause in transcription, as part of the attenuation process. Formation of the 1–2 stem loop occurs when a ribosome does not affiliate with the nascent *trp* operon leader mRNA. In the absence of an RNA-bound ribosome, regions 1 and 2 form a double-stranded stem. This leads, in turn, to subsequent formation of a 3–4 stem loop that terminates transcription.

The alternative to the 3–4 stem loop is the **2–3 stem loop**, which is the **antitermination stem loop**. This stem loop forms when region 1 is unavailable for immediate pairing with region 2, a situation that leads region 2 to pair with region 3. In turn, formation of the 2–3 stem loop precludes the formation of a 3–4 stem loop (**Figure 12.16b**). The antitermination stem loop allows RNA polymerase to continue transcription through the leader region and into the structural genes of the *trp* operon, beginning with the transcription of *trpE*. If transcription progresses past region 4, a polycistronic mRNA spanning the five *trp* genes is produced. Translation of the five enzymes required for tryptophan synthesis follows.

Each mRNA transcribed from the *trpL* operon eventually forms either a 2–3 stem loop or a 3–4 stem loop, but what determines the type of stem loop an mRNA will form? The coupling of transcription and translation that is a prominent feature of bacterial gene expression plays a critical role in deciding this outcome. Transcription of the *trpL* region begins at the +1 nucleotide after RNA polymerase initiates

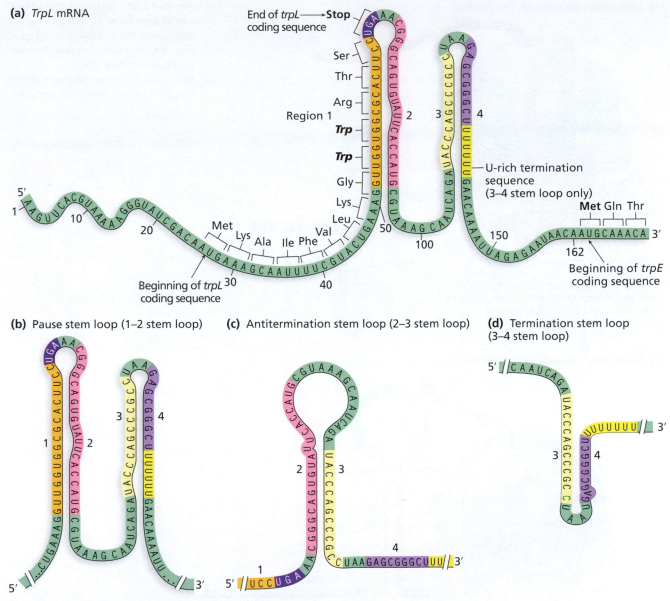

Figure 12.15 **The *trpL* attenuator region mRNA transcript. (a)** The *trpL* attenuator contains 162 nucleotides that include a 14-amino acid coding sequence and four inverted repeat sequences that encode regions 1 through 4 in *trpL* mRNA. **(b–d)** Three alternative stem loops can form in *trpL* mRNA.

transcription. Transcription across repeat regions 1 and 2 can lead to formation of a 1–2 stem loop that temporarily pauses the progress of RNA polymerase. The pause is only momentary, however; it lasts just long enough for a ribosome to bind at the start codon in *trpL* and begin translation of the 14–amino acid polypeptide starting with the AUG codon identified in Figure 12.15. Translation initiation breaks the 1–2 stem loop, RNA polymerase resumes transcription, and the ribosome and RNA polymerase begin their coupled progression.

Notice three features of the leader mRNA depicted in Figures 12.15 and 12.16: (1) The polypeptide-coding sequence overlaps the entirety of leader region 1, and the stop codon is immediately adjacent to region 2; (2) codons 10 and 11 of the mRNA specify tryptophan, making completion of translation dependent on tryptophan availability; and (3) region 4 is followed immediately by a poly-U string, a feature associated with intrinsic termination of transcription. As coupled transcription and translation proceed, the relative positions of RNA polymerase and the ribosome are determined by how efficiently the ribosome can progress along the mRNA. This process, in turn, is tied directly to the availability of tryptophan and the rapidity with which tryptophan is inserted into the nascent polypeptide chain. When the cell has an adequate supply of tryptophan, the ribosome makes steady progress along *trpL* mRNA until it arrives at the stop codon, where it partially overlies region 1 and region 2. Simultaneously, RNA polymerase is transcribing

(a) Tryptophan abundance: Termination

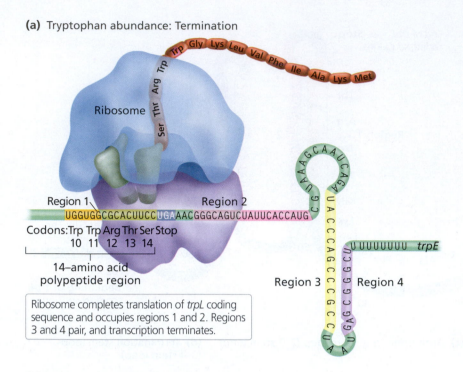

Ribosome completes translation of *trpL* coding sequence and occupies regions 1 and 2. Regions 3 and 4 pair, and transcription terminates.

(b) Tryptophan starvation: Antitermination

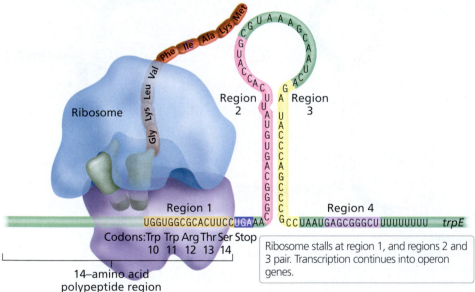

Ribosome stalls at region 1, and regions 2 and 3 pair. Transcription continues into operon genes.

Figure 12.16 Determination of *trpL* mRNA stem loop. **(a)** In tryptophan abundance, the 3–4 (termination) stem loop terminates transcription after the poly-U string. **(b)** In tryptophan starvation, the 2–3 (antitermination) stem loop leads to polycistronic mRNA synthesis.

Q If codons 10 and 11 shown in (b) were GGG (Gly) instead of UGG (Trp), would antitermination still occur at a low level of tryptophan? Why or why not?

region 3, followed by region 4. With a portion of region 2 occupied by the ribosome and unavailable for pairing in a stem loop, region 3 forms a stem loop with region 4, the only available complementary segment of the mRNA. The 3–4 stem loop, being immediately followed by a poly-U string, causes transcription to spontaneously terminate at the end of region 4 by the intrinsic process. Formation of the 3–4 stem loop (the termination stem loop) stops transcription of the *trp* operon in the leader sequence before RNA polymerase reaches the beginning of the *trpE* gene. Transcription thus ceases only when the system senses that no additional tryptophan is needed to supply translation.

When the cell is starved for tryptophan, the supply of charged tRNA^Trp is low. The ribosome is forced to pause momentarily at codons 10 and 11 to await the arrival of a charged tryptophan tRNA that will incorporate tryptophan into the nascent polypeptide. As the ribosome pauses, its mass covers region 1. Meanwhile, RNA polymerase continues to transcribe *trpL*. As RNA polymerase transcribes region 3, the region 3 mRNA finds a complementary partner in region 2, leading to 2–3 stem-loop formation. Region 3 is not followed by a poly-U string, making intrinsic termination impossible. Transcription continues through region 4 and on into the structural gene region of the operon to produce the polycistronic mRNA transcript of the operon. Formation of a 2–3 stem loop (the antitermination stem loop) thus permits transcription and translation of the enzymes necessary to synthesize tryptophan when the system senses that the available supply of tryptophan is insufficient to support translation.

Each *trpL* mRNA makes a molecularly based "decision" about whether to form a 3–4 or a 2–3 stem loop, depending on the availability of charged $tRNA^{Trp}$ at the moment $tRNA^{Trp}$ is needed by ribosomes. It is likely that at any given moment in time, a single bacterial cell contains a mixture of *trpL* mRNAs with 2–3 stem loops and *trpL* mRNAs with 3–4 stem loops. The balance shifts in the direction of more 3–4 stem loops and fewer 2–3 stem loops at higher levels of tryptophan concentration and shifts in the opposite direction—more 2–3 stem loops and fewer 3–4 stem loops—as tryptophan concentration falls. The resulting fine-tuning allows each cell to maintain a relatively steady concentration of tryptophan by turning tryptophan synthesis up or down to meet the needs of the cell.

Attenuation Mutations

The attenuation model is supported by mutagenesis experiments. For example, experiments altering one or both of the two adjacent tryptophan codons (in positions 10 and 11 of the *trpL* mRNA) by missense mutation to specify another amino acid have provided evidence of the importance of the back-to-back tryptophan codons in the *trpL* transcript. Mutation of one tryptophan UGG codon affects the attenuator responsiveness to tryptophan. If both tryptophan codons are altered by missense mutation, the attenuator no longer senses tryptophan concentration and instead senses the availability of the amino acid encoded by the mutated codons. Mutagenesis experiments have also targeted regions 3 and 4 of the leader sequence (**Figure 12.17**). Base substitutions that reduce the percentage of complementary base pairs binding these two regions destabilize the termination stem loop and reduce the efficiency of the mutated operon system in repressing structural gene transcription. **Genetic Analysis 12.2** examines mutations of the *trp* operon.

Remainder of
trpL mRNA
Nucleotide position 110
Poly-U string
140
UUUUUU
Region 3
Region 4
Mutations that reduce complementarity
125

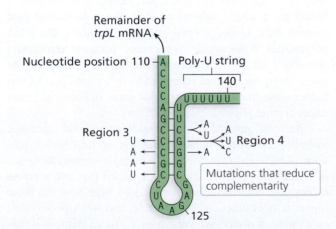

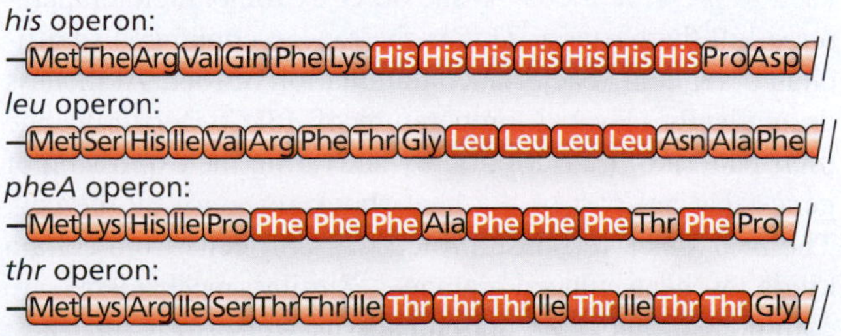

Figure 12.17 Mutations of *trpL*. Mutational analyses identify 10 base-pair substitutions in regions 3 and 4 of *trpL* that each decrease the efficiency of transcriptional regulation in the attenuator region by disrupting formation of the 3–4 stem loop.

Attenuation in Other Amino Acid Operon Systems

Attenuation represses transcription of structural genes in several amino acid operon systems in bacteria such as *E. coli* and *Salmonella typhimurium*. Like the *trp* operon, these other amino acid operons also contain multiple codons for the target amino acid in their leader transcripts (**Figure 12.18**). For example, the leader polypeptide of the *E. coli* histidine operon contains a run of seven consecutive histidine residues in the attenuator. Similarly, the phenylalanine leader polypeptide contains seven phenylalanine residues in a span of nine amino acids in the attenuator region. Like the *trp* operon, these operons use attenuation based on the formation of antitermination stem loops to regulate operon gene transcription.

12.5 Bacteria Regulate the Transcription of Stress Response Genes and Also Translation

The need on the part of bacteria to respond rapidly to changing environmental conditions suggests that transcriptional regulation must accommodate both common and rare circumstances, and also that the regulation of translation must be available under certain circumstances. This section presents examples of transcriptional regulation in bacteria under rarely encountered conditions and then describes how bacteria regulate translation.

Alternative Sigma Factors and Stress Response

The operon mechanisms described to this point are examples of the regulatory strategies employed by bacterial cells under conditions they encounter routinely. In response to rare or unusual environmental circumstances, however,

his operon:
Met The Arg Val Gln Phe Lys His His His His His His His Pro Asp
leu operon:
Met Ser His Ile Val Arg Phe Thr Gly Leu Leu Leu Leu Asn Ala Phe
pheA operon:
Met Lys His Ile Pro Phe Phe Phe Ala Phe Phe Phe Thr Phe Pro
thr operon:
Met Lys Arg Ile Ser Thr Thr Ile Thr Thr Thr Ile Thr Ile Thr Thr Gly

Figure 12.18 Four bacterial amino acid operons with attenuator control of transcription. The regulatory amino acid for each operon is shown in bright red.

PROBLEM Describe the effects on attenuation and on tryptophan synthesis of the following mutations of the tryptophan codons (UGG) in the attenuator region of the *trp* operon.

a. The tryptophan codons are mutated to UAGUGG.
b. The tryptophan codons are mutated to UUGUUG.

> **BREAK IT DOWN:** You should be able to define *attenuation* and to describe how the presence of two tryptophan codons in the *trp* operon leader transcript participates in determining whether the termination (3–4) stem loop or the antitermination (2–3) stem loop forms in the transcript. See Figure 12.16 (p. 458).

Solution Strategies	Solution Steps
Evaluate	
1. Identify the topic this problem addresses and the nature of the required answer.	1. This problem concerns the consequences of mutations to the UGG (tryptophan) codons in the attenuator region of the *trp* operon. The answer requires a description of mutational consequences for tryptophan regulation and synthesis.
2. Identify the critical information given in the problem.	2. The mutant codon sequences are given.
Deduce	
3. Examine the nature of the mutation in part (a).	3. The base substitution in mutant (a) creates a stop codon in place of the first tryptophan codon.
4. Examine the nature of the mutation in part (b).	4. Two base substitutions are seen in mutant (b). Each creates a leucine codon in place of a tryptophan codon.
Solve	Answer a
5. Describe the consequence of the mutation in part (a).	5. UAG is a stop codon that halts translation of the polypeptide. The location of this stop codon will prevent the ribosome from covering repeat region 2. The 2–3 stem loop is the only regulatory configuration that can form, and it will lead to constitutive tryptophan synthesis.
TIP: Compare the transcription of the wild-type operon to that of this mutant operon (see Figures 12.15 and 12.16).	Answer b
6. Describe the consequence of the mutation in part (b).	6. Both mutant codons in this case encode leucine. These mutational changes will prevent attenuation of the *trp* operon in response to tryptophan level. Instead, tryptophan synthesis will attenuate in response to the level of leucine, since the availability of leucine to add to the polypeptide will determine which stem loop will form.

For more practice, see Problems 7, 15 and 25.   Visit the Study Area to access study tools.   **Mastering Genetics**

---

bacteria switch gene transcription patterns to use genes that are not normally expressed. The response of *E. coli* to heat stress illustrates how expression of an *alternative sigma* (σ) *factor* alters gene transcription by activating the transcription of specialized heat stress response genes.

Escherichia coli grow vigorously at 37°C and can tolerate only narrow temperature variation. At low temperatures, their growth slows—an important reason refrigeration is used to preserve foods. At the other extreme, high temperatures kill the bacteria. This is the reason cooking is so efficient at reducing bacterial contamination of food. At the less dramatically elevated temperature of 45°C, *E. coli* change their pattern of transcription by activating the expression of genes that are part of the heat shock response by the cell. The heat shock response protects *E. coli* cells from certain kinds of heat-induced damage. Similar mechanisms are common in other microorganisms as well as in fruit flies, plants, and animals, including humans.

Heat shock response in bacteria involves expression of an **alternative sigma (σ) subunit** that changes the promoter-recognition capacity of the RNA polymerase core enzyme. Recall that the RNA polymerase core enzyme is bound by a sigma subunit to form the holoenzyme (see Section 8.2). Under normal growth conditions, the RNA polymerase holoenzyme recognizes bacterial promoters containing an AT-rich Pribnow box at the -10 site. The common sigma subunit, identified as σ^{70}, forms part of this holoenzyme that transcribes a wide array of bacterial genes under normal physiological conditions.

Bacteria grown at 45°C undergo several changes, including initiation of the expression of heat shock proteins, which are expressed only at high temperature, and of chaperone proteins, a class of proteins that either refold or degrade other proteins damaged by high heat. At these higher temperatures, σ^{70} is unstable, and RNA polymerase containing it functions very poorly. To explain the transcription of heat shock proteins in the presence of poorly functioning σ^{70}-containing RNA polymerase, researchers proposed and quickly found genetic evidence pointing to an alternative, high-temperature σ subunit.

(a) Promoter sequences recognized by different sigma factors

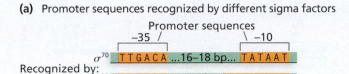

(b) Events at elevated temperature

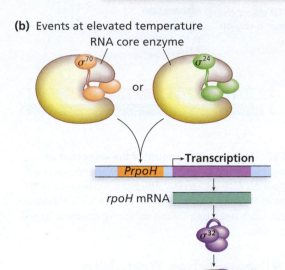

Figure 12.19 **Alternative sigma factors for heat shock genes.** (a) Promoter sequences recognized by σ^{70}- and σ^{32}-containing RNA polymerase. (b) At elevated temperature, σ^{70} and σ^{24} transcribe *rpoH*, which encodes σ^{32} that in turn joins the RNA core enzyme to transcribe heat shock genes.

The evidence came from studies of mutant, temperature-sensitive *E. coli* that grow normally at 37°C but fail to grow at 45°C. This temperature sensitivity is a conditional lethal mutation affecting a gene called *rpoH*, which encodes an alternative sigma subunit known as σ^{32}. When σ^{32} binds an RNA polymerase core enzyme, the resulting holoenzyme recognizes different promoter sequences than are recognized by holoenzymes containing σ^{70} (**Figure 12.19**). In contrast to the AT richness that characterizes the Pribnow box sequence of bacterial promoters, the −10 region of promoters recognized by σ^{32}-containing RNA polymerase is rich in G–C base pairs.

The promoter for *rpoH* is recognized by σ^{70}-containing RNA polymerase when the temperature is elevated. The sigma factor translated from *rpoH* mRNA (that is, σ^{32}) is very active in stimulating transcription of heat shock genes. In addition, transcription of a third sigma subunit known as σ^{24}, which is normally present in *E. coli* cells at a very low level, is greatly increased at elevated temperatures. The RNA polymerase holoenzyme containing σ^{24} also recognizes the *rpoH* promoter and transcribes the gene at elevated temperatures that inactivate σ^{70}.

A second transcriptional change that occurs as a consequence of high heat is a change in the chaperon proteins. At normal growth temperatures, several chaperon proteins bind the small amount of σ^{32} present in the cell to inhibit its ability to form holoenzyme. At high temperatures, chaperone proteins release σ^{32}, leaving it free to join an RNA polymerase core enzyme and form a holoenzyme. Free chaperon proteins are redirected to bind heat-damaged cellular proteins instead. In this role, chaperon proteins either degrade the proteins they bind or assist in refolding the proteins.

Several additional examples of the use of alternative sigma factors in bacteria have been described. For example, *Bacillus subtilis* is a bacterium that normally propagates by vegetative growth, but poor growth conditions switch the growth mode to sporulation by activating the expression of alternative sigma factors. The gene transcription evidence shows that as growth conditions deteriorate, transcription of the common sigma factor is replaced by the transcription of two alternative sigma factors. The new sigma factors recognize the promoters for genes used only in sporulation. A broad array of evidence shows that switching transcription from the normal sigma factor to alternative sigma factors induces a genome-wide change in the pattern of gene expression that silences previously active genes and initiates transcription of specialized genes that are used only under restrictive or extreme growth conditions. Table 12.7 compares the mechanisms of gene regulation in bacterial systems.

Translational Regulation in Bacteria

Transcriptional regulation is far and away the predominant mode of controlling gene expression in bacteria, but bacteria are also capable of translational regulation. Translational regulation takes place by two mechanisms, one that binds

Table 12.7	Mechanisms of Transcription Regulation in Bacteria	
Mechanism	**Actions and Outcomes**
Operon-specific control	Inducer substances, such as lactose, and negative feedback mechanisms, such as tryptophan availability, regulate gene transcription in coordinately controlled operons.
CAP–cAMP control	CAP–cAMP is utilized as a positive regulator of transcription for genes in several different operons, including the *lac* operon.
Alternative sigma factors	Extreme growth conditions, such as heat stress and starvation, induce transcription of alternative sigma factors.

protein to an mRNA to prevent its translation and another that pairs complementary *antisense RNA* with the mRNA to block its translation.

Translation repressor proteins regulate translation by binding mRNA in the vicinity of the Shine–Dalgarno sequence. Protein binding in this location interferes with recognition of the Shine–Dalgarno sequence by the 16S rRNA in the small ribosomal subunit and so blocks translation initiation. One of the clearest examples of this kind of regulatory protein–mRNA interaction is seen in the translational regulation of ribosomal proteins in *E. coli*. The ribosomal proteins are encoded in a series of operons that produce polycistronic mRNAs. These operons are under a certain degree of transcriptional regulation, but the most prominent control of production of ribosomal proteins is at the translational level. One of the protein products from each ribosomal protein operon can bind that operon's polycistronic mRNA near the 5'-most Shine–Dalgarno sequence, thus preventing binding of the small ribosomal subunit to the polycistronic mRNA and inhibiting synthesis of the proteins encoded by the operon.

Bacterial translation can also be inhibited by the activity of **antisense RNA**, an RNA molecule that is complementary to a portion of a specific mRNA. The binding of an mRNA by an antisense RNA prevents ribosome attachment to the mRNA and blocks translation. Several examples of bacterial translational regulation by antisense RNA have been described. One of the first-discovered mechanisms of antisense control of translation comes from the regulation of transposase production by the bacterial insertion sequence *IS10*. Transposase is the enzyme that drives the movement of transposable genetic elements in genomes (see Section 11.7). Transposase cuts DNA for transposable element removal and insertion. A low level of transposition can be tolerated by bacterial genomes and may even be advantageous. Excessive transposase expression, however, leads to excessive transposition, which may cause lethal mutations due to transposon insertion into critical genes.

The *IS10* insertion sequence contains two promoters. One, called P_{IN}, is relatively weak and controls transcription of the DNA strand coding for active transposase. The second promoter, P_{OUT}, is much stronger. This promoter is embedded in the transposase gene and directs transcription of the noncoding strand of the gene, producing an antisense RNA that is complementary to the 5' end of transposase mRNA and covers up the Shine–Dalgarno sequence of the mRNA, preventing its recognition by the small ribosomal subunit (**Figure 12.20**). As a consequence of the stronger P_{OUT} promoter, *IS10* antisense RNA is more abundant than transposase mRNA. This results in most of the transposase mRNA being bound by antisense RNA and effectively prevents translation of nearly all transposase mRNA. Nevertheless, an occasional transposase mRNA escapes antisense binding and undergoes translation, generating a low level of transposase that initiates the rare event of *IS10* transposition within the bacterial genome.

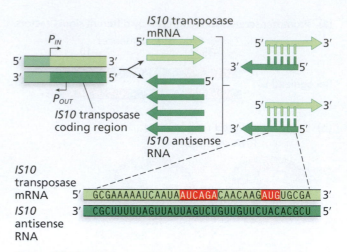

Figure 12.20   Antisense RNA control of the expression of *IS10* transposase. Two promoters each drive the synthesis of a transcript from the *IS10* transposon. The transposase gene mRNA transcript (from P_{IN}) can hybridize with the antisense RNA transcript (from P_{OUT}) to block production of the transposase enzyme by preventing translation.

12.6 Riboswitches Regulate Bacterial Transcription, Translation, and mRNA Stability

In the early 2000s, multiple researchers identified a new gene-regulating mechanism in bacteria. In this regulatory mechanism, called a **riboswitch**, a segment of the mRNA binds a small regulatory molecule. Riboswitches are common in bacteria, regulating the expression of about 5% of genes, including genes that synthesize amino acids, nucleotides, vitamins, and other essential molecules. Bacterial riboswitches regulate transcription and translation and can alter the stability of mRNA. In the years since the discovery of riboswitches in bacteria, suspected riboswitches have been found or proposed in archaeal genomes and in the genomes of fungi, algae, and plants.

Riboswitch Regulation of Transcription

The most common type of riboswitch in bacteria is exemplified by the production of thiamin, also known as vitamin B₁. The active form of the vitamin is a compound known as thiamin pyrophosphate (TPP). Bacterial TPP is produced by a biosynthetic pathway whose genes are located in the thiamin (*thi*) operon. In *Bacillus subtilis*, the *thi* operon uses TPP and a riboswitch located in the 5' UTR of mRNA to produce mRNAs in two configurations that are dependent on TPP concentration. When TPP concentration is low, the amount of TPP is inadequate for binding the riboswitch regulatory sequence of mRNA (**Figure 12.21a**). This leads to the formation of an antitermination stem-loop that allows transcription to progress through the 5' UTR region and into the *thi* operon genes. Transcription generates a polycistronic

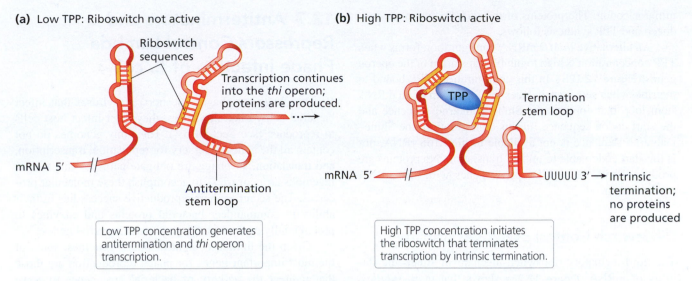

Figure 12.21   Transcriptional regulation by a riboswitch mechanism. (a) Transcription of *thi* operon genes in *Bacillus subtilis* occurs when TPP concentration is low. **(b)** At high TPP concentration, TPP binds to riboswitch sequences, resulting in transcription termination.

mRNA that produces the enzymes used in TPP synthesis. Alternatively, when TPP concentration is high, TPP binds to the riboswitch regulatory sequence (**Figure 12.21b**). This generates a termination stem loop that is immediately followed by a poly-U sequence, leading to intrinsic termination of transcription before RNA polymerase reaches the *thi* operon genes. Because the genes of the *thi* operon are not transcribed, no polycistronic mRNA is generated, and no protein production occurs. The TPP riboswitch is an attenuation mechanism that is able to sense the concentration of TPP so as to produce more when the concentration is low and less as the concentration rises.

Riboswitch Regulation of Translation

The regulation of TPP synthesis in *E. coli* also uses a riboswitch, but in this bacterium TPP production is controlled at the level of translation. The *thiMD* operon in *E. coli* contains genes used for TPP synthesis. When TPP concentration is low, the 5′ UTR region of mRNA folds into a secondary structure that contains a Shine–Dalgarno **antisequestor stem loop** (**Figure 12.22a**). The antisequestor stem loop allows the Shine–Dalgarno sequence to bind to 16S rRNA in the small ribosomal subunit (see Figure 9.7). This places the start codon (AUG) in position to act as the translation

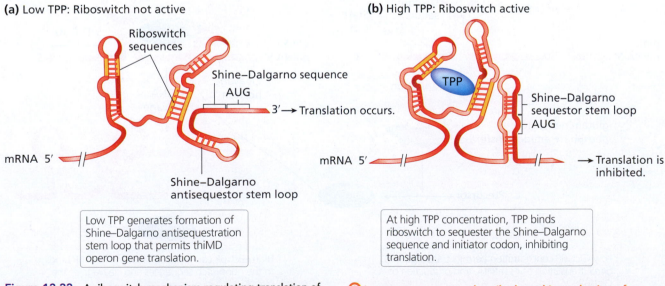

Figure 12.22   A riboswitch mechanism regulating translation of mRNA. (a) TPP is produced by translation of *E. coli thiMD* mRNA at low TPP concentration. **(b)** At high TPP concentration, translation is inhibited by TPP binding to riboswitch sequences.

🔵 **In a sentence or two, describe how this mechanism of riboswitch transcriptional regulation differs from the mechanism illustrated in the previous figure (Figure 12.21).**

initiator codon. The proteins of the *thiMD* operon are produced and TPP synthesis follows.

An alternative *thiMD* mRNA configuration forms when TPP concentration is high to inhibit translation of the operon genes (**Figure 12.22b**). In this configuration, TPP bound to the riboswitch sequence induces the formation of an mRNA stem loop that contains the Shine–Dalgarno sequence and the start codon sequence. In this configuration, the Shine–Dalgarno sequence is not available to bind 16S rRNA, nor is the start codon able to initiate translation. No proteins are produced from the *thiMD* operon genes with this mRNA configuration.

Riboswitch Control of mRNA Stability

The third regulatory riboswitch mechanism affects the stability of mRNA. **Figure 12.23a** shows that in *B. subtilus*, transcription and translation of the *glmS* gene produces the enzyme called glutamine:fructose-6-phosphate amidotransferase. This enzyme participates in the production of a sugar abbreviated as GlcN6P. Transcription of *glmS* and translation of its mRNA occur when the cellular concentration of GlcN6P is low and more is needed in the cell. The riboswitch regulatory activity occurs when GlcN6P concentration is high and no more need be produced. Under this circumstance, GlcN6P binds to the riboswitch sequences in the 5′ UTR of *glmS* mRNA (**Figure 12.23b**). This induces cleavage of the mRNA that prevents it from attaching to a ribosome and undergoing translation.

12.7 Antiterminators and Repressors Control Lambda Phage Infection of *E. coli*

Bacteriophage (or phage, for short) are viruses that infect bacterial cells. Like all viruses, they must infect host cells to reproduce (see Section 6.4). Their tiny genomes do not contain all the genes necessary for replication, transcription, and translation, so phage are obligate parasites that use an ingenious array of tricks to accomplish these molecular processes. The secret to their reproductive success lies in their ability to commandeer bacterial proteins and enzymes to preferentially express phage genes over bacterial genes.

Given the limited content of phage genomes, some of the most important genes for phage reproduction are those that redirect the activity of bacterial host genes to serve phage requirements. Successful phage infection requires (1) that genetic regulatory switches be controlled through phage gene expression to redirect the action of host genes and (2) that phage gene expression initiate a sequence of events leading the bacterium to participate in the expression of phage genetic information. In no bacteriophage is there a clearer picture of the processes that control regulatory genetic switching than in lambda (λ) phage.

Recall that all bacteriophage are capable of infecting and reproducing within the host bacterial cell. The infection ends with the lysis of the host cell, in a process called the lytic cycle (see Figure 6.16). But certain bacteriophage

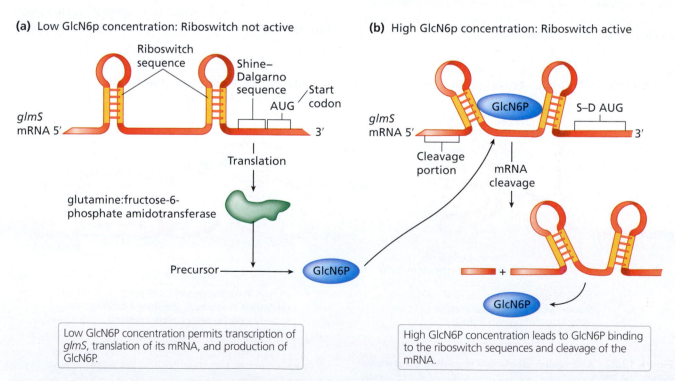

(a) Low GlcN6p concentration: Riboswitch not active

Low GlcN6P concentration permits transcription of *glmS*, translation of its mRNA, and production of GlcN6P.

(b) High GlcN6p concentration: Riboswitch active

High GlcN6P concentration leads to GlcN6P binding to the riboswitch sequences and cleavage of the mRNA.

Figure 12.23   Control of mRNA stability by a riboswitch. (a) Transcription and translation lead to production of GlcN6P in *B. subtilis* when GlcN6P concentration is low. **(b)** When GlcN6P is in high concentration, it binds to riboswitch sequences and generates mRNA cleavage.

known as temperate phage, of which λ phage is an example, are also capable of a lysogenic cycle, or lysogeny. The lysogenic cycle is characterized by integration of the phage into the host chromosome. With integration into a host chromosome, the phage DNA is identified as a *prophage*. Lysogenic integration is site specific, meaning it occurs at a sequence shared by the phage and the bacterial host. The phage enzyme integrase is responsible for lysogenic integration. In this section, we discuss the two life cycles of λ phage, examining the regulatory proteins that control which life cycle a particular infection will undertake, as well as the actions of the proteins that control each life cycle.

The Lambda Phage Genome

The λ phage genome is composed of approximately 48 kb of linear, double-stranded DNA that encodes nearly 60 genes (**Figure 12.24a**). Its injection into a host bacterial cell leads to an immediate circularization inside the host cell that is accomplished by the joining of two single-stranded **cohesive (*cos*) ends** that are each 12 nucleotides in length (**Figure 12.24b**). A host DNA ligase seals the two gaps that are left when the cohesive ends join and produces a circularized λ phage that is ready to begin gene expression.

The λ phage genome is organized as a series of operons. The genes in each operon are expressed in a well-defined sequence. Expression of genes in certain operons begins immediately after circularization. The specific order of gene expression is critical to the ability of λ phage to carry out successful infection of its bacterial host. Consequently, **immediate early genes** are expressed shortly after circularization, **delayed early genes** are expressed next, and **late genes** are expressed later in the infection cycle. These groups of genes are clustered into operons, and each cluster has a shared regulatory region that controls transcription. The transcription of immediate early, delayed early, and late gene regions is determined by binding of two regulatory proteins, one known as an **antiterminator**, whose binding permits gene transcription by preventing transcription termination, and the other protein acting as a repressor that blocks additional transcription.

Immediately following circularization of the λ phage chromosome, **early promoters** and **early operators** control transcription of genes whose protein products interact to determine whether the phage undergoes the lytic cycle or the lysogenic cycle. The lytic cycle results in a rapidly progressing infection leading to lysis (rupture) of the host cell and release of scores of progeny phage. In the lysogenic life cycle, on the other hand, the phage chromosome integrates into the host chromosome, as noted above. Expression of genes in the integrated phage chromosome (the prophage) is minimal; only the genes necessary to maintain lysogeny are expressed. Replication of the bacterial chromosome produces daughter cells that carry a copy of the prophage. Lysogeny continues until the prophage excises itself from its integration site, reactivating phage gene expression and the lytic cycle.

Early Gene Transcription

Upon circularization of the phage chromosome, the two immediate early λ phage genes *N* and *cro* are transcribed, and the N and Cro proteins are translated. Transcription and translation of these genes, as well as all of the other genes we mention, is accomplished by bacterial host proteins and ribosomes because the λ phage genome does not encode these functions. The N protein is the antiterminator protein mentioned above, and the Cro protein is the repressor. These two proteins engage in a molecular tug-of-war for control of a genetic switch that determines whether the infection will result in the lytic cycle or the lysogenic cycle. The early promoter P_R controls rightward transcription of immediate early genes, beginning with the *cro* gene (for control of *r*epressor and *o*thers; **Foundation Figure 12.25** ❶ and Figure 12.24a). The immediate early promoter P_L controls leftward transcription beginning with the *N* gene, whose protein product blocks transcription termination and allows delayed early and late genes to be transcribed ❶.

The antitermination protein N binds to three transcription-terminating DNA sequences: t_L, t_{R1}, and t_{R2} (see Foundation Figure 12.25 ❷). When not bound by N protein, termination sequence t_L acts to block leftward transcription beyond *N*. In the other direction, t_{R1} and t_{R2} prevent rightward transcription beyond *cro* or beyond three other early genes—*cII*, *O*, and *P*. When N protein binds t_L, t_{R1}, and t_{R2}, however, delayed early genes leftward of t_L and rightward of t_{R1} and t_{R2} are transcribed. One of the proteins produced by leftward transcription is integrase (the product of the *int* gene), which is required for prophage integration into the bacterial chromosome. In the other direction, rightward transcription produces protein cII, which forms a complex with protein cIII, one of the products of leftward transcription ❸. Together, the cII/cIII complex binds to the promoter P_{RE} (for *r*epressor *e*stablishment). This promoter initiates leftward transcription of the *cI* gene, producing the cI protein, which is also known as the λ repressor protein (Foundation Figure 12.25 ❹ and ❺).

Before the lytic cycle or the lysogenic cycle of infection can begin, two critical molecular "decisions" have to be made. The first of these decisions involves determining whether bacteria are actively growing. With active bacterial growth, lysis is favored because new progeny phage will readily find new host cells. If bacteria are growing poorly, however, lysogeny is favored. In this state, the prophage can remain quiescent until growth conditions improve.

The protein cII is critical to this first molecular decision. Protein cII is sensitive to bacterial proteases, enzymes that degrade proteins. Proteases are in abundance when bacterial growth conditions are favorable, but they are sparse under starvation conditions. If bacteria are actively growing in good conditions, cII is degraded, it never forms a complex with cIII, and little λ repressor protein is produced. If, on the other hand, bacterial growth conditions are poor, cII persists and forms a complex with cIII, and λ repressor protein is produced.

Figure 12.24 The map of the λ (lambda) phage genome. (a) The λ phage genome is organized into operons that function at defined times during infection of a host cell. (b) The cohesive (cos) site is the region that enables the linear phage chromosome to circularize when it enters the host bacterial cell. Immediate early, delayed early, and late genes are expressed in order.

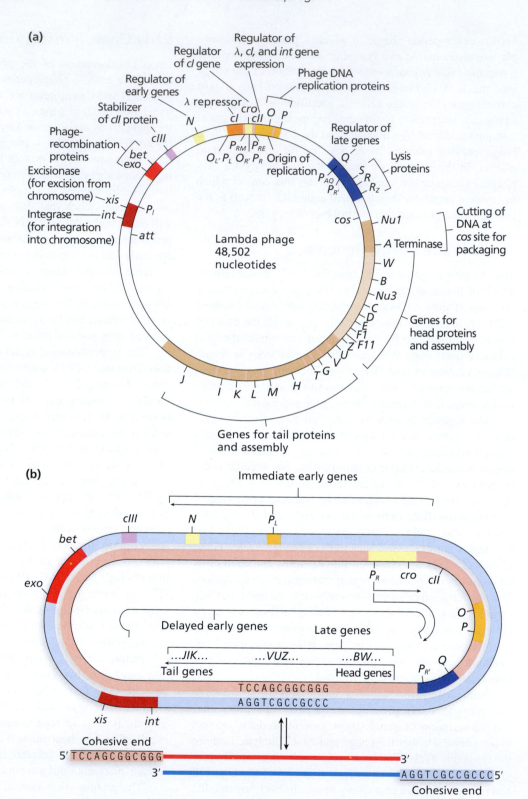

(a)

(b)

The second molecular decision to be made involves direct competition between the Cro protein and the λ repressor protein. They compete for binding to operator sites, with the winning molecule determining whether the lytic cycle or the lysogenic cycle is established. In the following discussion, we focus on the competitive binding between λ repressor protein and Cro protein.

Cro Protein and the Lytic Cycle

Entry into the lytic cycle requires the transcription of late genes that are regulated by **late promoters** and **late operators**. These genes are rightward of P_R, and are involved in the synthesis of head and tail proteins, as well as products that lyse the host cell. The genetic switch governing whether

Regulation of Bacteriophage Entry into the Lytic or Lysogenic Cycle

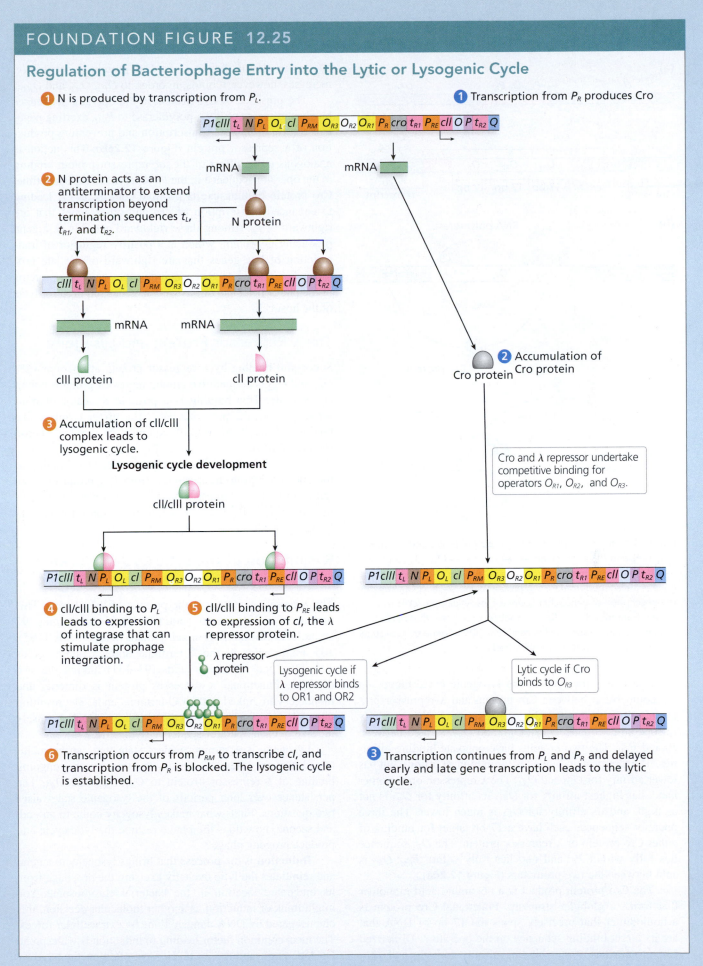

1 N is produced by transcription from P_L.

1 Transcription from P_R produces Cro

2 N protein acts as an antiterminator to extend transcription beyond termination sequences t_L, t_{R1}, and t_{R2}.

mRNA

N protein

mRNA

clll protein

cll protein

Cro protein

2 Accumulation of Cro protein

3 Accumulation of cll/clll complex leads to lysogenic cycle.

Lysogenic cycle development

cll/clll protein

Cro and λ repressor undertake competitive binding for operators O_{R1}, O_{R2}, and O_{R3}.

4 cll/clll binding to P_L leads to expression of integrase that can stimulate prophage integration.

5 cll/clll binding to P_{RE} leads to expression of cl, the λ repressor protein.

λ repressor protein

Lysogenic cycle if λ repressor binds to OR1 and OR2

Lytic cycle if Cro binds to O_{R3}

6 Transcription occurs from P_{RM} to transcribe cl, and transcription from P_R is blocked. The lysogenic cycle is established.

3 Transcription continues from P_L and P_R and delayed early and late gene transcription leads to the lytic cycle.

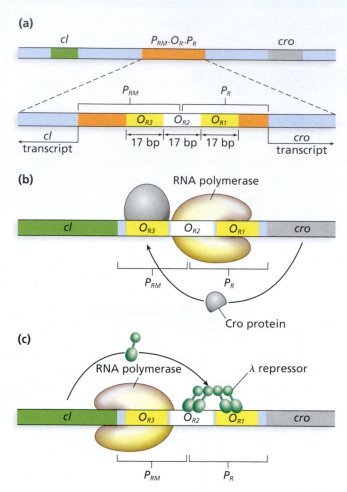

Figure 12.26 **Transcription of λ phage genes *cro* and *cl*.** **(a)** Promoters P_R and P_{RM} overlap three operator sites—O_{R1}, O_{R2}, and O_{R3}—that are competitively bound by regulatory proteins. **(b)** The *cro* gene is transcribed from P_R. Cro protein binds O_{R3} and O_{R2}, leading to transcription of genes that generate the lytic cycle. **(c)** The *cl* gene is transcribed from P_{RM} to produce λ repressor that binds to O_{R1} and drives additional *cl* transcription. Other gene transcription is blocked, and lysogeny is established.

λ phage enters the lytic or the lysogenic cycle hinges on the competition between Cro protein and λ repressor protein. Both Cro protein and λ repressor protein have affinity for operator sequences O_{R1}, O_{R2}, and O_{R3}, located between P_R and P_{RM}. The two proteins have opposite binding affinities. The Cro protein binds O_{R3} with highest affinity but has lower affinity for O_{R2} and O_{R1}. The λ repressor, on the other hand, has highest affinity for O_{R1}. Its affinity for O_{R2} is not as high, and its affinity for O_{R3} is much lower. The three operator sequences each have a 17-bp target for binding of either Cro protein or λ repressor protein. The O_{R1} sequence lies fully within P_R, and O_{R3} lies fully within P_{RM}; O_{R2} is split between the two promoters (**Figure 12.26a**).

The Cro protein product is a 66–amino acid monomer that forms a globular structure. Functional Cro protein is a homodimer that precisely spans the 17 bp of DNA that are its target binding sequence on the operators. Dimerized Cro protein has strong binding affinity for O_{R3} and O_{R2},

but lower affinity for O_{R1}. As Cro protein concentration increases, however, it binds, in order, to O_{R3}, O_{R2}, and O_{R1}.

The presence of Cro protein at the operator sequences blocks the access of RNA polymerase to P_{RM}, exerting negative control of *cl* gene transcription and preventing production of λ repressor protein (**Figure 12.26b**). This action is analogous to the effect of the *lac* repressor protein binding to the operator sequence in the *lac* operon. At the same time, Cro protein binding exerts positive control on P_R, leading to enhanced transcription of *cro* and other genes that are rightward of P_R. Among these rightward genes is *Q*, a gene producing Q protein, which is a positive regulator of transcription of late genes that are rightward of the late promoter P_R'. These late genes include genes encoding proteins of the phage head and tail as well as genes required for lysis of the host cell.

The λ Repressor Protein and Lysogeny

Successful binding by λ repressor protein at operator sites O_{R1} and O_{R2} is cooperative among repressor proteins bound at each site. This binding is a positive regulator of transcription from the promoter P_{RM}. The effect is much like binding of the CAP–cAMP complex in the *lac* operon (**Figure 12.26c**).

Under the influence of λ repressor protein binding to the operator region, transcription from P_{RM} produces more repressor protein. Repressor binding also prevents transcription from P_R, effectively blocking *cro* transcription, and lysogeny results.

Resumption of the Lytic Cycle Following Lysogeny Induction

The λ repressor protein is the product of the *cl* gene. This protein is a 236–amino acid polypeptide containing 92 amino acids in the C-terminal domain (amino acids 1–92), 105 amino acids in the N-terminal domain (amino acids 132–236), and 39 amino acids (93–131) linking the two domains. Functional λ repressor protein is dimeric, and monomers are linked at their C-terminal ends. The resulting dimers have a dimension that spans 17 bp of DNA, precisely the size of each operator sequence (**Figure 12.27a**).

Lysogeny is a semipermanent state that can be maintained for an extended period of time by the ongoing binding of λ repressor protein to O_{R1}, O_{R2}, and O_{R3}. The persistence over long periods of the lysogenic state raises two questions. First, what makes lysogeny come to an end, and second, how does the phage resume the lytic cycle and produce progeny phage?

Induction is the process that brings lysogeny to an end and reinitiates the lytic cycle by excising the prophage from its integrated location in the bacterial chromosome. You might think of induction as another molecular decision, this one triggered by DNA damage done by extracellular forces. The most common factor leading to induction is widespread DNA damage, and the mutagen most often encountered by

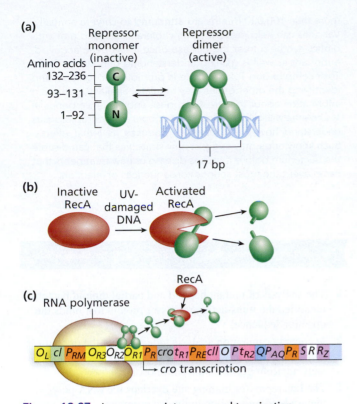

(a)

Amino acids

Repressor monomer (inactive)

Repressor dimer (active)

132–236 — C

93–131 —

1–92 — N

17 bp

(b)

Inactive RecA → UV-damaged DNA → Activated RecA →

RecA

(c)

RNA polymerase

O_L cI P_{RM} O_{R3} O_{R2} O_{R1} P_R cro t_{R1} P_{RE} cII O P t_{R2} Q P_{AQ} P_R' S R R_Z

→ *cro* transcription

Figure 12.27 Lysogeny maintenance and termination.
(a) A homodimeric λ repressor protein binds to 17-bp operator sequences to regulate its own transcription and maintain lysogeny. **(b)** UV light and other DNA-damaging agents activate RecA, which cleaves λ repressor monomers to inactivate repressor protein. **(c)** Lysogeny ends with the removal of λ repressor protein from operator sequences and the initiation of transcription of *cro*.

bacteria is ultraviolet light (UV), whose effects on DNA we described in Section 11.3. UV-induced DNA damage activates many proteins involved in DNA repair. Among the

numerous proteins activated in the DNA repair cascade is the protein RecA, whose role in mutation repair is to activate recombination.

When bacterial DNA is damaged by UV light, however, the protease (protein-destroying) activity of RecA protein is also activated. Among other targets of this protease activity is the amino acid segment of λ repressor monomers that joins the N- and C-terminal regions of each protein (**Figure 12.27b**). The C terminus is clipped off each monomer, effectively breaking apart repressor dimers. This causes the N-terminal ends to fall off DNA. With λ repressor no longer bound to DNA, the O_{R1}, O_{R2}, and O_{R3} sequences are exposed, and positive regulation of *cI* transcription ends, as does the negative regulation of *cro* transcription. A consequence of the removal of λ repressor from the operator region is the renewed production of Cro protein (**Figure 12.27c**). The Cro protein binds to the operators no longer occupied by repressor protein. This leads to the expression of *xis*, producing the enzyme excisionase that removes the lysogen from its integrated location. This event triggers the resumption of the lytic cycle and ultimately results in host cell lysis and the release of progeny phage.

In summary, λ phage is an elegant regulatory system that facilitates a molecular decision controlling whether a genetic switch is flipped in favor of the lytic cycle or the lysogenic cycle. The crucial interaction is between the protein products of the early genes *cro* and *cI* that compete for binding to operator sequences O_{R1}, O_{R2}, and O_{R3}. If Cro protein prevails by successfully binding to O_{R2} and O_{R3}, expression of *cI* is repressed, and the synthesis of late genes leading to completion of the lytic cycle is assured. On the other hand, if λ repressor protein prevails, its early occupation of O_{R1} and O_{R2} prevents transcription of late genes, ensuring that the lysogenic cycle will proceed.

CASE STUDY

Vibrio cholerae—Stress Response Leads to Serious Infection Through Positive Control of Transcription

Cholera is a severely debilitating and potentially fatal disease caused by infection with the intestinal bacterium *Vibrio cholerae*. It is a major public health problem in developing countries where sanitation and supplies of clean water are inadequate or following disasters that disrupt normal sanitation and supplies of clean water. The bacterium is transmitted from person to person through contact with infected fecal material. The ingestion of fecal-contaminated water is the most common way of contracting cholera. Many ingested bacteria are killed by the highly acidic environment of the stomach, but *V. cholerae* in particular can survive in greater numbers than most bacteria by undertaking a rapid switch in gene regulation that shuts down the expression of some genes and activates the expression of stress response genes. Unfortunately for infected humans, the *V. cholerae* stress response produces toxins that can rapidly lead to

degradation of the mucosal cells lining the intestines and to excessive leakage of water from the damaged cells. The leakage of water and electrolytes disturbs the osmotic balance of the cells; to compensate, they secrete more water, initiating a repeating cycle of ion leakage and water release that produces watery diarrhea and severe dehydration. Unless immediate antibiotic treatment and rehydration therapy are started, death can occur within hours.

VIBRIO CHOLERAE TOXINS In *V. cholerae*, three genes—*toxS*, *toxR*, and *toxT*—exert positive control over the transcription of genes producing virulence (active bacterial growth that causes disease). The expression of *toxS* and *toxR* genes is stimulated by the environmental cues encountered by *V. cholerae* in the hostile environment of the stomach. A protein complex formed by the products of these genes activates transcription of *toxT*. The polypeptide product of *toxT* is a transcription-activating protein that binds to the promoter P_{ctx} that controls transcription of an operon containing the two genes *CtxA* and *CtxB* (abbreviations for "cholera toxin A" and "cholera toxin B"). The polypeptide products of *CtxA* and *CtxB* are the cholera toxins that initiate the series of actions leading to cholera symptoms.

PREVENTING AND STUDYING THE DISEASE PROCESS

Preventing cholera is an obvious public health priority. According to the World Health Organization, between 3 million and 5 million people contract cholera each year, and more than 100,000 deaths are attributed to cholera annually. Vaccines can help prevent some cholera cases, and oral antibiotics can help treat the disease once it has been acquired. Important as well is gaining understanding of how the ToxS–ToxR complex and ToxT operate in promoter recognition, and identifying the other genes they regulate. Similarly, gathering information about the stress response and virulence genes in *V. cholerae* will help medical practitioners and microbiologists understand how the bacterium produces its lethal effects. Such knowledge may suggest new strategies that can disable the bacterium before it causes disease or new treatments that can prevent the most serious consequences of infection.

SUMMARY

Mastering Genetics For activities, animations, and review quizzes, go to the Study Area.

12.1 Transcriptional Control of Gene Expression Requires DNA–Protein Interaction

▌ Regulated genes are under transcriptional control, whereas constitutive genes are not regulated.

▌ In negative control of transcription, regulatory proteins bound to DNA reduce or eliminate transcription.

▌ Regulatory proteins, also called repressors, have a DNA-binding domain to bind regulatory DNA sequences and an allosteric domain to bind a regulatory molecule.

▌ An inducer molecule binds to the repressor molecule at an allosteric site to inhibit its action.

▌ In positive regulatory control, activator proteins bind DNA at promoters and other regulatory sequences and initiate or increase transcriptional efficiency.

12.2 The *lac* Operon Is an Inducible Operon System under Negative and Positive Control

▌ Bacterial operons transcribe two or more genes under the coordinated regulatory control of shared promoters, operators, and other regulatory elements.

▌ The lactose (*lac*) operon is an inducible operon system that produces three proteins—β-galactosidase (*lacZ*), permease (*lacY*), and transacetylase (*lacA*) that are required to metabolize lactose and its by-products. Its regulatory control center contains a promoter and an operator sequence (*lacO*).

▌ Negative control of *lac* operon gene transcription is exerted by a repressor protein (*lacI*) that binds to the *lacO* region to block transcription. Allolactose inactivates the repressor protein by changing its conformation and preventing it from binding to the operator.

▌ Positive control of transcription of *lac* operon genes is exerted by the CAP–cAMP complex that forms in the absence of glucose and binds to the CAP site of the *lac* promoter.

12.3 Mutational Analysis Deciphers Genetic Regulation of the *lac* Operon

▌ Mutation studies determined the order of *lac* operon genes as *lacZ–lacY–lacA*.

▌ The analysis of mutant haploid and partial diploid bacteria identified the trans-acting repressor protein that binds the operator sequence.

▌ *lac* operator mutation analysis indicates that the operator is a cis-acting element that controls transcription of immediately adjacent genes on the chromosome.

▌ The Lac repressor binding site overlaps the RNA polymerase binding location in the *lac* promoter.

▌ Lac repressor protein binding induces DNA loop formation that prevents RNA polymerase binding at the promoter.

▌ The CAP–cAMP complex binds to the CAP binding site of the *lac* promoter and facilitates RNA polymerase binding.

12.4 Transcription from the Tryptophan Operon Is Repressible and Attenuated

▌ The tryptophan (*trp*) operon is a repressible operon that produces five polypeptides that participate in tryptophan synthesis.

▌ *trp* operon transcription is inhibited by a feedback mechanism involving tryptophan as a corepressor.

▌ *trp* operon gene expression is attenuated to maintain the cellular concentration of tryptophan at a steady state. Many of the amino acid operons are regulated by an attenuation mechanism.

▌ The *trpL* (leader) region contains an attenuator sequence of four DNA repeats that form three alternative mRNA stem loops, two of which are central to attenuation.

▌ The 2–3 (antitermination) stem loop formed by mRNA permits transcription of five *trp* operon structural genes in a polycistronic mRNA.

▌ The 3–4 (termination) stem loop of mRNA terminates transcription before RNA polymerase binds to the structural genes of the operon.

12.5 Bacteria Regulate the Transcription of Stress Response Genes and Also Translation

▌ Alternative sigma factors are used to generate RNA polymerases that recognize promoters of genes not transcribed by the common bacterial RNA polymerase.

- Genes transcribed using alternative sigma factors are required only under specialized circumstances, such as in response to heat shock.
- The translation of bacterial mRNA can be blocked by RNA-binding translation repressor proteins or by antisense RNA that binds to mRNA from specific genes.

12.6 Riboswitches Regulate Bacterial Transcription, Translation, and mRNA Stability

- A riboswitch is a regulatory mechanism that uses riboswitch sequences located on mRNA to bind small regulatory molecules.
- Riboswitches can regulate the transcription of specific genes, the translation of certain mRNAs, or the stability and degradation of certain mRNAs.

12.7 Antiterminators and Repressors Control Lambda Phage Infection of *E. coli*

- Early genes of the bacteriophage λ genome produce proteins that compete to bind at the same regulatory region. The protein that prevails determines whether the phage infection will follow the lytic cycle or the lysogenic cycle.
- Completion of the lytic cycle requires the expression of late λ phage genes.
- Lysogen integration and maintenance requires ongoing expression of the λ repressor protein, which regulates its own transcription.
- Lysogen integration is reversed by environmental changes that lead to induction and to resumption of the lytic cycle.

PREPARING FOR PROBLEM SOLVING

In addition to the list of problem-solving tips and suggestions given here, you can go to the Study Guide and Solutions Manual that accompanies this book for help at solving problems.

1. Understand the functioning and the biological significance of inducible and repressible transcriptional regulatory mechanisms in bacteria.

2. Be prepared to describe the operation of transcriptional regulatory mechanisms.

3. Be prepared to describe the experimental analysis of transcription-regulating mechanisms and to interpret

the effects of mutations on the functioning of these mechanisms.

4. Understand the operation of attenuation in the production of proteins.

5. Be prepared to interpret the effects of mutations on attenuation.

6. Understand the mechanisms and effects of antisense regulation on protein production.

7. Know the normal functions of lac operon genes and regulatory sequence and the consequences of their mutation.

PROBLEMS

Mastering Genetics Visit for instructor-assigned tutorials and problems.

Chapter Concepts

For answers to selected even-numbered problems, see Appendix: Answers.

1. Bacterial genomes frequently contain groups of genes organized into operons. What is the biological advantage of operons to bacteria? Identify the regulatory components you would expect to find in an operon. How are the expressed genes of an operon usually arranged?

2. Transcriptional regulation of operon gene expression involves the interaction of molecules with one another and of regulatory molecules with segments of DNA. In this context, define and give an example of each of the following:
   a. operator
   b. repressor
   c. inducer
   d. corepressor
   e. promoter
   f. positive regulation
   g. allostery
   h. negative regulation
   i. attenuation

3. Why is it essential that bacterial cells be able to regulate the expression of their genes? What are the energetic and evolutionary advantages of regulated gene expression? Is

the expression of all bacterial genes subject to regulated expression? Compare and contrast the difference between regulated gene expression and constitutive gene expression.

4. Identify similarities and differences between an inducible operon and a repressible operon in terms of
   a. the transcription-regulating DNA sequences.
   b. the presence and action of allosteric regulatory molecules.
   c. the organization of structural genes of the operon.

5. The transcription of β-galactosidase and permease is inducible in *lac*+ bacteria with a wild-type *lac* operon. Explain the mechanism by which lactose gains access to the cell to induce transcription of the genes.

6. Is attenuation the product of an allosteric effect? Is attenuation the result of a transcriptional or a translational activity? Explain your answers.

7. The *trpL* region contains four repeated DNA sequences that lead to the formation of stem-loop structures in mRNA. What are these stem-loop structures, and how do they affect transcription of the structural genes of the *trp* operon?

8. The CAP binding site in the *lac* promoter is the location of positive regulation of gene expression for the operon. Identify what binds at this site to produce positive regulation, under what circumstances binding occurs, and how binding exerts a positive effect.

9. What role does cAMP play in transcription of *lac* operon genes? What role does CAP play in transcription of *lac* operon genes?

10. How would a *cap*⁻ mutation that produces an inactive CAP protein affect transcriptional control of the *lac* operon?

11. Explain the circumstances under which attenuation of operon gene expression is advantageous to a bacterial organism. Would you expect attenuation to be found in a single-celled eukaryote? In a multicelled eukaryote?

12. Consider the transcription of genes of the *lac* operon under two conditions: (1) when both glucose and lactose are present and (2) when glucose is absent and lactose is present. Describe the comparative levels of transcription of *lac* operon genes under these conditions, and explain the molecular basis for the difference.

13. Describe the lytic and lysogenic life cycles of λ bacteriophage. What roles do λ repressor and Cro protein play in controlling transcription from P_R and P_{RM}, and how are these roles linked to lysis and lysogeny?

14. Define *antisense RNA*, and describe how it affects the translation of a complementary mRNA. Why is it more advantageous to the organism to stop translation initiation than to inactivate or destroy the gene product after it is produced?

Application and Integration

For answers to selected even-numbered problems, see Appendix: Answers.

15. Attenuation of *trp* operon transcription is controlled by the formation of stem-loop structures in mRNA. The attenuation function can be disrupted by mutations that alter the sequence of repeat DNA regions 1 to 4 and prevent the formation of mRNA stem loops. Describe the likely effects on attenuation of each of the following mutations under the conditions specified.

Mutated Region	Tryptophan Level
a. Region 1	Low
b. Region 1	High
c. Region 2	Low
d. Region 2	High
e. Region 3	Low
f. Region 3	High
g. Region 4	Low
h. Region 4	High

16. In the *lac* operon, what are the likely effects on operon gene transcription of the mutations described in a–e?
   a. Mutation of consensus sequence in the *lac* promoter
   b. Mutation of the repressor binding site on the operator sequence

   c. Mutation of the *lacI* gene affecting the allosteric site of the protein
   d. Mutation of the *lacI* gene affecting the DNA-binding site of the protein
   e. Mutation of the CAP binding site of the *lac* promoter

17. Identify which of the following *lac* operon haploid genotypes transcribe operon genes inducibly and which transcribe genes constitutively. Indicate whether the strain is *lac*⁺ (able to grow on lactose-only medium) or *lac*⁻ (cannot grow on lactose medium).
   a. $I^+ P^+ O^+ Z^+ Y^-$
   b. $I^+ P^+ O^C Z^- Y^+$
   c. $I^- P^+ O^+ Z^+ Y^+$
   d. $I^+ P^- O^+ Z^+ Y^+$
   e. $I^+ P^+ O^+ Z^- Y^+$
   f. $I^+ P^+ O^C Z^+ Y^-$
   g. $I^+ P^+ O^C Z^+ Y^+$

18. Complete the accompanying table, indicating whether functionally active β-galactosidase and permease are produced in the presence and absence of lactose. Use "+" to indicate the presence of a functional enzyme and "−" to indicate its absence. Indicate whether the partial diploid strain is *lac*⁺ (able to grow on lactose-only medium) or *lac*⁻ (cannot grow on lactose medium).

Genotype	β-Galactosidase		Permease		Phenotype
	Lactose	No Lactose	Lactose	No Lactose	
Example: $I^+ P^+ O^+ Z^+ Y^+$	+	−	+	−	lac⁺
a. $I^S P^+ O^+ Z^+ Y^+/I^- P^+ O^+ Z^+ Y^+$					
b. $I^- P^+ O^+ Z^- Y^+/I^+ P^+ O^C Z^+ Y^-$					
c. $I^+ P^+ O^+ Z^- Y^+/I^+ P^- O^+ Z^+ Y^-$					
d. $I^- P^+ O^C Z^+ Y^+/I^+ P^- O^+ Z^+ Y^+$					
e. $I^+ P^+ O^C Z^+ Y^-/I^+ P^+ O^+ Z^+ Y^-$					
f. $I^+ P^+ O^+ Z^- Y^+/I^S P^+ O^+ Z^+ Y^-$					
g. $I^S P^+ O^+ Z^- Y^+/I^+ P^+ O^C Z^+ Y^-$					

19. List possible genotypes for *lac* operon haploids that have the following phenotypic characteristics:

    a. The operon genes are constitutively transcribed, but the strain is unable to grow on a lactose medium. List two possible genotypes for this phenotype.

    b. The operon genes are never transcribed above a basal level, and the strain is unable to grow on a lactose medium. List two possible genotypes for this phenotype.

    c. The operon genes are inducibly transcribed, but the strain is unable to grow on a lactose medium. List one possible genotype for this phenotype.

    d. The operon genes are constitutively transcribed, and the strain grows on lactose medium. List two possible genotypes for this phenotype.

20. Suppose each of the genotypes you listed in parts (a) and (b) of Problem 19 are placed in a partial diploid genotype along with a chromosome that has a fully wild-type *lac* operon.

    a. Will the transcription of operon genes in each partial diploid be inducible or constitutive?

    b. Which partial diploids will be able to grow on a lactose medium?

21. Four independent *lac⁻* mutants (mutants A to D) are isolated in haploid strains of *E. coli*. The strains have the following phenotypic characteristics:

    Mutant A is *lac⁻*, but transcription of operon genes is induced by lactose.
    Mutant B is *lac⁻* and has uninducible transcription of operon genes.
    Mutant C is *lac⁺* and has constitutive transcription of operon genes.
    Mutant D is *lac⁺* and has constitutive transcription of operon genes.

    A microbiologist develops donor and recipient varieties of each mutant strain and crosses them with the results shown below. The table indicates whether inducible, constitutive, or noninducible transcription occurs, along with *lac⁺* and *lac⁻* growth habit for each partial diploid. Assume each strain has a single mutation.

Mating	Transcription and Growth
A × B	*lac⁻*
A × C	*lac⁺*, inducible
A × D	*lac⁺*, constitutive
B × C	*lac⁺*, inducible
B × D	*lac⁺*, constitutive
C × D	*lac⁺*, constitutive

    Use this information to identify which *lac* operon gene is mutated in each strain.

22. Suppose the *lac* operon partial diploid *cap⁻ I⁺ P⁺ O⁺ Z⁻ Y⁺/cap⁺ I⁻ P⁺ O⁺ Z⁺ Y⁻* is grown.

    a. Will this partial diploid strain grow on a lactose medium?

    b. Is transcription of β-galactosidase and permease inducible, constitutive, or noninducible?

    c. Explain how genetic complementation contributes to the growth habit of this strain.

23. What is a riboswitch? Describe the riboswitch mechanism that regulates transcription of the *thi* operon in *B. subtilus*. What parallels can you see between this mechanism and the regulation of transcription of the *trp* operon in *E. coli*?

24. A repressible operon system, like the *trp* operon, contains three genes, *G*, *Z*, and *W*. Operon genes are synthesized when the end product of the operon synthesis pathway is absent, but there is no synthesis when the end product is present. One of these genes is an operator, one is a regulatory protein, and the other is a structural enzyme involved in synthesis of the end product. In the table below, "+" indicates that the enzyme is synthesized by the operon, and "−" means that no enzyme synthesis occurs. Use this information to determine which gene corresponds to each operon function.

Genotype	Enzyme Synthesis	
	End Product Present	End Product Absent
G⁺ Z⁺ W⁺	−	+
G⁻ Z⁺ W⁺	+	+
G⁺ Z⁻ W⁺	−	−
G⁺ Z⁺ W⁻	+	+
G⁻ Z⁺ W⁺/G⁺ Z⁻ W⁻	+	+
G⁺ Z⁻ W⁺/G⁻ Z⁺ W⁻	+	+
G⁻ Z⁻ W⁻/G⁺ Z⁺ W⁺	−	+
G⁺ Z⁺ W⁻/G⁻ Z⁻ W⁺	−	+

25. What is the likely effect of each of the following mutations of the *trpL* region on attenuation control of *trp* operon gene transcription? Explain your reasoning.

    a. Region 3 is deleted.

    b. Region 4 is deleted.

    c. The entire *trpL* region is deleted.

    d. The start (AUG) codon of the *trpL* polypeptide is deleted.

    e. Two nucleotides are inserted into the *trpL* region immediately after the polypeptide stop codon.

    f. Twenty nucleotides are inserted into the *trpL* region immediately after the polypeptide stop codon.

    g. Ten nucleotides are inserted between regions 2 and 3 of *trpL*.

    h. Two nucleotides are inserted immediately following the polypeptide start codon.

    i. The entire polypeptide coding sequence of *trpL* is deleted.

    j. The eight uracil nucleotides immediately following region 4 are deleted.

26. Suppose that base substitution mutations sufficient to eliminate the function of the operator regions listed below were to occur. For each case, describe how transcription or life cycle would be affected.

    a. *lacO* mutation in *E. coli*

    b. O_{R1} mutation in λ phage

    c. O_{R3} mutation in λ phage

27. Two different mutations affect P_{RE}. Mutant 1 decreases transcription from the promoter to 10% of normal. Mutant 2 increases transcription from the promoter to ten times greater than the wild type. How will each mutation affect the determination of the lytic or lysogenic life cycle in mutant λ phage strains? Explain your answers.

28. How would mutations that inactivate each of the following genes affect the determination of the lytic or lysogenic life cycle in mutated λ phage strains? Explain your answers.

    a. *cI*   c. *cro*   e. *cII* and *cro*
    b. *cII*   d. *int*   f. *N*

29. The bacterial insertion sequence *IS10* uses antisense RNA to regulate translation of the mRNA that produces the enzyme transposase, which is required for insertion sequence transposition. Transcription of the antisense RNA gene is controlled by P_{OUT}, which is more than 10 times more efficient at transcription than the P_{IN} promoter that controls transposase gene transcription.

    a. If a mutation reduced the transcriptional efficiency of P_{OUT} so as to be equal to that of P_{IN}, what is the likely effect on the transposition of *IS10*?
    b. If a mutation of P_{IN} eliminates its ability to function in transcription, what is the likely effect on the transposition of *IS10*?

30. For an *E. coli* strain with the *lac* operon genotype $I^+ P^+ O^+ Z^+ Y^+$, identify the level of transcription of the operon genes in each growth medium listed. Specify transcription as "none," "basal," or "activated" for each medium, and provide an explanation to justify your answer.

    a. Growth medium contains lactose and glucose.
    b. Growth medium contains glucose but no lactose.
    c. Growth medium contains lactose but no glucose.

31. How could antisense RNA be used as an antibiotic? What types of genes would you target using this scheme?

32. Section 9.4 describes the function of tRNA synthetases in attaching amino acids to tRNAs (see Figure 9.16). Suppose the tRNA synthetase responsible for attaching tryptophan to tRNA is mutated in a bacterial strain with the result that the tRNA synthetase functions at about 15% of the efficiency of the wild-type tRNA synthetase.

    a. How would this mutation affect attenuation of the tryptophan operon? Explain your answer.
    b. Would formation of the 3–4 stem loop structure in mRNA be more frequent or less frequent in the mutant strain than in the wild-type strain? Why?

33. The following hypothetical genotypes have genes *A*, *B*, and *C* corresponding to *lacI*, *lacO*, and *lacZ*, but not necessarily in that order. Data in the table indicate whether β-galactosidase is produced in the presence and absence of the inducer for each genotype. Use these data to identify the correspondence between *A*, *B*, and *C* and the *lacI*, *lacO*, and *lacZ* genes. Carefully explain your reasoning for identifying each gene.

Genotype	β-Galactosidase Production	
	Inducer Present	Inducer Absent
1. $A^- B^+ C^+$	+	+
2. $A^+ B^+ C^-$	+	+
3. $A^- B^+ C^+/A^+ B^+ C^+$	+	+
4. $A^+ B^+ C^-/A^+ B^+ C^+$	+	−

Collaboration and Discussion

34. Northern blot analysis is performed on cellular mRNA isolated from *E. coli*. The probe used in the northern blot analysis hybridizes to a portion of the *lacY* sequence. Below is an example of the gel from northern blot analysis for a wild-type *lac*⁺ bacterial strain. In this gel, lane 1 is from bacteria grown in a medium containing only glucose (minimal medium). Lane 2 is from bacteria in a medium containing only lactose. Following the style of this diagram, draw the gel appearance for northern blots of the bacteria listed below. In each case, lane 1 is for mRNA isolated after growth in a glucose-containing (minimal) medium, and lane 2 is for mRNA isolated after growth in a lactose-only medium.

For answers to selected even-numbered problems, see Appendix: Answers.

    a. *lac*⁺ bacteria with the genotype $I^+ P^+ O^C Z^+ Y^+$
    b. *lac*⁻ bacteria with the genotype $I^+ P^+ O^+ Z^- Y^+$
    c. *lac*⁻ bacteria with the genotype $I^+ P^- O^C Z^+ Y^+$
    d. *lac*⁺ bacteria with the genotype $I^- P^+ O^C Z^+ Y^+$
    e. *lac*⁻ bacteria with the genotype $I^+ P^+ O^+ Z^- Y^+$ that has a polar mutation affecting the *lacZ* gene
    f. *lac*⁻ bacteria with the genotype $I^+ P^+ O^C Z^- Y^-$
    g. *lac*⁻ bacteria with the genotype $I^+ P^+ O^+ Z^+ Y^+$ and a mutation that prevents CAP–cAMP binding to the CAP site

35. A bacterial inducible operon, similar to the *lac* operon, contains three genes—*R*, *T*, and *S*—that are involved in coordinated regulation of transcription. One of these genes is an operator region, one is a regulatory protein, and the third produces a structural enzyme. In the table below, "+" indicates that the structural enzyme is synthesized and "−" indicates that it is not produced. Use the information provided to determine which gene is the operator, which produces the regulatory protein, and which produces the enzyme.

Lane

1   2

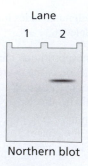

Northern blot

Genotype	Enzyme Synthesis	
	Inducer Present	Inducer Absent
$R^+ S^+ T^+$	+	−
$R^- S^+ T^+$	−	−
$R^+ S^- T^+$	+	+
$R^+ S^+ T^-$	+	+
$R^- S^+ T^+/R^+ S^- T^-$	+	+
$R^+ S^- T^+/R^- S^+ T^-$	+	+
$R^+ S^+ T^-/R^- S^- T^+$	+	−

36. For the following *lac* operon partial diploids, determine whether the synthesis of *lacZ* mRNA is "constitutive," "inducible," or "uninducible," and indicate whether the partial diploid is *lac*⁺ or *lac*⁻ (able or not able to utilize lactose).

Genotype	*lacZ* mRNA Synthesis	*lac* Phenotype
a. $I^- P^+ O^+ Z^+ Y^+/I^+ P^+ O^+ Z^+ Y^+$		
b. $I^+ P^+ O^C Z^+ Y^+/I^+ P^+ O^+ Z^- Y^+$		
c. $I^S P^+ O^+ Z^+ Y^+/I^+ P^+ O^+ Z^+ Y^+$		
d. $I^+ P^+ O^+ Z^- Y^+/I^+ P^- O^+ Z^+ Y^+$		
e. $I^+ P^+ O^+ Z^+ Y^-/I^+ P^+ O^+ Z^+ Y^-$		

37. The electrophoresis gel shown in part (a) is from a DNase I footprint analysis of an operon transcription control region. DNA sequence analysis of a 35-bp region is shown in part (b). The control region, labeled with ³²P at one end, is shown in a map in part (c). Separate samples of control-region DNA are exposed to DNase I, and the resulting DNase I–digested DNA is run in separate lanes of the electrophoresis gel. Unprotected DNA is in lane 1, DNA protected by repressor protein is in lane 2, and RNA polymerase–protected DNA is in lane 3. The numbers along the electrophoresis gel correspond to the 35-bp sequence labeled on the map in part (c). Use the information provided to solve the following problems.

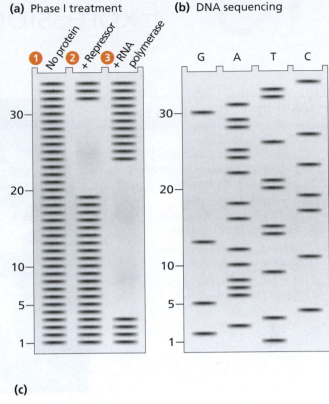

(a) Phase I treatment   (b) DNA sequencing

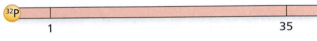

(c)

a. Determine the DNA sequence of the 35-bp region examined.
b. Locate the regions of the sequence protected by repressor protein and by RNA polymerase.

13 Regulation of Gene Expression in Eukaryotes

CHAPTER OUTLINE

13.1 Cis-Acting Regulatory Sequences Bind Trans-Acting Regulatory Proteins to Control Eukaryotic Transcription

13.2 Chromatin Remodeling and Modification Regulates Eukaryotic Transcription

13.3 RNA-Mediated Mechanisms Control Gene Expression

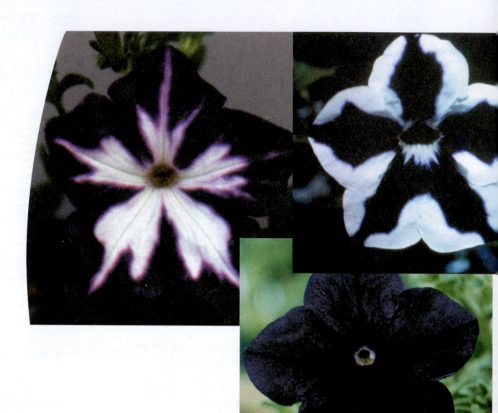

ESSENTIAL IDEAS

- Regulatory DNA sequences bind regulatory proteins to control the initiation or silencing of transcription in eukaryotes.

- Chromatin remodeling and modification regulates gene transcription by shifting the position or changing the chemical composition of nucleosomes.

- The structure of chromatin varies among different types of cells and sets the gene-expression program for distinct cell types.

- RNA-mediated mechanisms regulate eukaryotic gene expression by posttranscriptional interactions with mRNA.

Wild-type petunia flowers have solid color due to expression of a chromosomal pigment gene. Transgenic petunias with an extra copy of the pigment gene have colorless (white) regions due to co-suppression, a process in which regulatory RNAs inactivate both the chromosomal copy and the transgenic copy of the pigment gene.

I f the 46 chromosomes in a single nucleus from any cell in your body were stripped of their associated proteins and laid end to end, they would span almost 2 meters. Yet in their normal, compacted state, these chromosomes can fit inside a nucleus that is about 5 microns (5 millionths of a meter) in diameter and still leave room for DNA replication, transcription, pre-mRNA processing, and numerous other activities to take place. This efficient packaging and access to DNA are made possible by the chromatin structure of the genome and the dynamic changes of which chromatin is capable throughout the cell cycle.

The genomes of eukaryotic organisms—yours included—are considerably larger on average than those of bacterial and archaeal species, and they are packaged much differently as well. One major packaging difference is the localization of chromosomes in a nucleus in eukaryotic cells. Nuclear localization sequesters the chromosomes and encapsulates DNA replication, transcription, and the various RNA-processing activities. A second difference is the incorporation of DNA into chromatin.

The process of chromatin condensation is initiated at the beginning of prophase and culminates in fully condensed chromosomes in metaphase. This condensation is an essential predecessor of efficient chromosome separation in anaphase. Chromatin condensation also plays a pivotal role in permitting or blocking transcription. No cell in your body expresses all 20,400 or so protein coding genes of the human genome. Instead, most human cell types express only a few thousand genes, while the other genes are transcriptionally silent. In recent decades, cell biologists studying the close connection between structural changes in chromatin

and the transcription of eukaryotic genes have succeeded in uncovering many crucial details.

The processes that regulate gene expression in eukaryotes (see Chapters 8 and 9) are more varied and multifaceted than those governing gene expression in bacterial genomes (**Figure 13.1**). In the present chapter, we point out similarities to prokaryotic gene regulation while giving special attention to elements that do not occur in prokaryotes and yet are central to the regulation of transcription and gene expression in eukaryotes. The latter include (1) the organization of regulatory sequences other than promoters that contribute to the regulation of transcription; (2) mechanisms that remodel chromatin or reconfigure the association between nucleosomes and DNA to regulate transcription; (3) epigenetic mechanisms that exert transcriptional regulatory control over the course of an organism's development; (4) the transmission of epigenetic states from one generation of cells to another to exercise long-term control of

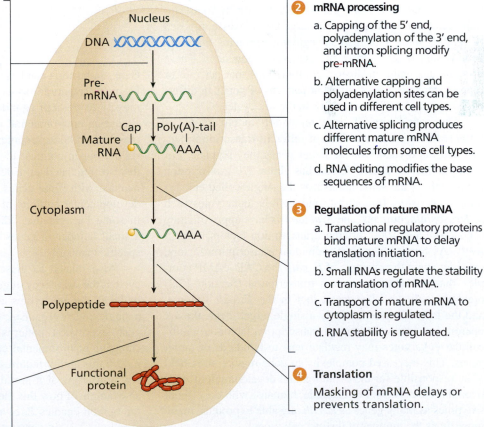

① Transcriptional regulation

  a. Regulatory proteins and transcription factors bind to consensus DNA sequences (promoter regions) to facilitate transcription.

  b. Additional regulatory DNA sequences (enhancers and silencers) bind regulatory proteins to facilitate transcription of specific genes in each cell type.

  c. Open chromatin structure, favorable for transcription, is formed by protein action.

  d. Alternative promoters are utilized in different cell types to produce different pre-mRNA molecules.

  e. Methylation of DNA inhibits transcription.

⑤ Post-translation

  a. Polypeptides are processed and modified in the Golgi body before transportation out of cell.

  b. Regulatory molecules bind to a polypeptide to alter its function.

  c. Protein stability is regulated.

② mRNA processing

  a. Capping of the 5′ end, polyadenylation of the 3′ end, and intron splicing modify pre-mRNA.

  b. Alternative capping and polyadenylation sites can be used in different cell types.

  c. Alternative splicing produces different mature mRNA molecules from some cell types.

  d. RNA editing modifies the base sequences of mRNA.

③ Regulation of mature mRNA

  a. Translational regulatory proteins bind mature mRNA to delay translation initiation.

  b. Small RNAs regulate the stability or translation of mRNA.

  c. Transport of mature mRNA to cytoplasm is regulated.

  d. RNA stability is regulated.

④ Translation

  Masking of mRNA delays or prevents translation.

Figure 13.1   An overview of gene regulation mechanisms in eukaryotes.

🔍 What aspects of eukaryotic gene expression differ from those of bacterial gene expression?

differential gene expression; and (5) RNA-based mechanisms operating posttranscriptionally to regulate the availability of mature mRNA for translation and therefore the ability to produce polypeptides.

13.1 Cis-Acting Regulatory Sequences Bind Trans-Acting Regulatory Proteins to Control Eukaryotic Transcription

Despite the considerable differences between eukaryotes and bacteria, the basic mechanisms controlling transcription are broadly similar in both groups of organisms. Gene regulation is dependent on specific DNA–protein interactions to activate or repress transcription. Trans-acting *activator proteins* bind cis-regulatory sequences to stimulate transcription (positive regulation of transcription), whereas *repressor proteins* bind other regulatory sequences to hinder transcription (negative regulation of transcription). Unlike their counterparts in bacteria, however, eukaryotic transcription activators and repressors, collectively known as transcription factors, are often found in large complexes composed of a large number of distinct regulatory proteins that bind a wide and diverse array of regulatory sequences. These proteins aggregate in diverse combinations that activate or repress transcription of different patterns of genes in different tissues and at different times in the life cycle.

The complexity of gene regulation in eukaryotes is reflected both in the numbers of different transcription factors and the diversity of the target genes they regulate. For example, the bacterium *E. coli* has about 270 transcription factors, about the same number as the single-celled eukaryote *S. cerevisiae*. In contrast, multicellular eukaryotes such as *Drosophila*, humans, and *Arabidopsis* have approximately 600, 1400, and 1900 different transcription factors, respectively. As for the targets of individual transcription factors, consider again the example of *E. coli*: the CAP–cAMP complex that activates *lac* operon transcription (Section 12.2) regulates only about a dozen loci in the *E. coli* genome, and the Lac repressor has only a single target locus, the *lac* operon. In contrast, individual transcription factors in multicellular eukaryotes may regulate tens to hundreds of target genes. This increased complexity in gene regulation is held to be responsible for the evolution and development of multicellular eukaryotes. For example, humans, with only about five times as many genes as *E. coli,* are able to produce many more times the number of distinct cell types.

Other differences in gene regulation between bacteria and eukaryotes, especially complex multicellular ones, are tied to differences in their ecology and life cycles (**Figure 13.2**).

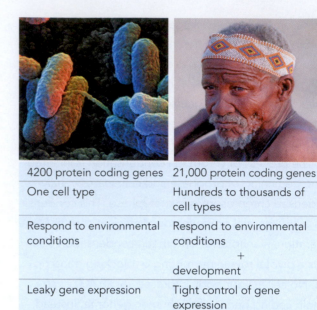

4200 protein coding genes	21,000 protein coding genes
One cell type	Hundreds to thousands of cell types
Respond to environmental conditions	Respond to environmental conditions + development
Leaky gene expression	Tight control of gene expression
Housekeeping types of gene regulatory control inducible (cell-type-specific in sporulation)	Housekeeping types of gene regulatory control inducible; developmental; cell-type-specific

Figure 13.2   Comparison of bacterial and eukaryotic gene expression.

Genes in bacteria can largely be categorized as either housekeeping (required for basic cellular function and constitutively expressed) or inducible (activated in response to a change in environmental conditions). Multicellular eukaryotes harbor housekeeping and inducible genes like bacteria do, but in contrast to bacteria, they also possess genes that are regulated in a developmental or cell-type–specific manner, with some genes utilized multiple times in precise developmental patterns of expression. (Note, however, that in some bacteria that "differentiate" into dormant spores, a small number of genes are also regulated in a cell-type–specific manner.)

Also related to these differences in ecology and life cycle is the stringency of gene regulatory control exercised in multicellular eukaryotes as compared with bacteria. *E coli*, a single-celled organism, depends on being able to change gene expression patterns rapidly to respond quickly to changing environmental conditions. The mechanism giving *E. coli* this ability requires that even when a gene is "off," a few transcripts of it are always present in the cell. We saw an example of how this "leaky" regulation in the case of the *lac* operon enables *E. coli* to sense the presence of lactose (Section 12.2). In contrast, in multicellular eukaryotes with hundreds to thousands of different cell types, genes encoding proteins that are required only in specific cell types need to be tightly regulated. This stricter control, in which genes that are "off" are essentially transcriptionally silent, is mediated by the packaging of chromatin into an inactive state, a subject we will explore in this chapter, after we first discuss the role of transcription factors in eukaryotic gene regulation.

Overview of Transcriptional Regulatory Interactions in Eukaryotes

To repeat, the regulatory sequences required for eukaryotic gene regulation are similar to those described for bacteria—a binding site for RNA polymerase and regulatory sequences that bind either activators or repressors. RNA polymerase II (pol II) and various general transcription factors (GTFs) are recruited to and bind to the *core promoter region* (see Section 8.3). This region contains the TATA box along with other sequences and lies immediately adjacent to the start of transcription (**Figure 13.3**).

Transcriptional activator proteins and transcriptional repressor proteins that bind to **enhancer** and **silencer sequences** (or **enhancers** and **silencers**) provide both quantitative and qualitative control of gene expression. Enhancers and silencers are typically composed of binding sites for a number of transcription factors, and this allows them to integrate the activities of different sets of transcription factors to produce different outputs. Often such a group of transcription factor binding sites is referred to as an enhancer or silencer module. In a broad sense, enhancer and silencer

activity controls the timing and location of eukaryotic gene transcription to help ensure the proper function and development of organisms (for example, by making a polypeptide available at crucial times or in specific cells or tissues).

Unlike core promoter elements, which are invariably located upstream of and close to the genes they regulate, enhancer and silencer modules can be upstream or downstream of genes they regulate and may reside in introns and even, occasionally, *within* coding regions. In multicellular eukaryotes, some enhancer and silencer sequences are close to the genes they regulate, but others are great distances, thousands to tens of thousands of nucleotides, away from the genes they regulate (Figure 13.3), though DNA loop formation can bring even very distant sequences together. In contrast, enhancers and silencers in yeast are usually situated relatively close to the genes they regulate. Some genes contain various *proximal elements* that lie upstream of the core promoter and that are often involved in quantitative gene regulation.

All of the regulatory regions described here are **cis-acting regulatory sequences**, which means they regulate transcription of genes located *on the same chromosome* that the regulatory sequence is on. In contrast, all of the proteins that bind these sequences are **trans-acting regulatory proteins**: they are able to identify and bind target regulatory sequences on *any* chromosome. RNA polymerase II, for example, is able to bind any core promoter region if the right general transcription factors are also present. Similarly,

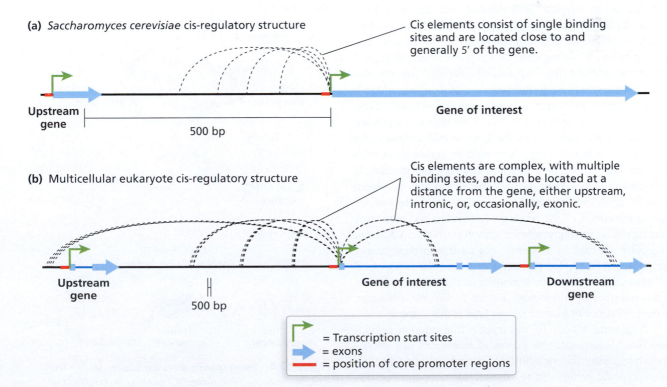

(a) *Saccharomyces cerevisiae* cis-regulatory structure

Cis elements consist of single binding sites and are located close to and generally 5′ of the gene.

Upstream gene

500 bp

Gene of interest

(b) Multicellular eukaryote cis-regulatory structure

Cis elements are complex, with multiple binding sites, and can be located at a distance from the gene, either upstream, intronic, or, occasionally, exonic.

Upstream gene

500 bp

Gene of interest

Downstream gene

= Transcription start sites
= exons
= position of core promoter regions

Figure 13.3   Cis-element regulatory structures in eukaryotes. (a) Typical cis-regulatory structure of a *Saccharomyces cerevisiae* gene. **(b)** Typical cis-regulatory structure of a gene of a multicellular eukaryote.

transcription activator and repressor proteins can bind their target regulatory sequences and can influence transcription with equal efficiency no matter where the sequence occurs.

In addition to the regulatory proteins that bind regulatory DNA in a sequence-specific manner, there are also many proteins that combine through protein–protein interactions to form larger complexes that then bind to regulatory DNA (as mentioned at the start of this section). At enhancers, for example, aggregation of multiple proteins (proteins binding other proteins and some also binding the enhancer sequence) forms a large protein complex known as an **enhanceosome**. Enhanceosomes direct DNA bending into loops that bring the enhanceosome into contact with RNA polymerase and transcription factors bound at the core promoter and to proximal promoter elements (see Figure 8.13). The DNA loops can be small or large, in keeping with the observation that enhancers may be close to or quite distant from the genes they regulate. Repressor proteins act in a similar manner, with some proteins binding DNA in a sequence-specific manner and recruiting additional proteins into a larger repressor complex.

Integration and Modularity of Eukaryotic Regulatory Sequences

The overview we presented above described the regulatory sequences that bind activators and repressors as if each sequence must either be an enhancer or a silencer. In reality, many regulatory modules bind both activators and repressors and thus act to integrate both positive and negative signals into a single output. As an analogy, consider the regulatory sequences of the *lac* operon, which could be viewed as a module consisting of binding sites for a repressor (the Lac repressor) and an activator (the CAP–cAMP complex). Transcription of the *lac* operon results from integration of the effects of binding the activator and repressor proteins; in this case, the repressor is dominant, since when it is bound, the operon is repressed regardless of the presence of the CAP–cAMP complex. An example of a eukaryotic regulatory module, consisting of multiple binding sites for both activator and repressor proteins, is presented in **Figure 13.4**. As with the *lac* operon, the output from the eukaryotic regulatory module represents the integration of the effects of the binding of activators and repressors (and repressors often prevail over activators), but via a different molecular mechanism. However, not all transcription factors are equal—some, called **pioneer factors** are the first to bind regulatory modules, and their binding facilitates the binding of additional transcription factors (Figure 13.4b). We will return to the importance of pioneer factors later in this chapter.

A general model of eukaryotic transcription regulation must incorporate the action of enhancers and silencers while taking the variability of their locations and their tissue-specific patterns of regulation into account. The different regulatory proteins present in different types of cells lead to tissue-specific patterns of expression of the target gene, producing a different set of polypeptides in each case.

The model depicted in **Figure 13.5**, for the *Sonic hedgehog* (*SHH*) gene, shows two distant enhancers controlling transcription of the same gene in a tissue-specific manner. Similar models depicting the binding of repressor proteins to silencer sequences describe how distant silencers can inhibit transcription of targeted genes in a tissue-specific manner.

In humans and other mammals, *SSH* directs the development of limbs, including the production of five digits (fingers or toes) on each appendage. It also plays a role in brain organization. Figure 13.5 compares the transcription

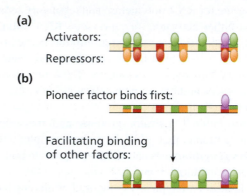

(a) Activators:
Repressors:

(b) Pioneer factor binds first:

Facilitating binding of other factors:

Figure 13.4 Eukaryotic enhancer and silencer module. (a) Modules consist of multiple binding sites for both activators and repressors, with the output from the module resulting through integration of the effects of all the bound factors. **(b)** Pioneer factors bind first, allowing the binding of additional transcription factors.

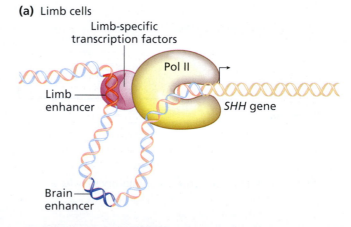

(a) Limb cells

Limb-specific transcription factors

Pol II

Limb enhancer

SHH gene

Brain enhancer

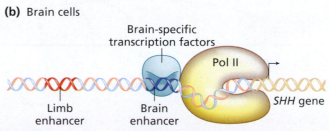

(b) Brain cells

Brain-specific transcription factors

Pol II

Limb enhancer

Brain enhancer

SHH gene

Figure 13.5 Tissue-specific enhancer action. (a) The limb-specific enhancer binds different, limb-specific transcription factors to express *SHH* differently in limb cells. **(b)** A different brain-specific enhancer is bound by brain-specific transcription factors and activates *SHH* transcription in brain cells.

of the *SHH* gene in brain tissue and in limb cells. Transcription in these tissues is controlled by different regulatory proteins and transcription factors produced in each cell type. One combination of regulatory proteins binds one enhancer in brain cells, whereas a different combination of regulatory proteins binds an alternative enhancer in limb cells. The limb enhancer of the *SHH* gene is 1 million base pairs (1 megabase) away from the gene. Genomic sequencing analysis reveals that this *SHH* enhancer is actually located in an intron of a neighboring gene (see Figure 16.17).

This model illustrates an important aspect of eukaryotic transcription regulation. Only when all of the necessary transcription factors and regulatory proteins are present in a cell can the assembly of protein complexes required for the tissue-specific or development-stage–specific pattern of transcription take place. The protein complexes assembled at regulatory sequences direct patterns of gene expression by activating transcription of certain genes while blocking transcription of other genes. This modularity of transcriptional regulation in eukaryotes can provide the flexibility that multicellular organisms need for regulation of differential gene expression. The polypeptides that are ultimately produced in each cell or at each stage of development drive the processes that make cells distinctive and lead to the observed developmental changes.

Our previous discussions of mutations have described numerous ways in which changes in DNA can result in abnormal polypeptides or abnormal levels of polypeptide production. The modularity of regulatory sequences means that changes in gene expression can also occur due to mutations in an enhancer module. As an example, the *SHH* limb enhancer is mutated in certain cases of a condition called polydactyly, in which extra fingers and toes can form during development. The extra digits result from abnormal expression of the *SHH* gene. In studies of certain human families with polydactyly, single base substitutions in the *SHH* enhancer have been identified. In addition, studies in mice in which a deletion of the *SHH* enhancer has occurred reveal significant abnormalities of limb development. Changes in gene regulation are held to be a significant driver in the evolution of morphological complexity. Moreover, the modularity of regulatory elements allows evolutionary changes in gene expression without loss of protein function. For example, since the coding sequences of chimp and human genes are nearly identical, it is likely that most differences between the two species are due to differences in gene regulation rather than to functional differences in protein products.

Locus Control Regions

The human β-globin gene produces the β-globin polypeptide, two copies of which join with two α-globin polypeptides produced by the α-globin gene to form the heterotetrameric hemoglobin molecule. The β-globin gene is, however, only one of six very closely related globin genes forming the β-globin complex on human chromosome 11 (**Figure 13.6a**).

(a) β-globin gene complex and LCR

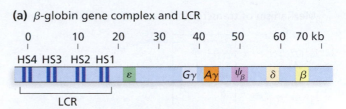

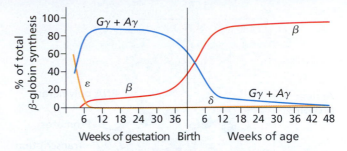

(b) Developmental expression of β-globin–complex genes

Figure 13.6 Locus control and developmental expression of human β-globin–complex genes. **(a)** The locus control region (LCR) of the human β-globin complex contains four regulatory segments (HS1 to HS4). **(b)** The LCR regulates the expression of five genes (Ψβ is an unexpressed pseudogene) in a developmental pattern matched to gestational age.

Located close to the β-globin complex is a regulatory region known as a **locus control region (LCR)**. LCRs are highly specialized enhancer elements that regulate the transcription of multiple genes packaged in complexes of related genes. The LCR regulating transcription of genes in the β-globin complex contains four distinct cis-acting regulatory sequences, designated HS1 to HS4. Together these elements orchestrate the sequential developmental expression of the β-globin–complex genes as a fetus develops during gestation. The LCR and the six genes it regulates occupy a little more than 70 kb.

Each gene of the β-globin complex produces a distinct globin polypeptide that imparts a different oxygen-carrying capacity to hemoglobin. During gestation, the oxygen requirements of the developing fetus change as its size increases and its organs develop. As gestation proceeds, transcription of the genes of the β-globin complex is switched from one to the next to produce hemoglobin molecules that have the oxygen-carrying capacity required by the developing fetus. The order of expression of β-globin–complex genes during development matches the order in which they occur on the chromosome. **Figure 13.6b** shows the expression profile of these genes during development. The HS1 to HS4 components of the β-globin–complex LCR bind regulatory proteins that direct the formation of small DNA loops, and these serve as a bridge to the promoters of the β-globin–complex genes (**Figure 13.7**). The composition of enhanceosomes bound to the LCR varies during development to vary the resulting loops and thus produce the developmentally regulated pattern of gene expression from the β-globin complex. A similar LCR drives transcription of a smaller number of genes in the α-globin complex.

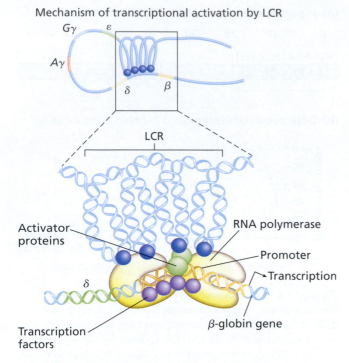

Mechanism of transcriptional activation by LCR

Gγ

ε

Aγ

δ

β

LCR

Activator proteins

RNA polymerase

Promoter

Transcription

δ

Transcription factors

β-globin gene

Figure 13.7 **Human β-globin–complex locus control region.** In combination with regulatory proteins that vary with developmental stage, the LCR forms DNA loops that also vary with developmental stage, allowing the LCR to activate transcription of specific genes of the complex. The RNA polymerase on the left transcribes the δ globin gene and the RNA polymerase on the right transcribes the β globin gene.

Recent genome-wide mapping studies in humans suggest that many disease-susceptibility alleles reside in noncoding sequences that may be regulatory. Some of the known examples are enhancer mutations, such as those causing certain cases of *thalassemia,* a kind of hereditary anemia in which mutation leads to an imbalance of production of α-globin and β-globin polypeptides. The imbalance reduces the amount of functional hemoglobin, since each hemoglobin molecule needs an equal number of both polypeptides. Distinct types of thalassemia result from different mutations of the α-globin or β-globin genes, but in some thalassemia patients, no mutations of either globin gene or of their promoters are detected. In several of these cases, the thalassemia is due to deletion or chromosome-rearrangement mutations that alter the LCR of one of the

globin gene complexes, resulting in enhancer mutations that alter the level of transcription of affected genes and lead to an imbalance of polypeptide production.

Enhancer-Sequence Conservation

Comparisons among species reveal DNA-sequence conservation in some enhancers. This implies that natural selection is operating to retain enhancer function, that is, to retain the capacity to bind specific regulatory proteins by conserving sequence composition. **Figure 13.8** shows enhancer sequences for the β-interferon gene in several mammals; the abbreviations at the top of each column represent the enhancer-binding proteins whose binding relies on certain sequences. The species listed on the left side of the figure share a common ancestor from which their different lineages diverged approximately 100 million years ago.

Genomic sequence analysis indicates evolutionary constraint on the diversification of some enhancer sequences. This constraint is demonstrated in enhancer elements that regulate key genes controlling the development of the vertebrate body plan and that have been conserved throughout vertebrate evolution. (We will resume the topic of genomics approaches to identifying conserved regulatory sequences in Chapter 16.) In contrast, certain enhancer module sequences have been observed to evolve quite rapidly and yet not produce significant differences in outcome. Since the output from an enhancer module is a result of the integration of several inputs, different combinations of activators and repressors can still result in similar outputs.

Yeast as a Simple Model for Eukaryotic Transcription

The yeast *Saccharomyces cerevisiae* provides a simple model for illustrating some principles of eukaryotic transcriptional regulation. For example, the regulation of transcription by enhancer sequences is well understood in *Saccharomyces cerevisiae* for the transcription of genes involved in the galactose utilization pathway. When the monosaccharide galactose is the only sugar in the growth medium, strains of *gal⁺* yeast will induce the transcription of four enzyme-producing genes, *GAL1, GAL2, GAL7,* and *GAL10,* that together import extracellular galactose (the role of *GAL2*) and, through a short series of biochemical

		Bound protein					
	ATF	Jun	IRF	IRF	IRF	IRF	NF-κB
Human	AAATGTAAATGACA	TAGG	AAAAC	TGAAAGGG	AGAAGTGAAAGT	GGGAAATTC	CTCTGAAT
Mouse	......AAATGACA	TAGG	AAAAC	TGAAAGGG	AGAACTGAAAGT	GGGAAATTC	CTCTGA..
Rat	......AAATGACG	TAGG	AAAAGT	GAAAGGG	AGAACTGAAAGT	GGGAAATTC	CTCTGA..
Swine	......AAATGACA	TAGG	AAAAC	TGAAAGGGG	AGAACTGAAAGT	GGGAAATTC	CTCTGAA.
Horse	.AATGTAAATGACA	TAGG	AAAAC	AGAAAGGG	AGAACTGAAAGT	GGGAAATTC	CTCTGAA.
Bovine2	.....TAAATGACA	TAGG	AAAAC	TGAAAGGG	AGAACTGAAAGT	GGGAAATCC	CTCC....
Bovine	....TAAATGACA	TAGG	AAAAAT	GAAAGCG	AGAACTGAAAGT	GGGAAATTC	CTCT....

Figure 13.8 **Conservation of enhancer sequences.** The enhancer sequence of β-interferon contains multiple sequences (colored boxes) conserved among mammalian species. Highlighted sequences are crucial to binding of specific regulatory proteins.

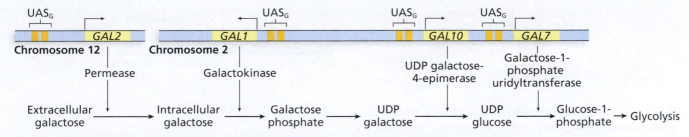

Figure 13.9   Galactose utilization in *S. cerevisiae*. Galactose utilization requires the action of products of each of four galactose-utilization (*GAL*) genes.

reactions, break down intercellular galactose into glucose-1-phosphate for glycolysis (*GAL1, GAL7,* and *GAL10*; **Figure 13.9**). Each of the four genes has its own promoter, but transcription of the genes is regulated by another gene, *GAL4*, which encodes Gal4, a regulatory protein. This is a transcription activator protein that binds to an enhancer element—called an **upstream activator sequence (UAS)** in yeast—located upstream of each of the four *GAL* genes. The Gal4 regulatory protein is continuously available in yeast cells and interacts with Gal80, encoded by the *GAL80* gene. When Gal80 protein binds to Gal4 protein, it inactivates Gal4 and blocks its ability to activate transcription.

The UAS$_G$ sequences are cis-acting regulatory elements, and Gal4 protein is a trans-acting regulatory protein. Each UAS$_G$ element contains two 17-bp repeat sequences that are the binding sites for Gal4 protein. In its active, DNA-binding form, Gal4 is a homodimeric protein composed of two identical polypeptides that form two active domains. The DNA-binding domain, at one end of the Gal4 dimer, targets the 17-bp repeats of UAS$_G$. The activation domain, at the opposite end, is a target for binding by the protein Gal80. Since Gal4 and Gal80 are each constitutively produced, they are normally bound to one another at the UAS$_G$ of Gal4. In this configuration, the activation domain of Gal4 is inactive, and transcription of *GAL* genes is blocked (**Figure 13.10a**). Conversely, when galactose is present, galactose and Gal3, the protein product of another *GAL* gene, binds to Gal80. Binding of the galactose–Gal3 complex alters Gal80 and causes it to release Gal4. The free Gal4 dimer then activates *GAL* gene transcription (**Figure 13.10b**).

In the *GAL* gene system, Gal4 acts as an activator protein, initiating transcription. Its target DNA sequence is UAS$_G$, an enhancer sequence that is separated from *GAL* gene promoters by a large number of nucleotides. Gal4 binding leads to the formation of a multiprotein complex known as **Mediator**, which is an enhanceosome that forms after Gal4 binds UAS$_G$. Mediator induces the formation of a DNA loop, and in so doing makes contact with the general transcription apparatus—including TFIID (transcription factor II D) and RNA polymerase II (pol II)—at a *GAL* gene promoter (see Figure 8.13). In sum, the transcription of *GAL*

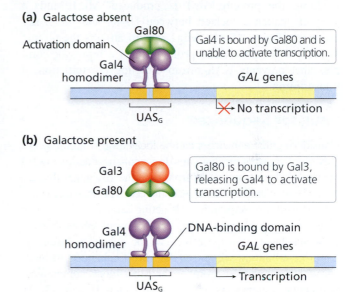

Figure 13.10   Regulation of *GAL* gene transcription. **(a)** When galactose is absent, Gal80 protein binds the activation domain of Gal4 to inactivate that protein and block *GAL* gene transcription. **(b)** When galactose is present, Gal3 protein binds Gal80 protein to prevent it from binding Gal4 protein. The activation domain of Gal4 protein is then available to initiate *GAL* gene transcription.

genes by RNA polymerase II is dependent on transcription activation by Gal4 binding to UAS$_G$ elements and causing the formation of Mediator. Distant silencers use the same kind of DNA loop formation to regulate transcription of targeted genes.

A common mode by which repressor proteins inhibit transcription in bacteria is to bind to operator sequences that overlap promoters, blocking the binding of RNA polymerase (see Chapter 12). In eukaryotes, this mechanism of transcription inhibition is not seen. However, among the mechanisms by which eukaryotic repressors do inhibit transcription is the binding of eukaryotic repressors to silencer sequences, indirectly preventing enhancer-mediated transcription. The galactose-utilization genes in yeast offer an example of this mechanism of transcription repression. When glucose is present in the yeast growth

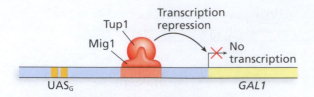

Figure 13.11   Transcription repression of the yeast *GAL1* gene. The proteins Mig1 and Tup1 bind to the Mig1 site to repress transcription when glucose is available in the growth medium.

medium, the protein Mig1 is produced. Mig1 binds a silencer sequence located between UAS$_G$ and the *GAL1* promoter (**Figure 13.11**). Mig1 in turn attracts the protein Tup1, and together these proteins form a repressor complex that prevents UAS$_G$ from directing the initiation of transcription.

Insulator Sequences

Considering that enhancers can be located far from the genes they regulate, what mechanisms direct enhancer action toward the intended gene and away from other nearby genes that are not to be regulated by the same enhancer? The answer, in part, lies in **insulator sequences**, cis-acting sequences located so as to separate enhancers from promoters of genes that are to be insulated from the effects of the enhancer. Insulators are protein-binding sequences that direct enhancers to interact with the intended promoter and that block communication between enhancers and other promoters (**Figure 13.12**). The mechanism of this activity may consist of allowing the formation of DNA loops containing enhancers and their intended promoter targets while preventing the formation of DNA loops containing an enhancer and a promoter that is not its intended target. The action of insulators partitions the genome into "neighborhoods" within which gene regulation can occur independently of the activity in adjacent neighborhoods. Mutations of insulator sequences have been associated with genetic defects in humans.

Up to this point our description of eukaryotic gene regulation has analogies to that of gene regulation in bacteria. First, in both lineages, specific sequences upstream of the transcription start site are required for recruitment of an RNA polymerase. Second, the transcriptional output is a result of the combinatorial activities of activator and repressor transcription factors bound to regulatory sequences that promote or facilitate RNA polymerase activity. For example, the *lac* operon in *E. coli* is positively regulated by the CAP–cAMP complex binding to upstream regulatory sequences and negatively regulated via the Lac repressor protein, with repression being dominant over activation—a situation similar in concept if not molecular mechanism to a gene regulatory module in eukaryotes. Where the analogies end and eukaryotic and bacterial gene regulation are most different has to do with the packaging of DNA, the subject of the next section.

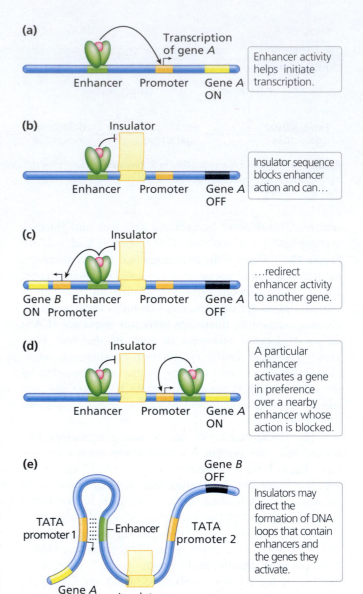

Figure 13.12   Insulator and enhancer interactions.

What might be the effect of a mutation in the insulator binding site?

13.2 Chromatin Remodeling and Modification Regulates Eukaryotic Transcription

Recall from Chapter 10 that eukaryotic chromatin can be broadly divided into two categories based on its extent of compaction: euchromatin, which is loosely compacted and available for transcription, and heterochromatin, which is more densely compacted and is transcriptionally inert. Some regions of the genome are always heterochromatic, referred to as **constitutive heterochromatin**, whereas others switch back and forth between being euchromatic and heterochromatic, and are referred to as **facultative heterochromatin**. These latter regions often contain genes that are active only at specific times or in certain tissues—genes involved in development or active in specific cell types. When DNA that is normally euchromatic is placed—through induced or accidental mutation—in the vicinity of heterochromatin, the heterochromatic character may spread into the normally euchromatic region, silencing gene expression, a phenomenon called position effect variegation (PEV; see Section 10.6). Analysis of mutations that affect the frequency or intensity of PEV in *Drosophila* provided the first insights into how euchromatic and heterochromatic states are established and maintained.

PEV Mutations

Genetic analysis of eukaryotic genomes reveals PEV to be a widespread phenomenon, suggesting that mechanisms controlling chromatin structure are important in the control of gene expression. In *Drosophila,* mutations modifying PEV have led to the identification of several genes and proteins that play a direct role in establishing and maintaining chromatin structures associated with gene expression and gene silencing. The starting point was a mutant line in which the eye color is variegated wild-type red and mutant white, due to an inversion placing the white gene in the vicinity of centromeric heterochromatin (see Figure 10.28). Mutations in which the variegation is either enhanced or suppressed were then identified. Mutations known as **E(var) mutations**, where *E(var)* is short for *e*nhancers of position effect *var*iegation, increase or enhance the appearance of the mutant white-eye phenotype by encouraging the spread of heterochromatin beyond its normal boundaries. (Note that the use of "enhancer" in this context refers to a genetic interaction, and is different from the concept of enhancers as regulatory sequences.) The effect of *E(var)* mutation is to produce a greater number of eye cells lacking pigment (**Figure 13.13**). In contrast, **Su(var) mutations**, where *Su(var)* is short for *su*ppressors of position effect *var*iegation, restrict the spread of heterochromatin or interfere with its formation. *Su(var)* mutations increase the extent of normally pigmented regions of the eye by suppressing the emergence of white patches.

Several dozen *E(var)* and *Su(var)* mutations are known in *Drosophila*, and they have proven especially valuable in the identification of genes and proteins that modulate chromatin structure. Genetic analysis of *E(var)* and *Su(var)* mutations supports the hypothesis that chromatin structure is dynamic and is associated with gene expression. In fact, chromatin structure appears to oscillate: Sometimes it is in a highly condensed state in which gene transcription is silenced (i.e., heterochromatic), and sometimes it is in a more loosely condensed state that allows transcription (i.e., euchromatic), but it can also exist in an intermediate state of condensation.

The analysis of one prominent group of *Su(var)* mutations exemplifies how the detection of defective proteins can

Variegated eye	*Su(var)* mutations	*E(var)* mutations
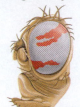	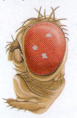	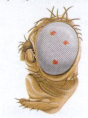
Red patches are produced by cells in which *w⁺* is transcribed, and white patches by cells in which *w⁺* is inactivated by heterochromatin spread.	Mutations block efficient formation of heterochromatin and leave most cells with active *w⁺* transcription.	Mutations enhance heterochromatin formation and restrict *w⁺* expression to small patches.

Figure 13.13   *E(var)* and *Su(var)* mutations. Mutations in genes whose protein products participate in chromatin modification are detected by enhancement or suppression of position effect variegation.

elucidate normal functions. Some *Su(var)* mutations are loss of function of heterochromatin protein-1 (HP-1), a protein found in association with centromeres, telomeres, and other constitutively heterochromatic chromosome locations in *Drosophila*. Comparison of *Su(var)* mutants with wild types reveals that HP-1 is a nucleosome-binding protein that binds lysine amino acids in position 9 of histone H3 if they carry a methyl group. Methylation of lysine 9 of H3 is one of the most common epigenetic modifications of histones in constitutively heterochromatic regions. The absence of HP-1 interferes with heterochromatin formation and suppresses variegation.

A second group of *Su(var)* mutations affects genes encoding histone methyltransferases (HMTs), enzymes responsible for catalyzing the addition of methyl groups to amino acids of histone proteins. Histone methyltransferases appear to target methylation-specific basic amino acids (e.g., arginine and lysine) in nucleosomes, attaching methyl groups to these amino acids as part of epigenetic marking of histones. As noted above, the lysine residue in position 9 of histone protein H3 is a frequent target for methylation. Upon methylation, this location is described as H3K9me, which is short for *h*istone *3*, lysine (one-letter abbreviation *K*), position *9*, and *me*thylation. If HMTs are not functioning properly, epigenetic methylation is not established, and heterochromatin formation is inhibited.

The identification of the activities affected by these two groups of *Su(var)* mutations led to a simple model of HP-1 and HMT function predicting that specific histone locations in nucleosomes (e.g., H3K9) are methylated by HMTs and then act as sites of HP-1 binding that helps condense chromatin structure to silence gene expression (**Figure 13.14**). According to this model, the *Su(var)* mutants, defective in their silencing of *w⁺*, could carry an HMT gene mutation

Heterochromatin

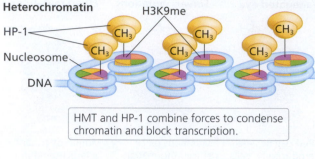

HMT and HP-1 combine forces to condense chromatin and block transcription.

Euchromatin

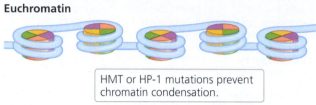

HMT or HP-1 mutations prevent chromatin condensation.

Figure 13.14 **HMT and HP-1 modify chromatin.** *Mutation analysis identifies the proteins HMT and HP-1 as drivers of heterochromatin formation. HMT or HP-1 mutations prevent chromatin modification.*

that leads to the failure to properly methylate nucleosomes or could carry a mutation of the *HP-1* gene and be rendered unable to remodel chromatin to a tightly condensed form. We now know that activity of HMT and HP-1 to produce and recognize H3K9me is a signature of constitutive heterochromatin, but as we will see below, similar systems operate to mark euchromatin and facultative heterochromatin.

Collectively, the experimental analyses of suppressors and enhancers of PEV identify genes that make epigenetic "marks" on histone proteins, causing attachment and detachment of chemical moieties (methyl, acetyl, and phosphoryl groups) to amino acids of the histones. These epigenetic marks are associated with chromatin remodeling that leads to gene transcription or gene silencing. The patterns of methylation and demethylation, acetylation and deacetylation, and phosphorylation and dephosphorylation are maintained on histones and may be passed through successive generations of cells, as we explore more closely in later pages. Five important features of epigenetic modification have been identified by researchers: (1) Epigenetic modifications alter chromatin structure, (2) they are transmissible during cell division, (3) they are reversible, (4) they are directly associated with gene transcription, and (5) they *do not* alter DNA sequence. We turn now to a discussion of how chromatin architecture is remodeled and modified and then explore examples of how changes in chromatin structure lead to activation or repression of gene expression.

Overview of Chromatin Remodeling and Chromatin Modification

The defining feature of eukaryotic DNA is its packaging into chromatin. A major question to be considered, then, is how do the activator and repressor transcription factors bind to regulatory DNA if it is packaged into chromatin? There are three basic mechanisms by which trans-acting proteins access specific regulatory sequences in eukaryotic DNA.

First, some regulatory sequences are not tightly bound by histones, which thus allow more or less direct entry to the regulatory DNA. These sequences include the "linker" sequences between nucleosomes and sequences with specific characteristics that prevent histones from binding efficiently.

Second, proteins called *chromatin remodelers* can enzymatically change the distribution or composition of nucleosomes (histone octamers). Chromatin-remodeling enzymes are recruited to specific sites in the chromatin by trans-acting factors that bind to specific DNA sequences.

As a third mechanism of access, proteins called *chromatin modifiers* can enzymatically modify histones by adding or removing methyl or acetyl groups at specific amino acid residues, most commonly lysines, of histone proteins. Addition of acetyl groups in conjunction with the addition of methyl groups to specific lysine residues is associated with gene activation and is typically found in euchromatin. In contrast, removal of acetyl groups and the addition of methyl groups to different lysine residues than in euchromatin are associated with gene repression and typically found in heterochromatin. As with chromatin-remodeling enzymes, chromatin-modifying enzymes are recruited to specific sites in chromatin by trans-acting factors that bind to specific DNA sequences.

Chromatin remodeler and modifier activities act together to determine the relative access of trans-acting transcription factors to cis-acting DNA sequences in particular cells, at different times of organismal development, and under certain physiological conditions. Thus, chromatin remodelers and chromatin modifiers mediate the reversible transition from inactive heterochromatic DNA to active euchromatic DNA.

Open and Covered Promoters

The terms *open promoter* and *covered promoter* describe two extremes along a continuum of types of nucleosome association with promoter sequences in DNA. In reality, most promoters fall somewhere between these two extremes with respect to their association with nucleosomes, but a discussion of how the two types differ can help us understand how chromatin structure contributes to transcription regulation.

Open promoters are associated with constitutively active genes, such as housekeeping genes encoding proteins vital for basic cellular functions. Open promoters have a **nucleosome-depleted region (NDR)**, which is a 100- to 150-bp region containing few nucleosomes that lies immediately upstream of the start of transcription. These promoters do not generally contain a TATA box. Instead, a region rich in adenine and thymine, known as a poly A/T tract, is located in the NDR, near the transcription start site (**Figure 13.15a**).

The poly A/T tract contains enhancer sequences (ES) that attract transcription activators (ACT). This binding region is usually flanked by sequences that help position two nucleosomes, one upstream and one downstream, of the NDR. The downstream nucleosome, identified as the +1 nucleosome, is placed at the transcription start site. This +1 nucleosome contains a variant histone 2A protein known as H2A.Z that is readily modified for removal from the transcription start site at transcription initiation, allowing RNA polymerase II to bind and access the transcription start sequence.

Covered promoters, on the other hand, are characteristic of genes whose transcription is regulated, in either an inducible, a developmental, or a cell-type–specific manner. Transcription of these genes is blocked until nucleosomes are displaced or removed from the promoter to allow transcription activators to bind to the necessary sequences, an event that leads in turn to RNA polymerase II binding and transcription initiation (**Figure 13.15b**). These promoters generally contain TATA boxes. At covered promoters, there is active competition between nucleosomes and transcription-activating factors for binding. As a result, regulatory mechanisms are required that remodel chromatin to give activator proteins access to binding sequences to initiate transcription.

Mechanisms of Chromatin Remodeling

Chromatin remodeling refers to chromatin modifications that reposition nucleosomes in such a way as to open or close promoters and other regulatory sequences (e.g., enhancer modules). Moving nucleosomes off regulatory sequences improves the availability of those sequences to transcription-activating regulatory proteins. **Open chromatin** is chromatin in which the association of DNA with nucleosomes is relaxed in regions containing regulatory sequences, allowing access by regulatory proteins. Modifications that cause regulatory DNA to be covered by nucleosomes, thus restricting the access of regulatory proteins to the sequences, produce **closed chromatin**. In closed chromatin, regulatory sequences cannot be efficiently accessed by regulatory proteins, and genes are transcriptionally silent.

Molecular biologists can determine experimentally whether a region of DNA contains closed chromatin or open chromatin by assessing the sensitivity of the region to the DNA-digesting enzyme DNase I. This enzyme randomly

cuts DNA in open chromatin regions but is not able to do so where chromatin is closed. Regions of open chromatin, sensitive to DNase I digestion, are known as **DNase I hypersensitive sites**. Where DNase I hypersensitivity is detected, genes are potentially transcribable. The experimental analysis of DNA for DNase I hypersensitivity is

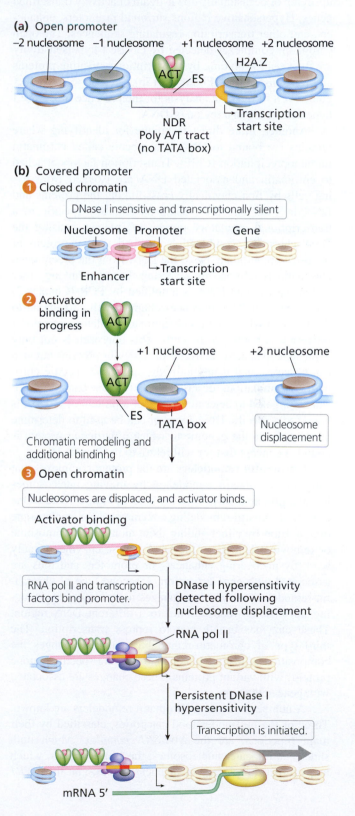

Figure 13.15 Transcription of open and covered promoters. **(a)** Open promoters have a nucleosome-depleted region (NDR) and no TATA box. Activator proteins (ACT) are attracted to enhancer sequences (ES) to recruit RNA polymerase II for transcription. **(b)** With covered promoters, transcription is activated by activator-protein binding and displacement of nucleosomes. Closed chromatin ❶ is inaccessible to transcription factors and insensitive to DNase I digestion, whereas following activator binding and nucleosome displacement ❷, the resulting open chromatin ❸ binds transcription factors and is DNase I hypersensitive.

much like DNA footprint protection analysis described in Research Technique 8.1 (pages 288–289). Fragments of DNA created by exposure to DNase I are separated and analyzed by gel electrophoresis.

DNase I hypersensitivity occurs in the immediate vicinity of transcribed genes and can also appear 1000 bp or more upstream or occasionally downstream of actively transcribed genes. Hypersensitive regions surround promoters, enhancers, and other transcription-regulating sequences. The open chromatin complexes detected by DNase I hypersensitivity are the sites for binding by transcription-activating proteins and for transcription (Figure 13.15b). Genetic Analysis 13.1 guides you through an analysis for the presence of DNase I hypersensitivity in a region of DNA.

Another, more direct technique for identifying where proteins are bound to DNA is a process called chromatin immunoprecipitation (ChIP). Transcription factors attached to chromatin and associated DNA are isolated from living cells by first chemically cross-linking the proteins and DNA together and then, using an antibody specific to a transcriptional regulatory protein of interest, causing the DNA–chromatin combination attached to that protein of interest to precipitate. Next, the DNA from the precipitated chromatin is released by reversing the cross-linking, after which the isolated DNA is amplified by PCR (Chapter 7) and sequenced. The sequences obtained will correspond to the DNA to which the transcriptional regulatory protein of interest was bound in the cells. This approach is not only applicable to specific activator or repressor proteins but also can be performed using antibodies targeting specific chromatin modifications described later in this chapter. ChIP can be targeted to determine whether a protein of interest is bound to a specific DNA locus or can be used to determine all the sites in the genome to which a particular protein is bound, a concept that we will return to in Chapter 16.

Chromatin remodelers are the protein complexes that carry out chromatin remodeling by moving nucleosomes in three principal ways (two are seen in **Figure 13.16**). One type of chromatin-remodeling enzyme changes nucleosome organization by either sliding them along the chromosome or removing them from the DNA. These enzymes usually work by uncovering enhancers or promoters and thus are associated with gene activation. A second type of chromatin-remodeling enzyme reorganizes nucleosomes by inducing nucleosome repositioning to a different DNA region. These enzymes usually act to repress transcription. The third type of chromatin-remodeling enzyme changes the composition of histone octamers, replacing specific histone proteins with variant proteins. These changes are associated with gene activation.

A number of distinct chromatin remodelers are known. Three of the best-understood categories, classified by their main functions, are the *SWI/SNF complex,* which both slides and relocates nucleosomes; the *ISWI complex,* which helps direct the placement of nucleosomes; and the *SWR1*

complex, which substitutes the variant histone protein H2A.Z in nucleosomes in place of the more common H2A protein.

The SWI/SNF Complex The **SWI/SNF complex** (pronounced "swee-sniff" or "swy-sniff") was first described in yeast and is now known to operate in all eukaryotes. Its name comes from yeast mutants unable to switch (SWI) mating types and from sucrose-nonfermenting mutants (SNF). The composition of this complex varies somewhat among eukaryotic species, but in each species it functions to open chromatin structure by displacing or ejecting nucleosomes. These actions expose promoter and other regulatory sequences to allow binding of transcription factors or activators that help initiate transcription (**Figure 13.17 ❶**).

The ISWI Complex Chromatin remodelers of the **ISWI** (*i*mitation *swi*tch) **complex** primarily function to control the placement of nucleosomes into an arrangement that causes the region to be transcriptionally silent. These proteins have the ability to "measure" the length of linker DNA between bound nucleosomes in order to place the nucleosomes at regular intervals where they will cover promoters, thus preventing regulatory proteins from having access to the TATA box and other regulatory sequences (see Figure 13.17 ❷). There is some evidence that certain nucleosome modifications can block ISWI activity, by a process that could be related to the opening of promoter and chromatin structure.

The SWR1 Complex The **SWR1 complex** (*s*witch *r*emodeling *1*) is responsible for replacing the common histone 2A protein of nucleosomes with a variant form known as H2A.Z that differs from the more common form by amino acid differences internal to the protein and in the amino terminal (N-terminal) protein tail. The differences found in H2A.Z alter its pairing with other H2A proteins and its interactions with H3/H4 tetramers in the nucleosome. H2A.Z is found primarily at the so-called +1 nucleosome that is affiliated with the start of transcription. Functional analyses in several species suggest that the role of H2A.Z is in the creation of unstable nucleosomes that might then be displaced, ejected from DNA, or modified to regulate transcription (see Figure 13.17 ❸).

It is important to note that chromatin remodeling complexes do not bind to DNA on their own but are recruited to specific chromosomal locations by sequence-specific binding activator or repressor transcription factors. Recruitment of chromatin remodelers can lead to the transition of closed chromatin to open chromatin and vice versa (Figure 13.15).

Chemical Modifications of Chromatin

In contrast to chromatin remodelers that move nucleosomes, the proteins called **chromatin modifiers** chemically modify histone proteins in the nucleosomes by adding or removing

(a) Nucleosome sliding

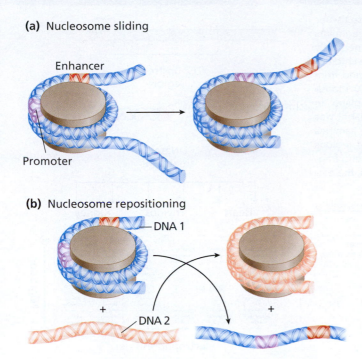

(b) Nucleosome repositioning

Figure 13.16 **Two of the modes of nucleosome displacement to expose regulatory sequences.** **(a)** Nucleosomes can be displaced by sliding or **(b)** can be repositioned to other DNA sequences.

specific chemical groups. These modifications alter the strength of association between nucleosomes and DNA. The changes can cause chromatin structure to relax, leading to open promoters and to transcription activation (euchromatin), or they can lead to closed structures that inhibit transcription (heterochromatin). The principal chemical modifications to nucleosomes take place through the addition and removal of acetyl groups ($COCH_3$) and methyl groups (CH_3) at specific amino acids in the N-terminal (amino terminal) region of histones.

Because different patterns of modifications of histone tails lead to greater or lesser amounts of transcription by contributing to the opening and closing of chromatin structures, molecular biologists Thomas Jenuwein and C. Davis Allis suggested that a "histone code" exists. This hypothesized code consists of different combinations of chemical modifications in histone N-terminal tails, resulting in different changes to the chromatin structure. Supporting this idea, studies examining different aspects of chromatin complexity in evolutionarily distant eukaryotes suggest chromatin exists in only a limited number of distinct states (**Figure 13.18**). These examinations of the complexity of chromatin modification patterns in *Drosophila* and *Arabidopsis* identified four prominent chromatin states. Thus, despite the potential for an enormous number of different chromatin states, it appears that only a limited number exist in vivo.

Enzymes that add chemical groups are collectively known as "writers," whereas those that remove groups are known as "erasers" (**Figure 13.19a**). Proteins that recognize the modified histones are called readers. Writers and erasers are recruited to specific chromatin locations by sequence-specific DNA-binding proteins, such as activators and repressors. Readers, as their name implies, can bind directly to the modified histones. The role of readers is to "read" the chromatin structure and act to maintain it in either an active or inactive state.

The recruited writers and erasers modify the histone tails, producing an opening or condensing of chromatin structure at the locus. The acetyl and methyl groups are added to or removed from lysine (K) residues in the N-terminal tail of histone 3. Three lysines, K4, K9, and K27, are particularly important targets for writers and erasers (**Figure 13.19b**).

Histone acetyltransferases (HATs) are chromatin-modifying writers that add acetyl groups. Acetyl groups are removed by **histone deacetylases (HDACs)**, which act as erasers (**Figure 13.20**). In their unacetylated form, positively charged amino acids such as lysine promote nucleosome

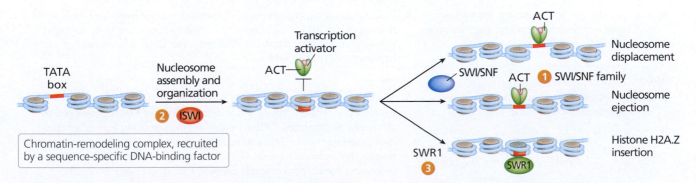

Figure 13.17 **The actions of chromatin-remodeling complexes.** ❶ The SWI/SNF family opens chromatin structure and helps initiate transcription by either displacing nucleosomes away from regulatory sequences or ejecting nucleosomes. ❷ ISWI assembles and organizes nucleosomes in a regular pattern and contributes to transcription repression. ❸ SWR1 inserts the modified histone protein H2A.Z into nucleosomes to help facilitate displacement.

Q How does the ISWI complex work to prevent binding of regulatory proteins?

PROBLEM The tissue enzyme TE2 is expressed in various mouse tissues at different times during the life cycle. Identical chromosome segments were isolated at different times in the cycle from a region immediately upstream of *TE2* and analyzed for DNase I hypersensitivity. The chromo-

> BREAK IT DOWN: DNase I cuts in regions of open chromatin but not condensed chromatin (p. 487–488).

some segments were collected from embryonic (E) and adult (A) mouse heart, kidney, and thymus gland. In the analysis, a radioactive label was attached to one end of each chromosome fragment, and the samples from each tissue were exposed to DNase I to determine if the regions upstream of *TE2* were DNase I hypersensitive. When the resulting fragments from each sample were separated by gel electrophoresis, the pattern shown at right was obtained.

a. Based on the gel results, is there evidence that chromatin remodeling plays a role in the expression of *TE2*? Explain your reasoning.

b. In which tissue(s) and at what times during development do the results indicate the expression of *TE2* was most likely taking place?

> BREAK IT DOWN: Chromatin remodeling is the process by which nucleosome position or identity is altered (p. 490).

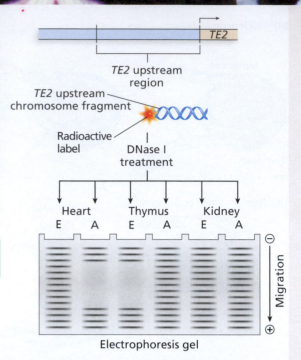

Solution Strategies	Solution Steps
Evaluate	
1. Identify the topic of this problem and the kind of information the answer should contain.	1. This problem concerns an experimental analysis for DNase I hypersensitivity in the region upstream (i.e., the promoter region) of *TE2*. The answers require interpretation of experimental results with respect to chromatin structure and gene expression.
2. Identify the critical information given in the problem.	2. Gel electrophoresis results are given for identical chromosome fragments from embryonic and adult heart, thymus, and kidney. All chromosome fragments were exposed to DNase I.

> TIP: DNase I hypersensitivity is detected when chromatin structure is open and potentially accessible to transcription-activating proteins. Closed chromatin is not hypersensitive to DNase I.

Deduce	
3. Compare and contrast the meaning of the continuous series of bands in some lanes of the gel versus lanes in which gaps are seen between bands.	3. A continuous series of DNase I–digested bands indicates DNase I hypersensitivity. Hypersensitivity correlates with open chromatin that is accessible to transcription. Gaps between gel bands indicate that certain regions of chromosomes are not fragmented by DNase I treatment. This result signals the absence of DNase I hypersensitivity in those regions and suggests closed chromatin structure and no transcription.
4. Evaluate the gel, and describe the patterns of DNase I–digestion bands for each sample.	4. Discontinuous band patterns are observed in adult heart and embryonic thymus gland DNA. This absence of DNase I hypersensitivity suggests closed chromatin structure. Each of the other DNA samples indicates hypersensitivity to DNase I.
Solve	Answer a
5. Determine whether the gel data indicates chromatin modification near *TE2*.	5. The DNase I hypersensitivity results indicate differential patterns of *TE2* expression in different tissues and at different times of development due to chromatin modifications. DNase I hypersensitivity resulting from open chromatin appears in embryonic and adult kidney, in embryonic heart, and in adult thymus chromosomal material. Hypersensitivity is not seen in adult heart or in embryonic thymus chromosomal material, indicating closed chromatin.
	Answer b
6. Name the tissues in which *TE2* is expressed, and describe the developmental timing.	6. *TE2* expression is likely to occur at embryonic and adult stages in the kidney, in the embryonic heart, and in the adult thymus gland. *TE2* expression is unlikely to occur in adult heart or in embryonic thymus gland.

For more practice, see Problem 20.

Visit the Study Area to access study tools. **Mastering Genetics**

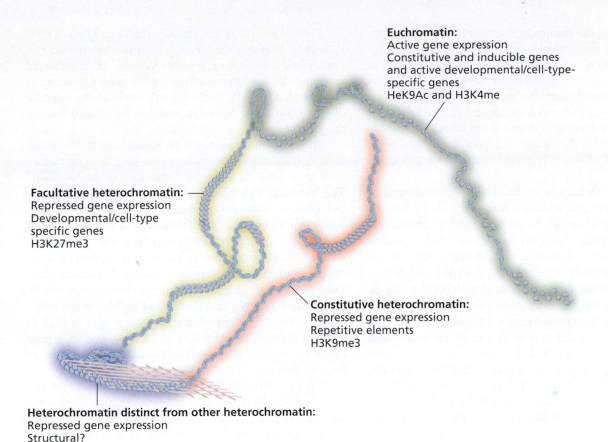

Euchromatin:
Active gene expression
Constitutive and inducible genes
and active developmental/cell-type-
specific genes
HeK9Ac and H3K4me

Facultative heterochromatin:
Repressed gene expression
Developmental/cell-type
specific genes
H3K27me3

Constitutive heterochromatin:
Repressed gene expression
Repetitive elements
H3K9me3

Heterochromatin distinct from other heterochromatin:
Repressed gene expression
Structural?

Figure 13.18   Chromatin states, gene content, and characteristic histone modifications.

adherence to negatively charged DNA. Acetylation neutralizes the positive charge and relaxes the tight hold the nucleosomes have on DNA. Thus, acetylation of K9 of histone 3, designated H3K9ac, is associated with an opening of the chromatin and active transcription (Figure 13.20). HATs are recruited to the chromatin by activator proteins (**1**), leading to the formation of euchromatin and active transcription (**2**). Conversely, HDACs are recruited by repressors (**3**), resulting in the formation of transcriptionally inactive heterochromatin (**4**).

The addition of methyl groups is accomplished by chromatin-modifying **histone methyltransferases (HMTs)**, which act as writers. Again, lysine is the frequent target for methylation, and residues can be mono- (me), di- (me2), or trimethylated (me3). Depending upon the K residue, methylation can play a role in converting open euchromatin to closed heterochromatin in conjunction with deacetylation; H3K9 is the residue methylated in the case of constitutive heterochromatin and H3K27 is the residue in the case of facultative heterochromatin. Conversely, methylation can contribute to forming open chromatin, as in the case of H3K4 methylation in conjunction with H3K9 acetylation (see Figure 13.19b). Demethylation is carried out by **histone demethylases (HDMTs)**, which act as erasers. HMTs and HDMTs are recruited to the chromatin by activators and repressors in a manner similar to that depicted for HATs and HDACs in Figure 13.20.

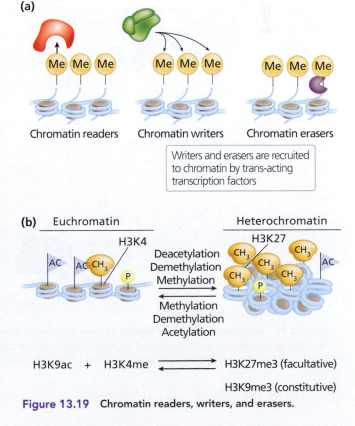

(a)

Chromatin readers   Chromatin writers   Chromatin erasers

Writers and erasers are recruited to chromatin by trans-acting transcription factors

(b)   Euchromatin   Heterochromatin

H3K4   H3K27

Deacetylation
Demethylation
Methylation

Methylation
Demethylation
Acetylation

H3K9ac + H3K4me ⇌ H3K27me3 (facultative)

H3K9me3 (constitutive)

Figure 13.19   Chromatin readers, writers, and erasers.

In summary, the chromatin state can be reversibly converted between euchromatin (active) and heterochromatin (inactive) through the combined action of transcription factors and chromatin modifiers. Multiple chemical modifications of N-terminal amino acids are required to convert from a closed to an open structure and vice versa. No single acetylation or methylation event changes chromatin structure; rather the change is accomplished through a coordinated set of events localized to a gene or regions of a gene.

Thus, the alternation of facultative heterochromatin between an open euchromatic state and a closed heterochromatic state is driven by an interplay of chromatin-modifying enzymes recruited by activator or repressor proteins. In many eukaryotes, this interplay between the opposing activities of writers and erasers involves a protein complex called the Polycomb group (PcG) acting in gene repression and another protein complex called Trithorax (Trx) acting to maintain gene expression. PcG and Trx complexes are recruited to specific loci by repressors and activators, respectively. The PcG complex acts to maintain a chromatin state that is marked with H3K27me3 and not acetylated; that is, it has an H3K27 HMT and an HDAC. In contrast, the Trx complex has a HAT and an H3K27 HDMT. (We will explore how these complexes work in an example below.)

Perhaps you recall from the original description of PEV in Section 10.6 that the *white* gene was relocated next to centromeric constitutive heterochromatin. In contrast to facultative heterochromatin, this type of heterochromatin is characterized by H3K9me3. We will return to the question of how constitutive heterochromatin is maintained later in this chapter.

At this point, you might be wondering: If chromatin is in an inaccessible heterochromatic state, how do factors bind to its DNA to initiate the transition to euchromatin? The transition can occur through the activity of a special class of transcription factors called pioneer factors, which can access and bind DNA even in heterochromatin (**Figure 13.21**). Pioneer factors may be a single protein. In other cases, a combination of factors that on their own are not pioneer factors can sometimes form a pioneer complex. One role of pioneer factors is to open up heterochromatin by first binding to DNA and then recruiting chromatin modifier and remodeling complexes. Another role is to bind to DNA to prepare the chromatin in such a way that a gene can be rapidly induced when additional transcription factors become available.

Finally, although it is convenient for the sake of discussion to divide chromatin states into active euchromatin and inactive heterochromatin, many genes do not fit neatly into those categories but instead are found along a

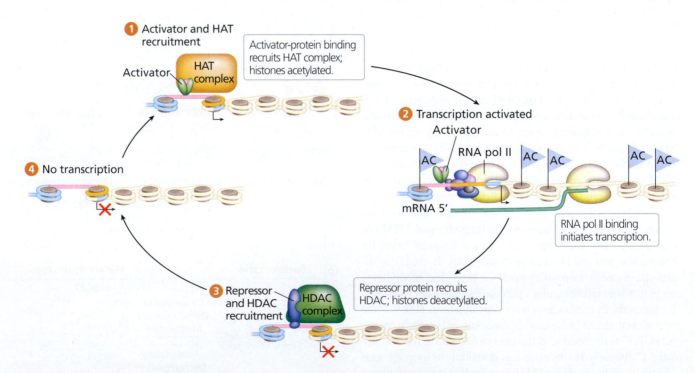

Figure 13.20 **Acetylation and deacetylation in open and closed chromatin structure.** Histone deacetylases (HDACs) deacetylate amino acids in N-terminal histone protein tails and close the chromatin structure. Histone acetyltransferases (HATs) acetylate N-terminal amino acids and help open the chromatin structure to activate transcription.

How are the HAT and HDAC complexes directed to specific chromosomal loci?

(a) Comparison with other transcription factors

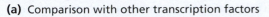

Most transcription factors cannot access their binding sites in heterochromatin

Pioneer transcription factors can access their binding sites in heterochromatin.

(b) Attributes

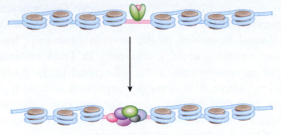

Can have an active role in opening heterchromatin.

Partially bound, inactive enhancer module

+ additional activators for induction

Fully bound, active enhancer module

Can have a role poising inducible genes for rapid induction.

Figure 13.21 **Pioneer factors.**
(a) Comparison with nonpioneer transcription factors. **(b)** Attributes of pioneer factors.

⊙ **What property makes pioneer factors special?**

continuum. Genes expressed in developmental and cell-type–specific patterns are tightly regulated and reside at the ends of the spectrum, whereas constitutive genes are always euchromatic. Other genes may carry both active and inactive chromatin marks that keep them poised to be expressed, allowing for rapid changes in gene expression.

An Example of Inducible Transcriptional Regulation in *S. cerevisiae*

To illustrate the role of chromatin modifications in the regulation of an inducible gene, we turn to transcription regulation of the *PHO5* gene in the yeast species *S. cerevisiae*. Our discussion of this particular example is based on numerous studies that collectively paint a comprehensive picture of the actions associated with chromatin modification in *PHO5* transcription initiation and regulation.

PHO5 is an inducible gene encoding an acid phosphatase that removes phosphate groups from other proteins. In yeast, *PHO5* transcription is activated by phosphate starvation, but it is repressed when phosphate level is high. In the repressed state, access of transcription factors and RNA polymerase II to the promoter's TATA box is blocked by a nucleosome labeled −1 in **Figure 13.22a**. Similarly, access of transcription activator proteins to a UAS element labeled UASp2 is blocked by a nucleosome labeled −2. In the repressed state, the transcription activator protein Pho2 and the acetylase protein NuA4 are present upstream of the promoter at a UAS element labeled UASp1. Upstream of these are nucleosomes labeled −3 and −4. There is a low level of acetylation of nucleosomes −1 to −4 in the repressed state. Together, the presence

(a) High phosphate results in transcription repression

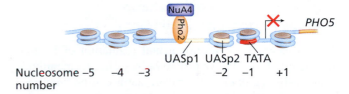

Nucleosome −5   −4   −3   −2   −1   +1
number

(b) Low phosphate results in transcription activation

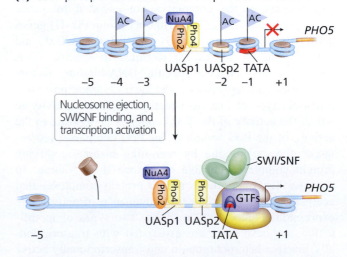

Nucleosome ejection, SWI/SNF binding, and transcription activation

Figure 13.22 **Transcription control of *PHO5* in *Saccharomyces cerevisiae*.** **(a)** Transcription is repressed in high-phosphate conditions. **(b)** In low-phosphate conditions, Pho4 joins Pho2 at UASp1, and NuA4 directs acetylation of nearby nucleosomes. The SWI/SNF complex attaches, leading to the ejection of nucleosomes −1 to −4. RNA polymerase II and general transcription factors initiate *PHO5* transcription.

of the nucleosomes −1 to −4 blocks access of activator protein and transcription factors to *PHO5* regulatory sequences.

Transcription of *PHO5* occurs when phosphate level falls. The activator, Pho4, is translocated to different locations within the cell depending on the level of phosphate: Under high-phosphate conditions Pho4 is phosphorylated and exported from the nucleus, whereas under low-phosphate conditions Pho4 is unphosphorylated and imported into the nucleus. Under low-phosphate conditions, the nuclear-localized Pho4 protein binds to Pho2, forming a protein complex that begins transcription activation (**Figure 13.22b**). Additional acetylation of the −1 to −4 nucleosomes takes place under the direction of NuA4. The Pho4–Pho2 complex then initiates chromatin modification by displacing nucleosome −2, making UASp2 available for binding by the Pho4 protein. The SWI/SNF protein complex assembles, and additional chromatin modification displaces nucleosomes −1 (that previously covered the TATA box), −3, and −4. With chromatin opened by nucleosome displacement, general transcription factor proteins and RNA polymerase II are able to bind the promoter and initiate transcription of the *PHO5* gene.

Facultative Heterochromatin and Developmental Genes

For an example of developmental regulation of facultative heterochromatin we turn to *Drosophila*. As mentioned previously, facultative heterochromatin can be converted to euchromatin and vice versa via the activities of large protein complexes known as Trithorax and Polycomb. Components of the complexes are encoded by genes known, respectively, as the Trithorax group (TrxG) genes and the Polycomb group (PcG) genes. Both the TrxG and PcG protein complexes are recruited to specific DNA sequences by sequence-specific DNA-binding factors (activators and repressors), and each complex possesses a distinct type of histone-3-methyltransferase activity in which the activity of the TrxG complex is opposite to the activity of the PcG complex. The PcG complexes repress target gene expression by recruiting histone-modifying protein complexes capable of histone deacetylation. In contrast, TrxG complexes recruit protein complexes that acetylate histone, leading to maintenance of active gene expression (**Figure 13.23a**). These two types of modification, we have seen, are associated with transcriptionally inactive heterochromatin and transcriptionally active euchromatin, respectively. As with chromatin remodelers, TrxG and PcG complexes are recruited to the cis-acting regulatory sequences of *Hox* genes by activators and repressors, respectively, to "lock" the chromatin into a particular form, allowing maintenance of either active or silent states of gene expression. *Hox* genes will be described in detail in Chapter 18, but for the present

discussion, it is sufficient to understand that these genes are involved in patterning the anterior-posterior axis of animal embryos.

For example, during *Drosophila* embryogenesis, the *Ubx* gene is initially activated in specific cells toward the posterior end of the embryo (**Figure 13.23b**). In wild-type embryos this pattern is maintained throughout embryogenesis. However, in PcG mutants, the *Ubx* gene later on becomes activated in cells of the anterior part of the embryo, where normally it is not expressed. This indicates that expression of the PcG complex is required for the continued normal repression of the gene in those cells later on during embryogenesis. Conversely, in TrxG mutants, *Ubx* gene expression fails to be maintained in the posterior region, where it is normally expressed in wild-type embryos. It is thought that the initial posterior activators and anterior repressors regulating *Ubx* expression recruit TrxG and PcG complexes, respectively, to maintain expression of *Ubx* through later stages of embryogenesis, even after the initial regulatory transcription factors are no longer present.

How does this occur mechanistically? Once the chromatin has been demarcated as heterochromatin, the H3K27me3 reader within the PcG complex can recognize the mark in heterochromatin, and the H3K27 methylase of the complex can write the mark on nearby octamers. The euchromatic state can be maintained by the TrxG complex in a similar manner. In this way, these proteins provide a type of epigenetic cellular memory that is propagated through cell divisions occurring long after the initial activators of *Hox* gene expression patterns have disappeared. We will revisit the role of these complexes in the development of a multicellular organism in Chapter 18.

Epigenetic Heritability

Activating the transcription of an individual gene requires a confluence of regulatory proteins that remodel or modify chromatin to provide enhancer and promoter access to transcription factors that initiate and carry out transcript synthesis. Mechanisms controlling differential chromatin-state formation and maintenance produce patterns of gene expression in different types of cells that are required for the growth and development of complex organisms. In a broad sense, these regulatory processes are the reason a single fertilized egg can develop and produce many distinct types of cells (liver cells, muscle cells, brain cells, and so on).

Among the trillions of somatic cells in your body are scores of different cell types, and yet all these cells contain the same genetic information. The differences of morphology and function between cell types are genetically controlled, as evidenced by the fact that daughter cells have the same structures and functions as parental cells, but DNA sequence variability *is not* the reason for those differences. Instead, the differences between somatic cells

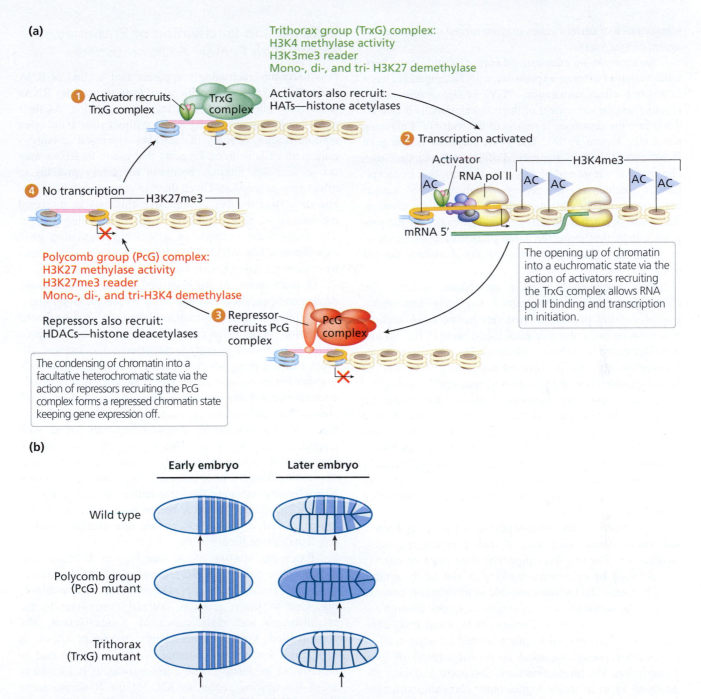

(a)

Trithorax group (TrxG) complex:
H3K4 methylase activity
H3K3me3 reader
Mono-, di-, and tri- H3K27 demethylase

1 Activator recruits TrxG complex

TrxG complex

Activators also recruit:
HATs—histone acetylases

2 Transcription activated

Activator

RNA pol II

H3K4me3

mRNA 5'

4 No transcription

H3K27me3

The opening up of chromatin into a euchromatic state via the action of activators recruiting the TrxG complex allows RNA pol II binding and transcription in initiation.

Polycomb group (PcG) complex:
H3K27 methylase activity
H3K27me3 reader
Mono-, di-, and tri-H3K4 demethylase

Repressors also recruit:
HDACs—histone deacetylases

3 Repressor recruits PcG complex

PcG complex

The condensing of chromatin into a facultative heterochromatic state via the action of repressors recruiting the PcG complex forms a repressed chromatin state keeping gene expression off.

(b)

	Early embryo	Later embryo
Wild type		
Polycomb group (PcG) mutant		
Trithorax (TrxG) mutant		

Figure 13.23 **Antagonistic activities of PcG and TrxG complexes in facultative heterochromatin. (a)** Activator proteins recruit the TrxG complex to the chromatin, resulting in erasing of repressive histone marks and writing of positive histone marks. HAT complexes are also often recruited to add positive acetyl marks. Conversely, repressor proteins recruit the PcG complex to the chromatin, resulting in erasing of positive histone marks and writing of repressive histone marks. HDAC complexes are also often recruited to erase positive acetyl marks. **(b)** *Ubx* expression (blue) is activated and maintained posteriorly in wild-type *Drosophila*, but its repression is lost in PcG mutants and its maintenance is lost in TrxG mutants.

Q **How do PcG and TrxG complexes provide a "memory"?**

are **epigenetic**, resulting from the distinct chromatin states affecting gene transcription in specific types of cells.

Epigenetic patterns are often heritable through mitosis from one generation of cells to the next, causing daughter cells to have the same patterns of gene expression as their parent and sibling cells—a cellular memory. Some epigenetic changes occur in the course of normal growth and development, in some cases resulting from different physiological conditions. These changes are potentially reversible and variable during the life cycle of an organism; the transcription of certain genes may be turned on and later off again, or vice versa.

An example we encountered earlier of mitotically heritable variation of gene expression with an epigenetic basis is position effect variegation (PEV) in *Drosophila,* which results from the movement of the transcriptionally active w^+ allele into the centromeric region of the fruit-fly X chromosome (see Figure 10.28). The DNA sequence of the gene is not altered. Instead, the spread of heterochromatin closes chromatin structure and blocks gene transcription by an epigenetic mechanism. The repressed transcriptional state is then maintained in daughter cells through mitotic division. The result is patches of cells descendant from original progenitor cells that share the same pattern of inactivation of w^+ expression. These cells form regions of white in the eye of the fly.

How is epigenetic control maintained in cells? For cellular memory to be maintained, any acetyl and methyl groups that are present on histones before DNA replication must be maintained or established on both the old and new histones after DNA replication. The specific molecular mechanics of this process are not entirely clear, but the partial disassembly and subsequent reassembly of nucleosomes is an essential component. Recall that chromatin structure is broken down as the replication fork passes (see Figure 10.27). Nucleosomes are separated from the parental DNA strands so the latter can serve as templates for the synthesis of daughter strands. The nucleosomes partially break apart, and old nucleosome segments along with newly synthesized nucleosome segments are reassembled on both new duplexes.

Immediately after DNA replication, the newly formed nucleosomes carry only part of their previous epigenetic information. The original epigenetic state must be quickly reestablished by epigenetic marking of the newly synthesized histones. Old histones are able to modify new histones to have the same pattern of epigenetic marks through the activities of the readers and writers of PcG and TrxG complexes. This process takes place among adjacent nucleosomes, thus preserving local epigenetic control of gene transcription. The interaction must also occur over long distances so as to maintain higher-order chromatin structure, such as that characterizing inactivated X chromosomes (see below).

In contrast to the formation and differentiation of specialized tissues and cells in the body, the formation of germline cells (cells that give rise to the next generation), must clear the replicating chromatin of the majority of accumulated epigenetic marks. Thus, most epigenetic marks added during the lifetime of an organism are erased during meiosis, resetting the epigenetic landscape for the next generation. However, there is evidence that some epigenetic differences *can* be heritable through meiosis, passing from one generation of the organism to the next, a topic we will explore in the Case Study.

lncRNAs and Inactivation of Eutherian Mammalian Female X Chromosomes

It is becoming increasingly apparent that a class of RNA molecules in eukaryotic cells called **long noncoding RNAs (lncRNAs)** play critical roles in gene regulation. As their name implies, they are long RNAs without substantial open reading frames. A study of lncRNAs expressed in embryonic stem cells in mice suggests that many lncRNAs may act as scaffolds linking chromatin regulatory proteins to affect gene expression. Given that the genomes of mammals encode a large number of lncRNAs, this may be a critical mechanism of gene regulation in the mammalian lineage. The best-known example of a lncRNA regulating gene expression is *Xist,* which is involved in X chromosome inactivation in eutherian female mammals.

X-inactivation, as we discussed in Section 3.6, is the dosage compensation mechanism by which eutherian mammalian females achieve the correct balance of X-linked gene expression. Mammalian females undergo random X inactivation in each nucleus early in gestational development, the precise timing being species specific. Recall that random X inactivation leaves one active X chromosome that is largely euchromatic and one inactive X chromosome that is almost entirely heterochromatic in each nucleus. The heterochromatic X chromosome is almost completely silent with respect to gene expression. This highly heterochromatic X chromosome forms a Barr body in the nucleus. All cells descending from the ones that originally underwent random X inactivation maintain the same active (euchromatic) and inactive (heterochromatic) X chromosomes, leading to the mosaic pattern of cells characteristic of eutherian mammalian females (see Figure 3.26).

Extensive studies of X inactivation in mice and humans have detected about a dozen genes on the heterochromatic (inactive) X chromosome that escape silencing. One of these genes is critically important to the establishment and maintenance of X-inactivation. The gene, called *X-inactivation-specific transcript* (*Xist*), is *active* on the heterochromatic X chromosome and is *inactive* on the euchromatic chromosome. It is located in the X-inactivation center, or XIC, of the X chromosome (**Figure 13.24**). The *Xist* gene is transcribed only on the heterochromatic chromosome, where it is active; it is not transcribed on the euchromatic X chromosome, where it is inactive. The gene transcript is a specialized RNA transcript called *Xist* RNA that never leaves the nucleus and is never translated. Instead, *Xist* RNA exclusively coats the X chromosome that produces it.

One idea of how the modification is accomplished is that the *Xist* RNA may act as a molecular bridge between the inactive chromatin and the repressive chromatin-modifying complexes such as PcG, whose associated HMTs and HDACs methylate (H3K27me3) and deacetylate histones, respectively. These epigenetic modifications are

Heterochromatic X chromosome

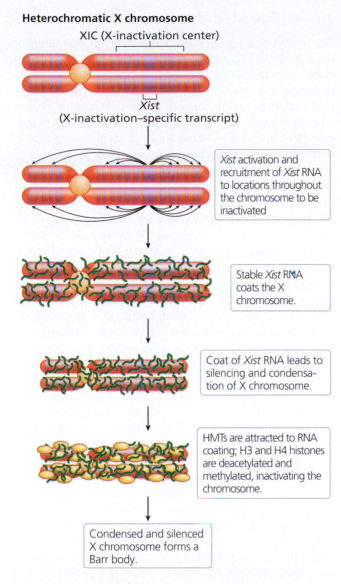

Figure 13.24 **The X-inactivation center (XIC).** The XIC contains *Xist*, which is transcribed to produce a specialized RNA that coats the X chromosome. This mechanism is responsible for random inactivation in eutherian mammals.

linked directly to transcriptional silencing of genes. The *Xist* RNA coating, subsequent methylation and deacetylation, and other protein-driven modifications inactivate one X chromosome and condense it into a heterochromatic state in each eutherian mammalian female nucleus. This would ensure that the patterns of chromatin modifications of the X chromosome established in embryogenesis are maintained throughout the lifetime of the organism. Note, however, that X-inactivation is reversible in eutherian mammalian female germ-line cells, ensuring that the process starts over each generation.

Genomic Imprinting

A specialized example of epigenetic regulation occurs in certain mammalian and flowering plant genes in a mechanism known as **genomic imprinting**. For the small number of mammalian genes subject to genomic imprinting, both copies of the gene are functional but just one is expressed. In mammals, two copies of each autosomal gene are inherited—one copy is on a chromosome inherited from the mother, and the other copy is on the homologous chromosome from the father—and usually both gene copies are expressed. For a small number of genes whose expression is subject to genomic imprinting, however, this pattern does not hold. Instead, one copy of the gene is actively expressed while the other copy is silent. The expressed gene copy is always inherited from a particular parent (for some genes it is the mother, for others it is the father), and the silent copy is the one inherited from the other parent.

The best-studied examples of genomic imprinting are two human genes encoded very near one another on chromosome 11. The insulin growth factor 2 (*IGF2*) gene on the paternally derived copy of the chromosome is expressed, whereas the *IGF2* gene on the maternally derived chromosome is silent. The opposite is the case for the *H19* gene, which is expressed from the maternally derived chromosome 11 but is silent on the paternal copy. These two genes are in a region of chromosome 11 containing several other genes that are also imprinted. They are among the few dozen human genes whose transcription is controlled by genomic imprinting.

Two regulatory sequences are responsible for these two instances of genomic imprinting. One is an enhancer downstream of *H19*; the other is an insulator sequence, called the **imprinting control region (ICR)**, located between *H19* and *IGF2* (**Figure 13.25**). In the maternal chromosome,

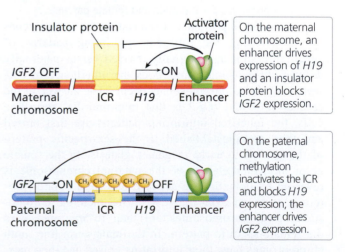

Figure 13.25 **Differential genomic imprinting of chromosome 11 in humans.**

activator proteins bind the enhancer sequence and direct transcription of *H19* by interacting with transcription factors and RNA polymerase II at the promoter. The ICR in the maternal chromosome is bound by an insulator protein that blocks the enhancer from affecting *IGF2*. On the paternal chromosome, on the other hand, extensive methylation of the ICR and *H19* prevents insulator protein binding and blocks transcriptional protein binding at the *H19* promoter. In the absence of the insulator protein, the enhancer stimulates transcription of *IGF2*.

Genomic imprinting silences expression of paternal *H19* and maternal *IGF2* and directs transcription of paternal *IGF2* and maternal *H19* in all somatic cells. This pattern is essential for normal development, and any other pattern produces profound abnormalities. A genetic condition called Beckwith–Wiedemann syndrome, characterized by an overgrowth of tissues, results if the both the maternally and paternally inherited chromosomes display the expression patterns normally associated with the paternally inherited locus. Conversely, if both inherited chromosomes display the typical maternal expression pattern, a genetic condition called Russell–Silver syndrome, characterized by underweight infants that fail to grow appropriately, results.

Why might these genes be imprinted in mammals? The reason may be related to the reproductive biology involving placentation, whereby the female bears the physiological burden for nurturing the young. *IGF2* encodes a growth factor promoting development—its expression promotes growth of the embryo. One hypothesis is that male mammals profit from promoting maximum growth in all their offspring, whereas female mammals profit more from balancing the growth of multiple offspring over the mother's lifetime. Thus, the active *IGF2* allele inherited from the father promotes embryo growth, while the female's inactive allele counterbalances the excess activity provided by the male. The evolution of imprinting in both mammals and flowering plants is likely due to their both being placental organisms, with different selectives pressures for the male and female parents.

Given the importance of imprinting for certain genes and considering the different imprinting patterns of gene expression in maternally derived versus paternally derived chromosomes, how does the inheritance of correctly imprinted chromosomes occur? The answer in the case of *H19* and *IGF2* is that in primordial germ-line cells, the inherited imprinting patterns are first erased and then are reestablished in the sex-specific pattern of the germ line early in gametogenesis. In the female germ line, methylation of the paternal chromosome is reversed by demethylase activity, and the insulator protein is removed from the ICR on the maternal chromosome. Both chromosomes are then re-imprinted with the female-specific pattern. In the male germ line, both chromosomes have their imprinting erased and then reestablished in the male-specific pattern. These processes ensure that each parent passes a properly imprinted chromosome during reproduction.

Nucleotide Methylation

The methylation pattern identified in genomic imprinting of the ICR and *H19* gene is a type of methylation that is associated with repression of gene expression in many plants and vertebrates, particularly mammals, that differs from the methylation of amino acids in N-terminal histone protein tails. In this case, methyl (CH_3) groups are attached to specific DNA *nucleotides*, not to amino acids in histone protein tails. Nucleotide methylation is performed by specialized DNA methyltransferases that add methyl groups primarily to cytosines located in **CpG dinucleotides**, side-by-side cytosine and guanine nucleotides in the same DNA strand. The *p* in CpG represents the single phosphoryl group in the phosphodiester bond connecting the nucleotides. Complementary strands of DNA containing CpG dinucleotides each have 5'-CG-3'. In plants, other C nucleotides may be methylated—the ones in 5'-CNG-3' and 5'-CNN-3' configurations, for example.

Much of the cytosine-methylated DNA in eukaryotic genomes is in transposable element sequences and noncoding sequences and is associated with a transcriptionally silent chromatin state. Just as with chromatin-remodeling enzymes, the DNA methyltransferases are recruited to specific loci by transcription factors when DNA methylation is being established. Also paralleling nucleosome modification, the pattern of cytosine-methylated sites is usually mitotically stable but can be reset during meiosis. A simple modification of Sanger sequencing in which the DNA is first treated with bisulfite, which converts cytosine to uracil but leaves methylcytosine untouched, allows the direct determination of the methylation status of DNA.

Recall from Section 11.2 that deamination of a methylated cytosine creates a thymine, which generates a mismatch that is repaired either to a C-G or a T-A base pair at approximately equal frequencies. Thus, in organisms with a significant amount of cytosine methylation, such as in vertebrates, where most of the cytosines in CpG dinucleotides are methylated, over time the number of CpG dinucleotides is reduced. In these species, sequences rich in CpG, called **CpG islands**, are regions of the genome in which there is strong selection for maintenance of cytosines, reflecting a functional role for such regions. As a result, CpG islands can be used to identify potentially functional genomic regions such as gene regulatory sequences.

13.3 RNA-Mediated Mechanisms Control Gene Expression

In the past several years, RNA has emerged as a key component in the regulatory control of eukaryotic gene expression. Largely unknown before the mid-1990s, RNA-mediated regulatory mechanisms have rapidly become a major focus of research in plants and animals. This important area of inquiry emerged unexpectedly from experiments designed to produce a more colorful petunia.

In the early 1990s, Richard Jorgensen and his colleagues were attempting to deepen the color of petunias by introducing into the petunia genome a pigment-producing gene under the control of an active promoter. The researchers hoped that active transcription of this recombinant gene would dramatically deepen flower color. To Jorgensen's surprise, however, rather than exhibiting more intense color overall, many of the resulting flowers were variegated (see the chapter opener photo). Some flowers had stripes of deep pigment and stripes lacking pigment, and some flowers were almost entirely white. The researchers called this phenomenon **cosuppression** because expression of both the introduced pigment gene and the petunia's natural pigment-producing gene was suppressed.

By 1995, similar gene-silencing phenomena had been documented in numerous plant species, in the fungus *Neurospora crassa*, in the nematode worm *Caenorhabditis elegans*, and in the fruit fly *Drosophila*. The fundamental mechanism behind this form of regulation was identified in 1998 by a research team led by Andrew Fire and Craig Mello. Fire and Mello found that double-stranded RNA (dsRNA) molecules were taking part in a posttranscriptional regulatory mechanism now known universally as **RNA interference (RNAi)**. Fire and Mello received the Nobel Prize in Physiology or Medicine in 2006 for their work.

Gene Silencing by Double-Stranded RNA

RNA interference silences gene expression either by blocking transcription of targeted genes or by blocking gene expression posttranscriptionally. Posttranscriptional silencing occurs following binding of small regulatory RNAs to mRNA targets by complementary base pairing. The binding of these regulatory RNAs either can lead to the destruction of the target mRNAs or can block their translation. Alternatively, some regulatory RNAs enter the nucleus, where they bind DNA to block transcription of targeted genes. Any of these regulatory processes first require that small regulatory RNA molecules use complementary base pairing to bind their targets.

The regulatory RNAs in RNAi are derived from various sources that produce double-stranded RNAs. An enzyme known as **Dicer** (**Figure 13.26**) cuts the double-stranded RNA into 21- to 25-bp fragments. These fragments are then bound by a protein complex called the **RNA-induced silencing complex (RISC)** that denatures the double-stranded RNAs into single strands of 21 to 25 nucleotides. The RNA single strands produced by RISC are identified as the **guide strand**, which is biologically active, and the passenger strand, which is usually degraded. The guide strand remains bound to RISC, and the complex directs one of three gene-silencing processes (numbers 1 through 3 in the figure): ❶ The complex uses complementary base

pairing to attach the guide strand to mRNA, and the mRNA is destroyed; ❷ the RISC–guide RNA binds to complementary mRNAs and blocks their translation; or ❸ the complex directs chromatin-modifying enzymes to the nucleus, where they silence transcription of selected genes.

What is the origin of the dsRNA? It can be produced from endogenous genes or from the transcription of other endogenous nongene sequences (e.g., transposons), or it can come from exogenous sources. In many eukaryotes, genes encode precursors of dsRNA ❹ that are processed into 21- to 24-nucleotide **microRNAs (miRNAs)** at a Dicer complex. Most genes encoding miRNAs are transcribed by RNA polymerase II, and the resulting transcript folds back on itself into a dsRNA. The targets of miRNAs are endogenous mRNAs that are then either cleaved or have their translation blocked subsequent to activity mediated through RISC.

Another type of dsRNA is **small interfering RNA (siRNA)**. In contrast to miRNAs, siRNAs are usually not derived from genes but rather come from exogenous sources or from other endogenous transcription. For example, if both strands of a genomic region happen to be transcribed, dsRNA can form. Transcription from opposite strands of repetitive elements, such as transposons, can also lead to dsRNA production ❺. In the latter case, the two strands do not have to be derived from the same genomic location. Some eukaryotes possess RNA-dependent RNA polymerases, which can produce dsRNA using single-stranded RNA as a template.

The endogenous sources of dsRNAs can direct either posttranscriptional silencing, through the destruction of target mRNAs or inhibition of their translation, or transcriptional silencing of target genes that takes place by chromatin-modifying processes. Finally, exogenous sources of dsRNA can include RNA viruses ❻ that trigger virus-induced gene silencing.

Cleaving dsRNA The general mechanism of action by which Dicer cleaves dsRNA into fragments of the proper size involves the enzyme's dsRNA-binding site (called PAZ) and its two RNase domains, separated from the PAZ site by a distance corresponding to the length of the resulting dsRNA fragments. Dicer repeats the cleaving action, each time behaving as a molecular ruler measuring off precisely sized dsRNAs. The spacing between the PAZ site and RNase domains varies among species and appears to correlate with species-specific differences in the lengths of siRNAs produced by subsequent RISC processing of dsRNAs.

Precursor transcripts of miRNAs and siRNAs are synthesized in the nucleus of a cell and are processed into miRNAs and siRNAs by Dicer activity. In the case of miRNAs, the precursor transcript is called a primary microRNA (pri-miRNA). The pri-miRNA folds to form a double-stranded stem typically containing 65 to 70 nucleotides and having free ends on one side and a single-stranded loop on the other side (**Figure 13.27**). In animals, the **Drosha** enzyme complex cuts pri-miRNA near the middle of the stem and produces

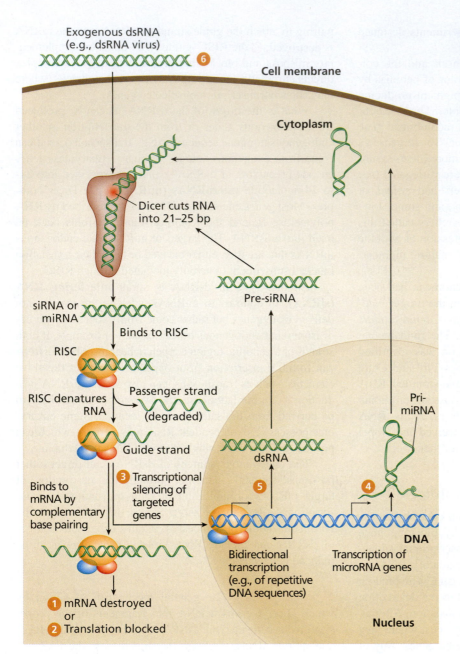

Figure 13.26 Gene silencing by RNAi. Dicer cuts dsRNA into 21- to 25-bp siRNA or miRNA segments that are then denatured by RISC. RISC–guide strand complexes can degrade targeted mRNAs, block translation of target mRNAs, or enter the nucleus to modify chromatin.

two segments, one of which, now called precursor microRNA (pre-miRNA), contains the remainder of the upper stem, which is approximately 21 to 25 bp, and the terminal loop ❶. The pre-miRNA is transported to the cytoplasm, where Dicer removes the terminal loop, leaving dsRNA of approximately 21 to 25 bp ❷. RISC then binds the dsRNA and separates the strands to create miRNAs ❸. In contrast to animals, plants use a single Dicer enzyme to perform all the miRNA processing activities. The creation of siRNA is similar.

RISC and Argonaute The newly produced siRNA or miRNA remains bound by RISC to act as a guide strand. Within the RISC is a protein of the **Argonaute** gene

family that plays a central role in how the RISC–guide strand silences gene expression. Many species encode multiple Argonaute proteins—humans encode eight, for example—and each seems to direct a somewhat different activity by RISC–guide strand.

The best-understood mechanism of gene silencing by RISC–guide strand involves complementary binding of the guide strand to a target mRNA. If the percentage of base-pair complementation is high enough, this binding forms a structure that allows an RNase domain of Argonaute to cut the targeted mRNA strand near the middle of the guide strand–mRNA duplex, thus causing cleavage of the mRNA. When the guide strand–mRNA base pairing is less well

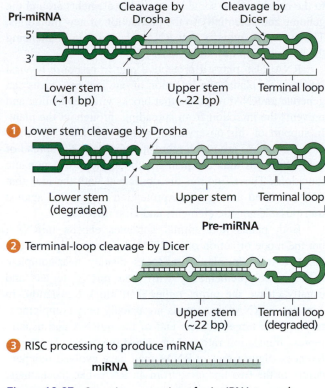

Figure 13.27 **Stepwise processing of pri-miRNA to produce miRNA.**

matched—that is, when only a core of complementary base pairs are present in the guide strand–mRNA duplex—the RNase domain of Argonaute is unable to cut the duplex. Instead, the duplex retains its double-stranded form, causing translation to be blocked.

Constitutive Heterochromatin Maintenance

For the third mechanism by which the RISC–guide strand complex silences gene expression, we return to the topic of chromatin modification. Details of how small RNAs contribute to the maintenance of heterochromatin were worked out in the yeast *Schizosaccharomyces pombe*. The first evidence of a role for RNAi in chromatin modification came from the study of centromeric heterochromatin in *S. pombe*. The centromeres of *S. pombe,* like those of other complex eukaryotes, contain a central element surrounded by repeat sequences. The histones in the centromeric region have a low level of acetylation, and lysine 9 of the N-terminal tail of H3 (that is, H3K9) is methylated. Both types of modification are consistent with the formation of a closed chromatin structure and the spread of constitutive heterochromatin to silence nearby genes.

S. pombe possesses single genes for Dicer and for Argonaute, and mutation of either gene disrupts RNAi activity in the cell. The surprising finding, however, was that *S. pombe* with Dicer or Argonaute mutations also lacks

methylation of H3K9 and does not have gene silencing around the centromere. The explanation for these additional deficiencies is that in *S. pombe*, both strands of the centromeric repeat sequences are transcribed by RNA polymerase II (Figure 13.28 ❶). The resulting mRNAs are complementary

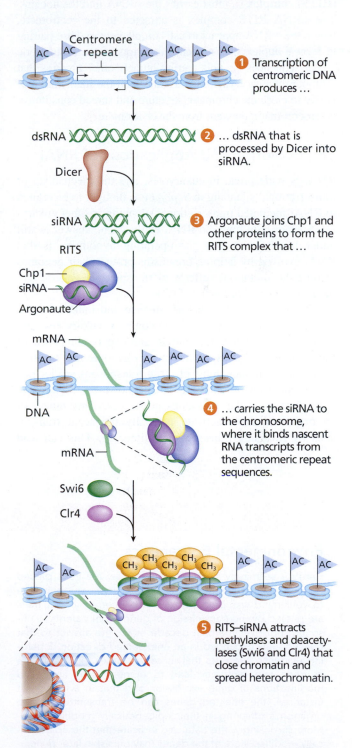

Figure 13.28 **RNA-induced transcriptional silencing (RITS) in yeast.**

Q **Compare and contrast the action of RITS with that of RISC.**

and form double-stranded RNAs that Dicer cuts ❷. The siRNA fragments produced by this process are then separated into single strands that bind to Argonaute, which then joins a protein known as Chp1 and other proteins to form a RISC-like complex called the **RNA-induced transcriptional silencing (RITS) complex** (❸) that carries the siRNA into the nucleus. The siRNA–RITS complex is attracted to the centromere, where the siRNA appears to use complementary base pairing to form a duplex with nascent transcripts of the centromeric repeat sequences ❹. This pairing attracts other proteins that promote the deacetylation of histones and the methylation of H3K9 to close the chromatin structure and spread constitutive heterochromatin outward from the centromere ❺.

The Evolution and Applications of RNAi

RNAi is widespread in eukaryotes, and the mechanism of transcriptional silencing in *S. pombe* is thought to be related to RNAi-mediated transcriptional silencing in other eukaryotic species. But how did RNAi evolve? The answer is still under investigation, but the operating hypothesis is that RNAi evolved by helping organisms protect their genomes against the mutational effects of transposable genetic elements (described in Section 11.7).

Transposable elements are diverse and make up large percentages of the genomes of complex eukaryotes. For example, almost half the human genome is composed of transposable elements. In the human genome and in other eukaryotic genomes, most of these transposons are located in heterochromatin and are silent; however, researchers have discovered that mutations in the RNAi machinery of an organism can reactivate normally quiescent transposons by reversing transcriptional silencing. This can lead to the movement of some transposable elements around the genome and potentially to the production of new mutations. The evidence suggests that RNAi plays a role in silencing the transcription of transposons.

RNAi also plays a protective role in response to viral infection. In plants, the infection of one leaf by a virus can generate an RNAi response that blocks viral replication and prevents the infection from spreading throughout the plant. In support of this observation, plants with Dicer or Argonaute mutations are much more susceptible to the spread of viral infections than are plants without Dicer or Argonaute mutations. These findings are consistent with the idea that RNAi evolved as a genome-protection mechanism against transposable genetic elements and viral infection.

Both plants and animal genomes encode miRNAs, but the mode of action of miRNAs differs slightly between the two taxa. In plants, miRNAs display near-complete sequence complementarity with their mRNA targets and usually cleave the target rather than block translation. In contrast, miRNAs in animals are usually only complementary to their targets at one end of the miRNA and usually repress translation rather than cleave the target. These differences suggest that miRNAs may have evolved independently in the two lineages, from an RNAi-like mechanistic precursor.

RNAi is also a powerful research tool that can be used in a multitude of ways. One frequent application of RNAi in research is the use of siRNAs to "knock down," or obstruct, the expression of selected genes. Researchers can then examine how phenotype is altered in the absence of the obstructed genes and in this way discover the genes' usual effects. We discuss other experimental applications of RNAi in Section 14.3.

CASE STUDY

Environmental Epigenetics

Here's a seemingly simple question: How are traits passed from one generation to the next? The first answer that came to your mind was probably (and not incorrectly) that traits are passed by the transmission of genes from parents to offspring. But over the past decade or so, the answer to that question has expanded in an unexpected direction. Emerging evidence suggests that in certain cases, an organism's nutrition and diet may lead to epigenetically controlled modifications of gene expression and that in a few select instances, the affected genes can be transmitted to the organism's offspring in their epigenetically modified form. More surprisingly, the data also indicate that the epigenetically modified state of the genes may persist in later generations. In other words, it may be possible for the nutritional experience of grandparents to affect gene expression in their grandchildren—an idea reminiscent of the theories of Lamarck, who proposed the inheritance of traits acquired within a lifetime!

HONEYBEE DESTINY Three lines of evidence suggest a role for nutrition and dietary history in the epigenetic modification of gene expression. The first comes from studies in honeybees, where it has been shown that genetically identical larvae can develop into either fertile queens or sterile worker bees following differential feeding with royal jelly, the compound fed to larvae that become queens. Experimental analysis led by Ryszard Maleszka in 2008 reveals that silencing the expression of the DNA methyltransferase *Dnmt3* by knocking down translation of the Dnmt3 transcript by RNA interference leads to the development of fertile queens. In other words, blocking a major histone methylation pathway led to the expression of genes that are typically expressed only when a larva is fed royal jelly. The implication is that methylation is an important epigenetic mechanism for repressing gene expression and directing the development of worker bees. Methylation and the resulting transcriptional repression are subverted by feeding royal jelly to produce the development of fertile queen bees.

EVIDENCE IN MICE The second line of evidence comes from multiple studies of the connection between environmentally generated methylation of genes and variation in gene expression in rats and mice. In one study, genetically identical mice carry a modified *agouti* gene that produces yellow coat color and extreme obesity when the gene is expressed, whereas the normal brown coat color and normal body weight are produced if the modified gene is not expressed. The coat color and body weight of genetically identical mouse pups carrying this modified gene are determined by the diet of the mother in the weeks before impregnation and during pregnancy and lactation.

In controlled experiments, mothers that will transmit the modified *agouti* gene to their pups are fed either a diet enriched with three compounds that each act as donors of methyl groups to DNA—folic acid (vitamin B_{12}), choline chloride, and anhydrous betaine—or a diet without these compounds. The controlled dietary period begins 2 weeks before mating and continues through pregnancy and lactation. The pups produced are genetically identical, and after they are weaned, they are all fed the same diet. At 3 weeks of age, however, the appearance of the pups is dramatically different. Mice produced by mothers who were fed the enriched diet have brown coat color and normal body weight, whereas genetically identical mice produced by mothers not fed the enriched diet have yellow coat color and are obese. The difference indicates that the modified *agouti* gene is expressed when it is transmitted from mothers that were not fed the diet enriched with methyl donors. If the modified gene is transmitted from mothers receiving the enriched diet, however, the modified *agouti* gene is methylated and silenced.

INHERITANCE OF FAMINE EFFECTS The third line of evidence comes from an unfortunate event during World War II. A severe famine occurred in German-occupied Netherlands between November 1944 and May 1945. The famine reduced daily caloric intake to 500 to 800 calories per day, much less than the body needs to fuel its normal metabolic activities. Long-term studies have been performed on Dutch people who were conceived or born during the famine and on their descendants. Studies of the health effects of the famine find that so-called famine babies were often born severely underweight. As the famine babies grew into adults and aged, they suffered increased risk of cardiovascular disease, diabetes, and obesity compared with peers who had not been affected by the famine. The proposed explanation is that the restricted nutritional conditions in the womb caused alterations of gene expression, producing an energetically "thrifty" metabolism. More surprising, however, was that among the children of the famine babies, there is also an elevated risk of cardiovascular and other diseases. The explanation proposed for this second-generation effect is epigenetic modification of gene expression that is transmitted through multiple generations.

A 2008 study by Bastiaan Heijmans on the methylation pattern of the *IGF2* gene on chromosome 15 confirms the epigenetic control mechanism that we discussed previously in connection with genomic imprinting, Prader–Willi syndrome, and Angelman syndrome. Heijmans and colleagues found that *IGF2* in certain famine babies (now in their sixties) still bears the marks of famine. The *IGF2* genes of those exposed to famine during the first 10 weeks of gestation are marked by significantly fewer methyl groups than are the genes of their same-sex siblings not exposed to famine conditions. These results support the idea that prenatal conditions can impart specific epigenetic patterns to genes and that environmental factors contributing to epigenetic patterns may play an important role in modifying gene expression over multiple generations.

SUMMARY

Mastering Genetics For activities, animations, and review quizzes, go to the Study Area.

13.1 Cis-Acting Regulatory Sequences Bind Trans-Acting Regulatory Proteins to Control Eukaryotic Transcription

❙ Promoters, proximal elements, and enhancer modules are cis-acting DNA sequences that bind trans-acting regulatory proteins to regulate transcription.

❙ The effects of activators and repressors binding to enhancer/silencer modules integrate to produce an output, with repressors often dominant.

❙ Enhancer sequences can be strongly conserved, indicating they perform essential functions.

❙ Upstream activator sequences (UASs) in yeast are enhancer-like elements that regulate the expression of genes such as those involved in galactose utilization.

❙ Locus control regions (LCRs) are specialized enhancers that control the sequential expression of sets of genes such as those in the developmentally regulated human β-globin gene complex.

❙ Insulators block enhancer influence on nearby genes and direct that influence to other genes.

13.2 Chromatin Remodeling and Modification Regulates Eukaryotic Transcription

❙ Heterochromatin has a closed chromatin structure and is transcriptionally silent, whereas euchromatin has an open structure that is transcriptionally active.

❙ Open promoters are constitutively transcribed (often housekeeping genes), whereas transcription from covered promoters is regulated.

❙ Chromatin-remodeling complexes displace nucleosomes to allow transcription initiation by RNA pol II and general transcription factors.

❙ Chromatin is modified by writers and erasers, and read by readers. Writers and erasers are recruited by transcription factors to open and close the chromatin by adding and removing acetyl and methyl groups at specific amino acids in the N-terminal tails of histone proteins.

❙ Polycomb group and Trithorax group complexes act to transform facultative heterochromatin into euchromatin and vice versa.

- Epigenetic states of chromatin are heritable in somatic cells that divide by mitosis and may be reset in germ-line cells that divide by meiosis.
- Genomic imprinting in mammalian genomes involves nucleotide methylation and the action of enhancer and insulator sequences.
- A specific form of regulatory RNA directs mammalian X-inactivation.

- Small interfering RNAs (siRNAs) and microRNAs (miRNAs) are principal regulatory RNA molecules.
- The Dicer protein complex processes dsRNAs into small RNAs.
- RISC carries regulatory RNAs to RNAs targeted for destruction or for blockage of translation.
- RITS acts to maintain constitutive heterochromatin.

13.3 RNA-Mediated Mechanisms Control Gene Expression

- RNA interference (RNAi) is an RNA-mediated mechanism for regulating gene expression in eukaryotes.

PREPARING FOR PROBLEM SOLVING

In addition to the list of problem-solving tips and suggestions given here, you can go to the Study Guide and Solutions Manual that accompanies this book for help at solving problems.

1. Familiarize yourself with the mechanistic differences between bacterial and eukaryotic gene expression.

2. Understand that enhancer/silencer modules integrate inputs of several transcription factors into a single output.

3. Review the roles of chromatin remodelers and chromatin modifying enzymes in eukaryotic gene expression.

4. Familiarize yourself with the functions of TrxG and PcG complexes in facultative heterochromatin.

5. Review the different classes of chromatin and their relation to gene expression, for example, the types of genes they are likely to contain.

6. Acquaint yourself with the sources and processing of dsRNAs and their subsequent roles in modulating gene expression.

PROBLEMS

Mastering Genetics Visit for instructor-assigned tutorials and problems.

Chapter Concepts

For answers to selected even-numbered problems, see Appendix: Answers.

1. Devoting a few sentences to each, describe the following structures or complexes and their effects on eukaryotic gene expression:
   a. promoter
   b. enhancer
   c. silencer
   d. RISC
   e. Dicer

2. Describe and give an example (real or hypothetical) of each of the following:
   a. upstream activator sequence (UAS)
   b. insulator sequence action
   c. silencer sequence action
   d. enhanceosome action
   e. RNA interference

3. What is meant by the term *chromatin remodeling*? Describe the importance of this process to transcription.

4. What general role does acetylation of histone protein amino acids play in the transcription of eukaryotic genes?

5. Describe the roles of writers, readers, and erasers in eukaryotic gene regulation.

6. Outline the roles of RNA in eukaryotic gene regulation.

7. What are the roles of the Polycomb and Trithorax complexes in eukaryotic gene regulation?

8. Most biologists argue that the regulation of gene expression is considerably more complex in eukaryotes than in bacteria. List and describe the four factors that in your view make the largest contribution to this perception.

9. Compare and contrast the transcriptional regulation of *GAL* genes in yeast with that of the *lac* genes in bacteria.

10. The term *heterochromatin* refers to heavily condensed regions of chromosomes that are largely devoid of genes. Since few genes exist there, these regions almost never decondense for transcription. At what point during the cell cycle would you expect to observe the decondensation of heterochromatic regions? Why?

11. Compare and contrast promoters and enhancers with respect to their location (upstream versus downstream), orientation, and distance (in base pairs) relative to a gene they regulate.

12. What are the different chromatin classifications, and what is their relationship to gene expression?

13. Define epigenetics, and provide examples illustrating your definition.

14. What is one proposed role for lncRNAs?

15. What are the sources of dsRNA? Diagram the mechanisms by which dsRNAs are produced and processed into small RNAs.

16. How does dsRNA lead to posttranscriptonal gene silencing?

Application and Integration

For answers to selected even-numbered problems, see Appendix: Answers.

17. A hereditary disease is inherited as an autosomal recessive trait. The wild-type allele of the disease gene produces a mature mRNA that is 1250 nucleotides (nt) long. Molecular analysis shows that the mature mRNA consists of four exons that measure 400 nt (exon 1), 320 nt (exon 2), 230 nt (exon 3), and 300 nt (exon 4). A mother and father with two healthy children and two children with the disease have northern blot analysis performed in a medical genetics laboratory. The results of the northern blot for each family member are shown here.

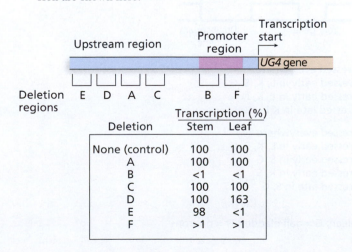

a. Identify the genotype of each family member, using the sizes of mRNAs to indicate each allele. (For example, a person who is homozygous wild type is indicated as "1250/1250.")

b. Based on your analysis, what is the most likely molecular abnormality causing the disease allele?

18. The *UG4* gene is expressed in stem tissue and leaf tissue of the plant *Arabidopsis thaliana*. To study mechanisms regulating *UG4* expression, six small deletions of DNA sequence upstream of the gene-coding sequence are made. The locations of deletions and their effect on *UG4* expression are shown here.

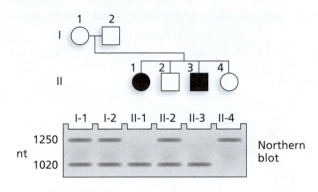

Deletion	Transcription (%)	
	Stem	Leaf
None (control)	100	100
A	100	100
B	<1	<1
C	100	100
D	100	163
E	98	<1
F	>1	>1

a. Explain the differential effects of deletions B and F on expression in the two tissues.

b. Why does deletion D raise *UG4* expression in leaf tissue but not in stem tissue?

c. Why does deletion E lower expression of *UG4* in leaf tissue but not in stem tissue?

19. Diagram and explain how the inducibility of a gene—for instance in response to an environmental cue—could be mediated by an activator. Then show how it could be mediated by a repressor.

20. A muscle enzyme called ME1 is produced by transcription and translation of the *ME1* gene in several muscles during mouse development, including heart muscle, in a highly regulated manner. Production of ME1 appears to be turned on and turned off at different times during development. To test the possible role of enhancers and silencers in *ME1* transcription, a biologist creates a recombinant genetic system that fuses the *ME1* promoter, along with DNA that is upstream of the promoter, to the bacterial *lacZ* (β-galactosidase) gene. The *lacZ* gene is chosen for the ease and simplicity of assaying production of the encoded enzyme. The diagram shows bars that indicate the extent of six deletions the biologist makes to the *ME1* promoter and upstream sequences. The blue deletion labeled D is within the promoter whereas the gray bars span potential enhancer/silencer modules. The table displays the percentage of β-galactosidase activity in each deletion mutant in comparison with the recombinant gene system without any deletions.

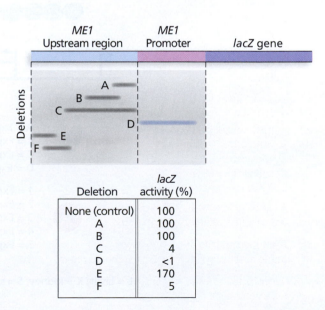

Deletion	*lacZ* activity (%)
None (control)	100
A	100
B	100
C	4
D	<1
E	170
F	5

a. Does this information indicate the presence of enhancer and/or silencer sequences in the *ME1* upstream sequence? If so, where is/are the sequences located?

b. Why does deletion D effectively eliminate transcription of *lacZ*?

c. Given the information available from deletion analysis, can you give a molecular explanation for the observation that *ME1* expression appears to turn on and turn off at various times during normal mouse development?

Collaboration and Discussion

For answers to selected even-numbered problems, see Appendix: Answers.

21. Using the components in the accompanying diagram, design regulatory modules (i.e., enhancer/silencer modules) required for "your" gene to be expressed only in differentiating (early) and differentiated (late) liver cells. Answer the three questions presented below by describing the roles that activators, enhancers, repressors, silencers, pioneer factors, insulators, chromatin remodeling complexes, and chromatin readers, writers, and erasers will play in the regulation of expression of your gene, that is, what factors will bind and be active in each case? Specify which transcription factors need to be pioneer factors.

a. How will the gene be activated in the proper cell type?

b. How will its expression be maintained?

c. How will expression be prevented in other cell types?

22. The majority of this chapter focused on gene regulation at the transcriptional level, but the quantity of functional protein product in a cell can be regulated in many other ways as well (see Figure 13.1). Discuss possible reasons why transcriptional regulation or posttranscriptional regulation may have evolved for different types of genes.

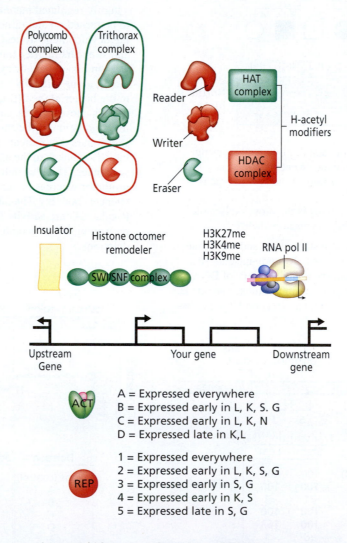

A = Expressed everywhere
B = Expressed early in L, K, S. G
C = Expressed early in L, K, N
D = Expressed late in K,L

1 = Expressed everywhere
2 = Expressed early in L, K, S, G
3 = Expressed early in S, G
4 = Expressed early in K, S
5 = Expressed late in S, G

L = Liver; K = kidney; S = spleen; G = gall bladder; N = neurons

Analysis of Gene Function by Forward Genetics and Reverse Genetics

14

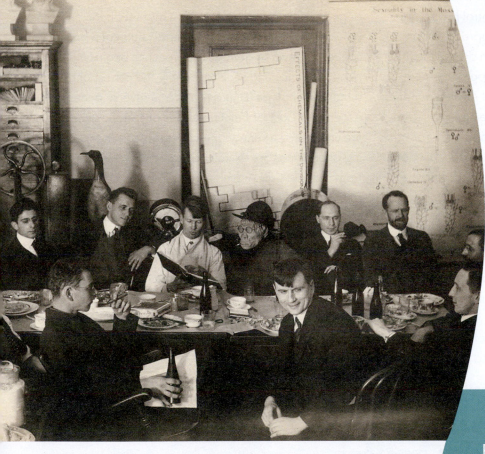

CHAPTER OUTLINE

14.1 Forward Genetic Screens Identify Genes by Their Mutant Phenotypes

14.2 Genes Identified by Mutant Phenotype Are Cloned Using Recombinant DNA Technology

14.3 Reverse Genetics Investigates Gene Action by Progressing from Gene Identification to Phenotype

14.4 Transgenes Provide a Means of Dissecting Gene Function

Thomas Hunt Morgan's fly room (he is at far right, back row) was the site of the original mutagenesis experiments. The first screens for mutations were limited by their reliance on spontaneous mutants, but the discovery by Hermann Muller (second from right, back row) that X-rays are mutagenic turned genetic screens into routine and powerful tools to uncover gene function. Also visible in this photo are Calvin Bridges (third from left, back row), who used observations of nondisjunction to prove the chromosome theory of heredity, and Alfred Sturtevant (middle front row), who constructed the first genetic map.

A central goal of biology is to understand the molecular and genetic bases of physiology and development. Beginning with Mendel and resuming in the first part of the 20th century, geneticists attempted to dissect the rules of heredity by connecting phenotypes to genetic loci. The discovery of DNA as the hereditary material indicated that genes are specific DNA sequences and that allelic differences reflect differences in those sequences. In the 1970s, discoveries stemming from the study of bacteria and their phages led to

ESSENTIAL IDEAS

- Forward genetic screens induce mutations to identify genes involved in a biological process; subsequent cloning sheds light on their molecular function.

- DNA sequences of specific genes can be discovered using recombinant DNA technology.

- Reverse genetics techniques start with a gene sequence and then proceed to the identification of a mutant phenotype.

- Phenotypes of transgenic organisms can provide information on gene function.

the development of tools to manipulate DNA in vitro. With these tools, collectively referred to as *recombinant DNA technology*, geneticists could for the first time obtain the precise DNA sequences of specific genes and alleles, thus identifying the molecular basis of phenotypic differences.

The exploration of how genes control physiological and developmental processes is approached in two ways that attack the problem from diametrically opposite directions. These opposite approaches are known as *forward genetic analysis* and *reverse genetic analysis*. The goals of forward and reverse analysis are the same: to identify the genes responsible for hereditary variation, to determine the structure and function of wild-type alleles controlling traits, and to describe how mutant alleles generate abnormal phenotypes. However, the two strategies begin at different ends of the process of gene identification.

Forward genetic analysis starts with a **genetic screen** that identifies specific phenotypic abnormalities in a population of organisms that have been mutagenized—**mutagenesis** being the intentional introduction of mutations into the genome of an organism. The abnormal phenotype is then studied to identify the

nature of the hereditary abnormality and, by inference, the normal functions of an associated gene. Ultimately, the sequence of the gene responsible for the abnormality is determined and may suggest the molecular function of the corresponding gene product (**Figure 14.1a**). In contrast to forward genetics approaches, which begin genetic investigation with a mutant phenotype and proceed toward the identification of a gene sequence, **reverse genetics** approaches begin with a gene sequence and seek to identify the corresponding mutant phenotype (**Figure 14.1b**). In a reverse genetics experiment, loss-of-function alleles of specific genes are created by a variety of techniques, and the resulting phenotypes are examined to see how they differ from the wild type. Reverse genetic analysis has risen to prominence as a result of the enormous quantity of DNA sequence data made available since the late 1990s and of the ability of recombinant DNA technology to manipulate DNA sequences in vitro and in vivo.

In this chapter, we discuss forward and reverse genetic analyses from a conceptual viewpoint, and in Chapter 15 we present details of the recombinant DNA technology used to conduct this research.

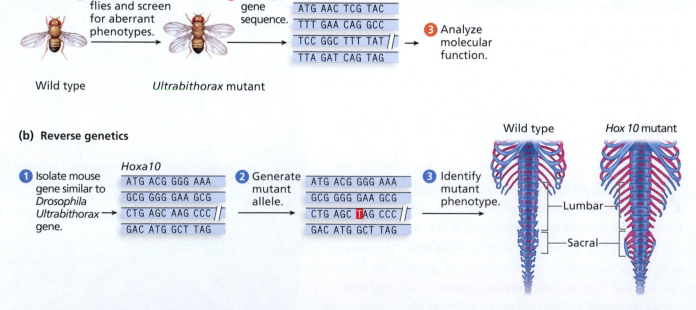

Figure 14.1 General strategies of forward and reverse genetics.

Ⓠ **Does this figure suggest a way in which the approaches of forward and reverse genetics complement one another?**

14.1 Forward Genetic Screens Identify Genes by Their Mutant Phenotypes

With the discovery by Hermann Muller that ionizing radiation induces mutations (see Section 11.3), geneticists realized that mutant organisms could be generated at will and systematically screened for phenotypes of interest. Mutant phenotypes provide information on the function of the wild-type allele and insight into biological processes. The earliest example of this logic is the work of Archibald Garrod, who in 1908 connected the human autosomal recessive hereditary condition alkaptonuria to the lack of a specific biochemical activity, the metabolism of homogentisic acid (see Figure 4.17b). He suggested that the wild-type version of the gene encodes the enzyme responsible for this biochemical activity. After Muller brought the mutagenic powers of X-rays to their attention (see Section 11.3), geneticists began to employ systematic genetic screens to dissect other biological processes, and the genetic bases for entire biochemical pathways were elucidated.

The designing of genetic screens to identify genes involved in specific biological processes is limited only by the imagination of the geneticist. An example is the research by Seymour Benzer that led to the field of behavioral genetics in the 1970s. Benzer believed mutations could be identified that specifically affect behavioral processes, such as one you are using now, the process of learning and memory. At the time, behavior was thought by many to be too complex to be dissected genetically. However, Chip Quinn, a graduate student in Benzer's lab, built on previous ideas and designed an ingenious screen to identify learning- and memory-deficient mutants in *Drosophila*. Wild-type flies could be taught that a pulse of odor would be followed by a shock; later, when the flies smelled the odor, they would take evasive action. When Quinn and Benzer subjected a mutagenized population of *Drosophila* to this genetic screen, they identified mutant strains of flies that could perceive the odor but seemed unable to associate the odor with the stimulus; either they did not learn or could not remember.

Two mutant genes identified in the study, *dunce* and *rutabaga*, were later shown to encode proteins involved in the production or degradation of the small signaling molecule cyclic adenosine monophosphate (cAMP). At the time, signaling via a cAMP pathway was known to be required for learning in the sea hare, *Aplysia*. Since both *Drosophila* mutants were defective in cAMP physiology, other genes that encoded proteins involved in cAMP signaling and response were also investigated for roles in learning. Ultimately, a transcription factor called *creb* (*cAMP response element–binding* protein), which activates or represses genes in response to cAMP signaling, was shown to be critical for storing memories in flies. Remarkably, *creb* is widely conserved in animal species, and mouse mutants lacking *creb* activity also fail to remember. A similar gene

is found in our genome, and there is great interest in the role of this gene in human memory.

A great strength of forward genetic screens is that they are unbiased; no prior knowledge of the molecular function of the encoded gene product is required. In a sense, by performing a mutagenesis, the geneticist is allowing the organism to reveal how its biological processes operate. Once genes in particular physiological or developmental processes have been identified by mutation, clues to the molecular function of the gene product can be obtained using recombinant DNA technology.

General Design of Forward Genetic Screens

Forward genetic screens often require the mutagenesis of thousands of individuals, followed by screening large numbers of their progeny for mutant phenotypes. Each progeny may contain multiple mutations, but only a small fraction of the progeny will have a mutant phenotype of interest. For example, in their screens to identify auxotrophs, Beadle, Tatum, and colleagues screened many thousands of individual mutant lines to find the few arginine auxotrophs that were produced. Although some screens necessitate the visual inspection of all progeny, others are specifically designed to highlight certain mutants of interest against the background of all other mutants. The designing of such screens is an art.

Perhaps the most dramatic screen is one in which application of a simple selection technique allows mutants of interest to survive while those not of interest die. Examples include the isolation of bacteria resistant to antibiotics, insects resistant to insecticides, and plants resistant to herbicides. Similarly, isolation of mutants resistant to analogs of cellular chemicals or to high levels of naturally occurring hormones has proven useful in genetic screens. Often in such cases, mutations identify genes encoding proteins involved in the metabolism or signaling pathways of the respective chemicals.

Even when strong selection criteria cannot be applied, knowledge of the biological process of interest can influence the design of the screen. For example, in research on the genetic control of embryonic development (described in Section 18.2), Eric Wieschaus and Christiane Nüsslein-Volhard designed a screen for *Drosophila* embryogenesis mutants based on the assumption that the mutations of interest were all likely to be lethal to the larva. Thus they could limit their intensive analysis to mutant lines in which larval lethality was evident.

Specific Strategies of Forward Genetic Screens

Forward genetic screens begin with a mutagenesis: An organism is treated with a mutagen to create mutations randomly throughout the genome. A typical goal is to induce mutations in every gene in a population of mutagenized individuals, an approach called **saturation mutagenesis**. The mutagenized population is then screened for phenotypic defects in whatever biological process is being studied, and the mutants are collected and propagated for further analysis. Strategies for mutagenesis depend on the biological process of interest, which dictates the experimental organism to use, the choice of mutagen, and the screening procedure to identify mutations.

Choosing an Organism The attributes that make an organism a good genetic model (see back endsheets) also make it a good choice for a mutagenesis experiment: The organism must be able to progress through its entire life cycle in the laboratory, have a short generation time (for eukaryotic models, the time it takes to produce sexually mature progeny and complete the sexual life cycle), and produce a reasonable number of progeny. In addition, researchers must be able to manipulate it to produce specific genetic crosses. Organisms that are diploid usually have a starting genotype (the genotype to be mutagenized) that is inbred—in other words, for the most part homozygous at all loci. Such a genotype allows newly induced mutations to be readily identified, without interference from the confounding effects of polymorphisms. Finally, it is advantageous to use the simplest organism possible for the biological process under study. Because *Saccharomyces cerevisiae* has a rapid life cycle and is easily manipulated in the laboratory, it is often used to investigate biological processes common to all eukaryotes. The principles elucidated in *S. cerevisiae* can often be extended to other eukaryotes, including humans.

Choosing a Mutagen The choice of mutagen is dictated by both the organism and the type of mutant alleles desired; different mutagens have different advantages and disadvantages (Table 14.1). Mutagens inducing different types of changes in DNA sequences were described in Section 11.3.

Treatment with chemical mutagens can induce hundreds of mutations in a single individual, allowing saturation to be reached with only a few thousand mutagenized individuals. However, the cloning of genes identified by chemical mutagenesis can be laborious. In contrast, mutagens that result specifically in insertions of DNA, such as transposons, result in far fewer mutations per individual, making saturation difficult. But these mutagens have the advantage of being able to provide a DNA "tag" that facilitates finding and cloning the mutated genes.

In all mutageneses used for forward genetic screens, care must be taken to "outbreed" mutants of interest by crossing them with the wild-type progenitor strain. This will ensure that the collected mutant lines have only the mutation of interest and not others that were also induced during the mutagenesis.

Strategy for Identifying Dominant and Recessive Mutations The overall goal of mutagenesis is to identify multiple independent mutant alleles of each gene involved in the biological process of interest. Let us consider the identification of dominant and recessive mutations in a typical animal example.

Most animals spend most of their life cycle in the diploid state. Their germ cells are set aside early in development and do not contribute to the somatic development of the remainder of the animal body. When animals are treated with a mutagen—for example, by feeding males ethyl methanesulfonate (EMS), a potent mutagen that causes a spectrum of mutant alleles (see Table 14.1)—only the mutations induced in the germ cells are heritable and will be passed to the progeny of the mutagenized animals.

Breeding these mutagenized males with wild-type females will allow newly induced dominant mutations to be identified in the resulting F_1 generation (Figure 14.2a). However, only a small fraction of all the mutagenized flies will harbor a dominant mutation, since they are rare. This rarity is due to the low probability that any change in the DNA sequence of a gene will produce a gain in function for the encoded gene product, either qualitatively or quantitatively.

Table 14.1	Common Mutagens Used for Mutagenesis		
Mutagen	Mutation Spectrum	Mutation Rate per Locus	Allele Spectrum
Chemical			
Ethyl methanesulfonate (EMS)	mostly G → A (C → T) transitions Stop codons created: TGG → TAG Splice sites destroyed: AG → AA	High	Usually loss-of-function (null, hypomorphic), hypermorphic (rare)
Radiation			
Fast-neutron X-ray Gamma-ray	Rearrangements (deletions, inversions, translocations)	Moderate	Usually loss-of-function (often null), but can be gain-of-function
Insertional			
Transfer DNA Transposons	Insertions	Low	Usually loss-of-function (often null)

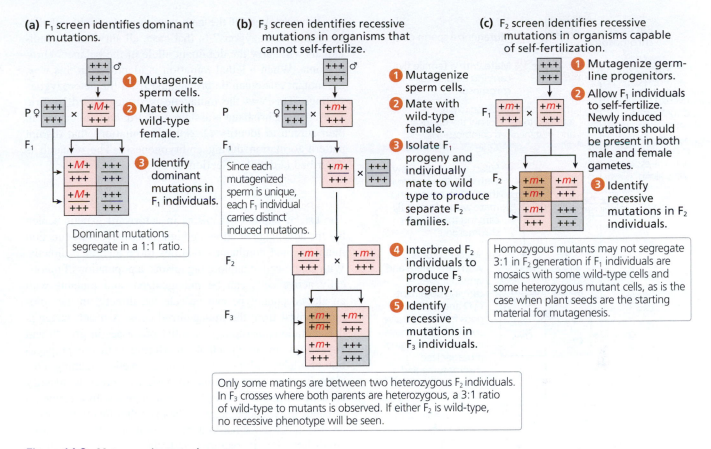

(a) F_1 screen identifies dominant mutations.

(b) F_3 screen identifies recessive mutations in organisms that cannot self-fertilize.

(c) F_2 screen identifies recessive mutations in organisms capable of self-fertilization.

Figure 14.2 Mutagenesis strategies.

Mutations that result in a loss of function are more common, but loss-of-function mutations are usually recessive and do not result in an observable phenotype in the F_1 generation. Therefore, further breeding must be performed, to produce homozygous loss-of-function mutants. Specifically, recessive mutations are identified in an F_3 screen (**Figure 14.2b**). In this screen, each F_1 individual derived from the mating of mutagenized males with wild-type females carries unique mutations. The F_1 individuals are then crossed with wild-type females, producing an F_2 generation in which half of the individuals will carry the newly induced mutations. The F_2 siblings are interbred, producing an F_3 population segregating for individuals that are homozygous for the induced mutation. The interbreeding of the F_2 to produce homozygous mutant F_3 is inefficient, since only half of the F_2 are heterozygous for the induced mutation. Nonetheless, such mutagenesis strategies are employed with many species, such as mice and zebrafish.

Identification of recessive mutations is somewhat simpler in organisms that self-fertilize, such as *Caenorhabditis elegans* and many plants (e.g., *Arabidopsis* and maize). In these organisms, F_1 individuals are self-fertilized to produce an F_2 generation from which recessive mutations can be identified. An example of an F_2 screen is shown in **Figure 14.2c**. In either an F_2 or F_3 screen, mutations resulting in homozygous lethality can be maintained in heterozygous siblings.

Use of Balancer Chromosomes for Tracking Mutations

The inefficiency of an F_3 screen can be circumvented using chromosomes that are marked so they can be followed through generations. **Balancer chromosomes** developed in *Drosophila* allow specific chromosomes to be transmitted intact and followed through multiple generations.

Balancer chromosomes have three general features: (1) one or more inverted chromosomal segments, within which meiotic recombinants are not transmitted (see Section 10.5 for a review); (2) a recessive allele that results in lethality, so an individual cannot be homozygous for the balancer chromosome; and (3) a "mark" in the form of a dominant mutation conferring a visible nonlethal phenotype, so the segregation of the chromosome can be followed through generations. An example of a balancer chromosome is the ClB chromosome used by Hermann Muller to demonstrate that X-rays induce mutations (see Experimental Insight 10.1, page 382).

Balancer chromosomes are available for all of the *Drosophila* chromosomes and can be used to identify mutations on specific chromosomes (**Figure 14.3**). Male flies are fed EMS to induce mutations and then are mated with females containing a balancer chromosome. Note that while mutations are induced throughout the genome, only those on the homolog of the balancer chromosome are analyzed. Male F_1 progeny are selected that inherit a mutagenized chromosome from their father and the balancer chromosome from

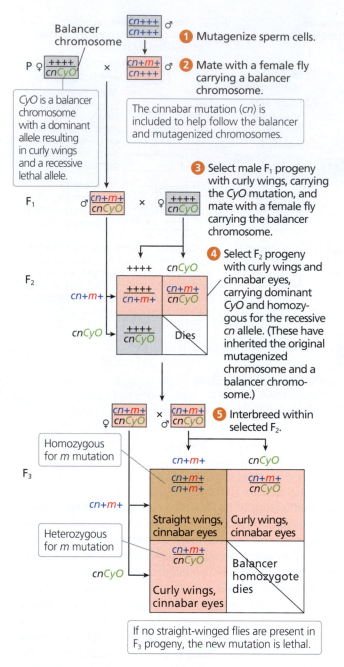

Figure 14.3 Identifying recessive mutations in *Drosophila* using a balancer chromosome.

What happens if the new mutation results in lethality when it is homozygous? In that case, all surviving F$_3$ individuals will carry the dominant allele of the balancer chromosome. When a lethal mutation is identified in this way, the mutant allele can be propagated from the heterozygous siblings. This was the mutagenesis strategy used by Eric Wieschaus, Christiane Nüsslein-Volhard, and colleagues in their screen to identify *Drosophila* mutations that disrupt pattern formation during embryogenesis. The research is described in detail in Section 18.2.

Screening for Conditional Alleles in Haploid Organisms

The use of haploid organisms in a forward genetic screen has the advantage of allowing both recessive loss-of-function mutations and dominant mutations to be identified directly. With single-celled haploid organisms, a population of mitotically active cells can be mutagenized, and mutants with an altered phenotype can be selected directly in the colonies derived from the mutagenized cells. A disadvantage is that mutations disrupting essential processes in growth and physiology are often lethal, interfering with the propagation of alleles and thus complicating genetic screening. Fortunately, it is often feasible to design a screen to identify conditional mutant alleles of essential genes. In conditional mutants, the encoded gene product is either functional or not needed under one environmental condition—the **permissive condition**—but is required and either inactive or absent under another—the **restrictive condition**).

With some lethal mutations, the mutant phenotype can be rescued by addition of a needed substance to the growth medium. For example, histidine auxotrophic mutants can grow only when histidine is present in the growth medium. In a screen for conditional mutants of this type, the mutagenized population is initially grown under permissive conditions—in this case, in a medium containing histidine—so that both mutant and wild type will grow. This mutagenized population is then replica plated, and the population is screened for phenotypic defects (e.g., lethality) when grown under the restrictive condition (e.g., a lack of histidine). Such genetic screens were performed by Beadle and Tatum to identify auxotrophs in *Neurospora* in the research that established biochemical genetics and produced the one gene–one enzyme theory (see Section 4.3).

Some kinds of mutants can be rescued not by supplying a certain substance to the medium but by altering other kinds of environmental conditions instead. In temperature-sensitive mutants, the stability of the polypeptide product of a mutant allele differs with temperature (see Section 4.1), often as a result of a missense mutation.

This type of conditional lethal allele in the yeasts *S. cerevisiae* and *Schizosaccharomyces pombe* led to a molecular genetic understanding of the cell cycle, a biological process shared by all eukaryotes. Mutagenized yeast were grown at a permissive temperature to allow propagation, and then the mutant lines were exposed to a restrictive temperature, causing an arrest in growth

their mother. Next, the selected males are mated to females of the balancer stock, producing F$_2$ progeny. The F$_2$ generation consists of both males and females heterozygous for the induced mutation and can be interbred to produce F$_3$ progeny. In the F$_3$ generation, 25% should be homozygous for the induced mutation and will not carry the dominant allele of the balancer chromosome; 50% will be heterozygous for the newly induced mutation and also carry the dominant allele; and the remaining 25% will die due to homozygosity for the balancer chromosome. The homozygous progeny lacking the dominant allele from the balancer chromosome can be screened for an aberrant phenotype.

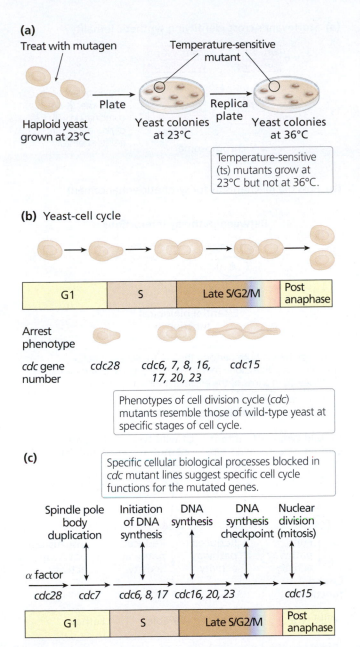

Figure 14.4 An example of identification and analysis of conditional alleles.

⊙ What are the advantages (and disadvantages) of working with a haploid organism?

progression through various stages of the cell cycle (**Figure 14.4c**). The studies in yeast provided the foundation for understanding the role of cell cycle regulation in cancer (see Section 3.1).

Analysis of Mutageneses

Typically, the initial analysis of mutants obtained by mutagenesis will focus on three key questions: (1) Are mutant alleles dominant or recessive with respect to the wild-type allele? (2) How many different genes have been identified in the mutagenesis? (3) How many different mutant alleles of each gene have been identified?

Determining Dominance or Recessiveness The answer to the first question provides insight into whether the mutant allele likely represents a loss of function or a gain of function (see Sections 4.1 and 11.1 for descriptions of these categories). Dominance or recessiveness is assessed during the mutagenesis (see Figure 14.2) and then confirmed using the same approach Mendel employed. Individuals homozygous wild-type, heterozygous mutant, and homozygous mutant for the new mutations, which can be generated by intercrossing two heterozygous mutants, can be compared to see whether the mutant phenotype is dominant or recessive.

Determining the Number of Genes Identified The answer to the second question—about the number of different genes revealed—provides clues to how many genes are involved in the biological process of interest. The most straightforward method of determining the number of genes represented by a new collection of mutants that produce similar mutant phenotypes is to perform complementation tests between different pairs of the mutant lines. If the progeny produced by crossing two recessive mutant lines exhibit a mutant phenotype, then the two mutations are in the same gene, whereas if the progeny exhibit a wild-type phenotype, then the two mutations are in different genes (see Section 4.4). In practice, we can limit the number of crosses by recognizing that complementation is transitive; that is, if mutation A is allelic to mutation B, and mutation B is allelic to mutation C, then mutations A and C are allelic. In some special cases, such as with mutations that are dominant or gametophytically lethal (lethal in a haploid stage of the life cycle, e.g., in pollen; see Section 4.1), complementation experiments cannot easily be performed, and other methods to ascertain allelism, such as mapping (see Section 5.2), may be employed.

Determining the Number of Mutant Alleles Identified for a Gene The answer to the third question should follow from the complementation analysis. Obtaining multiple mutant alleles of each gene is useful for two reasons. Comparing mutant phenotypes of multiple alleles allows an assessment of the range of phenotypic variation that

of some of the mutant strains (**Figure 14.4a**). Surprisingly, in some mutant lines, growth was arrested at specific stages of the cell cycle, rather than randomly along the continuous spectrum of growth (the latter would be expected if the mutation had disrupted a metabolic pathway). These yeast mutants fell into discrete phenotypic categories defined by the stage of the cell cycle at which they were arrested. One possible explanation was the existence of specific checkpoints in the cell cycle (**Figure 14.4b**), and, indeed, some of the genes identified by these mutations were found to regulate the cell's

can be obtained by mutation of the gene in question (see Section 4.1). The recovery of multiple alleles for each gene also provides information on the saturation of the genetic screen; in other words, it suggests what percentage of the genes that could be identified have in fact been identified. When a mutagenesis experiment is shown to have produced multiple independent mutations in each gene identified, most genes in the process of interest have likely been mutated.

Genetic Analysis 14.1 challenges you to design a screen that identifies genes involved in a particular biological process.

Identifying Interacting and Redundant Genes Using Modifier Screens

Generally, mutant phenotypes reflect the response of the organism to a loss or change of a particular gene product. However, individual genes do not act in isolation. The activity of other genes may modify, by either enhancing or suppressing, the phenotypic defects caused by the loss of a gene product. One approach to discovering genetic interactions is to carry out a genetic **modifier screen** to see if mutations in a second gene can enhance or suppress the phenotype of the first mutation. For example, starting with a *Drosophila* mutant with slightly curled wings, a modifier screen could be carried out to identify second-site mutations that result either in more severely curled wings or in a wing morphology that is restored to a wild-type phenotype. Genes identified in modifier screens are often involved in the same or closely related genetic pathways. An **enhancer screen** is a modifier screen in which mutations in a second site enhance the phenotype of the initial mutant. A **suppressor screen** is a modifier screen designed to identify second-site mutations that suppress the phenotype of the initial genotype. Note that both types of screens can be performed simultaneously. Enhancer–suppressor screening strategies are almost limitless in number and sophistication and have the potential to identify genes that function in interacting genetic pathways.

Modifier screens can identify double mutants that display an unexpected phenotype, one that is not simply the combination of the phenotypes of the two single mutants. In perhaps the most dramatic form of enhancement, termed **synthetic lethality**, the two single mutants are viable but the double mutant is inviable.

Synthetic lethality, or synthetic enhancement, was first noted by *Drosophila* geneticists who observed that some pairwise combinations of mutant alleles were inviable. For example, when Alfred Sturtevant crossed *prune* (*pn*) mutant females (*pn* is on the X chromosome) with males from a stock of separate origin called S/E-S, he noted that the progeny consisted solely of *pn*⁺ females and no viable males (**Figure 14.5a**). Sturtevant determined that the S/E-S males carried an autosomal dominant mutation, which he called *Prune-killer* (*K-pn*), that in combination with *pn* results in lethality, but he noted that flies

(a) Sturtevant's cross identifying synthetic lethality

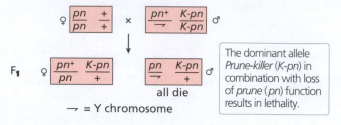

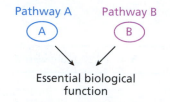

The dominant allele *Prune-killer* (*K-pn*) in combination with loss of *prune* (*pn*) function results in lethality.

⟶ = Y chromosome

(b) Possible mechanisms for synthetic enhancement

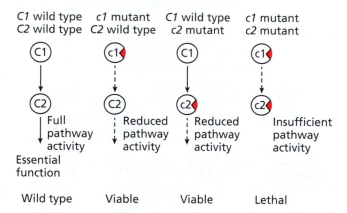

Figure 14.5 Synthetic enhancement.

🔴 **What kind of modifier screen can uncover genetic redundancy?**

homozygous for *K-pn* mutation alone did not have an aberrant phenotype. In his cross, all male progeny inherited a *pn* allele from their mother and a *K-pn* allele from their father, and therefore these progeny died. In contrast, the female progeny were viable, since despite inheriting a *K-pn* allele from their father, they also inherited a *pn*⁺ allele from their father. In this example, both *pn* mutants and *K-pn* mutants are viable, but the *pn*, *K-pn* double mutant results in lethality.

PROBLEM In all eukaryotic organisms, proteins to be secreted from the cell or embedded in the plasma membrane are translated at the endoplasmic reticulum and travel via the Golgi apparatus to reach the plasma membrane. Outline a genetic screen for identifying genes involved in protein secretion.

> BREAK IT DOWN: The posttranslational processing steps can be reviewed in Section 9.4 (p. 336).

> BREAK IT DOWN: In planning a mutagenesis, consider what type of organism and mutagen are appropriate.

Solution Strategies	Solution Steps
Evaluate	
1. Identify the topic this problem addresses and the nature of the required answer.	1. This problem is about designing a genetic screen to find a certain type of gene. The answer should describe a genetic screen to identify mutations in genes that function in protein secretion.
2. Identify the critical information given in the problem.	2. Information is given about protein secretion in cells, a universal process among eukaryotes.
Deduce	
3. Consider any information given about genes involved in the secretory process.	3. Since we have not been given any information about the genes involved in protein secretion, a forward genetic screen would be a good approach, because forward genetic mutageneses do not depend on prior knowledge about biochemical functions or gene sequences.
TIP: Consider experimental approaches that do not require prior knowledge of gene function.	
4. Based on the chapter discussion of forward genetic screens, choose an appropriate organism.	4. Since secretory systems in all eukaryotes are similar, they are likely to be homologous, that is, inherited from a common ancestor. Thus we can choose any eukaryote amenable to genetic analysis. *Saccharomyces cerevisiae* would be a good choice because many genetic tools already exist for this model genetic organism.
TIP: In which organisms does the biological process occur?	
5. Based on the chapter discussion of designing a forward genetic screen and on the phenotypic consequence of a loss of protein secretion, pick a strategy for identifying desirable mutant alleles.	5. Because complete loss of a functioning secretory system is likely to be lethal to any organism, we should use a strategy to identify conditional mutant alleles. Thus we should use a mutagen that induces point mutations.
PITFALL: Avoid the possibility of mutations that are lethal under all growth conditions.	
Solve	
6. Design an approach for a genetic screen based on Solution Steps 3–5.	6. A good design would be one similar to the procedure used to identify temperature-sensitive mutant alleles in genes of the cell cycle in *S. cerevisiae*. Mutagenesis of haploid cells could be performed at a permissive temperature (e.g., 25°–30°C), followed by screening for mutant phenotypes at a restrictive temperature (e.g., 39°C).
7. Describe how you would identify mutations specifically affecting secretion.	7. A method to monitor secretion is required. One approach would be to select a protein known to be secreted into the growth media of wild-type *S. cerevisiae* and look for mutants that do not secrete that protein (i.e., the protein is not detected in the medium in which they are growing).

For more practice, see Problems 17, 20, 21, 22, 25, 26, and 28. Visit the Study Area to access study tools. **Mastering Genetics**

Figure 14.5b shows two possible mechanisms to explain synthetic lethality. In one mechanism, the two genes in question act in parallel complementary pathways. In this scenario, mutations resulting in the loss of either pathway can be compensated for by the activity of the remaining pathway. However, when both pathways are disrupted, a dramatic enhancement in mutant phenotype is observed. An alternative mechanism is possible when both genes are acting in the same pathway: A reduction in function of one component of the pathway results in a mild phenotype, but when two components are disrupted, the pathway no longer

functions effectively. Note that in the latter scenario, hypomorphic alleles can result in synthetic enhancement, but null alleles cannot.

The first scenario, where two genes act in parallel, is an example of **genetic redundancy**, where the loss of the function of either gene alone is compensated for by the activity of the other, nonmutant gene. Only when both genes are mutant would a conspicuous mutant phenotype be evident. In such a case, a 15:1 segregation ratio could be expected in the F_2 of a cross between the two recessive single mutants (see the discussion of duplicate gene action in Section 4.3). In the most obvious case of genetic redundancy, two genes encode very similar proteins that can function interchangeably. In many instances, the activities of the two genes do not fully compensate for one another, so that single mutations, in either gene alone, result in a mild phenotype, while a severe phenotype is seen when both genes are mutant. Genetic redundancy caused by the presence of duplicate genes can arise in a species through small-scale duplications or through whole-genome duplications. As we explore in detail in Chapter 16, genome sequences of eukaryotes show such duplications to be very common.

Genetic redundancy can also arise from the compensatory action of genes that have little or no sequence similarity and encode biochemically different activities. This type of genetic redundancy is difficult to predict on the basis of the DNA sequences of the genes, but it too can be uncovered by enhancer–suppressor screens. Enhancer–suppressor screens have been performed on many organisms, including *Drosophila*, *C. elegans*, *Arabidopsis*, and mice (see Section 14.3), and are extremely successful at identifying interacting genetic pathways (see Section 18.3).

14.2 Genes Identified by Mutant Phenotype Are Cloned Using Recombinant DNA Technology

Although genes can be identified by genetic screens, determination of the specific DNA sequences of the wild-type and mutant alleles requires the use of recombinant DNA techniques to manipulate DNA molecules in vitro and in vivo. In this section, we discuss the theoretical foundations of how cloning of specific genes is achieved. Recombinant DNA technology is touched on in this chapter but discussed in detail in Section 15.1.

To appreciate the magnitude of the task of cloning a specific gene, consider that the goal is to single out the particular gene responsible for the mutant phenotype from among the thousands (or tens of thousands, in the cases of many eukaryotes) in the organism's genome, the proverbial needle in a haystack. Because both the biology and the ease of manipulation vary depending on the organism, different approaches have been developed for different species. In this section, we describe two of those approaches.

We begin by identifying two fundamental aspects of recombinant DNA technology that are required for cloning genes. First, gene sequences created in vitro can be introduced into the genome of a living organism. Such genes are termed **transgenes**, and the resulting organism is a **transgenic organism**. Because this process is similar to the transformation of bacteria—that is, the uptake of free DNA from outside the cell to inside the cell (see Section 6.3)—the creation of a transgenic organism is also referred to as transformation. The ease with which this process is accomplished varies significantly between organisms and thus

influences strategies for gene cloning and subsequent analyses of gene function.

A second key aspect is the creation of libraries, collections of clones of DNA fragments, derived from the total DNA or mRNA isolated from an organism. A library is a set of recombinant DNA molecules that collectively includes clones of all the relevant DNA sequences of an organism.

Genomic libraries are collections of cloned DNA fragments that as a group represent the entire genome of an organism, including repetitive and noncoding sequences. Genomic libraries usually consist of tens to hundreds of thousands of clones, each carried within an individual **cloning vector**—usually a plasmid (see Section 6.1) or bacteriophage (see Section 6.5) that has been modified to accommodate the insertion of exogenous fragments of DNA and that can be stably maintained in a host, such as *E. coli*. Some cloning vectors are specialized for carrying small (2–10 kb) pieces of genomic DNA and other cloning vectors are specialized for carrying large pieces (greater than 100 kb). After the fragments of a genome have been inserted into vectors, the vectors containing the genomic DNA are propagated in bacteria. A collection of many thousands to millions of bacterial colonies, each of which harbors copies of a different piece of genomic DNA, makes up the genomic library.

In contrast to genomic libraries, **complementary DNA libraries (cDNA libraries)** are collections of cloned DNA fragments that represent mRNA produced by an organism or cell type. In other words, only the portion of the genome that is transcribed is represented in a cDNA library. The clones of a cDNA library are also placed in cloning vectors, such as specially modified plasmids, and introduced into bacteria so that the complete cDNA library is composed of a large number of bacterial colonies, each of which harbors a different cDNA clone derived from the mRNA population.

Within a library, clones containing specific DNA sequences can be identified through complementary base pairing. With awareness of these tools, we can now consider the two approaches that are the focus of this section and whose purpose is to physically identify specific genes.

❙ First, genes can be identified by introducing a wild-type copy of a gene to complement a recessive mutant phenotype.

❙ Second, advances in DNA sequencing technology have made it feasible to find genes identified in genetic screens by directly comparing the genome sequence of the mutant with that of the wild-type strain from which it was derived.

Cloning Genes by Complementation

The most direct approach to identifying specific genes is to detect genetic complementation of a mutant phenotype by an introduced wild-type gene. This approach is restricted to cases in which large numbers of transgenic organisms can be generated. Consider the yeast temperature-sensitive cell-cycle mutants described in Section 14.1. If clones of a yeast cDNA expression library are transformed into a yeast cell-cycle mutant, any clones that complement the mutant phenotype so that the cells grow normally should contain wild-type alleles of the mutated gene (**Figure 14.6**).

In a procedure of this type, the yeast strain would first be transformed and grown at the permissive temperature. The resulting yeast colonies would then be transferred to an environment maintained at the restrictive temperature. Only the yeast colonies receiving a clone encoding a wild-type version of the mutant gene in question would be able to continue growth at the restrictive temperature; in those colonies, the mutant phenotype would have been complemented by the added gene.

Complementation experiments can also be used to identify similar genes from other species, if there is sufficient conservation of protein function. For example, research in which a yeast cell-cycle mutant was transformed using a human cDNA expression library (one in which the human cDNA clones were first fused with sequences allowing for their transcription and translation in yeast) has led to identification of human genes similar in function to the mutated yeast genes. The fact that both human and plant genes can complement these yeast mutants demonstrates the universality of the cell-cycle machinery and indicates that such proteins were present in the common ancestor of eukaryotes.

Genome Sequencing to Determine Gene Identification

Cloning genes by complementation is not applicable to all organisms, as it relies on a high efficiency of transformation—that is, a high frequency of successful transformation events in a host population (available in many bacteria and some fungi). When this is not feasible, as in most multicellular eukaryotes, how do biologists find the DNA sequence for a gene that is known only by its mutant phenotype? The most direct way to identify the molecular nature of mutations might seem to be to compare the genome sequence of the mutant line with that of the wild-type strain from which it was derived.

In theory, comparison of wild-type and mutant sequences should be straightforward, but there are both technical and physiological obstacles. First, in organisms like humans, it is difficult to distinguish between causative mutations and widespread polymorphisms. Second, even in inbred laboratory animals, typical mutagenesis protocols produce up to several hundred new mutations in each mutagenized gamete, introducing the need to backcross new mutant lines with their wild-type parental strain, as described earlier in this chapter, to isolate the causative mutation from the background of other mutations induced during the mutagenesis.

These obstacles can be overcome in inbred laboratory organisms by examining the genome sequences of many mutant individuals simultaneously after backcrossing. The details of how genome sequencing is accomplished are described in Section 16.1, but a conceptual outline of its application to identify a gene originally defined by a mutant phenotype is presented in **Figure 14.7**. First, the newly identified mutant line is backcrossed with the wild-type strain from which it was derived. The resulting F_1 individuals are interbred to produce an F_2 generation from which homozygous mutants can be selected. DNA is isolated from a number of homozygous mutants in the F_2 and is then pooled and sequenced in amounts sufficient to ensure that, on average, every nucleotide in the genome of each individual will be sequenced. The idea is that the causative mutation will be homozygous in all F_2 individuals selected, while other mutations will not. Mutations that are not linked to the causative mutation will segregate in a Mendelian fashion in the F_2, and this pattern will be reflected in the genome sequences. Mutations that *are* linked will segregate according to how closely they are linked to the causative mutation.

The concept behind using a large number of F_2 progeny is that, although in a single F_2 individual the probability of

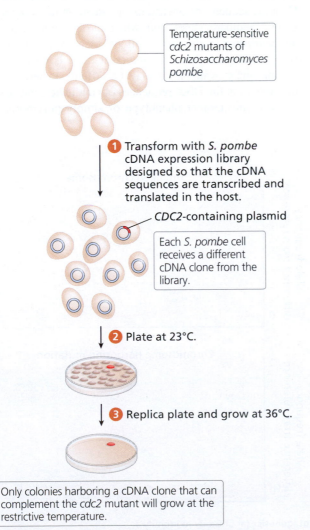

Temperature-sensitive *cdc2* mutants of *Schizosaccharomyces pombe*

① Transform with *S. pombe* cDNA expression library designed so that the cDNA sequences are transcribed and translated in the host.

CDC2-containing plasmid

Each *S. pombe* cell receives a different cDNA clone from the library.

② Plate at 23°C.

③ Replica plate and grow at 36°C.

Only colonies harboring a cDNA clone that can complement the *cdc2* mutant will grow at the restrictive temperature.

Figure 14.6 An example of cloning by complementation.

recombination between the causative mutation and another, closely linked mutation will be low, in a large population some level of recombination will occur between the causative mutation and most unlinked mutations. For example, if 50 homozygous mutant F_2 individuals are examined, 100 meiotic events are being assayed (since meiosis will have occurred to produce each of the gametes in the F_1 parents), providing a resolution of approximately 1 cM. Knowing

the genome sizes of the model genetics organisms and their genetic map length (see back endsheets), a researcher can approximate the likelihood of identifying only a small number of candidate mutations. Due to inexpensive DNA-sequencing technologies, this approach for going from mutant phenotype to gene identification is becoming commonplace in *Drosophila*, *C. elegans*, and *Arabidopsis*.

How does one prove that the causative mutation has been identified? In organisms amenable to transformation, the "gold standard" of gene identification is to complement the mutant phenotype by introducing a copy of the wild-type allele into the mutant background. This approach is similar to cloning by complementation described earlier, except the number of candidate genes is reduced from the entire set of genes in the genome to only the candidate gene(s) identified by genome sequencing. Transformation experiments are routine in many model genetic organisms and are described in more detail in Section 15.2.

In organisms not amenable to transformation (e.g., humans), other approaches must be used to identify causative mutations conclusively. For example, having multiple independent mutant alleles can facilitate gene identification. Genome sequencing of each independent mutant may reveal many candidate genes, but when the genome sequences are compared, they should all be seen to contain mutations of the same gene. However, if there is only a single mutant allele available, it may be difficult to tell whether differences in the DNA sequences of candidate genes are the cause of the mutant phenotype or simply polymorphisms

(a)

1 Cross new homozygous mutant with wild-type strain from which it was derived. The only differences in DNA sequence should be those introduced during mutagenesis.

2 Interbreed F_1 individuals.

3 Select a large number of homozygous mutant F_2 individuals.

4 Isolate DNA from 25–100 homozygous mutant F_2 individuals.

5 Pool DNA, and sequence such that, on average, every nucleotide is sequenced for each of the pooled individuals.

Closely linked mutations will segregate with causative mutations.

Causative mutation will be present in all sequences.

Unlinked mutations at distant sites on the same chromosome or on other chromosomes should segregate in a Mendelian manner.

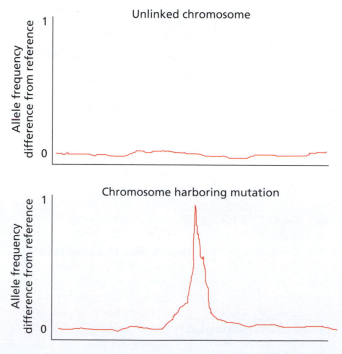

Figure 14.7 Genomics approach to gene identification following mutagenesis. (a) Strategy to identify a mutant gene via genomic sequencing. **(b)** Example from *Arabidopsis*.

existing in the population. In this case, candidate mutations must be assessed by additional approaches, such as examining whether the corresponding gene is expressed in a pattern consistent with the mutant phenotype.

14.3 Reverse Genetics Investigates Gene Action by Progressing from Gene Identification to Phenotype

Forward genetics was for a long time the primary—and for much of the 20th century, the only—approach to uncovering gene function. Now, however, the development of molecular methods for gene and genome manipulation and advances in sequencing technologies are making reverse genetics approaches increasingly valuable and common.

The reasons for shifting toward reverse genetics are twofold. First, the enormous amount of genomic sequence available has increased by orders of magnitude the number of known gene sequences, and only a fraction of them have been assigned a function by forward genetics. For example, when the *E. coli* genome was fully sequenced, 4288 protein-coding genes were identified, only 1853 of which had been previously identified through forward genetic screens. Second, genomic sequencing and reverse genetic screens have uncovered a degree of gene duplication not previously suspected. Gene duplications often result in genetic redundancy. In forward genetic screens, such duplicated genes would not be identified, since mutation of only one of the genes would not usually result in a conspicuous mutant phenotype. However, reverse genetics approaches, where the functions of both duplicates can be disrupted in an individual organism, are particularly suited in these situations to provide evidence of gene function.

Reverse genetics begins with the creation of a mutant allele for a gene identified only by its sequence (see Figure 14.1). The selection of mutational tools is largely dependent on the biology of the experimental organism. We describe here four technologies for reverse genetics, including one that is presently revolutionizing the field of genetics.

Genome Editing

You may not realize it, but you are living through a revolution in genetics due to advances in technologies to manipulate DNA sequences in the genomes of living cells. A dream of geneticists for many decades was to have the ability to "edit" the genome—precisely changing the nucleotide sequence at a specific chromosomal locus to any desired sequence. Remarkably, this dream has become reality in the past few years. The general concept is to design a DNA endonuclease to target a specific genomic location. The endonuclease creates a double-strand break at the site, which can be subsequently repaired by endogenous repair

mechanisms, either through nonhomologous end joining (NHEJ) or homologous recombination (see Section 11.5). If the double-strand break is repaired by NHEJ, then small deletions often remain at the site of the break, leading to possible loss- or gain-of-function alleles, depending on what sequences are lost. Alternatively, the break may be repaired by homologous recombination, either with endogenous sequence from the homologous chromosome in a diploid cell or with exogenously supplied DNA sequences. In the latter case, if the exogenously supplied DNA has been constructed in such a way that it contains the desired change, a specific sequence change in the chromosome may be accomplished.

Two different approaches have been designed used to cause the nuclease to target a specific site in the genome of living cells. First, the nuclease can be translationally fused to a sequence-specific DNA binding domain that recognizes only the site in the genome to be targeted (translational fusion is discussed in Section 14.4). Second, the nuclease can be incorporated into a complex with an RNA molecule, which provides specificity via complementary base pairing with the target sequence of interest. This latter approach is based on reengineering a bacterial system called CRISPR–Cas9, which has become the system of choice due its ease of use, its flexibility, and the fact that it is inexpensive.

CRISPR–Cas9 The CRISPR story begins in the 1990s in the salt marshes along the Mediterranean coast of Spain, where scientists were investigating an extremely salt tolerant archaeal microbe, *Haloferax mediterranei*. They noted that an enigmatic array of repetitive DNA in its genome—unique spacer sequences alternating with a repeat sequence—seemed to change with changing environmental conditions. It soon became obvious from studies by numerous other scientists that related archaeal species and bacteria also possessed similar arrays but with distinct sequences. The repeats were termed CRISPR, for *c*lustered *r*egularly *i*nterspaced *pal*indromic *r*epeats, describing the nature of the repetitive sequences (**Figure 14.8a**). Additionally, in each case, adjacent genomic loci encoded related sets of genes, termed CRISPR-associated (*cas*) genes. The *cas* genes encode a DNA endonuclease, either as a single protein or as a protein complex depending on the species. Given that genes in prokaryotes are often organized into operons, it became apparent that the repeats and associated genes (CRISPR–*cas*) had a common function, but it was not until the early 2000s that the function was determined.

A range of accumulated experimental evidence indicated that the **CRISPR–*cas*** system acts as a defense mechanism against invading nucleic acids. The unique spacer sequences in the CRISPR repeat were found to be derived from the genomes of phage (see Section 6.5) and to act as guides directing the Cas endonuclease to a specific sequence of an invading phage. The CRISPR sequences are transcribed into a noncoding RNA and processed into individual repeat

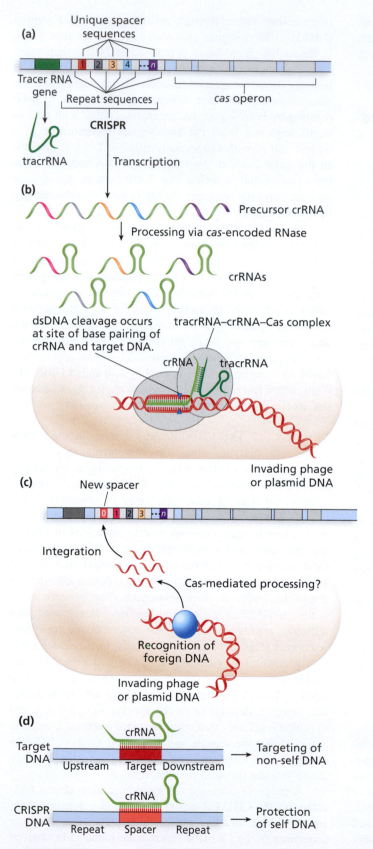

(a)

Unique spacer sequences

Tracer RNA gene

Repeat sequences

CRISPR

tracrRNA

cas operon

Transcription

(b)

Precursor crRNA

Processing via *cas*-encoded RNase

crRNAs

dsDNA cleavage occurs at site of base pairing of crRNA and target DNA.

tracrRNA–crRNA–Cas complex

crRNA   tracrRNA

Invading phage or plasmid DNA

(c)

New spacer

Integration

Cas-mediated processing?

Recognition of foreign DNA

Invading phage or plasmid DNA

(d)

crRNA

Target DNA

Upstream   Target   Downstream

Targeting of non-self DNA

crRNA

CRISPR DNA

Repeat   Spacer   Repeat

Protection of self DNA

Figure 14.8 **Structure and mechanism of CRISPR–*cas* in microbes.**

How is memory of past infections retained in the CRISPR–*cas* system?

units, called **crRNAs**, by *cas*-encoded RNases. Each crRNA has a repeat sequence and a unique sequence. The tracer RNA gene is also transcribed into a small noncoding RNA (**tracrRNA**), part of which binds to the Cas endonuclease to form an RNA–protein complex. The other part of the tracrRNA is complementary to the repeat section of the crRNAs. Thus, a complex linking the Cas endonuclease to a unique crRNA sequence is established, enabling the Cas nuclease to introduce double-strand (ds) breaks in DNA molecules (of invading phages or plasmids) at sites determined by the unique sequence of the crRNA (Figure 14.8a). New spacer sequences may be added to the array if a microbe survives a phage infection, and in this manner the CRISPR sequences in the microbe can increase over time and be passed on to its progeny (**Figure 14.8b**). As with all immune systems, a conundrum arises as to how to distinguish self from nonself, because the endogenous genomic CRISPR locus could also be targeted by the crRNAs it encodes. In at least some species it seems that discrimination between self and nonself targets is mediated by the extent of potential base pairing between the repetitive region of the crRNAs and the target DNA (**Figure 14.8c**).

Soon after the mechanistic details of the CRISPR–Cas system in microbe immunity were elucidated, multiple scientists realized that the system could be reengineered to target any DNA sequence of interest and "edit" the genome of a living cell (**Figure 14.9**). The general idea is to replace the unique sequence of a crRNA with a sequence that targets your sequence of interest. The system of *Staphylococcus* was found to have a single Cas protein, Cas9, that was sufficient for endonuclease activity. Moreover, the tracrRNA and crRNA sequences could be fused into a single sequence, termed a **guideRNA**, thus reducing the system to two components. The combined tracrRNA–crRNA then forms a complex, and the unique crRNA sequence guides the complex to a specific site in the genome. A double-strand break introduced into a chromosomal location will undergo repair, often by NHEJ, in which case deletions of a single base pair or longer are often introduced at the site of cleavage (**1**). This tendency to cause deletions makes the CRISPR–Cas9 system potentially very efficient at introducing mutations at a specific site in the genome. At the same time, mismatches of only a single base pair between crRNA and the target genome sequence can reduce or eliminate the efficiency of cleavage by CRISPR–Cas9.

Often the goal of genome editing is not to make random mutations at a specific locus but rather to change the sequence of a single base pair. This can be accomplished by introducing

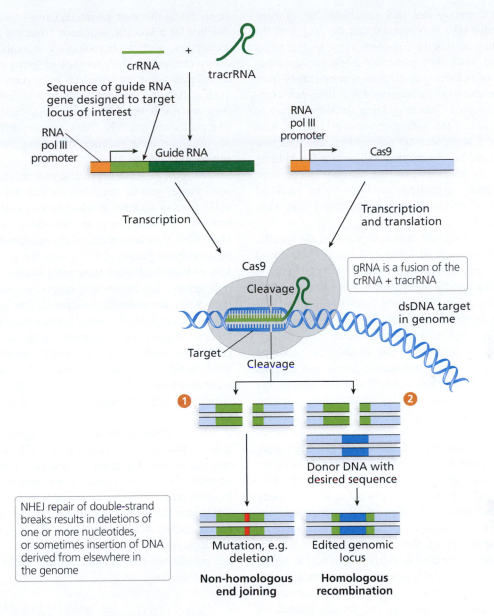

Figure 14.9 Reengineering CRISPR–*cas* for genome editing.

a fragment of DNA containing the desired base change along with the CRISPR–Cas9 components (**2**). A fraction of the time, the CRISPR–Cas9 complex will create a double-strand break in the DNA that will be repaired by homologous recombination using the supplied DNA fragment. The end result is a genome in which a single base pair has been edited.

The development of CRISPR–Cas for genome editing provides a striking example of how discoveries in basic curiosity-driven science that appear to have little immediate application (e.g., the study of salt-tolerant archaea) can lead to technologies that have a profound effect on biology, including that of human health.

Application of CRISPR–Cas9 The application of the CRISPR–Cas9 system in different organisms depends on the biology of the organism in question. For example, the two components of the system could be introduced either as transgenes or, in some instances, protein, or RNA could be directly injected into a cell. If the components are introduced as transgenes, they will be heritable, whereas if only protein or RNA (or both) are supplied into single cells, the effect will be transient, and over time, daughter cells of the injected cell will not contain either component.

In an approach similar to the endogenous scenario, where the CRISPR loci encode multiple crRNAs, multiple guideRNA genes can be introduced into a single cell to target multiple chromosomal loci simultaneously. Target-site selection must take into account that the length of the guideRNA sequence that is complementary to the target is about 20 base pairs. Any particular 20-bp sequence has the probability of occurring at random approximately once every 10^{12} base pairs ($\frac{1}{4}^{20}$, assuming equal base pair composition in a genome). This may seem sufficiently rare to be acceptable even in the human genome of 3×10^9 base pairs, but genome sequences are not random, and therefore a target site should be chosen that will reduce the binding at "off-targets" as much as possible. Having the genome sequences for many organisms available to be searched makes the task of choosing appropriate target sites simpler (see Chapter 16).

The ability of CRISPR technology to create specific mutations in the genome of a live cell has revolutionized reverse genetic approaches to the study of gene function and given rise to a rapidly proliferation of applications. One obvious application that we explore further in Section 15.3 is gene therapy, in which a mutant allele in the cells of an individual is "corrected" to a functional state.

Applications in agriculture that modify the genotype and hence phenotype of domesticated plants and animals have the potential to accelerate creation of new breeds and varieties for specific purposes or for adaptation to changing climates. Such technologies can be designed to ensure that the resulting organisms do not carry any exogenous genes and thus are nontransgenic. The technology has been used, for example, to create hornless cattle, obviating the need for painful "dehorning," and to produce pigs that are resistant to swine flu. Further demonstrating what is feasible using CRISPR systems, geneticists targeted 62 endogenous retrovirus loci in a pig embryo for simultaneous mutation, thereby eliminating all of these elements from the pig genome. The rationale behind this experiment was to generate a pig breed suitable for temporary xenotransplantation of organs into humans while they await a more permanent human donor organ. Also pushing the present boundaries of accomplishment, DNA from a woolly mammoth, a species that went extinct 4000 years ago, was spliced into the DNA in a cell of an elephant, raising the prospect of one day recreating now-extinct plants and animals. As can be seen from these applications, there are significant ethical considerations to examine before such modified organisms can be released from the confines of the laboratory.

Use of Homologous Recombination in Reverse Genetics

Although CRISPR–Cas has dramatically transformed how reverse genetics is approached, other previously established methods are still in use. Another powerful technique for producing loss-of-function alleles, for example, is to utilize the endogenous mechanisms of recombination to integrate exogenous DNA fragments into the genome. Conceptually, the simplest way to construct a loss-of-function allele would

be to delete the gene of interest from the genome, but the deletion of a specific sequence from the genome requires techniques, such as homologous recombination, that precisely manipulate the genomes of living organisms. These techniques are very efficient in certain microorganisms, such as bacteria, archaea, and some simple eukaryotes, but they are much less efficient in more complex eukaryotes like plants and animals. Thus, various different approaches are used in reverse genetics, depending on the nature of the organism (Table 14.2).

Reverse genetics approaches for most of the commonly used model genetic organisms utilize **knockout libraries**, collections of mutants in which most or all genes have been mutated by inactivating, or "knocking out," their expression. Most knockout mutants are produced by the insertion of exogenous pieces of DNA into the genome to generate loss-of-function alleles; thus, most alleles in the libraries are null alleles. *Saccharomyces cerevisiae* and *E. coli* geneticists have, for example, systematically generated loss-of-function alleles of all known *S. cerevisiae* and *E. coli* genes by homologous recombination. In these knockout library collections, each strain has a single mutation in a different gene. In this subsection we discuss the use of homologous recombination, and in the next we discuss applications in which the DNA is integrated at random locations in the genome.

If DNA that is introduced into an organism has no origin of replication, it undergoes one of two fates: enzymatic degradation or integration into the host genome. Enzymatic degradation, accomplished by nucleases that are common in cells, will eliminate the introduced DNA. Integration of DNA into the host genome, in contrast, allows the introduced nucleic acid to persist in the host cell. Integration is accomplished by either of two distinct mechanisms of recombination: illegitimate recombination or homologous recombination.

Table 14.2	Reverse Genetics Approaches in Model Genetic Organisms
Species	**Reverse Genetics Tools**
Escherichia coli	Knockouts by homologous recombination
Saccharomyces cerevisiae	Knockouts by homologous recombination
Arabidopsis thaliana	CRISPR; random T-DNA and transposon insertions; TILLING; RNAi
Drosophila melanogaster	CRISPR; random *P* element insertion lines; RNAi
Caenorhabditis elegans	CRISPR; RNAi loss-of-function alleles
Mus musculus	CRISPR; knockouts by homologous recombination; RNAi

Illegitimate recombination integrates introduced DNA at a random, nonhomologous location. This form of recombination does not require any homology between the introduced DNA and the genomic DNA into which the former is integrated. In contrast, the second mechanism for integration of introduced DNA, **homologous recombination** between the introduced DNA and the host genomic sequence, requires a significant length of DNA sequence in common between the two recombining molecules. The relative frequencies with which these mechanisms occur depend on the species into which the DNA is introduced. In most plant and animal species, illegitimate recombination is the more common fate, but techniques exist to select for individuals in which homologous recombination has occurred (as described later in this chapter). In bacterial and fungal species, introduced DNA is often recombined in the genome in a homologous manner.

For example, fragments of DNA introduced into the yeast, *S. cerevisiae*, have a propensity to undergo homologous recombination with the yeast chromosome if sequence homology is present. An introduced circular molecule of DNA can recombine by either a single crossover or a double crossover (**Figure 14.10a**). In a single crossover, the entire molecule of introduced circular DNA is integrated into the yeast genome with no loss of any genomic DNA. If recombination of a circular molecule occurs by double crossover, however, only DNA between the homologous flanking sequences is integrated into the recipient genome, and the integration is accompanied by a concomitant loss from the genome of the DNA between the homologous sequences. Thus, recombination with two crossovers results in replacement of the genomic DNA with the introduced DNA flanked by the homologous sequences.

Introducing a linear rather than circular molecule of DNA favors retrieval of recombinants produced by double crossover, since a single crossover will cause a deletion event resulting in recombinant molecules lacking a large portion of the original chromosome and therefore likely

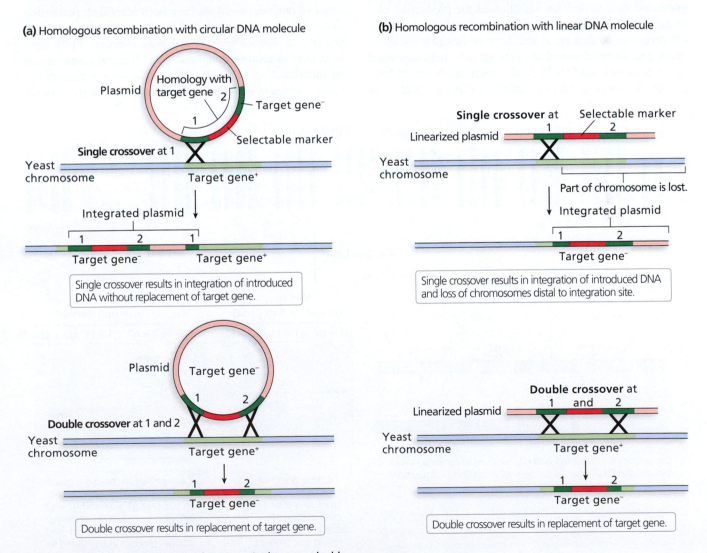

(a) Homologous recombination with circular DNA molecule

(b) Homologous recombination with linear DNA molecule

Figure 14.10 **Homologous recombination: single versus double crossovers.**

Why is linear DNA more efficient for obtaining mutants through homologous recombination?

to be lethal (**Figure 14.10b**). Linearized DNA molecules recombine at a higher frequency than circular ones, making the introduction of linear molecules the method of choice for homologous recombination experiments.

Taking advantage of this tendency for homologous recombination to occur in yeast, yeast geneticists create recombinant yeast both through gene insertion and gene replacement. Loss-of-function alleles are created by replacing the target gene with heterologous DNA, often a selectable marker gene, thus eliminating the production of functional wild-type protein by the target gene. Gene insertions that result in a deletion of the entire coding region of the gene create null alleles that produce no protein product. Such insertion alleles are often called **gene knockouts** because the insertion "knocks out" the function of the gene (as explained above in the definition given for knockout libraries), creating a recessive loss-of-function allele. Conversely, inserting a functional gene, often creating a gain-of-function allele, is called a knock-in.

The ease with which homologous recombinants are generated in *S. cerevisiae* has allowed the production of a large number of yeast strains for genetic analysis of biological processes in this organism. Loss-of-function alleles of every gene in the *S. cerevisiae* genome have been generated and can be ordered from a stock center. Such stocks have greatly facilitated genetic research by relieving scientists of

the need to produce mutations in the genes of interest at the start of every new genetic experiment.

Use of Insertion Mutants in Reverse Genetics

In many model genetic organisms, homologous recombination frequencies are very low, and thus it is not technically simple or economically feasible to systematically generate loss-of-function mutants for all the genes. However, if an organism is easy to transform, populations of random mutant organisms can be generated by transposon insertions or, in the case of plants, T-DNA insertions (see Section 15.2 for details). These populations can then be screened for mutations in specific genes, using PCR-based techniques with a primer that is specific to the gene of interest and a primer that is specific to the insertional mutagen used (**Figure 14.11**).

For some model genetic systems, such as *Drosophila* and *Arabidopsis*, the precise genomic locations of thousands of random insertions have been identified, permitting mutations in specific genes to be ordered directly from stock centers. In *Drosophila*, *P* elements (Section 11.7) have been used as an insertional mutagen. These *P* elements can be mobilized—by crossing flies possessing a nonautonomous *P* element with flies possessing an active transposase

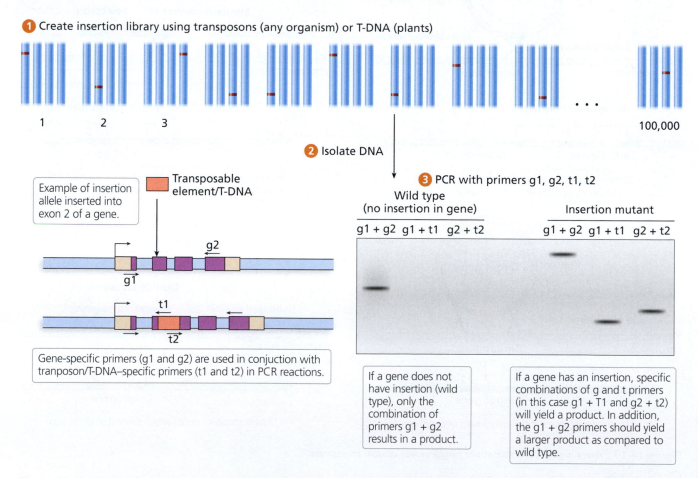

Figure 14.11 Reverse genetics using insertional mutagenesis.

gene—to create additional local insertions, as the majority of transposition events are transpositions to nearby genomic locations. In this manner, a large number of mutant alleles at a specific locus can be generated. In *Arabidopsis*, more than 100,000 T-DNA and transposon lines in which the insertion site is precisely known are available. Such knockout libraries are an invaluable resource for large-scale reverse genetics experiments that aim to elucidate the function of every gene in the model genetic organism (see Section 16.4). An example of an application of reverse genetics to determine the function of closely related genes in *Arabidopsis* is described in the Case Study at the end of this chapter.

RNA Interference in Gene Activity

Another approach to producing loss-of-function phenotypes is to harness the endogenous system of RNA interference (RNAi). As described in Section 13.3, double-stranded RNA (dsRNA) can act as a trigger for the degradation not only of the double-stranded RNA itself but also of any RNA molecules that are complementary to the double-stranded RNA. A primary role of this gene-silencing system is to silence repetitive DNA. Transcription from several different copies of repetitive elements often generates double-stranded RNA molecules, since collectively both strands of the repetitive DNA are often transcribed. In addition, RNAi protects cells against double-stranded RNA viruses. Thus, dsRNA-mediated gene silencing acts as a genomic immune system to silence both repetitive DNA sequences and invading nucleic acids.

To take advantage of endogenous RNAi activity as a way of silencing genes, scientists utilize double-stranded RNA that is complementary in sequence to the target gene. The mRNA of the target gene will then be degraded through the action of Dicer and Argonaute enzymes (described in Section 13.3), causing a loss-of-function phenotype of the target gene (**Figure 14.12**). The efficiency of silencing can approach that of a null allele, although often the phenotypes induced represent a range of partial loss-of-function phenotypes.

Loss-of-function phenotypes induced by RNAi can be heritable if the source of the dsRNA is a transgene integrated into the genome. However, double-stranded RNA can also be introduced directly into cells or organisms by injection of double-stranded RNA or indirectly by infection with a double-stranded RNA virus, and in these cases the effects are transient, disappearing when the source of the dsRNA is removed. In animals, transient introduction of double-stranded RNA into cell cultures has been successful. One of the methods for introducing double-stranded RNA into *C. elegans* is surprisingly simple. *Caenorhabditis elegans* normally eats *E. coli* as food, and, remarkably enough, when *C. elegans* is fed *E. coli* that is producing double-stranded RNA, the double-stranded RNA will be taken up into *C. elegans* and will silence genes in many organs of the *C. elegans* body. Although in this case the RNAi-induced phenotype is not indefinitely heritable, the phenotypic effects can be seen in several subsequent

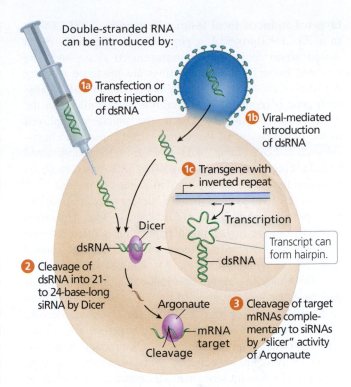

Figure 14.12 Reverse genetics using RNAi.

Ⓠ **What are the exogenous and endogenous sources of dsRNA in RNAi?**

generations produced by self-fertilization of the worm that was fed the *E. coli*. This persistence is due to the activity of RNA-dependent RNA polymerases that exist in *C. elegans*. Such enzymes are not present in many animals, but in plants RNA-dependent RNA polymerases act in the immune system to detect and destroy invading dsRNA viruses.

The advantages of the RNAi approach to reverse genetics include the ease and rapidity of applying the method. It allows large-scale reverse genetic screens to be conducted in cell cultures and whole organisms without the laborious preparatory task of creating mutagenized populations. In addition, transient RNAi-mediated gene silencing offers an alternative means of applying reverse genetics in species for which stable transformation protocols do not exist, but for which techniques to introduce dsRNA are available.

In a related approach, synthetic microRNAs have been created to target the degradation of specific mRNAs. Like RNAi-mediated gene silencing, synthetic microRNA–mediated gene silencing takes advantage of endogenous gene-silencing machinery (see Section 13.3). The synthetic microRNAs are designed according to principles derived from known microRNAs but are customized to block the translation or direct the mRNA cleavage of the gene of interest.

Reverse Genetics by TILLING

Another approach to reverse genetics that can often be applied when species cannot be transformed easily is

targeted induced local lesions in genomes (TILLING). In a TILLING protocol, a population of organisms of an inbred strain is randomly mutagenized throughout the genome. Enough independent lines are produced to bring the level of mutagenesis to near saturation, so that, ideally, each gene is represented by multiple mutant alleles in the mutagenized population. Often, the mutagen employed in the development of the mutagenized lines is a chemical such as EMS (Table 14.1). DNA from the mutagenized lines is screened systematically using PCR-based methods to search for mutations in a particular gene of interest.

For each individual of the mutagenized population, both progeny and DNA are collected. The generation derived from the mutagenized population is often referred to as the M_1 generation (**Figure 14.13a**). DNA is isolated from M_1 individuals or from M_2 families of organisms. Any DNA carrying a mutation induced in the mutagenesis will be either heterozygous (if the DNA was derived from an M_1 individual) or segregating (if the DNA was derived from an M_2 family). A region of the target gene is chosen for PCR-based amplification. The PCR products generated in this analysis are expected to contain both the wild-type sequence and mutant sequence. Those that consist solely of the wild-type allele can be distinguished from those consisting of a mixture of the wild-type allele and a mutant allele as follows.

The PCR products are first denatured and allowed to reanneal, creating some homoduplex DNA, in which the strands are fully complementary because they are derived from the same allele, and some heteroduplex DNA (**Figure 14.13b**). Heteroduplex DNA is composed of strands that are largely complementary but contain one or more mismatched base pairs, indicating that the strands are derived from DNA containing different alleles. Heteroduplex DNA can be distinguished from homoduplex DNA by either a difference in migration of the products during electrophoresis or by differential susceptibility to an endonuclease that cleaves heteroduplex DNA at mismatched base pairs. Heteroduplex DNA forms only in DNA samples in which a mutation in the target gene is present. Screening progeny from several thousand mutagenized individuals often allows identification of multiple mutant alleles of the target gene. Individuals homozygous or heterozygous for the mutant allele can then be identified in the appropriate M_2 family.

When chemical mutagenesis is used to produce TILLING alleles, it results in both null alleles and partial loss-of-function alleles. The spectrum of phenotypes produced by alleles obtained through TILLING approaches is often of use in dissecting gene function, even in organisms where gene knockouts are available. Although TILLING was developed for studies in model genetic species, it is suitable for any organism that can be mutagenized and genetically analyzed. It is currently being applied to several crop plants.

Genetic Analysis 14.2 tests your understanding of the reverse genetics analytical techniques discussed in this section.

(a) Seeds are mutated to produce M_1 generation. Each M_1 plant is heterozygous for mutations in different genes (colors).

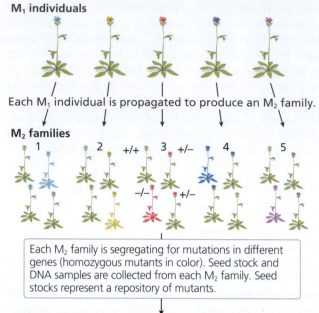

Each M_2 family is segregating for mutations in different genes (homozygous mutants in color). Seed stock and DNA samples are collected from each M_2 family. Seed stocks represent a repository of mutants.

(b) Mutations in specific genes are identified by analyzing DNA isolated from each M_2 family. For example, one representative M_2 family has a red mutant segregating.

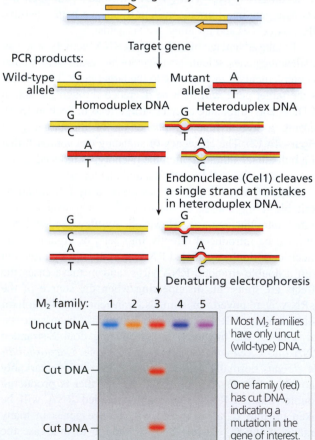

Figure 14.13 Reverse genetics by TILLING.

PROBLEM In searching the mouse genome, you identify three mouse orthologs similar to the single *hedgehog* gene of *Drosophila*. (Orthologs are genes descended from a single gene in the common ancestor of two or more species and therefore often have similar functions in those species; for more detailed discussion see Section 16.2.) The mouse genes are *Sonic hedgehog*, *Indian hedgehog*, and *Desert hedgehog*. Describe the research design you would use to learn the function of each of the genes and whether that gene function is unique or redundant in the mouse.

> **BREAK IT DOWN:** When genes in different species are highly similar, they are likely to have originated from a single ancestral gene in a common ancestor.

> **BREAK IT DOWN:** You are starting with gene sequences and wish to know gene functions. Which genetics approach, forward or reverse, is most appropriate?

Solution Strategies	Solution Steps
Evaluate	
1. Identify the topic this problem addresses and the nature of the required answer.	1. This problem is about designing research to identify the functions of genes known only by sequence and to discover whether those functions are unique or redundant.
2. Identify the critical information given in the problem.	2. While only one *hedgehog* gene exists in *Drosophila*, three "hedgehog" gene sequences exist in the mouse, raising the question of whether the three mouse genes have different functions or whether there is any sharing of function.
Deduce	
3. Consider possible approaches to discovering the functions of genes known only by sequence.	3. Functions of genes known only by sequence can be determined by reverse genetics approaches.
4. Consider possible approaches to reverse genetics available for use with mice.	4. CRISPR–Cas9 approaches can be used to produce loss-of-function mutations in mice. Other reverse genetics approaches, such as homologous recombination or RNAi, could also be used, but CRISPR–Cas9 is the preferred method.
Solve	
5. Describe a genetics approach to determine whether the genes have unique or redundant functions.	5. First, use CRISPR–Cas9 to create loss-of-function knockout alleles of each of the three genes. Homozygous mutant lines can then be bred and the phenotypes of each of the three single knockouts examined. Interbreeding the single-mutant lines will lead to the creation of strains in which combinations of two or more genes are inactive. Comparison of phenotypes of single mutants with those of multiple mutants allows an assessment of whether the genes exhibit unique or redundant functions.

> TIP: Reverse genetics approaches can be used for functional analysis (p. 521).

> TIP: Consider the methods appropriate for creating mutations in mice (see Table 14.2).

For more practice, see Problems 14, 16, 29, and 31. Visit the Study Area to access study tools. **Mastering Genetics**

14.4 Transgenes Provide a Means of Dissecting Gene Function

Transgenes have other uses in the study of gene function, in addition to the creation of loss-of-function alleles. For example, chimeric genes, which are transgenes composed of regulatory sequences from one gene and coding sequences from a second gene or of coding sequences from two different genes, provide a means to create gain-of-function alleles, as well as to monitor gene expression patterns. This section describes in greater detail the ways transgenes can reveal genetic function.

Although an almost limitless array of transgenes can be constructed for genetic analysis, many fall into one of two categories. One category consists of **reporter genes**, used to investigate gene regulation because they produce a visual output of gene expression patterns. Fusion of the regulatory sequences of a gene of interest to coding sequences of a reporter gene provides information about where, when, and how much a gene is expressed. Some reporter genes facilitate live imaging and monitoring of gene expression in real time.

The second category of transgenes useful for genetic analysis consists of gain-of-function alleles generated by placing coding regions from one gene under control of regulatory sequences derived from another gene. An allele constructed in this way often results in ectopic expression, meaning expression observed at times or in places where the gene is not normally expressed. The use of either or both of these types of transgenes can complement analyses of loss-of-function alleles by providing information on how genes are normally expressed and the phenotypic consequences of changing their normal expression pattern.

Monitoring Gene Expression with Reporter Genes

A gene can act as a reporter if its product can be detected directly or is an enzyme that produces a detectable product. The regulatory sequences of a gene under study are used to drive the expression of the reporter gene. Two types of reporter gene fusions can be constructed: transcriptional and translational (**Figure 14.14**).

In a *transcriptional fusion*, regulatory sequences directing transcription of the gene of interest are fused with the reporter gene so as to direct transcription of the coding sequences of the reporter gene. In this case, the reporter gene will be transcribed in the pattern directed by the regulatory sequences to which it is fused. Note that the transcriptional fusion shown in Figure 14.14 is idealized and that regulatory sequences may reside in regions other than immediately 5′ upstream of the gene of interest. In *translational fusion*, not only the regulatory sequences but also the coding sequence of the gene of interest are fused to the reporter gene in such a way that the reading frame for translation is maintained for both the gene of interest and the reporter gene. As a result, the reporter *protein* will be translationally fused with the protein of interest, and the location of the reporter protein will provide information not only on the spatial and temporal transcriptional expression pattern but also on the subcellular location of the fusion protein. In translational fusions, care must be taken to ascertain whether the fusion protein is still functional, since the addition of the reporter protein could interfere with the proper folding or activity of the protein of interest.

Some frequently used reporter genes are represented in **Figure 14.15**. The choice of reporter gene depends on the biological question being addressed. With some reporter genes, the assay to monitor gene expression requires sacrificing the organism, whereas the expression of other reporter genes can be traced in a living organism. To be detected, reporter gene products sometimes require substrates that must penetrate into the tissues or cells where the reporter genes are expressed. In addition, reporter genes vary in their sensitivity.

One of the first reporter genes to be developed emerged from research on the *lac* operon in *E. coli* (see Section 12.2). To purify and study the activity of β-galactosidase, encoded by the *lacZ* gene, a number of β-galactosides were synthesized and tested as substrates. Two β-galactosides, abbreviated X-gal and ONPG, were found to be useful. β-galactosidase cleaves the colorless substrate, ONPG, into a yellow product. This assay is typically used for in vitro measurement of β-galactosidase activity. In contrast, X-gal, also colorless, is cleaved by β-galactosidase into a blue product. This assay can be used in bacteria in vivo, since bacterial cells can take up the X-gal substrate without a reduction in viability.

The *lacZ* gene can be used in conjunction with the substrate X-gal as a reporter gene in animal systems (Figure 14.15a). However, because plants have an endogenous β-galactosidase activity, *lacZ* is not suitable for studying plant systems. An alternative option is the *E. coli uidA* gene encoding β-glucuronidase, which enzymatically cleaves a colorless precursor, X-gluc, into a blue product (Figure 14.15b). Conversely, because animals have endogenous β-glucuronidase activity, the *uidA* gene cannot be

Gene in eukaryotic genome

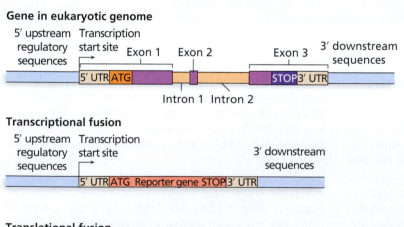

Transcriptional fusion

Translational fusion

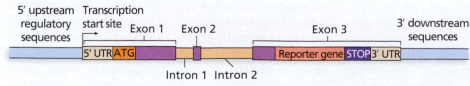

Figure 14.14   Transcriptional versus translational gene fusions.

Q What different types of information are derived from transcriptional versus translational fusions?

(a) *Lin-3* regulatory sequences driving *lacZ* reporter gene in *C. elegans*

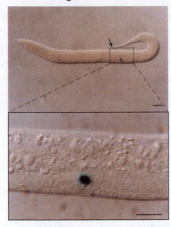

(b) *PHABULOSA* regulatory sequences driving *uidA* reporter gene in *Arabidopsis*

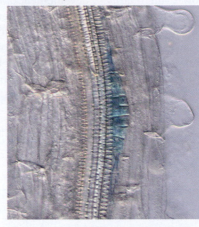

(c) *CaMV 35S* regulatory sequences driving luciferase reporter gene in tobacco

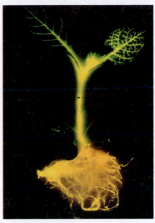

(d) *RHODOPSIN* regulatory sequences driving *GFP* reporter gene in *Mus musculus*

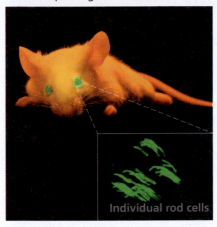

Individual rod cells

(e) *Mus musculus* neurons expressing three different fluorescent reporter genes, derived from modifying GFP

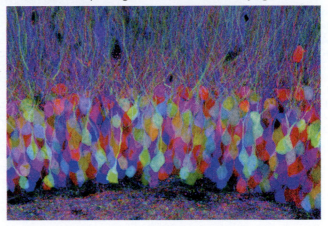

Figure 14.15 Reporter genes.

used as a reporter in animals. A limitation of both of these reporter genes in organisms other than bacteria is that in order for the substrate to be taken up effectively into internal tissues, the tissue to be stained must be bathed in a solution that kills the cells.

Research into reactions that cause the natural emission of light in some animals has led to the development of reporter genes that cause light to be produced in living cells. For example, luciferase, the enzyme responsible for the glow of fireflies, catalyzes a reaction between the substrate luciferin and ATP that results in the emission of light. Transgenic plants expressing the luciferase gene will emit a yellow-green glow if supplied with the substrate (Figure 14.15c). However, luciferin is not delivered to all cells of the plant in equal measure, which in many cases limits the usefulness of the luciferase gene as a reporter.

The development of **green fluorescent protein (GFP)** led to great strides both in genetics and cell biology by providing a noninvasive means of visualizing gene and protein expression patterns in living organisms (Figure 14.15d). The *GFP* gene, derived from the jellyfish *Aequoria victoria*, is the source of the natural bioluminescence of this species. Its wild-type protein product, consisting of 238 amino acids, fluoresces green (a 509-nm wavelength) when illuminated with UV light (a 395-nm wavelength), which in this case is the "substrate," delivered by laser.

Because UV light, with its short wavelength, can be harmful to organisms (e.g., causing thymine dimers to form in DNA, as described in Section 11.3), the wild-type *GFP* gene was mutated to produce variants that respond to lower-energy wavelengths. A major improvement was a mutation that shifted the excitation wavelength to 488 nm, corresponding to blue light and minimizing the potential damage to cells being illuminated. Subsequent modification of the GFP protein sequence has led to the production of variants that emit other colors (e.g., yellow, cyan, blue). Genes encoding fluorescent reporter proteins have also been isolated from marine corals and other jellyfish. The availability of multiple fluorescent reporter genes makes it possible to visualize the expression of several genes simultaneously in a single organism (Figure 14.15e). Osamu

Shimomura, Martin Chalfie, and Roger Y. Tsien received the 2008 Nobel Prize in Chemistry for their discovery and development of GFP.

Reporter genes can be used to dissect regulatory DNA sequences and identify specific sequences required for particular aspects of gene regulation. The general approach is to start with a clone in which all the regulatory sequences required for proper gene expression are present and then

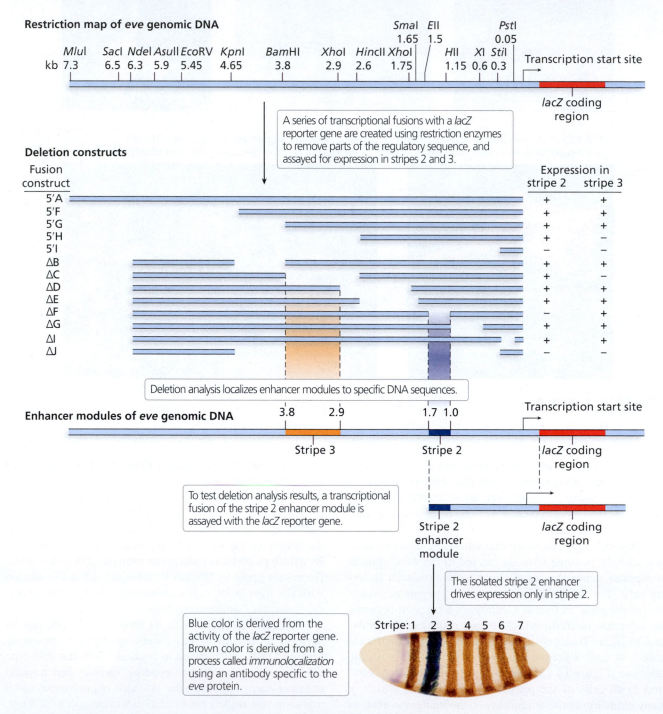

Figure 14.16   Use of reporter gene in promoter analysis of the *even-skipped* (eve) gene.

to assay the effects of deleting or changing specific portions of the clone. An example of such an analysis of the *Drosophila even-skipped* (*eve*) gene, which is expressed in seven stripes in the segmentation pattern of the embryo, is shown in **Figure 14.16**. Overlapping deletions spanning large regions are assayed first. Then regions identified as important for gene regulation are dissected with smaller deletions. The concept is similar to that described earlier for deletion mapping (see Sections 6.5 and 10.4). When specific sequences required for proper gene expression are deleted, expression of the reporter gene will be correspondingly altered.

If genomic sequence is available from two or more related species, regulatory elements may be predicted by searching for sequences that are conserved between the related species, using a method known as *phylogenetic footprinting* (discussed in Chapter 16). Such initial genomic sequence analyses can direct subsequent experimental tests that use reporter genes to analyze expression in transgenic organisms.

Enhancer Trapping

Enhancer trapping uses a variation of an insertional library to identify genes based on expression patterns. This approach combines the generation of a large number of random insertion mutants with the expression of a reporter gene (**Figure 14.17**). In its simplest application, a population of transgenic organisms is generated by random insertion of a transposon (or T-DNA) containing the coding sequence of a reporter gene fused with a core promoter region for RNA polymerase II transcription (see Section 13.1). If the insertion occurs near enhancer or silencer regulatory sequences that can act in conjunction with the minimal promoter of the reporter gene, the reporter can be expressed in a pattern that reflects the regulatory capability of the nearby genomic DNA sequences. The enhancers (or silencers) of the adjacent genomic DNA are co-opted, or "trapped," by the insertion to drive expression of the reporter gene. Thus, from the expression patterns of the inserted reporter gene, researchers can infer the existence of regulatory sequences, presumably from adjacent genes, that drive gene expression in the observed patterns. While reporter gene expression may not precisely reflect the expression of the adjacent gene, the expression of the reporter often at least partially reflects the normal gene expression pattern of the adjacent gene. Enhancer trapping techniques were first pioneered in *Drosophila* and have now been adapted to other systems. Because they identify genes by gene expression patterns, enhancer trapping techniques complement forward genetic screens.

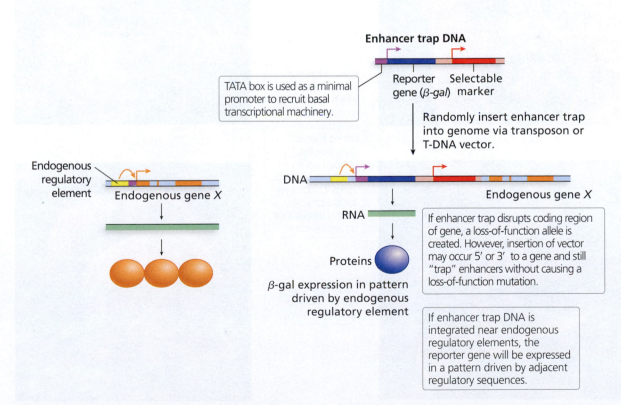

Figure 14.17 **Enhancer trapping to reveal expression patterns of endogenous genes.** Strategy for generation of enhancer trap lines.

Investigating Gene Function with Chimeric Genes

A **chimeric gene**, as mentioned earlier, is one in which regulatory and coding sequences derived from two or more different genes are recombined in a novel manner. For example, combining the regulatory sequences from one gene with the coding sequences from another gene often results in a gain-of-function allele due to ectopic expression of the gene represented by the coding sequences.

Figure 14.18 shows one way experimenters can take advantage of this potential to obtain information on gene function. This example makes use of the *eyeless* gene of *Drosophila*, so named because recessive loss-of-function mutations in this gene result in a failure of eyes to develop in the fly.

The *eyeless* gene is normally expressed in the eye imaginal discs during *Drosophila* development. Imaginal discs are groups of precursor cells that are set aside during embryonic development. They grow by mitotic proliferation during larval life and later differentiate into adult body tissues during metamorphosis. However, a gain-of-function *eyeless* allele can be created by constructing a chimeric gene in which expression of the *eyeless* coding sequences is driven by regulatory sequences active in *all* imaginal discs. If the *eyeless* gene is ectopically expressed in noneye imaginal discs, such as those that would normally give rise to the antennae or legs, the imaginal discs will differentiate as eye tissue instead. This outcome indicates that cells in any imaginal disc are capable of differentiating into eyes and that the *eyeless* gene product can promote the development of eyes from any imaginal disc. Thus, when the *eyeless* allele is ectopically expressed as a gain-of-function mutation in inappropriate imaginal discs, the resulting phenotype is the converse of the phenotype of the loss-of-function *eyeless* allele—ectopic eyes as opposed to an absence of eyes.

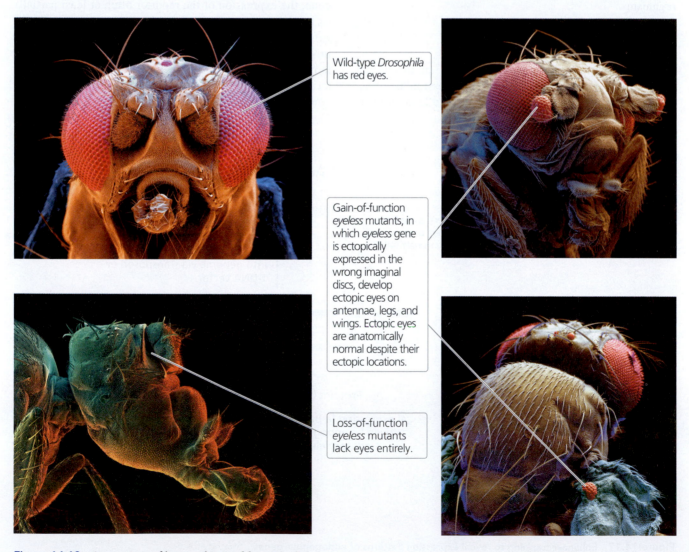

Wild-type *Drosophila* has red eyes.

Gain-of-function *eyeless* mutants, in which *eyeless* gene is ectopically expressed in the wrong imaginal discs, develop ectopic eyes on antennae, legs, and wings. Ectopic eyes are anatomically normal despite their ectopic locations.

Loss-of-function *eyeless* mutants lack eyes entirely.

Figure 14.18 Comparison of loss- and gain-of-function alleles.

In cases where the gain-of-function and loss-of-function phenotypes are complementary, interpretation of the effects of ectopic expression is straightforward. Thus, in the preceding example, *eyeless* is revealed to be a master control gene for the differentiation of eyes in *Drosophila*. However, ectopic expression of genes can also lead to enigmatic phenotypes that are more difficult to interpret. For example, ectopic expression of *eyeless* during embryogenesis leads to embryonic lethality, a phenotype that is not easily reconciled with the loss-of-function phenotype. Therefore, when considering gain-of-function alleles generated by ectopic expression, we must remember that the phenotypes represent what the gene is capable of doing when expressed in particular contexts and may not reflect the normal function of the gene.

CASE STUDY

Reverse Genetics and Genetic Redundancy in Flower Development

In this case study, we see an example of how forward genetics and reverse genetics work together to provide a broader view of both gene function and evolution. The story begins with forward genetics—the isolation of a mutation that alters flower development and the subsequent identification of the mutant gene sequence using recombinant DNA technology. The gene is then cloned and used as a probe for cloning genes of similar sequence. Finally, reverse genetics approaches are applied to identify mutant alleles of related genes, and their biological function is inferred based on the mutant phenotypes.

FORWARD GENETICS REVEALS GENES OF INTEREST In flowering plants, the types of floral organs that develop are decided by the expression of a set of transcription factors. (For further description of this activity, see Section 18.5.) The identity of *Arabidopsis* reproductive organs (stamens and carpels) is determined in part by the activity of the *AGAMOUS* gene. Recessive null loss-of-function *agamous* alleles lead to the development of petals in the positions usually occupied by stamens and of an additional flower in the position usually occupied by carpels. Homozygotes for *agamous* are sterile and do not produce gametes (hence the name *AGAMOUS*). In forward genetic screens aimed at identifying genes involved in *Arabidopsis* flower development, *agamous* mutant alleles induced by either EMS or T-DNA have been isolated (**Figure 14.19**, step ❶).

The T-DNA–induced allele proved a useful tool for cloning the *AGAMOUS* gene because the T-DNA "tagged" the gene (step ❷). Since the mutation of the *AGAMOUS* gene was caused by the insertion of T-DNA, the presence of a T-DNA sequence in a region of *Arabidopsis* DNA was an indication that the sequences encoding the *AGAMOUS* gene were adjacent. Recombinant DNA techniques described in Section 15.1 were used to find those sequences.

Subsequently, the genomic clone encoding *AGAMOUS* could be used to identify *AGAMOUS* cDNA clones from a library constructed with mRNA from wild-type flowers. Sequencing of the *AGAMOUS* cDNA clones revealed that the encoded protein had a similarity to known eukaryotic transcription factors. This conclusion was based on the similarity between a 60–amino acid domain of the AGAMOUS protein and DNA-binding domains in yeast and mammalian transcription factors ❸.

IDENTIFICATION OF HOMOLOGOUS GENES When the *AGAMOUS* cDNA is used to probe a Southern blot of restriction-enzyme–digested *Arabidopsis* genomic DNA, sequences related to the *AGAMOUS* gene sequence can be identified ❹ (see Section 1.4 to review Southern blotting). The same *AGAMOUS* cDNA can be used as a probe on the flower cDNA library to identify clones of related genes. Genes related to *AGAMOUS* were called *AGAMOUS-LIKE*, or *AGL*, genes. These related genes possess the same highly conserved DNA-binding domain but differ in the rest of their protein sequences. To determine how the *AGL* genes are related to *AGAMOUS* and to each other, a phylogenetic tree can be constructed ❺ (see Section 1.5 to review phylogenetic trees).

REVERSE GENETICS REVEALS FUNCTIONS OF HOMOLOGOUS GENES Since the related genes are known by gene sequence only, a reverse genetics approach can be undertaken to determine gene function. CRISPR– or T-DNA–induced mutant alleles of many of the *AGL* genes in *Arabidopsis* can be identified in available knockout libraries ❻ (see Section 14.3).

Researchers were initially surprised to find that plants homozygous for loss-of-function alleles of many single genes did not display an aberrant phenotype. Hypothesizing that the more closely related the genes, the more similar their functions would be, researchers crossed mutants to obtain organisms containing multiple loss-of-function alleles of closely related genes ❼. For example, *sep1* mutants—having mutations of the *SEPALLATA1* gene—were crossed with *sep2* mutants, after which *sep1 sep2* double mutants were identified in the F_2 generation. Disappointingly, the *sep1 sep2* double mutants did not differ significantly from wild-type plants. However, *sep1 sep2 sep3* triple-mutant plants proved to have flowers consisting solely of sepals, which indicates that these genes have a function related to floral organ specification but distinct from the role of *AGAMOUS*.

Genetic redundancy due to gene duplications is extensive in most eukaryotic genomes (see Section 16.3). Immediately following an occurrence of gene duplication, the duplicate genes often have identical DNA sequences and expression patterns, and they are therefore genetically redundant. Over time, however, the functions of the two genes may diverge due to the accumulation of mutations that lead to changes in protein sequence and expression pattern. Yet, because the genes are evolutionarily related, they often function in similar biological processes. Reverse genetics approaches can facilitate the analysis of closely related genetically redundant genes.

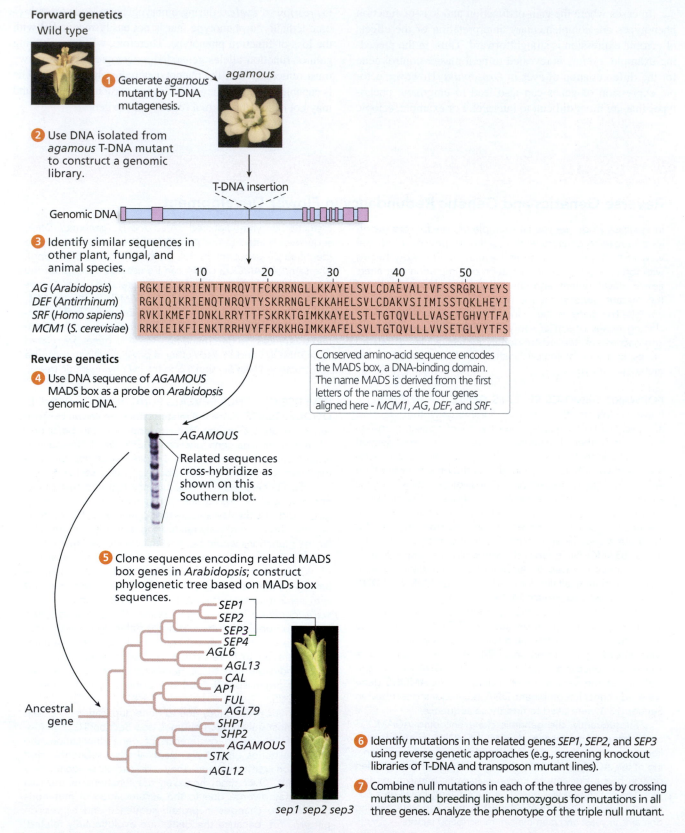

Forward genetics
Wild type

agamous

❶ Generate *agamous* mutant by T-DNA mutagenesis.

❷ Use DNA isolated from *agamous* T-DNA mutant to construct a genomic library.

T-DNA insertion

Genomic DNA

❸ Identify similar sequences in other plant, fungal, and animal species.

	10	20	30	40	50

AG (*Arabidopsis*)   RGKIEIKRIENTTNRQVTFCKRRNGLLKKAYELSVLCDAEVALIVFSSRGRLYEYS
DEF (*Antirrhinum*)   RGKIQIKRIENQTNRQVTYSKRRNGLFKKAHELSVLCDAKVSIIMISSTQKLHEYI
SRF (*Homo sapiens*)   RVKIKMEFIDNKLRRYTTFSKRKTGIMKKAYELSTLTGTQVLLLVASETGHVYTFA
MCM1 (*S. cerevisiae*) RRKIEIKFIENKTRRHVYFFKRKHGIMKKAFELSVLTGTQVLLLVVSETGLVYTFS

Reverse genetics

❹ Use DNA sequence of *AGAMOUS* MADS box as a probe on *Arabidopsis* genomic DNA.

Conserved amino-acid sequence encodes the MADS box, a DNA-binding domain. The name MADS is derived from the first letters of the names of the four genes aligned here - *MCM1*, *AG*, *DEF*, and *SRF*.

AGAMOUS

Related sequences cross-hybridize as shown on this Southern blot.

❺ Clone sequences encoding related MADS box genes in *Arabidopsis*; construct phylogenetic tree based on MADs box sequences.

SEP1
SEP2
SEP3
SEP4
AGL6
AGL13
CAL
AP1
FUL
AGL79
SHP1
SHP2
AGAMOUS
STK
AGL12

Ancestral gene

❻ Identify mutations in the related genes *SEP1*, *SEP2*, and *SEP3* using reverse genetic approaches (e.g., screening knockout libraries of T-DNA and transposon mutant lines).

❼ Combine null mutations in each of the three genes by crossing mutants and breeding lines homozygous for mutations in all three genes. Analyze the phenotype of the triple null mutant.

sep1 sep2 sep3

Figure 14.19 **Use of forward and reverse genetics to determine gene function.**

14.1 Forward Genetic Screens Identify Genes by Their Mutant Phenotypes

■ Forward genetic screens are designed to identify genes by creation of a mutant phenotype, often allowing researchers to infer the biological function of a gene.

■ Complementation tests are used to discover the number of alleles and the number of genes affected in a forward genetic screen.

■ Mutations resulting in lethality can be identified in genetic screens for conditional alleles.

■ Enhancer and suppressor genetic screens identify genes that act in related or redundant pathways.

14.2 Genes Identified by Mutant Phenotype Are Cloned Using Recombinant DNA Technology

■ Some genes can be cloned by complementation of a mutant phenotype.

■ Advances in sequencing technologies facilitate direct identification of mutant genes.

■ Candidate genes can also be identified by expression analyses, DNA sequence analyses of multiple mutant alleles, or complementation experiments.

14.3 Reverse Genetics Investigates Gene Action by Progressing from Gene Identification to Phenotype

■ Reverse genetics approaches, in which determination of biological function proceeds from gene sequence to mutant phenotype, make use of collections consisting of mutants that are each defective in a different defined gene.

■ CRISPR–Cas9–mediated genome editing has revolutionized reverse genetic approaches and enabled unprecedented manipulation of genome sequences in vivo.

■ Collections of insertion alleles, the TILLING process, and RNAi-mediated gene silencing all contribute to the reverse genetics analysis of model organisms.

14.4 Transgenes Provide a Means of Dissecting Gene Function

■ Reporter genes are used to monitor gene-expression patterns in transgenic organisms and for the dissection of regulatory sequences. Some reporter genes, such as the green fluorescent protein, can be visualized in real time in living organisms.

■ Chimeric genes represent novel alleles that can provide clues to gene function.

PREPARING FOR PROBLEM SOLVING

In addition to the list of problem-solving tips and suggestions given here, you can go to the Study Guide and Solutions Manual that accompanies this book for help at solving problems.

1. Be familiar with mutagenesis strategies employed in forward genetics.

2. Know general strategies for analyzing collections of mutants generated in forward genetic screens.

3. Review the approaches to cloning genes known only by a mutant phenotype.

4. Review the different approaches employed in reverse genetics and the reasons for choosing one approach over another.

5. Know different ways in which CRISPR–Cas can be utilized for genome editing.

6. Be acquainted with different types of reporter genes.

7. Understand how chimeric genes can be used to investigate gene function.

PROBLEMS   Mastering Genetics   Visit for instructor-assigned tutorials and problems.

Chapter Concepts

For answers to selected even-numbered problems, see Appendix: Answers.

1. What are the advantages and disadvantages of using *GFP* versus *lacZ* as a reporter gene in mice, *C. elegans*, and *Drosophila*?

2. You conduct a study in which the transcriptional fusion of regulatory sequences of a particular gene with a reporter gene results in relatively uniform expression of the reporter gene in all cells of an organism. A translational fusion with the same gene shows reporter gene expression only in the nucleus of a specific cell type. Discuss some biological causes for the difference in expression patterns of the two transgenes.

3. Discuss the similarities and differences between forward and reverse genetic approaches, and when you would choose to utilize each of the approaches.

4. Using the data inside the back cover of the book, calculate the average number of kilobase (kb) pairs per centimorgan in the six multicellular eukaryotic organisms.

How would this information influence strategies to clone genes known only by a mutant phenotype in these organisms?

5. What are the advantages and disadvantages of using insertion alleles versus alleles generated by chemicals (as in TILLING) in reverse genetic studies?

6. You have cloned the mouse ortholog (see Genetic Analysis 14.2 for definition) of the gene associated with human Huntington Disease (HD) and wish to examine its expression in mice. Outline the approaches you might take to examine the temporal and spatial expression pattern at the cellular level.

7. Diagram the mechanism by which CRISPR–Cas functions in the immune system of bacteria and archaea.

8. Describe how CRISPR–Cas has been modified to create a genome-editing tool.

9. Discuss the advantages (and possible disadvantages) of the different approaches to reverse genetics.

10. Discuss the advantages (and possible disadvantages) of the different mutagens in Table 14.1.

Application and Integration

For answers to selected even-numbered problems, see Appendix: Answers.

11. You have identified a gene encoding the protein involved in the rate-limiting step in vitamin E biosynthesis. How would you create a transgenic plant producing large quantities of vitamin E in its seeds?

12. You have identified a recessive mutation that alters bristle patterning in *Drosophila* and have used recombinant DNA technology to identify a genomic clone that you believe harbors the gene. How would you demonstrate that your gene is on the genomic clone?

13. The *CBF* genes of *Arabidopsis* are induced by exposure of the plants to low temperature.
    a. How would you examine the temporal and spatial patterns of expression after induction by low temperature?
    b. Can you design a method that would reveal these changes in gene expression in a way that a farmer could recognize them by observing plants growing in the field?

14. When the *S. cerevisiae* genome was sequenced and surveyed for possible genes, only about 40% of those genes had been previously identified in forward genetic screens. This left about 60% of predicted genes with no known function, leading some to dub the genes *fun* (function unknown) genes.
    a. As an approach to understanding the function of a certain *fun* gene, you wish to create a loss-of-function allele. How will you accomplish this?
    b. You wish to know the physical location of the encoded protein product. How will you obtain such information?

15. Translational fusions between a protein of interest and a reporter protein are used to determine the subcellular location of proteins in vivo. However, fusion to a reporter protein sometimes renders the protein of interest nonfunctional because the addition of the reporter protein interferes with proper protein folding, enzymatic activity, or protein–protein interactions. You have constructed a fusion between your protein of interest and a reporter gene. How will you show that the fusion protein retains its normal biological function?

16. In humans, Duchenne's muscular dystrophy is caused by a mutation in the *dystrophin* gene, which resides on the X chromosome. How would you create a mouse model of this genetic disease?

17. How would you perform a genetic screen to identify genes directing *Drosophila* wing development? Once you have a collection of wing-development mutants, how would you

analyze your mutagenesis to learn how many genes are represented and how many alleles of each gene? How would you discover whether the genes act in the same or different pathways, and if in the same pathway, how do you discover the order in which they act? How would you clone the genes?

18. In enhancer trapping experiments, a minimal promoter and a reporter gene are placed adjacent to the end of a transposon so that genomic enhancers adjacent to the insertion site can act to drive expression of the reporter gene. In a modification of this approach, a series of enhancers and a promoter can be placed at the end of a transposon so that transcription is activated from the transposon into adjacent genomic DNA. What types of mutations do you expect to be induced by such a transposon in a mutagenesis experiment?

19. In Genetic Analysis 14.1, we designed a screen to identify conditional mutants of *S. cerevisiae* in which the secretory system was defective. Suppose we were successful in identifying 12 mutants.
    a. Describe the crosses you would perform to determine the number of different genes represented by the 12 mutations.
    b. Based on your knowledge of the genetic tools for studying baker's yeast, how would you clone the genes that are mutated in your respective yeast strains? What is an approach to cloning the human orthologs (see Genetic Analysis 14.2 for definition) of the yeast genes?

20. How would you design a genetic screen to find genes involved in meiosis?

21. The eyes of *Drosophila* develop from imaginal discs, groups of cells set aside in the fly embryo that differentiate into the adult structures during the pupal stage. Despite their importance in nature, eyes are dispensable for fruit-fly life in the laboratory.
    a. Devise a genetic screen to identify genes directing development of the fly eye.
    b. What complications might arise from genetic screens targeting an organ that differentiates late in development?

22. Given your knowledge of the genetic tools for studying *Drosophila*, outline a method by which you could clone the *dunce* and *rutabaga* genes identified by Seymour Benzer's laboratory in the genetic screen described at the beginning of this chapter.

23. Mutations in the *CFTR* gene result in cystic fibrosis in humans, a condition in which abnormal secretions are present in the lungs, pancreas, and sweat glands. The gene was mapped to a 500-kb region on chromosome 7 containing three candidate genes.
    a. Using your knowledge of the disease symptoms, how would you distinguish between the candidate genes to decide which is most likely to encode the *CFTR* gene?
    b. How would you prove that your chosen candidate is the *CFTR* gene?

24. How would you clone a gene that you have identified by a mutant phenotype in *Drosophila*?

25. How would you conduct a screen to identify recessive mutations in *Drosophila* that result in embryo lethality? How would you propagate the recessive mutant alleles?

26. In land plants, there is an alternation of generations between a haploid gametophyte generation and a diploid sporophytic generation. Both generations are typically multicellular and may be free-living. The male (pollen) and female (embryo sac) gametophytes are the haploid generation of flowering plants.
    a. How would you conduct a screen to identify genes required for female gametophyte development in *Arabidopsis*?
    b. How would you conduct a screen to identify genes required for male gametophyte development?

27. The *Drosophila even-skipped* (*eve*) gene is expressed in seven stripes in the segmentation pattern of the embryo. A sequence segment of 8 kb 5′ to the transcription start site (shown as +1 in the accompanying figure) is required to drive expression of a reporter gene (*lacZ*) in the same pattern as the endogenous *eve* gene. Remarkably, expression of most of the seven stripes appears to be specified independently, with stripe 2 expression directed by regulatory sequences in the region 1.7 kb 5′ to the transcription start site. To further examine stripe 2 regulatory sequences, you create a series of constructs, each containing different fragments of the 1.7-kb region of 5′ sequence. In the lower part of the figure, the bars at left represent the sequences of DNA included in your reporter gene constructs, and the + and – signs at right indicate whether the corresponding *eve*-*lacZ* reporter gene directs stripe 2 expression in *Drosophila* embryos transformed through *P* element mediation. How would you interpret the results—that is, where do the regulatory sequences responsible for stripe 2 expression reside?

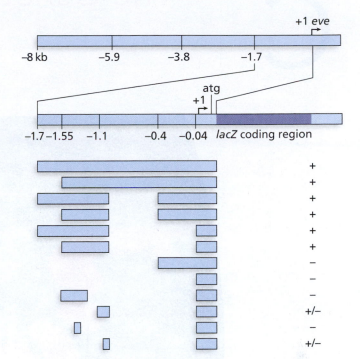

28. Most organisms display a circadian rhythm, a cycling of biological processes that is roughly synchronized with day length (e.g., jet lag occurs in humans when rapid movement between time zones causes established circadian rhythms to be out of synch with daylight hours). In *Drosophila*, pupae eclose (emerge as adults after metamorphosis) at dawn.
    a. Using this knowledge, how would you screen for *Drosophila* mutants that have an impaired circadian rhythm?
    b. In most plants, such as *Arabidopsis*, genes whose encoded products have roles related to photosynthesis have expression patterns that vary in a circadian manner. Using this knowledge, how would you screen for *Arabidopsis* mutants that have an impaired circadian rhythm?
    c. In each case, how would you clone the genes you identified by mutation?

29. As shown in Figure 14.1, mutations in the *Drosophila Ultrabithorax* (*Ubx*) gene result in wings developing from two thoracic segments, rather than just one as in wild-type flies. In the mouse genome there are two *Ubx* orthologs (see Genetic Analysis 14.2 for definition). How would you determine whether the two mouse genes have distinct or redundant functions?

Collaboration and Discussion

For answers to selected even-numbered problems, see Appendix: Answers.

30. How would you edit a specific nucleotide in a genome?

31. Through a forward genetics screen in *Arabidopsis* you have identified a mutation that results in leaves curling upward, rather than being flat as in wild type. You have cloned the corresponding gene and note that it is a member of a small gene family composed of three additional members in *Arabidopsis*. How will you determine if the other three members of the gene family have similar or distinct functions as compared with the gene you first identified?

32. The CRISPR–Cas9 complex directs the Cas9 endonuclease to a specific genomic locus. If the endonuclease domain is inactivated and replaced with a transcriptional activator (or repressor) domain, what would be the functional consequence of directing such a complex to a specific chromosomal location?

33. Describe how enhancer screens can be used to uncover genetic redundancy.

34. How might you use CRISPR–Cas9 to create a large deletion?

The Genetics of Cancer

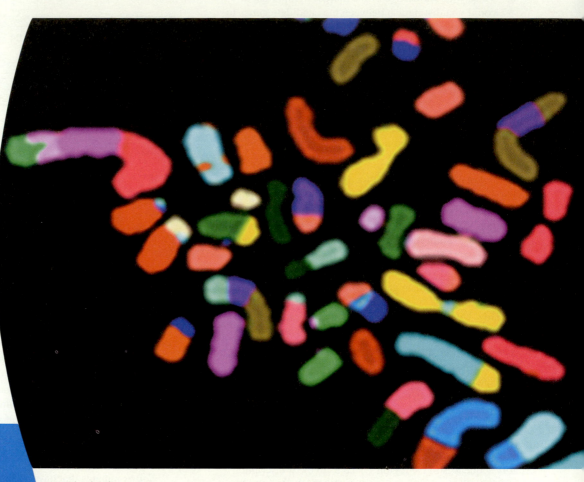

Multiple chromosome mutations, including duplications, deletions, inversions, and translocations, are common in cancer cells. Chromosome-specific fluorescent stains reveal translocations, which produce mutant chromosomes stained two or more colors. Other data and observations reveal the other chromosome mutations.

In summer 2015, former President Jimmy Carter was diagnosed with metastatic melanoma, an aggressive and potentially lethal cancer that often starts on the skin but can occur in other tissues as well. In Carter's case, the melanoma had metastasized to his liver and his brain. (*Metastasize* means to spread from the original tumor to one or more new locations.) Carter underwent surgery to remove the liver tumors and received radiation treatments that focused directly on his brain tumors. He was also given the drug that goes by the trade name Keytruda (its compound name is pembrolizumab) that targets a process cancer cells often use to evade detection by the immune system. Fortunately for Carter, his case was caught early enough in the metastatic process to be treatable. According to some cancer treatment specialists, the combination of surgery and radiation might have been sufficient to control the cancer; but the addition of

Keytruda, which Carter has continued to take since his diagnosis, may also have played a significant role.

Keytruda is one of a class of new drugs known as checkpoint inhibitors that have been approved to treat cancer since 2014. Working similarly to another drug in this class, Opdivo (compound name nivolumab), Keytruda operates on a checkpoint inhibitor receptor protein known as PD-1 residing on the immune system cells known as T-cells. T-cells have the ability to attack cancer cells. Cancer cells can evade destruction by T-cells, however, by producing the protein PD-L1, which binds to PD-1 and prevents T-cell recognition of cancer cells. Keytruda and Opdivo prevent the binding of PD-L1 to PD-1, allowing T-cells to attack cancer cells.

Since the first approval of these checkpoint inhibitor drugs for cancer treatment, they have proven effective in treating a wide range of cancers, including those affecting the lung, stomach, colon, and skin. With variation depending on the type of cancer treated, they are effective in about 25 to 40% of cases, prolonging life beyond what would be expected with chemotherapy and surgery alone. They are not universally effective, however, and cancer may recur even with successful initial treatment. In addition, treatment with these drugs can be very expensive—up to $150,000 per year. On balance, however, these drugs represent the start of a new wave of cancer treatments that target the immune system in various ways as a defense mechanism against existing cancer. The goal of these immune system–based cancer treatments is to stimulate immune system cells, most often T-cells, to fight cancer the way they fight invading bacterial cells in an infection: identify an abnormal cell, attach to it, and destroy it.

Several avenues of investigation have converged to aid in developing and targeting these immune system–based cancer therapies. From a genetic perspective, research over the past 25 years that has investigated mutations in cancer cells and more recently has focused on deciphering the genome sequences of cancer cells has proven enormously helpful both in understanding the biology of cancer and in helping to devise effective treatment approaches. Former President Carter is one of a large number of cancer patients alive today who have benefitted from this recent research and from new therapeutic approaches that seek to change the way medicine treats and manages cancer.

According to data published by the United States Centers for Disease Control, cancer is the second most common cause of death in the nation, following heart disease. The American Cancer Society reports that in the United States there were 1,685,210 new cases of cancer diagnosed in 2016 and 595,690 deaths due to cancer—a rate of 1627 deaths a day. Worldwide, according to the International Agency for Research on Cancer (IARC), 14.1 million cases of cancer were reported in 2012, and more than 13 million deaths due to cancer. IARC estimates that by 2030, the number of cancer cases annually will exceed 21.6 million.

Cancer is not a single disease. Rather, it is two hundred or more different diseases, affecting almost all organ systems, tissues, and types of cells. Table C.1 lists the ten most common types of cancer. Among these ten, lung cancer, prostate cancer, cancer of the uterus or ovary, and breast cancer are the cancers most often identified as causes of death.

The past 25 years have seen major advancements in the understanding of cancer screening, in research into and knowledge about cancer biology, and in the development of cancer treatment. These advancements have led to decreases in the rates of some cancers, to the ability to discover many cancers at earlier stages when they are more amenable to treatment, and to new targeted therapies to more effectively treat cancer. The overall result has been a decline of more than 20% in the rate of cancer deaths since the 1980s. Not all the news is good, however. Death rates from some cancers are higher, and some that were once relatively rare are now more common. The potentially fatal cancer melanoma is an example.

Table C.1	Incidence of the Ten Most Common Cancers[a]
Cancer	**Cases per 100,000 People**
Breast (female)	122.2
Prostate (male)	105.3
Lung and bronchus	60.4
Colon and rectum	38.9
Reproductive system (female)	25.7
Bladder	20.2
Melanoma of the skin	19.9
Non-Hodgkins lymphoma	18.5
Kidney	15.9
Thyroid	14.3

[a]U.S. Centers for Disease Control (2013).

Research on cancer in recent decades has demonstrated that cancer is a genetic disease at the level of the cell. It is now well established that the biological abnormalities found in cancer cells are the result of multiple gene mutations and chromosome mutations that alter the protein products of genes and disrupt a number of key activities and functions in cancer cells.

The study of cancer, like many areas of inquiry in genetics, is increasingly molecular in its focus. Particularly prominent are genome sequencing approaches that make it feasible to sequence the entire genome of cancer cells to achieve a full picture of the abnormalities present. These approaches are also leading to new insight concerning potential treatments of certain cancers, including those described in the chapter introduction. This chapter presents a general discussion of the current biological view of cancer, describing selected examples of the role gene mutations and chromosome mutations play in cancer development, outlining cancer cell genome sequencing strategies, and surveying new drug-based and immune system–based approaches to cancer treatment.

C.1 Cancer Is a Somatic Genetic Disease that Is Only Occasionally Inherited

One of the most important advances in understanding cancer is the recognition of cancer as a genetic disease that usually results from the occurrence of multiple gene mutations in somatic cells of the body. Somatic cells are all the cells of the body except the sex cells, sperm and egg. It is estimated that 90 to 95% of cancer cases develop in this way. Like those cancers, the remaining 5 to 10% require the presence of multiple mutations, but in this smaller group, one or more of the mutations is inherited, making the pathway

to cancer considerably shorter than in the large majority of cases. We discuss some examples of inherited mutations that predispose individuals to cancer in a later section.

The trillions of somatic cells in your body are each derived by mitotic division from parental cells. Recall from the discussion in Chapter 3 that mitosis produces two daughter cells that are genetically identical to one another and genetically identical to the parental cell from which they are derived. In thinking about gene mutations and cancer, this means that if a cell acquires a gene mutation, the mutation is passed to its daughter cells. If in a later generation a descendant cell acquires a second mutation, then that line of cells carries two mutations. Such a cell lineage might acquire a third mutation, and a fourth mutation, and so on. The multiple gene mutations required for a cell to become cancerous accumulate over time measured in decades. This is the principal reason why cancer is almost never the result of a single mutation and why cancer occurs more often in older people than in younger people. Age is the greatest of all risk factors for cancer.

C.2 What Is Cancer and What Are the Characteristics of Cancer?

Rather than being a single disease, cancer is a category comprising many diseases that differ by the gene mutations responsible for their origin and the cell types in which they occur. Even cancers affecting the same tissue in different people will have different mutations. These differences are manifested in dissimilarities in cancer growth rates, degrees of invasiveness, ages of onset, responsiveness to treatment, and prognosis. Nevertheless, all cancer cells can be described as differing from normal cells in four general ways. First, whereas most normal somatic cells are highly specialized (i.e., they have characteristic sizes and shapes and perform or interact in characteristic ways), cancer cells are **dedifferentiated**. This means that in comparison with normal somatic cells from the same tissue, cancer cells look different and behave differently—more like primordial cells than specialized cells. Second, compared with normal cells, cancer cells have a higher rate of **proliferation**. In other words they divide and grow much more quickly than normal cells of the same tissue. Third, cancer cells are larger than their normal counterparts and also have larger nuclei. Finally, cancer cells are poorly organized as they grow. Whereas normal cell growth is confined to the boundaries of each type of tissue and restricted by cell-to-cell contact, cancer cells not only lose their cell-to-cell sensitivity but have the propensity to overgrow their normal confines and invade surrounding tissues.

Progression of Abnormalities

Cancer cell lineages evolve through mutations from normal cells. As they do so, they often progress through a series of stages that appear to be progressively abnormal (**Figure C.1**).

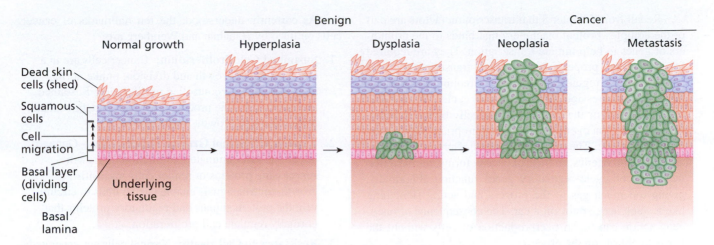

Figure C.1 Abnormal tissue growth and cancer development. Abnormal tissue growth commonly follows a pattern of increasing, but noncancerous, abnormality beginning with hyperplasia that can progress to dysplasia. Neoplasia (cancer) can follow, and metastasis can occur if neoplastic growth invades normal tissue.

Before they become cancerous, cells begin to look abnormal and grow abnormally. The abnormality can first appear as **hyperplasia**, meaning extra growth, and progress to **dysplasia**, meaning disorganized growth. Hyperplastic and dysplastic cells can form **tumors**, masses of abnormal cells, but in these early stages the tumors are classified as **benign tumors**, meaning they are noncancerous, are usually well encapsulated by surrounding tissues or membranes. Benign tumors are considered "precancerous." They are composed of abnormal cells that can grow excessively, but they do not invade surrounding normal tissue. If they are accessible, benign tumors can often be removed relatively easily by surgical or other treatments. For example, abnormal growths on the skin can be removed quickly and simply by spraying the growth with liquid nitrogen ($-321°F$, or $-196°C$) to kill the abnormal cells by freezing. Abnormal growths in the colon detected during colonoscopy can be removed surgically during the screening procedure.

Dysplastic cells can progress, however, to **neoplasia**, a state of growth in which they are now cancer cells proliferating in large numbers and in a highly disorganized manner. In this state, the masses are classified as **malignant tumors**, which are not confined in their growth. If malignant tumor growth continues it can enter **metastasis**, a state in which the tumor invades normal tissues (such as the basal lamina and underlying tissue seen in Figure C.1) and in which cancer cells may be carried in blood or lymphatic circulation to new locations, where they can seed new tumors.

New cancer research, driven by genetics, has altered the understanding of the nature of tumors and the characteristics of cancer. In years past, a tumor was thought to be a mass of millions of cells that were essentially genetically identical to one another, having been generated as a cell lineage derived by mitotic division from an original cancer cell. In this sense, a tumor was thought to be clonal. Today, cancer biologists understand that a tumor is a complex mixture of cells, some malignant but many others normal, containing cancer cells that can have different genetic profiles. and with a biology as complex as that of most other tissues. The current view describes cancer as a progressive disease that develops through stages proceeding from normal to malignant, as Figure C.1 illustrates.

The Hallmarks of Cancer Cells and Malignant Tumors

Cancer cells are profoundly abnormal cells, malignant tumors are profoundly abnormal tissues, and cancer is a profoundly abnormal biological state, the endpoint of a long series of genetic and biological changes that have occurred within the affected cell lineage over the life span of a person. Despite the many differences distinguishing the various types of cancer, these extreme genetic and biological abnormalities of cancer cells and malignant tumors do have certain hallmark features.

As an introduction to the hallmarks of cancer, it helps to be familiar with two conceptual categories of genes that have been used to describe how mutations often contribute to cancer development. These categories classify some genes as *proto-oncogenes* and some genes as *tumor suppressor genes*. Both categories contain large numbers of genes, and all the genes in each category are genes we all carry that perform essential functions in cells. It is when these genes are mutated and have aberrant function, no function, or excessive activity that they contribute to cancer development.

The **proto-oncogenes** are a broad array of normal genes stimulating cell division and progression through the cell cycle (see Chapter 3 for a discussion of the cell cycle). As a group, proto-oncogenes encode transcription factor proteins and cell-cycle regulating proteins. You can think of proto-oncogenes as the "gas" that propels the transcription of other genes in cells or drives the cell cycle forward.

Recall from Chapter 8 that transcription factors are part of the complex protein machinery that binds to the promoters of genes to help initiate transcription. They are required for normal and proper control of gene transcription. Similarly, cell-cycle regulatory proteins are required for normal, controlled progression through the cell cycle. Proteins that fail to function or that function incorrectly owing to mutations of proto-oncogenes result in inappropriate progression of the cell cycle. The mutated versions of proto-oncogenes are called **oncogenes**. In their oncogene forms, transcription factor or cell-cycle regulatory genes function abnormally, giving too much gas to the process and acting something like a stuck accelerator on a car. The consequence of oncogene action can be an overproduction of cells without the normal controls on the process.

Tumor suppressor genes are a large and varied group of normal genes whose protein products largely function at cell cycle checkpoints, such as the transition from G_1 to S phase or from S phase to G_2, or function in other ways during the cell cycle to pause it until conditions are right to continue. Tumor suppressor genes can also express proteins that function in the normal process for bringing on the death of aged or damaged cells. Tumor suppressor genes can be thought of as the "brake" that controls the speed and pace of cell proliferation. Mutations of tumor suppressor genes are like brake failure in a car. In this case, the normal controls on cell proliferation are missing, and either the cell cycle moves forward too quickly or cells that should undergo cell death evade the process.

The maintenance of normal tissue and organ size, boundaries, and cell numbers is achieved by a balance between the mitotic production of new cells and the death of old cells. The many genes in the proto-oncogene and tumor suppressor gene categories interact in complex ways to preserve that balance. If important players in that balancing process are mutated, causing excess cell proliferation and the insufficient elimination of old cells by cell death, the balance can break down.

The concepts of proto-oncogenes and tumor suppressor genes are helpful but have proven to be incomplete for describing the genetic abnormalities driving cancer development and progression. A major advancement in understanding the cancer process has come from the identification of ten hallmarks of cancer that represent the various ways in which the biological and genetic controls required in normal cells are lost or altered in cancer cells.

In 2000, Douglas Hanahan and Robert Weinberg synthesized the large amount of research literature on cancer and created a list of six hallmarks of cancer. Their paper outlined supporting data and examples and provided cancer researchers with a well-organized way to view and investigate the biology of cancer. In 2011, Hanahan and Weinberg added four additional hallmarks developed largely through the collection and analysis of cancer cell genomic sequences and the assessment of gene mutations in cancer cells.

As currently understood, the ten hallmarks of cancer cells outlined by Hanahan and Weinberg are

1. **Sustained Cell Proliferation:** Cancer cells are in a chronic state of growth and division, unlike normal cells that undergo controlled proliferation. Sustained proliferation can be produced by gene mutations that drive excessive growth.

2. **Evasion of Normal Growth Suppression**—Gene mutations that eliminate the function of growth-suppressing proteins or render cells insensitive to growth-control signals enable cancer cells to circumvent the protein signals and regulatory proteins that normally regulate cell proliferation.

3. **Resistance to Cell Death:** Normal cells are generated through mitotic division, age during their active phase, and then enter senescence and undergo a process known as apoptosis, during which they die. Cancer cells in contrast generally live much longer than normal cells, owing to gene mutations that, by interfering with the normal mechanisms and signals leading to apoptosis, enable cancer cells to delay or bypass cell death.

4. **Cellular Immortality:** In addition to bypassing induced cell death, cancer cells also live much longer than is normal for cells that do not undergo apoptosis. Many are effectively rendered immortal by mutations that stabilize cells or modify the indicators of cell aging in a manner that allows them to grow and divide perpetually.

5. **Angiogenesis Induction: Angiogenesis** is the development of new blood vessels. Malignant tumors require blood vessels to supply the growing tumor with oxygen and compounds needed for growth. A number of normal cell types are recruited by the tumor to form blood vessels. These are among of the cadre of normal cells that are part of a tumor.

6. **Activation of Invasion and Metastasis:** The growth of normal cells usually requires the presence of other cells, partly because contact with other cells exercises control over that growth, keeping each tissue confined to a limited area. In cancer, a succession of gene mutations alters normal growth restrictions, allowing tumors to grow in size and invade surrounding tissues. Additional gene mutations, coupled with cellular immortality, can enable single cancer cells to break away from the original tumor, plant themselves in a new location, and proliferate to produce a new malignant tumor. This is the process of metastasis.

7. **Reprogramming of Energy Metabolism:** The active proliferation of malignant tumors requires a disproportionate amount of energy. Thus, in addition to stimulating angiogenesis to supply itself with oxygen, the tumor must reprogram its cellular metabolism to meet its energy needs.

8. **Immune System Avoidance:** The immune system is responsible for detecting and eliminating foreign microbes and cells that may do harm to the body. In addition, the immune system monitors the body for abnormal cells and helps eradicate precancerous and cancer cells before they develop into tumors. For newly forming tumors to proliferate, it is now thought that they must evade immune system detection. This notion is related to another emerging theory that links inflammatory processes in the body to the proliferation of cancer cells and malignant tumor formation.

9. **Tumor-promoting Inflammation:** Cancerous tumors attract immune system cells deployed by the immune system to attack and eradicate cancer cells. This causes an inflammatory reaction within tumors that, paradoxically, helps promote some aspects of tumor growth, such as angiogenesis. Inflammation can also help supply the tumor with growth factors that in turn promote growth and survival factors, helping cancer cells evade destruction.

10. **Genome Instability and Mutation:** Cancer cells are highly unstable and rapidly acquire new mutations of various kinds. This frequently gives them a growth advantage that allows them to proliferate much faster than surrounding normal cells. Large numbers of individual gene mutations are present in cancer cells, and a great deal of research activity is devoted to identifying which of these mutations are "drivers" of cancer cell proliferation (i.e., which mutations actively promote tumor growth) and which mutations are "passengers" (i.e., mutated due to cancer cell genome instability but not essential for tumor growth). These mutations can be identified by cancer cell genome sequencing.

Cancer cell genome instability can be observed visually. Cancer cell chromosomes typically contain large numbers of duplications, deletions, and chromosome rearrangements, in addition to frequent changes in chromosome number (see Chapter 10 for discussion of chromosome mutations). The chapter opener micrograph shows the chromosomes of a cancer cell stained by a method that produces a distinct fluorescent color for each homologous chromosome pair. Normally, each chromosome should be a single color, but notice that many of them instead contain two or three colors. This is direct evidence of chromosome translocations, and further inspection of these chromosomes would reveal chromosome deletions, duplications, and inversions.

Underlying many of the hallmarks of cancer is another layer of abnormality, consisting of the disruption of normal epigenetic regulation in cancer cells and of mutations that disrupt epigenetic writers, readers, and erasers (see Section 13.2). Among the cancer hallmarks to which epigenetic changes are known to contribute are the effects on cancer cell metabolism and cancer immunology. In hematologic cancers, where the data are strongest, associations have been found between three epigenetics-regulating genes and cancer. The DNA methyltransferase gene *DNMT3A* is one of several genes whose protein products help to methylate chromatin as part of gene silencing. Mutations of *DNMT3A* appear to occur early in certain leukemias, altering gene expression patterns and causing genome instability in the form of chromosome deletions and rearrangements. Other DNA methylation genes, including *TET2* and *IDH*, are also associated with abnormal methylation patterns in cancer cells. In addition, mutations of these genes are associated with disruption of the expression of certain chromatin modifier genes. As a whole, the information on epigenetic alterations in cancer suggests that epigenetic dysregulation is a major contributor to cancer development and proliferation.

C.3 The Genetic Basis of Cancer

To review, most cases of cancer result from the accumulation in somatic cells of multiple and diverse gene mutations that combine to gradually but progressively transition normal cells into cancerous ones. These cases are classified as **sporadic** because they can potentially affect anyone and because they result from mutations that occur at random during the lifetime of the affected individual. Based on the current state of knowledge, and taking into account the many different types of cancer under study, 90% or more of all cases of cancer are thought to fall into the sporadic category.

In this section, however, we shift our focus away from the large majority of cancers that are sporadic toward those that either have a simpler pathway to malignancy or that develop in part through the inheritance of a mutation that significantly increases the likelihood that an individual will develop cancer. We examine certain rare cancers for which the disease is the result of mutation of a single gene, and we look at inherited susceptibility to cancer through the inheritance of **germ-line mutations**, meaning mutations that occur in sperm or eggs and are passed to offspring during reproduction. Germ-line mutations that predispose to the development of cancer tend to cluster in families as a result of hereditary transmission. This pattern of cancer is identified as a **familial** or **hereditary cancer** Certain of these cancers develop through the mutation of a single gene by de novo mutation (new mutation). These mutations that hit a critical gene are followed by a second mutation that leads to cancer.

Single Gene Mutations and Cancer Development

In this section, we describe two types of cancer that usually result from de novo mutations and two other cancers that can be due either to de novo mutations or to the inheritance of a predisposing mutation from a parent. All these rare cancers can be traced to changes in a single gene, but the first two arise from chromosome rearrangements that lead to the

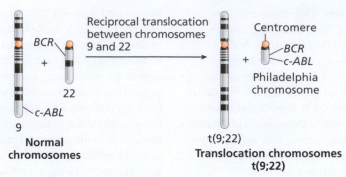

Figure C.2 Reciprocal translocation in chronic myelogenous leukemia. Reciprocal translocation between chromosomes 9 and 22 [t(9;22)] moves the *c-ABL* gene from chromosome 9 into the *BCR* gene region on chromosome 22, forming a *c-ABL–BCR* fusion gene on the shortened copy, called the Philadelphia chromosome, of chromosome 22. The chimeric c-ABL–BCR protein produces CML.

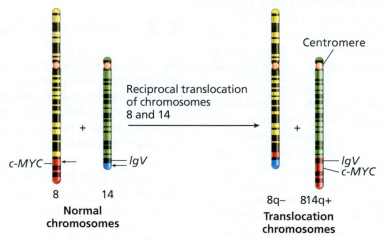

Figure C.3 Example of reciprocal translocation in Burkitt's lymphoma. Translocation of the *c-MYC* gene from chromosome 8 that has lost a portion of its long arm (8q–) to the *IgV* immunoglobulin gene region on chromosome 14 that has gained a portion from chromosome 8 containing c-MYC (14q+). The translocation overproduces c-MYC protein to cause Burkitt's lymphoma.

altered gene expression. In both of these cancers, the chromosome rearrangement occurs so frequently that it is effectively diagnostic for the particular type of cancer.

Chronic Myelogenous Leukemia **Figure C.2** shows a reciprocal translocation between one copy of chromosome 9 and one copy of chromosome 22 that is seen in most cases of chronic myelogenous leukemia (CML). This mutation is usually a de novo mutation. Leukemias (there are many types) are cancers of the blood in which the bone marrow produces certain white blood cells in an uncontrolled manner. In CML, the white blood cells known as granulocytes are overproduced. The chromosome translocation that is typical of CML leads to the production of an abnormal protein.

The nuclei of cancer cells in patients with CML have one normal copy of each of the chromosomes 9 and 22 along with a copy of chromosome 9 and a copy of chromosome 22 that have undergone reciprocal translocation. The translocation produces a short version of chromosome 22 known as the Philadelphia chromosome. It is named after the city in which cancer researcher Janet Rowley was working at the

time she discovered the chromosome in cell samples from CML patients. A gene known as *c-ABL*, located on chromosome 9, is translocated into the chromosome 22 region containing the gene *BCR*. The result of the translocation produces a *c-ABL–BCR* "fusion gene." Expression of this fusion gene produces a chimeric BCR–c-ABL protein. Normal BCR protein is part of a cell signaling pathway. It normally transfers cell growth signals from the external environment to the cell nucleus to stimulate cell proliferation. The chimeric BCR–c-ABL protein continuously stimulates cell division, even in the absence of an external growth signal. The capability for sustained growth is an example of cancer hallmark 1 (sustained proliferation) described above.

Since the specific cause of CML is known, it was an early focus of targeted cancer therapy, involving a drug treatment aimed at controlling the aberrant chimeric protein activity. This effort has been successful, and today CML can be effectively treated, as discussed in a Section C.4.

Burkitt's Lymphoma Another cancer resulting from a de novo chromosome rearrangement is Burkitt's lymphoma (**Figure C.3**). In Burkitt's lymphoma, a reciprocal translocation takes place between chromosome 8, which breaks in a region containing the *c-MYC* gene, and chromosome 2, 14, or 22. The breaking of chromosome 1, 14, or 22 occurs in regions containing genes that encode immunoglobulin proteins, which are part of the immune system. Immunoglobulin genes are very actively transcribed on these chromosomes.

The protein product of *c-MYC* is a transcription factor that plays a role in regulating the transcription of about 15% of all the genes in the human genome. Among the genes it regulates are genes involved in cell cycle progression and apoptosis. A translocation moving *c-MYC* into the region of immunoglobulin genes takes *c-MYC* out of a location where its expression is carefully regulated and puts it in a chromosome region where it is continuously expressed. There is no mutation of the MYC protein produced in Burkitt's lymphoma, because it is identical to normal MYC protein. The abnormality is overexpression of *c-MYC* that produces much more MYC protein than normal, driving excessive cell division and thus causing the disease. This regulatory abnormality in Burkitt's lymphoma is another example of cancer hallmark 1 (sustained proliferation) described above.

Retinoblastoma Retinoblastoma is a rare cancer of the retina that occurs in a few out of every 100,000 newborn infants and very young children. Under normal circumstances, structures of the eye develop during gestation and continue to develop in the first months after birth; but once development is complete in the retina, intercellular signaling stops the division of cells, and they divide no more. Several other types of cells in the body follow a similar course, including cells in bones known as osteocytes. These bone cells divide during childhood and adolescent growth and development and then receive signals to stop growing.

Sporadic retinoblastoma is a retinoblastoma resulting when both copies of an autosomal gene known as *RB1*, located on chromosome 13, are mutated in the same somatic cell. These cells are homozygous for mutant copies of RB1. This form of retinoblastoma is called "sporadic" because there is no family history of the cancer, and both mutations are de novo in their origin. Any cell in either developing retina can acquire a mutation of one copy of *RB1*. During the proliferation of the lineage of this cell by mitosis, the occurrence of a second somatic mutation affecting the other copy of *RB1* in one of the descendants makes that descendant cell homozygous for *RB1* mutations.

The protein product of *RB1*, called pRB, plays an essential role in controlling cell division. **Figure C.4** illustrates the action of pRB in normal cells. A complex forms between pRB and a transcription activator protein known as E2F, and it in turn binds to a complex known as cyclin–CDK. This binding prevents E2F from being available to bind to DNA, where it would stimulate the transcription of other genes. A biochemical process can cause the release of E2F, freeing it to bind to DNA and thus activate the transcription of genes whose protein products are required for cell cycle progression.

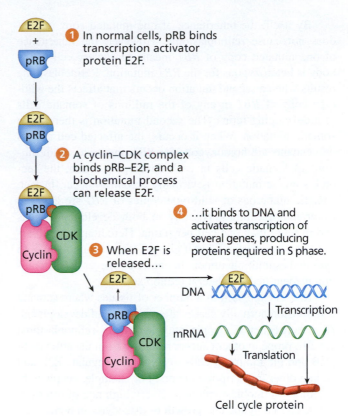

1. In normal cells, pRB binds transcription activator protein E2F.

2. A cyclin–CDK complex binds pRB–E2F, and a biochemical process can release E2F.

3. When E2F is released...

4. ...it binds to DNA and activates transcription of several genes, producing proteins required in S phase.

Cell cycle protein

Figure C.4 The functional role of pRB. The pRB protein product of *RB1* joins with transcription factor E2F and then with the cyclin–CDK complex. When E2F is released from the complex, the E2F binds to DNA and drives the transcription of genes whose expression is required for cell cycle progression. The absence of pRB leads to cell division that is not turned off at the right time in retinal cells and certain other cells.

Homozygosity for mutations of *RB1* removes pRB and prevents the inactivation of E2F. Retinal cells lacking pRB therefore have active transcription factor proteins that continually drive retinal cell division past the point at which their division would normally be halted by pRB expression. The result is significant overgrowth of retinal cells and the development of retinoblastoma. The likelihood of somatic mutations occurring in both homologous copies of *RB1* in a cell is extremely low. As a consequence, sporadic retinoblastoma is always confined to just one eye and occurs as a single tumor in that eye. This condition is identified as unilateral retinoblastoma.

Another form of retinoblastoma, **hereditary retinoblastoma**, usually occurs in both eyes and often produces multiple tumors in each affected eye. Alfred Knudson, a physician and medical researcher, studied hereditary retinoblastoma and in 1971 devised an explanation for it known as the **two-hit hypothesis**. Knudson's proposal was that both copies of a certain gene (Knudson didn't know the gene was *RB1*) had to be mutated to cause retinoblastoma. He suggested that the development of hereditary retinoblastoma begins with the inheritance of one mutant copy of the gene, either in sperm or egg. Consequently, the fertilized egg is initially heterozygous for the mutation, that is, $RB1^+/RB1^-$.

By itself, the inheritance of one mutated copy of *RB1* does not cause retinoblastoma. However, the inheritance of one mutated copy of *RB1* means that every cell in the body is heterozygous for the *RB1* mutation. Retinoblastoma results when a second mutation occurs that affects the wild-type copy of *RB1* in any of the millions of somatic cells in a developing retina. The second mutation is therefore a somatic mutation. When it occurs, the affected cell and its descendants are homozygous for *RB1* mutations. With millions of somatic cells in each developing retina, the second, somatic mutation is virtually certain to occur. In fact, somatic mutations of wild-type copies of *RB1* are likely to occur multiple times, possibly in both developing retinas and in more than one cell per retina. Hereditary retinoblastoma can be unilateral, but it also presents as tumors in both eyes and as multiple tumors in one or both eyes. This condition is identified as bilateral retinoblastoma.

RB1 is expressed in a number of tissues where somatic cell division normally ceases after growth and development. As a consequence, people with hereditary retinoblastoma are also prone to other cancers resulting from the absence of pRB and the failure of cells to be able to regulate E2F and certain other transcription factors. For example, people with hereditary retinoblastoma have a very high rate of osteosarcoma, caused by the overgrowth of osteocytes in bone.

Li–Fraumeni Syndrome Our final example of cancer caused by mutation of a single gene is a cancer-prone condition called Li–Fraumeni syndrome (LFS) that is named after the researchers who first described it. LFS is passed from one generation to the next in a manner that matches the transmission pattern of autosomal dominant inheritance (**Figure C.5**). This is seen in the successive transmission of cancer from one generation to the next and in the occurrence of cancer in members of both sexes about equally. In addition to the apparent hereditary transmission of cancer in this syndrome, what is also notable is that the cancer cases in LFS families typically involve different organs and tissues. Notice that the family members illustrated in Figure C.5 have breast cancer, brain cancer, leukemia, sarcoma, and other cancers.

The key to understanding LFS came from molecular genetic studies of gene mutations in LFS families. Researchers discovered that more than 70% of people with LFS have a mutation of the *TP53* gene, which normally produces a protein known as TP53. This protein is a transcription factor that helps stimulate or repress the transcription of more than 50 other genes.

TP53 is a critically important protein in cells. It is normally produced continuously but most of it is rapidly destroyed; thus, it is usually present in only low levels in cells. Several kinds of stress to cells can block the rapid breakdown of TP53 and increase its cellular concentration. These cellular stresses include a high level of damage to DNA caused by exposure to a mutagen or accumulated due to aging.

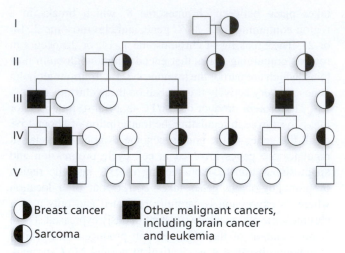

Breast cancer

Sarcoma

Other malignant cancers, including brain cancer and leukemia

Figure C.5   Li–Fraumeni syndrome. Inherited mutations of the *TP53* gene are transmitted in an autosomal dominant pattern in families with Li–Fraumeni syndrome. Various cancers such as breast cancer, brain cancer, sarcomas, leukemia, and others occur often in such families.

TP53 can initiate two responses to DNA damage. First, it blocks the cell cycle to give the cell time to repair the damage. Too long a pause of the cell cycle, however, triggers the other action of TP53, the initiation of apoptosis and destruction of the cell. Apoptosis is common among older cells since they have the highest rates of DNA damage.

Mutations of *TP53* prevent the gene from producing functional TP53. In the absence of TP53 protein, cells have great difficulty pausing the cell cycle to allow DNA damage repair to take place; in addition, cells lacking functional TP53 protein cannot efficiently initiate apoptosis, even when high levels of DNA damage are present. As a result, cells lacking functional TP53 progress through the cell cycle and divide despite the presence of damaged DNA, and they are prone to acquiring new gene mutations, stemming from the earlier damage, as the cycles of replication and division continue. Thus, cells lacking functional TP53 have high mutation rates and are very likely to become malignant. The presence of many different types of cancer in LFS families is a consequence.

Cases of LFS that are not caused by mutation of *TP53* are most often caused by mutation of *CHEK2* (checkpoint kinase 2). Like *TP53*, *CHEK2* is activated when DNA is damaged, and it too normally acts to prevent the cell from progressing in the cell cycle. The protein product of *CHEK2* interacts with TP53, suggesting that both mutations disrupt the same general cellular pathway.

The Genetic Progression of Cancer Development and Cancer Predisposition

Despite the relative rarity of the cancers caused by single-gene mutations, they do illustrate the pivotal role gene mutations play in cancer development. Nevertheless, it bears repeating that the vast majority of cancers result from the accumulation of a large number of somatic mutations. As the mutations accrue, the once-normal cells are gradually converted to an abnormal state and eventually develop into cancer cells.

One of the clearest examples of this process comes from the study of gene mutations in the development of colon and rectal cancer. Studies of the genetic abnormalities in this type of cancer offer both a glimpse into the process of somatic mutation leading to cancer development and a lesson on how the inheritance of germ-line mutations can predispose individuals to develop cancers like colon and rectal cancer. Colorectal cancer is a good example of a condition brought on by multiple somatic mutations because most cases progress very slowly, through stages of progressive cellular abnormality over several decades. The abnormal cells that develop prior to the formation of colon and rectal cancer are not cancerous. They occur in clusters on the epithelial surface lining the colon and rectum. These early abnormal growths are known clinically as "adenomas" or, more commonly, as "polyps." They can easily be visualized by colonoscopy, and their removal prevents the potential development of colon or rectal cancer (see the progression of benign and cancerous stages depicted in Figure C.1).

The genetic progression that takes cells from a normal to a malignant state is not a fixed series of specific steps in any cancer. What is often observed, however, is that mutations in certain genes are found much more commonly than mutations in other genes. These often-mutated genes are likely to be the "drivers" of cancer development, i.e. the mutations that are most directly tied to the development of cancer and to the hallmarks of cancer. The acquisition of these commonly occurring mutations correlates with progression from one stage of abnormality to the next, as **Figure C.6** illustrates for different stages of colorectal cancer development. The process begins with the excessive proliferation of abnormal tissue. It then progresses to the production of adenomas (polyps), the larger, easily detected clusters of abnormal tissue. A small proportion of adenomas that continue to grow can become cancerous and produce colon or rectal cancer.

The figure identifies four specific genes that frequently, but not universally, are found to be mutated in association with the transition from one particular stage of abnormality to the next. These mutations are common, occurring in about 25 to 75% of cases, but progression can also occur

without mutation of these genes. Mutation of the *APC* gene is a common first step in the transition from normal colon epithelium to abnormally proliferating epithelium. The protein product of the *APC* gene limits the growth of epithelial cells that are in contact with other cells. As adenomas form and advance, mutation of the *KRAS* gene frequently occurs. This gene normally produces a cell division signal transduction protein that responds to external signals and conveys a message to the nucleus that drives cell division. The deletion of a gene known as *DCC* results in the loss of a protein that suppresses cell growth. This mutation allows adenomas to generate finger-like outgrowths (villi) that advance the spread of the adenoma. The transition to a cancerous state often occurs with the mutation of the *TP53* gene. As was described above for Li–Fraumeni syndrome, mutation of *TP53* leads to failure of cell cycle pausing for DNA damage repair and also severely impairs the initiation of apoptosis in heavily damaged and aged cells. These gene mutations, common but not always present in colorectal cancer, are usually accompanied by mutations in other genes as well; in fact, other genes must mutate if the colorectal cancer lesion is to become metastatic.

About 75 to 80% of people developing colorectal cancer have sporadic disease that occurs as a result of the acquisition of these or other gene mutations in somatic cells. The remaining 20 to 25% of colorectal cancers are linked to inheritance of a germ-line mutation that predisposes a person to develop cancer. These inherited mutations do not by themselves lead to cancer, since several additional somatic mutations must still occur to drive the progression of tissue through the adenomatous stages to cancer.

Many of the gene mutations inherited in colorectal cancer–prone families are not known or are not fully characterized, but one gene, *APC*, is known to be transmitted in mutated form in some families prone to colorectal cancer. About 1 to 2% of colorectal cancer cases result from genetic predisposition to a cancer known as **familial adenomatous polyposis (FAP)**. FAP is a hereditary form of cancer in which affected family members inherit a mutated copy of *APC*. As with sporadic colorectal cancer, germ-line transmission of *APC* mutations leads to the development of adenomas in the colon. Since all the cells of a person inheriting one mutated copy of *APC* are heterozygous for the mutation, the formation of colonic polyps in such a person is prolific. In some cases, hundreds to thousands of polyps may form as early as the teenage years or in a person's early twenties.

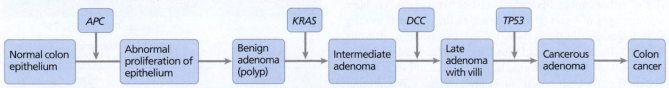

Figure C.6 **Mutation acquisition in familial adenomatous polyposis.** FAP features the development of hundreds of colonic polyps that can become cancerous. Mutational analysis identifies at least four genes that are frequently, but not universally, mutated as polyps progress toward malignancy.

Table C.2	Selected Cancers with Inherited Predispositions
Cancer Type	**Predisposing Gene Mutation[a]**
Early-onset familial breast cancer	BRCA1, BRCA2
Familial adenomatous polyposis	APC
Familial melanoma	CDKN2
Gorlin syndrome	PTCH1
Lynch syndrome	MSH2, MSH6
Li–Fraumeni syndrome	TP53, CHEK2
Multiple endocrine neoplasia, type 1	MEN1
Multiple endocrine neoplasia, type 2	RET
Neurofibromatosis, type 1	NF1
Neurofibromatosis, type 2	NF2
Retinoblastoma	RB1
Von Hippel–Lindau syndrome	VHL
Wilms tumor	WT1

[a]Go to http://www.ncbi.nlm.nih.gov/omim and enter the gene abbreviation in the Search box at the top of the page to get gene identity and information on gene function and mutations.

These polyps do not necessarily progress to a cancerous state any more often than sporadically occurring polyps do, but since there are so many of them, the progression of one or more to a cancerous state is a virtual certainty.

In FAP, inheritance of a mutated copy of APC represents the first step of a multistep mutational process that can lead to cancer. FAP was one of the first of several types of cancer to be shown to in some cases result from an inherited predisposition (Table C.2). In FAP and in some of the other cancers in Table C.2, the inherited mutation is one that is also commonly found in sporadic cases.

Breast and Ovarian Cancer and the Inheritance of Cancer Susceptibility

Between 90 and 95% of all cases of breast and ovarian cancers are sporadic. Less than 10% are attributable to the inheritance of gene mutations that increase a woman's lifetime risk of either cancer. Sporadic breast or ovarian cancers have average ages of onset (the age at which the cancer is usually first diagnosed) in the sixties. These cases occur in just one breast or in one ovary, and thus they are classified as unilateral. As with retinoblastoma, however, bilateral cancer also occurs (i.e., in both breasts or in both ovaries). When bilateral cancer occurs, or when breast or ovarian cancer occurs at a much younger than average age of onset—in the thirties or forties or earlier—inherited susceptibility to cancer can be suspected. In addition to people with bilateral cancers or

cancers with an early age of onset, families in which large numbers of breast or ovarian cancer occur or in which the pattern of cancer occurrence is similar to autosomal dominant inheritance can also be suspected of having inherited susceptibility. Similarly, contralateral breast cancer (cancer in the second breast subsequent to cancer developing in the first breast) is strongly influenced by inherited susceptibility.

Two genes have each been shown to have mutations that dramatically affect the risk of breast and ovarian cancer. The first discovery of a gene whose mutation increased susceptibility to breast and ovarian cancer, a gene called BRCA1 (breast cancer 1), occurred in the late 1990s. This was followed by the identification of a second gene, BRCA2 (breast cancer 2), a few years later, and by determination of the normal roles these genes play in cells. Each gene was first located and mapped to a human chromosome. Subsequently, research determined that both BRCA1 and BRCA2 are DNA damage repair genes normally operating in pathways that identify and repair DNA damage that generates point mutations such as base pair substitutions.

BRCA1 and BRCA2 are genes that all humans carry. In their normal state, they help screen DNA for damage and repair the damage that is detected. The increased risk of cancer with which they are connected derives from certain mutations of these genes that significantly reduce or eliminate the ability of their protein products to function normally. The most accurate estimates of the risk of breast or ovarian cancer associated with a mutation of BRCA1 or BRCA2 come from long-term prospective studies that follow women with a mutation over an extended period of time. A 2013 study by Nasim Mavaddat and a large number of colleagues followed nearly 1900 British women with a mutation of either BRCA1 or BRCA2 for 10 years (Table C.3). The researchers estimated that with a BRCA1 mutation, the average cumulative risk of cancer by age 70 was 60% for breast cancer, 59% for ovarian cancer, and 83% for contralateral breast cancer. The cumulative risk of cancer by age 70 with a BRCA2 mutation was 55% for breast cancer, 16% for ovarian cancer, and 62% for contralateral breast cancer. The results reported by this study are similar to those of other studies. Collectively, they point to mutations of either gene as conferring significantly increased risks of cancer.

Whereas mutation of BRCA1 or of BRCA2 significantly increases the risk that a woman will develop breast or ovarian

Table C.3	Increased Cancer Risk with BRCA1 or BRCA2 Mutation		
	Cancer Risk by Age 70[a]		
Cancer	**General Population**	**Mutation of BRCA1**	**Mutation of BRCA2**
Breast	11%	60%	59%
Ovary	1–2%	59%	16%
Contralateral breast	<1%	83%	62%

[a]Mavaddat, N. et al. 2013. *J. Natl. Cancer Inst.*, 105:812–822.

cancer, neither mutation guarantees the development of cancer. Other mutations and, perhaps, specific nongenetic events must also occur for cancer to develop. Stated another way, a woman with one of these mutations has about a 40% of *not* experiencing breast cancer, a roughly 40 to 84% chance of *not* experiencing ovarian cancer, and a roughly 17 to 38% chance of *not* having a second breast cancer in the healthy breast after the other breast has become diseased. The involvement of other genes and, perhaps, of nongenetic factors is a principal reason why cancer cell genomes have been so aggressively investigated. One outcome of this avenue of investigation for breast and ovarian cancer is that genetic testing is now available for more than two dozen other genes whose mutations make small but meaningful contributions to the overall risk of breast and ovarian cancer development.

C.4 Cancer Cell Genome Sequencing and Improvements in Therapy

With continuous advances improving the accuracy, reducing the cost, and dramatically increasing the speed of genome sequencing, several major studies have sequenced the genomes of multiple types of cancer cells and identified the mutations present in each of them. Collectively, these studies have sequenced the genomes of several thousand malignant tumors of more than two dozen kinds of cancer.

Major goals of these studies are to discover the identity of mutated genes, the frequency of individual gene mutations, and the driver mutations likely to be of significance to the disease process, separating them from the "passenger" mutations that do not make a significant contribution to cancer development and proliferation (see hallmark 10 of the hallmarks of cancer cells listed earlier in this chapter). For example, one large study in 2013 sequenced the genomes of 3,281 tumors from 12 major cancer types. The study identified more than 617,000 somatic mutations in the tumors examined. The number of mutations varied widely across the tumor types. On average, each tumor had two to six mutations, although some had many more than that. The relatively low average number of mutations suggests that the number of driver mutations is relatively small. By comparing the genomes of sequenced tumors and taking into account known gene functions, the study identified 127 driver mutations that appear to play a significant role in the development of one or more tumor types.

Of these 127 significant driver mutations, the most commonly mutated gene in cancer cells was found to be *TP53*. Approximately 42% of all tumors studied carried a *TP53* mutation. Given the dual functions of TP53 protein in pausing the cell cycle for DNA damage repair and the role of TP53 in initiating apoptosis in heavily damaged cells, it makes sense that a mutation of *TP53* would frequently play an important role in cancer development. The *KRAS* gene and a second gene known as *PTEN* are commonly mutated in some, but not all, tumor types studied. *KRAS* mutation permits excessive cell proliferation, as described above for colorectal cancer. *PTEN* produces a protein product that normally acts similarly to TP53. It helps regulate cell cycle progression and also participates in apoptosis. Mutations of numerous other genes were found to be more or less common in individual types of tumors. This and other studies like it make three features of cancer mutations clear: (1) no two tumors of the same type have exactly the same profile of mutations, (2) some mutations are common to multiple types of cancer, and (3) specific types of cancer often, but not always, contain certain mutations.

The Cancer Genome Atlas

A comprehensive approach to cancer genome sequencing has emerged in recent years as part of an international effort to understand the genetic basis of cancer. This program, called the Cancer Genome Atlas (TCGA) is compiling genome sequence and analysis of somatic genetic mutations in thousands of tumors of many types, with the goals of achieving a complete understanding of cancer genetic abnormalities, identifying different categories of cancer occurring within a single organ or tissue, and helping to develop more effective detection and treatment options. The 2013 study described above is part of TCGA.

Pancreatic cancer is among the most lethal of all malignancies. In 2015, researchers participating in TCGA accomplished the complete genome sequencing analysis of 100 patients with pancreatic cancer. Genomes from pancreatic tumor cells and normal cells from the same patients were sequenced to fully identify mutations present in cancer cells. Chromosome rearrangements were common in cancer cells, and mutations of several genes, including *TP53, BRCA1*, and *BRCA2*, were frequently detected. Based on the complete set of gene mutations and chromosome rearrangements, the researchers were able to classify the pancreatic cancers examined into four subtypes. Each subtype had its own set of commonly occurring mutations and chromosome rearrangements, although there was some overlap of mutations in various subtypes. One of the subtypes, called "unstable," had an array of mutations that suggested the disease might be responsive to a particular type of chemotherapy. Of five patients with the unstable type of pancreatic cancer who received this chemotherapy, four showed substantial responsiveness to the treatment.

Epigenetic Irregularities

Other recent genomic research on cancer has focused on epigenetic dysregulation and the role it plays in the development and proliferation of cancers, especially hematologic cancers (as described in Section C.2). The largest of these studies to date found that the integrity of epigenetic processes is disrupted in cancer in the two ways. First, epigenetic regulation can be abnormal, and second, mutation of epigenetic readers, writers, and erasers can alter epigenetic patterns in cells, leading to irregularities of gene expression. Mutations affecting methylases and demethylases, for example, can lead to alterations of normal methylation patterns of the genome in cancer cells.

Several studies identify global hypomethylation as a cause of genome instability, including chromosome deletions and rearrangements. The studies also find a significant degree of hypomethylation of microRNA (miRNA) genes. In addition, studies find that hypermethylation in cancer appears to play an important role in silencing tumor suppressor genes, particularly by hypermethylating CpG islands in promoters. Examples of cancer hypermethylation have been identified in tumor suppressor genes such as *RB1, BRCA1,* and *MutL*.

Targeted Cancer Therapy

The 2015 study of pancreatic cancer genomics adds to a growing list of cancers that can be classified by their patterns of mutations. This information can then be used to target the cancer with specific kinds of chemotherapy. The first successful example of the use of chemotherapy to target the specific malfunction in a cancer was for chronic myelogenous leukemia (CML).

Recall that CML is caused by a chromosome translocation that forms a fusion *c-ABL–BCR* gene. The resulting c-ABL–BCR chimeric protein continuously activates cell proliferation. The problem with the chimeric protein is that it is always in an active state and it cannot be inactivated. In the late 1990s, researchers looking for chemicals that might be able to block the continuous activation of c-ABL–BCR tried a drug named imatinib and found that it bound to c-ABL–BCR in a manner that could inhibit the protein from activating cell proliferation. Under the trade name Gleevec, the drug was initially administered to 54 CML patients in the early 2000s, and the cancer almost or completely vanished in 53 of the 54 patients. Gleevec has now been used for more than 15 years and has proven to be a highly effective targeted treatment for CML. Similar kinds of success are now achieved with targeted cancer chemotherapy in some lung cancers, melanoma skin cancers, colon cancers, and breast cancers. The targeted cancers carry mutations of specific genes, making them responsive to targeted cancer therapy by chemical treatment.

Most recently, targeted cancer therapy has turned in a new direction, using genetically modified cells from a cancer patients own immune system to attack cancer cells that otherwise evade immune system detection. A study published in 2015 reported the results of treating patients diagnosed with terminal acute lymphoblastic leukemia (ALL) and non-Hodgkins lymphoma. Each of the patients in the study had been nonresponsive to other chemotherapy approaches or had a relapse of cancer. Life expectancy under either circumstance is a few months.

Researchers first isolated a type of immune system cell called T cells from each patient. T cells normally carry molecules on their surfaces that target specific proteins on foreign cells and destroy those foreign cells. The isolated T cells were then genetically modified with a chimeric antigen receptor (CAR), a protein that allows modified T-cells to target leukemia cells with the antigen CD-19 on the surface. The modified T cells were grown in the laboratory. The modified T-cells, called CAR-T cells, and injected back into the patient, where they attack and destroy cells with the CD-19 antigen.

The preliminary results of this targeted cancer therapy were very encouraging. Of 29 ALL patients, 27 were free of all traces of cancer following treatment. Additional studies were undertaken and a total of 63 children with treatment-resistant ALL or ALL that had relapsed were treated with the CAR-T therapy. Fifty-two of the 63 children (83%) had cancer remission within three months—a high rate, given that these cases are usually quickly fatal. In August 2017 the U.S. Food and Drug administration approved this CAR-T cell therapy for the treatment of ALL in patients up to age 25 with treatment-resistant ALL or ALL relapse. The therapy is named Kymriah and the genetically-modified CAR-T cells are made by Novartis.

Kymirah therapy can have severe potential side effects and it is very expensive. patients are treated just once with Kymirah therapy and the cost is approximately $475,000. The long-term survival of these patients remains to be determined. Despite these drawbacks, targeted cancer therapies made possible by cancer genome sequencing point to positive advances and new directions in the understanding and treatment of cancer. The development of such approaches is one of the goals of genome sequencing, which seeks to make personalized medicine a reality in the coming decades. Along with the apparent success of Keytruda and other drugs that improve patients' immune response to cancer indicates that continued pursuit of immune system stimulation may offer new avenues of cancer treatment.

Other new additions to the anticancer arsenal of drugs are those that aim at counteracting mutations affecting cancer cell epigenetics. To date, epigenetic therapies have been limited to the use of DNA methyltransferase inhibitors and histone deacetylase inhibitors. The U.S. Food and Drug Administration has recently approved drugs in both categories for use in treating T-cell lymphoma and multiple myeloma.

PROBLEMS

Mastering Genetics Visit for instructor-assigned tutorials and problems.

For answers to selected even-numbered problems, see Appendix: Answers.

1. Identify the normal functions of the following genes whose mutations are associated with the development of cancer.
   a. *RB1* (retinoblastoma)
   b. *c-MYC* (Burkitt's lymphoma)
   c. *p53* (Li–Fraumeni syndrome)
   d. *APC* (familial adenomatous polyposis)
   e. Which of these genes would you classify as a proto-oncogene and which as a tumor suppressor gene? Explain your categorization for each gene.

2. A tumor is a growing mass of abnormal cells.

   a. Describe the difference between a benign tumor and a malignant tumor.

   b. Give an example from this chapter of a benign tumor that becomes a malignant tumor.

   c. What must happen for a benign tumor to become malignant?

3. For the retinal cancer retinoblastoma, the inheritance of one mutated copy of *RB1* from one of the parents is often referred to as a mutation that produces a "dominant predisposition to cancer." This means that the first mutation does not produce cancer but makes it very likely that cancer will develop.

   a. Define the "two-hit hypothesis" for retinoblastoma.

   b. Explain why cancer is almost certain to develop with the inheritance of one mutated copy of *RB1*.

   c. Using $RB1^+$ for the normal wild-type allele and $RB1^-$ for the mutant allele, identify the genotype of a cell in a retinoblastoma tumor.

   d. What is the genotype of a normal cell in the retina in a person who has sporadic retinoblastoma? What is the normal cell genotype if the person has hereditary retinoblastoma? Explain the reason for the difference between the genotypes.

4. Explain the following processes involving chromosome mutations and cancer development.

   a. How the chromosome mutation producing the Philadelphia chromosome leads to CML.

   b. How the chromosome mutation producing Burkitt's lymphoma generates the disease.

5. In March 2011 an earthquake measuring approximately 9.0 on the Richter scale struck Fukushima, Japan. Several nuclear reactors at the Fukushima Daichii nuclear plant were damaged, and nuclear core meltdown occurred. A massive release of radiation accompanied damage to the plant, and 5 years later the incidence of thyroid cancer in children exposed to the radiation was determined to be well over 100 times more frequent than expected without radiation exposure. DNA damage and mutations resulting from radiation exposure are suspected of causing this increased cancer rate.

   a. What gene discussed in this chapter might be responsible for pausing the cell cycle of dividing cells long enough for radiation-induced damage to be repaired in cells?

   b. Do you think it is possible that significant increases in the incidence of other types of cancer will occur in the future among people who were exposed to the Fukushima radiation? Why?

6. Radiation is frequently used as part of the treatment of cancer. The radiation works by damaging DNA and components of the cell.

   a. How can radiation treatment control or cure cancer?

   b. Is there a risk of damage to noncancer cells?

   c. Under what circumstances do you think radiation treatment is a good choice to treat cancer?

7. Based on what you read in this chapter

   a. Can a tumor arise from a single mutated cell? Are all the cells in a tumor identical?

   b. Why do most cancers require the mutation of multiple genes?

8. The inheritance of certain mutations of *BRCA1* can make it much more likely that a woman will develop breast or ovarian cancer in her lifetime.

   a. Can you say with certainty that a woman inheriting a mutation of *BRCA1* will definitely develop breast or ovarian cancer in her lifetime? Why or why not?

   b. In addition to inheriting a *BRCA1* mutation, what else must happen for a woman to develop breast or ovarian cancer?

9. Go to the website http://www.cancer.gov and scroll down to the box labeled "Find a Cancer Type." Select "B" and then select "Breast Cancer." Scroll down to "Causes and Prevention" and then select "BRCA1 and BRCA2: Cancer Risk and Genetic Testing." Use the information on this page to answer the following questions.

   a. What are the approximate percentage increases in risk of having breast cancer and of having ovarian cancer for women inheriting harmful mutations of *BRCA1* and *BRCA2* compared with the risks in the general population?

   b. What features of family history increase the likelihood that a woman will have a harmful mutation of *BRCA1* or *BRCA2*?

   c. With regard to the results of genetic testing for *BRCA1* and *BRCA2* mutations, what is meant by a "positive result"?

   d. Are there measures a woman with a positive result can take to lessen her chances of developing cancer or to catch a cancer early in its development?

   e. As a special project, instead of selecting "Breast Cancer" from the list of types of cancer select another cancer you would like to know more about and produce a short summary of what you find.

10. What kind of information will be made available by the Cancer Genome Atlas (TCGA)? What sort of role do you think TCGA information will play in cancer diagnosis and cancer treatment in the future?

11. Go to the website http://www.ncbi.nlm.nih.gov/omim and enter "Lynch syndrome" in the Search box at the top of the page. From the list of options given, select "#120435—Lynch Syndrome." Use the information you retrieve to answer the following questions.

   a. There are two types of Lynch syndrome, what are they?

   b. What genes are most commonly mutated in Lynch syndrome?

   c. Provide a brief summary of the normal functions of the protein products of these genes.

   d. What are the approximate rates of cancer that develop in people carrying a mutation of one of these genes?

12. Genetic counseling has not been discussed in this chapter, but it is a service provided by trained professional counselors who also have detailed knowledge of medical genetics, as described in Application Chapter A. Genetic counselors provide details about gene mutations and have knowledge of most of the details of diseases associated with genetic abnormalities. With regard to genetic testing to identify one's personal risk of cancer, what are the three or four topics you think are most important to be able to discuss with a genetic counselor?

15 Recombinant DNA Technology and Its Applications

CHAPTER OUTLINE

15.1 Specific DNA Sequences Are Identified and Manipulated Using Recombinant DNA Technology

15.2 Introducing Foreign Genes into Genomes Creates Transgenic Organisms

15.3 Gene Therapy Uses Recombinant DNA Technology

15.4 Cloning of Plants and Animals Produces Genetically Identical Individuals

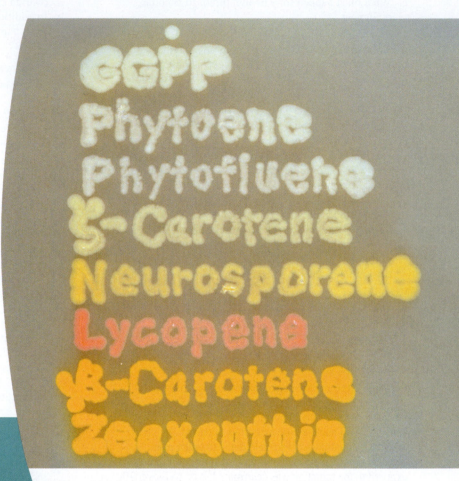

ESSENTIAL IDEAS

▌ DNA can be amplified by either molecular cloning or the polymerase chain reaction.

▌ In molecular cloning, DNA fragments are inserted into a cloning vector, which in turn is replicated in a live host.

▌ Libraries are collections of clones of DNA fragments, derived from the DNA or mRNA isolated from cells or an organism.

▌ Transgenic organisms are created by harnessing biological vectors to introduce genes into organisms.

▌ Recombinant DNA technology in humans is a pathway to the development of gene therapy.

▌ Cloning of plants and animals produces genetically identical individuals.

The writing in this image consists of transgenic *E. coli* expressing the genes for the carotenoid biosynthetic pathway, derived from plants. Carotenoid pigments, responsible for the red and orange colors of tomatoes, peppers, and oranges, act as a buffer system to absorb excess electrons and radicals produced during photosynthesis.

The advent of recombinant DNA technology for recombining, copying, and analyzing genetic sequences opened the way to studying gene function at the molecular level. This aspect of genetic exploration began with a set of basic strategies for the in vitro manipulation of DNA and for identifying the sequence of any given gene. The next step after that achievement was to invent methods for the precise manipulation of gene action in living organisms.

One of the central technical developments propelling that latter advance was development of the ability to create *transgenic organisms*—organisms that have had genes from other organisms inserted into their genomes. The methodology, now routine in genetic analysis, can be adapted to an almost limitless number of experimental approaches. It is a powerful tool for manipulating the activity of specific genes, observing the resultant phenotypes, and in this way acquiring new insight into biological processes.

Collectively, the techniques of recombinant DNA technology have permitted the sequencing of the entire genomes of many species, including our own, providing an unprecedented view of life. Increasingly sophisticated techniques have enabled both in vitro and in vivo manipulation of DNA sequences, shedding light on the molecular basis for development and physiology and for genetic variation both within and between species. Recently, genome-editing techniques have transformed both the study of gene function and the development of applications for specific medical, agricultural, or industrial purposes. If used wisely, this knowledge can be applied to better the human condition as well as the condition of the planet.

In this chapter, we discuss these applications of recombinant DNA technology while focusing on the methods used to create transgenic organisms and manipulate gene activity. These discussions furnish the nuts-and-bolts details of how reverse genetics is accomplished in different model organisms.

15.1 Specific DNA Sequences Are Identified and Manipulated Using Recombinant DNA Technology

Recombinant DNA technology is the set of techniques developed for amplifying, maintaining, and manipulating specific DNA sequences in vitro and also in vivo. This technology, which is based on advances in microbiology—particularly in understanding the life cycles of bacteria and their viruses, the bacteriophages—has revolutionized the study of genetics. With the ultimate goal of studying specific genes and their functions, biologists use recombinant DNA techniques to (1) fragment DNA into easily managed pieces and then separate and purify these fragments; (2) create many copies of DNA molecules of identical sequence; (3) combine DNA fragments to construct chimeric, or

recombinant, DNA molecules; (4) determine the exact sequence of specific DNA molecules; (5) identify fragments of DNA containing complementary sequences; (6) introduce specific DNA molecules into living organisms; (7) precisely edit the genomes of organisms; and (8) assay the phenotypic effects of the genetic changes.

The major challenges of recombinant DNA technology are the identification of specific DNA sequences and their manipulation in vitro. To see these challenges in perspective, consider that each of your cells contains two copies each of 22 autosomes and 2 sex chromosomes. Collectively, a haploid set of 23 chromosomes contains 3 billion base pairs and carries some 20,400 or so genes. A typical gene encodes an mRNA transcript consisting of a few thousand bases, although the mRNA may be transcribed from a region that spans millions of base pairs. Molecular analysis of genes and of allelic variation is possible only by distinguishing a gene of interest from others in the genome.

Recombinant DNA technology allows researchers to divide the genome into smaller segments that can then be analyzed and reassembled to provide a molecular view of genes and the genome. In the following sections we survey the development of recombinant DNA technology tools and their application to identify specific DNA sequences. We begin with discoveries in the 1970s that have led to increasingly sophisticated methods for manipulating genomic sequences.

Restriction Enzymes

Restriction enzymes, which cut DNA at specific sequences, have become a basic tool of recombinant DNA technology. Each type of restriction enzyme recognizes a particular sequence at which it cuts both strands of the sugar-phosphate backbone of the DNA, cleaving the restriction sequence in the same way each time it is encountered. Restriction enzymes were originally discovered in bacterial cells, where they protect the bacteria from invasions of nucleic acids, such as the injected genomes of bacteriophages, by digesting foreign DNA. They were given the name *restriction enzymes* because they restrict the growth of the bacteriophages. Bacterial cells also contain **restriction–modification systems**, which modify the restriction sequences in the bacterial DNA by the addition of methyl groups and thus protect the bacteria's own DNA from being digested by endogenous restriction enzymes. Experimental Insight 15.1 explains how restriction enzymes and restriction-modification systems were identified and how they became an indispensable part of molecular biology.

Restriction enzymes are common in bacteria. The names given these enzymes are generally derived from the first letter of the bacterial genus and first two letters of the species moniker, followed by a Roman numeral. For example, *Eco*RI is derived from *Escherichia coli* (*E. coli*); the letter R denotes the strain from which the enzyme was

From Bacteriophage to Restriction Enzymes: Basic Research Spawned a Biological Revolution

Basic biological research aims to discover and understand phenomena from every part of the spectrum of life. Thousands of biologists engage in this research every day, and most have specialties that may seem obscure or trivial to nonscientists. Nevertheless, their discoveries can not only revolutionize research but affect how we view the world.

In the mid-1960s, Werner Arber was studying a bacterial phenomenon called *host-controlled restriction and modification*, which acts as a simple immune system for bacteria invaded by bacteriophages. He showed that *E. coli* produces two enzymes that affect the same short palindromic DNA sequence (meaning a sequence that has the same 5′-to-3′ base sequence in both of its antiparallel DNA strands). One enzyme, called a *restriction endonuclease*, cleaves DNA at that sequence, like a pair of molecular scissors. The second enzyme, called a *modification enzyme*, adds methyl groups (CH_3) to DNA, thereby preventing restriction endonucleases from binding to and cleaving the DNA.

In 1970, Hamilton Smith extended Arber's work by studying a restriction endonuclease from *Haemophilus influenzae*. Smith isolated the restriction endonuclease, now called *Hind*II, and determined that it cleaves at the sequence

$$5'-GTPyPuAC-3' \qquad 5'-GTPy \quad PuAC-3'$$
$$3'-CAPuPyTG-5' \rightarrow 3'-CAPu \quad PyTG-5'$$

*Hind*II cleaves both strands of its target sequence between the central purine (Pu = A or G) and pyrimidine (Py = T or C), leaving blunt ends on either side of the cut (blunt ends are discussed on page 559).

Smith's work on *Hind*II identified some important characteristics of restriction enzymes. First, *Hind*II cleaves foreign DNA into large fragments, but it does not affect *H. influenzae* DNA. This confirmed Arber's idea that bacterial DNA is protected from the action of the bacteria's own restriction enzymes.

Second, each resulting DNA fragment has the same three base pairs at its ends, indicating that cleavage occurs only at the target sequence. Smith also discovered that restriction enzymes cleave every copy they encounter of their target sequence.

In 1971, Daniel Nathans pioneered the use of restriction endonucleases to address genetic and genomic questions. Nathans used *Hind*II to digest the small genome of the Simian virus SV40 and found that 11 DNA fragments were formed. In 1973, Nathans digested SV40 with two newly discovered restriction endonucleases. He then used the three sets of restriction fragments to create the first *restriction map* of the SV40 genome, by determining the number of restriction sites for each enzyme and their order in the genome and assembling the information into a map (as demonstrated elsewhere in this chapter).

By the time Nathans completed his SV40 genome map, biologists were already looking for other restriction enzymes. Within 5 years, more than 100 more restriction enzymes were discovered. Many formed "sticky" ends on digested DNA (described on this page), and Paul Berg realized that DNA fragments from different organisms could be joined together if they had complementary sticky ends. This finding led to his creating the first recombinant DNA molecule, in 1975.

Arber, Smith, and Nathans shared the Nobel Prize in Physiology or Medicine in 1978 for their work on restriction enzymes, and Berg won the prize in 1980 for the development of recombinant DNA. Since then, restriction enzymes have become a ubiquitous tool in genetic and genomic research. Arber's initial study of an obscure event in bacteria had spawned a revolution as momentous as Watson and Crick's description of DNA structure or Mendel's description of the laws of heredity.

---

obtained (RY13), and the numeral (I) indicates it was the first enzyme identified. *Eco*RI recognizes the palindromic sequence

$$5'-GAATTC-3'$$
$$3'-CTTAAG-5'$$

Recall that a palindrome has the same 5′-to-3′ base sequence in both of its antiparallel DNA strands. Most restriction enzymes recognize palindromic sequences. *Eco*RI cuts the sugar-phosphate bond between the G and the adjacent A residues in both strands, and the staggered cut results in two products, each ending with a four-base, single-stranded sequence:

$$5'-G \quad AATTC-3'$$
$$3'-CTTAA \quad G-5'$$

The single-stranded segments at the ends of each *Eco*RI fragment are referred to as **sticky ends** because they can "stick" to a complementary base-pair sequence by hydrogen bonding. Production of sticky ends facilitates the combining of DNA fragments generated with restriction enzymes, and complementary base pairing plays a role in almost all recombinant DNA techniques. The principle is that if two DNA molecules produced by restriction enzyme digestion have complementary sticky ends, they can be combined by complementary base pairing.

Another enzyme, *Eco*RI methylase, protects the *E. coli* genome from being itself digested by the *Eco*RI endonuclease. *Eco*RI methylase does this by adding a methyl group to the A adjacent to the T in both strands of the DNA. This is the "modification" performed by the *Eco*RI restriction–modification system.

Hundreds of restriction enzymes have been isolated from bacteria and are commercially available. Although many restriction enzymes produce sticky ends, either with 5′ overhangs (as produced by *Eco*RI) or with 3′ overhangs, some restriction enzymes leave **blunt ends** that lack a single-stranded segment. Blunt-ended DNA molecules can also be recombined, by techniques discussed later in this chapter (see page 559).

Some restriction enzymes recognize 4-bp sequences, others recognize sequences of 5 bp or 6 or 8 bp. The length of the recognition sequence influences how frequently a given enzyme will cut DNA. If an organism had DNA consisting of 25% A, 25% T, 25% G, and 25% C and the bases were randomly distributed, then a restriction enzyme that had a 4-bp recognition sequence would be expected to cut the DNA once every 256 bp $\left(\frac{1}{4} \times \frac{1}{4} \times \frac{1}{4} \times \frac{1}{4} = \frac{1}{256}\right)$. Likewise, a restriction enzyme that recognized a 6-bp sequence would cut the DNA once every 4096 bp $\left(\frac{1}{4^6}\right)$ on average, and a restriction enzyme that recognized an 8-bp sequence would cut the DNA once every 65,536 bp $\left(\frac{1}{4^8}\right)$ on average. In reality, genomes of most organisms do not consist of equal amounts of each of the four bases. For example, most genomes of multicellular eukaryotes are AT-rich (that is, their genomes have a higher content of A and T than of G and C), and so restriction enzymes that recognize a GC-rich sequence would cut less frequently on average than would enzymes that recognize an AT-rich sequence.

Scientists use data from restriction experiments, including the number of restriction sites and the number of base pairs between the sites, to create maps of specific DNA sequences. These **restriction maps** provide a foundation for further manipulation of the DNA fragments—for example, by suggesting where to further subdivide cloned fragments in order to clone still smaller fragments in a process known as **subcloning**.

Let's use the genome of *E. coli* lambda phage in an example of the restriction mapping process. The DNA of the phage genome can be isolated by purifying the phage and removing its protein coat. If this is done gently, the isolated nucleic acid will be the entire lambda chromosome, which is a linear molecule 48,502 bp in length. Electrophoresis of the chromosome in an agarose gel containing a fluorescent stain for DNA would reveal a single fluorescent 48.5-kb band (first lane in **Figure 15.1**). If the purified lambda chromosome is first digested with *Apa*I, two fragments, one measuring 10.1 kb and the other 38.4 kb, are generated, indicating that *Apa*I must cut the genome once. This allows us to begin drawing the restriction map as shown below

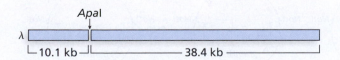

If we digest the purified lambda chromosome with *Xho*I, two fragments, one 33.5 kb and one 15 kb, are generated, indicating that *Xho*I must also cut the genome once:

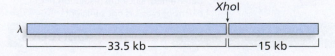

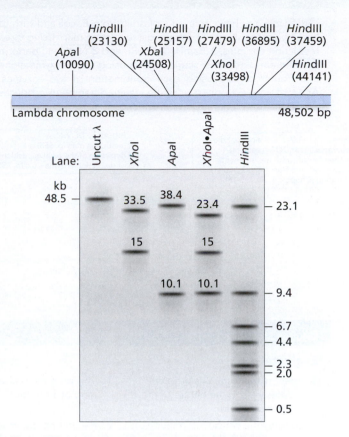

Figure 15.1   **Restriction mapping of lambda phage.**

However, two orientations are possible for the *Xho*I restriction map relative to the *Apa*I restriction map drawn above. It could also be drawn as shown below.

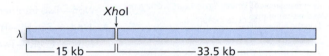

To determine which order is correct, we need to perform a double digest, in which both enzymes are used simultaneously to cut the lambda genome. This experiment generates three pieces: 10.1 kb, 15 kb, and 23.4 kb. Since the 15-kb *Xho*I fragment remained intact but the 33.5-kb *Xho*I fragment was cut into two fragments (10.1 kb and 23.4 kb) by *Apa*I, we conclude that the map must be:

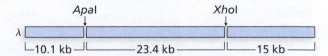

The other possible map can be eliminated as incorrect since it would generate fragments of 4.9, 10.1, and 33.5 kb:

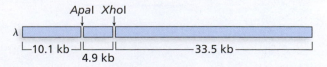

Genetic Analysis 15.1 provides additional practice at constructing a restriction map.

β-Carotene

PROBLEM You have isolated a plasmid from *E. coli* and wish to begin your analysis of it by making a restriction map. Using three restriction enzymes, **1** *Bam*HI, **2** *Eco*RI, and **3** *Not*I, you perform six different digestions: single digests using each enzyme alone and double digests using each combination of two enzymes. Agarose gel electrophoresis of the resulting fragments produces the results shown here. Draw a restriction map of the plasmid.

> **BREAK IT DOWN:** A plasmid is a circular DNA molecule (Chapter 6, p. 189). Cut once, it becomes linear; cut twice, it forms two fragments; and so on.

> **BREAK IT DOWN:** Gel electrophoresis separates linear DNA fragments by their length, with the fragments moving farthest from the origin of migration (Chapter 1, pp. 15-16).

> **BREAK IT DOWN:** A restriction map (p. 555) is a depiction of the relative positions of restriction-enzyme sites (p. 553).

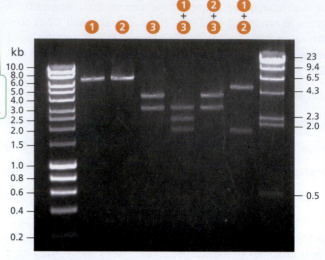

Solution Strategies	Solution Steps
Evaluate	
1. Identify the topic this problem addresses and the nature of the required answer.	1. This problem is about restriction mapping and asks you to construct a restriction map of a plasmid.
2. Identify the critical information given in the problem.	2. Electrophoresis results are given for three single digests and the three possible double-digest combinations.

Deduce

3. Identify the sizes of each of the fragments of the single digests, and determine how many times each enzyme cuts plasmid.

> TIP: Compare the sizes of fragments in the sample lanes with the sizes of the standards in the outer lanes.

4. Identify the sizes of each of the fragments of the double digests.

5. Compare single- and double-digest results for similarities and differences.

> TIP: In analyzing double digests, the relative position of restriction sites can be determined by observing which fragments remain intact and which are cut into smaller fragments.

> PITFALL: If two sites are very close to one another, there will be fewer fragments than expected in the double digest.

3. *Bam*HI—A single 7-kb fragment. Since plasmids are circular, *Bam*HI must cut the plasmid only once.
   *Eco*RI—A single 7-kb fragment. One site in the plasmid.
   *Not*I—Two fragments: 3 kb and 4 kb. *Not*I must cut the plasmid at two sites.

4. *Not*I + *Bam*HI—Three fragments: 3 kb, 2.3 kb, 1.7 kb.
   *Not*I + *Eco*RI—Two fragments: 4 kb, 3 kb.
   *Bam*HI + *Eco*RI—Two fragments: 5.3 kb, 1.7 kb.

5. *Not*I + *Bam*HI—Three fragments, with the 3-kb *Not*I fragment intact, suggesting the *Bam*HI site is within the 4-kb *Not*I fragment.
   *Not*I + *Eco*RI—Two fragments, with both the 4-kb and 3-kb *Not*I fragments intact, suggesting the *Eco*RI site is adjacent to one of the *Not*I sites.
   *Bam*HI + *Eco*RI—Two fragments, indicating the two sites are separated by 1.7 kb (or 5.3 kb the long way around the plasmid).

Solve

6. (a) Draw a restriction map with *Not*I sites. (b) Add in the *Bam*HI site. (c) Add in the *Eco*RI site.

> TIP: Drawing of the restriction map does not require the three enzymes to be examined in any particular order.

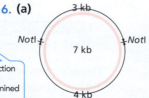

Digestion with *Bam*HI cuts the 4-kb *Not*I fragment into 2.3-kb and 1.7-kb fragments.

The *Eco*RI site must be adjacent to one of the *Not*I sites and is 1.7 kb from the *Bam*HI site. The relative order of the *Eco*RI and adjacent *Not*I sites cannot be determined, since the resolution of gel electrophoresis is not sufficient.

For more practice, see Problems 16, 18, 19, 20, and 21. Visit the Study Area to access study tools. **Mastering Genetics**

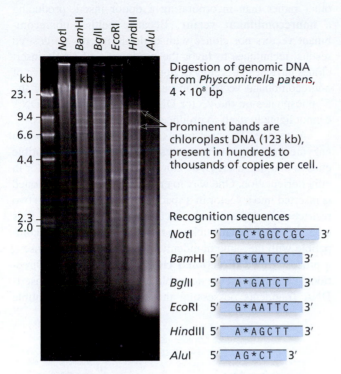

Figure 15.2 **Restriction-enzyme digestion of genomic DNA.**

Digestion of genomic DNA from *Physcomitrella patens*, 4×10^8 bp

Prominent bands are chloroplast DNA (123 kb), present in hundreds to thousands of copies per cell.

Recognition sequences

*Not*I   5′ GC*GGCCGC 3′

*Bam*HI 5′ G*GATCC 3′

*Bgl*II   5′ A*GATCT 3′

*Eco*RI 5′ G*AATTC 3′

*Hind*III 5′ A*AGCTT 3′

*Alu*I   5′ AG*CT 3′

To analyze DNA from organisms with large genomes, researchers must fragment the genomes into more manageable pieces. For example, the genome of the moss *Physcomitrella patens* consists of 400 million base pairs, so digestion with a restriction enzyme like *Eco*RI that cuts on average every 4096 bp produces approximately 100,000 different DNA fragments. When this digested DNA is electrophoresed through an agarose gel, the fragments making up the resulting "smear" seen in **Figure 15.2** range from greater than 20 kb down to smaller than 100 bp. The smeared appearance results because, although the enzyme cuts every 4096 bp on average, the distances between *Eco*RI sites will vary due to variation in the genome sequence, and the resolving power of agarose gel electrophoresis is not sufficient to separate all of the different-sized fragments into discrete bands. This lack of resolution is compounded with larger genomes, such as ours, where digestion with *Eco*RI produces approximately 730,000 pieces (3,000,000,000/4096).

Molecular Cloning

After a genome under study has been reduced to smaller pieces by restriction enzymes, the individual pieces must be reproduced in large amounts—generally, either by molecular cloning or by the polymerase chain reaction (PCR)—so that each of them can be analyzed in greater detail. Molecular cloning arose from discoveries in bacterial enzymology and utilizes bacteria and their plasmids or phages to amplify and propagate specific fragments of DNA.

In molecular cloning, isolated DNA fragments are inserted into a **vector,** a carrier fragment of DNA with

attributes that will allow amplification (replication) in a biological system. Then the recombinant DNA molecule is introduced into a biological system (a living organism) that amplifies the DNA, making many identical copies called **DNA clones.** Molecular cloning produces a large quantity of identical DNA molecules that can be analyzed by a variety of techniques, including restriction enzyme analysis and DNA sequencing.

Molecular cloning has three general steps:

1. The joining together of the cloning vector and a donor DNA fragment to produce a **recombinant DNA molecule**

2. Screening to select recombinant vectors containing copies of the DNA segment of interest

3. Amplification (cloning) of the recombinant DNA molecule in a biological system

In the rest of this section, we first describe how DNA fragments are combined in vitro, the attributes of some common cloning vectors, and the means of their amplification. We then describe how DNA libraries—collections of cloned DNA fragments, usually derived from a single DNA source—are constructed.

Creating Recombinant DNA Molecules One common method of producing recombinant DNA for cloning is to digest DNA from the donor source and DNA of the cloning vector with the same restriction enzyme. The resulting linear fragments from the two DNA sources can then be annealed at their complementary sticky ends. **Figure 15.3** illustrates restriction digestion by *Eco*RI of both the vector DNA—a plasmid, in this case—and DNA from the human genome. Mixing the two DNAs in a test tube allows the sticky ends to hybridize to one another by complementary base pairing, after which the remaining single-stranded nicks are sealed ("ligated") with DNA ligase (see Section 7.4), resulting in a recombinant DNA molecule. In this case, a recombinant plasmid containing human DNA is formed.

Although it is common to cut both source and vector DNA with the same enzyme, variations on this theme are frequently employed. For example, two different restriction enzymes that create complementary sticky ends are sometimes used. When different restriction enzymes are used to digest vector and donor DNA, complementary sticky ends are called **cohesive compatible ends.** For example, *Bam*HI recognizes the 6-bp sequence

$$5'-GGATCC-3'$$
$$3'-CCTAGG-5'$$

and leaves sticky ends

$$5'-G \qquad GATCC-3'$$
$$3'-CCTAG \qquad G-5'$$

*Sau*3A recognizes the 4-bp sequence

$$5'-GATC-3'$$
$$3'-CTAG-5'$$

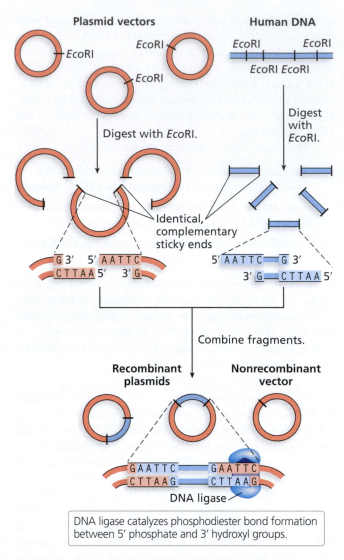

Figure 15.3 **Making recombinant DNA molecules.**

DNA ligase catalyzes phosphodiester bond formation between 5′ phosphate and 3′ hydroxyl groups.

and leaves sticky ends

$$5'-\text{N} \qquad\qquad \text{GATCN}-3'$$
$$3'-\text{NCTAG} \qquad\qquad \text{N}-5'$$

(where N represents any nucleotide). Since the sticky ends created by the two enzymes are the same ($5'-\text{GATC}-3'$), the ends of a *Bam*HI- and a *Sau*3A-digested fragment can combine to create recombinant DNA molecules. However, in this case, the resulting ligated products will often lack an intact *Bam*HI site, since the 5′ Ns from the *Sau*3A site may not be Gs.

Usually the goal of this process is to create recombinant DNA molecules in which a single piece of source DNA is combined with a single cloning vector molecule. However, because digested DNA from both sources is mixed together in a test tube, a variety of recombinant molecules may arise. For example, some recombinants may have a single donor-DNA insert, whereas others may have two or more donor fragments that join together and then insert into the vector. In addition, the sticky ends of vectors can rejoin each

other rather than incorporating a donor insert, producing a **nonrecombinant vector**. Because neither nonrecombinant vectors nor clones with multiple inserts are desired results, techniques to favor the production of single-insert clones have been developed. For example, the occurrence of nonrecombinant vectors can be reduced by removal of the 5′ phosphates on the vector DNA, so that the vector DNA cannot ligate to itself to produce nonrecombinant clones.

A feature of experiments using a single restriction enzyme or using two enzymes with cohesive compatible ends is that the insert DNA can be ligated into the vector in either orientation. One way to ensure that DNA to be cloned is inserted into a vector in a specific orientation is to use two restriction enzymes that each cut a different sequence, thus creating two different sticky ends on the vector that are compatible with the same nonidentical sticky ends of the insert, a process called **directional cloning** (**Figure 15.4**). Directional cloning has three desirable features. First, only insert-DNA fragments possessing the two different compatible

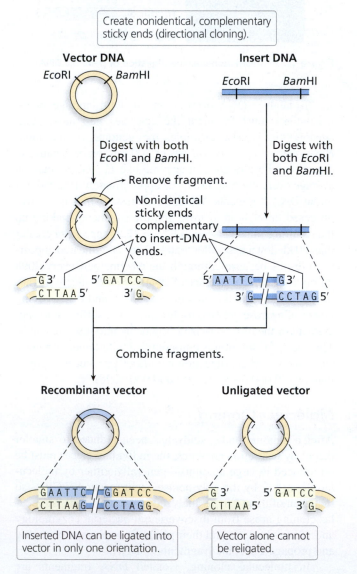

Figure 15.4 **Directional cloning of DNA molecules.**

ends will be efficiently inserted into the vector. Second, the inserted fragments are ligated in a particular orientation dictated by the cohesive compatible ends. And third, due to the incompatibility of the two ends of the digested vector DNA, the vector cannot re-ligate to itself, thus minimizing the creation of nonrecombinant vectors.

Although hundreds of restriction enzymes are commercially available, cohesive compatible ends are not always possible to produce at the positions necessary for constructing the desired recombinant DNA molecules. One approach to creating compatible ends in such a case is to generate blunt ends—ends without any overhang—that can then be ligated to form a recombinant molecule.

Some restriction enzymes naturally create blunt ends, but any restriction enzyme site can be converted into a blunt end. There are two general strategies (**Figure 15.5**). For example, DNA polymerase (see Section 7.2) can use a 5′ overhang as a template and add dNTPs to the recessed 3′ end until a blunt end has been produced. Alternatively, 3′ overhangs can be made blunt by a DNA exonuclease (see Section 7.4) that degrades only single-stranded DNA and "chews back" the 3′ overhang. Some procedures use shearing force rather than restriction enzymes (for example, by passing DNA through a fine needle), producing random DNA fragments whose ends can then be blunted by treatment with a DNA polymerase and exonuclease. Conversely, blunt ends can be converted into sticky ends by ligation of short oligonucleotides (nucleic acid molecules composed of a relatively small number of nucleotides) onto the blunt-ended DNA molecules. The oligonucleotides can be synthesized to have sequences for any restriction enzyme desired, thus adding any specific restriction site to the end of any DNA molecule. Oligonucleotides of this type are called **linkers**.

Plasmids as Cloning Vectors Plasmids are circular DNA molecules that replicate autonomously in bacteria and usually carry nonessential genes. The F-factor involved in *E. coli* conjugation (see Section 6.2) is a plasmid. Plasmids used as cloning vectors replicate independently of the bacterial chromosome and, unlike the F-factor, which can recombine into the *E. coli* chromosome, always remain separate from it. Most plasmids used as cloning vectors have been modified in the laboratory to possess several features that facilitate the production of recombinant DNA molecules (**Figure 15.6a**). For example, plasmids have an *origin of replication* (*ori*) that drives efficient replication of the plasmid within the bacterial host. They also contain a gene conferring a trait that permits bacteria harboring the plasmid to be selectively grown. Genes conferring resistance to antibiotics are commonly used as selectable markers.

Two types of plasmids, identified as pUC-based plasmids and pBR-based plasmids, are most frequently used in constructing recombinant plasmids capable of transforming competent bacteria. Both types have many different forms, developed through extensive genetic engineering in the

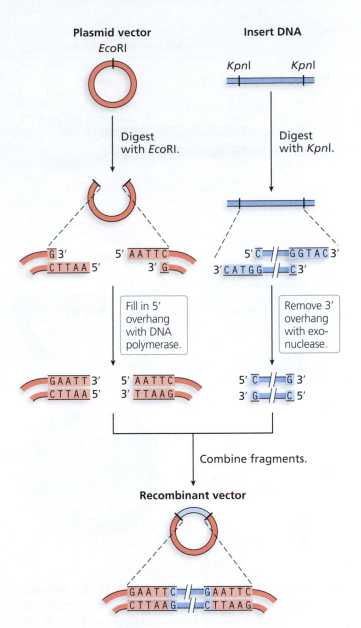

Figure 15.5 **Connecting blunt ends to create recombinant DNA molecules.**

laboratory. In these vectors, the *bla* gene for β-lactamase, which confers resistance to ampicillin, is often used as the selectable marker. The origin of replication was derived from a naturally occurring *E. coli* plasmid called the ColE1 plasmid. The ColE1 *ori* allows these plasmids to be maintained at a high copy number of 100–200 plasmids per cell.

Both pUC and pBR plasmids also contain a **multiple cloning site (MCS)** that has several different restriction enzyme sites into which DNA can be inserted. These restriction enzyme sites occur only within the MCS and nowhere else in the plasmid. In pUC-based plasmid cloning vectors, the MCS is embedded in the *lacZ* gene, which encodes β-galactosidase, an arrangement that provides a colorimetric assay for determining which bacteria harbor vectors with

(a)

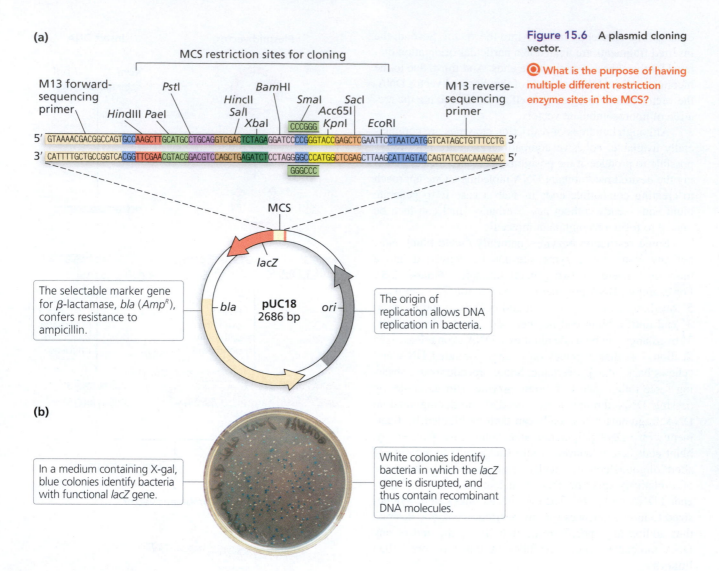

Figure 15.6   A plasmid cloning vector.

🔴 **What is the purpose of having multiple different restriction enzyme sites in the MCS?**

(b)

In a medium containing X-gal, blue colonies identify bacteria with functional *lacZ* gene.

White colonies identify bacteria in which the *lacZ* gene is disrupted, and thus contain recombinant DNA molecules.

an insertion of DNA into the MCS (**Figure 15.6b**). Although the normal substrate for β-galactosidase is lactose, the enzyme can also cleave lactose analogs, such as X-gal. When the colorless substrate X-gal is added to the growth medium, bacteria with a functional *lacZ* gene producing β-galactosidase will convert X-gal to a blue product (see Section 14.4). When a fragment of DNA is inserted into the MCS, the *lacZ* gene is disrupted and rendered nonfunctional. Bacteria then will appear as white colonies, whereas bacteria harboring a cloning vector that does not contain a fragment of DNA inserted in the MCS are blue. This difference allows rapid identification of colonies harboring vectors with inserts in the MCS. Thus, selection based on antibiotic resistance allows identification of bacteria that have been transformed, and *blue versus white* screening allows identification of bacteria harboring plasmid vectors with an insertion of recombinant DNA.

Amplifying Recombinant DNA Molecules For amplification—that is, replication of the recombinant DNA molecules in large numbers—the recombinant molecules are

introduced into *E. coli* by transformation, the same process described by Griffiths and by Avery, MacLeod, and McCarty in their early investigations of the hereditary function of DNA (**Figure 15.7**; also see Section 6.3). In modern laboratories, DNA is mixed with *E. coli* in a test tube. The bacteria are chemically treated with either divalent cations (such as Ca^{2+}) or an electrical shock to open pores in their membranes, thus making the bacteria "competent" to take up exogenous DNA by transformation. For safety purposes, the bacterial strains used in recombinant DNA experiments are chosen for characteristics that do not allow them to survive well outside of the laboratory.

The concentrations of DNA used to transform competent bacteria are those determined empirically to be concentrations at which individual bacterial cells are likely to take up no more than one DNA molecule. After transformation, the bacteria are allowed to recover for a short period of time and are then plated on growth medium that selects for cells containing the selectable marker gene, conferring resistance to an antibiotic, encoded on the DNA vector. When the transformed bacteria are plated on media containing the

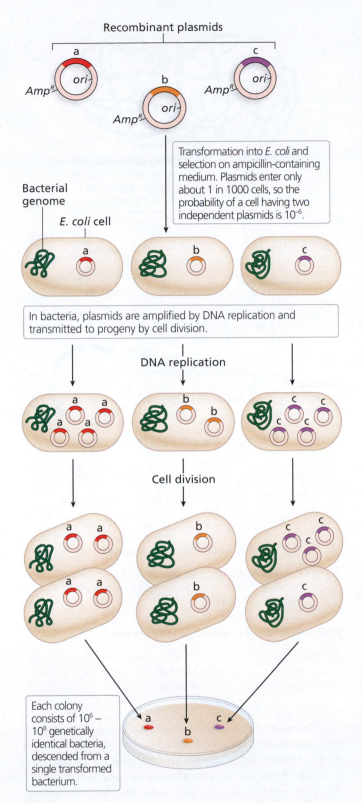

Figure 15.7 **Amplification of recombinant DNA molecules in bacteria.**

antibiotic, only those bacteria harboring vector DNA will survive.

Recombinant DNA molecules introduced into microbial cells are amplified by repeated cycles of DNA replication

within the bacteria. Since the recombinant vector has an origin of replication, it will amplify by autonomous replication using bacterial enzymes. After that, the next time the bacterium divides, each of its progeny will receive copies of the recombinant DNA molecule. Because a single bacterium with a recombinant DNA molecule can grow into a colony consisting of some 10^8 bacteria, each with multiple copies of the recombinant DNA molecule, billions of identical copies of DNA molecules are made.

The use of plasmid vectors for cloning large DNA fragments is limited, mainly because large plasmids (more than 20 kb) are not efficiently maintained in a high copy number. This limitation restricts the usefulness of plasmids in cloning eukaryotic genomic DNA. Eukaryotic genomes can be large (the human genome is 3×10^9 bp), with individual genes that are often much longer than 20 kb and therefore cannot be cloned in a single plasmid. To overcome these limitations of plasmids, vectors capable of handling larger clones have been developed. Two general approaches have been employed to propagate larger DNA fragments. In one approach, vectors based on the life cycle of bacteriophages accommodate larger fragments of DNA. The second approach harnesses chromosomal origins of replication to efficiently propagate larger recombinant DNA molecules. We look now more closely at this second approach.

Artificial Chromosomes Vectors called artificial chromosomes are frequently used to carry larger DNA fragments than can be carried in plasmids. These were developed through accumulated knowledge of how chromosomes propagate in bacteria.

Bacterial artificial chromosomes (BACs) have an insert-size capacity of 100–200 kb and are the preferred artificial chromosome for use as a cloning vector, largely because of the ease of using *E. coli* as a host. Like plasmids, BAC vectors contain an origin of replication, a selectable marker gene, and an MCS. However, the origin of replication in BAC vectors is derived from the F-factor plasmid. Unlike replication via the ColE1 origin, replication via the F-factor origin is strictly controlled, producing only one or two copies of the F-factor per cell. This difference allows large plasmids, such as BACs, to be maintained in the bacterial cell, making the F-factor origin a good choice for use in bacterial artificial chromosomes.

The utility of BAC cloning vectors becomes apparent when we consider the typical sizes of eukaryotic genes. For example, whereas individual globin genes in the β-globin locus are about 1.4 kb in length, the regulatory sequences controlling the cluster of globin genes span about 70 kb of genomic DNA. The entire β-globin locus can be contained in a single BAC but would not be contained in a single smaller plasmid clone. However, some eukaryotic genes, such as the gene for Duchenne's muscular dystrophy in humans, span more than a megabase and are unlikely to be contained within a single BAC clone.

DNA Libraries

A **DNA library** is a collection of cloned fragments of DNA, usually derived from the nucleic acids of a single source (recall our use of *library* in Section 14.2). DNA libraries come in two varieties: those derived from the genomic DNA of an organism are called **genomic libraries**, and those derived from mRNA are called **complementary DNA (cDNA) libraries**. Since the source of nucleic acids for each type of library differs, the kinds of sequences represented in each type also differ.

In theory, genomic libraries should contain all the sequences found in the genome of the source organism. For example, a human genomic library would contain all 3×10^9 bp in the haploid genome sequence. This would include the exons and introns of genes, the regulatory sequences controlling gene expression, the intergenic sequences (noncoding sequences between genes), and repetitive sequences (centromeres, telomeres, ribosomal DNA, transposons, retroelements, etc.). By contrast, cDNA libraries are derived from mRNA and thus represent the DNA sequences that are transcribed in the tissue from which the mRNA is derived. Since only a fraction of the genes present in the genome are likely to be expressed in any particular tissue, and even those are expressed at different levels, only a fraction of the genes are represented, and in different amounts, in any cDNA library. Thus, the number of times a specific sequence is represented in a library differs significantly between genomic and cDNA libraries.

Constructing Genomic Libraries Genomic libraries are collections of individual clones derived from the genomic DNA of an organism. To construct a genomic library, genomic DNA, usually from a single individual, is isolated and fragmented into smaller pieces that are then ligated into cloning vectors (**Figure 15.8**). The recombinant vectors are transformed into bacteria that grow into colonies that collectively contain clones representing the entire genome.

A genomic library contains each sequence in the genome at approximately the same frequency. Thus, sequences representing the exons and introns of genes, the regulatory sequences controlling their expression, and repetitive and intergenic sequences are all approximately equally represented in the genomic library. However, in practice, some sequences are not efficiently maintained in the host cells and will be underrepresented, so the entire genome is not fully represented in any typical genomic library. For example, repetitive DNA tends to be underrepresented due to its propensity to undergo intragenic recombination that results in deletion of DNA sequences within clones.

Three desirable attributes for a genomic library are that (1) the genomic clones are broadly representative of DNA of the entire genome, (2) the genomic clones are large enough to be useful for sequencing and subcloning, and (3) the genomic clones are roughly similar in size. Let's look at how these attributes are achieved.

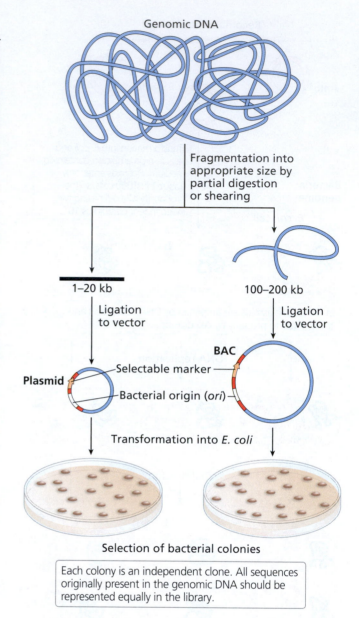

Genomic DNA

Fragmentation into appropriate size by partial digestion or shearing

1–20 kb

Ligation to vector

100–200 kb

Ligation to vector

BAC

Plasmid — Selectable marker — Bacterial origin (*ori*)

Transformation into *E. coli*

Selection of bacterial colonies

Each colony is an independent clone. All sequences originally present in the genomic DNA should be represented equally in the library.

Figure 15.8 **Construction of genomic libraries.**

How many BAC clones of 100 kb would be required to harbor the genome of *E. coli*? Or the genome of you? See back endpapers for genome sizes of model organisms.

To ensure that a genomic library is broadly representative, care must be taken to fragment it into random pieces of an appropriate and relatively uniform size for cloning into a vector. Random fragmentation is accomplished by two different methods. In one technique, the DNA is *partially digested* with an enzyme that cuts very frequently (e.g., a restriction enzyme that has a 4-bp recognition sequence). Partial digestion refers to the use of *less* restriction enzyme than would be needed to cut the DNA at every restriction sequence the enzyme recognizes, resulting in cuts at some of the restriction sequences but not all of them. Since a 4-bp recognition sequence should occur every 256 bp on average, partial digestion of DNA in which, on average, only one in 400 recognition sequences are cut, should result in DNA fragments of approximately 100 kb. Thus, partial digestion with an enzyme that otherwise cuts frequently will generate random, large genomic DNA fragments with sticky ends, as desired. The second technique for obtaining random fragmentation of DNA is random shearing of genomic DNA with subsequent enzymatic treatment to create blunt ends. In theory, either technique should provide random representation of genomic DNA from the entire genome.

The size of DNA clones in genomic libraries results from technical choices that seek a balance between, on the one hand, the difficulty of isolating, cloning, and propagating large molecules of DNA and, on the other hand, the greater number of smaller fragments that would have to be cloned to span the entire genome. As we discuss in Section 16.1, however, a set of genomic libraries that each have a different-sized insertion can be useful for determining the sequence of an entire genome.

Constructing cDNA Libraries The starting material for a cDNA library is mRNA, often derived from a specific tissue or cell type. Messenger RNA cannot be cloned directly because it is single stranded and is of course RNA, not DNA. Cloning of mRNA sequences can be accomplished by synthesizing a double-stranded cDNA copy of the mRNA and then ligating the cDNA into a vector. cDNA libraries are especially useful for working with eukaryotic organisms whose gene sequences are interrupted by many long introns.

The concept and development of cDNA libraries required advances in understanding the life cycle of retroviruses and the movement of retrotransposons (see Section 11.7). The availability of the enzyme **reverse transcriptase**, found in RNA-containing retroviruses, and of retrotransposons, which use single-stranded RNA as a template to produce a complementary strand of DNA, makes cloning from mRNA possible. Reverse transcriptase creates cDNA by first transcribing a single-stranded DNA molecule complementary to mRNA acting as a template. The poly-A tail added to RNA polymerase II transcripts in eukaryotes facilitates the construction of cDNA libraries from such mRNA, since the first strand of cDNA can be synthesized using an oligo dT primer (a single-stranded sequence of deoxythymine, dT; **Figure 15.9**). The mRNA template is then enzymatically removed, and the second strand of DNA is synthesized by DNA polymerase, using the first cDNA strand as a template.

The composition of a cDNA library reflects the level of expression of different genes active in the tissue from which the mRNA was extracted. Genes that are highly expressed are represented in the mRNA at a higher frequency than genes expressed at a lower level, and genes not expressed in the tissue of origin are not represented. In contrast to genomic libraries, which represent all genes at approximately equal frequency, the frequency with which any particular gene will be represented in a cDNA library is

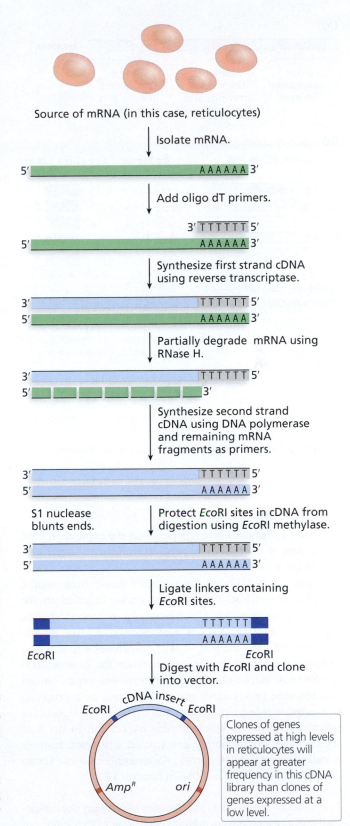

Source of mRNA (in this case, reticulocytes)

Isolate mRNA.

Add oligo dT primers.

Synthesize first strand cDNA using reverse transcriptase.

Partially degrade mRNA using RNase H.

Synthesize second strand cDNA using DNA polymerase and remaining mRNA fragments as primers.

S1 nuclease blunts ends.

Protect *Eco*RI sites in cDNA from digestion using *Eco*RI methylase.

Ligate linkers containing *Eco*RI sites.

*Eco*RI   *Eco*RI

Digest with *Eco*RI and clone into vector.

cDNA insert

*Eco*RI   *Eco*RI

Amp^R   ori

Clones of genes expressed at high levels in reticulocytes will appear at greater frequency in this cDNA library than clones of genes expressed at a low level.

Figure 15.9   Construction of cDNA libraries.

(a)

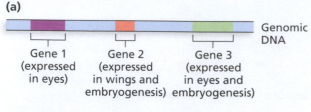

(b)

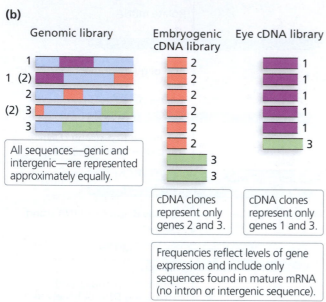

Figure 15.10 Content of genomic versus cDNA libraries.

🔎 **With respect to the three genes in this figure, what would be the composition of a cDNA library made from mRNA isolated from wing tissue?**

difficult to estimate, since it depends on the expression level of the gene in the mRNA population from which it was created (**Figure 15.10**).

Since cDNA libraries are usually made from mature cytoplasmic mRNA, the only sequences included in the cDNA clones are the 5′ untranslated region (5′-UTR), the exons, and the 3′-UTR (see Section 8.1 for discussion of UTRs and the poly-A tail); the clones will lack any intronic and intergenic sequences. Since the genetic code is universal, cDNA clones derived from one organism can be expressed in any other organism as long as appropriate transcriptional (e.g., promoter) and translational signals are inserted to promote efficient gene expression in the host organism. A cDNA library constructed with such features is called an *expression library*. An example of a use for an expression library is described in Section 14.2.

The Uses of Libraries DNA libraries have many uses, especially as a resource from which genomic or cDNA clones of specific genes can be identified and then employed in subsequent experiments. For example, clones from a library can be manipulated to create reporter genes or to produce novel alleles (e.g., chimeric genes) that can then be used in the creation of transgenic organisms (see Section 14.4). In addition,

library construction is the starting point for most protocols performing next-generation sequencing of the genomes or mRNA content of organisms, which we will explore in greater detail in Chapter 16.

Advances in Altering and Synthesizing DNA Molecules

Often, the wild-type version of a gene is the one that geneticists wish to express as a transgene. But we have seen that in some cases, it is desirable to express a modified version in which specific nucleotides have been changed. One reason it is sometimes desirable to alter the sequence of an encoded protein is to render the protein either more or less active. For example, changes in the identities of specific amino acids can sometimes cause an enzyme to be constitutively active or to be more stable at high or at low temperatures. A second reason to change the nucleotide sequence of a gene is to improve its expression in a species with a different codon bias than that of the species from which the gene was derived (a situation discussed further in Section 15.2).

In the past, making specific changes to a DNA sequence was a laborious process. However, technology for chemically synthesizing DNA molecules has improved significantly in recent years in terms of both accuracy and cost, making the synthesis of any DNA sequence feasible. Today oligonucleotides tens to hundreds of bases in length are inexpensive to construct via PCR-based approaches. More recently, chemical syntheses of DNA molecules up to 50,000 bases in length have become feasible. Geneticists are able to design a DNA molecule from scratch and synthesize it for subsequent use in living organisms. This approach is useful when multiple changes would otherwise be required in a DNA molecule before its introduction into a transgenic organism. As with sequencing technologies, advances in chemical synthesis of large DNA molecules have the potential to transform biotechnology and biological research. In 2008, the entire 582,970-bp genome of *Mycoplasma genitalium* was chemically synthesized in vitro and propagated in *Saccharomyces cerevisiae*. The synthetic genome was then transplanted into a receptive *Mycoplasma* cytoplasm, generating a cell that would use the genetic information contained on the synthetic chromosome. In 2017, all 16 chromosomes of the *S. cerevisiae* genome were chemically synthesized and introduced back into yeast where the endogenous chromosomes were subsequently selectively eliminated, with the resulting synthetic yeast strain phenotyically normal. The synthetic yeast genome included several modifications including deletions, insertions, and base substitutions facilitating investigations of chromosome structure, stability, and evolution. The ability to synthesize genome-sized nucleic acid molecules could revolutionize experimental biology; for example, synthesis of genomic segments of extinct animals, such as the wooly mammoth, has been proposed to understand more about this species.

The recombinant DNA technology described in this section, combined with the techniques of DNA sequencing, and the polymerase chain reaction (PCR) described in Section 7.5, enable sophisticated in vitro manipulation and characterization of DNA molecules. However, biology is "in vivo," and the questions geneticists ask pertain to how genes behave in the context of the living cell or organism. Thus, techniques have been developed to introduce in vitro–constructed DNA molecules into living organisms.

15.2 Introducing Foreign Genes into Genomes Creates Transgenic Organisms

The introduction of a gene from one organism into the genome of another organism creates a **transgenic organism**. The introduced gene is known as a **transgene**; if the introduced gene comes from a different species, it is a heterologous transgene. The two principal challenges to creating a transgenic organism are (1) the need to introduce DNA into a cell in such a way that the DNA integrates into the genome and (2) the need to provide appropriate regulatory sequences so that the transgene will be properly expressed.

Because cells of different organisms differ in the ability to import DNA from their environment and in their propensity to recombine exogenous DNA into their genomes, protocols for introducing transgenes vary according to the organism. Nevertheless, the production of transgenic organisms is surprisingly straightforward, perhaps because naturally occurring mechanisms have evolved in most lineages of life for the uptake or delivery of DNA. Many organisms or cells will absorb DNA from their environment, and once inside the cell, one potential fate of the DNA is to recombine into the genome. Recall our discussion of certain naturally occurring versions of this process, including gene transfer by Hfr donors into recipient bacteria, transduction of genes from a bacterial donor to a recipient, and gene transfer between and within species by transformation (see Chapter 6).

Although the designing of transgenes utilizes techniques of recombinant DNA technology, the expression of transgenes is like the expression of any gene: The gene sequence must first be transcribed into mRNA and then translated into a polypeptide. The universality of the genetic code permits the translation of coding sequences even when they have been transferred between the most distantly related organisms—even when one of them is bacterial or archaeal and the other a eukaryote. However, regulatory sequences and their molecular interactions with transcriptional and translational machinery vary significantly among organisms, and they are not interchangeable between distantly related organisms. Thus, for transgenes to be efficiently expressed, they must be combined with host regulatory sequences.

In contrast to situations where exogenous DNA is introduced into the genome of an organism, creating a transgene, the use of CRISPR–Cas9–mediated genome editing (see Section 14.3) often does not involve the introduction of exogenous DNA. In cases where no exogenous DNA has been added, the United States Agriculture Department has deemed the resulting organisms to be nontransgenic. The discussions that follow in this section primarily describe methods to construct transgenic organisms, but they will also at times refer to CRISPR–Cas9–mediated genome editing.

Expression of Heterologous Genes in Bacterial and Fungal Hosts

Bacterial transformation by a recombinant plasmid is the primary method for generating transgenic bacteria. As seen in Section 15.1, foreign DNA can be introduced into bacteria, such as *E. coli,* using a plasmid vector possessing sequences required for DNA replication and also possessing a selectable marker, such as antibiotic resistance, to facilitate the identification of transformants.

Expression vectors are vectors that have been furnished with sequences capable of directing efficient transcription and translation of transgenes (**Figure 15.11**). For transgenes to be properly expressed in *E. coli*, regulatory sequences compatible with the transcription and translation machinery in *E. coli* need to be present in the vector.

E. coli **expression vector**

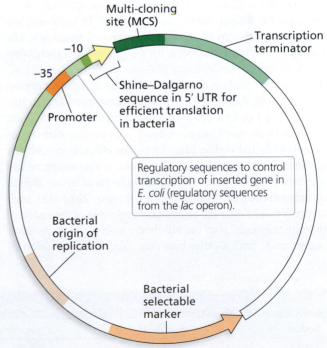

Figure 15.11 **Typical features of expression vectors for *E. coli.***

🔴 How would you design a eukaryotic expression vector—that is, what regulatory elements would you need to include?

Expression vectors for use in *E. coli* are constructed from plasmids that have been equipped with promoter sequences that bind RNA polymerase upstream of the multi-cloning site (MCS) of the plasmid. Recall that the MCS is a cluster of unique restriction sites into which the gene to be expressed is inserted in recombinant clones. Efficient translation of mRNA in *E. coli* also requires the presence of a Shine–Dalgarno sequence in the 5′ untranslated region of the mRNA, another feature that is built into *E. coli* expression vectors. In addition, since mRNA-splicing machinery does not exist in bacteria, eukaryotic transgenes must be free of introns if they are to be properly translated in bacteria. This requirement necessitates the use of cDNAs as eukaryotic transgenes in *E. coli* expression systems.

Expression of the heterologous gene carried by an expression vector can be either constitutive ("on" all the time) or regulated by the addition or removal of inducer compounds. An example of the latter approach is the use of the regulatory apparatus of the *lac* operon of *E. coli* to induce expression of transgenes: Fusion of the *lac* operator and CAP binding sites of the *lac* operon to the RNA polymerase binding site allows the transgene to be controlled in the same inducible manner as the genes of the *lac* operon (the *lac* operon is described in Section 12.2).

Two kinds of variation in the genetic mechanisms of living organisms can hamper the efficient production of functional transgenic products. The first complication affects the efficiency of translation. Although the universal genetic code does indeed allow the translation of heterologous transgenes, organisms vary in the degree to which they use specific codons when the genetic code contains more than one for a given amino acid or signal. In most species, synonymous codons are not used with equal frequency. For example, glycine is encoded by GGN, with N representing any nucleotide, but GGA and GGG are rarely used in *E. coli*, whereas these codons are commonly used in the other organisms listed in **Table 15.1**. The tRNAs corresponding to frequently used codons are expressed at higher levels than are the tRNAs for rarely used codons. This preferential use of codons is called **codon bias**. Thus, for efficient production of heterologous proteins in *E. coli*, the codon usage within the heterologous gene sequences may have to be altered to approximate the codon bias in *E. coli*. Note that such changes do not alter the amino acid sequence of the encoded protein; they only alter the efficiency with which translation occurs in *E. coli*. Codon bias can affect the expression of

heterologous transgenes in any case where genes are being transferred between distantly related species.

A second possible obstruction to the production of functional heterologous proteins in *E. coli* is presented by the posttranslational modifications many proteins must undergo to function. Posttranslational modifications of proteins differ between species, in particular between eukaryotes and bacteria. For example, carbohydrate and lipid groups are added to many kinds of eukaryotic proteins. In addition, the functions of proteins may be modified by phosphorylation, acetylation, or methylation of amino acid residues; other posttranslational polypeptide processing; and specific protein-folding activities. Most of these processes either do not occur in bacterial cells or they occur but with significant differences. In such cases, eukaryotic cells, such as yeast or cells in tissue culture, and eukaryotic expression vectors must be used. **Eukaryotic expression vectors** have the eukaryotic features analogous to the features found in bacterial expression vectors, including sequences for the regulation of transcription (such as a TATA box for binding of RNA polymerase II), enhancer sequences for qualitative and quantitative control of transcription, and polyadenylation and transcription-termination signals.

Production of Human Insulin in *E. coli*. A gene encoding insulin was among the first human genes to be expressed in *E. coli*, and human insulin was the first protein manufactured from recombinant DNA technology for therapeutic use in humans. Insulin, a protein hormone, regulates sugar metabolism in animals by stimulating liver and muscle cells to take in glucose, and fat cells to take in lipids, from the blood. Individuals who are unable to produce insulin, or whose cells cannot respond to it, have diabetes, an often debilitating disease that affects millions of people worldwide.

Insulin is cyclically produced in the pancreas by specialized cells in the islets of Langerhans and is released into circulating blood in response to the ingestion of sugar-containing carbohydrates. The pancreatic cells initially synthesize a 110–amino acid precursor protein called preproinsulin that is not secreted and does not have hormonal function until it is proteolytically processed. Twenty-four N-terminal amino acids—the "pre" amino acids of preproinsulin—are cleaved from the precursor to produce proinsulin, an event followed by the cleavage of an additional 35 amino acids—called the "pro" segment—from the middle

Table 15.1	Preference in Different Organisms for Specific Glycine Codons			
Codon	*E. coli*	*S. cerevisiae*	*H. sapiens*	*A. thaliana*
GGA	0%	23%	23%	37%
GGG	2%	12%	26%	15%
GGC	38%	20%	33%	14%
GGT	59%	45%	18%	34%

of the protein (Figure 9.17). Further cleavage generates two amino acid chains, called the A chain and the B chain, that are 21 and 30 amino acids, respectively, in length. The A chain is joined to the B chain by disulfide bonds between cysteine residues to produce insulin.

The amino acid sequence of insulin was determined by Fred Sanger in the early 1950s (**Figure 15.12**, ❶), but the human gene encoding insulin was not identified until the late 1970s. Even before the human insulin gene was cloned, however, molecular biologists began experiments

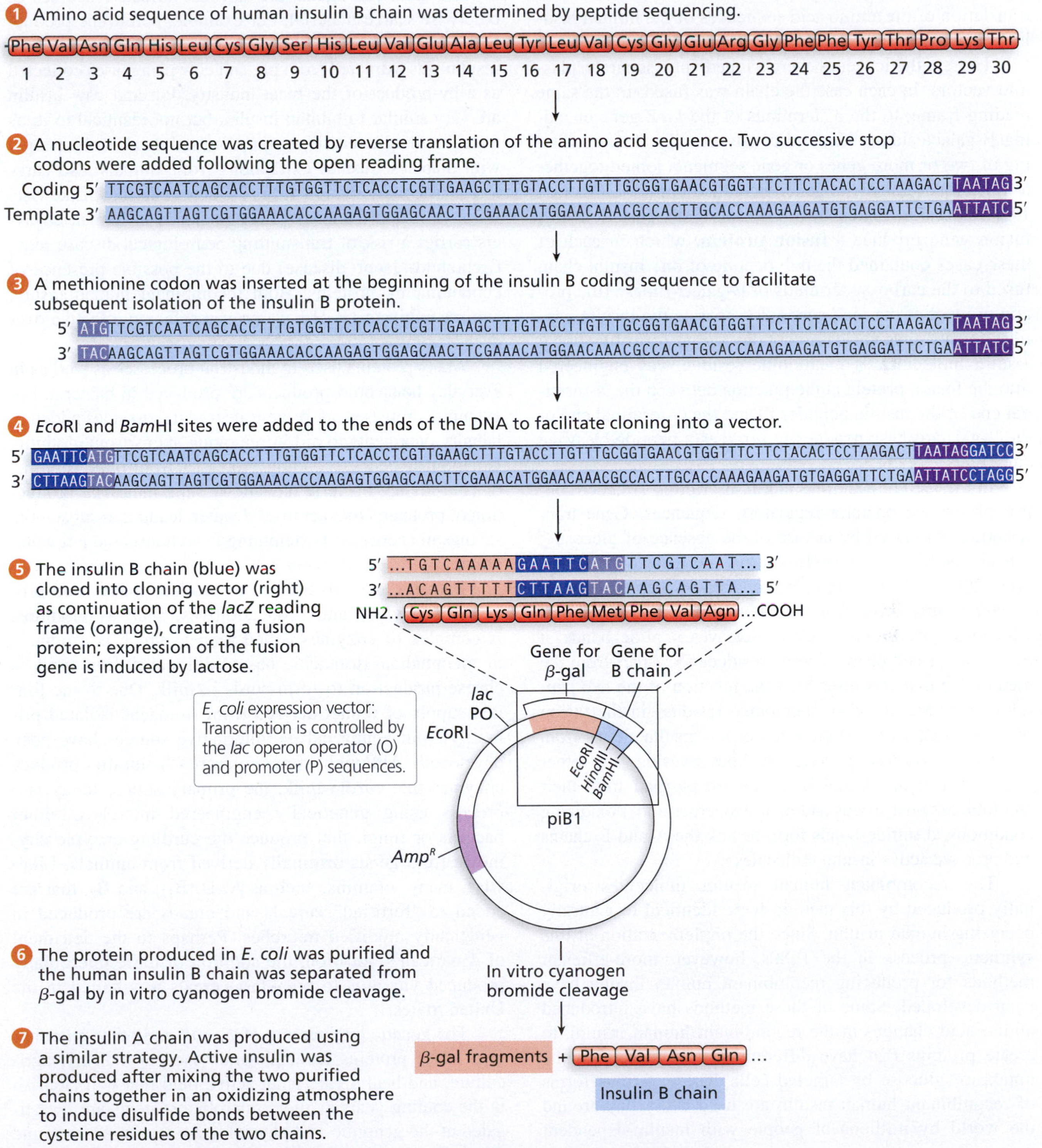

❶ Amino acid sequence of human insulin B chain was determined by peptide sequencing.

Phe Val Asn Gln His Leu Cys Gly Ser His Leu Val Glu Ala Leu Tyr Leu Val Cys Gly Glu Arg Gly Phe Phe Tyr Thr Pro Lys Thr
1   2   3   4   5   6   7   8   9 10 11 12 13 14 15 16 17 18 19 20 21 22 23 24 25 26 27 28 29 30

❷ A nucleotide sequence was created by reverse translation of the amino acid sequence. Two successive stop codons were added following the open reading frame.

Coding 5′ TTCGTCAATCAGCACCTTTGTGGTTCTCACCTCGTTGAAGCTTTGTACCTTGTTTGCGGTGAACGTGGTTTCTTCTACACTCCTAAGACTTAATAG 3′
Template 3′ AAGCAGTTAGTCGTGGAAACACCAAGAGTGGAGCAACTTCGAAACATGGAACAAACGCCACTTGCACCAAAGAAGATGTGAGGATTCTGAATTATC 5′

❸ A methionine codon was inserted at the beginning of the insulin B coding sequence to facilitate subsequent isolation of the insulin B protein.

5′ ATGTTCGTCAATCAGCACCTTTGTGGTTCTCACCTCGTTGAAGCTTTGTACCTTGTTTGCGGTGAACGTGGTTTCTTCTACACTCCTAAGACTTAATAG 3′
3′ TACAAGCAGTTAGTCGTGGAAACACCAAGAGTGGAGCAACTTCGAAACATGGAACAAACGCCACTTGCACCAAAGAAGATGTGAGGATTCTGAATTATC 5′

❹ EcoRI and BamHI sites were added to the ends of the DNA to facilitate cloning into a vector.

5′ GAATTCATGTTCGTCAATCAGCACCTTTGTGGTTCTCACCTCGTTGAAGCTTTGTACCTTGTTTGCGGTGAACGTGGTTTCTTCTACACTCCTAAGACTTAATAGGATCC 3′
3′ CTTAAGTACAAGCAGTTAGTCGTGGAAACACCAAGAGTGGAGCAACTTCGAAACATGGAACAAACGCCACTTGCACCAAAGAAGATGTGAGGATTCTGAATTATCCTAGG 5′

❺ The insulin B chain (blue) was cloned into cloning vector (right) as continuation of the *lacZ* reading frame (orange), creating a fusion protein; expression of the fusion gene is induced by lactose.

5′ ...TGTCAAAAAGAATTCATGTTCGTCAAT... 3′
3′ ...ACAGTTTTTCTTAAGTACAAGCAGTTA... 5′
NH2...Cys Gln Lys Gln Phe Met Phe Val Agn...COOH

E. coli expression vector: Transcription is controlled by the *lac* operon operator (O) and promoter (P) sequences.

Gene for β-gal   Gene for B chain
lac PO
EcoRI
EcoRI / HindIII / BamHI
piB1
Amp^R

❻ The protein produced in *E. coli* was purified and the human insulin B chain was separated from β-gal by in vitro cyanogen bromide cleavage.

In vitro cyanogen bromide cleavage

❼ The insulin A chain was produced using a similar strategy. Active insulin was produced after mixing the two purified chains together in an oxidizing atmosphere to induce disulfide bonds between the cysteine residues of the two chains.

β-gal fragments + Phe Val Asn Gln ...
Insulin B chain

Figure 15.12 Producing human insulin in *E. coli*. This strategy was used in the late 1970s by the City of Hope National Medical Center and the biotechnology company Genentech to produce human insulin in *E. coli*. The entire DNA fragment was chemically synthesized.

designed to produce human insulin in *E. coli* by constructing recombinant plasmids containing chemically synthesized DNA encoding human insulin. An experimental strategy called the two-chain method utilized two synthetic genes, one encoding the A chain and the other encoding the B chain. Each synthetic gene was constructed from oligonucleotides whose sequence was based on the reverse translation of the amino acid sequences of the human insulin gene chains ❷.

The synthetic genes were cloned into separate plasmid vectors. In each case the chain was fused, in the same reading frame, to the 3′ terminus of the *lacZ* gene encoding β-galactosidase. Genetic constructs like this, consisting of two or more genes or gene segments joined together to form a new, artificial gene, are called chimeric (Section 14.4) or **fusion genes**. Transcription and translation of a fusion gene produce a **fusion protein**, which in each of these cases contained the polypeptide of one insulin chain fused to the carboxyl terminus of β-galactosidase (the protein product of the *lacZ* gene). To separate the insulin peptides from β-galactosidase peptides and to form functional insulin molecules, a methionine residue was engineered into the fusion protein at the junction between the N-terminal end of the insulin peptides ❸ and the C-terminal end of the β-galactosidase peptides to serve as a peptide cleavage site ❹.

In the recombinant plasmid, transcription is under control of the *lac* operator regulatory sequences. Gene transcription is induced by lactose in the absence of glucose ❺ (see also Section 12.2). Under appropriate growth conditions, up to 20% of the total protein produced by the recombinant *E. coli* strains is the fusion protein. Treatment of proteins with cyanogen bromide (CNBr) cleaves peptide bonds at the carboxyl end of methionine residues ❻. Apart from the methionine that was inserted at the junction of the two peptides, there are no other methionine residues in the fusion protein, so CNBr treatment releases the insulin chains from the β-galactosidase peptides without causing any other breaks. When the A and B chains are purified from their recombinant host strains and mixed together under oxidizing conditions, disulfide bonds form to link the A and B chains and produce active insulin molecules ❼.

The recombinant human insulin molecules originally produced by this method were identical to naturally occurring human insulin. Since the implementation of this synthetic process in the 1980s, however, more-efficient methods for producing recombinant human insulin have been developed. Some of these methods have introduced amino acid changes in the recombinant human insulin, to create proteins that have different desired effects on the uptake of glucose by targeted cells. These various forms of recombinant human insulin are used every day around the world by millions of people with insulin-dependent diabetes.

The ease and economy of working with bacteria compared with eukaryotes have made it practical to produce many eukaryotic proteins in bacteria for medical, industrial, and agricultural applications. For example, in addition to human insulin, proteins such as human growth hormone (HGH) and erythropoetin (which induces red blood cell formation) are produced in bacterial systems. The recombinant systems used to produce these and many other pharmaceutical and industrial agents are safe and effective sources of otherwise scarce material. For example, before the production of human insulin by recombinant DNA technology, insulin was extracted from pig and cow pancreases collected as a by-product of the meat industry. Pig and cow insulin are very similar to human insulin, but not identical to it; as a result, allergic reactions compromised their use by people with diabetes. Insulin extractions from animals also carry a risk of contamination from the source tissues. Likewise, HGH extracted from the pituitary glands of human cadavers carries a risk of transmitting neurological disease (e.g., Creutzfeldt–Jacob disease) due to the possible presence of contaminating proteins. Both recombinant human insulin and recombinant HGH have proven safe and effective over decades of use.

Many proteins used in industrial processes as well as in everyday household products are produced in bacteria. For example, proteases are protein-degrading enzymes added to laundry detergents to aid in removing stains from clothing. Isolation of genes encoding proteases from psychrophilic, or cold-loving, bacteria has allowed the industrial production of proteases that act in cold water, leading to substantial savings in energy costs stemming from household hot water usage.

Bacteria are also utilized to produce many food-processing enzymes and food additives, such as vitamins. A complex of enzymes called rennet, which is produced in mammalian stomachs, has traditionally been used in cheese production to form curds in milk. Due to the limited supply of rennet derived from stomachs isolated primarily from young calves, alternative sources have been developed. Although some microbes naturally produce enzymes that curdle milk, the primary source today is a process using genetically engineered microbes, either bacteria or fungi, that produce the curdling enzyme chymosin from genes originally derived from animals. Likewise, many vitamins, such as A, D, B_{12}, and B_2, that are added to "fortified" cereals and breads are produced in genetically modified microbes. Perhaps to the detriment of American's nutrition, the addition of these microbially produced vitamins to breakfast cereals was halted in the United States.

The genetic engineering of *E. coli* and other microbes to produce proteins or compounds used in industry, agriculture, and health care is an active field that will flourish in the coming years as more microbial systems are investigated at the genomic and physiological levels. An example of the transfer of an entire biochemical pathway into *E. coli* to produce a medically important compound is described in Experimental Insight 15.2.

EXPERIMENTAL INSIGHT 15.2

Plant-Derived Antimalarial Drugs Produced in *E. coli*

The production of amorphadiene in *E. coli* exemplifies the use of genetic engineering to produce a high-value pharmaceutical product. Amorphadiene is the immediate precursor to artemisinin, a potent antimalarial drug. Artemisinin has been touted as the next-generation antimalarial drug because it is effective at treating multiple stages of malarial infection and exhibits no cross-resistance with existing antimalarial drugs, such as chloroquine and quinine. Chloroquine and quinine have been used to fight malarial infection for several decades, but their effectiveness is decreasing due to the evolution of resistant strains of *Plasmodium*, the malaria parasite.

OBSTACLES TO ARTEMISININ PRODUCTION

Like many modern drugs, artemisinin was originally discovered in plant extracts. Currently the drug is extracted and purified from the sweet wormwood plant, *Artemisia annua*. The logistics of growing *Artemisia* are limiting factors, however, and the cost of producing large amounts of artemisinin from its natural source is also prohibitive. Production of artemisinin in a fermentable biological system such as *E. coli* could increase drug supply, conserve natural resources, and dramatically lower production costs.

Artemisinin is a complex terpene molecule produced in several biosynthetic steps. All plants produce the precursors of the terpene pathway, isopentenyl pyrophosphate (IPP) and dimethylallyl pyrophosphate (DMAPP), but the specific terpenes produced from them by each plant species vary. The final two steps in artemisinin biosynthesis, from farnesyl pyrophosphate (FPP) to artemisinin, are catalyzed by enzymes encoded by genes specific to *Artemisia*. Although *E. coli* naturally produces IPP and DMAPP, the pathway is subject to feedback inhibition, preventing large quantities of these molecules from accumulating.

SUCCESS THROUGH GENETIC ENGINEERING

This obstacle to producing large quantities of amorphadiene in *E. coli* is circumvented by use of a combination of eight genes from *Saccharomyces cerevisiae* and *E. coli* to recreate the biosynthetic pathway leading to FPP production. ❶ A mutant *E. coli* strain is used in which the normal feedback inhibition of the FPP biosynthetic pathway is lacking. ❷ Expression of the eight *S. cerevisiae* genes is coordinated by distribution of the genes into two operons—one containing three genes and one containing five—controlled by *lac* operon regulatory sequences (see Section 12.2 for a description of the *lac* operon system). In this way, gene expression is induced in the presence of either lactose or the synthetic inducer isopropyl-β-D-thiogalactopyranoside (IPTG). ❸ The amorphadiene synthetase (*ADS*) gene is cloned from *Artemisia* and placed under the control of *lac* operon regulatory sequences.

In initial experiments with this system, the levels of ADS protein produced in *E. coli* were disappointingly low. The reason was discovered to be differences in codon bias between *Artemisia* and *E. coli*. When codons preferred by *Artemisia* were replaced with synonymous codons preferred by *E. coli*, the production of ADS protein in *E. coli* became much more efficient. ❹ Now the bacteria produced a large quantity of amorphadiene, which could be converted into artemisinin either by chemical synthesis or in vivo by the introduction of the artemisinin synthetase gene from *Artemisia*. Although the initial proof-of-principle production of artemisinin was performed in *E. coli*, the production was subsequently shifted to similarly genetically engineered yeast (*Saccharomyces cerevisiae*).

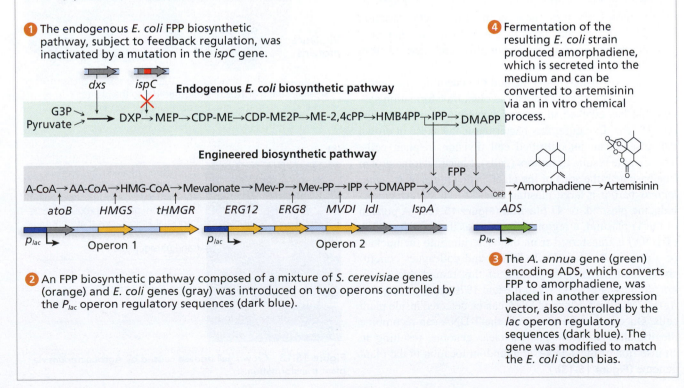

❶ The endogenous *E. coli* FPP biosynthetic pathway, subject to feedback regulation, was inactivated by a mutation in the *ispC* gene.

❹ Fermentation of the resulting *E. coli* strain produced amorphadiene, which is secreted into the medium and can be converted to artemisinin via an in vitro chemical process.

❷ An FPP biosynthetic pathway composed of a mixture of *S. cerevisiae* genes (orange) and *E. coli* genes (gray) was introduced on two operons controlled by the P_{lac} operon regulatory sequences (dark blue).

❸ The *A. annua* gene (green) encoding ADS, which converts FPP to amorphadiene, was placed in another expression vector, also controlled by the *lac* operon regulatory sequences (dark blue). The gene was modified to match the *E. coli* codon bias.

Yeast Plasmids Transgenes can be introduced into fungal cells in a manner similar to the techniques described for bacteria, using a plasmid system developed for the fungus *Saccharomyces cerevisiae* (baker's yeast). In addition, DNA can be readily integrated into the genomes of many fungi by homologous recombination, making direct manipulation of the fungal genome feasible (see Figure 14.10).

Some strains of *S. cerevisiae* harbor a circular 6.3-kb plasmid that, because of its approximately 2-μm diameter, is known as the 2-micron plasmid. This plasmid can be modified into a recombinant plasmid by the insertion of transgenes. An *E. coli* origin of replication and appropriate selectable markers are also introduced into the 2-micron plasmid, which already contains the *S. cerevisiae* origin of replication. With these additions, the plasmid becomes a **shuttle vector**, a vector that can replicate in two species—in this case, both *E. coli* and *S. cerevisiae*—and thus can be used to shuttle DNA sequences between them. With this shuttle vector, DNA sequences can be manipulated in *E. coli*, where manipulation is easier, after which the modified plasmids can be shuttled into yeast for heterologous protein expression.

Transformation of Plant Genomes by *Agrobacterium*

Our food is mainly derived from plants, and humans have been genetically modifying plants since the beginning of agriculture, nearly 10,000 years ago. For most of this history, genetic improvement was limited to interbreeding wild and domesticated species to select for traits already present in nature. The recently developed techniques for introducing DNA from many sources into plants have added a new dimension to the genetic modification of plants for agricultural purposes. By these new means, the genetic variation available in plants has been extended to include not only genes from other plant species but also genes derived from animals, fungi, and bacteria.

The most widely used method of generating transgenic plants takes advantage of a natural plant transformation system that has evolved in the soil bacterium *Agrobacterium tumefaciens*. In nature, this bacterium is the cause of crown gall disease, an uncontrolled cell division in plant cells. This disease results in tumors (galls), typically at the crown (the base near the soil) of the plant. Wild strains of *A. tumefaciens* harbor a large plasmid (200 kb) called the tumor-inducing plasmid, or **Ti plasmid** (Figure 15.13a). A portion of the Ti plasmid, a region referred to as the **transfer DNA (T-DNA)** is transferred from the bacterium into the nucleus of a plant cell. Mary-Dell Chilton and colleagues conclusively demonstrated the nature of this remarkable cross-kingdom transfer of DNA in the late 1970s by showing that *Agrobacterium* Ti plasmid DNA can be detected inside plant cells. Once inside the plant cell, the T-DNA can recombine illegitimately with the plant nuclear genome, resulting in an insertion of the T-DNA at a random location in the plant genome (Figure 15.13b).

(a)

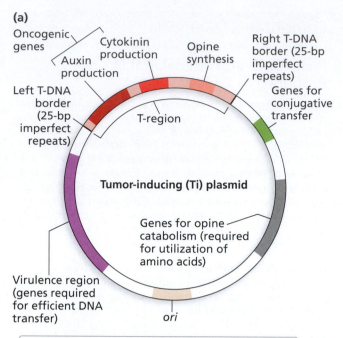

Tumor-inducing (Ti) plasmid

Transfer DNA (T-DNA) contains auxin and cytokinin biosynthetic genes and genes for amino acid biosynthesis.

(b) ***Agrobacterium tumefaciens*** (1–2 microns wide)   **Plant cell** (5–50 microns wide)

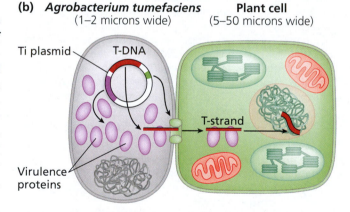

A single strand of T-DNA is transferred into the plant cell and is integrated into the plant nuclear genome.

(c)

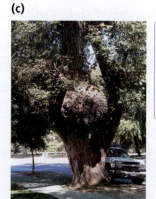

Expression of auxin and cytokinin biosynthetic genes leads to uncontrolled cell division and gall formation; gall cells produce the unusual amino acids that *Agrobacterium* uses as carbon and nitrogen sources.

Figure 15.13 Crown gall disease caused by *Agrobacterium* via plant transformation.

From the bacterial perspective, the outcome of this natural transformation event is the expression of genes in the T-DNA that encode proteins causing plant cells to (1) divide in an uncontrolled manner and (2) produce amino acids only the bacterium can utilize as an energy source. *Agrobacterium* essentially reprograms the plant cells into food factories for the bacteria. Bacterial genes encoding plant-hormone–biosynthesizing enzymes cause transformed plant cells to produce high levels of two plant hormones, auxin and cytokinin, which in turn cause uncontrolled division of plant cells, resulting in tumor formation (**Figure 15.13c**). The other genes on the T-DNA encode opine-biosynthesizing enzymes. Opines, such as nopaline and octopine, are amino acids that do not naturally occur in plants; therefore, plants do not produce any enzymes capable of metabolizing opines. *Agrobacterium* does have such enzymes, however; consequently, the opines produced by the plant cells can be used as carbon and nitrogen sources by the bacteria. Other genes on the Ti plasmid, but not located within the T-DNA region, encode enzymes required for the transfer of the T-DNA to the plant cell. In nature, the transfer of T-DNA into a plant genome usually occurs in somatic cells and is thus not transmitted to the next generation. However, we know of at least one case in which the T-DNA has entered the germ line and now forms part of the genome of a species—the sweet potato, *Ipomoea batatas*. It is estimated that the transfer occurred at least 8000 years ago, since the T-DNA is found in both cultivated and wild varieties, making the sweet potato a naturally transgenic food crop.

Sequence analysis has revealed that the genes involved in the transfer of T-DNA are evolutionarily related to those involved in the transfer of the F-factor in *E. coli* (see Section 6.2). Thus, *Agrobacterium* has evolved a mechanism to transfer DNA into plant cells by adapting genes originally involved in bacterial conjugation. A striking aspect of this cross-kingdom gene transfer is that the genes on the T-DNA have evolved to be transcribed and translated efficiently in plant cells instead of in bacterial cells. In nature, *Agrobacterium* normally transforms plants only; but in the laboratory, the bacterium has the ability to transfer DNA into almost any eukaryotic cell, including human cells.

Creating Transgenic Plants Scientists can use *Agrobacterium* to transfer any gene of interest into plants. To do so, they remove the opine- and tumor-producing genes normally found in the T-DNA and replace them with DNA encoding the gene of interest. The T-DNA then transfers the gene of interest into the plant cell, where it becomes integrated into the genomic DNA of the plant.

To repeat, the general strategy for modifying the Ti plasmid for transformation procedures starts with deletion of the tumor-inducing and opine genes, producing what is called a "disarmed" Ti plasmid. Then the gene of interest is inserted between the two ends of the T-DNA region, referred to as the left and right borders. These border regions contain sequences required for efficient transfer. Proteins encoded by genes of the Ti plasmid outside of the T-DNA recognize specific sequences in the left and right border and catalyze the transfer of a single strand of T-DNA from the bacterium to the plant cell; when this occurs, the gene of interest that has been inserted between the two border sequences will be transferred as well. As with any other protocol for constructing transgenic organisms, a selectable marker is included (between the left and right borders) in addition to the gene of interest to allow efficient selection of transformed plants. For experiments with plants, genes conferring resistance to either antibiotics (which inhibit translation in the chloroplast) or herbicides may be employed as selectable markers. The selectable marker genes are usually expressed using a promoter that confers constitutive expression, so that transgenic plants can be selected at any stage of their development.

Because the Ti plasmid is too large to be easily manipulated, most experimental protocols that use *Agrobacterium* construct a strain harboring two plasmids: One is a disarmed Ti plasmid, and the second is a plasmid that contains left and right border sequences flanking the DNA of interest (**Figure 15.14a**). This strategy, separating the functional elements of the Ti plasmid into two plasmids, is referred to as the binary approach. It results in the efficient transfer of the DNA of interest into the plant cell and its subsequent integration into the plant genome (**Figure 15.14b**).

Unlike bacteria and yeast, which are single-celled organisms, transformed plant cells must be regenerated into an entire plant to reveal the effects of transgenes on the plant phenotype. Traditionally, scientists have taken advantage of a unique feature of plant development, the **totipotency** of most plant cells: Under the appropriate environmental and hormonal conditions, an entire normal plant can be regenerated from a single isolated plant cell. Thus, after infection of plant cells with the modified *Agrobacterium* strain and selection of transformed cells on the basis of the selectable marker gene, progeny plants can be regenerated from the individual transformed cells (**Figure 15.14c**). This technique has been successfully applied to a wide variety of flowering plant species, including crop species such as rice, maize, and tomatoes.

Plant researchers using *Arabidopsis* as a model system for studying basic biological processes sought an easier method of transformation that would not require regeneration from a single transformed cell. After several different techniques were attempted, they discovered that the simple technique of dipping *Arabidopsis* flowers into a culture of *Agrobacterium* works surprisingly well. It allows the T-DNA to be transferred directly from *Agrobacterium* to the egg cell of the female gametophyte. In this protocol, transgenic plants are selected from seed produced by the plant exposed to *Agrobacterium*.

Many plant species are susceptible to *Agrobacterium*-mediated transformation. If they are not, DNA can be directly introduced into their cells. The cell walls of isolated plant cells are first removed enzymatically, after which the

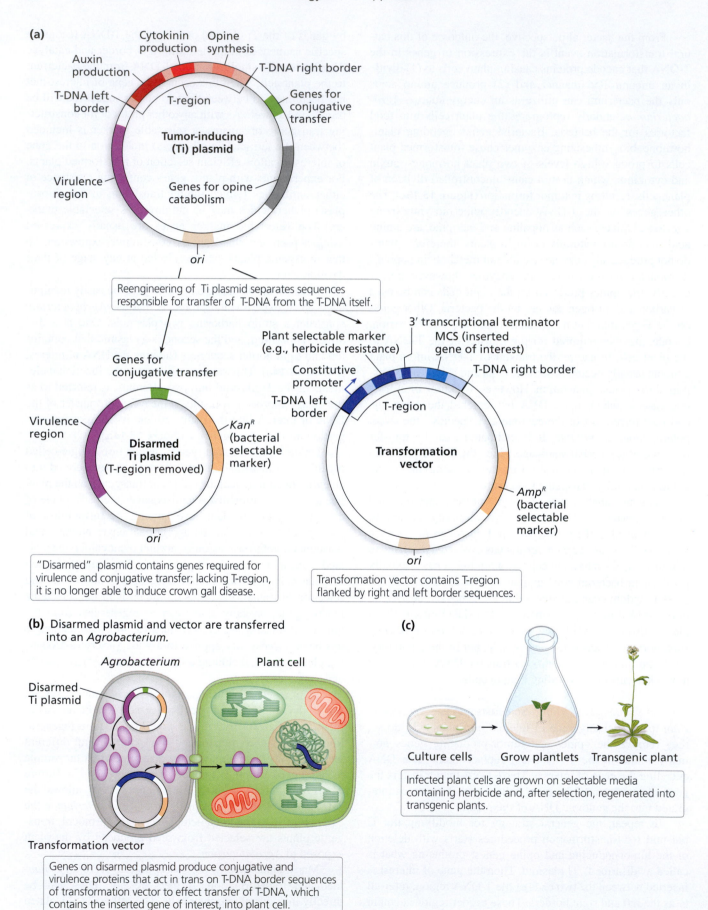

(a)

Tumor-inducing (Ti) plasmid
- Cytokinin production
- Opine synthesis
- Auxin production
- T-DNA left border
- T-DNA right border
- T-region
- Genes for conjugative transfer
- Virulence region
- Genes for opine catabolism
- *ori*

Reengineering of Ti plasmid separates sequences responsible for transfer of T-DNA from the T-DNA itself.

Disarmed Ti plasmid (T-region removed)
- Genes for conjugative transfer
- Virulence region
- *Kan^R* (bacterial selectable marker)
- *ori*

"Disarmed" plasmid contains genes required for virulence and conjugative transfer; lacking T-region, it is no longer able to induce crown gall disease.

Transformation vector
- Plant selectable marker (e.g., herbicide resistance)
- 3′ transcriptional terminator
- MCS (inserted gene of interest)
- Constitutive promoter
- T-DNA right border
- T-DNA left border
- T-region
- *Amp^R* (bacterial selectable marker)
- *ori*

Transformation vector contains T-region flanked by right and left border sequences.

(b) Disarmed plasmid and vector are transferred into an *Agrobacterium*.

Agrobacterium
- Disarmed Ti plasmid
- Transformation vector

Plant cell

Genes on disarmed plasmid produce conjugative and virulence proteins that act in trans on T-DNA border sequences of transformation vector to effect transfer of T-DNA, which contains the inserted gene of interest, into plant cell.

(c)
Culture cells → Grow plantlets → Transgenic plant

Infected plant cells are grown on selectable media containing herbicide and, after selection, regenerated into transgenic plants.

Figure 15.14 Reengineering the Ti plasmid to create transgenic plants.

cells are mixed with heterologous DNA and given a heat or electrical shock to depolarize the membrane and facilitate the entry of DNA. Once in the cell, the DNA has the same fate as described above for DNA transferred into fungi. In plants, homologous recombination is rare relative to illegitimate recombination, so the most common outcome is the insertion of the heterologous DNA into a random location in the genome. In another technique, DNA is introduced into plant cells by particle gun bombardment, the use of high pressure to fire microscopic particles coated with DNA into plant cells. The particles are propelled with enough force to penetrate the cell wall and plasma membrane. Both of these techniques can be applied to any plant species.

Transgenic Plants in Agriculture The two most common traits engineered into transgenic crops grown today are herbicide resistance and insect resistance. With herbicide-resistant crops—for example, the varieties sold as Roundup Ready—farmers can apply herbicide to a field to clear the ground of weeds and other noncrop plants without damaging the crop itself. This reduces the amount of tilling done to plow weeds under at the beginning of the season. Less tilling results in less soil loss and also saves on the use of fossil fuels.

Cotton and maize crops resistant to insect herbivory are two of the most widely grown transgenic crops. Insect resistance is usually conferred by the expression of genes derived from the bacterium *Bacillus thuringiensis*. Genes encoding approximately 100 insect toxins, known as Bt toxins, have been identified in different strains of *B. thuringiensis*. The toxins work by perforating the guts of different insect species, and different toxins have different "host" specificity. Transgenic plants expressing genes encoding Bt toxins are less palatable to insects and exhibit reduced insect herbivory. As a consequence, transgenic plants expressing Bt toxin genes require significantly less application of insecticides than do nontransgenic plants, thus reducing the insecticide load in the environment.

Although Bt toxins are clearly toxic to insects, other herbivores, such as humans, are impervious to the compounds. The properties of Bt toxins have been appreciated for some time. Organic farmers routinely spray *B. thuringiensis* directly on their crops to act as a "natural" insecticide. Millions of acres of transgenic maize, cotton, and potatoes expressing Bt genes and of herbicide-resistant soybeans are presently cultivated in the United States and several other countries.

Golden Rice Although many transgenic crops thus far used in agriculture have primarily benefited farmers in the developed world, the humanitarian potential for crop modification in aid of subsistence farmers in developing countries is exemplified by techniques for biofortifying staple foods with vitamins or minerals. In some crops, an increase in nutritional content can be accomplished by conventional breeding or by genome editing of endogenous genetic pathways, but in other cases, a transgenic approach, exemplified by Golden Rice, is required.

Rice (*Oryza sativa*) is the major staple food for much of the world. Because oil tends to become rancid, especially in tropical climates, rice is often milled until its oil-rich outer layer has been removed. Unfortunately, the remaining edible grain, the endosperm, lacks several micronutrients, including provitamin A, a vitamin A precursor. (Vitamin A can be obtained directly through consumption of animal products or indirectly from plants that produce carotenoids, which are converted to vitamin A after ingestion and are therefore termed provitamin A.)

Vitamin A deficiency results in blindness and increased disease susceptibility, thus contributing to childhood mortality in many developing countries. It is estimated that vitamin A deficiency affects between 140 million and 250 million preschool children worldwide, leading to 250,000 to 500,000 cases of blindness per year. Because no wild or domesticated cultivars of rice produce provitamin A in the endosperm, recombinant technologies, rather than a conventional breeding program, are required to produce rice that has an endosperm containing provitamin A.

Scientists knew that rice endosperm synthesizes geranylgeranyl diphosphate (GGPP), a precursor in the synthesis of carotenoids. Study of the carotenoid biosynthetic pathway in plants suggested that five plant-derived enzymes are needed to convert GGPP to β-carotene. However, the discovery that a single bacterial enzyme (CRTI) could replace three of the plant enzymes (PDS, ZDS, CRTISO) simplified the genetic engineering strategy (**Figure 15.15a**). Then, in 2000, Ingo Potrykus, Peter Beyer, and colleagues reported that the addition of only two genes, a daffodil-derived gene called *PSY* and the bacterial gene called *CRTI*, resulted in the production of β-carotene in rice endosperm (**Figure 15.15b**). This outcome was surprising because a gene called *LCY* was expected to be necessary as well, but apparently the endogenous rice *LCY* gene is already expressed in endosperm.

Subsequently, work has focused on tailoring the process so that (1) the transgenes would be expressed only during endosperm formation and only in endosperm, (2) the β-carotene synthesis could be increased using different versions of the genes, (3) the selectable marker could be removed from the transgenic lines, and (4) the transgenes could be introduced into rice cultivars that are typically used by subsistence farmers in southeast and south central Asia and Africa. These improvements have led to transgenic lines that could provide part of the required daily intake of provitamin A (**Figure 15.15c**).

The funding for the research to produce Golden Rice was public, in part from the Rockefeller Foundation, but patents on many of the techniques and tools used to generate the transgenic rice are held by biotech companies. Fortunately, these companies agreed to license the inventors of Golden Rice to provide the technology free of charge for humanitarian use in developing countries. Golden Rice is an example of how customized crops could be developed

(a) Synthesis of beta-carotene

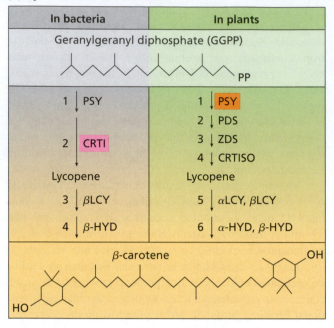

(b) Recombinant plasmids

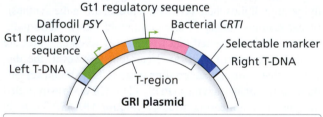

First-generation golden rice (GRI): Daffodil phytoene synthase gene (*PSY*) and bacterial CRTI gene from *Erwinia uredovora* are driven with rice glutelin-1 (Gt1) endosperm regulatory sequences (green).

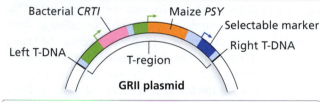

Second-generation golden rice (GRII): A maize *PSY* gene was exchanged for the daffodil *PSY* gene, boosting the production of β-carotene.

(c) Appearance of wild-type and transgenic rice

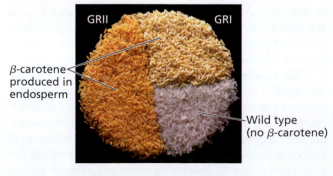

Figure 15.15   The generation of Golden Rice.

to address specific nutritional needs and public health problems caused by dietary deficiencies.

One potential hurdle for the introduction of genetically modified biofortified crops is that they are usually, at least initially, produced in only a single genetic background, or genotype, that may or may not be suited to local growing conditions or tastes. This obstacle, which is also often a problem with conventionally bred new varieties, can be overcome by conventional breeding to cross the desired trait into different genetic backgrounds, or by introduction of the transgene directly into locally favored genotypes.

Transgenic plants have been largely accepted in some parts of the world, but many concerns have been raised about their introduction. Some critics fear that transgenes could be adverse to human health—for example, that people may have allergic reactions to the protein product of a transgene. Another concern is that the transgenes may "escape" into the environment if transgenic crop plants interbreed with related species growing nearby. The likelihood of this occurrence can be reduced by not growing transgenic crops in environments harboring related species that have potential to interbreed. Transgenic crops must be tested to allay these concerns, but we must also recognize that, although the concerns about transgenic agricultural crops are valid, they are equally applicable to the cultivation of crops developed by traditional breeding methods.

Transgenic Animals

Protocols for the generation of transgenic animals are similar to those described for fungi and plants, but as with plants, homologous recombination occurs much less frequently than illegitimate recombination (i.e., recombination not based on sequence homology). Totipotency is not characteristic of most animal cells; thus, methods to produce transgenic animals rely on the injection of DNA into eggs, embryos, or cells that will give rise to gametes, with the hope that the injected DNA will be integrated into the genome either by homologous or illegitimate recombination.

Where injection directly into gametes is not feasible, DNA can be injected into isolated cells that are subsequently transplanted into an embryo. The embryo then develops as a **genetic mosaic**, an organism in which some cells have a different genotype than others, and will transmit transgenes to progeny only if the embryonic germ cells carry a copy of the transgene.

As with the protocols utilized in fungi and plants, methods for the production of transgenic animals vary depending on the biological characteristics specific to each type of organism. Here we provide examples of the various methods available for creation of transgenic animals. We focus on *Drosophila melanogaster* and *Mus musculus* (mice), two widely used genetic model animals.

Drosophila   In the 1980s, Gerald Rubin and Allan Spradling demonstrated that *P* transposable elements, a class of transposons, offered an efficient means of creating transgenic *Drosophila,* in most cases inserting only one copy of the DNA being transferred (see Section 11.7 for a description of *P* elements). Their idea was to use the endogenous activity of *P* elements to transpose transgenes into the genome (**Figure 15.16**).

Based on their knowledge of *P* element transposition, Rubin and Spradling reasoned that they could replace much of the *P* element DNA with exogenous DNA as long as (1) transposase, the enzyme that controls *P* element movement, was provided; and (2) the *P* element ends were retained, since these are required for recognition by the transposase. In

their method, two DNA molecules, one a modified *P* element and the other a DNA molecule encoding the transposase but lacking the sequences required for transposition, are co-injected into a *Drosophila* embryo. The modified *P* elements are induced to insert into the genome at random positions by the action of the transposase. Typically, only a single *P* element is inserted. This strategy resembles the use of *Agrobacterium* to transform plants in that it too utilizes a biological system that has evolved to recombine DNA into a host genome.

Since *P* elements transpose only in the germ-line cells of *Drosophila,* the injection is made into an early-stage embryo, targeting those cells that will give rise to the germ line. Early-stage *Drosophila* embryos are syncytial (consisting of a single, multinucleate cell; Section 18.2), and nuclei at the posterior end of the syncytium are most likely to give rise to the germ cells. The fly derived from the injected embryo is therefore a mosaic in which most soma (the parts of the organism other than germ cells) and some gametes are wild type, but some soma and gametes are transgenic. When the injected fly is mated with an uninjected fly of the same strain, gametes into whose genomes a *P* element was inserted will produce transgenic progeny.

A commonly used selectable marker in *Drosophila* is the *rosy* (*ry*) gene. In the procedure under discussion, the embryos to be injected are ry^-/ry^- and have rosy eyes, rather than the wild-type red eyes. A wild-type, ry^+, copy of the gene is included in the modified *P* element, in addition to the DNA to be transformed into the fly. Although flies derived from the injected embryos will have rosy eyes, some of the progeny of those flies, derived from transgenic gametes of the injected embryo, will have red eyes due to the action of the dominant ry^+ allele on the inserted *P* element. As is characteristic of transposons, *P* elements insert into the genome at random locations.

***Mus musculus* and Other Vertebrates** A general approach to creating transgenic vertebrates is to inject DNA directly into the nucleus of a fertilized egg cell. The injected DNA can become integrated into the genome at random positions by illegitimate recombination. Because the DNA integrates randomly into the genome, the transgene becomes inserted at different locations in the genomes of different individual animals. In organisms such as salmon, each injected egg has the potential to develop into a transgenic individual (**Figure 15.17**).

Transgenic Atlantic salmon containing a Chinook salmon growth hormone gene driven by regulatory sequences from ocean pout (*Zoarces americanus*) exhibit a size phenotype similar to that of the transgenic coho salmon generated by a similar approach in Figure 15.17. Treatment of the transgenic salmon eggs causes them to be triploid, making the salmon sterile and thus reducing the risk of their interbreeding with wild-type salmon. These transgenic fish have been approved for aquaculture and sale to U.S. (2015) and Canadian (2016) consumers.

Two features of this method lead to variability in the expression of the transgene. First, the transgenes are

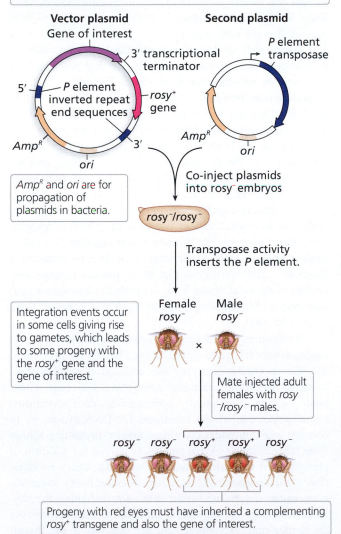

Figure 15.16 *P* element–mediated transformation in *Drosophila.*

Q **Why does the *rosy*⁺ phenotype not segregate 1:1 in the second generation?**

Endogenous sockeye salmon growth hormone gene

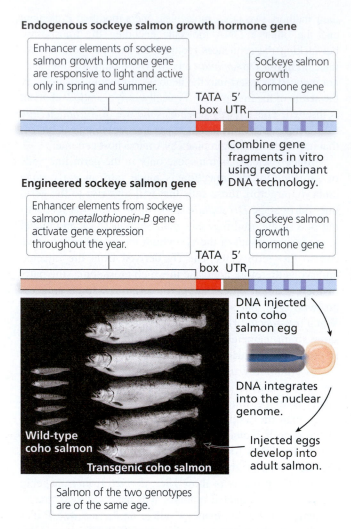

Enhancer elements of sockeye salmon growth hormone gene are responsive to light and active only in spring and summer.

TATA box

5′ UTR

Sockeye salmon growth hormone gene

Combine gene fragments in vitro using recombinant DNA technology.

Engineered sockeye salmon gene

Enhancer elements from sockeye salmon *metallothionein-B* gene activate gene expression throughout the year.

TATA box

5′ UTR

Sockeye salmon growth hormone gene

DNA injected into coho salmon egg

DNA integrates into the nuclear genome.

Wild-type coho salmon

Transgenic coho salmon

Injected eggs develop into adult salmon.

Salmon of the two genotypes are of the same age.

Figure 15.17 Creation of transgenic salmon through injection of DNA into salmon eggs.

integrated as multicopy concatemers—that is, multiple tandem copies of the inserted DNA—often resulting in abnormal levels of gene expression. Second, the expression of the transgene can be abnormal because of the chromosomal environment in which it is located. For example, if the transgene is inserted into heterochromatin, gene expression may be altered as described for position effect variegation in *Drosophila* (see Section 13.2).

Note that the problem of transgene position effects is shared by all transgenic organisms in which the transgene is integrated into the genome by illegitimate recombination; but whereas position effects can pose problems in *Drosophila* and plants, they are exacerbated in vertebrates, like salmon and mice, due to the larger average size of vertebrate genes and the larger amount of heterochromatin in vertebrate genomes. The mouse (*Mus musculus*) is an important genetic model for human diseases and human physiology, so it was important to overcome the problems of variability in transgene expression by developing methods to more precisely insert transgenes into mice.

Two general approaches are available for creating transgenic mice, a targeted approach and a nontargeted approach. The nontargeted approach, in which the transgene is randomly inserted into the genome through illegitimate recombination, is similar to that illustrated for salmon in Figure 15.17. In contrast, targeted approaches insert the transgene into a specific locus in the genome, either through homologous recombination or CRISPR–Cas9–mediated genome editing. The targeted methods have transformed the study of mouse biology by allowing for the creation of mice with specific loss-of-function (or knockout) and gain-of-function alleles. In 2007, Mario Capecchi, Martin Evans, and Oliver Smithies shared the Nobel Prize in Medicine or Physiology for their work leading to the development of knockout mice via homologous recombination. Today most studies would employ CRISPR–Cas9–mediated genome editing, but for historical reasons we look at the technique of homologous recombination here. The CRISPR–Cas9–mediated genome editing approach is presented in the next section.

The overall strategy for producing knockout mice by homologous recombination is similar to that described for homologous recombination in yeast. The transformation vector contains two regions of DNA homologous to the target locus flanking a positive selectable marker—meaning a gene that enables its host to survive the screening process (**Figure 15.18a**). An example of a positive selectable marker is the *Neomycin* (*Neo*) gene, whose product metabolizes the drug G418, which blocks translation and is lethal to mammalian cells. A vector containing the homologous regions is capable of integration into the genome by homologous recombination, but more than 99% of integrations will occur by illegitimate recombination. To select against nonhomologous recombination events, a negative selectable marker—a gene that by its presence suppresses growth or survival of the host—is added to the vector *outside* one of the regions of homology to the target gene (Figure 15.18a).

A commonly used negative selectable marker is a *thymidine kinase* (*tk*) gene derived from a herpes simplex virus. Thymidine kinase catalyzes the addition of a phosphate to deoxythymidine, forming deoxythymidine monophosphate, which is eventually converted to deoxythymidine triphosphate, one of the substrates for DNA synthesis. In contrast to mammalian thymidine kinase, thymidine kinase from herpes simplex virus can also catalyze the addition of phosphate to thymidine analogs that cause chain termination when incorporated into DNA. Because the endogenous mammalian thymidine kinase does not recognize the thymidine analogs as substrates, only those cells expressing the herpes simplex virus *tk* gene are sensitive to the thymidine analogs. Thus, cells harboring the viral *tk* gene will be selected against when plated on media containing the thymidine analog ganciclovir. Such thymidine analogs are also used as potent antiviral medications, since only cells harboring the virus are sensitive to the analog.

(a) Create knockout allele by homologous recombination in embryonic stem cells.

(b) Generate knockout mouse from ES cells.

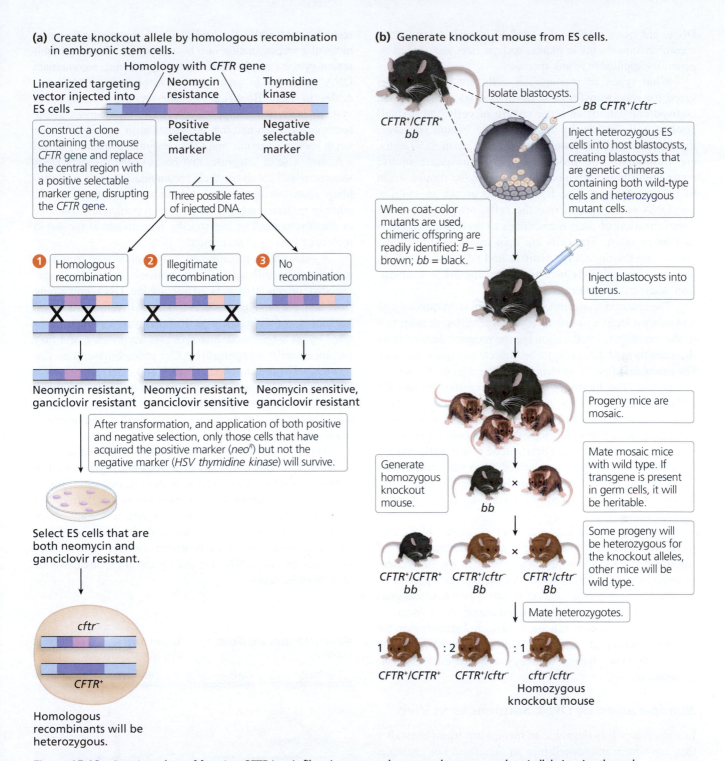

Figure 15.18 **Creating a loss-of-function *CFTR* (cystic fibrosis transmembrane conductance regulator) allele in mice through homologous recombination.** Mutations in the human ortholog are the cause of cystic fibrosis.

For transformed mouse cells to survive, they must acquire the positive marker and must lose the negative marker. The occurrence of a homologous recombination event between the negative and positive markers is one possible way in which the introduced DNA can be integrated to produce a cell that possesses the positive and lacks the negative marker. Selection for this type of transformation is called **positive–negative selection**. A related protocol, negative–positive–negative selection, where negative selectable markers are positioned at each end of the introduced

DNA, has been successfully used to identify homologous recombination events in plants, such as rice, and should be generally applicable to any species.

What types of mammalian cells are typically targeted for gene transfer? The blastocyst-stage mammalian embryo consists of an outer sphere of cells and a small pool of cells inside the sphere. At the blastocyst stage, the internal cells, known as embryonic stem (ES) cells, are totipotent. The production of a transgenic mouse starts with the isolation of ES cells from the mouse strain to be transformed. The ES cells are grown in culture, and DNA is introduced into the cells, often by transient depolarization of their membranes to make the cells permeable to DNA. The cells are then transferred to media containing the agents for positive and negative selection, and transformed cells in which homologous recombination occurred are selected.

The selected transformed ES cells are reintroduced into a blastocyst from a mouse of a genotype different from that of the transformed cells, allowing the progeny derived from the transformed ES cells to be detected (**Figure 15.18b**). For example, alleles conferring differences in coat color are often used. The blastocyst, now carrying transformed ES cells, is implanted into a surrogate female mouse. Because only some of the ES cells in the host blastocyst are transgenic, the mouse that develops from the embryo in which the transformed cells were introduced is a genetic mosaic in which some tissues are derived from the transformed ES cells and other tissues are derived from host ES cells. Mosaic animals can be readily identified by their variegated coat color.

It is hoped that at least some of the gametes of the chimeric offspring of the host mouse will be derived from the transformed ES cells, so that some mice in the subsequent generation will be heterozygous for the mutation caused by the homologous recombination event. If two heterozygous offspring of this generation are interbred, mice homozygous for the mutation can be produced. Technologies for the construction of other transgenic mammals, including sheep, cats, cows, horses, monkeys, and rats, follow a similar protocol.

Manipulation of DNA Sequences in Vivo

In some cases it is desirable to manipulate transgenes after they have been introduced into an organism. For example, the ability to remove the positive selectable marker gene after selection of transformants mitigates one of the concerns raised by critics of transgenic plants, as we discuss below. In addition, in vivo manipulation of transgenes facilitates the production of conditional alleles of genes whose null allele is lethal. The ability to specifically recombine DNA molecules makes in vivo manipulation of transgenes feasible.

Several bacteriophages use **site-specific recombination** systems during their life cycle, either for intramolecular recombination within the bacteriophage genome or for intermolecular recombination into host genomes. These recombination systems can be harnessed for producing recombinant DNA molecules in vitro and for recombining DNA molecules in vivo. Bacteriophage site-specific recombination systems have two components: (1) DNA sequences in the bacteriophage genome that are identical to sequences in the target bacterial genome and (2) an enzyme, commonly called a recombinase or integrase, that binds to the identical DNA sequences and catalyzes their recombination. Two bacteriophage recombination systems, one in bacteriophage λ and the other in bacteriophage P1, have proven particularly valuable in the development of site-specific recombination for use in molecular biology experiments.

A site-specific recombination system derived from bacteriophage P1 utilizes Cre recombinase, a bacteriophage-encoded protein that acts to recombine DNA containing *loxP* sequences (**Figure 15.19**). The *loxP* sites are 34-bp sequences consisting of two 13-bp inverted repeats separated by an 8-bp spacer that provides asymmetry, and they are specifically recognized by Cre recombinase. The Cre recombinase binds to two *loxP* sites and catalyzes a recombination event between them. If the two *loxP* sites are direct repeats, the intervening DNA is deleted, whereas if the two *loxP* sites are inverted relative to one another, the intervening sequence is inverted.

The Cre–*lox* recombination system has been adapted to recombine DNA in vivo in transgenic organisms. For example, *loxP* sites are added to the ends of the DNA to be deleted or inverted and the construct is then introduced as a transgene into an organism. Later, a second transgene encoding the Cre recombinase is also introduced into the same organism. In cells where the Cre recombinase is expressed, the DNA flanked by the *loxP* sites will be deleted or inverted.

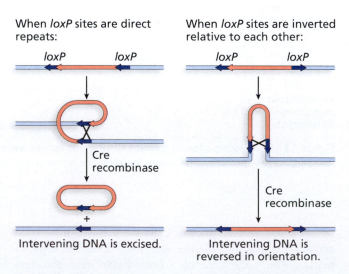

When *loxP* sites are direct repeats:

When *loxP* sites are inverted relative to each other:

Cre recombinase

Cre recombinase

Intervening DNA is excised.

Intervening DNA is reversed in orientation.

Figure 15.19 **Bacteriophage site-specific recombination systems.**

One reason a geneticist might want to delete a transgene after having introduced it into the genome is to assess the function of the gene at specific times and in specific tissues during development. For example, if a null loss-of-function allele results in embryonic lethality, the role of the gene at later developmental stages is difficult to assess. One approach to determining the postembryonic function of such genes is to complement a loss-of-function mutant with a functional copy of the gene flanked by *loxP* sites. Then, Cre recombinase can be supplied in specific cells or tissues of interest. In cells where the Cre recombinase is active, the transgene will be deleted, causing these cells and their descendants to have a mutant genotype. If the Cre recombinase is driven by a promoter that confers inducible expression or expression that is temporally or spatially restricted, a genetic chimera can be created, allowing an assessment of gene function in specific tissues.

A second application of site-specific recombination is the removal of selectable markers in transgenic organisms. An objection to the use of transgenic organisms in agriculture is that some transgenic strains contain a selectable marker providing resistance to antibiotics, which might spread into the natural population. The antibiotic-resistant marker genes were used to select the transgenic organism but are no longer needed once the transgenic organism has been identified. One strategy for eliminating the selectable marker is to flank the unwanted transgene with *loxP* sites in a direct repeat orientation. A plant containing this transgene is then crossed with another transgenic plant expressing the Cre recombinase, and the unwanted transgene is deleted in the F$_1$. It is then possible, by selective breeding, to segregate the transgene encoding the Cre recombinase away from the desired transgene in subsequent generations.

Genetic Analysis 15.2 asks you to put some of these ideas to work by designing a mouse model of a human disease.

15.3 Gene Therapy Uses Recombinant DNA Technology

The use of genes as therapeutic agents to cure or alleviate disease symptoms is termed **gene therapy**. The ultimate technology for gene therapy would be the ability to precisely change DNA sequences in the genome in vivo. Remarkably, this has now become available with the advent of CRISPR–Cas systems. (It is also the ultimate approach for investigation of gene function, as discussed earlier in the chapter and in Section 14.3.) Two types of gene therapy, classified as somatic gene therapy and germinal gene therapy, are feasible.

Two Forms of Gene Therapy

Somatic gene therapy targets somatic cells, whose descendants will not give rise to germ cells. Any genetic alterations induced in the targeted cells will be passed to daughter cells by mitosis, but the alteration will not be inherited by progeny of the individual undergoing somatic gene therapy. The specific somatic cells to be targeted depend on the disease in question. For example, in individuals with cystic fibrosis, the epithelial cells of the lungs represent a logical target, since lungs are severely affected in cystic fibrosis. On the other hand, for diseases of the blood, cells of the various hemopoietic lineages are the target cells; they can be removed from bone marrow, treated, and returned to the same individual. Somatic gene therapy turns the treated individual into a genetic chimera that has the transgene present in the target cells but not in other somatic cells or in germ cells. Somatic gene therapy can potentially be used to treat several genetic diseases whose phenotype becomes apparent early in childhood.

In essence, gene therapy involves extracting cells from an organism, correcting the genetic defect, and then reinserting the cells back into the body in a manner that permits them to function appropriately. Each gene therapy procedure is accompanied by technical difficulties that depend on the specific circumstances of the disease. In some cases—for example, in hemopoietic diseases—the cells to be treated can be extracted from the body, treated in vitro, and then injected back into the body. However, in other cases—for example, cystic fibrosis, in which lung epithelial cells are the target—the cells must be treated in situ because they cannot be removed from the patient.

The alternative strategy for gene therapy, **germinal gene therapy**, targets cells of the germ line, which give rise to gametes. Because germinal gene therapy alters germ-line cells, the therapeutic transgene is transmitted to the progeny of the treated individual. Both types of gene therapy have been successful in animal systems; but for ethical reasons, only somatic gene therapy has been attempted in humans. In the following paragraphs, we discuss somatic gene therapy using embryonic stem cells in humans and describe modifications of these protocols suggested by successful somatic gene therapy experiments in mice.

Somatic Gene Therapy Using ES Cells

The ideal somatic gene therapy would be one that corrects the specific mutation causing the genetic disease rather than just compensating for the mutant allele. Advances in understanding the biology of embryonic stem (ES) cells have brought new forms of somatic gene therapy that may approach this ideal for some genetic diseases. Embryonic stem cells are normally found only in developing embryos, hence their name, and are the undifferentiated cells that will go on to develop into the mammalian body. Embryonic stem cells are totipotent, meaning they have the potential to differentiate into any cell type in the body. In addition, as discussed in Section 15.2, the genome of an ES cell can be edited using CRISPR–Cas9. Thus, if ES cells can be isolated from an individual, gene mutations within the cells could perhaps be corrected, and the cells could then be

β-Carotene

PROBLEM Mouse models of human diseases are valuable research tools that can be used to test therapies and drugs. How would you make a transgenic mouse model of Huntington disease, which is caused by an autosomal dominant mutation consisting of an expanded sequence of trinucleotide repeats?

BREAK IT DOWN: Review the discussion on p. 575 of procedures for creating transgenic mice.

BREAK IT DOWN: Review the defining features of an autosomal dominant mutation/CORE (see Section 4.1).

Solution Strategies	Solution Steps
Evaluate	
1. Identify the topic this problem addresses and the nature of the required answer.	1. This problem about recombinant DNA technology asks how to construct a specific strain of transgenic mouse.
2. Identify the critical information given in the problem.	2. The desired disease model is of Huntington disease (HD), described as an autosomal dominant mutation that consists of an expanded sequence of trinucleotide repeats. The transgenic mouse is to be used to test therapies and drugs.
Deduce	
3. Inheritance patterns are always a key consideration in genetic research designs. Identify the inheritance pattern of the HD phenotype.	3. Since HD is dominant, a phenotype should be evident if a single mutant allele is introduced into the genome.
4. Evaluate the ways in which the *HD* allele can be transferred into mice.	4. Transgenic mice can be generated by random integration of a transgene or, alternatively, by homologous recombination that replaces the endogenous gene with a mutant version.
5. Choose the method of generating a transgenic mouse that will come closest to modelling the disease of interest. PITFALL: Randomly integrated transgenes may exhibit variation in expression patterns.	5. Because we want the transgene to be expressed in the same pattern as the wild-type mouse *HD* gene, homologous recombination is the best approach, because the mutant *HD* gene will then be in the same genomic context and will be expressed in the same pattern as the wild-type gene.
Solve	
6. Design a strategy to replace the wild-type mouse *HD* gene with a mutant version of the human *HD* gene. PITFALL: Since a functional allele is desired, the positive selectable marker must not interfere with *HD* transgene function.	6. The positive–negative selection approach outlined in Figure 15.18 to produce a transgenic mouse by homologous recombination results in a loss-of-function allele. This approach must be modified to create a gain-of-function allele.
	a. Construct a vector in which a human mutant *HD* gene is flanked by mouse *HD* regulatory sequences (5′ and 3′ of the *HD* gene).
	b. The positive selective marker gene can be placed downstream of the *HD* gene, in a position not likely to interfere with HD gene expression, or could be removed using the Cre–*lox* approach outlined in Figure 15.19.
	c. A second type of transgenic mouse, expressing the wild-type human gene driven by the same regulatory sequences, would provide a useful control to compare with the specific phenotypic effects induced by the expression of the mutant allele.

For more practice, see Problems 7, 8, 11, 27, and 30.   Visit the Study Area to access study tools.   **Mastering Genetics**

induced to differentiate into the appropriate cell type to treat the genetic disease. As illustrated in the mouse experiment described below, the ability to create and manipulate ES cells provides a means of isolating cells from an individual, correcting mutations in the cells, and reintroducing the "corrected" cells into the body.

Creating ES Cells From Differentiated Cells of the Adult Body In many cases, the diagnosis of a genetic disease is not made until early childhood, when the body no longer possesses any ES cells, because they form only during early embryogenesis. How can ES cells be obtained from a person who has none? The answer is to create ES cells from other cells of the body. In 2006 and 2007, a series of experiments demonstrated that mouse or human fibroblasts, a type of cell occurring in connective tissue, could be reprogrammed in vitro to behave like stem cells. These reprogrammed cells have been called *induced pluripotent stem cells*, or *iPS cells*. (The word *pluripotent* is used because scientists do not yet know if the iPS cells are totipotent.)

The reprogramming of differentiated cells was accomplished by expressing a combination of three to four transcription factors (choices included Oct4, Sox2, c-Myc, and Klf4). These transcription factors are normally expressed in ES cells and appear to be sufficient to induce reprogramming of the transcriptional networks of differentiated somatic cells into networks characteristic of ES cells. These four transcription factors act in combination as pioneer factors to activate embryonic gene expression and indirectly repress the genetic program of the differentiated cell via reprogramming of the epigenetic marks on the chromatin (see Section 13.2). Although it is not clear whether the epigenetic marks in iPS cells and ES cells are identical, iPS cells appear to be essentially equivalent to ES cells. The four factors are sometimes referred to as *Yamanaka factors*, after Shinya Yamanaka, who shared the 2012 Nobel Prize in Medicine with John B. Gurdon for their discovery that adult differentiated cells could be reprogrammed to be pluripotent.

One impediment to all strategies of gene therapy is the challenge of delivering genes or gene products to the cells of interest. For example, after you isolate fibroblast cells, how do you introduce the four transcription factors into the cell? Gene therapy methods often take advantage of viruses that have evolved mechanisms to enter specific cell types. Essentially, viruses are harnessed to transduce the transgene into the target cells the way that bacteriophages accomplish the transduction of DNA between bacteria (see Section 6.4). The viruses can be "disarmed" so that they no longer have the ability to cause the diseases associated with their wild-type relatives. Several types of viral vectors have been used, including gamma-retroviruses, lentiviruses, and adenoviruses.

Many viral vectors deliver transgenes by integrating into the genome of the target cell. Integration provides a mechanism for stable gene transfer and thus permanent correction of the defect. Integration of the vector into the genome is not without risks, however; the insertion may cause a detrimental mutation, a problem that has plagued most human gene therapy experiments to date.

Another problem associated with the use of iPS cells is that the continued expression of the Yamanaka factors predisposes cells to become cancerous. Thus, methods are needed to stop the expression of the Yamanaka factors once they have induced iPS cell formation. One such method is to flank the genes encoding the Yamanaka factors with *lox* sites so the genes can later be excised from the genome by providing the iPS cells with Cre recombinase.

Gene Therapy Proof of Principle: Curing Sickle Cell Disease in Mice These advances in iPS cell biology have set the stage for the use of iPS cells in gene therapy. Proof of principle (a phrase used by scientists to mean proof that the general idea is valid) was provided using a mouse model for sickle cell disease (**Figure 15.20**). The basic strategy being tested consisted of harvesting adult cells ❶, reprogramming adult cells into iPS cells ❷, repairing the genetic defect ❸, differentiating the iPS cells into hemopoietic precursors in vitro ❹, and transplanting the corrected cells into bone marrow of affected mice ❺.

The starting point for this test of somatic gene therapy was the creation of a "humanized" mouse model for sickle cell anemia by substituting human α-globin genes for the endogenous mouse α-globin genes and substituting human β^S (sickle) globin genes for the mouse β-globin genes. Mice homozygous for the β^S-globin allele (β^S/β^S) exhibited typical disease symptoms, including severe anemia and erythrocyte sickling. Fibroblasts isolated from the tail of β^S/β^S mice were infected with retroviruses encoding the Oct4, Sox2, and Klf4 transcription factors and with a lentivirus encoding the c-Myc transcription factor. Expression of these four transcription factors resulted in the reprogramming of the fibroblast cells into iPS cells. On either side of the *c-Myc* gene on the lentivirus, *lox* sites had been placed, to allow the gene to be excised from the genome when the cells were infected with an adenovirus encoding Cre recombinase. Although the other three transgenes were not removed in this experiment, their removal by a similar mechanism is also recommended.

In the original experiment in 2007, homologous recombination–based gene replacement was used to correct the β^S-globin allele (see Figure 15.18). However, in Figure 15.20 we illustrate how CRISPR–Cas9 genome editing would be employed for that purpose, since that is now the method of choice. The components of the CRISPR–Cas9 system—the guideRNAs and either mRNA encoding Cas9 or the Cas9 protein itself—can be injected directly into iPS cells. To correct the defect, a linear DNA template encoding the wild-type version of the gene is injected along with the CRISPR–Cas9 components. In some cases, two guideRNAs are used, one on each side of the site to be repaired, to create double-strand breaks flanking the site. Following the formation of double-strand breaks, homologous recombination of the wild-type template results in correction of the defect (i.e., genome editing). Unlike homologous recombination, where the resulting iPS cells are heterozygous, the approach illustrated here permits genome editing to occur on both chromosomes, resulting in homozygosity of the wild-type allele.

The β^A/β^A iPS cells can then be differentiated into hemopoietic progenitors (HPs, cells that have the potential to differentiate into any of the hemopoietic lineages) by infection with another retrovirus encoding the *HoxB4* gene, which induces the differentiation of ES cells into HPs when incubated with cytokines secreted from bone marrow cells.

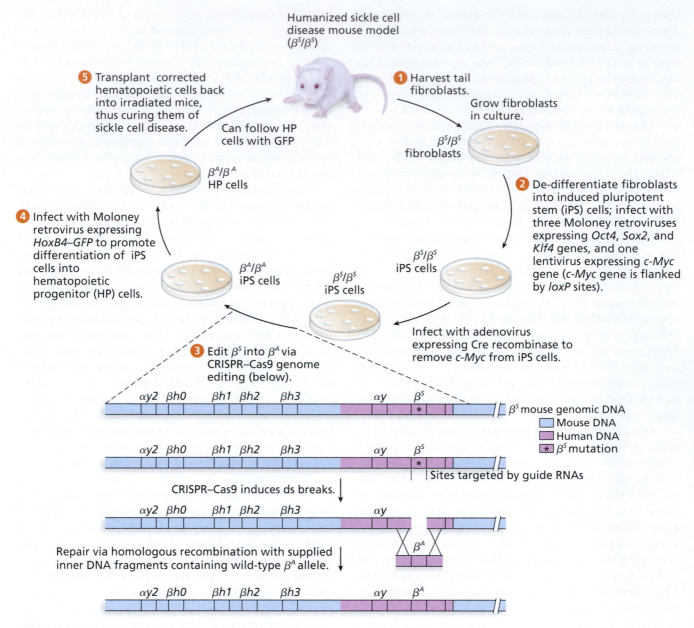

Figure 15.20 Genetic therapy for mice with sickle cell disease.

The β^A/β^A HPs are next transplanted back into β^S/β^S mice in which the endogenous β^S/β^S bone marrow cells have been eliminated by irradiation, so that now the β^A/β^A HPs constitute the primary source of hemopoietic cells. In the original 2007 experiment, the *HoxB4* coding sequence was translationally fused with that of green fluorescent protein (GFP), so the activity of the HP cells could be monitored by the presence of GFP^+ cells in the blood. Subsequently, by all physiological tests, the mice receiving the corrected HPs were cured of sickle cell disease.

These experiments in mice suggest there is promise in the use of ES or iPS cells for gene therapy, but at least two facets of gene therapy procedures continue to cause concern. Problems associated with using retroviruses and oncogenes for reprogramming need to be resolved before

implementing such a protocol in humans. For example, due to their insertion in the genome retroviruses can cause unintended mutations and the introduction of an oncogene has the potential to cause cancer (see Application Chapter C). In addition, researchers have yet to ascertain whether iPS cells are truly totipotent or still contain an epigenetic memory of their origin. Because an individual's own cells are used as the raw material for genetic modification, there is no problem of immune system incompatibility. However, this approach is limited to diseases, such as blood disorders, in which cells can be isolated, genetically corrected, and reintroduced into the body.

In recent years other approaches combining elements of the method described above have been investigated for treating genetic diseases unrelated to the blood. For example,

Duchenne muscular dystrophy (DMD) is a progressive muscle-wasting disease caused by loss-of-function alleles in the *DYSTROPHIN* gene. The gene has 79 exons, but even if some internal exons are skipped, the encoded protein can still function as long as the two ends are intact. A majority of DMD patients have mutations in middle exons and thus could benefit if the mutant exon were skipped (shortening the resulting encoded polypeptide) but the ends remained intact. Three groups used CRISPR–Cas9 genome editing to delete mutant exon 23 from a mouse model of DMD. In this model, the mutant exon harbors a nonsense mutation consisting of an in-frame stop codon (**Figure 15.21**). An adenovirus, injected intramuscularly, was used to carry the genome-editing components into the muscle cells. In some of the muscle cells, exon 23 was specifically deleted, and those cells began to produce functional dystrophin. Among other results of this research was the demonstration that editing could occur in muscle stem cells. The treated mice exhibited restored muscle structure and function. These studies hold promise for development of a somatic treatment for muscular dystrophy.

A second example is hemophilia B, caused by loss-of-function alleles of a gene encoding clotting factor IX, which is normally produced in the liver and then exported into the bloodstream. Two adenovirus vectors, one carrying the CRISPR–Cas9 components, with Cas9 being fused to enhancer modules driving expression only in the liver, and the second vector containing a human factor IX cDNA, were introduced into mice carrying mutations in their factor IX gene. The resulting genome editing led to a chimeric mouse–human factor IX gene driven by the endogenous mouse regulatory sequences, effectively "curing" the mice of hemophilia B.

15.4 Cloning of Plants and Animals Produces Genetically Identical Individuals

Many plants have the capacity for vegetative (asexual) propagation in addition to sexual propagation. Poplar and aspen (*Populus* sp.) groves often consist of vegetatively propagated clones, all genetically identical. Some of these clonal groves are estimated to be at least 10,000 years old. Humans, taking advantage of the ability of plants to reproduce vegetatively, have been clonally propagating plants for centuries in agricultural practices. The bananas that you eat are an example, all propagated via vegetative cuttings. In this case, the vegetative propagation is necessary because the cultivated bananas are triploid and therefore do not produce viable seed—the black specks you see embedded in the flesh of the fruit are the aborted seeds (see Section 10.3 for discussion of the effects of triploidy). With these techniques, heterozygous genotypes of agriculturally desirable specimens can be propagated intact, without the segregation of alleles that occurs during sexual reproduction; this maintains the consistency of desirable traits while promoting the hybrid vigor that can result in higher yields in comparison with inbred varieties (a topic also discussed in Section 10.3).

Perhaps the most conspicuous example of agricultural vegetative propagation is the cultivation of grapes (*Vitis vinifera*), which were domesticated 6000 to 7000 years ago. Most grape cultivars are highly heterozygous; that is, they have two different alleles at many genomic loci. Thus, when they are self-fertilized or crossed with another cultivar, extensive segregation of genotypes and phenotypes is observed in the progeny. Because this presents an obstacle

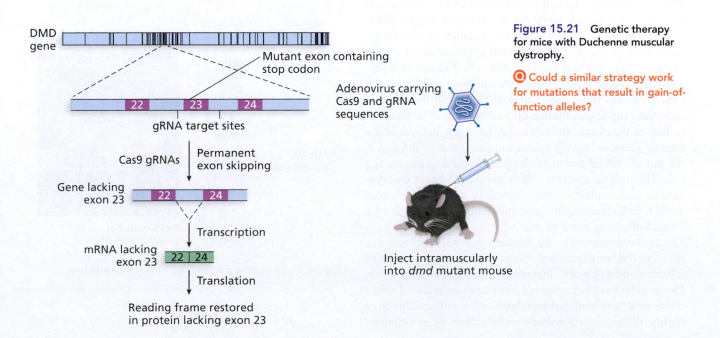

Figure 15.21 Genetic therapy for mice with Duchenne muscular dystrophy.

Could a similar strategy work for mutations that result in gain-of-function alleles?

DMD gene

Mutant exon containing stop codon

22 23 24

gRNA target sites

Cas9 gRNAs — Permanent exon skipping

Gene lacking exon 23 — 22 24

Transcription

mRNA lacking exon 23 — 22 | 24

Translation

Reading frame restored in protein lacking exon 23

Adenovirus carrying Cas9 and gRNA sequences

Inject intramuscularly into *dmd* mutant mouse

to controlling the properties of grape plants through breeding, cultivars that possess favorable phenotypes are propagated by cuttings (that is, additional plants are grown from pieces of source plants). In most vineyards, the vines are chimeric: The shoots are all genetically identical and chosen on the basis of their fruit phenotype, and the roots, also identical to one another, are of a different genotype that is chosen for being well adapted to local soil conditions.

Several wine grape cultivars can be traced back to the Middle Ages, and some are likely to be even older. For example, Pinot was first described in Roman times and is thought to be at least 2000 years old. Although clonal propagation has allowed maintenance of specific genotypes, somatic mutations—due, for example, to errors in DNA replication and transposable element activity—can accumulate over time and have led to phenotypic variation. For example, a mutation in a gene required for pigment synthesis led to the formation of Pinot blanc, a white-berry cultivar, from Pinot noir, the ancestral black-berry cultivar.

Unlike plants, most animals do not readily propagate clonally in nature—but there are exceptions. For example, some aphid species undergo multiple parthenogenetic (clonal) generations in the spring and summer, followed by sexual reproduction in the autumn. Since most animal cells are not totipotent (embryonic stem cells excepted), animals do not readily regenerate from single cells. Thus, techniques for cloning animals, and in particular mammals, from single differentiated cells are considerably more complicated than those for cloning plants.

Dolly, a sheep, born in July 1996, was the first cloned mammal. In the protocol used to produce Dolly, a diploid nucleus is isolated from a differentiated cell of the animal to be cloned (**Figure 15.22**). This nucleus, containing all the nuclear genetic information of the animal from which it was taken, is injected into an egg cell that has had its own nucleus removed. The egg cell can be derived from the animal to be cloned (if it possesses egg cells) or from a different individual. If the nuclear transplantation is successful, the genome of the donor nucleus will direct the development of the embryo derived from the egg cell. The use of a diploid donor nucleus means that fertilization with a sperm cell is not required to produce a diploid nucleus in the embryo; thus, the genetic constitution of the embryo will be identical to that of the donor. Bear in mind, however, that while the nuclear genome is genetically identical to that of the donor, the mitochondrial genome is derived from the surrogate egg cell. The diploid egg cell is then induced to begin embryogenesis and implanted into a surrogate mother. If all goes well, it will develop into a normal embryo, and birth of a normal offspring will follow.

In most mammals, the frequency of success with this protocol has been quite low. Dolly's was the only one out of 270 implanted egg cells that resulted in the birth of a sheep. Donor cells have been derived from adult animals—Dolly's donor cell was a mammary gland cell—and are therefore highly differentiated somatic cells rather than totipotent

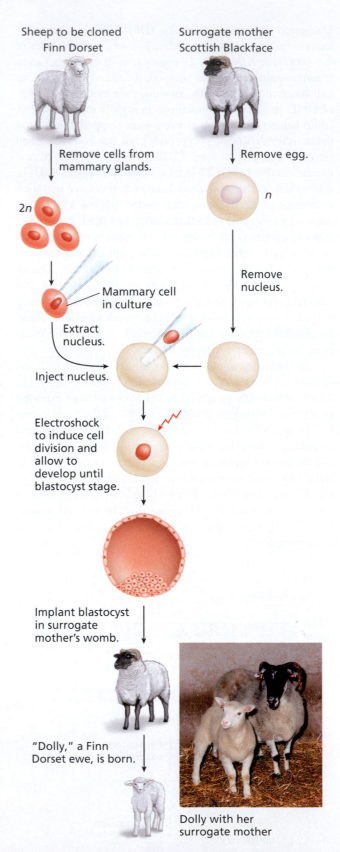

Figure 15.22   **Cloning animals by nuclear implantation.**

embryonic stem cells. In differentiated somatic cells, such as those of the mammary gland, the patterns of facultative heterochromatin (see Section 13.2) are vastly different from those of embryonic stem cells. In other words, although the sequences of nucleotides in the genomes of differentiated and embryonic stem cells are identical, the epigenetic modifications of the histones and DNA methylation patterns differ. The low frequency of success in the initial attempts to clone mammals was likely due to deficiencies in reprogramming the genetic material of the injected nucleus to mimic the epigenetic modifications characteristic of an embryonic stem cell. However, although Dolly's life span

was about half that of the average sheep in captivity, there is no evidence that a failure in epigenetic reprogramming contributed to her shortened life span. Rather, she died of lung cancer caused by a virus, a not uncommon cause of mortality in sheep kept indoors.

In the past decade, advances in knowledge of ES cell biology, in particular the discovery of the Yamanaka factors and their use to reprogram differentiated cells into iPS cells, suggest that the cloning of mammals will improve over time. Already, many different mammals besides sheep have been successfully cloned, including mice, cows, horses, donkeys, cats, and dogs.

CASE STUDY

Gene Drive Alleles Can Rapidly Spread Through Populations

In Chapter 2 we learned that during sexual reproduction in diploid organisms, each of the two alleles at any locus is inherited by 50% of the offspring. However, in some rare cases, genetic elements called *gene drives* circumvent this Mendelian pattern of segregation by increasing the frequency of inheritance of the gene drive allele over the wild-type allele (**Figure 15.23a**). Gene drive alleles induce biased inheritance patterns either by converting the wild-type allele to a gene drive allele or by reducing the fitness of the wild-type allele in some manner. The former mechanism entails the gene drive element copying and inserting itself into the wild-type locus. This mechanism is described in more detail below. Regardless of mechanism, if gene drive elements are highly efficient, they have the potential to spread through a population even if they impose a fitness cost on the organism. Although gene drive alleles exist in nature, they are usually inefficiently propagated such that they are not often rapidly spread throughout a population.

A GENE DRIVE ELEMENT CREATED WITH CRISPR–Cas
For a gene drive allele to function, it must first recognize the homologous wild-type allele and copy itself into that location. The insertion of a copy requires both the creation of a double-strand break in the target DNA and, if the target DNA is the homologous locus, the ability to recognize that sequence. These faculties, while rarely found in nature, can be engineered using the CRISPR–Cas9 genome editing complex; the Cas9 protein harbors the endonuclease activity and a guideRNA provides the required sequence specificity (**Figure 15.23b**).

To examine how this works in practice, envision a target locus in the genome for which you design a complementary guideRNA. A vector is constructed in which the Cas9 gene and your guideRNA gene are placed in tandem, and flanking the two genes is included sequence identical to the genome sequence flanking your target site ❶. When this construct is introduced into a cell, the CRISPR–Cas9 complex will cut the genomic target, creating a double-strand break ❷. The double-strand break can be repaired by homologous recombination using the DNA construct that was introduced, creating an allele in which the Cas9 and guideRNA genes are inserted into the genomic target site ❸. This allele is a gene drive because it has the capacity to convert the homologous allele on the second chromosome into a drive allele in a similar

manner ❹. The Cas9 and guideRNA genes from the first allele will produce a CRISPR–Cas9 complex that can induce double-strand breaks in the second allele ❺ that can be repaired via homologous recombination using the first allele as a template ❻. The end result is a homozygous individual in which both alleles are now gene drive alleles.

If the Cas9 and guideRNA genes are driven constitutively, alleles in all somatic and germ-line cells can be converted into gene drive alleles. If an individual with a gene drive allele is crossed with a wild-type individual, the gene drive allele has the capacity to convert the allele inherited from the wild-type parent into a gene drive allele (Figure 15.23a) in the same manner as the homologous chromosome was in Figure 15.23b. Thus, the gene drive allele has the potential to spread throughout an interbreeding population. The speed and extent of spread is dictated by the efficacy of the gene drive allele at converting homologous alleles and by the nature of the breeding population.

Note that each time an allele is converted to a gene drive allele, it also encodes both the Cas9 and guideRNA genes, because they are located between the regions of genomic homology. The original construct could be modified to include additional genes as well, often referred to as cargo genes (**Figure 15.23c**), and as the gene drive allele spreads through a population, the cargo genes would also be disseminated. If either the gene drive allele itself or a cargo gene confers a phenotype, this will also be propagated throughout the population.

APPLICATIONS Among the potential applications of gene drives, the most commonly mentioned are to control the spread of vector-borne diseases, to suppress populations of agricultural pest species, and to reduce populations of environmentally destructive invasive species. Proof of principle has been obtained in two approaches to controlling the spread of mosquito-borne malarial parasites. Cargo genes encoding anti-*Plasmodium falciparum* (the Apicomplexan malarial parasite) effector proteins were disseminated in one approach. The other approach was aimed at spreading recessive loss-of-function alleles for three genes to produce female sterility. Both approaches led to rapid spread of the desired alleles in laboratory populations of the *Anopheles* mosquitos, the hosts for *P. falciparum*.

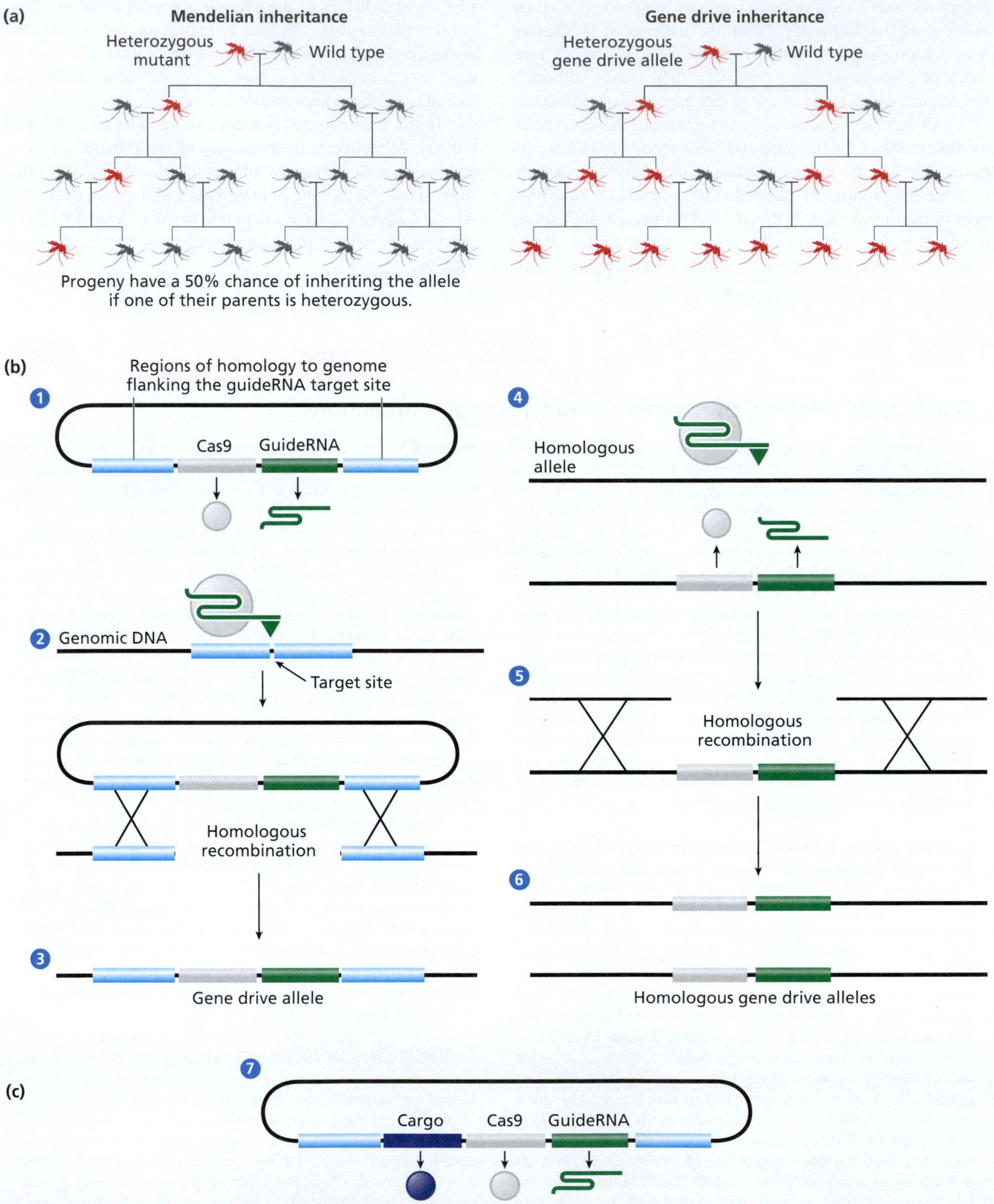

(a)

Mendelian inheritance

Heterozygous mutant — Wild type

Progeny have a 50% chance of inheriting the allele if one of their parents is heterozygous.

Gene drive inheritance

Heterozygous gene drive allele — Wild type

(b)

1 Regions of homology to genome flanking the guideRNA target site

Cas9   GuideRNA

2 Genomic DNA

Target site

Homologous recombination

3 Gene drive allele

4 Homologous allele

5 Homologous recombination

6 Homologous gene drive alleles

(c)

7

Cargo   Cas9   GuideRNA

Figure 15.23 **How gene drive alleles can spread through populations.**

⊙ How would the efficiency of gene drive be affected if the Cas9 gene were located on a different chromosome than the guideRNA target locus?

Gene drives for reducing populations of invasive species or agricultural pests could utilize various strategies. For example, the gene drive allele could be targeted to an essential gene, one in which phenotypic defects are minimal in heterozygotes but are severely deleterious in homozygotes. If the drive allele is only active (e.g., Cas9 is expressed) during meiosis, then heterozygous animals will be phenotypically normal but would pass the drive allele to a high proportion of their gametes. This pattern of inheritance would eventually lead to spread of the allele and a collapse of the population. Alternatively, in an organism with an XY sex chromosome system often found in animals, gene drives could selectively target destruction of a sex chromosome. For example, if a gene drive allele that targets sequences on the X chromosome leading to X-chromosome destruction is located on the Y chromosome, and its expression limited to spermatogenesis, it would target the destruction of the X chromosome in gametes. Thus, the only viable gametes produced would be ones harboring the Y chromosome, bringing about a reduction in viable females and eventually a population crash.

CONCERNS Given the potential of gene drive alleles to affect entire populations of organisms, with ripple effects spreading through entire ecosystems, there is great concern about how, or if, to deploy such systems as biological control agents. Because of this concern, the U.S. National Academy of Sciences convened a meeting to discuss both the potential applications of gene drive alleles and the containment protocols that must be in place when they are used, even in laboratory settings.

Containment would be needed at both the molecular and ecological levels. For example, a required molecular control would be to separate the Cas9 gene from the gene drive allele so that the gene containing the guideRNA and target site locus would be apart from (not linked to) and able to segregate from the Cas9 gene. Because the guideRNA would not be able to act as a gene drive allele without a supply of Cas9, the spread through a population would be greatly reduced and eventually extinguished. More sophisticated multicomponent systems are being tested to examine whether they would act through only a fixed number of generations and thereby perform as transient gene drive systems for local population control.

These new scientific possibilities raise some unprecedented ethical issues. From the earliest days in the development of recombinant DNA technologies, the potential ethical problems and possible environmental and other concerns have been the subject of intense debate. In 1975, following an initial self-imposed moratorium, scientists met at Asilomar Conference Grounds, in California, to draw up a set of guidelines addressing many of the safety concerns. Potential ethical problems raised by gene drive technology will need to be addressed by similar public debates.

SUMMARY

Mastering Genetics For activities, animations, and review quizzes, go to the Study Area.

15.1 Specific DNA Sequences Are Identified and Manipulated Using Recombinant DNA Technology

- Restriction enzymes, which cut at specific DNA sequences, are used to fragment large DNA molecules into defined smaller pieces.
- A restriction map of a DNA molecule can be constructed by analyzing patterns of DNA fragments after restriction enzyme digestion.
- DNA fragments can be ligated to create recombinant DNA molecules, usually composed of a vector that can be amplified in a biological system and a target DNA insert to be amplified.
- Although cohesive compatible ends facilitate the creation of recombinant DNA molecules, any two DNA fragments can be ligated if their ends are made blunt.
- Amplification of recombinant DNA molecules in a biological system allows the production of DNA clones.
- Bacterial artificial chromosomes allow the cloning of large DNA molecules.
- Genomic libraries are collections of cloned DNA fragments that represent the entire genome of an organism.
- cDNA libraries are collections of cloned DNA fragments that represent the mRNA population of an organism or tissue.

15.2 Introducing Foreign Genes into Genomes Creates Transgenic Organisms

- Genes introduced into an organism are called transgenes. Genes introduced from another species are termed heterologous transgenes.
- Transgenes can be introduced into microbes by homologous recombination into the chromosome.
- *Agrobacterium* and its tumor-inducing plasmid can be harnessed to create transgenic plants in which the transfer DNA carries the desired transgene.
- Transgenic *Drosophila* are created by injection into embryos of a *P* element transposon carrying the transgene.
- Transgenes are introduced into mice by direct injection of DNA into isolated cells. The injected DNA can be integrated either by homologous recombination or using CRISPR–Cas9–induced DNA breaks.
- Differentiated mammalian cells can be converted into pluripotent iPS cells by the activity of the Yamanaka transcription factors.
- Bacteriophage recombination systems can be used to manipulate DNA sequences in vitro and transgenes in vivo.

15.3 Gene Therapy Uses Recombinant DNA Technology

▌ Gene therapy is the application of recombinant DNA technology and transgenesis to treat human diseases.

▌ In somatic gene therapy, transgenes are targeted to somatic cells and are not heritable. In germinal gene therapy, transgenes are targeted to germ cells and are thus heritable.

▌ Recent approaches to gene therapy involve genome editing using CRISPR–Cas9.

15.4 Cloning of Plants and Animals Produces Genetically Identical Individuals

▌ Many plants reproduce clonally in nature, whereas clonal reproduction in animals is rare.

▌ Clonal reproduction in mammals requires reprogramming of differentiated somatic cells into stem cells.

PREPARING FOR PROBLEM SOLVING

In addition to the list of problem-solving tips and suggestions given here, you can go to the Study Guide and Solutions Manual that accompanies this book for help at solving problems.

1. Be familiar with the basic techniques of recombinant DNA technology. Understand how DNA molecules are manipulated in vitro and how clones are propagated in bacterial hosts

2. Know the similarities and differences between genomic and cDNA libraries.

3. Know the different techniques by which exogenous DNA (e.g., transgenes) are introduced into different organisms.

4. Know the approaches to somatic gene therapy using CRISPR–Cas9.

5. Recognize how the ways plants can be cloned differ from the ways animals can be cloned.

PROBLEMS

Mastering Genetics Visit for instructor-assigned tutorials and problems.

Chapter Concepts

For answers to selected even-numbered problems, see Appendix: Answers.

1. What purpose do the *bla* and *lacZ* genes serve in the plasmid vector pUC18?

2. The human genome is 3×10^9 bp in length.
   a. How many fragments would be predicted to result from the complete digestion of the human genome with the following enzymes: *Sau*3A (˘GATC), *Bam*HI (G˘GATCC), *Eco*RI (G˘AATTC), and *Not*I (GC˘GGCCGC)?
   b. How would your initial answer change if you knew that the average GC content of the human genome was 40%?

3. Ligase catalyzes a reaction between the 5′ phosphate and the 3′ hydroxyl groups at the ends of DNA molecules. The enzyme calf intestinal phosphatase catalyzes the removal of the 5′ phosphate from DNA molecules. What would be the consequence of treating a cloning vector, before ligation, with calf intestinal phosphatase?

4. You have constructed four different libraries: a genomic library made from DNA isolated from human brain tissue, a genomic library made from DNA isolated from human muscle tissue, a human brain cDNA library, and a human muscle cDNA library.
   a. Which of these would have the greatest diversity of sequences?
   b. Would the sequences contained in each library be expected to overlap completely, partially, or not at all with the sequences present in each of the other libraries?

5. Using the genomic libraries in Problem 4, you wish to clone the human gene encoding myostatin, which is expressed only in muscle cells.
   a. Assuming the human genome is 3×10^9 bp and that the average insert size in the genomic libraries is 100 kb, how frequently will a clone representing myostatin be found in the genomic library made from muscle?
   b. How frequently will a clone representing myostatin be found in the genomic library made from brain?
   c. How frequently will a clone representing myostatin be found in the cDNA library made from muscle?
   d. How frequently will a clone representing myostatin be found in the cDNA library made from brain?

6. The human genome is 3×10^9 bp. You wish to design a primer to amplify a specific gene in the genome. In general, what length of oligonucleotide would be sufficient to amplify a single unique sequence? To simplify your calculation, assume that all bases occur with an equal frequency.

7. Using animal models of human diseases can lead to insights into the cellular and genetic bases of the diseases. Duchenne muscular dystrophy (DMD) is the consequence of an X-linked recessive allele.
   a. How would you make a mouse model of DMD?
   b. How would you make a *Drosophila* model of DMD?

8. Compare methods for constructing homologous recombinant transgenic mice and yeast.

9. Chimeric gene-fusion products can be used for medical or industrial purposes. One idea is to produce biological therapeutics for human medical use in animals from which the products can be easily harvested—in the milk of sheep or cattle, for example. Outline how you would produce human insulin in the milk of sheep.

10. Why are diseases of the blood simpler targets for treatment by gene therapy than are many other genetic diseases?

11. Injection of double-stranded RNA can lead to gene silencing by degradation of RNA molecules complementary to either strand of the dsRNA. Could RNAi (see Sections 13.3 and 14.3) be used in gene therapy for a defect caused by a recessive allele? A dominant allele? If so, what might be the major obstacle to using RNAi as a therapeutic agent?

12. Compare and contrast methods for making transgenic plants and transgenic *Drosophila*.

13. It is often desirable to insert cDNAs into a cloning vector in such a way that all the cDNA clones will have the same orientation with respect to the sequences of the plasmid. This is referred to as directional cloning. Outline how you would directionally clone a cDNA library in the plasmid vector pUC18.

14. A major advance in the 1980s was the development of technology to synthesize short oligonucleotides. This work both facilitated DNA sequencing and led to the advent of the development of PCR. Recently, rapid advances have occurred in the technology to chemically synthesize DNA, and sequences up to 10 kb are now readily produced. As this process becomes more economical, how will it affect the gene-cloning approaches outlined in this chapter? In other words, what types of techniques does this new technology have potential to supplant, and what techniques will not be affected by it?

Application and Integration

For answers to selected even-numbered problems, see Appendix: Answers.

15. The bacteriophage lambda genome can exist in either a linear form (see Figures 15.1 and 15.8) or a circular form.
    a. How many fragments will be formed by restriction enzyme digestion with *Xho*I alone, with *Xba*I alone, and with both *Xho*I and *Xba*I in the linear and circular forms of the lambda genome?
    b. Diagram the resulting fragments as they would appear on an agarose gel after electrophoresis.

16. The restriction enzymes *Xho*I and *Sal*I cut their specific sequences as shown below:

*Xho*I	5'–C	TCGAG–3'
	3'–GAGCT	C–5'
*Sal*I	5'–G	TCGAC–3'
	3'–CAGCT	G–5'

Can the sticky ends created by *Xho*I and *Sal*I sites be ligated? If yes, can the resulting sequences be cleaved by either *Xho*I or *Sal*I?

17. The bacteriophage φX174 has a single-stranded DNA genome of 5386 bases. During DNA replication, double-stranded forms of the genome are generated. In an effort to create a restriction map of φX174, you digest the z-stranded form of the genome with several restriction enzymes and obtain the following results. Draw a map of the φX174 genome.

PstI	5386		*Pst*I + *Psi*I	3078, 2308
PsiI	5386		*Pst*I + *Dra*I	331, 1079, 3976
DraI	4307, 1079		*Psi*I + *Dra*I	898, 1079, 3409

18. To further analyze the *CRABS CLAW* gene (see Problems 19 and 20), you create a map of the genomic clone. The 11-kb *Eco*RI fragment is ligated into the *Eco*RI site of the MCS of the vector shown in Problem 18. You digest the double-stranded form of the genome with several restriction enzymes and obtain the following results. Draw, as far as possible, a map of the genomic clone of *CRABS CLAW*.

*Eco*RI	11.0, 3.0		
*Eco*RI + *Xba*I	4.5, 6.5, 3.0	*Xba*I	4.5, 9.5
*Eco*RI + *Xho*I	10.2, 3.0, 0.8	*Xho*I	13.2, 0.8
*Eco*RI + *Sal*I	6.0, 5.0, 3.0	*Sal*I	6.0, 8.0
*Eco*RI + *Hind*III	9.0, 3.0, 1.5, 0.5	*Hind*III	12.0, 1.5, 0.5

What restriction digest would help resolve any ambiguity in the map?

19. You have isolated a genomic clone with an *Eco*RI fragment of 11 kb that encompasses the *CRABS CLAW* gene (see Problem 18). You digest the genomic clone with *Hin*dIII and note that the 11-kb *Eco*RI fragment is split into three fragments of 9 kb, 1.5 kb, and 0.5 kb.

   a. Does this tell you anything about where the *CRABS CLAW* gene is located within the 11-kb genomic clone?

   b. Restriction enzyme sites within a cDNA clone are often also found in the genomic sequence. Can you think of a reason why occasionally this is not the case? What about the converse: Are restriction enzyme sites in a genomic clone always in a cDNA clone of the same gene?

20. You have identified a 0.80-kb cDNA clone that contains the entire coding sequence of the *Arabidopsis* gene *CRABS CLAW*. In the construction of the cDNA library, linkers with *Eco*RI sites were added to each end of the cDNA, and the cDNA was inserted into the *Eco*RI site of the MCS of the vector shown in the accompanying figure. You perform digests on the *CRABS CLAW* cDNA clone with restriction enzymes and obtain the following results. Can you determine the orientation of the cDNA clone with respect to the restriction enzyme sites in the vector? The restriction enzyme sites listed in the dark blue region are found only in the MCS of the vector.

*Eco*RI	0.8, 3.0
*Hin*dIII	0.3, 3.5
*Eco*RI + *Hin*dIII	0.3, 0.5, 3.0

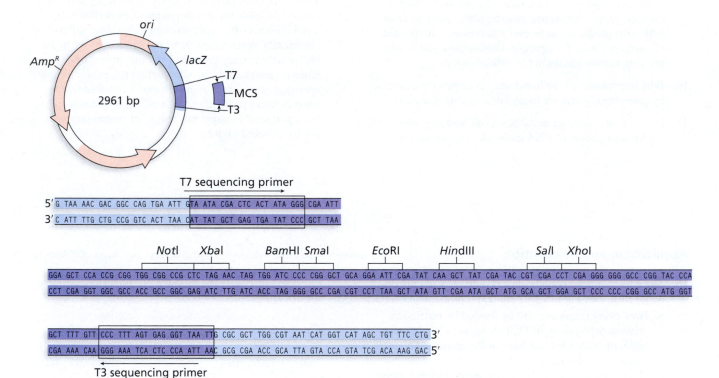

21. You have isolated another cDNA clone of the *CRABS CLAW* gene from a cDNA library constructed using the vector shown in Problem 20. The cDNA was directionally cloned using the *Eco*RI and *Xho*I sites. You sequence the recombinant plasmid using primers complementary to the T7 and T3 promoter sites flanking the MCS (the positions of these sequences are shown in the figure in Problem 20). The first 30 to 60 bases of sequence are usually discarded since they tend to contain errors.

   a. Which of the sequences shown below represents the 5′ end of the gene? Which sequence represents the 3′ end of the gene?

   b. Will the long stretch of T residues in the T3 sequence exist in the genomic sequence of the gene?

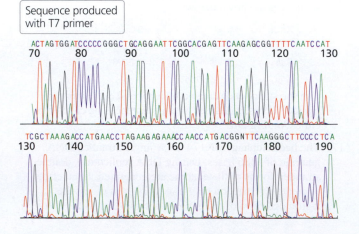

Sequence produced with T7 primer

Genomics: Genetics from a Whole-Genome Perspective

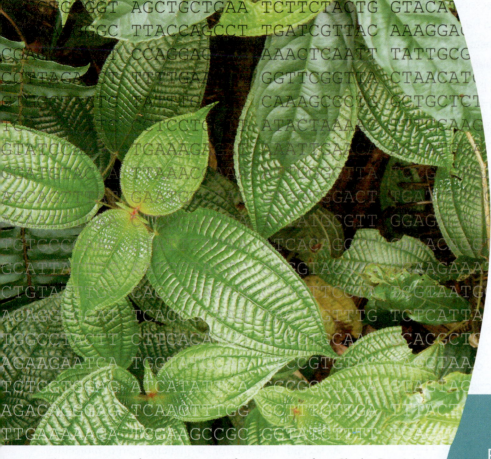

CHAPTER OUTLINE

16.1 Structural Genomics Provides a Catalog of Genes in a Genome

16.2 Annotation Ascribes Biological Function to DNA Sequences

16.3 Evolutionary Genomics Traces the History of Genomes

16.4 Functional Genomics Aims to Elucidate Gene Function

ESSENTIAL IDEAS

▌ The goal of sequencing the human genome stimulated technological advances that enabled its realization. In addition to the human genome, researchers have now sequenced the genomes of hundreds of bacteria and archaea and scores of eukaryotes.

▌ The evolutionary history of a species is written in its genome and can be read both from its gene content and its chromosome architecture.

▌ Genome-wide analyses of gene expression, protein–protein interactions, protein–DNA interactions, and genetic interactions provide insights into the biological functions of the genes.

The sequencing of entire genomes of many species from Charles Darwin's "tangled bank" has clarified evolutionary relationships of life on Earth and provided the genetic blueprints that define organisms, although the precise functions of most genes are presently unknown.

Genomics, the scientific study of biological processes from the perspective of the whole genome, originated in the Human Genome Project (HGP). This audacious project was initiated in the 1980s to sequence and analyze the human genome. At the time, neither the technologies for generating large amounts of DNA sequence nor the computing power to analyze such large amounts of data existed.

Although a primary goal of the HGP was to sequence the human genome, several model genetic organisms were also sequenced under its auspices, including those that have appeared most often in the pages of this book: *Escherichia coli*, *Saccharomyces cerevisiae*, *Caenorhabditis elegans*, *Drosophila melanogaster*, *Arabidopsis thaliana*, and *Mus musculus*. The genome sequences of these model organisms have contributed to our understanding of the organisms themselves as well as to interpretations of human genome structure, function, and evolution. Since then, the genomes of thousands of other bacteria, hundreds of other eukaryotes, and many archaea have also been sequenced. Due to ever-decreasing costs and ever-improving technologies, genome sequencing is now so affordable and routine that it is becoming part of your medical record. In the future, species may be defined by characteristics of their genomic sequence.

In the initial analyses of the genomes of model organisms, two findings stand out. First, even in well-studied organisms, only a fraction of genes identified by genome sequencing had been previously identified by forward genetic analysis; this brings up the question of the function of all the previously unknown genes. Second, genomic analyses have also revealed the highly dynamic nature of genomes, providing insights into the extent of differences between individuals of a species and between species, and also into the rates at which DNA sequences evolve.

This chapter provides an overview of genomics by describing three of its major subdivisions. **Structural genomics** is concerned with the sequencing of whole genomes and the cataloging, or annotation, of sequences within a given genome. It provides a parts list of the genetic tool kit of an organism. **Evolutionary genomics** is the comparison of genomes, both within and between species. It illuminates the genetic bases of similarities and differences between individuals or species. **Functional genomics** uses genomic sequences to understand gene function in an organism. Together, these three approaches contribute to the ultimate goal of understanding the role of every gene a given genome contains.

16.1 Structural Genomics Provides a Catalog of Genes in a Genome

Genomes vary enormously in size, from several hundred kilobases in some bacterial species to several thousand megabases in some vertebrate and plant species (**Table 16.1**).

Genomes may consist of a single DNA molecule, as in many bacterial and archaeal species, or of hundreds of chromosomes, as in some eukaryotic species. From a broad perspective, gene number generally increases with organismal complexity. However, genomes also vary in their proportions of coding versus noncoding DNA sequences, and in multicellular eukaryotes, genome size can increase much more than gene number due to a disproportionate increase in noncoding DNA.

Ideally, one would start sequencing a genome from one end of each chromosome and proceed to the other end. In reality, this ideal is not yet possible. Even the smallest bacterial genomes are thousands of times longer than the 600 to 900 bp that can be sequenced in a traditional single dideoxy sequencing reaction, and longer than the "sequence reads" (sequenced DNA fragments) that can be generated with third-generation sequencing (see Chapter 7). Clearly, to sequence any genome would require many iterations of these procedures.

There are two basic strategies for sequencing large DNA molecules. The first technique, **primer walking** (**Figure 16.1a**), relies on the successive synthesis of primers based on the progressive attainment of new sequence information. The DNA sequence information obtained in the first dideoxy sequencing reaction provides a foundation for the design of a second primer. If the second primer is 600 to 800 bases from the first primer, the second dideoxy sequencing reaction can extend the known sequence up to 1800 bases from the first primer. Reiterations of this process allow technicians to "walk" along a long DNA molecule, designing new primers every 600 to 800 bases. The speed with which a molecule is sequenced by this method is limited by its reiterative nature.

A second method for sequencing large molecules of DNA is **shotgun sequencing**, an approach that relies on redundant sequencing of fragmented target DNA in the hope that all regions will be sequenced at least a few times. In this technique, a large DNA molecule (e.g., a BAC clone of 100 kb or an entire genome) is fragmented into smaller pieces (**Figure 16.1b**). The fragments may be generated by partial restriction enzyme digestion or by shearing the DNA. The key here is that fragmentation is done in such a way as to produce random and hence overlapping pieces of the original molecule. The ends of these fragments can then be sequenced using a primer based on vector sequences if the fragments are ligated into cloning vectors, or based on the added linker sequence if a next-generation sequencing approach is being used (see Figure 7.31). The collection of fragments can be considered a *library* of sequences from the larger DNA molecule. The strategy is to sequence enough fragments to assemble a complete contiguous sequence on the basis of overlaps in the generated sequences. Computer algorithms are available to perform much of this task, allowing data from millions of sequencing reactions to be assembled

Table 16.1	Examples of Sequenced Genomes					
Organism	Description	Genome Size (Mb)[a]	Predicted Number of Protein-Encoding Genes[b]	Number of Genes in Multigene Families[c]	Number of Genes with Assigned Molecular Function[d]	Predicted Number of Genes/Mb
Escherichia coli	Gram-negative gammaproteobacterium	4.64	4262	3372	1824	919
Synechocystis sp.	Single-celled cyanobacterium	3.57	3482	2459	1094	975
Chlamydia trachomatis	Obligate intracellular parasitic bacterium	1.04	895	614	361	861
Sulfolobus solfataricus	Single-celled archaean	3.0	2981	1889	974	994
Chlamydomonas reinhardtii	Single-celled chlorophyte alga	112	14,404	8660	4570	129
Arabidopsis thaliana	Multicellular flowering plant	136	27,352	24,241	10,257	201
Oryza sativa	Multicellular flowering plant (rice)	427	62,904	38,416	14,670	147
Saccharomyces cerevisiae	Single-celled fungus (baker's yeast)	12.2	6728	4827	2823	551
Neurospora crassa	Multicellular fungus (bread mold)	41	9780	6830	3528	239
Caenorhabditis elegans	Multicellular nematode worm	103	20,452	15,027	6814	199
Drosophila melanogaster	Multicellular insect (fruit fly)	169	14,217	11,079	5853	84
Danio rerio	Multicellular fish (zebrafish)	1464	27,187	25,210	14,219	19
Nematostella vectensis	Multicellular sea anemone	450	24,768	18,513	8708	55
Gallus gallus	Multicellular bird (chicken)	1230	15,789	14,698	8313	12.8
Ornithorhynchus anatinus	Multicellular monotreme (platypus)	2073	21,122	17,441	9695	10.2
Mus musculus	Multicellular mammal (mouse)	2731	22,322	21,229	11,843	8.2
Pan troglodytes	Multicellular mammal (chimpanzee)	2996	18,693	17,665	9794	6.2
Homo sapiens	Multicellular mammal (human)	3101	20,972	19,900	10,924	6.8

[a]Genome sizes given for most multicellular eukaryotes are estimates because sequences of the heterochromatic regions of the genomes are often unknown.
[b]Gene number estimates are based on 2015 annotations and will change with new experimental evidence.
[c]Gene families are evolutionarily related genes.
[d]Molecular function is defined as the predicted function of the protein at a biochemical level, not necessarily the biological function.

quickly. Thus, in shotgun sequencing, the sequencing of the many different fragments proceeds simultaneously ("in parallel"), allowing long DNA molecules to be sequenced rapidly.

Clearly the more efficient way to sequence DNA molecules (i.e., chromosomes) millions of bases in length is to employ a shotgun sequencing strategy, breaking the long DNA fragments into smaller ones and sequencing the fragments in parallel. Computer algorithms are then used to assemble the sequences of the fragments into a single **contiguous sequence (contig)**. Two basic approaches to this general mode of attack differ only in the starting DNA to be fragmented and sequenced. In one approach, called **whole-genome shotgun (WGS) sequencing**, DNA representing the entire genome is fragmented into smaller pieces, and a large number of fragments are chosen at random and sequenced.

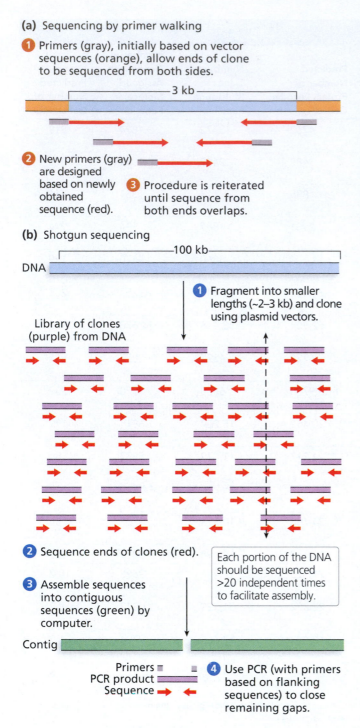

(a) Sequencing by primer walking

1 Primers (gray), initially based on vector sequences (orange), allow ends of clone to be sequenced from both sides.

├─── 3 kb ───┤

2 New primers (gray) are designed based on newly obtained sequence (red).

3 Procedure is reiterated until sequence from both ends overlaps.

(b) Shotgun sequencing

├────100 kb────┤

DNA

1 Fragment into smaller lengths (~2–3 kb) and clone using plasmid vectors.

Library of clones (purple) from DNA

2 Sequence ends of clones (red).

3 Assemble sequences into contiguous sequences (green) by computer.

Contig

Each portion of the DNA should be sequenced >20 independent times to facilitate assembly.

Primers ▪   ▪
PCR product ▬▬▬   ▬▬▬
Sequence ➡   ⬅

4 Use PCR (with primers based on flanking sequences) to close remaining gaps.

Figure 16.1 **Primer walking versus shotgun sequencing approaches.**

In the second approach, often called **clone-by-clone sequencing**, each chromosome is first broken into overlapping clones that are then arranged in linear order to produce a physical map of the genome. Each clone in the map is then sequenced separately. The WGS approach is applicable to any genome and is the approach in widespread use today. The clone-by-clone approach, which has been supplanted by the WGS approach, relies on the availability of specific genetic resources (such as genetic and physical maps) and thus was applicable only to some model organisms.

Whole-Genome Shotgun Sequencing

The WGS approach sequences genomic DNA by the shotgun method without prior construction of a physical map. For this reason, WGS can be applied to any genome. Once the genomic DNA is broken into fragments and sequenced, the sequences are assembled into contigs based on sequence overlaps (Figure 16.1b). To ensure enough overlapping of sequences for this purpose, technicians commonly generate sequences totaling approximately 30 to 40 times the actual length of the genome (this degree of overlap is called 30–40× coverage); thus, any one sequence occurs in multiple reads, minimizing the chance of sequencing errors. The ease with which sequences are assembled into contigs depends on the lengths of the sequencing reads, and these vary between technologies (see Section 7.5). Prior to the development of third-generation sequencing technologies, sequence reads were limited to less than 1000 bp in length, but now reads many kilobases in length may be utilized in WGS approaches.

Repetitive DNA presents an obstacle in the assembly of WGS sequencing data. Dispersed repetitive DNA sequences (for example, transposons and retrotranposons) interfere with genome assembly, as explained in **Figure 16.2**, because they can map to multiple locations within the genome. Consequently, the assembled sequence often remains broken at repetitive sequences. One way of circumventing this problem is to use *paired-end sequence* data to bridge the gaps. In **paired-end sequencing**, sequence is generated from both ends of genomic DNA fragments of known size. The paired-end sequences, some of which are on the ends of fragments containing a repetitive element, can then be used to assemble the fragments into a **scaffold**, a set of contigs that are physically linked by paired-end sequences. The relative orientations of paired-end sequences and their distance from one another can be incorporated into assembly algorithms to construct the scaffold and ultimately show the locations of repetitive elements. Despite the high rate of errors with third-generation sequencing technologies, the use of their long reads to facilitate assembly of contigs into scaffolds is becoming commonplace.

Let's examine how scaffold assembly works. Typically, several genomic libraries are generated, each containing cloned DNA fragments of a different size (**Figure 16.3**)—for example, one library of 2- to 3-kb clones, a second of 6- to 8-kb clones, and a third of larger clones (20 to 30 or more kilobases). Paired-end sequence data generated from clones in the different libraries provide information on whether two particular sequences are physically linked and the approximate distance between the two sequences. Even if repetitive DNA occurs between the paired-end sequences, they can still be linked into a scaffold. Dispersed repetitive DNA in the genome often consists either of simple, short repeats

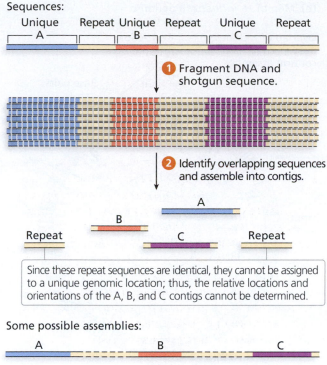

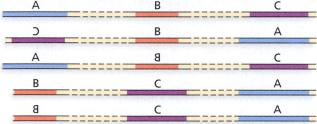

Figure 16.2 **The problem of repetitive DNA.**

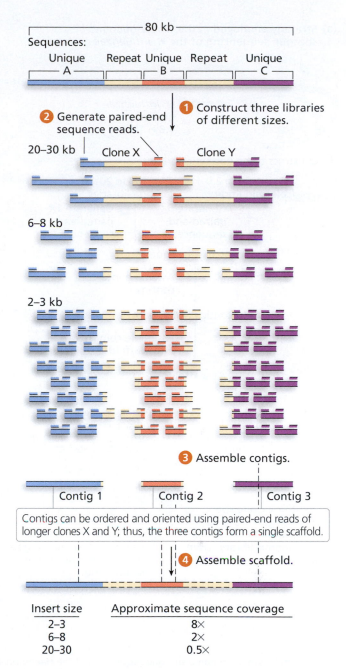

Insert size	Approximate sequence coverage
2–3	8×
6–8	2×
20–30	0.5×

Figure 16.3 **Paired-end shotgun sequencing strategy.**

(microsatellites or minisatellites) or transposable element sequences (up to 10,000 bp). Most repeat sequences will be flanked by paired-end sequence from at least one of the differently sized libraries. However, repetitive sequences longer than the largest available clones (for example, centromeric repeat sequences, in many eukaryotes) cannot be spanned using this approach and thus cause gaps to remain between certain contigs.

For an idea of how the WGS approach works in practice, let us consider two examples, a small bacterial genome with little repetitive DNA and a large eukaryotic genome containing a significant proportion of repetitive DNA.

WGS Sequencing of a Bacterial Genome The first genome to be sequenced by a paired-end WGS approach (at The Institute for Genomic Research, or TIGR, in 1995) was that of *Haemophilus influenzae*, a Gram-negative bacterium whose natural host is humans. The *H. influenzae* genome is 1.8×10^6 bp and has relatively few dispersed repetitive elements. Paired-end sequences were generated from three genomic libraries: one plasmid library and two libraries composed using lambda (λ) bacteriophage chromosomes (in a manner similar to using bacterial chromosomes) as vectors (**Figure 16.4a**). The sequence data from the three

libraries were assembled into 140 contigs whose relative orders and orientations were unknown. Since the *H. influenzae* genome is a single circular chromosome, the assembled sequence had 140 gaps for which sequence information was lacking. However, with information on the physical linkage of paired-end reads, the gaps could be divided into two categories: 98 were **sequence gaps** within a scaffold, meaning gaps for which a clone was available for further sequencing that could close the gap; and 42 were **physical gaps** between scaffolds, meaning gaps for which there was no clone to supply the sequence.

Sequence gaps were closed by sequencing of spanning clones identified through paired-end sequencing. Two

(a) Strategy employed in the whole-genome shotgun sequencing of the *H. influenzae* genome

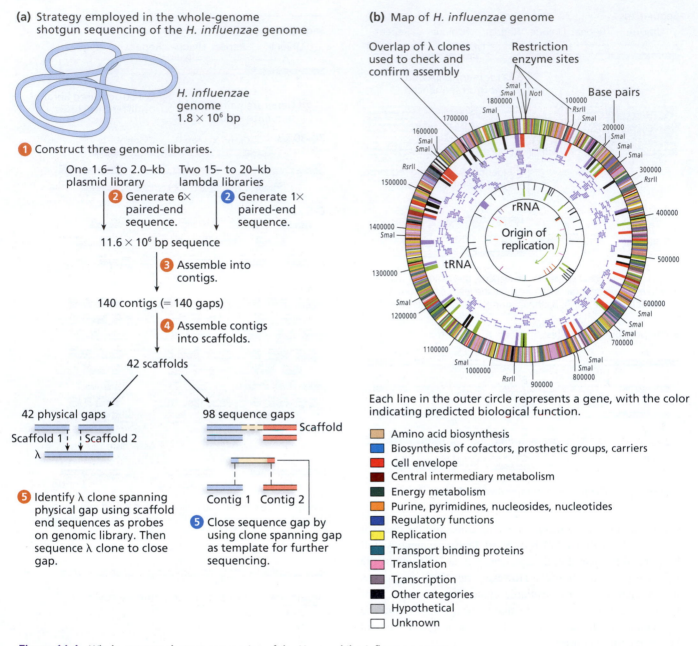

(b) Map of *H. influenzae* genome

Figure 16.4 **Whole-genome shotgun sequencing of the *Haemophilus influenzae* genome.**

approaches were combined to close the physical gaps. First, the lambda genomic libraries were probed with sequences derived from the ends of the scaffolds: If a single genomic clone hybridized with ends of two scaffolds, the clone should span the gap between the two scaffolds. Second, polymerase chain reaction (PCR) methodology, using combinations of primers specific to sequences at the ends of scaffolds, was employed to amplify spanning sequences. With this combination of approaches, the entire 1,830,137-bp sequence of the *H. influenzae* genome was assembled into a single contig (**Figure 16.4b**).

WGS Sequencing of a Eukaryotic Genome The genome of *Drosophila* was the first large eukaryotic genome containing a significant fraction of repetitive DNA to be sequenced using a WGS approach. The *Drosophila* genome is approximately 170 Mb, of which 120 Mb is considered to be euchromatic and the remaining 50 Mb heterochromatic. Because centromeric heterochromatic DNA is not efficiently cloned, owing to its highly repetitive nature, only the euchromatic portion of the genome was initially sequenced, using the Sanger sequencing method (see Section 7.5).

Paired-end sequencing was accomplished using three genomic libraries, of 2 kb, 10 kb, and 130 kb (**Figure 16.5**). The 10-kb clones were large enough to span most of the dispersed repetitive elements (such as transposons and retrotransposons) found in the *Drosophila* genome, whereas the 130-kb clones provided long-range linking information

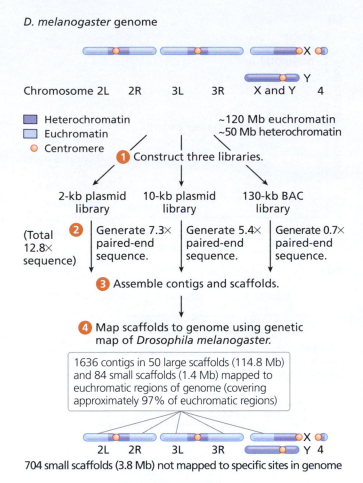

D. melanogaster genome

Chromosome 2L   2R   3L   3R   X and Y   4

■ Heterochromatin   ~120 Mb euchromatin
□ Euchromatin   ~50 Mb heterochromatin
○ Centromere

① Construct three libraries.

2-kb plasmid   10-kb plasmid   130-kb BAC
library   library   library

(Total
12.8×
sequence)

② Generate 7.3×   Generate 5.4×   Generate 0.7×
paired-end   paired-end   paired-end
sequence.   sequence.   sequence.

③ Assemble contigs and scaffolds.

④ Map scaffolds to genome using genetic
map of Drosophila melanogaster.

1636 contigs in 50 large scaffolds (114.8 Mb)
and 84 small scaffolds (1.4 Mb) mapped to
euchromatic regions of genome (covering
approximately 97% of euchromatic regions)

2L   2R   3L   3R   X   Y   4

704 small scaffolds (3.8 Mb) not mapped to specific sites in genome

Figure 16.5 Whole-genome shotgun sequencing of the *Drosophila melanogaster* genome.

from which to infer overall structure in the sequence assembly. Most of the 12×-coverage sequence generated could be assembled into 50 scaffolds representing almost 115 Mb of the euchromatic portion of the genome. The remaining sequence was assembled into almost 800 additional scaffolds representing about 5 Mb; thus, the assembled *Drosophila* genome sequence had several hundred physical gaps. Genetic and physical maps of *Drosophila* were used to assign the 50 large scaffolds and an additional 84 scaffolds to specific regions of the four chromosomes, corresponding to most of the euchromatic regions of the chromosome arms.

The WGS sequencing of the *Drosophila* genome benefited from the genetic resources that *Drosophila* geneticists had constructed throughout the 20th century, such as genetic maps of morphological and molecular markers. These tools allowed sequences to be assigned to specific chromosomal locations. They also provided a benchmark for assessing the completeness of the assembled sequence: Of the 2783 previously known genes of *Drosophila*, 2778 could be found in the scaffolds, thus accounting for an estimated 97.5% of the euchromatic DNA. Subsequently, next-generation and third-generation sequencing technologies (see Section 7.5) have

been used to sequence the *Drosophila* genome at greater depth, leading to more complete coverage and assembly into scaffolds representing chromosomes or chromosome arms. The most up-to-date assembly of the *Drosophila* genome can be found at www.flybase.org.

The Human Genome The U.S. Human Genome Project (HGP) began officially in 1990 with a projected timescale of 15 years and a budget of $3 billion. This government-funded project took a clone-by-clone approach to sequencing the human genome; therefore, it started by developing tools to build a physical map. In 1998, however, the newly founded Celera Corporation announced that it would provide a human genome sequence in just 3 years by using a WGS sequencing approach. Competition from this private company increased the pace of the publicly funded project, so that the genome sequencing was completed 4 years ahead of schedule.

In 2000, then-President Bill Clinton, appearing at a press conference with J. Craig Venter, the president of Celera, and with Francis Collins, the director of the Human Genome Sequencing Consortium, announced the completion of a "draft" of the human genome sequence. In fact, there were two draft sequences—one furnished by the HGP clone-by-clone approach and one by the Celera WGS approach—and both had numerous gaps. In subsequent years, a "complete" sequence of the human genome has been generated by targeted sequencing of specific regions of the genome to connect adjacent contigs and ensure that the error rate is less than 1/10,000. The gaps between the scaffolds and contigs were closed by the same approaches described above for the *H. influenzae* and *Drosophila* genomes, resulting in a genomic sequence consisting of approximately one contig for each chromosome arm.

Reference Genomes and Resequencing

It is convenient to speak of "sequencing the genome of a species" as though one genome represents all members of that species, but logic tells us that this is not the case. Allelic differences, defined by polymorphisms in DNA sequences, are the ultimate cause of phenotypic differences between individuals of a species. And this genetic diversity, the raw material on which natural selection can act, is seen in intraspecific comparisons of the genomes of any two individuals that are not clones.

The study of allelic distributions is the foundation of population genetics (the subject of Chapter 20). Just as the evolutionary history of life in general is written in the genomes of the different species, the evolutionary history of a species is reflected in the distribution of polymorphic alleles among populations. The field of population genetics has been established and active for many decades, but it is just beginning to examine genetic diversity from a genomic perspective. We explore this theme further in regard to humans in Application Chapter D: Human Evolutionary Genetics.

The sequences representing the genomes of model organisms were derived from either a haploid individual or an inbred (homozygous at most or all loci) laboratory strain of a diploid organism and thus lack polymorphisms. The DNA sequence of the individual or individuals used to construct the initial complete genome sequence is called the **reference genome sequence**. Once a reference genome sequence is constructed, polymorphisms in the species can be identified by comparing the reference genome sequence with the genome sequences of different strains collected from different populations derived from the wild. This allows the reference genome sequence to be refined and enhanced to reflect genetic variation not displayed in the originally sequenced genome. The use of next-generation sequencing technologies, as well as the use of the reference genome sequence to expedite the assembly of WGS sequence data from each new subject, makes such "resequencing" of genomes relatively inexpensive. Thus, thousands of human genome sequences have now been produced and used to augment and improve understanding of the reference human genome sequence.

Genetic variation ranges from differences in the identity of a single nucleotide—that is, single nucleotide polymorphisms (SNPs)—to larger-scale structural variations, such as insertions and deletions—collectively called *indels*—and inversions. These indels and inversions are in turn—collectively called "structural variants," and their prevalence—was previously unknown until large-scale sequencing studies brought them to light, because they are too small to be detectable by karyotype analysis. A specific type of indel, called a **copy-number variant (CNV)**, is a repeated section of genome where each repeat is greater than 1 kb in length (**Figure 16.6a**). Although many CNVs are small, some are hundreds of kilobases long, span several genes, and result in differences in gene dosage. The larger deletions that occur as structural variations are often in chromosomal regions that are present in more than one copy due to previous duplications, suggesting that genes in the deleted segments would have been redundant. A likely origin of indels is the occurrence of unequal crossing over after mispairing during meiosis via misalignment of repetitive sequences (**Figure 16.6b**). An unexpected observation from sequencing multiple genomes from a single species is that individuals can vary substantially in gene content, including genes present in some individuals but not in others, due to CNVs. The **pangenome** is the entire set of genes present in a species, with the core genome being genes present in all individuals and the variable genome composed of genes present in only some individuals.

Studies analyzing genome sequences of parents and their offspring indicate that 8–25 kb of CNV variation accumulates due to mutation in each individual's germ cells in each generation. Likewise, studies analyzing genome sequences of parents and their offspring indicate that SNP variation accumulates due to mutation at the rate of about 30 to 50 new SNPs in each individual's germ cells in each generation. This is a rate of about 1 change in every 10^8 bp, a figure remarkably similar to that observed in similar

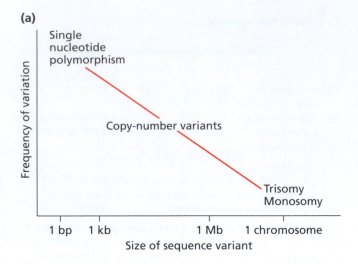

(a)

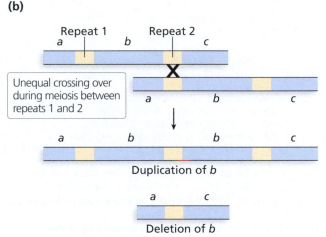

(b)

Figure 16.6 Copy-number variants. (a) Relationship between size of DNA polymorphisms and their frequency. **(b)** CNVs can be formed during meiosis by unequal crossing over mediated by repetitive DNA.

⊙ **Explain how CNVs can change in length.**

experiments in the flowering plant *Arabidopsis*, suggesting this error rate may be near the limit of DNA replication fidelity. We will explore human genetic variation further in Application Chapter D.

Metagenomics

In both the number of individual organisms and their total mass, microbial populations constitute the majority of life on Earth. However, unlike model genetic organisms, which are convenient for scientists to study, only a small fraction of microbes can be cultivated in the laboratory. How can we begin to understand microbial diversity without being able to grow the necessary range of microorganisms in the lab? One approach is to apply WGS sequencing to DNA isolated from entire natural communities consisting of a range of organisms. The genetic material or data derived from such a sequencing project is called a **metagenome**.

One of the first metagenomics projects provides an example. It was an environmental genomic shotgun sequencing of DNA isolated from microorganisms from the Sargasso Sea, a region of ocean bounded by the Gulf Stream off the southeast coast of the United States. In this study, approximately 265 Mb of sequence was generated and assembled into a large number of contigs, representing an estimated 1800 different genomes. However, none of the estimated 1800 genomes was complete, and many were represented by only one or a few contigs. This situation highlights a complication arising in metagenomic studies: Species in any given environmental sample are not equally represented, and so data from common species are over-weighted relative to those of scarcer ones. Consequently, any complete genome sequences that are produced are likely to belong to very common species, whereas genomes of rare species are represented by only a small number of contigs.

Despite such limitations, metagenomic analyses provide information on species diversity and relative population levels in an environmental setting and also contribute to the identification of gene sequences of organisms living in a particular environment. Such analyses have been applied, for example, to ecological communities living in acidic mine tailings, contaminated groundwater, and drinking-water systems and also to more "natural" (less human-influenced) ecosystems such as soils, oceans, and hot springs. The sequencing of ancient DNA (i.e., DNA from long-dead organisms) can also be considered a metagenomics task, given the inevitable contamination of the ancient sample with microorganisms over the years (often millenia) since the organism of interest was alive.

EXPERIMENTAL INSIGHT 16.1 presents the results of metagenomic analyses of several microbial biomes of humans, including the gut, mouth, and skin, revealing that, collectively, our microbial biomes possess a comparable number of genes with that of our own genome. The same analytical approaches can be applied to any biological system

EXPERIMENTAL INSIGHT 16.1

Our Communities Within and Upon

When we look in the mirror, we like to think we are looking at just ourselves, but the number of microbes within and upon us, primarily bacteria, is about the same as the number of our own cells, though the microbes comprise only about 1 kg of our weight. Perhaps the first to recognize that we are host to our own microbiome was Antonie van Leeuwenhoek, who, scraping "gritty matter" from between his teeth, observed the "animalcules," or bacteria, in his dental plaque in 1683. Subsequently, bacterial culturing techniques demonstrated that microbes inhabit many parts of our bodies; but as has since been revealed by the application of metagenomic shotgun sequencing, only a small fraction of the microbial diversity in and on our bodies was culturable. Metagenomics has revolutionized our thinking on this topic, leading to the present view that each of us has our own private ecosystems, complete with diverse habitats and ecology.

DIGESTIVE MICROBIOME

Our inner mucosal surfaces (gastrointestinal tract and mouth) and skin are dominated by four phyla of bacteria: Actino-bacteria, Firmicutes, Bacteroidetes, and Proteobacteria. It is becoming apparent that the makeup of our gut microbial community, in particular, influences our health and well-being, and its composition is influenced by our diet. Metagenomic sequencing of the gut microbiomes from hundreds of individuals revealed that these microbiomes fall into three general types of gastrointestinal bacterial communities, or enterotypes, corresponding strongly to long-term dietary habits. For example, high protein and animal fat consumption is correlated with the *Bacteroides* enterotype, and a high carbohydrate diet is correlated with a *Prevotella* enterotype, suggesting there is feedback between diet and habitat favoring growth of specific bacterial groups.

A striking example of how diet can influence our resident microbes is the occurrence of a unique lateral gene transfer event in Japanese individuals who eat substantial amounts of red algae, the "wrapping" used in sushi. In this case, genes encoding enzymes that break down red algal polysaccharides have been transferred from bacteria that normally live on the red algae to *Bacillus* species resident in the human gut. Thus, the bacteria in people who consume quantities of red algae evolve to better utilize this food source.

We obtain our initial gut microbiome from our mother's birth canal and subsequently from her milk. Those born by caesarean section miss out on these potentially important contributions. Short-term changes in diet do not appear to induce changes in gut microbial communities, but major perturbations, such as antibiotic usage, can alter them. Normally, the ecology of the gastrointestinal community is robust and rebounds to its former composition even after major insults. However, sometimes new communities, often detrimental to the health of their host, take over, and these may be resistant to removal by antibiotics. A seemingly radical method of displacing these unwanted microbes by doing a fecal transplant from a healthy individual appears to be highly effective, suggesting that similar transplant approaches may be capable of replacing "bad" microbiota with "good." Several disease states, including Crohn's disease, colorectal cancer, and irritable bowel syndrome, are associated with alterations of the gut microbiome, highlighting the critical relationship we share with our ecosystems.

SKIN MICROBIOME

Our skin offers about 1.8 m^2 of diverse habitats colonized by microbes. Despite our bathing and shedding of skin cells, our bacterial communities remain relatively constant and are dominated by the same four phyla as our guts, but with Actinobacteria more abundant.

(continued)

Three distinct skin habitats—moist, dry, and sebaceous—are created by variations in skin thickness, folds, and density of glands and hairs. The three habitat types are colonized by distinct bacterial communities, with greater similarity arising from similar habitat type than from topographic proximity. In transplant experiments where forehead (sebaceous) and forearm (dry) habitats were populated with tongue bacteria, the tongue bacteria remained for some time at the forearm site but were quickly replaced by "native" bacteria on the forehead. This research and temporal monitoring of bacterial communities indicate that the moist and sebaceous habitats have more stable communities than the dry skin areas. In contrast, the dry skin areas, such as the forearm, heel, and buttock, having more exposure to the surrounding environment, may be colonized opportunistically by a broader range of bacteria. If we are born by the normal birth process, we acquire a coating of primarily *Lactobacillus* in our mother's birth canal. This is replaced by habitat-characteristic communities in the first years of our life.

Although it is not yet clear how many of our microbes are commensal, symbiotic, or pathogenic in relation to us or each other, it is becoming clear that they exert a significant influence on our health and well-being. In particular, the proper development of our immune system, both when it is being established during infancy and later when protecting our internal mucosal system, is influenced by the composition of our microbiome. Experiments manipulating the gut microbiomes of mice suggest that intestinal microbiota can even influence brain chemistry and behavior. Thus, next time you look in the mirror, ponder the ecosystem you are cultivating and how its denizens are contributing to your life.

from which purified DNA belonging to a single species is difficult to obtain. In addition, an application of metagenomics is presented in the Case Study at the end of this chapter.

16.2 Annotation Ascribes Biological Function to DNA Sequences

The genome sequence can be considered the finest-scale physical map of the genome, and in it are encoded all the genes of the organism. Genome annotation identifies the location of genes and other functional sequences within the genome sequence.

Annotation is the process of attaching biological functions to DNA sequences, and gene annotation describes the biochemical, cellular, and biological function of the gene products the genome encodes. Until annotated, a genome sequence is nothing but a very long string of As, Ts, Cs, and Gs. Annotation describes both structural and functional features of a gene. Its goal, moreover, is not only to identify known genes, regulatory sequences, and so on, but also to identify sequences that are likely to be genes though their function, if they are genes, is as yet unknown. Annotations may be based on experimental evidence—the gold standard—or on computational analysis, which then must be confirmed experimentally.

Experimental Approaches to Structural Annotation

Structural annotation aims to identify genes and their structural components, including transcribed, coding, and regulatory sequences. Experimental approaches to identifying transcribed sequences in a genome make use of complementary DNA (cDNA). Comparison of cDNA sequences with genomic sequences identifies the parts of the genome that undergo transcription leading to production of RNA molecules (see Section 14.2 for a review of cDNA and genomic libraries).

In theory, a complete set of transcribed sequences representing all the genes from an organism would allow complete annotation of the transcribed regions of its genome. In practice, though, complete sets of such sequences are not available, due to both variability in expression levels and variation in structure and processing of different transcripts (see Section 8.4 for a discussion of mRNA splicing). Nevertheless, for many organisms, a large amount of cDNA sequence is available, allowing the partial or complete assembly of gene transcripts. Comparing these transcribed sequences with the genomic sequence allows accurate annotation of gene exons and introns, including alternative splicing and other mRNA variants (**Figure 16.7**).

Computational Approaches to Structural Annotation

The genomes of multicellular eukaryotes often contain tens of thousands of genes, for many of which little or no experimental data have been collected. In the absence of experimental data concerning the existence or function of a gene, computational approaches are used to identify possible genes within genome sequences. The use of computational approaches to decipher DNA-sequence information is termed **bioinformatics**.

Bioinformatic annotation algorithms predict gene structure by identifying **open reading frames (ORFs)**, sequences that appear to possibly code for polypeptides. Most of these algorithms initially search for ORFs larger than a minimum size, such as 50 amino acids, since ORFs of at least that size are less likely to occur at random. Data derived from known cDNA sequences of the organism under analysis can be used to fine-tune the algorithms. Even so, predictions are not infallible, especially with large eukaryotic genomes, where

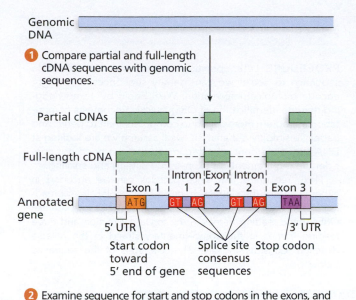

Genomic DNA

1 Compare partial and full-length cDNA sequences with genomic sequences.

Partial cDNAs

Full-length cDNA

Intron Exon Intron
Exon 1 1 2 2 Exon 3

Annotated gene
ATG GT AG GT AG TAA

5′ UTR 3′ UTR

Start codon toward 5′ end of gene

Splice site consensus sequences

Stop codon

2 Examine sequence for start and stop codons in the exons, and splice site consensus sequences at the ends of the introns.

Figure 16.7   Experimentally acquired evidence for gene annotation.

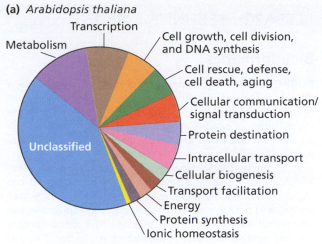

(a) *Arabidopsis thaliana*

Transcription
Metabolism
Cell growth, cell division, and DNA synthesis
Cell rescue, defense, cell death, aging
Cellular communication/ signal transduction
Protein destination
Unclassified
Intracellular transport
Cellular biogenesis
Transport facilitation
Energy
Protein synthesis
Ionic homeostasis

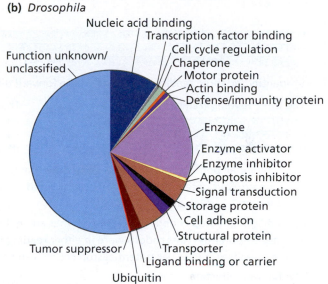

(b) *Drosophila*

Nucleic acid binding
Transcription factor binding
Cell cycle regulation
Chaperone
Motor protein
Actin binding
Defense/immunity protein
Function unknown/ unclassified
Enzyme
Enzyme activator
Enzyme inhibitor
Apoptosis inhibitor
Signal transduction
Storage protein
Cell adhesion
Structural protein
Tumor suppressor
Transporter
Ligand binding or carrier
Ubiquitin

Figure 16.8   Genome annotation of predicted biological function. Genes are categorized with presumed functions based on similarity to known genes. When the *Arabidopsis* and *Drosophila* genomes were first annotated in 2000, many genes (blue) had no similarity to genes of known function. However, in the past decade significant progress has been made to functionally characterize these genes, either using functional or comparative approaches.

exons are often small relative to introns and are dispersed over large distances. Thus, bioinformatic algorithms are generally less successful than experimental data in correctly predicting exons, but they can provide enough information to assist in the design of experimental approaches for clarifying gene structures. Furthermore, because searching for ORFs is not helpful for recognizing genes that code for RNA molecules, experimental or comparative genomic approaches are usually required for annotating genes whose products are noncoding RNA. The process by which genes are predicted is explored further in **Research Technique 16.1**.

Another bioinformatic method of gene annotation is to compare genome sequences of related species. As we discuss in a later section, this and other forms of comparative genomic analysis are becoming increasingly powerful as the genome sequences of more species become available. Remember, though, that after genes are predicted computationally, either from algorithms or phylogenetic comparisons, they must then be confirmed experimentally.

Functional Gene Annotation

In addition to pinpointing genes and their structural components, gene annotation aims to describe biochemical and biological function. Let us consider the *lacI* gene, which encodes the Lac repressor protein of *E. coli*. The biochemical function of the encoded protein is to bind to DNA and allolactose, and its cellular function is to regulate transcription of the *lac* operon (see Section 12.2). The biological function of the *lacI* gene is regulation of gene expression in response to sugar availability in the environment. In this case, the annotation we make can be quite detailed, since we know a great deal about the *lacI* gene.

Genes that are similar to each other in sequence are assumed to encode gene products with similar biochemical functions. Genes similar in sequence to the *lacI* gene, for example, are likely to encode transcription factors that regulate gene expression. However, the nature of the genes they regulate may not be easy to predict. In other words, their biochemical function may be predicted by sequence comparison, but determination of their biological function requires experimental analysis, the most powerful tool being a loss-of-function allele (see Chapter 14 for descriptions of approaches to mutant analysis). Initial annotation of the eukaryote genomes represented in **Figure 16.8** categorized many genes by their presumed biochemical or cellular function. At that time, only about half of the genes predicted for these species had either known biochemical and cellular functions (see Table 16.1), learned

RESEARCH TECHNIQUE 16.1

Bioinformatics

PURPOSE What do computer algorithms "look for" in a DNA sequence during annotation of a bacterial, archaeal, or eukaryotic genome? Often, the first step in annotation is the identification of open reading frames (ORFs). In bacteria and archaea, all ORFs that are translated into protein will have a start codon (ATG) and a stop codon (TAA, TAG, or TGA) with an uninterrupted open reading frame lying between. In eukaryotes, however, where genes may be separated into multiple exons, only the amino-terminal exon has a start codon, and only the last-coding exon has a stop codon, but all internal exons have the sequences that ensure proper splicing, as do the 3′ end of the first exon and the 5′ end of the last exon.

PROCEDURE Let's practice examining a nucleotide sequence to see if we can identify sequences that might encode biological information. We'll begin by acknowledging that the identification of ORFs quickly becomes a computational problem more suited to computers than to pencil and paper. To simplify our analysis, we'll assume we are looking at DNA sequence from a bacterium, so that we need not consider the requirements of exon–intron cutting and splicing.

Next, recognize that since proteins can be encoded in either strand of the double-stranded DNA molecule, six reading frames must always be considered in searches for potential ORFs: three reading frames in the forward direction and three reading frames in the complementary strand in the reverse direction. Consider the first 21 nucleotides of the sequence below.

```
5′ TTGCAGTATGGGCTAGACCAAAGAGAGAGTTGATAACTAGCCGAAACGAACCATGTTCGTCAATCAGCACCTTTGTGGTT
   CTCACCTCGTTGAAGCTTTGTACCTTGTTTGCGGTGAACGTGGTTTCTTCTACACTCCTAAGACTTAAGCTAGCTAAGTA
   TAGATGGCGAGGTGACACACACACACACAGGTAGATATTAA 3′
```

1 Identify the three reading frames (rf) in the forward direction and in the complementary strand.

The three reading frames in the forward direction

```
rf1 5′ / TTG CAG TAT GGG CTA GAC CAA / 3′
rf2 5′ / T TGC AGT ATG GGC TAG ACC AA / 3′
rf3 5′ / TT GCA GTA TGG GCT AGA CCA A / 3′
```

The three reading frames in the complementary strand

```
rf4 3′ / AAC GTC ATA CCC GAT CTG GTT / 5′
rf5 3′ / AA CGT CAT ACC CGA TCT GGT T / 5′
rf6 3′ / A ACG TCA TAC CCG ATC TGG TT / 5′
```

2 Highlight all potential start codons (ATG); note that these can occur in any of the six reading frames. There are four potential start codons, highlighted under step **3** below: rf2-1 (reading frame 2, first potential start codon), rf2-2, rf2-3, and rf4-1.

3 Highlight any stop codons (TTA, TAG, TGA) that are in the same reading frame as the four identified start codons. Since all potential start codons were in either reading frame 2 or 4, we need only look for potential stop codons in these reading frames. Six potential stop codons can be found in reading frame 2, and seven in reading frame 4.

The forward direction

```
                rf2-1      rf2                                    rf2                         rf2-2
5′ TTGCAGT ATG GGC TAG ACCAAAGAGAGAGTTGATAACTAG CCGAAACGAACC ATG TTCGTCAATCAGCACCTTTGTGGTT
   CTCACCTCGTTGAAGCTTTGTACCTTGTTTGCGGTGAACGTGGTTTCTTCTACACTCCTAAGACT TAA GCTAGC TAA GTA
                                                                       rf2          rf2
   TAG ATG GCGAGGT GAC ACACACACACACACAGGTAGATATTAA 3′
   rf2 rf2-3      rf2
```

The reverse complementary sequence

```
                                              rf4           rf4                     rf4
5′ TTAATATCTACCTGTGTGTGTGTGTGTCACCTCGCCATCTATACT TAG CTAGCT TAA GTCTTAGGAGTG TAG AAGAAACC
   ACGTTCACCGCAAACAAGGTACAAAGCTTCAACGAGG TGA GAACCACAAAGGTGC TGA TTGACGAAC ATG GTTCGTTTCG
                                         rf4                 rf4              rf4-1
   GC TAG TTATCAACTCTCTCTTTGGTC TAG CCCATACTGCAA 3′
      rf4                       rf4
```

4 Identify open reading frames and corresponding amino acid sequences.

> We find that the rf2-1, rf2-3, and rf4-1 potential start codons are followed almost immediately by in-frame stop codons, preventing the open reading frames from encoding more than 2, 3, or 5 amino acids. In contrast, the open reading frame commencing from rf2-2 is much longer.

The rf2-2 start codon is followed by an open reading frame of 93 nucleotides that could encode a protein of 31 amino acids:

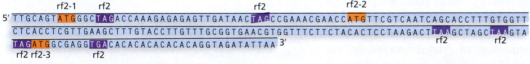

```
5′ TTGCAGT ATG GGC TAG ACCAAAGAGAGAGTTGATAAC TAG CCGAAACGAACC ATG TTCGTCAATCAGCACCTTTGTGGTT
                                                              M F L N Q H L C G S

   CTCACCTCGTTGAAGCTTTGTACCTTGTTTGCGGTGAACGTGGTTTCTTCTACACTCCTAAGACT TAA GCTAGC TAA GTA
   S H L V E A L Y L V C G E R G F F Y T P K T *

   TAG ATGGCGAGGT GA CACACACACACACAGGTAGATATTAA 3′
```

For more practice with bioinformatics concepts, see Problems 4, 5, and 6. Visit the Study Area to access study tools.

from previous experimental evidence, or a presumed biochemical function based on sequence similarity to known proteins. Functional genomics experiments, such as those described in Section 16.4, provide additional information for functional gene annotation.

Related Genes and Protein Motifs

Examination and comparison of whole-genome sequences have allowed researchers to recognize **gene families**, groups of genes that are evolutionarily related and share conserved sequences and gene structures (Table 16.1) that can aid in the process of annotation. Some gene families may be prominent in certain species, whereas others may be entirely absent. The 20,000 to 21,000 protein-coding genes of the human genome represent about 10,000 gene families. Although most mammals largely share this set of 10,000 gene families, only 3000 to 4000 of these gene families are found in all eukaryotes. Other lineages, such as fungi and plants, have their own sets of lineage-specific gene families.

Expansion and retention of particular gene families depends on the importance of their biological functions to the organism. For example, in mammals, the gene family encoding olfactory receptors is often the largest in the genome, frequently consisting of more than 1000 members. However, the olfactory receptor gene family is much larger in organisms that rely heavily on this sense (a mouse has more than 900 of these genes) than in species in which the sense of smell is diminished (humans have only 339). In humans, the largest gene family encodes proteins functioning in the immune system, but this family of genes is absent in both the plant *Arabidopsis* and the fungus *Saccharomyces*, where the largest gene families encode protein kinases.

Annotation can also be assisted by recognition of genome segments coding for conserved protein domains. Many eukaryotic proteins are modular, consisting of distinct protein domains joined together (**Figure 16.9**). Because many protein domains correlate with exon structure in genes—that is, one or more exons specifically encode a particular protein domain—a hypothesis has been advanced that composite genes (genes that encode multiple conserved protein domains) are generated by *exon shuffling*, a process in which one or more exons become part of a new gene through duplication, translocation, or inversion of DNA sequence or a combination of such events. The modular structure of proteins means that the number of genes is much larger than the number of unique functional protein domains. Exon shuffling creates novel arrangements of protein domains that can be co-opted to fulfill new biological roles. The available data indicate that the protein repertoires of multicellular eukaryotes are generally more complex, averaging more different domains per protein, than those of single-celled eukaryotes. Knowledge of conserved protein domains often provides insight into potential biochemical activities of proteins, but, again, understanding the biological function requires mutant analysis.

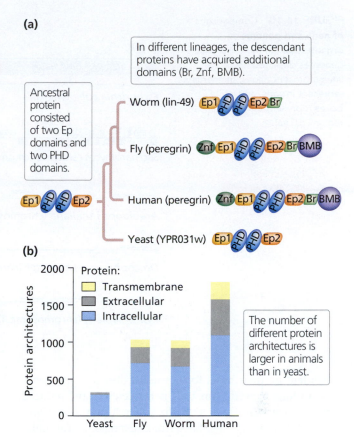

Figure 16.9 Modularity of protein domains. EPC-like protein, a protein type found in all eukaryotes, is used as an example. **(a)** Proteins are often modular, composed of discrete domains (e.g., Ep1, Ep2, PHD, Br, BMB, Znf). Complex proteins can evolve by mixing and matching of protein domains, usually through a process known as exon shuffling. **(b)** Multicellular eukaryotes have more complex protein architectures than single-celled eukaryotes.

Variation in Genome Organization among Species

Having obtained and compared genome sequences of bacteria and archaea and of eukaryotes (see Table 16.1), biologists can draw several general conclusions about genome organization (**Figure 16.10**). First, bacteria and archaea have fewer genes and much higher gene density than eukaryotes. This high gene density is attributable to the lack of introns, the more compact size of regulatory sequences, and the generally less complex structures of most encoded proteins in bacteria and archaea. Second, eukaryotes differ widely in both gene number and gene density, and the genomes of single-celled eukaryotes tend to encode fewer genes than those of multicellular eukaryotes. At the same time, groups of related eukaryotes—for example, mammals—often have similar numbers of genes, suggesting that gene regulation rather than number or type largely determines differences between related species. Third, species that have evolved to be obligate parasites often experience genome contraction. As parasites become

FIGURE 16.10 **Comparisons of gene and genome organization.** In the eukaryotic genomes depicted, thick lines represent exons, thinner lines represent introns, and white boxes represent untranslated regions (UTRs).

❓ **What is all the "extra" (i.e. non-protein coding) DNA in multicellular eukaryote genomes compared with bacterial genomes?**

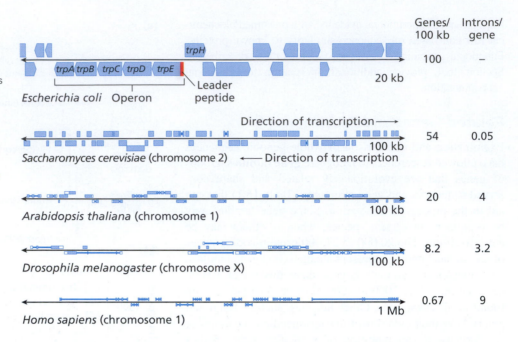

	Genes/100 kb	Introns/gene
Escherichia coli	100	–
Saccharomyces cerevisiae (chromosome 2)	54	0.05
Arabidopsis thaliana (chromosome 1)	20	4
Drosophila melanogaster (chromosome X)	8.2	3.2
Homo sapiens (chromosome 1)	0.67	9

dependent on their hosts for nutrients, they lose the genes they no longer need. This trait is reflected in the reduced genome size compared with the other bacteria of *Chlamydia trachomatis*, the bacterium responsible for chlamydia in humans (see Table 16.1).

Just as gene number and density vary among eukaryotes, so does the proportion of repetitive DNA in the genome. The human genome consists of more than 50% repetitive DNA: Approximately 45% consists of transposable elements (transposons, retrotransposons, and retroelements; see Section 11.7); a further 3% consists of microsatellite sequence; and about 5% contains recent gene duplications. Additional repetitive DNA is present in the centromeric and telomeric sequences. The repetitive DNA that is not centromeric or telomeric is often called *dispersed repetitive DNA* because it is distributed throughout the genome. The proportion of dispersed repetitive DNA, largely transposons, retrotransposons, and retroelements, in a genome is a significant factor influencing gene density. Some features of genome organization can be seen in human chromosome 21, shown in **Figure 16.11**.

The annotated genome sequences of model genetic organisms can be found at the websites provided on the back endsheets of this book. The host site for the human genome (http://genome.ucsc.edu/) also acts as a portal to the annotated genomes of several additional species.

Three Insights from Genome Sequences

Analyses of genome sequences from a range of bacteria, archaea, and eukaryotes have produced many insights into the nature of genomes, of which three are particularly important. First, genomic comparisons demonstrate that the genomes of all organisms are highly dynamic in nature. Transposable elements (see Section 11.7) are just one of the factors driving genome evolution; large- and small-scale chromosomal duplications as well as deletions and other rearrangements also contribute. Substantial genetic variation is seen even within species, thus providing raw material for natural selection and the evolution of new species.

Second, genome sequencing of model organisms reveals the limitations of forward genetic screens. Even in intensely studied species, such as *E. coli* and *S. cerevisiae*, forward genetic screens (see Section 14.1) identified only a fraction (one-third to one-half as many) of the genes identified by genome sequencing. What are the functions of all these previously unknown genes?

The third insight obtained from the analysis of genomes is the discovery that the number of genes in the human genome is comparable with that of various other multicellular eukaryotes. Over the past 25 to 30 years, the estimates of gene number in the human genome have steadily decreased. Having once estimated our genome to contain as many as 80,000 to 120,000 genes, we may find it humbling to discover that we and other animals have fewer genes than many plants. The currently estimated number of about 20,000 protein-coding genes in the human genome is typical for vertebrates, and it is not much higher than the 14,000 or so estimated for *Drosophila*. If some of us have "gene number anxiety," it should be assuaged by recognizing that gene number does not translate directly into protein number or organism complexity. Both exon shuffling and alternative splicing increase the complexity of proteins in eukaryotes, and these processes are much more prevalent in animals than in either fungi or plants. In the remaining pages of this chapter, we address these major insights in more detail.

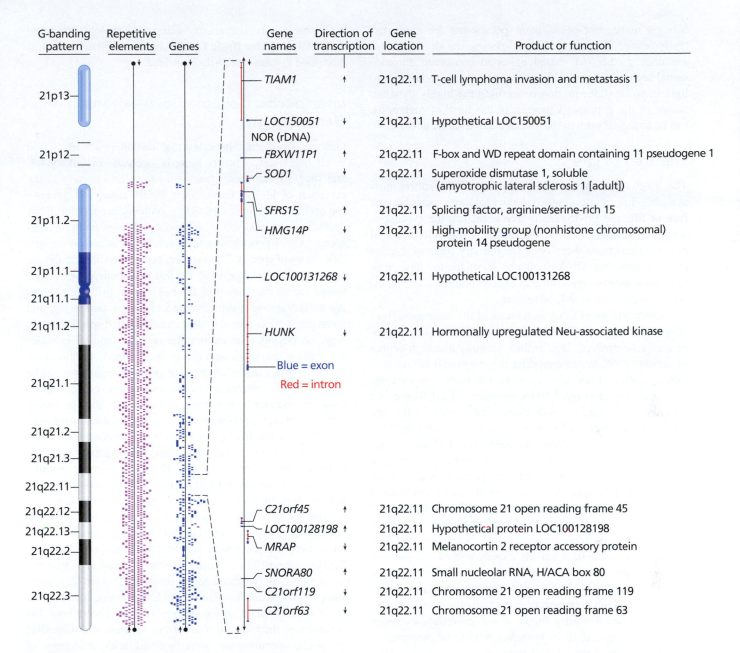

Figure 16.11 Genome annotation of human chromosome 21.

Are there more genes or more repetitive elements in human chromosome 21?

16.3 Evolutionary Genomics Traces the History of Genomes

Evolutionary genomics, sometimes called phylogenomics or comparative genomics, is the comparative study of genomes. **Interspecific comparisons** of genomes—comparisons between species—identify sequences conserved over evolutionary time and thus facilitate the annotation of genomes and provide insight into the evolution of genes and organismal diversity. In contrast, **intraspecific** **comparisons** identify sequence polymorphisms that are responsible for the genetic differences within populations of a single species. These differences are the raw material of evolution and form the basis of population genetics and the evolution of species.

The evolutionary history of each organism can be traced in its genome and in the composition of its chromosomes. Evolutionary genomics has revealed the striking fact that a large number of genes are shared by phylogenetically distant species, reaffirming that all life on Earth is related. Species that are more closely related to one another share a larger number of genes than species that are more distantly related. In closely related species, the similarities in sequence go beyond shared genes to conserved chromosomal segments. Evolutionary genomics has also brought to light important information concerning the highly dynamic nature of the genome. Changes, in the form of mutations, can be observed even in the time scale of a single generation.

The Tree of Life

The large amount of DNA sequence information now available has revolutionized how biologists perceive the **tree of life**, the phylogenetic tree depicting the evolutionary relationships between organisms. Morphological and physiological traits were once the primary basis of species classification, but DNA sequence comparisons have provided new clarity concerning questions that the older methods of study were unable to resolve.

Comparisons of DNA sequences of the same gene from different species are particularly useful for assessing phylogenetic relationships. Due to their ubiquity and high degree of conservation, genes encoding the ribosomal RNAs provide a universal set of sequences for such comparisons. By comparing ribosomal RNA sequences, Carl Woese and colleagues revealed through pioneering studies in the late 1970s that all forms of life on Earth fall into one of three distinct domains: Bacteria, Archaea, and Eukarya. Since then, relationships within many eukaryotic groups have been clarified using DNA sequence comparisons, allowing the basic architecture of the tree of life to be determined (**Figure 16.12**). Some surprising relationships have emerged. For example, the Fungi and Metazoans, which had traditionally been considered two separate "kingdoms" of life, were discovered to be relatively closely related and are now grouped with Amoebozoa in a clade called the Unikonts. Since animals and plants are the most conspicuous lifeforms from a human perspective, the tree presented in Figure 16.12 is biased toward a focus on the interrelationships in those two groups. If all its branches were to be presented in equal detail, the "tree" would more closely resemble a very dense bush.

The tree of life in Figure 16.12 was constructed using DNA sequence information (see Section 1.5) and comparison of the alignment of *homologous nucleotides* with ascertain phylogenetic relationships. **Homologous nucleotides** are those that are descended from the same nucleotide in the common ancestor of the two species being compared (Figure 1.18). Highly conserved protein-coding DNA sequences, some of which have been conserved over timescales of more than a billion years, are analyzed to identify ancient evolutionary branch points, or **nodes.** Conversely, rapidly evolving sequences are compared to clarify recent nodes in species evolution. Intron and intergenic sequences, on which there may be little selective pressure to maintain a specific sequence, can accumulate mutations and change rapidly over time. A strategy developed to search for homologous sequences, using a computer program called **BLAST**, for **Basic Local Alignment Search Tool**, is described in **Research Technique 16.2**.

Interspecific Genome Comparisons: Gene Content

Genome sequencing indicates that certain genes are found in all organisms, whether bacteria, archaea, or eukaryotes, and suggests that these genes must have arisen early in the evolution of life on Earth. Such highly conserved genes—for example, the genes encoding proteins needed for DNA synthesis—are involved in biological processes common to all species. Other genes have a more recent origin and define specific clades of species. For instance, genes encoding tubulin are found in all eukaryotes, implying that the tubulin gene evolved before the diversification of the eukaryotes. Still other genes are shared among more restricted clades of organisms, and some genes are confined to only closely related species. In this way, the phylogenetic distribution of gene families provides information on when specific genes evolved. Furthermore, the set of genes shared among any group of organisms can be considered to represent the minimum genomic content of the common ancestor of that group of organisms, thus providing information on the evolution of both genomes and organisms.

Because the first genomes to be sequenced were from phylogenetically diverse organisms, many genes appeared to be specific to particular taxa. However, as more genome sequences were determined, genes initially thought to be unique were found to have counterparts in the genomes of related species. Indeed, two closely related species may share almost their entire genome content, with the genomic differences between sister taxa defining the differences between the two species. For example, genome content is very similar in four closely related *Saccharomyces* species (*S. cerevisiae, S. paradoxus, S. mikatae,* and *S. bayanus*), all separated by 5 to 20 million years (**Figure 16.13**). Throughout the genomes of the four *Saccharomyces* species, just a handful of species-specific genes were detected, with an average of one unique gene for every 0.5 million years of evolutionary distance. Similarly, in *Drosophila melanogaster* and related species, the rate of the origin of new functional genes was estimated to be 5 to 11 genes per million years. It is not yet clear whether these rates are typical for other organisms. But it does bring up the question: How do new genes form?

The Births and Deaths of Genes In tracing the evolutionary history of genes by comparing genome sequences, geneticists obtain clues to the mechanisms through which new genes arise (**Figure 16.14**). These mechanisms include the following.

1. **Gene duplication by duplication of genomic DNA.**
   Duplication of genetic material can duplicate a portion of a gene, a single gene, a chromosome or chromosome segment, or the entire genome (see Chapter 10).

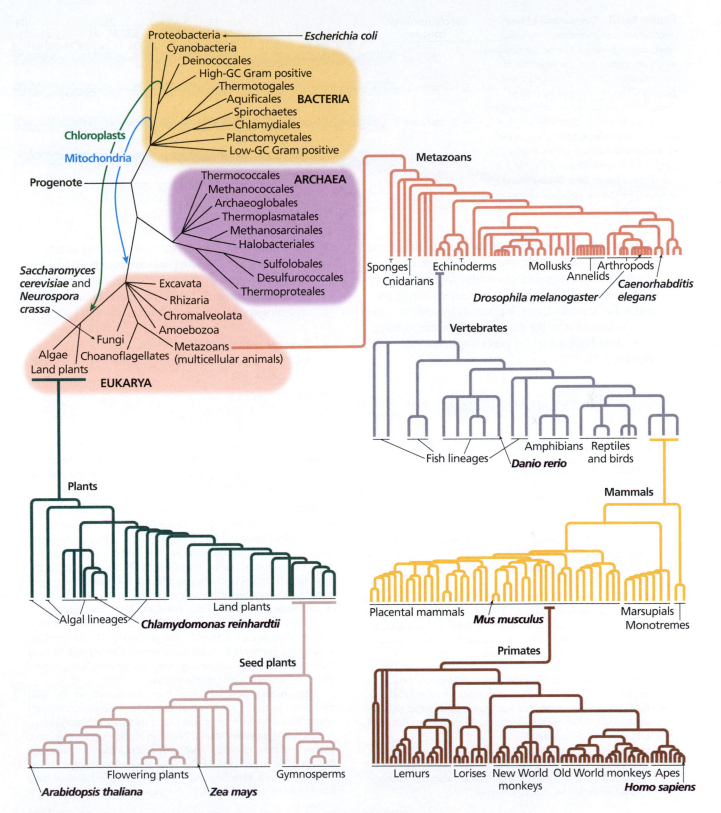

Figure 16.12 The tree of life, highlighting the phylogenetic relationships of model organisms discussed in this book.

Figure 16.13 **Comparison of four** *Saccharomyces* **genomes.** Predicted open reading frames (ORFs) are depicted as arrows pointing in the direction of transcription. Orthologous ORFs (see page 612) are connected by dotted lines. ORFs with a one-to-one correspondence are shown in blue; ORFs with a one-to-two correspondence are in red (*S. paradoxus* has two genes in place of gene 7 of *S. cerevisiae*); ORFs that are unmatched (gene 24 in *S. cerevisiae*) are in white. Sequence gaps are indicated by vertical black lines.

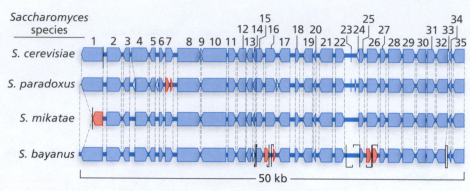

2. **Gene duplication by unequal crossover.** In a special case of gene duplication, one or more genes can be duplicated by unequal crossover due to misalignment of homologous chromosomes at synapsis during prophase I of meiosis. Gene duplication by unequal crossover is indicated by the detection of tandem repeats, or back-to-back copies, of genetic material (see Section 5.5).

3. **Exon shuffling.** During an exon-shuffling event, exons from two or more genes are combined in a new genomic context (see Figure 16.9a). The rearranging could occur through illegitimate recombination events or, alternatively, through retrotransposition events.

4. **Reverse transcription.** Reverse transcription of cellular RNAs using a retrotransposon-encoded reverse

RESEARCH TECHNIQUE 16.2

Basic Local Alignment Search Tool

PURPOSE Homologous genes are derived from a common ancestral gene and often have similar functions. A computer program called the Basic Local Alignment Search Tool (BLAST) was developed in 1990 by Stephen Altschul, David Lipman, and colleagues to search for homologous sequences. BLAST, perhaps the most widely used and most important tool employed in bioinformatic endeavors, allows scientists to search databases for sequences similar to any input sequence.

The BLAST program of the National Center for Biotechnology Information at the National Institutes of Health (http://blast.ncbi. nlm.nih.gov/Blast.cgi) enables searches of either DNA sequence similarity or protein similarity. Various types of searches can be performed. Here are three of the most common.

- **nucleotide blast (blastn):** A nucleotide query sequence is compared with nucleotide sequences in the database.
- **tblastn:** A protein query sequence is compared with the nucleotide databases, hypothetically translated into all six potential reading frames.
- **tblastx:** A nucleotide query sequence is translated into all six possible reading frames and compared against the nucleotide sequences in the database, also translated into all six possible reading frames.

PROCEDURE One of the first experiments researchers perform once they have determined the sequence of a gene is to "BLAST" their sequence against the GenBank database, where most DNA sequences determined anywhere in the world are deposited. To perform a search, the user enters an "input" nucleotide or protein sequence into a window,

and the BLAST program then searches chosen databases for similar sequences. Sequences are given a score based on the extent of similarity and relative to the probability that the sequences could be similar by chance.

CONCLUSION What information can be derived from this experiment? First, the results of the BLAST search can provide clues to the biological and biochemical function of the gene used as a query. Since homologous genes are descended from a common ancestor, they likely share biochemical activity if not biological context. Second, knowledge of the phylogenetic distribution of homologous genes allows inferences to be made about when the gene evolved. For example, if the query is a human gene and if genes homologous to it are detected in all eukaryotes, the protein is likely to perform a function conserved in all eukaryotes. Conversely, if only mammals have homologous genes, the gene is likely to perform a function specific to mammals.

Since related species often have conserved amino acid sequences but, due to the redundancy of the genetic code, possess different nucleotide sequences, a tblastn (or tblastx) search is often more sensitive than a blastn in identifying homologous sequences from distantly related species. When a researcher has no prior knowledge of the DNA sequence being used as a query, tblastx searches are particularly useful because they identify DNA sequences with the potential to encode similar proteins.

What if a BLAST search fails to find any other sequences in the database similar to the query sequence? If the sequence is known to encode a protein, the result suggests that the gene for the protein is unlikely to be conserved in a broad phylogenetic sense. Alternatively, if the sequence is noncoding DNA, a lack of similarity to other DNA sequences is not unexpected.

For more practice with bioinformatics concepts, see Problems 14 and 15. Visit the Study Area to access study tools.

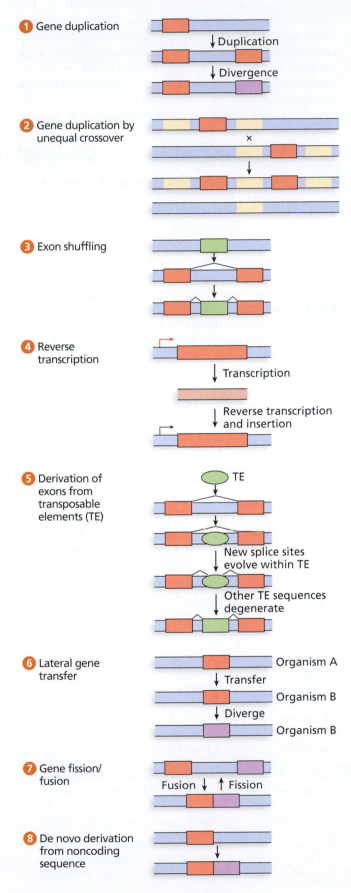

1 Gene duplication

↓ Duplication

↓ Divergence

2 Gene duplication by unequal crossover

×

3 Exon shuffling

4 Reverse transcription

↓ Transcription

↓ Reverse transcription and insertion

5 Derivation of exons from transposable elements (TE)

TE

New splice sites evolve within TE

Other TE sequences degenerate

6 Lateral gene transfer

Organism A

↓ Transfer

Organism B

↓ Diverge

Organism B

7 Gene fission/fusion

Fusion ↓ ↑ Fission

8 De novo derivation from noncoding sequence

Figure 16.14 **The birth of genes.**

Ⓠ **Which mechanisms of gene formation also duplicate associated regulatory sequences?**

transcriptase, and insertion of the cDNA products into the genome, often leads to the formation of **pseudogenes**, sequences recognizable as mutated gene sequences, but can also produce new genes. More than 10,000 pseudogenes have been recognized in the human genome, and many were derived from reverse transcription. In addition, the insertion of a retrotransposon into a new genomic location can alter the expression pattern of adjacent genes, potentially leading to new gene functions.

5. **Derivation of exons from transposons.** Transposons have sequences encoding a DNA-binding protein called transposase that is necessary for movement of the transposon. Transposase sequences can be made to perform a new function if fused with other exons derived from the genome. For example, the *RAG1* and *RAG2* genes of jawed vertebrates, whose protein products are involved in rearrangement of DNA sequences during the maturation of the immune system, were derived from sequences encoding a transposase.

6. **Lateral (horizontal) gene transfer.** The movement of genes from one species into the genome of another species is referred to as lateral gene transfer. Such events are common in bacteria and archaea, which may exchange genes with even distantly related organisms (see Section 6.6). Endosymbioses lead to large-scale lateral gene transfer events, as in the case of the mitochondrion and chloroplast. Although less common between eukaryotes, lateral gene transfer has been documented in some protists and plants.

7. **Gene fusion and gene fission.** Two genes can fuse into a single gene by deletion of the stop codon and transcription-termination signals that normally separate genes. Alternatively, a single gene may be split into two genes, each with its own regulatory sequences.

8. **De novo derivation.** Exons can be derived de novo from previously intronic or intergenic sequences that are incorporated into exons of adjacent genes.

Comparisons between the genomes of several related *Drosophila* species have provided insights into the origins of new genes in a multicellular eukaryote. The major source of new genes, slightly less than 80% of the time, was gene duplication, in which the duplicates were either tandemly arranged or dispersed at distant chromosomal locations. A further 10% of new genes were derived from retrotransposition events, and, surprisingly, approximately 12% arose de novo, from previously noncoding sequences.

Two mechanisms—gene duplication in eukaryotes and lateral gene transfer in bacteria and archaea—stand out as being the major mechanisms responsible for generation of genes. Let's consider each of these mechanisms in greater detail.

Gene Duplication The high rate of gene duplication is one surprising discovery arising from evolutionary genomics. Most genomes contain a mosaic of gene families derived from both ancient and more recent duplication events, indicating that genomes are dynamic and continuously changing over time. A study in 2000 by Michael Lynch and John Conery counted the duplicated genes in nine eukaryotic species and estimated the duplication rate: approximately 0.01 genes per million years. Thus, for an average eukaryotic genome with 10,000 to 30,000 genes, this research suggests that one gene duplicates and is maintained in the genome every 3000 to 10,000 years, a rate of gene formation higher than has been observed in the *Saccharomyces* species.

The fate of duplicated genes depends on the molecular basis of the duplication. If the entire gene including regulatory sequences is duplicated, both copies will be able to produce a functional protein product in the correct amount, time, and place. In this case, the duplicate genes are genetically redundant and are free to evolve new functions, as long as the composite functions of the two duplicate genes retain the function of the original gene. Fully redundant genes are not maintained over long time periods, usually because the duplicate genes undergo one of three likely fates (**Figure 16.15**). First, the vast majority of new genes degenerate into pseudogenes due to a lack of positive selection, without which mutations will slowly accumulate and render the genes nonfunctional. Pseudogenes form a significant fraction of the genomes of some organisms.

Second, mutations in each of the two copies—for example, mutations in two different tissue-specific enhancers, as in Figure 16.15—can result in the two genes having complementary activities such that their combined activity is the same as the activity of the gene before duplication,

a process called **subfunctionalization**. Third, in a process called **neofunctionalization**, a mutation in one of the duplicates could provide a function not performed by the original gene. In rare cases where the new function provides a selective advantage, the gene can be maintained and become fixed in the population. In the latter two cases, both copies remain functional, whereas in the first case, only a single copy retains activity.

Repeated duplication events produce families of related genes. Through gene duplications, gene losses, and speciation events, the relationships among these genes often become complex. Three terms describe different relationships of evolutionarily related genes. The broadest term is *homology*, which is defined as descent from a common ancestor. Thus, **homologous genes**, or **homologs**, have descended from a common ancestral gene and are said to constitute a gene family (**Figure 16.16**). Two other terms define specific relationships between homologous genes. **Paralogous genes**, or **paralogs**, are genes whose origin lies in a gene duplication event. No indication of the age of the duplication event leading to the paralogs is implied. Generally, paralogs perform biologically distinct but biochemically related functions. **Orthologous genes**, or **orthologs**, are genes whose origin lies in a speciation event. They are genes in different species that are derived from a single ancestral gene in two species' last common ancestor. Orthologs most often, but not always, have equivalent functions in the two organisms being compared. The globin genes in Figure 16.16 illustrate these evolutionary relationships. See Genetic Analysis 16.1 for practice in determining orthologous and paralogous relationships of evolutionarily related genes.

Gene duplication has been a key mechanism in generating new genes that over time have made possible the

Figure 16.15 The fates of duplicate genes.

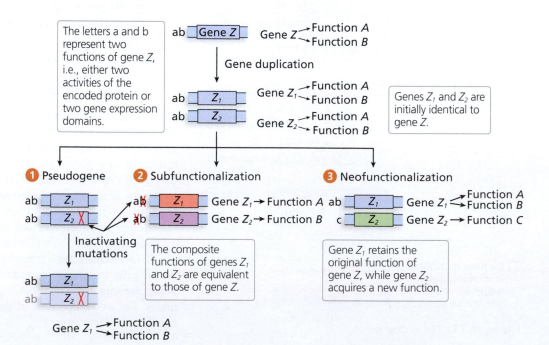

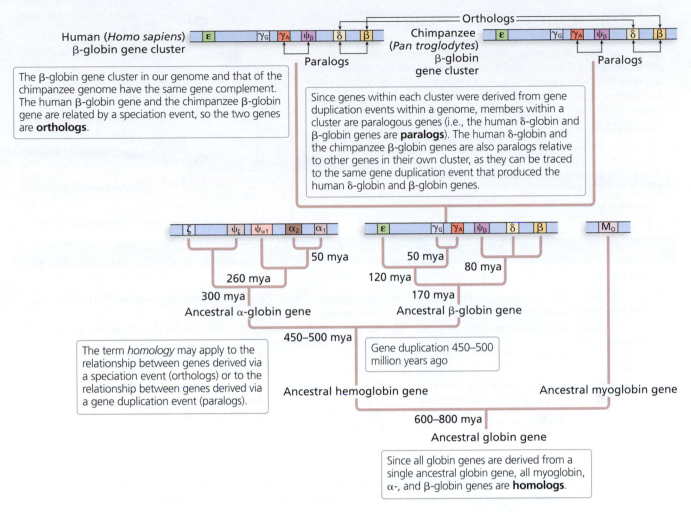

Figure 16.16 Orthology and paralogy, speciation events and gene duplications: Examples from the globin gene family.

evolution of complex organisms. During globin gene evolution, gene duplication has permitted specialization, which in turn has allowed greater physiological complexity. Both subfunctionalization and neofunctionalization can be seen within the globin gene family. Neofunctionalization can be seen in the gene duplication event that produced the hemoglobin and myoglobin genes, where hemoglobin functions to carry oxygen in the blood and myoglobin functions to bind oxygen in muscles. Subfunctionalization has also occurred in the globin genes, if an assumption is made that the ancestral β-globin was active throughout the life cycle of the organism. If so, subfunctionalization is now evident between the ε-globin and β-globin paralogs, where the ε-globin is active in the embryo and the β-globin is active in the adult. Other examples of gene duplication are seen in the duplications of an ancestral gene leading to the family of genes that allow trichromatic vision in some primate species, including humans (see Section 3.5), and in the creation of another gene family that specifies identity along the anterior–posterior axis of animals (see Section 18.2).

Lateral Gene Transfer Lateral gene transfer, also known as horizontal gene transfer, is the transfer of genetic material between two species. Lateral gene transfer may have been extensive early in the evolution of life, but as specialized genetic mechanisms evolved for control of gene expression, lateral gene transfer became less frequent within the eukaryotic lineage.

A common lateral gene transfer event occurs through the sharing of plasmids among bacterial species (see Chapter 6), but other lateral gene transfer events between bacterial species and between bacterial and archaeal species also have been documented. Based on comparison of the sequenced bacterial and archaeal genomes, an estimated 1.5 to 14.5% of genes in any genome are the result of lateral gene transfer. This is likely to be an underestimate, since ancient transfer events may not be detectable. In an extreme example of lateral gene transfer, hyperthermophilic bacterial species (bacteria able to live in extremely hot environments) have acquired genes from hyperthermophilic archaeal species. Nearly a quarter of the genes in the bacterium *Thermotoga maritima* are most similar to archaeal genes, indicating an archaeal origin. One acquired

PROBLEM Consider the phylogenetic tree of seven homologous eukaryotic genes derived from three species. What is the relationship between the human genes and the *Drosophila* gene—are they paralogs or orthologs? What are the relationships between the mouse and human *sonic hedgehog* genes, between the human *sonic hedgehog* and human *desert hedgehog* genes, and between the human *desert hedgehog* and mouse *indian hedgehog* genes? In each case, are the genes paralogs or orthologs?

BREAK IT DOWN: Recall that homologous genes are genes that have descended from a common ancestral gene (p. 612)

BREAK IT DOWN: Recall that orthologs are homologous genes produced by a speciation event, and paralogs are homologous genes produced by a gene duplication event within a species.

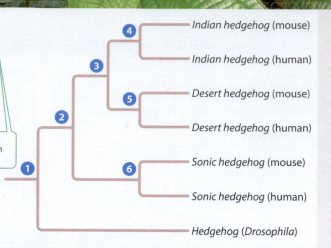

Solution Strategies	Solution Steps
Evaluate	
1. Identify the topic this problem addresses and the nature of the required answer.	1. This problem is about determining orthology and paralogy of homologous genes.
2. Identify the critical information given in the problem.	2. The phylogenetic tree provides information about how the genes are related to one another.
Deduce	
3. Consider the topology of the phylogenetic tree. First examine the relationship between the *Drosophila* gene and the mammalian genes. TIP: How many genes were in their common ancestor?	3. The node at the base of the tree represents the ancestral gene. Since all of the mammalian genes are more closely related to one another than they are to the *Drosophila* gene, the ancestral organism had only a single gene.
4. Examine the earliest node in the phylogenetic tree to see if it corresponds to a speciation event or a gene duplication event.	4. At the earliest node in the tree (node ❶), the divergence produced the *Drosophila* gene and a lineage of mammalian genes. Thus, this node is a speciation event, with the common ancestor of *Drosophila* and mammals speciating to produce a lineage leading to *Drosophila* and another leading to mammals.
5. Determine for each node in the tree whether it represents a speciation or gene duplication event.	5. Following the lineage leading to the mammalian genes (node ❷), the divergence produces two lineages, each containing both mouse and human genes. Thus, the duplication must have been a gene duplication and not a speciation. The divergence at node ❸ is similar to that of node ❷ and so must also be a gene duplication. In contrast, nodes ❹, ❺, and ❻ all diverge to produce a mouse gene and a human gene and thus represent the speciation event leading to mice and humans.
Solve	
6. What is the relationship between the *Drosophila* gene and the mammalian genes? TIP: Orthologs are produced by a speciation event and paralogs are produced by a gene duplication event.	6. Since we concluded that the divergence at node ❶ was a speciation event, the *Drosophila* gene is orthologous to all of the mammalian genes and vice versa.
7. What are the relationships between the human and mouse genes?	7. Let's consider three specific sets of genes. First, consider mouse *sonic hedgehog* and human *sonic hedgehog*—these two genes are related by a speciation even at node ❻ and are thus orthologs. Next, consider human *sonic hedgehog* and human *desert hedgehog*—these two genes are related by a gene duplication event at node ❷ and are thus paralogs. Finally, consider human *desert hedgehog* and mouse *indian hedgehog*—these two genes are related by a gene duplication event at node ❸ and are thus paralogs.

For more practice, see Problems 16 and 23.

Visit the Study Area to access study tools.

Mastering Genetics

archaeal gene encodes a reverse gyrase, a topoisomerase that induces positive supercoils in DNA and is required for adaptation to living at high temperatures.

Although genes encoding proteins with metabolic functions appear to have been donated in lateral gene transfer events, those that encode proteins for information processing (e.g., replication, transcription, and translation) are not commonly transferred. One possible explanation for this bias is that proteins with information processing functions often act in large complexes and are not easily incorporated into existing complexes in other species.

The rarity of lateral gene transfer between eukaryotes and also between eukaryotes and members of either of the other two domains, compared with its relative frequency among bacteria and archaea, is due in part to the differences between eukaryotic transcriptional and translational control mechanisms and those of bacteria and archaea. Even though the bacterium *Agrobacterium tumefaciens* transfers genes to plant cells (see Section 15.2), there is little evidence that those genes have entered the germ line of the transformed plants. Conversely, there is no evidence of transfer of genes from transgenic plants to soil bacteria. However, there is one prominent exception to this generalization: the transfer of genetic material from endosymbionts to their hosts. The most conspicuous examples are the large-scale transfers of genes from mitochondria and chloroplasts to the nucleus in eukaryotic cells (explored in greater detail in Section 17.5). Finally, although lateral gene transfer between two eukaryotes is not thought to be common, it has been documented—for example, between parasitic flowering plants and their flowering plant hosts as well as between fungi and aphids.

Interspecific Genome Comparisons: Genome Annotation

By comparing the genome sequences of related species, researchers are often able to refine their annotations of predicted genes whose existence has not been experimentally confirmed. If the predicted gene in fact functions as a gene, orthologous genes are likely to exist in related species.

Conserved Coding Sequences Comparative genomic analyses can facilitate the discovery of previously unannotated genes. Sequences that are conserved in the genomes of two or more species are more likely to be functional (e.g., encode genes) than sequences that are not conserved. Due to the redundancy of the genetic code, amino acid sequences of proteins are often more conserved than the nucleotide sequences that encode them. Thus, in searches for conserved coding sequences, the nucleotide sequences of each of the genomes are first translated into all six potential reading frames and the hypothetical amino acid sequences are compared (see tblastx in Research Technique 16.2). Conserved sequences can then be used to direct experimental examination of the predicted genes, leading to refinement of the genome annotation.

Gene annotation can be hampered by a lack of homology to known genes. This is especially the case with genes or exons of a small size (e.g., encoding proteins of less than 100 amino acids), as they are particularly difficult to predict. Consider that stop codons occur, on average, about once in 21 codons (3/64) in a random sequence. Thus, random ORFs of 63 amino acids occur frequently (approximately 5% of the time in any random 189-bp sequence). Furthermore, in multicellular eukaryotes, the coding sequences of genes are typically broken into small exons (often encoding fewer than 100 amino acids) dispersed over large distances, thus making their unambiguous identification a challenge. Annotation of such genes is typically feasible only with either experimental evidence or evidence of similar sequences in other genomes.

In the case of the *Saccharomyces* species (see Figure 16.13), comparisons between the four genomes led to prediction of more than 40 previously unannotated genes encoding proteins between 50 and 100 amino acids in length. Likewise, comparisons of the human genome with the genomes of other vertebrates have aided in the identification of exons and significantly refined the annotation of the human genome. This is one respect in which the genome sequencing of model genetic organisms has greatly increased our knowledge of our own genome.

Conserved Noncoding Sequences Besides helping to identify open reading frames, genome comparisons have also detected the presence of **conserved noncoding sequences (CNSs)**. Noncoding DNA was once called "junk" DNA (a term originally coined by Sydney Brenner) since junk, as opposed to garbage, is something we tend to keep even though it serves no identifiable purpose. Today, however, we know that at least some of this noncoding DNA is functional; it contains regulatory sequences and genes that produce functional noncoding RNAs, such as microRNA genes and lncRNAs (see Section 13.3 for discussion of these types of genes).

There are two methods for identifying conserved noncoding sequences, and they approach the task from opposite directions. In **phylogenetic footprinting**, conserved sequences are identified by searching for similar sequences in species separated *by large evolutionary distances*. Conversely, in **phylogenetic shadowing**, conserved sequences are identified by comparison of sequences *in closely related species*, after first eliminating sequences that are not conserved among them. Comparative sequence analyses of CNSs are now often the first step to predicting regulatory sequences, which are then tested by experiment (see Figure 14.18).

Regulatory sequences controlling expression of genes in most multicellular eukaryotes consist of enhancer modules spanning hundreds and potentially tens of thousands of base pairs (see Section 13.1). A large number of CNSs that correspond to regulatory sequences have been identified by phylogenetic footprinting using comparisons of

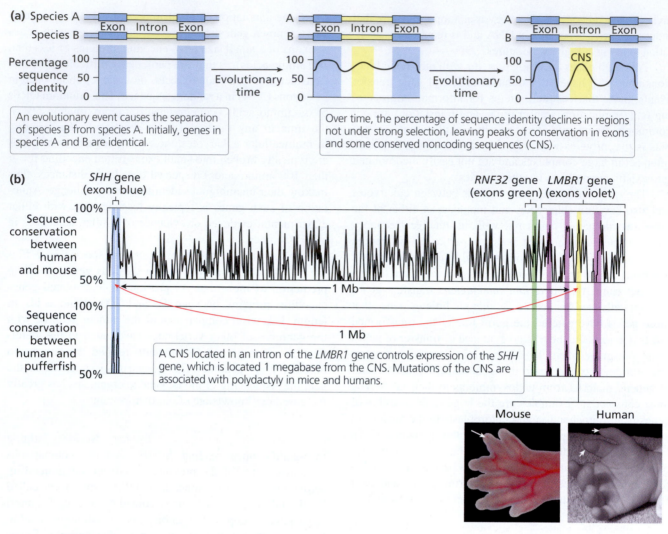

Figure 16.17 **Phylogenetic footprinting.** **(a)** Evolution of a conserved noncoding sequence (CNS). **(b)** A CNS associated with the *SHH* gene acts as an enhancer directing expression of the *SHH* gene in the developing limb bud.

mammalian and other vertebrate genomes (**Figure 16.17a**). Comparisons between mammals and fish have shown that enhancer modules can be conserved over large evolutionary distances (the lineages leading to fish and humans separated about 400 million years ago). Conserved noncoding sequences are often clustered in the genome, and they are often adjacent to evolutionarily conserved genes involved in basic developmental processes. For example, comparisons between the human, mouse, and fugu (pufferfish) genomes identified a CNS corresponding to an enhancer module approximately 1 megabase distant from the *sonic hedgehog* (*SHH*) gene (**Figure 16.17b**). When this CNS was tested for regulatory activity, it drove expression of a reporter gene in mice in a manner reminiscent of the endogenous *SHH* expression pattern in developing limb buds. This CNS is functionally important because mutations in this enhancer are associated with polydactyly in both mice and humans.

In contrast to phylogenetic footprinting, phylogenetic shadowing identifies conserved sequences via comparison of multiple closely related species. In this approach, sequences that are not conserved in at least one of the species are removed from consideration, whereas sequences that *are* conserved in all species are considered as potential functional sequences. Phylogenetic shadowing has identified functional sequences in the human genome by looking for sequences that have not changed in any of several primate species (**Figure 16.18**).

Interspecific Genome Comparisons: Gene Order

Just as the evolutionary history of organisms and genes can be traced by comparisons of genomes, so can the evolutionary histories of chromosomes. For example, humans have $2n = 46$ chromosomes, but our closest relatives (chimpanzees,

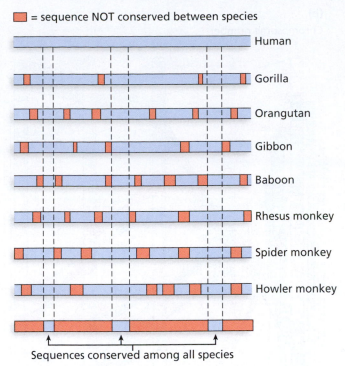

= sequence NOT conserved between species

Sequences conserved among all species

Figure 16.18 Phylogenetic shadowing of primate species.

Contrast the approach of phylogenetic shadowing with that of phylogenetic footprinting.

gorillas, orangutans) have an additional pair of chromosomes, $2n = 48$ (see Figure 10.30). Comparing the chromosomes of humans and these other primates for **synteny**—the conserved order of consecutive orthologous genes along the length of a chromosome or chromosomal segment—shows that a pair of chromosomes in our common ancestor fused to form a single chromosome, chromosome 2, in humans. Other minor differences among primate chromosomes can be accounted for by a small number of translocation and inversion events.

Synteny can also be observed in more distantly related mammals, such as between mouse and human lineages that diverged about 100 million years ago (**Figure 16.19**). Genome sequence information can provide detailed views of synteny between even more distantly related organisms. Even if chromosome synteny is not conserved, synteny at the level of only a few genes, referred to as **microsynteny**, can sometimes be detected. For example, such information has revealed relationships between the chromosomes of birds and mammals.

Even when synteny is conserved at a chromosomal level, comparative studies have revealed large numbers of small rearrangements between closely related species. In a sense, this can be considered a loss of microsynteny. The large amount of repetitive DNA in eukaryotic genomes coupled with unequal crossing over due to mispairing during meiosis provides a mechanism by which DNA rearrangements can

Figure 16.19 Synteny between human and mouse chromosomes.

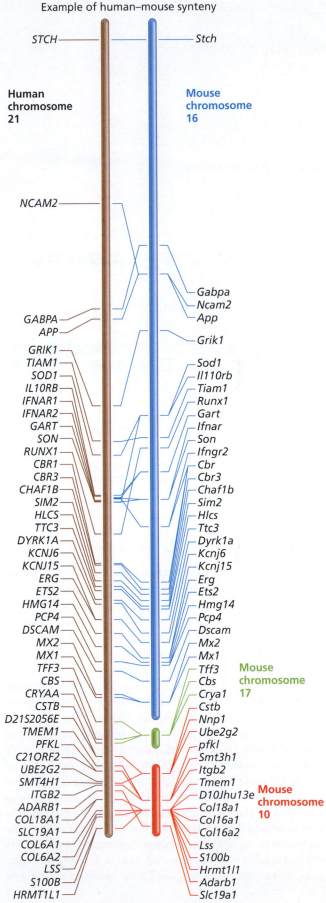

Example of human–mouse synteny

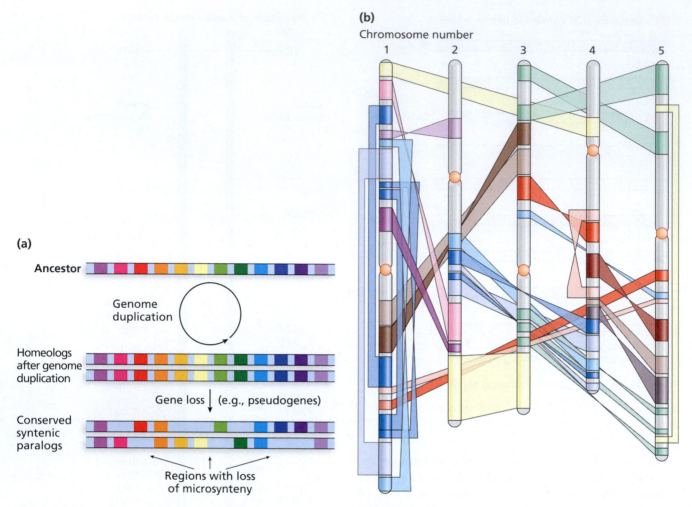

Figure 16.20 **Evidence of past whole-genome duplications.** **(a)** Following a whole-genome duplication, gene loss via pseudogene formation results in a "diploid" species. **(b)** Evidence of past whole-genome duplications in the *Arabidopsis* genome. Colored bands connect duplicated segments. Twisted bands connect duplicated segments having reversed orientations.

occur. The presence of numerous small deletions, duplications, and inversions suggests that chromosome structure is dynamic on a local scale. An example of a loss of micro-synteny can be seen in the loss of strict colinearity between the mouse and human chromosomes shown in Figure 16.19. As we discuss later in this chapter, small rearrangements are also found within individuals of a single species.

Another striking feature of most eukaryotic genomes examined to date is the evidence of past whole-genome duplications as well as smaller duplications involving only segments of chromosomes. Whole-genome duplications result in gene duplications on a massive scale and have contributed significantly to the evolution of many eukaryotic lineages. A whole-genome duplication instantly provides duplicate sets of genes, referred to as **homeologs**, that can subsequently undergo sub- and neo-functionalization, the latter a driver of evolution. Immediately following a whole-genome duplication, a previously diploid species is transformed into a tetraploid. However, over time, through duplicate genes evolving into

pseudogenes or becoming subfunctionalized, the initially tetraploid species evolves into one whose chromosomes behave as a diploid. This process has been termed diploidization (**Figure 16.20a**).

Evidence for both past whole-genome and smaller segmental duplications can be seen in the *Arabidopsis* genome in **Figure 16.20b**. Although whole-genome duplications (e.g., polyploidy) are particularly abundant in plants (see Section 10.3), they are not limited to plants. Evidence of past genome duplications is seen in fungal (e.g., *S. cerevisiae*) as well as vertebrate (e.g., *Danio rerio*) genomes.

16.4 Functional Genomics Aims to Elucidate Gene Function

Although the genome sequence supplies a catalog of genes for an organism, it does not directly provide an understanding of how the genes direct the organism's development and physiology. For this, we need to know when and where genes are expressed, the phenotypes of loss- and gain-of-function alleles, which other genes act in the same or redundant pathways, and which proteins each gene product interacts with. Functional genomics is the study of gene function from a whole-genome perspective.

High-throughput technologies, in which a large number of genes are analyzed simultaneously, have enabled genome-wide examination of RNA- and protein-expression patterns, genetic interactions, and protein–DNA as well as protein–protein interactions. In addition, high-throughput technologies have facilitated the creation of mutant alleles of all genes in the genome of some model genetic species. In this section, we describe some high-throughput technologies of functional genomics and consider what we have learned by applying them to model organisms.

Transcriptomics

One important clue to the function of a gene is when and where the gene is expressed. The study of gene expression from a genomic perspective is called **transcriptomics**, and the set of transcripts present in a cell or organism is called the **transcriptome**. Two high-throughput techniques used to analyze the transcriptome are high-throughput sequencing of cDNA and hybridization on DNA microarrays. High-throughput sequencing is becoming the dominant method, but DNA microarrays are still in widespread use. Below we describe the two techniques and illustrate their use in transcriptomic analyses.

Transcriptome Analysis by Sequencing High-throughput DNA sequencing techniques (see Section 7.5) provide a direct way of assaying the transcriptome. In this approach, RNA isolated from the cells of interest and converted into cDNA is fragmented and sequenced by high-throughput technology. The resulting sequence, often referred to as "RNA-seq," is then compared with the reference genome sequence to identify similar sequences that are present in the cDNA population as a whole (**Figure 16.21a**). The power to examine gene expression patterns through the use of sequencing is limited only by the degree to which mRNA can be extracted from specific cells or tissues and converted to cDNA, with the sequencing of mRNA from a single cell now possible.

The sequencing approach has two advantages over hybridization-based techniques used with microarrays. First, the sequencing approach has the potential to be more quantitative. Since millions of cDNA fragments can be sequenced, precise quantitative data on gene expression levels can be obtained. The number of times a sequence is detected in cDNA pool reflects the relative expression level of that sequence in the cDNA sample. Second, sequencing approaches can more easily distinguish between transcripts with similar sequences, such as alternative splice variants and SNPs, which are sometimes difficult to distinguish with hybridization techniques.

The first application of high-throughput sequencing to transcriptome analysis of the yeast genome was published in 2008. It provided precise descriptions of the 5′ and 3′ ends of transcripts and clarified gene annotations. Subsequent similar studies on other species followed, revealing the extent and nature of alternative splicing, which is prevalent in most multicellular eukaryotes. Such experiments have also facilitated gene annotation by identifying novel transcripts. Genes that had not yet been annotated using computational approaches have often been identified by using expression data.

One surprising result from the application of next-generation sequencing of transcriptomes was the large number of previously unidentified transcripts, many of them noncoding, present in the cells of many multicellular eukaryotes. Some of these have been shown to encode microRNAs or lncRNAs (see Section 13.3), but many others do not have any as-yet-known functions. The numbers of such transcripts range in the hundreds in some invertebrates to thousands in mammals, and an active area of research is to identify the functions, if any, for these RNA molecules.

DNA Microarrays **DNA microarrays** consist of collections of synthesized DNA fragments (oligonucleotides) attached to a solid support (**Figure 16.21b**). The DNA fragments are of a fixed length, usually 25 to 70 bases. The specific DNA sequences, representing sequences present in a genome, are chemically synthesized on a silicon substrate, called a chip, at high density—tens of thousands to millions of oligonucleotide sequences per array, each sequence located on a different spot in the array. Following hybridization with a fluorescent probe representing cDNA, the intensity of the signal from each of the spots reflects the concentration of the sequence complementary to the probe. One advantage of microarrays is that they can be custom designed, because the spots can be added independently. An **expression array** carries unique sequences from every annotated gene of the genome. Hybridization of an expression array with labeled cDNA probes produces quantitative information about the relative expression levels of the genes represented on the array.

Arrays can also be designed to identify binding sites and proteins bound to DNA, including transcription factor binding sites and histone modifications (see Section 13.2). This is accomplished by applying the technique of chromatin immunoprecipitation (ChIP) at a whole-genome level. As described in Chapter 13, DNA that is immunoprecipitated with antibodies to the protein of interest can be sequenced, revealing the genomic sequences to which the targeted protein was bound in the cell. This technique provides a genome-wide view of protein–DNA interactions and is known colloquially as "ChIP-seq" (bottom two lines in Figure 16.21a).

(a)

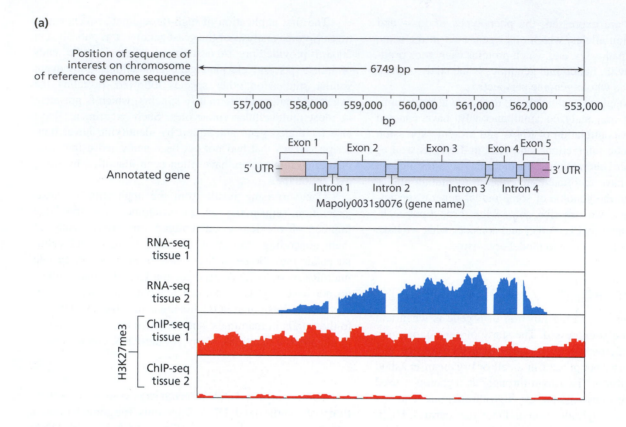

(b)

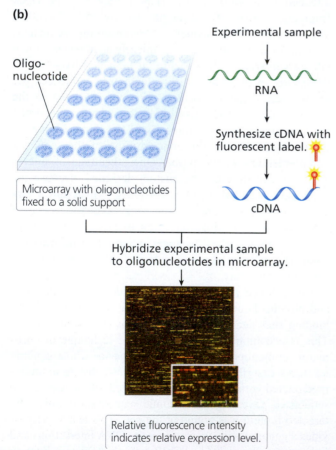

Oligo-
nucleotide

Microarray with oligonucleotides
fixed to a solid support

Experimental sample

RNA

Synthesize cDNA with
fluorescent label.

cDNA

Hybridize experimental sample
to oligonucleotides in microarray.

Relative fluorescence intensity
indicates relative expression level.

Figure 16.21 Transcriptome analysis. (a) Reads of RNA-seq
map primarily to exons and UTRs, as intronic sequence degrades
rapidly following splicing. In this example, gene expression is
inversely correlated with H3K27me3 marking (see Section 13.2),
mapped by ChIP-seq. **(b)** Oligonucleotide arrays. Each spot contains copies of a different sequence.

Example of Transcriptome Analysis An example from the budding yeast *S. cerevisiae* illustrates how microarray data can provide insight into the function of genes not previously identified by forward genetic approaches. Diploid yeast cells of *S. cerevisiae* produce haploid cells through the developmental process of sporulation, which consists of meiosis and spore morphogenesis. From forward genetic studies, approximately 150 genes were known to be involved in sporulation, and these could be classified into four groups defined by expression patterns and mutant phenotypes.

To examine genome-wide expression patterns during sporulation, diploid yeast cells were induced to sporulate, RNA samples were taken at seven time points spanning 11 hours, and their expression levels were compared to identify genes whose expression was either induced or repressed at those different times (**Figure 16.22**). More than 1000 genes exhibited significant changes in expression at some point during the sporulation process: In about 40% of these cases the genes became induced, and in the other 60% the genes became repressed. In other words, more than six times as many genes as had been identified previously were likely to play some role during sporulation.

The researchers categorized the induced genes by their expression patterns, expanding the four previously described patterns to at least seven. Genes with expression patterns similar to those of known genes could be hypothesized to have biological roles similar to those of the known genes. For example, some "Early I" genes (see Figure 16.22) are known to function in the synapsis of homologous chromosomes. By extrapolation, other Early I genes whose functions are unknown may also have roles in synapsis of chromosomes, suggesting areas for experimental study to support or refute the predicted roles. Similarly, comparisons of sequences upstream of coordinately regulated genes can provide information on gene regulation. For example, more than 40% of the Early I genes have a consensus upstream regulatory sequence (URS1) to which the transcription factor UME6 binds, suggesting that this set of genes is coordinately regulated by the same transcription factor. This research into temporal gene-expression patterns during sporulation has provided clues to the functions of hundreds of previously uncharacterized genes, some with homologs in humans.

Transcriptome analyses are routinely used in functional genomics studies, including many pertaining to the study of human cancers. In cancer studies, for example, they allow precise characterization of gene expression in morphologically similar but molecularly different cancers, facilitating the design of targeted treatments using drugs known to affect specific gene products.

Although transcriptomics can provide a broad overview of genome-wide gene expression, techniques in addition to transcriptomic approaches are often required for multicellular organisms, to provide details concerning genes that are expressed in a tissue- or cell-type–specific manner. Reporter genes (see Section 14.4) provide one approach to determining both temporal and spatial gene expression patterns at high resolution. Comparative genomic techniques to identify potential regulatory sequences (see Figures 16.17 and 16.18) can guide the design of reporter gene constructs. Confirmation of expression patterns revealed by reporter gene analysis can be obtained in a process analogous to a northern blot (see Section 1.4) but in which a labeled RNA probe is applied directly to tissue in which the mRNA is fixed in place rather than purified and separated by electrophoresis.

Other "-omes" and "-omics"

By the same logic that produced the terms *genomics* and *transcriptomics*, **proteomics** is the study of all the proteins—collectively known as the **proteome**—expressed in a cell, tissue, or individual. Whereas the biochemistry of nucleic acids is predictable—any nucleic acid can base-pair with any other nucleic acid, given complementary sequences—the biochemistry of the proteome is complicated by the much greater range of protein structures and functions. The study of proteins thus requires techniques tailored to specific subsets of proteins.

Multiple high-throughput technologies have been developed for proteomic analyses, including techniques to study protein expression, protein modification, and protein–protein interactions. Examples of the latter—techniques that reveal whether and how different proteins interact—provide information on the functioning of biological systems by identifying, for instance, sets of proteins that form a complex. Here we discuss one technique for identifying interacting proteins.

The **two-hybrid system** is a high-throughput method for discovering whether two proteins interact. This system is based on the modular nature of the Gal4 transcription factor from yeast that binds to the *GAL4* upstream activation sequence (or UAS_{GAL4}), which is an enhancer element, to activate the transcription of genes involved in galactose metabolism (see Section 13.1). One domain of the Gal4 protein, the DNA-binding domain, binds to the UAS_{GAL4} sequence; a second domain, the activation domain, activates transcription by interacting with RNA polymerase II as well as other chromatin factors (**Figure 16.23a**). The two domains can be physically separated.

To test whether two proteins interact, one of the proteins to be tested is translationally fused (see Section 14.4) to the Gal4 DNA-binding domain (BD), and the other protein to be tested is translationally fused to the Gal4 activation domain (AD). Both of these chimeric genes are then transformed into a single yeast strain. If the two proteins interact, the Gal4-BD and Gal4-AD will be brought together, and Gal4-activated genes will be transcribed. Conversely, if the two proteins do not interact, no transcription of the Gal4-activated reporter gene will be observed. To facilitate the screening process,

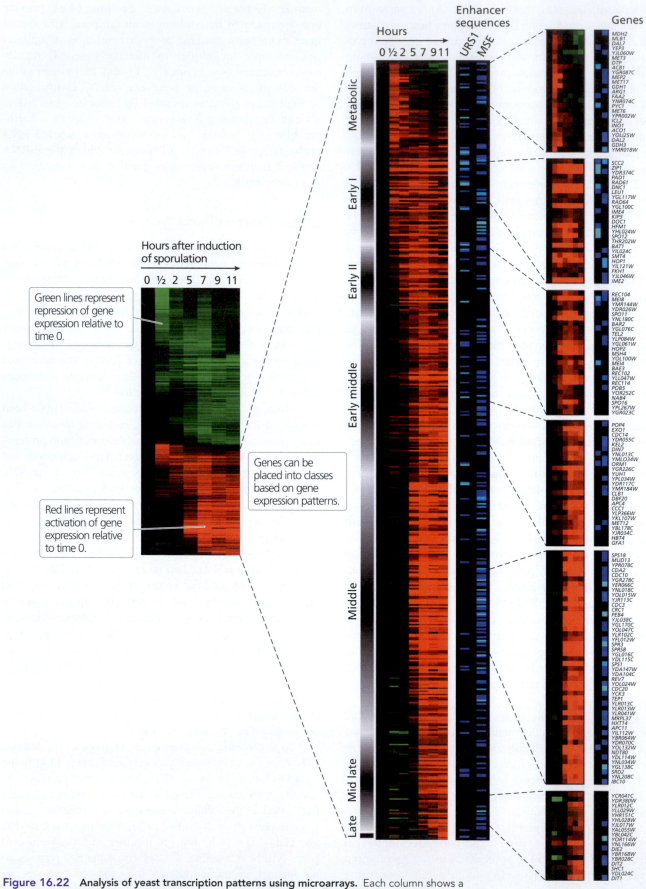

Figure 16.22 Analysis of yeast transcription patterns using microarrays. Each column shows a different pattern of gene expression, correlating to a different point in time in the sporulation process.

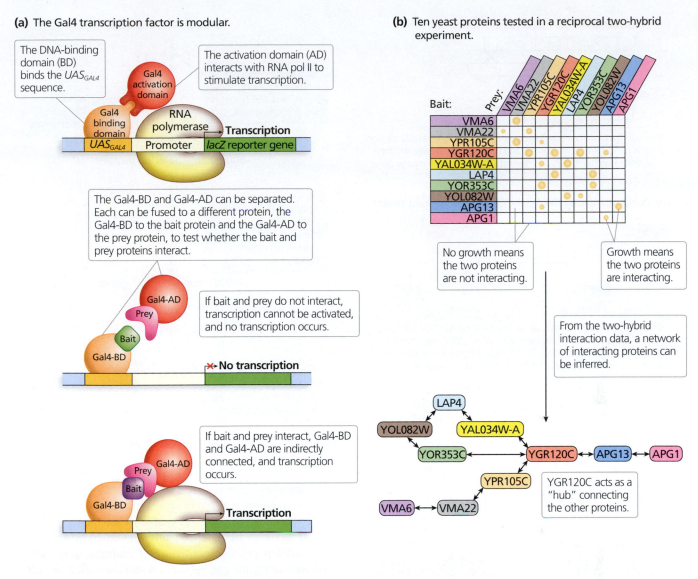

Figure 16.23 **Identifying protein–protein interaction networks. (a)** The two-hybrid system identifies interacting proteins. **(b)** Application of the two-hybrid system identifies networks of interacting proteins.

Q **Why might some proteins be incapable of being analyzed by the two-hybrid system?**

an auxotrophic yeast strain is often used in which UAS_{GAL4} drives expression of a gene that will complement the auxotrophic defect. For example, a *histidine* auxotroph with a UAS_{GAL4}:*HIS* transgene will not grow on media lacking histidine unless Gal4-mediated transcription is active. However, certain interactions cannot be detected with the standard two-hybrid system, including those in which the interacting proteins are not efficiently transported into the nucleus and those in which proteins require a third partner for interaction.

Two-hybrid approaches have been applied successfully to many model systems, providing information on their protein-interaction networks. In *S. cerevisiae*, all pairwise combinations of the more than 6000 proteins encoded in the genome have been tested, providing an overview of protein-interaction networks in the living yeast cell (see **Figure 16.23b**). The sum of all of the protein–protein interactions in an organism is known as the **interactome**.

Genomic Approaches to Reverse Genetics One surprising result of genome sequencing was the large number of genes identified by sequence analysis but not previously identified by forward genetic screens. Even in an intensely studied organism such as *S. cerevisiae*, only about 1000 of the more than 6000 genes in the genome had been identified by forward genetic screens. Of the remaining 5000 or so genes, about half had some sequence similarity to genes with a known or probable function, whereas the other half did not exhibit homology to any other known genes in other model systems. Analyses of other multicellular eukaryotic genomes had similar outcomes.

At the same time, the high-throughput techniques discussed above have limitations. They can provide information on gene expression patterns and protein–protein interactions, but to fully understand gene function, we must be able to analyze loss- and gain-of-function alleles.

(a) Construction of barcoded yeast deletion mutants

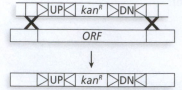

The coding regions of each gene were replaced by a selectable marker gene (e.g., kanamycin resistance), and barcodes unique to each gene were added upstream (UP) and downstream (DN) of the marker gene.

(b) Competitive growth of pools of deletion mutant strains

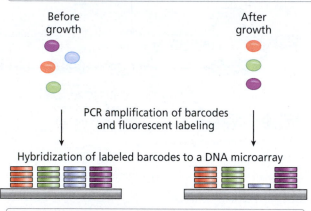

The barcoded mutant strains can be grown in competition with wild type or each other. In this example, the "blue" strain does not grow as well as the other three strains. DNA is isolated before and after growth, and each gene can be analyzed by using fluorescently labeled barcode primers.

Before growth — After growth

PCR amplification of barcodes and fluorescent labeling

Hybridization of labeled barcodes to a DNA microarray

The relative proportion of growth of each strain can be examined by hybridizing the products to a DNA microarray.

Figure 16.24 Barcoded knockout libraries for phenotypic analyses of mutants.

Reverse genetic approaches (see Section 14.3) provide an experimental avenue for exploring such alleles and, through them, the function of the many previously unidentified genes revealed by genome sequencing techniques.

A useful tool for genomic analysis by reverse genetics is a collection of mutant alleles for every gene in the genome, referred to as a **knockout library**. Such libraries are available for many model organisms, although for most they are not quite complete (see Section 14.3). In the case of *S. cerevisiae*, a knockout library containing deletion loss-of-function alleles of every gene is available. In the mutant strains, the entire target gene is replaced with a marker gene that confers resistance to the antibiotic kanamycin (**Figure 16.24**). In addition, in each deletion strain,

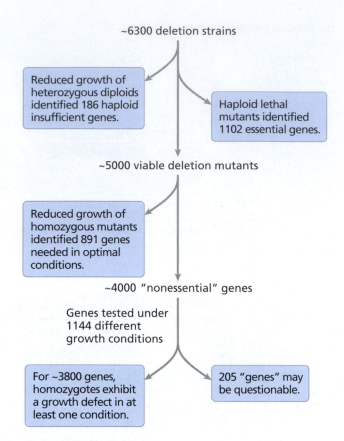

Figure 16.25 Global analysis of yeast deletion mutants.

the kanamycin gene is flanked by two 20-bp sequences, termed **barcodes**; a different set of barcodes is used for each deletion strain. The barcodes enable the abundance of each mutant strain to be independently quantified when grown in a mixed population consisting of multiple strains. Specific mutant strains can be verified and quantified by selective amplification of barcode sequences using PCR-based strategies.

Use of Yeast Mutants to Categorize Genes

A challenge for the future is to determine more precisely the molecular and biological roles of all genes, to illuminate why they are maintained in the genome. As an initial step in this direction, yeast deletion strains have been analyzed to categorize *S. cerevisiae* genes as either essential for life or nonessential.

The deletion strains are first constructed in diploid yeast. The heterozygous diploid deletion strain is then induced to undergo meiosis, allowing the phenotypes of deletion alleles to be analyzed in the haploid progeny. When mutations in each of the 6300 genes of *S. cerevisiae* were examined in this way, deletion alleles of 1102 genes were not recoverable in haploid progeny (**Figure 16.25**). These genes, about 20% of the yeast genome, define the essential gene set of *S. cerevisiae*, meaning that they are required for survival of the organism. In addition, 186 of the deletion mutants had a reduced-growth phenotype as heterozygotes before induction of meiosis, thus indicating haploinsufficiency of these genes. (Recall that haploinsufficiency is a dominant phenotype in diploid organisms that are heterozygous for a loss-of-function allele.) For the remaining 5000 genes, both haploid deletion mutants and homozygous diploid mutants were obtained. However, 891 of these mutant strains exhibited a slow-growth defect in rich media under optimal conditions, which indicates that the genes are required for vital biological processes in optimal growth conditions. This leaves about 4000 genes for which no obvious mutant phenotype is detected under optimal growth conditions. These genes are referred to as nonessential, but that classification is dependent on environment; in other words, the genes are nonessential under optimal laboratory growth conditions.

One possible explanation for the lack of conspicuous mutant phenotypes associated with 4000 nonessential *S. cerevisiae* genes is that the genes are required only under specific growth conditions. To test this hypothesis, each mutant strain was grown under a variety of environmental conditions, including variations in temperature, media composition, and the presence of antifungal compounds, salts, and other chemicals known to perturb specific biological processes. As a result, yeast geneticists discovered measurable growth defects under at least one environmental condition for 3800 of the 4000 genes previously identified as nonessential. Thus, these genes are required for efficient growth in at least one tested environmental condition; they are not really "nonessential" from an evolutionary perspective, because their presence is likely to provide a selective advantage. Growth defects were not found for only about 200 deletions, suggesting that either (1) these genes are authentically nonessential, (2) the conditions under which they confer an advantage were not among the ones tested, (3) that other genes serve the same function, or (4) designating them as genes is incorrect.

To further analyze the essential genes, conditional alleles are required. Traditionally, temperature-sensitive alleles isolated in forward genetic screens have been used. Various libraries of engineered conditional alleles of *S. cerevisiae* essential genes have also been constructed for this purpose. In one approach, each essential gene is placed under the control of a tetracycline-repressible promoter. In the absence of tetracycline, the gene is expressed, but upon addition of tetracycline, gene expression is repressed, creating a loss-of-function phenotype. In another approach, a short peptide tag that confers heat-inducible protein degradation is added to the coding regions of essential genes. Under the normal growth temperature of 30°C, the protein is stable, but at 37°C, the tagged proteins are degraded and lose the ability to function.

Other types of libraries that have been constructed provide additional tools for identifying potential gene functions in *S. cerevisiae*. For example, a library in which every gene is a translational fusion with green fluorescent protein (GFP) permits visual determination of the subcellular location of proteins.

Genetic Networks

Identification of genetic interactions can provide clues to gene function by revealing that two genes act in the same pathway or redundant pathways (see Section 14.1). Data derived from double mutants identify sets of interacting genes that define **genetic networks**.

An extreme example of a genetic interaction is *synthetic lethality*, where the mutation of either gene alone is not lethal but mutation of both genes together results in lethality (see Figure 14.5). A genome-wide estimate of the number of synthetic lethal interactions in *S. cerevisiae* was obtained by using mutants representing 132 genes and analyzing their genetic interactions. For genes whose single-mutant phenotype is inviability, conditional alleles were used; for nonessential genes, null alleles were used. Each of the 132 mutants was crossed with 4700 viable deletion mutants, and the double-mutant phenotypes were examined. Approximately 4000 different synthetic lethal interactions were identified, involving about 1000 different genes. The number of interactions per gene ranged from 1 to 146, with an average of 34. One striking feature of this genetic interaction study is that essential genes exhibited about five times as many interactions as did "nonessential" genes. These results suggest that genetic networks consist of a small number of essential genes participating in many interactions and a larger number of nonessential genes participating in fewer interactions (**Figure 16.26**).

If the same level of synthetic lethality exists for the remaining genes in the yeast genome, it is estimated that 200,000 different synthetic lethal interactions will occur among all yeast genes and that 1% of all double mutants will result in synthetic lethality. Thus, although only 1000 genes are essential under optimal laboratory growth conditions as defined by single-mutant phenotypes, additional genes become essential when organisms are compromised by a mutation in another gene. One explanation for the observed levels of synthetic lethality is that where there are multiple genetic pathways, some of the pathways buffer one another, creating stable genetic systems that are better able to withstand environmental and genetic perturbations.

Genetic networks defined by genetic interactions often identify groups of genes having similar molecular functions, such as translation, lipid metabolism, or DNA repair (see Figure 16.26). If a gene of unknown function belongs to a genetic network in which many genes have known roles—say, in lipid metabolism—experiments to identify the molecular function of the unknown gene might begin by investigating whether the gene in question also plays a role in lipid metabolism.

Genetic networks constructed on the basis of genetic interactions can be examined in comparison with groupings based on other gene attributes, such as their annotations,

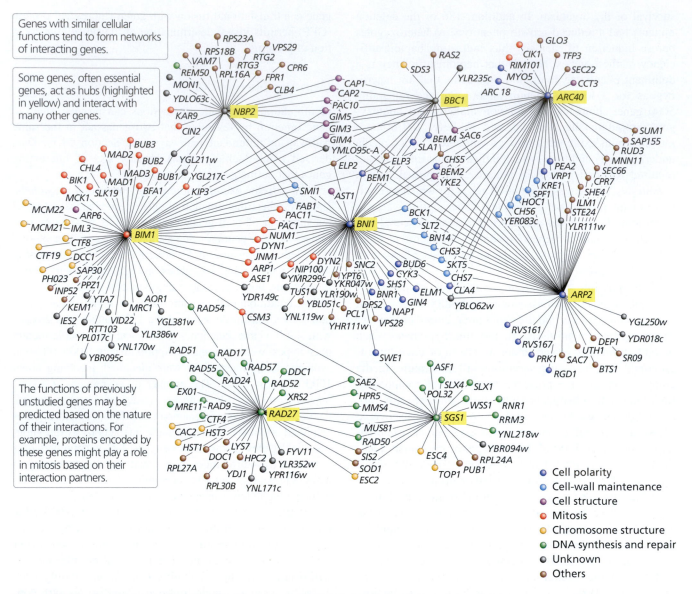

Genes with similar cellular functions tend to form networks of interacting genes.

Some genes, often essential genes, act as hubs (highlighted in yellow) and interact with many other genes.

The functions of previously unstudied genes may be predicted based on the nature of their interactions. For example, proteins encoded by these genes might play a role in mitosis based on their interaction partners.

- Cell polarity
- Cell-wall maintenance
- Cell structure
- Mitosis
- Chromosome structure
- DNA synthesis and repair
- Unknown
- Others

Figure 16.26 Genetic interactions identified through synthetic lethal analysis. Mutant alleles of eight genes (*BNI1*, *RAD27*, *SGS1*, *BBC1*, *NBP2*, *BIM1*, *ARP2*, and *ARC40*) were assayed for synthetic lethal interactions with the 5000 viable deletion mutants of yeast.

Q Compare and contrast genetic hubs with protein–protein interaction hubs.

expression patterns, or interactomes (discerned from protein–protein interaction data). The prediction of biological functions of genes based on correlations between different data sets is referred to as **systems biology**.

Genetic interaction data often correlate well with gene expression data, since genes that compensate for one another in function often exhibit similar expression patterns. In contrast, genetic interactions and protein–protein interactions overlap less often. One reason is that physically interacting proteins are likely to act in the same protein complex, whereas in genetic interactions involving null alleles, the proteins the genes encode often act in compensating pathways that would normally be composed of different protein complexes with related functions. For the most part, this generalization holds true only when null alleles are used

to test genetics interactions; however, when hypomorphic alleles are used, genetic interactions can reveal genes encoding proteins that act in the same complex or pathway (see Section 14.1).

The ultimate objective of functional genomics studies is to define the molecular function of every gene in an organism by compiling genomic data and searching for correlations that suggest hypotheses for further experimentation. The discussion here has focused on studies in *S. cerevisiae*, but similar approaches are being taken in other organisms. For example, enhancer–suppressor genetic screens described in Section 14.1 are a directed approach for uncovering genetic interaction networks and can be applied to most organisms regardless of the availability of knockout libraries.

CASE STUDY

Genomic Analysis of Insect Guts May Fuel the World

In metagenomic analysis, biologists study genomes collected from the multiple organisms that together inhabit a single environment. Two recent studies suggest that metagenomic analysis of insect digestive tracts could potentially have a significant impact on the production of biofuels.

Much of the current supply of ethanol for fuel is produced from cellulose that comes from the lignocellulose component of corn. Lignocellulose is a mixture of cellulose (a complex carbohydrate composed of glucose molecules) and lignin (the rigid structural material that protects cellulose). The production of corn ethanol requires high temperature, high heat, and the use of toxic chemicals to break down the lignin and hydrolyze the cellulose. This step is followed by microbial fermentation of the sugar and distillation of ethanol. Obtaining ethanol from corn in this way has adverse effects on the environment, consumes a great deal of energy, and may not be economically viable. These are principal reasons why the investigation of lignocellulose digestion in insects is attractive. Identification and characterization of the genes responsible for lignocellulose digestion may allow the development of new, biologically based methods of biofuel production.

In 2007, the microbiologist Falk Warnecke and colleagues conducted a metagenomic study of the microbes in the gut of the wood-eating termite species *Nasutitermes*. Termites are wood-digesting creatures whose ancestors have inhabited cellulose-rich environments for more than 100 million years. *Nasutitermes* has a bacteria-laden gut that acts like a tiny bioreactor for digesting the lignocellulose in wood. Lignocellulose provides energy for these microorganisms, which first break down lignin to liberate cellulose and then break down cellulose via hydrolysis driven by hydrolase enzymes.

Nasutitermes has a three-part stomach, the main part of which, designated P3, contains a rich microbial mixture of hundreds of bacterial species that are primarily responsible for wood digestion. Warnecke and his colleagues collected *Nasutitermes* in Costa Rica. Then, in the laboratory, they isolated and emptied P3 and found that its total volume in each insect is just 1 microliter (μL). They isolated and performed shotgun sequencing on the DNA from the P3 microbial mass.

Warnecke estimates that the DNA in this metagenomic analysis may come from as many as 300 bacterial species whose symbiotic relationship with the termite allows the termite to derive energy from wood. Gene-identification analyses indicate that many of the most frequently found genes in these bacteria produce glycoside hydrolases (GH) that hydrolyze lignocellulose. More than 700 different GH genes representing more than 45 different gene families were found in this study. A large group of previously unidentified genes was also found, and Warnecke speculates that these genes might be involved in various kinds of lignocellulose binding and digestion reactions.

Although Warnecke's study detected numerous bacterial genes that may carry out cellulose digestion, it did not identify any genes responsible for lignin digestion. However, a second study, published in 2008 by Scott Geib and colleagues, examined lignin digestion in the Asian longhorn beetle (*Anoplophora glabripennis*) and the Pacific dampwood termite (*Zootermopsis angusticollis*). Biochemical analysis of the digestive tracts and digestive products of both insects shows significant evidence of lignin digestion, suggesting either that the genomes of these organisms encode lignin-digesting enzymes or that the organisms carry symbiotic microbes whose genomes encode the enzymes. The researchers did not perform metagenomic analyses of the insect genomes or digestive system contents, but they did identify a single fungal species in the gut of the Asian longhorn beetle whose genome is likely to encode lignin-digesting enzymes.

A great deal of additional "bioprospecting" research will be necessary to characterize the genes that encode the enzymes driving lignin and cellulose digestion in insect guts. In the process, further genomic and metagenomic analyses may suggest ways these genes can be cloned and used to replace the costly current methods of lignocellulose-based ethanol production.

16.1 Structural Genomics Provides a Catalog of Genes in a Genome

- Genomes can be sequenced using a whole-genome shotgun approach.
- Paired-end sequencing facilitates assembly of scaffolds consisting of sequence fragments generated by shotgun sequencing.
- Metagenomics studies the genetic sequences of communities of organisms whose member species may be difficult to cultivate individually.

16.2 Annotation Ascribes Biological Function to DNA Sequences

- Genome annotation indicates the locations of genes and other functional sequences in a genomic sequence. It aims to ascribe biological function to sequence data.
- Biochemical functions of some annotated genes may be predicted based on sequence similarities with known genes as analyzed through computational approaches and bioinformatics, but experimental verification that includes analysis of mutant phenotypes is required to determine biological functions.

16.3 Evolutionary Genomics Traces the History of Genomes

- A phylogenetic tree of life can be constructed by comparing sequences of orthologous genes.
- New genes can be produced by gene duplication due to unequal crossing over or by larger-scale duplications of DNA, retrotransposition, and other mechanisms.
- Most new genes degenerate rapidly, but some are retained and may acquire new functions, driving the evolution of new species.

- Gene duplication has been a key feature in the evolution of complex organisms. Lateral gene transfer is a common mechanism of acquisition of new genes in bacteria and archaea, but it is less common in eukaryotes.
- By comparing genomes of related species, researchers can identify conserved genes and noncoding sequences and refine gene annotation. Conserved noncoding sequences often consist of gene regulatory sequences.
- Intraspecific genome comparisons identify genetic variation within a species and provide information about its evolutionary history and population dynamics. Both intra- and interspecific comparisons reveal that genomes are dynamic and can change rapidly on evolutionary timescales.

16.4 Functional Genomics Aims to Elucidate Gene Function

- High-throughput sequencing and DNA microarrays can reveal polymorphisms, global transcription patterns, and transcription-factor binding sites.
- Protein–protein interactions can be determined by using genetic tools developed from the study of yeast.
- Knockout libraries are used to perform genome-wide genetic screens that elucidate gene function. They have allowed classification of all yeast genes as essential or nonessential under specific growth conditions.
- Genes classified as essential under optimal growth conditions have on average more genetic interactions than those classified as nonessential.
- Genome-wide analyses of synthetic lethal interactions in yeast reveal large numbers of genes that are essential in genetically compromised organisms.
- Systems biology is a research approach that correlates data sets derived from functional genomics to define and elucidate gene function.

PREPARING FOR PROBLEM SOLVING

In addition to the list of problem-solving tips and suggestions given here, you can go to the Study Guide and Solutions Manual that accompanies this book for help at solving problems.

1. Familiarize yourself with the process of whole-genome shotgun sequencing and possible complications due to repetitive DNA.

2. Review how transcriptome sequences can be used to annotate genomic sequence.

3. Review how new genes can arise, and understand the possible fates of a duplicated gene.

4. Review how species become polyploid and then return to a state of diploidy.

5. Review how transcriptome data can be generated and used to examine gene function.

6. Review how knowledge of protein–protein interactions and genetic interactions provides insight into gene function.

Chapter Concepts

For answers to selected even-numbered problems, see Appendix: Answers.

1. You have discovered a new species of archaea from a hot spring in Yellowstone National Park.
   a. After growing a pure culture of this organism, what strategy might you employ to sequence its genome?
   b. How would your strategy change if you were unable to grow the strain in culture?

2. Repetitive DNA poses problems for genome sequencing.
   a. Why is this so?
   b. What types of repetitive DNA are most problematic?
   c. What strategies can be employed to overcome these problems?

3. When the whole-genome shotgun sequence of the *Drosophila* genome was assembled, it comprised 134 scaffolds made up of 1636 contigs.
   a. Why were there so many more contigs than scaffolds?
   b. What is the difference between physical and sequence gaps?
   c. How can physical gaps be closed?
   d. How can sequence gaps be closed?

4. How do cDNA sequences facilitate gene annotation? Describe how the use of full-length cDNAs facilitates discovery of alternative splicing.

5. How do comparisons between genomes of related species help refine gene annotation?

6. You are designing algorithms for the bioinformatic prediction of gene sequences. How might algorithms differ for predicting genes in bacterial versus eukaryotic genomic sequence?

7. You have sequenced a 100-kb region of the *Bacillus anthracis* genome (the bacterium that causes anthrax) and a 100-kb region from the *Gorilla gorilla* genome. What differences and similarities might you expect to see in the annotation of the sequences—for example, in number of genes, gene structure, regulatory sequences, repetitive DNA?

8. You have just obtained 100 kb of genomic sequence from an as yet unsequenced mammalian genome. What are three methods you might use to identify potential genes in the 100 kb? What are the advantages and limitations of each method?

9. The human genome contains a large number of pseudogenes. How would you distinguish whether a particular sequence encodes a gene or a pseudogene? How do pseudogenes arise?

10. Based on the tree of life in Figure 16.12, would you expect human proteins to be more similar to fungal proteins or to plant proteins? Would you expect plant proteins to be more similar to fungal proteins or human proteins?

11. When comparing genes from two sequenced genomes, how does one determine whether two genes are orthologous? What pitfalls arise when one or both of the genomes are not sequenced?

12. What is a reference genome? How can it be used to survey genetic variation within a species?

13. The two-hybrid method facilitates the discovery of protein–protein interactions. How does this technique work? Can you think of reasons for obtaining a false-positive result, that is, where the proteins encoded by two clones interact in the two-hybrid system but do not interact in the organism in which they naturally occur? Can you think of reasons you might obtain a false-negative result, in which the two proteins interact in vivo but fail to interact in the two-hybrid system?

Application and integration

For answers to selected even-numbered problems, see Appendix: Answers.

14. Go to http://blast.ncbi.nlm.nih.gov/Blast.cgi and follow the links to *nucleotide blast*. Type in the sequence below; it is broken up into codons to make it easier to copy.

```
5′ ATG TTC GTC AAT CAG CAC CTT TGT GGT
TCT CAC CTC GTT GAA GCTTTG TAC CTT GTT
    TGC GGT GAA CGT GGT TTC TTC TAC ACT
              CCT AAG ACT TAA 3′
```

As you will note on the BLAST page, there are several options for tailoring your query to obtain the most relevant information. Some are related to which sequences to search in the database. For example, the search can be limited taxonomically (e.g., restricted to mammals) or by the type of sequences in the database (e.g., cDNA or genomic). For our search, we will use the broadest database, the "nucleotide collection (nr/nt)." This is the nonredundant (nr) database of all nucleotide data (nt) in GenBank and can be selected in the "database" dialogue box. Other parameters can also be adjusted to make the search more or less sensitive to mismatches or gaps. For our purposes, we will use the default setting, which is automatically presented. Press "search." What can you say about the DNA sequence?

15. In the course of the *Drosophila melanogaster* genome project, the following genomic DNA sequences were obtained. Try to assemble the sequences into a single contig.

```
5′ TTCCAGAACCGGCGAATGAAGCTGAAGAAG 3′
5′ GAGCGGCAGATCAAGATCTGGTTCCAGAAC 3′
5′ TGATCTGCCGCTCCGTCAGGCATAGCGCGT 3′
5′ GGAGAATCGAGATGGCGCACGCGCTATGCC 3′
5′ GGAGAATCGAGATGGCGCACGCGCTATGCC 3′
5′ CCATCTCGATTCTCCGTCTGCGGGTCAGAT 3′
```

Go to the URL provided in Problem 14, and using the sequence you have just assembled, perform a blastn search of the "nucleotide collection (nr/nt)" database. Does the search produce sequences similar to your assembled sequence, and if so, what are they? Can you tell if your sequence is transcribed, and if it represents protein-coding sequence? Perform a tblastx search, first choosing the "nucleotide collection (nr/nt)" database and then limiting the search to human sequences by typing *Homo sapiens* in the organism box. Are homologous sequences found in the human genome? Annotate the assembled sequence.

16. Consider the phylogenetic trees below pertaining to three related species (A, B, C) that share a common ancestor (last common ancestor, or LCA). The lineage leading to species A diverges before the divergence of species B and C.

a. For gene *X*, no gene duplications have occurred in any lineage, and each gene *X* is derived from the ancestral gene *X* via speciation events. Are genes *AX, BX,* and *CX* orthologous, paralogous, or homologous?

b. For gene *Y*, a gene duplication occurred in the lineage leading to A after it diverged from that leading to B and C. Are genes *AY1* and *AY2* orthologous or paralogous? Are genes *AY1* and *BY* orthologous or paralogous? Are genes *BY* and *CY* orthologous or paralogous?

c. For gene *Z*, gene duplications have occurred in all species. Define orthology and paralogy relationships for the different *Z* genes.

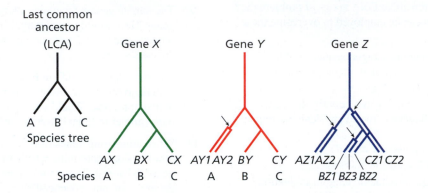

17. You have isolated a gene that is important for the production of milk and wish to study its regulation. You examine the genomes of human, mouse, dog, chicken, pufferfish, and yeast and note that all genomes except yeast have an orthologous gene.

a. How would you identify the regulatory elements important for the expression of your isolated gene in mammary glands?

b. What does the existence of orthologous genes in chicken and pufferfish tell you about the function of this gene?

18. When the human genome is examined, the chromosomes appear to have undergone only minimal rearrangement in the 100 million years since the last common ancestor of eutherian mammals. However, when individual humans are examined or when the human genome is compared with that of chimpanzees, a large number of small indels and SNPs can be detected. How are these observations reconciled?

19. *Symbiodinium minutum* is a dinoflagellate with a genome size that encodes more than 40,000 protein-coding genes. In contrast, the genome of *Plasmodium falciparum* has only a little more than 5000 protein-coding genes. Both *Symbiodinium* and *Plasmodium* are members of the Alveolate lineage of eukaryotes. What might be the cause of such a wide variation in their genome sizes?

20. Substantial fractions of the genomes of many plants consist of segmental duplications; for example, approximately 40% of genes in the *Arabidopsis* genome are duplicated. How might you approach the functional characterization of such genes using reverse genetics?

21. A modification of the two-hybrid system, called the one-hybrid system, is used for identifying proteins that can bind specific DNA sequences. In this method, the DNA sequence to be tested, the bait, is fused to a TATA box to drive expression of a reporter gene. The reporter gene is often chosen to complement a mutant phenotype; for example, a *HIS* gene may be used in a *his⁻* mutant yeast strain. A cDNA library is constructed with the cDNA sequences translationally fused to the GAL4 activation domain and transformed into this yeast strain. Diagram how trans-acting proteins that bind to cis-acting regulatory sequences can be identified using a one-hybrid screen.

22. A substantial fraction of almost every genome sequenced consists of genes that have no known function and that do not have sequence similarity to any genes with known function.

a. Describe two approaches to ascertaining the biological role of these genes in *S. cerevisiae*.

b. How would your approach change if the genes of unknown function were in the human genome?

23. In the globin gene family shown in Figure 16.16, which pair of genes would exhibit a higher level of sequence similarity, the human δ-globin and human β-globin genes or the human β-globin and chimpanzee β-globin genes? Can you explain your answer in terms of timing of gene duplications?

24. You are studying similarities and differences in how organisms respond to high salt concentrations and high temperatures. You begin your investigation by using

microarrays to compare gene expression patterns of *S. cerevisiae* in normal growth conditions, in high-salt concentrations, and at high temperatures. The results are shown here, with the values of red and green representing the extent of increase and decrease, respectively, of expression for genes *a–s* in the experimental conditions versus the control (normal growth) conditions. What is the first step you will take to analyze your data?

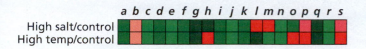

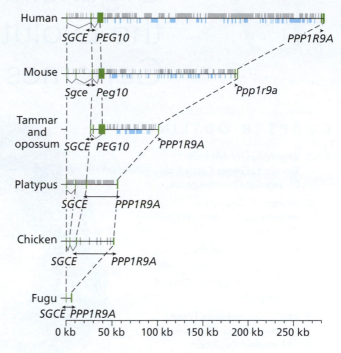

25. In conducting the study described in Problem 24, you have noted that a set of *S. cerevisiae* genes are repressed when yeast are grown under high-salt conditions.
    a. How might you determine whether this set of genes is regulated by a common transcription factor?
    b. How might you approach this question if genome sequences for the related *Saccharomyces* species, *S. paradoxus*, *S. mikatae*, and *S. bayanus*, were also available?

26. *PEG10* (paternally expressed gene 10) is a paternally expressed gene (meaning only the paternal allele is expressed) that has an essential role in the formation of the placenta of the mouse. In the mouse genome, the *PEG10* gene is flanked by the *SGCE* and *PPP1R9A* genes. To study the origin of *PEG10*, you examine syntenic regions spanning the *SGCE* and *PPP1R9A* loci in the genomes of several vertebrates, and you note that the *PEG10* gene is present in the genomes of placental and marsupial mammals but not in the platypus, chicken, or fugu genomes.

    The green bars in the figure indicate the exons of each gene. The gray bars represent LINEs and

SINEs, and the blue bars represent long terminal repeat (LTR) elements of retrotransposons. Solid black diagonal lines link introns, and dashed black lines connect orthologous exons. Arrowheads indicate direction of transcription.

Using the predicted protein sequence of *PEG10*, you perform a tblastn search for homologous genes and find that the most similar sequences are in a class of retrotransposons (the sushi-ichi retrotransposons). Propose an evolutionary scenario for the origin of the *PEG10* gene, and relate its origin to its biological function.

Collaboration and Discussion

For answers to selected even-numbered problems, see Appendix: Answers.

27. What is the difference between biochemical and biological function?

28. Using the two-hybrid system to detect interactions between proteins, you obtained the following results: A clone encoding gene *A* gave positive results with clones *B* and *C*; clone *B* gave positive results with clones *A*, *D*, and *E* but not *C*; and clone *E* gave positive results only with clone *B*. Another clone *F* gave positive results with clone *G* but not with any of *A–E*. Can you explain these results?

    To follow up your two-hybrid results, you isolate null loss-of-function mutations in each of the genes *A–G*. Mutants of genes *A, B, C, D*, and *E* grow at only 80% of the rate of the wild type, whereas mutants of genes *F* and

G are phenotypically indistinguishable from the wild type. You construct several double-mutant strains: The *ab, ac, ad*, and *ae* double mutants all grow at about 80% of the rate of the wild type, but *af* and *ag* double mutants exhibit lethality. Explain these results.

    How do the two-hybrid system and genetic interaction results complement one another? Can you reconcile your two-hybrid system and genetic interaction results in a single model?

29. Describe at least two mechanisms by which duplicate genes arise. What are the possible fates of duplicate genes? Does the mode of duplication affect possible fates?

17 Organellar Inheritance and the Evolution of Organellar Genomes

CHAPTER OUTLINE

17.1 Organellar Inheritance Transmits Genes Carried on Organellar Chromosomes

17.2 Modes of Organellar Inheritance Depend on the Organism

17.3 Mitochondria Are the Energy Factories of Eukaryotic Cells

17.4 Chloroplasts Are the Sites of Photosynthesis

17.5 The Endosymbiosis Theory Explains Mitochondrial and Chloroplast Evolution

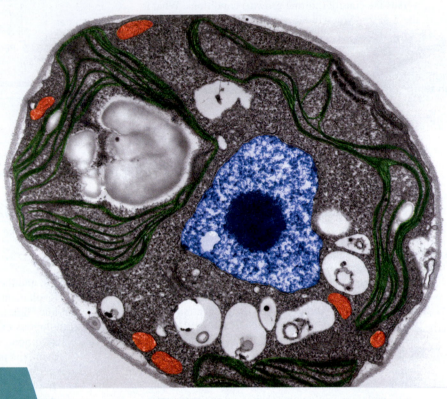

Cross section of *Chlamydomonas* showing three types of cellular compartments having their own genetic material: nucleus (blue), mitochondrion (red), and chloroplast (green).

ESSENTIAL IDEAS

- Mitochondria and chloroplasts possess their own genomes encoding a small number of genes.

- Eukaryotic cells may have many copies of organelle DNA, and multiple genotypes may coexist in a single cell.

- The inheritance of organellar genomes can be uniparental, as in maternal inheritance in mammals, or biparental.

- The organization and expression of organellar genomes reflect their evolutionary origins as symbiotic bacteria.

- Genes have been, and continue to be, transferred from the organellar genomes to the genome of the host cell.

Soon after the rediscovery of Mendel's laws in the early 1900s, Carl Correns and Erwin Baur, working independently, each noted a pattern of inheritance that was distinctly non-Mendelian. Both Correns and Baur were studying the inheritance in plants of a variegated phenotype in which individual branches had either white, green, or variegated leaves. Reciprocal crosses between flowers growing on white or green branches produced progeny that invariably exhibited the phenotype of the female parent in the cross.

The green coloration in land plants and green algae is due to the presence of the green pigment chlorophyll, which harvests light for photosynthesis. In plants, chlorophyll is found in **chloroplasts,** which are the organelles where photosynthetic reactions convert light energy and CO_2 into fixed organic carbon. The variegated and white phenotypes studied by Correns and Baur are caused by a failure of chloroplast development in some cells, which as a consequence remain colorless (white).

In the 1950s, studies demonstrated that chloroplasts contain their own genome. In combination with the observation that chloroplasts are strictly maternally inherited in many plants, this discovery suggested an explanation for the maternal inheritance seen by Correns and Baur: The mutations they were studying must reside on the chloroplast genome. As we will see, the cell's energy-producing and energy-capturing organelles—mitochondria and chloroplasts, respectively—each possess their own genome and may be either uniparentally or biparentally inherited depending on the species. Furthermore, uniparental inheritance may be maternal, paternal, or genetically determined. In this chapter, we explore the transmission of organelle genomes, the remarkable evolutionary events that led to the development of organelles, and the surprisingly dynamic interactions between the organelle and nuclear genomes of eukaryotes.

17.1 Organellar Inheritance Transmits Genes Carried on Organellar Chromosomes

Organellar inheritance refers to the transmission of genes on mitochondrial and chloroplast chromosomes—genes that are located in the cytoplasmic organelles as opposed to the nucleus. As with nuclear genes, expression of mitochondrial and chloroplast genes produces proteins and RNAs that perform specific functions in cells. However, genetic analysis of organellar inheritance differs from that of nuclear gene inheritance because within a fertilized egg the cytoplasm, in which the organelles are found, is not usually derived from equal contributions of both parental gametes.

In many eukaryotic species, the mitochondria and chloroplasts in fertilized eggs are **uniparental** in their origin. This means that just one parental gamete—often the maternal gamete—contributes all of the cytoplasm and cytoplasmic organelles. In some species, organelles are inherited in a uniparental manner even though equal amounts of cytoplasm are inherited from both parental gametes. In such cases, the organelles derived from one of the gametes are selectively destroyed. In still other species, both parental

gametes make contributions of cytoplasm and cytoplasmic organelles to the zygote; this pattern is termed **biparental.** Biparental cytoplasmic contributions are often *unequal* because one gamete contributes more of the cytoplasm and the other gamete makes a smaller contribution. Additional reasons that the study of organellar inheritance differs from the study of nuclear inheritance may be summarized as follows:

1. Multiple organelles may be present in eukaryotic cells.

2. Each mitochondrion or chloroplast may contain multiple copies of its chromosome. The potential presence of tens to hundreds of copies of organellar chromosomes in each cell stands in contrast to the two copies of nuclear genes present in the cells of diploid organisms, in terms of both number and variability.

3. The genome sizes (six to hundreds of kilobases), numbers (few to hundreds), and identities of the genes contained in the organellar genomes are variable from one species to another.

4. Traits controlled by organellar inheritance can also be influenced by nuclear genes. Most biological functions ascribed to mitochondrial or chloroplast genes are produced through the joint action of nuclear genes and organellar genes.

The Discovery of Organellar Inheritance

Erwin Baur and Carl Correns were working independently of one another in 1908—Baur on *Pelargonium* (geraniums) and Correns on *Mirabilis jalapa* (the four o'clock plant)—when each made his discovery of non-Mendelian inheritance. Baur was studying leaf-color inheritance in geraniums. He began his investigation by doing self-fertilization experiments and found that seeds derived from self-fertilization of flowers on green branches produced plants that contained only green leaves. Seeds derived from self-fertilization of flowers on white branches produced seedlings that had only white leaves. These latter seedlings grew poorly and never produced mature plants. The self-fertilization of flowers from branches with variegated leaves produced a mixture of progeny that were either variegated, had all white leaves, or had all green leaves.

These results led Baur to make reciprocal crosses between branches with different leaf colors. Using pollen from a flower located on a branch with one leaf color, he fertilized ovules from a flower located on a branch with a different leaf color. The results, as shown in **Figure 17.1**, were progeny that invariably exhibited the phenotype of the female parent in the cross. This is *not* the result predicted by Mendelian genetics (which predicts no difference in the results of reciprocal crosses), nor is it the result expected if leaf color were inherited on a sex chromosome. Instead, the outcome suggested that transmission of leaf color occurs through **maternal inheritance**—that is, through

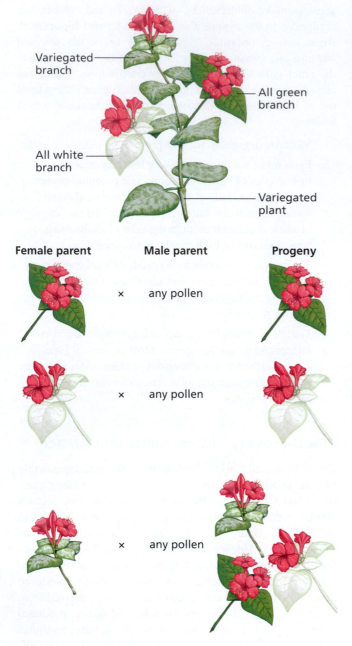

Figure 17.1 Reciprocal crosses demonstrating maternal inheritance of chloroplasts.

🔍 **Describe how a variegated mother can give rise to variegated, white, or green offspring.**

genes transmitted in the ovule. Leaf color in the geranium is controlled exclusively by maternal inheritance, and the male gamete (in the pollen) makes no contribution to the phenotype.

White leaves are produced when leaf cells contain mutant chloroplasts that lack the ability to produce chlorophyll. Variegated leaves are produced by plants whose cells contain a mixture of normal and mutant chloroplasts. The green patches of variegated leaves are composed of cells containing chloroplasts that can produce chlorophyll,

whereas the white leaf patches are composed of cells containing mutant chloroplasts that are unable to produce chlorophyll. Modern-day plant biology explains these results as a consequence of organellar inheritance and states that the allelic differences reside in a gene in the chloroplast genome. Correns's results with the four o'clock plant paralleled those obtained by Baur with geraniums.

In the 1950s, several decades after Baur and Correns described their observations of non-Mendelian inheritance in plants, Yasutane Chiba and colleagues suggested that mitochondria and chloroplasts contain their own genomes. This assertion was based on the results of staining with the compound Feulgen, which specifically stains DNA. In studying mitochondria and chloroplasts from a variety of plants and animals, Chiba detected Feulgen-positive spots in the cytoplasm of virtually all cells examined, and determined that the Feulgen-stained cytoplasmic DNA was contained within the organelles. This result is consistent with the presence of chromosomes in mitochondria and chloroplasts.

Homoplasmy and Heteroplasmy

Figure 17.1 illustrates that if an ovule is obtained from a flower on a branch with all green leaves, then it contains chloroplasts that produce chlorophyll, and its progeny plants will have only green leaves regardless of the leaf color of the pollen-producing plant. Similarly, an ovule obtained from an all-white-leafed branch contains mutant chloroplasts, and all progeny will have only white leaves due to the transmission of defective chloroplasts from the ovule. Ovules from variegated plants can produce progeny with green, white, or variegated leaves. This apparent departure from the maternal inheritance pattern for green and white leaves can be reconciled by the observation that each plant cell contains many copies of each chloroplast gene.

The amount of nuclear genetic material is constant: haploid cells have a single copy of each chromosome, and diploid cells have two copies of each chromosome. In contrast, the number of copies of organellar genes in each cell is much higher and varies significantly with both organism and cell type. Copy-number variation occurs at two levels. First, the number of organelles per cell can vary from one to hundreds, and second, the number of copies of the organelle genome per organelle also varies from one to many. Thus the terms *homozygous* and *heterozygous* are not applicable to alleles of genes on organelle genomes. Rather, a cell or organism in which all copies of a cytoplasmic organellar gene are the same is identified as **homoplasmic** and is said to exhibit **homoplasmy** for that gene (**Figure 17.2a**). On the other hand, if variation exists among the copies of an organellar gene, the cell or organism is **heteroplasmic** and exhibits **heteroplasmy**, carrying a mixture of alleles of an organellar gene. Note that in a heteroplasmic organism, some cells can be homoplasmic wild type, other cells homoplasmic mutant, and still others heteroplasmic. In cells with both wild-type and mutant genotypes, the wild-type allele can complement the mutant allele.

(a) Homoplasmic and heteroplasmic cells

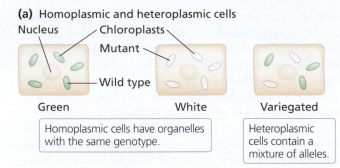

Homoplasmic cells have organelles with the same genotype.

Heteroplasmic cells contain a mixture of alleles.

(b) In maternal inheritance, phenotype of progeny depends only on the genotype of the maternal parent.

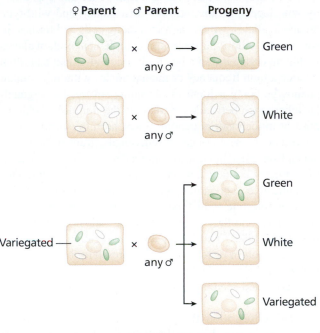

Figure 17.2   Homoplasmy and heteroplasmy in cells.

🄠 Describe the difference between homoplasmic or heteroplasmic organellar alleles and homozygous or heterozygous nuclear alleles.

Homoplasmic and heteroplasmic genotypes for chloroplast genes explain the maternal inheritance of variegation observed by Baur in geraniums (**Figure 17.2b**). Ovules derived from flowers on branches that contain green leaves are homoplasmic for wild-type chloroplast genes and transmit only wild-type chloroplasts to their progeny. In contrast, ovules derived from flowers on branches with white leaves are homoplasmic for a chloroplast mutation, and only mutant chloroplasts are passed to progeny.

The progeny phenotypes derived from flowers on variegated branches illustrate the complexity of organellar genetics. Consider an ovule produced on a variegated branch that consists of a mixture of cells. Some of them are heteroplasmic, inheriting a cytoplasm containing many chloroplasts, some that are wild type and others that harbor the mutant allele. During the mitoses and meiosis that produce egg cells, the chloroplasts are divided randomly

among daughter cells. If an egg cell inherits both wild-type and mutant chloroplasts, a heteroplasmic plant with variegated leaves develops. However, if by chance the organelles inherited by an egg cell are all wild type, the branches of the plant produced by fertilization of the egg will be green. Alternatively, chance might result in an egg cell inheriting chloroplasts that are all mutant, in which case the plant will have white leaves.

Genome Replication in Organelles

Organellar DNA is packaged into protein–DNA complexes in an area within the organelle called a **nucleoid**. Each nucleoid usually contains multiple copies of the organellar genome. There may be several nucleoids per organelle and multiple organelles per cell, resulting in a copy number for organelle genomes that is in the range of hundreds to thousands per cell. To better understand the transmission of mutations in organellar genomes, and their phenotypic effects, let us examine how organellar DNA is replicated.

A major difference between replication of the nuclear genome and that of an organelle is in their relationship to the cell cycle. Each of the nuclear chromosomes is duplicated once each mitotic cycle, so that daughter cells have exactly the same chromosome constitution as the parent cell following cell division. In contrast, the replication of organellar genomes is not tightly coupled to the cell cycle. Rather, the replication of organellar genomes depends on three factors (**Figure 17.3**). First, organellar transmission genetics depends on the growth, division, and segregation of the organelles themselves ("organelle division" in Figure 17.3). There appears to be a mechanism to ensure that each daughter cell receives approximately equal amounts of the organelles present in the mother cell. Second, the segregation of genes encoded in the organellar genome is connected to the division and segregation of nucleoids within an organelle ("nucleoid division" in Figure 17.3). Details of this process are still being discovered, but differences in the replication rate of nucleoids have been observed both between cells and between organelles. Third, organellar transmission genetics depends on the replication of the individual organellar genomes ("DNA replication" in Figure 17.3). There is evidence that DNA molecules within a nucleoid are related to each other; they are sometimes physically linked, which would suggest that they are products of DNA replication.

Replicative Segregation of Organelle Genomes

The variation in the numbers of organelles and of their genomes in different somatic cells and tissues can significantly influence the phenotypic effects of mutations in organellar genes. Consider again the case of the variegated leaves. If a cell is homoplasmic with regard to this trait, cells

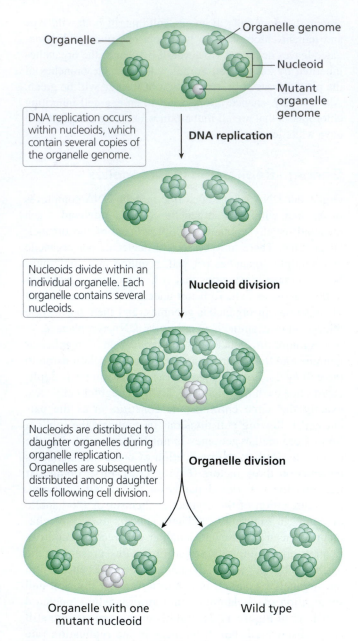

DNA replication occurs within nucleoids, which contain several copies of the organelle genome.

DNA replication

Nucleoids divide within an individual organelle. Each organelle contains several nucleoids.

Nucleoid division

Nucleoids are distributed to daughter organelles during organelle replication. Organelles are subsequently distributed among daughter cells following cell division.

Organelle division

Organelle with one mutant nucleoid

Wild type

Figure 17.3 Factors in replication of organelle genomes.

descended from this cell by division will also be homoplasmic. However, cells that are heteroplasmic can produce both heteroplasmic and homoplasmic descendants.

To see how this happens, imagine a plant cell in which a mutation occurs in a chloroplast genome. Through segregation of nucleoids during chloroplast division, chloroplasts in which all copies of the genome harbor the mutations can arise. Since chloroplasts within a cell do not fuse with one another, once a homoplastic mutant chloroplast arises, it does not acquire wild-type genomes from other chloroplasts within the cell. During cell division, the chloroplasts are randomly distributed to the daughter cells. If by chance all the organelles inherited by a daughter cell are of a single genotype, homoplasmic cells can be generated from a

heteroplasmic ancestral cell (see the cells at the bottom of the far-right columns in Figure 17.4). This random segregation of organelles during replication is termed **replicative segregation**. Replicative segregation is of great importance since it affects the proportion of mutant organellar genomes in a cell, thus influencing the severity (penetrance and expressivity) of phenotypes produced by mutations in organellar genomes. It can lead to genetically mosaic organisms with both "mutant" cells and "wild-type" cells; and, as we see with the variegated plants, it can influence transmission of mutant alleles to subsequent generations depending on the organellar genotype of the germ cells.

In heteroplasmic individuals, penetrance and expressivity will depend on the ratio between mutant and wild-type organelle alleles, which can vary among cells and tissues. In some cases, wild-type alleles can complement mutant alleles within an organelle, so a heteroplasmic individual can often tolerate a high frequency of mutant alleles without a mutant phenotype being evident or becoming severe. For organellar inheritance between generations, the number of chloroplast or mitochondrial genomes present in the germ cells is important. In heteroplasmic individuals, transmission will depend on what fraction of organellar genomes present in the gametes contain mutant versus wild-type alleles. Due to replicative segregation, gametes can be produced that are homoplasmic wild type, homoplasmic mutant, or heteroplasmic, and they can have varying ratios of mutant and wild-type alleles. Thus, replicative segregation can explain both variation in penetrance and expressivity between individuals and also variable transmission, where green, white, and variegated seedlings can all be derived from variegated plants.

The observation that mitochondria undergo frequent fusion and fission has implications for the segregation of mitochondrial DNA and creates the potential for genotypes within a cell's mitochondria to become mixed and homogenized. Thus, replicative segregation in mitochondria is more complicated than that described for chloroplasts.

Now that we have described some of the complexities of transmission of the organellar genomes, for the remainder of the chapter we will assume that individuals are homoplasmic, unless there is evidence that heteroplasmy exists.

17.2 Modes of Organellar Inheritance Depend on the Organism

The inheritance of organellar genomes occurs through two basic mechanisms. In many organisms, the transmission is biased toward whichever gamete contributes the bulk of the cytoplasm to the zygote. In this case transmission can be either uniparental (maternal or paternal) or biparental. Alternatively, inheritance is genetically determined: one gamete's organelles are destined to be transmitted to the progeny

Figure 17.4 Development of homoplasmy from heteroplasmy by replicative segregation.

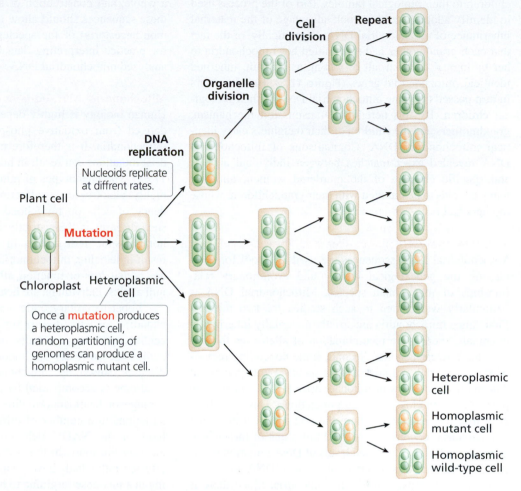

while the other gamete's organellar contributions are selectively destroyed. Even in cases where one gamete contributes most of the cytoplasm, genetic mechanisms may exist to eliminate the residual organellar contribution from the other gamete. Thus, the two mechanisms are not mutually exclusive. In this section, we explore three cases illustrating three different inheritance patterns, those of mammals, of the alga *Chlamydomonas reinhardii,* and of the yeast *Saccharomyces cerevisiae.*

Mitochondrial Inheritance in Mammals

Maternal inheritance of mitochondria is the norm in mammals because the egg contributes all of the cytoplasm and the sperm contributes primarily a nucleus during fertilization. Maternal inheritance of the mitochondrial genome in mammals has four important consequences that we examine in this section:

1. Predictions of inheritance of mitochondrial mutations can be made based solely on the genotype of the mother.

2. Maternal inheritance allows the maternal lineage of organisms to be examined specifically.

3. Since there is no paternal contribution, phylogenetic trees constructed using mitochondrial DNA sequences can be interpreted as maternal genealogies reflecting the maternal history of species.

4. Human genetic diseases due to mitochondrial mutations are maternally inherited.

Mother–Child Identity of Mitochondrial DNA In mammals, mothers and their children of both sexes share identical mitochondrial DNA (mtDNA). These identical genetic matches are put to many practical uses. One of the most dramatic examples in humans is the use of mitochondrial DNA to find matches between grandmothers and grandchildren who were separated during political unrest in Argentina during the 1970s. An Argentinean military dictatorship undertook a campaign of kidnapping and murder of political dissidents in the early 1970s. Among those kidnapped were pregnant women, who were allowed to give birth before they were murdered. The children of these women were adopted by unrelated families, and their identities were hidden from their biological families.

As the political environment in Argentina became less repressive, a group known as Las Abuelas de la Plaza de Mayo

(Grandmothers of the Plaza de Mayo) demanded an accounting of the murder of the dissidents and the return of the adopted children to their biological families. Part of the process used to identify adopted children took advantage of the maternal inheritance of mitochondrial DNA—specifically, of the fact that each grandmother had transmitted her mitochondria to her biological children, all of whom, as a result, inherited identical mitochondrial genes (**Figure 17.5**). Her daughters in turn passed the same mitochondrial DNA to their biological children. By this hereditary transmission mechanism, grandmothers and the children of their daughters carry identical mitochondrial DNA. Comparisons of mitochondrial DNA revealed exact matches between individual abuelas and specific children of the murdered women, allowing many abuelas to be reunited with their grandchildren, whose mothers had been "disappeared."

Mitochondrial DNA Sequences and Species Evolution

Mitochondrial DNA sequences are used as a tool for deciphering the genealogical history and evolutionary relationships of mammalian species. Mitochondrial DNA is particularly well suited to such studies for two reasons. First, since mitochondria are strictly maternally inherited in mammals, there is no recombination of alleles, as there is with the nuclear genome. Second, some noncoding regions of mitochondrial genomes evolve quickly, with the result that many differences in mitochondrial DNA sequence are present even in closely related populations. This is particularly true for mammals, where the rate of mutation in the mitochondrial genome is about 10 times that of the nuclear genome, reflecting decreased levels of DNA mutation repair in mitochondria versus repair of nuclear DNA or higher rates of DNA damage in the mitochondria. Since there is little selective pressure to maintain a specific sequence in noncoding regions, mutations in these regions accumulate at a relatively steady rate.

Once a mitochondrial mutation becomes homoplasmic in the germ cells of an individual female, the mutation is transmitted to all her progeny. Therefore, maternal lineages can be traced by following the mutational changes back in

time. The mitochondrial DNA sequences in the present population reflect the maternal genealogy of the population as a whole, and construction of a phylogenetic tree based on these sequences should allow the identification of the common ancestor(s) of the species. See Genetic Analysis 17.1 for practice interpreting data from a research project that analyzed mitochondrial DNA.

Mitochondrial Mutations and Human Genetic Disease

Human biology is highly dependent on the cellular energy derived from oxidative phosphorylation reactions in our mitochondria. It is therefore not surprising that mitochondrial mutations can result in human genetic diseases (**Figure 17.6a**). The phenotypes of mitochondrial diseases are often highly pleiotropic, a reflection of the ubiquitous dependency of cells on mitochondrial function. A hallmark of such diseases is their strictly maternal transmission. Since homoplasmic null alleles in mitochondrial genes would result in lethality, mitochondrial mutations in humans either are partial loss-of-function alleles (see Section 4.1) or, if null alleles, individuals are heteroplasmic.

Leber hereditary optic neuropathy (LHON) is a mitochondrial genetic disease in which degeneration of the central optic nerve results in blindness, usually in late adolescence to early adulthood (**Figure 17.6b**). Like most diseases caused by mitochondrial mutations, the LHON syndrome is accompanied by pleiotropic defects, primarily a range of heart abnormalities. LHON can be caused by mutations in a number of different genes that encode proteins of the NADH dehydrogenase subunit involved in electron transport. In the pedigree shown in Figure 17.6b, affected individuals have a single base-pair change, resulting in a missense (arginine to histidine) mutation in the subunit 4 gene, *ND4*.

Close inspection of the pedigree in Figure 17.6b reveals that, although all affected individuals have an affected mother, not all children of an affected mother exhibit LHON. If we assume strict maternal inheritance of the mitochondrial mutations, then the phenotype is not fully penetrant. There are three possible reasons for incomplete penetrance: the effects of heteroplasmy, the effects of genetic interactions with nuclear genes, and the effect of environmental factors interacting with mitochondrial gene mutations to produce a mutant phenotype. A discussion of mitochondrial gene–environment interactions appears in the Case Study at the end of this chapter, and an example of mitochondrial–nuclear interactions appears in Experimental Insight 17.1 on 651. Here we consider heteroplasmy as a cause for incomplete penetrance.

Heteroplasmy can lead to incomplete penetrance of a human hereditary disease because, as discussed earlier, each cell contains multiple mitochondria and each mitochondrion contains multiple copies of the mitochondrial genome. There is no fixed number of copies of organelle genomes in a cell. The numbers of organelles within a cell can influence expressivity, penetrance, and transmission of

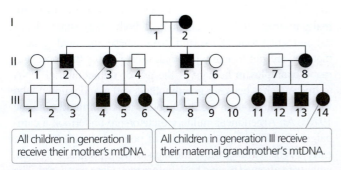

All children in generation II receive their mother's mtDNA.

All children in generation III receive their maternal grandmother's mtDNA.

Figure 17.5   Maternal inheritance of mitochondrial genes in mammals.

How would you distinguish maternal inheritance from sex-linked inheritance?

PROBLEM Although North American bison (*Bison bison*) and domestic cattle (*Bos taurus* and *Bos indicus*) descended from a common ancestor, they do not readily interbreed. However, because they still share the same chromosome number and structure, the production of fertile interspecific hybrids is possible. Male bison have been known to breed with female cattle, but not the converse. Twelve North American bison herds (numbered 1 through 12 at right) were examined for evidence of such interbreeding by a comparison of their mtDNA sequences with those of several cattle breeds and related species. A phylogenetic tree constructed from the comparisons is presented here. The numbers in the left half of the diagram represent confidence values for the particular relationships (100 is the maximum).

BREAK IT DOWN: How is mitochondrial DNA inherited in mammals?

BREAK IT DOWN: Phylogenetic trees reveal relatedness and suggest common ancestry.

a. Explain why mtDNA but not nuclear DNA is used to detect bison–domestic cattle interspecific hybrids.

b. Based on this phylogeny, identify which bison herds show evidence of interspecific breeding with domestic cattle.

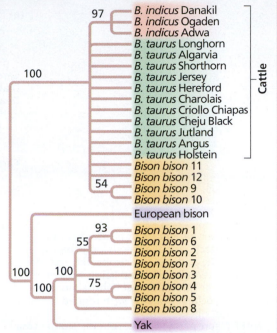

Solution Strategies	Solution Steps
Evaluate	
1. Identify the topic of this problem and the kind of information the answer should contain.	1. This problem presents a phylogenetic analysis of an mtDNA sequence in domestic cattle and in bison. We must explain why mtDNA was used rather than nuclear DNA, and then we must examine the phylogeny to identify bison herds that do and do not have bison–cattle hybridization in their lineage.
2. Identify the critical information given in the problem.	2. The phylogenetic tree depicts evolutionary relationships between cattle mtDNA and mtDNA samples from bison.
Deduce	
3. Examine the pattern of major clades in the phylogenetic tree and the membership of each clade.	3. The phylogeny has two major clades. The bottom clade contains eight North American bison herds (*Bison bison* 1 through 8) and two outside reference species, European bison and yak. The upper clade contains fourteen domestic cattle breeds (*Bos taurus* and *Bos indicus*) and four North American bison herds (*Bison bison* 9 through 12).
4. Identify the kind of phylogenetic evidence (based on mtDNA) that would be consistent with interspecific hybridization and also the kind that would be inconsistent with it.	4. If a clade consists either only of domesticated breeds or only of bison, then the animals in the clade, being more closely related to one another than they are to animals in other clades, do not have interspecific hybridization in their lineage. If a clade contains bison *and* domesticated cattle breeds, then there is a close relationship between the bison and the cattle in that clade.

TIP: In interspecies hybridization, bison mtDNA sequences would be more closely related to cattle sequences than they are to other bison sequences.

Solve

5. Explain why mtDNA but not nuclear DNA sequences were used in this phylogenetic analysis

TIP: In mammals, all mitochondrial DNA is maternally inherited.

Answer a

5. We are told that female cattle interbreed with male bison, but not the reverse. Since mtDNA is inherited maternally, the resulting hybrids would possess solely cattle mtDNA but would contain equal mixtures of cattle and bison nuclear DNA.

Answer b

6. Determine which bison are interspecies hybrids.

TIP: Bison of hybrid origin will harbor mtDNA more closely related to that of cattle than of bison.

6. Bison herds 9 to 12 are in the same clade as a number of breeds of domestic cattle, signifying that their mtDNA sequences are more closely related to domesticated cattle than to the wild bison and yak species. Thus these four herds have cattle mtDNA from interspecific hybridization in previous generations.

For more practice, see Problem 24.

Visit the Study Area to access study tools. **Mastering** Genetics

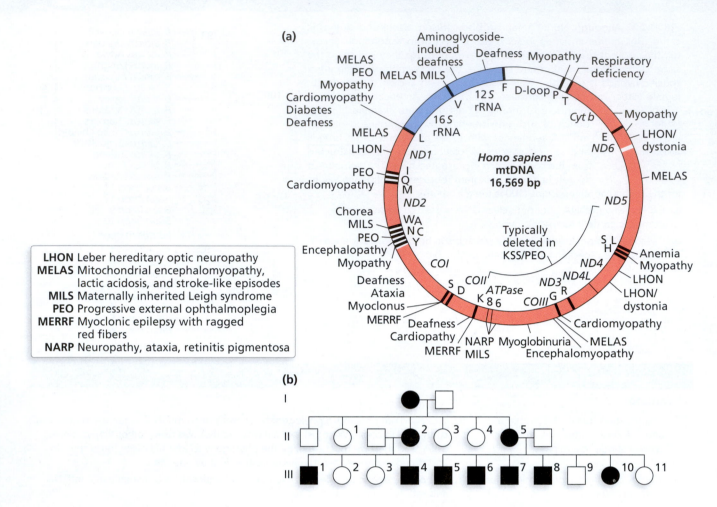

Figure 17.6   **Mutations in human mitochondrial genes leading to disease syndromes.** **(a)** Muscle functioning, hearing, and vision all require high levels of energy produced by mitochondria. **(b)** Pedigree showing maternal inheritance with incomplete penetrance of LHON.

Q Why do individuals III-2 and III-3 not exhibit disease symptoms? Will their offspring be affected?

mutant alleles in various ways. The numbers of copies of mitochondrial genomes in human cells vary from hundreds to hundreds of thousands, depending on the cell type and physiological state. In cells with both wild-type and mutant mitochondrial genotypes, the wild-type allele can complement the mutant allele.

In human pedigrees, heteroplasmic mothers can produce wild-type homoplasmic progeny, mutant homoplasmic offspring, or heteroplasmic offspring (**Figure 17.7a**). For mitochondrial transmission in mammals, the number of mitochondria present in the egg cell is what matters. Human oocytes typically have a small number (e.g., 10) of large mitochondria that are subsequently divided into many smaller mitochondria in the zygote. In humans, an egg cell contains up to 2000 mitochondrial genomes. In heteroplasmic individuals, replicative segregation can lead to variable penetrance, in which the ratio of mutant : wild-type mitochondrial genomes varies significantly between progeny (**Figure 17.7b**).

Furthermore, replicative segregation of mitochondrial mutations over the lifetime of an individual can lead

to variable ratios of mutant : wild-type mitochondrial genomes in different cells and tissues of the same heteroplasmic individual; and this too results in variable phenotypic penetrance. Disease symptoms will develop only when vulnerable cells contain a high proportion of mutant mitochondria. For example, in the case of another mitochondrial disease, called MERRF (myoclonic epilepsy with ragged red fibers), an individual who displayed the mutant genotype in 85% of his mitochondrial DNA did not exhibit a phenotype defect, whereas a cousin with 96% mutant mitochondria displayed a severe phenotype. See Genetic Analysis 17.2 for practice in analyzing a pedigree for evidence of various forms of nuclear and mitochondrial inheritance.

Mating Type and Chloroplast Segregation in *Chlamydomonas*

Chlamydomonas reinhardii is a single-celled green alga with a haploid nuclear genome that harbors a single, large chloroplast containing 50 to 100 genomes divided among

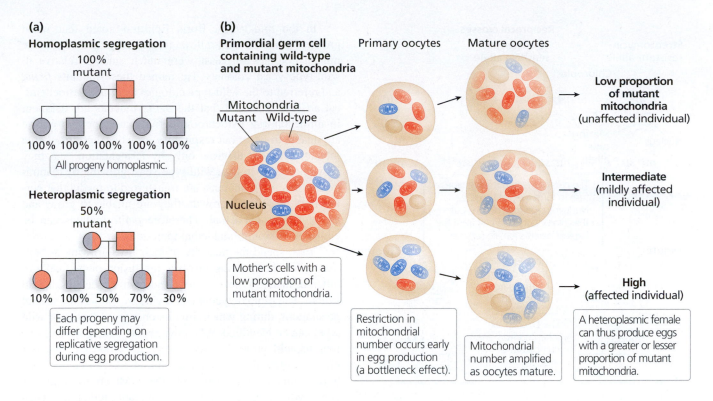

Figure 17.7 Variable penetrance of mitochondrial mutations.

Ⓠ Which organisms would be more likely to produce homoplasmic offspring, those with a single organelle in their egg cells or those with many organelles in their egg cells?

5 to 15 nucleoids. Haploid cells of *Chlamydomonas* also typically have about 50 copies of the mitochondrial genome distributed among a small number of mitochondria in the germ cells and a larger number of mitochondria at other stages of the life cycle.

Matings between *Chlamydomonas* cells of different mating types produce diploid algae that undergo meiosis to produce haploid progeny. Mating compatibility is determined by the genotype at the *mt* locus, and *mt*⁺ individuals mate only with *mt*⁻ individuals. Both mating types appear to contribute equally to the cytoplasmic content of the diploid zygote, but in approximately 95% of matings, the chloroplast genome is contributed by the *mt*⁺ mating type. In the remaining 5% of matings, chloroplast inheritance is biparental. The first mutation in a chloroplast gene discovered in *Chlamydomonas* was isolated by Ruth Sager in 1954 and confers resistance to the antibiotic streptomycin (str^R). Analogous to reciprocal crosses between four o'clock flowers of different leaf types, reciprocal crosses between streptomycin-resistant and streptomycin-sensitive *Chlamydomonas* strains of different mating types give different results, with the chloroplast genotype being contributed primarily by the *mt*⁺ parent (**Figure 17.8**). Remarkably, though the chloroplast genome is preferentially transmitted by the *mt*⁺ mating type, mitochondria are preferentially transmitted by the *mt*⁻ mating type. The genetic mechanisms by

which the different mating types preferentially transmit the different organellar genomes are presently unknown.

During the mating process in *Chlamydomonas*, the two cells of opposite mating type fuse, after which the chloroplast genome from the *mt*⁺ parent is selectively maintained, while that from the *mt*⁻ parent is degraded. As indicated above, the mechanism by which the *mt*⁻ cell's chloroplast genome is eliminated is not known, but it is likely to involve degradation of that genome at some point in the mating process. A similar process leads to the loss of the mitochondrial genomes contributed by the *mt*⁺ gamete. Perhaps the degradation of organelles or their genomes provides a possible source of organellar DNA that may be transferred between genomes—into the nuclear genome, for example. (We will return to this topic later in the chapter, when we discuss the evolution of the organelles and their genomes.) For the cases in which biparental inheritance occurs, the presence of the two types of chloroplast genomes in the same organelle allows the genomes to undergo recombination that may result in the segregation of recombinant and parental chloroplast genomes.

Biparental Inheritance in *Saccharomyces cerevisiae*

Saccharomyces cerevisiae is a single-celled yeast that can grow either aerobically (with oxygen) or anaerobically

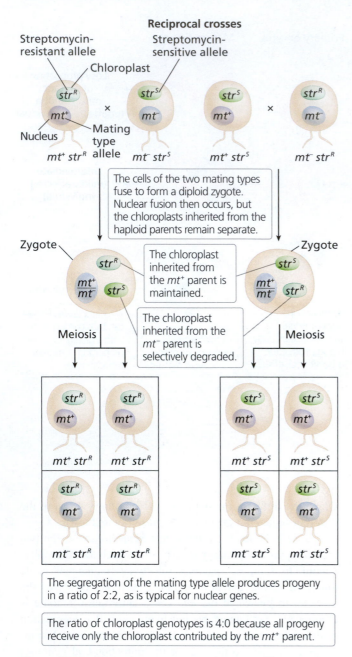

Figure 17.8 Chloroplast segregation determined by mating type in *Chlamydomonas*.

The cells of the two mating types fuse to form a diploid zygote. Nuclear fusion then occurs, but the chloroplasts inherited from the haploid parents remain separate.

The chloroplast inherited from the *mt*⁺ parent is maintained.

The chloroplast inherited from the *mt*⁻ parent is selectively degraded.

The segregation of the mating type allele produces progeny in a ratio of 2:2, as is typical for nuclear genes.

The ratio of chloroplast genotypes is 4:0 because all progeny receive only the chloroplast contributed by the *mt*⁺ parent.

(without oxygen). Mitochondria are not able to produce energy (ATP) when oxygen is unavailable; so under anaerobic growth conditions, yeast obtain their energy from fermentation, which does not require mitochondria. Under aerobic conditions, however, mitochondria-mediated aerobic respiration allows yeast to grow faster than they grow by fermentation. Thus mutations that eliminate mitochondrial function in yeast do not prevent growth, but they do cause the mutant yeast to grow at a slower pace than do wild-type yeast. This dual growth capacity makes *Saccharomyces* a versatile system for studying the genetics of mitochondrial biology.

In the mid-1950s, Boris Ephrussi noted that when grown on media that allow fermentative growth, some mutant colonies of yeast were much smaller relative to wild-type yeast colonies. He named these mutants *petite* and referred to the wild-type colonies as *grande*. Biochemical analyses revealed that the *petite* mutants are deficient in mitochondrial cytochrome activity and for this reason are unable to carry out respiratory growth. Therefore *petite* mutants are able to grow only by fermentation, and they grow more slowly than wild-type yeast growing by respiration. When *petite* mutants are transferred to media that permit only respiratory growth, they are unable to grow, and the mutations are lethal. Therefore *petite* mutants can be classified as conditional lethal mutations.

Yeast spend the majority of their lives growing as haploid cells. Their mating involves the fusion of two cells of different mating types, called **a** and **α**, to produce a diploid zygote. The diploid zygote can divide by mitosis for several generations, during which time its phenotype (petite or wild type) can be identified. When the zygote undergoes meiosis, four haploid progeny (ascospores) are produced, the four progeny referred to as a tetrad, and tetrads can be analyzed to determine the segregation of alleles. Mutations in nuclear genes will segregate in a 2:2 ratio (mutant : wild type) when mutant lines are mated with wild type (**Figure 17.9a**). Both **a** and **α** gametes contribute mitochondrial genomes to the zygote, making inheritance of organelles in *Saccharomyces* biparental.

Genetic analysis of *petite* mutants reveals that they fall into three distinct classes. One class, called *nuclear*, or *segregational*, *petites* (designated *pet⁻*), segregate 2:2 when crossed with the wild type (**Figure 17.9b**); *pet⁻* are mutations in nuclear genes. The existence of nuclear *petites* demonstrates that the functioning of the mitochondria depends not only on its own genome but also on genes contained in the nuclear genome. Both genomes encode genes whose products function in the organelle, as we discuss in a later section.

The other two classes of *petite* mutations—*neutral petites* and *suppressive petites*—do not show Mendelian inheritance and are the result of mutations in the mitochondrial genome. When *neutral petites* are crossed with wild-type yeast, the diploid zygote grows normally, and the tetrads contain only wild-type spores (**Figure 17.9c**). These are called "neutral" because the *petite* phenotype is lost after the initial mating with wild type. Examination of *neutral petite* mutants reveals that they lack virtually all mitochondrial DNA, and thus they obviously lack proper mitochondrial function. When *neutral petites* are mated to wild-type *Saccharomyces*, essentially all mitochondrial DNA is derived from the wild-type parent, resulting in phenotypically wild-type progeny.

When *suppressive petites* are crossed with wild-type yeast, the diploid zygote has respiratory properties intermediate between those of the *petite* and wild type. If the diploid zygotes are grown mitotically for several divisions, the diploids tend to become *petite* in phenotype, and the

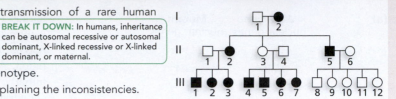

PROBLEM The pedigree presented here shows transmission of a rare human hereditary disorder.

> **BREAK IT DOWN:** In humans, inheritance can be autosomal recessive or autosomal dominant, X-linked recessive or X-linked dominant, or maternal.

a. Determine the most likely mode of inheritance.

b. Identify any individuals in the pedigree whose phenotype is inconsistent with the expected phenotype.

c. Justify your proposed mode of inheritance by explaining the inconsistencies.

Solution Strategies	Solution Steps
Evaluate	
1. Identify the topic of this problem and the kind of information the answer should contain.	1. This problem concerns the mode of inheritance of a hereditary abnormality in a human pedigree. The answer requires proposing a mode of inheritance, identifying family members whose phenotypes are inconsistent with the proposed mode, and explaining those inconsistencies in a manner that justifies the proposed mode.
2. Identify the critical information given in the problem.	2. The pedigree gives the phenotype of each family member in three generations.
Deduce	
3. Identify the possible modes of inheritance of the gene causing this abnormality. TIP: Human cells contain maternally inherited mitochondria in addition to nuclear chromosomes.	3. The possibilities are that the trait might be caused by the mutation of either a nuclear gene or a mitochondrial gene. If the mutated gene is nuclear, it might be either recessive or dominant and either autosomal or X-linked. If the mutation is mitochondrial, the transmission pattern will be maternal inheritance.
4. Examine the pedigree to see whether the pattern is generally consistent with autosomal recessive or X-linked recessive inheritance.	4. The pattern is inconsistent with X-linked recessive inheritance, in which many more males than females have the recessive phenotype. Here, the ratio of six females to four males is close to 1:1, so X-linked recessive inheritance is highly unlikely. Autosomal inheritance is unlikely, since siblings in generation III are either all affected or none affected within families.
5. Examine the pedigree to see whether the pattern is generally consistent with X-linked dominant or autosomal dominant inheritance.	5. In X-linked dominant inheritance, all daughters of males with the dominant-mutation are also expected to have the trait. II-5 does not transmit the trait to any of his three daughters, thus making X-linked dominant inheritance highly unlikely. Autosomal dominant inheritance is possible, where II-3 is nonpenetrant; but there is only a 1/32 chance $(1/2^5)$ that II-5 would have five children who do not have the trait.
6. Examine the pedigree to see whether the pattern is consistent with maternal inheritance.	6. The pedigree pattern is consistent with maternal (mitochondrial) inheritance. Affected individuals are all offspring of affected mothers (I-2, II-2) or of female II-3 (who may harbor the mutant allele but does not exhibit the phenotype).
Solve	Answers a and b
7. Determine the mode of transmission that is consistent with the pedigree data.	7. Maternal inheritance best explains the observed segregation pattern, but there is one inconsistency. Individual II-3 does not show the phenotype as expected under strict application of the rules of maternal inheritance.
	Answer c
8. Explain the presence of the anomalous individuals whose phenotypes are inconsistent with maternal inheritance. TIP: Heteroplasmy may occur among the multiple copies of mitochondrial chromosomes present in each cell. TIP: Proteins produced by mitochondrial genes interact with proteins produced by nuclear genes.	8. Lack of penetrance of the phenotype (as in II-3) may result from (1) variable penetrance owing to some individuals being heteroplasmic, since some could have a greater proportion of mutant mitochondria than others; (2) other genetic risk factors, such as alleles of nuclear genes (since females show variable penetrance, alleles of autosomal genes may be influencing the penetrance of the mitochondrial mutation, although common alleles of X chromosome genes cannot be ruled out); (3) environmental factors that influence the penetrance of the phenotype.

For more practice, see Problems 10, 12, 15, 16, 17, and 19.
Visit the Study Area to access study tools. **Mastering** Genetics

(a)

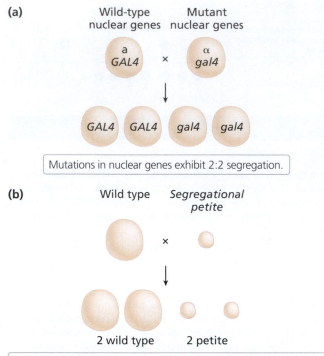

Mutations in nuclear genes exhibit 2:2 segregation.

(b)

Wild type   *Segregational petite*

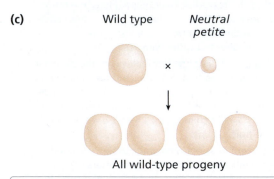

2 wild type   2 petite

Progeny of petite and wild-type phenotypes are produced in a 2:2 ratio, indicating that *segregational petite* mutations are in nuclear genes.

(c)

Wild type   *Neutral petite*

All wild-type progeny

Progeny do not exhibit the petite phenotype, indicating that *neutral petite* mutants are not transmitted. Examination of *neutral petite* mutants indicates that they lack most or all mitochondrial DNA.

(d)

Wild type   *Suppressive petite*

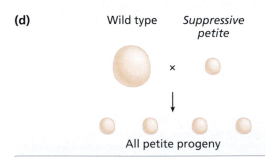

All petite progeny

Petite mitochondrial DNA dominates, and all progeny exhibit the petite phenotype. Examination of *suppressive petite* mutants indicates that they have deletions of only portions of their mitochondrial DNA.

Figure 17.9 **Transmission of *petite* phenotypes in *Saccharomyces cerevisiae*.**

tetrads contain all *petite* spores (**Figure 17.9d**). Thus the *suppressive petite* phenotype suppresses the wild-type phenotype, resulting in progeny that are all deficient in respiration. Analysis of the mitochondrial genome reveals that initially, *suppressive petites* have small deletions of mitochondrial DNA; but upon further growth, all copies of the mitochondrial DNA tend to become rearranged and duplicated. These gross defects in mitochondrial DNA lead to losses and disruptions of mitochondrial genes and to deficiencies in aerobic respiration.

Why do the mitochondria inherited from the *suppressive petite* parent overwhelm those of the wild-type parent? Two nonmutually exclusive possibilities are that (1) *suppressive petite* mitochondria replicate faster than wild-type mitochondria, perhaps due to having additional copies of a replication origin, and (2) the *suppressive petite* and wild-type mitochondria fuse, and the genomic rearrangements present in the *suppressive petite* mitochondrial genome induce rearrangements in the mitochondrial genomes inherited from the wild-type parent. The latter hypothesis has gained support from the observation that mitochondria within a cell often interact and fuse into a continuous mitochondrial network.

Summary of Organellar Inheritance

In sum, there are four primary modes of inheritance of organellar genes. Three of the modes are uniparental— the organelles are contributed primarily by a single parent—as in (1) the maternal inheritance of organelles in mammals and many flowering plants; (2) the paternal inheritance of organelles, which is seen in gymnosperms; and (3) selective degradation or silencing of organellar DNA during mating, as in *Chlamydomonas*. The fourth mode of inheritance is biparental; both parents contribute organelles and their genomes to the progeny, as in *Saccharomyces*.

As we learned in Section 17.1, mitochondria and chloroplasts contain their own genomes, composed of genes that are unique to the organelles and are expressed and replicated by mechanisms independent of those working on nuclear genes. The discussions that follow explore the structure, replication, function, and evolution of mitochondrial and chloroplast genomes.

17.3 Mitochondria Are the Energy Factories of Eukaryotic Cells

Enzymatically driven phosphorylation that transfers phosphates from adenosine triphosphate (ATP) to other molecules provides energy used by cells for many processes and functions. In most eukaryotes, mitochondria are the sites of ATP production, where electron transport is coupled to oxidative phosphorylation to generate this small, energy-transporting molecule. The protein complexes that produce ATP are composed of gene products encoded by both the mitochondrial and nuclear genomes. Thus, the synthesis and regulation of the protein complexes responsible for oxidative phosphorylation and other mitochondrial processes depend on coordination between the mitochondrial and nuclear genomes. In many species, mitochondrial genes also participate in other metabolic processes and biochemical reactions, including ion homeostasis and biosynthetic pathways.

The general structure of a **mitochondrion** can be described as two membranes surrounding a matrix (**Figure 17.10**). The enzyme complexes responsible for oxidative phosphorylation are found on the inner membrane. The mitochondrial matrix is the site of mitochondrial genome transcription, translation, and DNA replication. The mitochondrial genome is responsible for only a fraction of the genes needed to carry out these processes, however, and most of the proteins active in mitochondrial DNA replication, transcription, and translation are encoded in the nuclear genome.

Following their translation, nucleus-encoded mitochondrial proteins are transported into mitochondria. Examination of the mitochondrial genomes of different species reveals enormous diversity as to whether specific proteins are mitochondrial- or nucleus-encoded; only a few proteins are consistently encoded by the mitochondrial genome. This suggests that genes have moved from the mitochondrial genome to the nuclear genome at different times during evolution.

Mitochondrial Genome Structure and Gene Content

Genetic mapping studies and direct observation of mitochondrial chromosomes by electron microscopy indicate the chromosomes often have a circular structure (**Figure 17.11**). There is evidence, however, that circular mitochondrial genomes can assume a linear form and that the mitochondrial genomes of certain species are primarily linear. In the vast majority of species, the mitochondrial genome is a single molecule; but in a few species, the genome consists of more than one molecule. Thus, in some species, the mitochondrial genome consists of one (*Tetrahymena*) or more (*Amoebidium*) linear molecules that have terminal repeat sequences, which are reminiscent of telomeres.

Unlike the DNA in the nucleus, mitochondrial DNA is not packaged in chromatin composed of histones. Rather, the genomes are anchored to the inner membrane of the mitochondria, in a manner similar to that of bacterial chromosomes. These and other features described below give

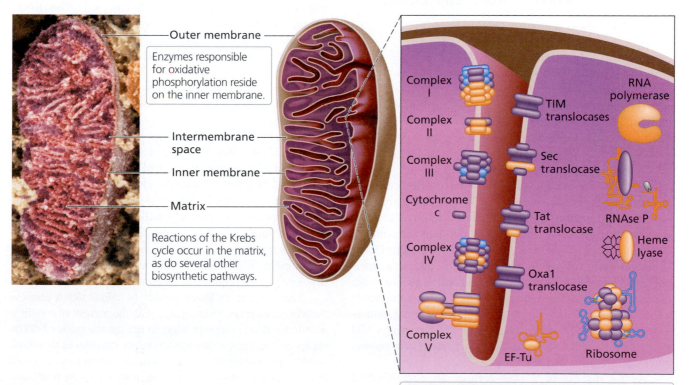

Enzymes responsible for oxidative phosphorylation reside on the inner membrane.

Outer membrane

Intermembrane space

Inner membrane

Matrix

Reactions of the Krebs cycle occur in the matrix, as do several other biosynthetic pathways.

Complex I
Complex II
Complex III
Cytochrome c
Complex IV
Complex V

TIM translocases
Sec translocase
Tat translocase
Oxa1 translocase
EF-Tu

RNA polymerase
RNAse P
Heme lyase
Ribosome

Ribosomal RNA and a few proteins (blue) are always encoded by the mitochondrial genome, other products (purple) are always encoded by the nuclear genome, and still others (orange) may be encoded by either genome depending on the species.

Figure 17.10 Mitochondrial structure and function.

(a)

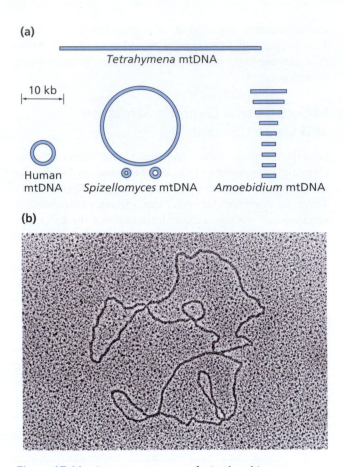

Tetrahymena mtDNA

10 kb

Human mtDNA   *Spizellomyces* mtDNA   *Amoebidium* mtDNA

(b)

Figure 17.11   Genome structures of mitochondria.

clues to the evolutionary origin of mitochondria, as we discuss further in a later part of this chapter.

The gene content and size of mitochondrial genomes vary substantially among eukaryotes (**Figure 17.12a**). Known genome sizes range from a low of 6 kb in the malarial parasite *Plasmodium* to hundreds or thousands of kilobases in flowering plants. However, as with nuclear genomes, the size in kilobases does not necessarily correlate with the number of genes. For example, the *Saccharomyces* mitochondrial genome is approximately five times as large as the human mitochondrial genome, but it contains only a few more genes. This is because much of the extra DNA, including some introns, is noncoding. In contrast to their nuclear genomes, mammalian mitochondrial genomes are particularly compact and have no introns and little noncoding DNA. Known gene numbers in mitochondrial genomes vary from a low of 6 in *Plasmodium* to a high of nearly 100 genes in certain jakobid flagellates such as *Reclinomonas americana* (**Figure 17.12b**).

As we discuss in a later section, all mitochondrial genomes are descended from a common bacterial ancestral genome that likely possessed thousands of genes. The differences between mitochondrial genomes in living organisms reflect differential losses of genes from the ancestral genome in the different lineages. Gene losses in parasites such as *Plasmodium,* which obtains its energy from its

hosts, are often extreme, owing to loss of the genes encoding proteins required for oxidative phosphorylation.

Mitochondrial Transcription and Translation

The mitochondrial genome is transcribed by an RNA polymerase similar to that found in bacteria (see Section 8.2). In some species, the mitochondrial RNA polymerase is encoded by a mitochondrial gene; in other species, it is encoded by a nuclear gene. Transcriptional regulation of mitochondrial gene expression also varies among species but in most cases has features reminiscent of bacterial operons. For example, transcription of the mammalian mitochondrial genome involves the production of just three polycistronic mRNA transcripts from only three promoters (**Figure 17.13**). All promoters are within the mitochondrial control region, and transcription is promoted in both directions, with the result that each strand of DNA is transcribed. Transcription of the two strands generates precursor RNA molecules encompassing the entire circumference of the mitochondrial genome that encode both RNAs and proteins. The rRNAs and mRNAs are flanked by tRNAs, which are cleaved from the precursor RNAs, thus releasing the rRNA and mRNA molecules.

Mitochondrial translation occurs on ribosomes that resemble bacterial ribosomes (see Section 9.2). The rRNAs utilized in mitochondria are always encoded by the mitochondrial genome, but the mitochondrial ribosomal proteins may be encoded by either the mitochondrial or nuclear genome. In *Reclinomonas americana,* Shine–Dalgarno sequences are present upstream of most protein-coding genes, but such sequences are not evident in the mitochondrial genes of most eukaryotes.

Most mitochondrial genomes encode many fewer than the 61 different tRNA genes that are theoretically required for translation of all codons. Recall that the genetic code contains 64 codons, of which 61 encode amino acids during translation. Each codon can be uniquely recognized by a complementary anticodon sequence in tRNA, but third-base wobble and the redundancy of the genetic code permit genomes to carry fewer than 61 unique tRNA genes. Consequently, only 32 different tRNA anticodon sequences (i.e., 32 different tRNA genes) are required to recognize the 61 codons.

The substantially lower number of unique tRNA genes in mitochondrial genomes compared with the number of codons is accommodated in different ways in the mitochondria of different species. In mammalian mitochondria, the rules of third-base wobble are more lenient than they are for nuclear genes. Certain mammalian tRNAs can read codons with any of the four bases in the third position, a system that reduces the number of different tRNA genes needed in mammalian mitochondria to 22.

In some mammalian species, not all mitochondrial tRNAs are encoded in the mitochondrial genome; instead, some nucleus-encoded tRNAs are imported into mitochondria. In extreme cases, such as *Plasmodium*, all tRNAs have

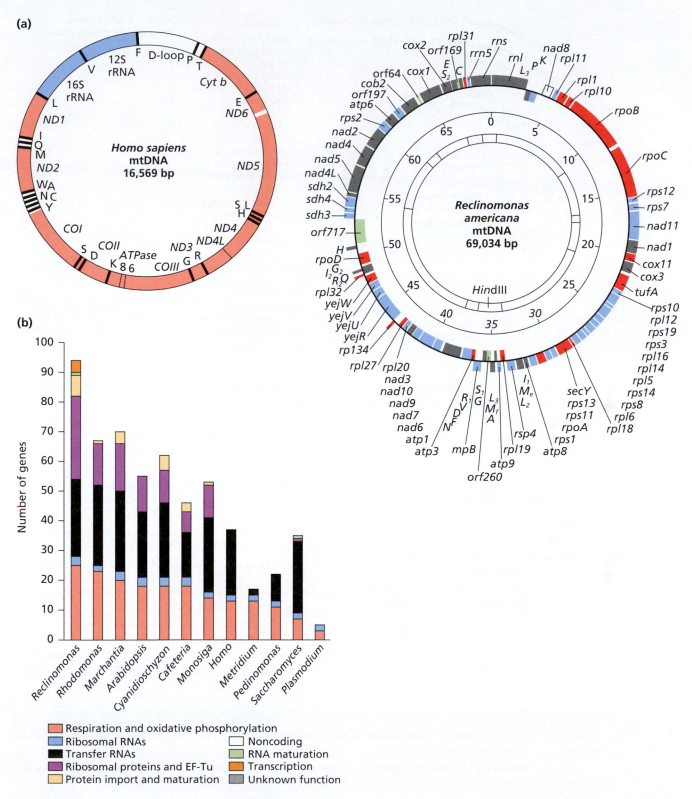

Figure 17.12 **Gene content of mitochondrial genomes.**

to be imported since none are encoded in the mitochondrial genome. In addition to mechanisms that reduce the total number of different tRNA genes encoded in mitochondria, there are differences between the mitochondrial genetic codes of certain animals, plants, and fungi (Table 17.1).

Still, in many species the mitochondrial genetic code is the same as the universal code, thus supporting the hypothesis that most of the changes listed in Table 17.1 occurred relatively late in the evolution of the major branches of eukaryotes. Some of the same differences have apparently evolved

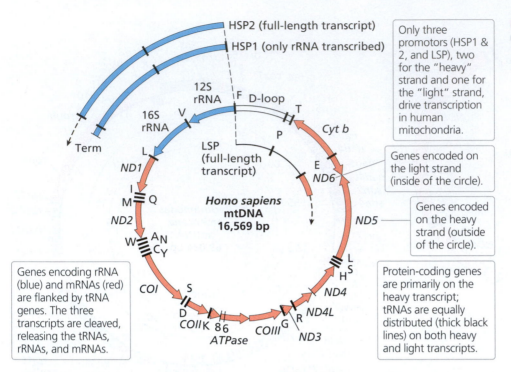

HSP2 (full-length transcript)
HSP1 (only rRNA transcribed)

Only three promotors (HSP1 & 2, and LSP), two for the "heavy" strand and one for the "light" strand, drive transcription in human mitochondria.

Genes encoded on the light strand (inside of the circle).

Genes encoded on the heavy strand (outside of the circle).

Genes encoding rRNA (blue) and mRNAs (red) are flanked by tRNA genes. The three transcripts are cleaved, releasing the tRNAs, rRNAs, and mRNAs.

Protein-coding genes are primarily on the heavy transcript; tRNAs are equally distributed (thick black lines) on both heavy and light transcripts.

Homo sapiens mtDNA 16,569 bp

Figure 17.13 Human mitochondrial transcription.

independently in multiple mitochondrial lineages, suggesting that certain changes may confer a selective advantage. It may be that the reduction in tRNA gene number in the mitochondrial genome is related to the relaxed evolution of the mitochondrial genetic code.

17.4 Chloroplasts Are the Sites of Photosynthesis

Chloroplasts—present in green plants, their algal relatives, and many other taxa that carry out photosynthesis—are only the most familiar of various organelles derived from a precursor organelle called a **plastid**. In the green tissues of plants, plastids differentiate into chloroplasts in response to light; but in nongreen tissues, plastids may differentiate into other types of specialized organelles. For example, tomatoes get their red color from pigments in a plastid derivative

called a chromoplast. Regardless of type, all plastids and their derivatives possess a genome.

Chloroplasts resemble mitochondria in being enclosed by a double-membrane system (**Figure 17.14**). However, chloroplasts also possess a third membrane system, the thylakoid membranes. These membranes reside in the stroma, the region equivalent to the matrix of the mitochondrion. The protein complexes that carry out photosynthetic reactions are embedded in the thylakoid membranes. As with mitochondria, most chloroplast proteins are encoded in the nuclear genome but are produced and regulated through interactions between the two genomes (plastid and nuclear).

Chloroplast Genome Structure and Gene Content

Many structural features of chloroplast genomes are similar to those of bacterial and mitochondrial genomes. For example, the chloroplast genome is anchored to the inner chloroplast

Codon	Universal	Mitochondrial					
		Vertebrate	Echinoderms	*Saccharomyces* (Yeast)	*Chondrus* (Red Algae)	Land Plants	Ciliates
UGA	Stop	Trp	Trp	Trp	Trp	—	Trp
AUA	Ile	Met	—	Met	—	—	—
CUN	Leu	—	—	Thr	—	—	—
AGG, AGA	Arg	Ser/Stop	Ser	—	—	—	—
CGN	Arg	—	—	—	—	—	—

Table 17.1   Examples of Differences in Mitochondrial Genetic Codes

N, any of the four bases A, G, U, C; —, no change from the universal code.

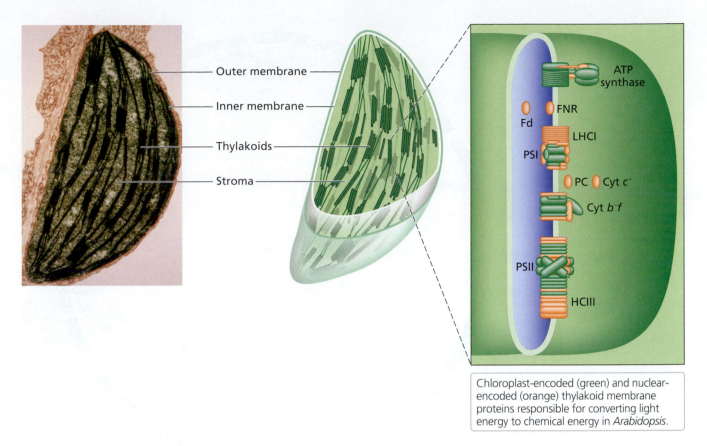

Chloroplast-encoded (green) and nuclear-encoded (orange) thylakoid membrane proteins responsible for converting light energy to chemical energy in *Arabidopsis*.

Figure 17.14   Chloroplast structure and function.

membrane, and chloroplast genomes are not packaged in chromatin composed of histones. Like mitochondrial genomes, chloroplast genomes are generally found to be circular, on the basis of genetic and molecular mapping as well as direct observation with the electron microscope. However, there is evidence that linear chloroplast genomes may also occur. The similarity of chloroplast genomes and bacterial genomes reflects the ancestral evolutionary relationship that we explore in Section 17.5.

Compared with mitochondrial genomes, chloroplast genomes are structurally less diverse. Chloroplast genomes range in size from 120 to 200 kb and usually encode 100 to 250 genes; the precise gene content varies between species. The chloroplast genome of *Marchantia polymorpha* is typical of many (**Figure 17.15a**). Whereas chloroplast ribosomal proteins may be encoded by either the chloroplast or nuclear genome, the rRNA is always encoded by the chloroplast genome, and the tRNA molecules are usually encoded by the chloroplast genome. Most of the remaining chloroplast genes with known functions encode proteins involved in photosynthesis.

One of the photosynthetic genes in the chloroplast genome encodes the large subunit of ribulose-1,-5-bisphosphate carboxylase/oxygenase, the enzyme responsible for the fixation of carbon from CO_2. The enzyme, often abbreviated RuBisCO, represents up to 50% of the protein content of green plants and is thus possibly the most abundant protein on the planet. RuBisCO is composed of two protein subunits, abbreviated rbcL and rbcS, for the large and small subunit, respectively. Whereas rbcL is encoded in the chloroplast genome (**Figure 17.15b**), rbcS is encoded in the nuclear genome, providing another example of the extensive coordination between the two genomes, which in this case must cooperate to produce appropriate quantities of the two subunits.

Chloroplast Transcription and Translation

Transcription and translation of chloroplast genes are similar to those of bacteria. Many chloroplast genes are arranged in operons and as a result are coordinately transcribed. The RNA polymerase resembles that found in bacteria and, as in bacteria, recognizes consensus sequences (similar to those of bacterial promoters) at −10 and −35 of chloroplast gene promoters (see Section 8.2). Like bacterial mRNAs, chloroplast mRNAs are neither capped at their 5′ end nor polyadenylated at their 3′ end. However, some RNA processing occurs, such as the removal of introns from a few genes and RNA editing in most land plants (a process described in more detail below). The ribosomes of chloroplasts are also similar to those of bacteria. For example, ribosome function is disrupted by aminoglycoside antibiotics, which also inhibit bacterial ribosome function.

From 30 to 35 different tRNAs are usually encoded by the chloroplast genome, and as a result all codons can be

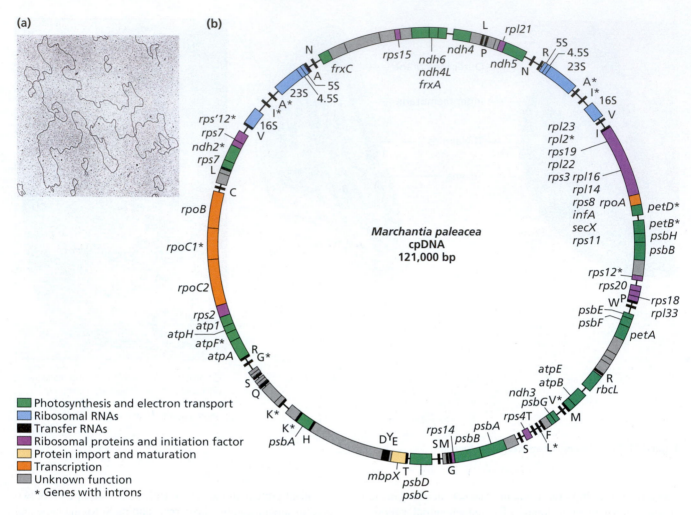

Figure 17.15 Chloroplast genome of (a) *Lactuca sativa* (lettuce) and (b) *Marchantia paleacea* (liverwort).

translated without the additional wobble found in mitochondria. The kinds of deviations from the universal genetic code that are seen in mitochondrial genes are not observed in chloroplasts.

Editing of Chloroplast mRNA

RNA editing is the process of altering the sequence of an RNA molecule after transcription from the DNA genome (see Section 8.4). RNA editing was first discovered in the mitochondria of trypanosomes, where insertion (or, less frequently, deletion) of U residues occurs in mitochondrial mRNAs. The mechanism by which this editing process occurs (described in Section 8.4) involves complementary guide RNAs that are encoded in the mitochondrial genome. The guide RNAs provide a template on which the changes to the target mRNA are made; there, enzymes either add or delete U residues from the mRNA.

RNA editing has also been noted in the mitochondria and chloroplasts of land plants, where the editing process results in C-to-U (or, less frequently, U-to-C) changes in organellar mRNAs. In contrast to the RNA editing to insert and delete bases, the RNA editing in the organelles of plants does not utilize a guide RNA. Rather, C-to-U editing is performed by an enzyme, C deaminase, which converts the C to a U, whereas U-to-C editing is presumably performed by the reverse reaction, the addition of an amine group to the U. Proper RNA editing in these cases requires the presence of specific sequences adjacent to the sites to be edited, suggesting that the adjacent sequences represent binding sites for trans-acting proteins.

Not surprisingly, given that the mRNAs of several genes encoding proteins involved in photosynthesis are edited, genetic screens designed to identify mutants in which photosynthesis is compromised have identified nuclear genes controlling chloroplast RNA editing. For example, mutations in the nuclear *CCR4* gene of *Arabidopsis* result in a loss of C-to-U editing of one nucleotide in the *ndhD* mRNA within chloroplasts; this editing normally generates a start codon, AUG, from the ACG encoded in the chloroplast genome (**Figure 17.16**).

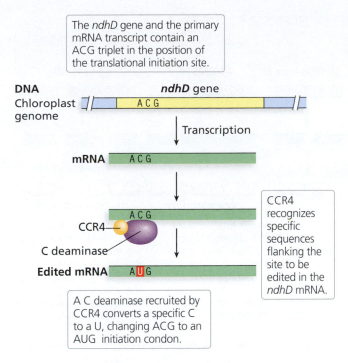

The *ndhD* gene and the primary mRNA transcript contain an ACG triplet in the position of the translational initiation site.

DNA   ***ndhD* gene**
Chloroplast   ACG
genome

Transcription

mRNA   ACG

CCR4
C deaminase

Edited mRNA   AUG

CCR4 recognizes specific sequences flanking the site to be edited in the *ndhD* mRNA.

A C deaminase recruited by CCR4 converts a specific C to a U, changing ACG to an AUG initiation condon.

Figure 17.16   A model for C-to-U RNA editing.

CCR4 encodes a member of the pentatricopeptide repeat (PPR) family of proteins. These proteins are thought to play diverse roles in RNA processing, including cleavage of RNA precursor molecules. Surprisingly, the other four edited sites in *ndhD* RNA are edited correctly in *ccr4* mutants. The nuclear genomes of land plants encode large numbers of *PPR* genes, and there is a strong correlation between the number of nucleus-encoded PPR proteins and the extent of organellar RNA editing. It appears that each edited site in organellar RNA is processed by a different trans-acting PPR protein! Studies in plant mitochondria have also identified PPR proteins as important components of RNA processing; in so doing, these studies have illuminated the mechanism of cytoplasmic male sterility, a phenotype used in plant breeding that is described in **Experimental Insight 17.1**.

17.5 The Endosymbiosis Theory Explains Mitochondrial and Chloroplast Evolution

Endosymbiosis is a symbiotic (interdependent, often mutually beneficial) relationship between organisms in which one organism inhabits the body of the other. Several lines of evidence indicate that the mitochondria and chloroplasts inhabiting modern animal and plant cells are the descendants of formerly free-living bacteria that took part in ancient infections of eukaryotic cells. These ancient invaders established endosymbiotic relationships with their hosts and have

evolved along with their hosts to produce the diversity we observe in organelles today. The principal lines of evidence supporting the **endosymbiosis theory** of mitochondria and chloroplast evolution, several of which are discussed below, including the following:

- The double-membrane system found in both organelles is derived from a similar membrane system found in bacteria.
- The organelles are similar in size to extant bacteria.
- Organellar DNA is packaged in a manner similar to the packaging of chromosomes in bacteria and dissimilar to that of DNA in the nuclear genome.
- The transcriptional and translational machinery of the organelles closely resembles that of bacteria.
- The protein-coding sequences of organellar genes are more like those of bacteria than like either the nuclear genes of eukaryotes or the sequences of archaea.

Separate Evolution of Mitochondria and Chloroplasts

The available genetic evidence indicates that mitochondria are monophyletic; that is, all mitochondria are descendants from a single common ancestor. Coupled with evidence that mitochondria bear strong similarities to bacteria, this finding suggests that the point of origin of all mitochondria was a single endosymbiotic event (**Figure 17.17**).

Based on the fossil record, the minimum age of the eukaryotes is approximately 1.5 to 2 billion years. One hypothesis concerning the origin of eukaryotes is that they evolved from an anaerobic ancestor that acquired an aerobic **endosymbiont** (the mitochondrial ancestor). This event was perhaps linked with the global rise in atmospheric oxygen that began about 2 billion years ago and that could have provided a selective environment for aerobic organisms. Based on similarity in gene sequences, the closest extant relatives of mitochondria are free-living **α-proteobacteria**. These living α-proteobacteria have genomes of 4 to 9 Mb of DNA encoding 4000 to 9000 genes, so it appears that extensive gene loss has characterized the evolution of mitochondrial genomes.

Chloroplasts are also monophyletic, having descended from a single endosymbiotic event that occurred, according to the fossil record, at least 1.2 billion years ago (see Figure 17.17). Based on similarity of gene sequences, the closest extant relatives of chloroplasts are free-living **cyanobacteria**. Existing cyanobacteria have genomes of 1.6 to 9.0 Mb of DNA encoding 1900 to 7400 genes, implying extensive gene loss in the evolution of the chloroplast genome as well. Phylogenetic evidence also suggests multiple secondary symbioses (discussed at the end of this section) in which some eukaryotes acquired a photosynthetic eukaryotic symbiont (see Figure 17.17). These events

Cytoplasmic Male Sterility in Flowering Plants

You probably do not think of sterility as a useful trait in a crop plant; however, male sterility in one parent plant provides an efficient mechanism for producing hybrid seed. This is possible because the male sterile plant can act as the female parent in a cross with a second variety. In a phenomenon called hybrid vigor, plants that are the progeny of crosses between two different varieties often exhibit higher yield than do either of the parents. Here we describe how hybrid seed can be produced by taking advantage of genetic interactions between specific nuclear and chloroplast genes.

In plants, male sterility is a failure to produce viable pollen. Some cases, called cytoplasmic male sterility (CMS), are maternally inherited and are due to mutations in the mitochondrial genome. However, the phenotypic defects of these mitochondrial mutations can often be suppressed by the presence of dominant alleles of nuclear genes, called *Restorer of fertility*, or *RF*, genes. The interaction between typical *CMS* and *RF* genes provides an example of how genetic interactions between nuclear and mitochondrial genotypes can influence phenotypes. It can be outlined as follows:

Female Parent	×	Pollen Parent	Progeny Genotype	Progeny Phenotype
CMS *rf/rf*		N *rf/rf*	CMS *rf/rf*	Male sterile
CMS *rf/rf*		N *Rf/Rf*	CMS *Rf/rf*	Male fertile

CMS = male sterile cytoplasm; N = wild-type cytoplasm; *Rf* = dominant nuclear *RF* allele; *rf* = recessive nuclear *RF* allele.

In this system, CMS cytoplasm in an *rf/rf* background makes a male sterile, but a dominant *RF* allele, *Rf*, is sufficient to restore fertility. Many different CMS mutants are known, and they exhibit exclusive relationships with particular nuclear *RF* genes, thus indicating several distinct nuclear–mitochondrial genome interactions. The *RF* loci may act either sporophytically, in which case all pollen produced from *Rf/rf* plants is fertile, or gametophytically, in which case only half of the pollen produced by a heterozygote is viable. Since most plants produce a vast excess of pollen, these latter plants are considered male fertile.

CMS mitochondrial genes (*MG* in the figure ❶) usually have novel open reading frames (ORFs) that combine sequences of unknown origin with mitochondrial gene-coding sequences. Expression of the novel ORFs is driven by adjacent mitochondrial promoter sequences ❷. Since most plants harboring CMS-causing ORFs have a full complement of normal mitochondrial genes, the CMS ORFs can be considered gain-of-function mutations.

Several *RF* genes encode proteins of the pentatricopeptide repeat (PPR) family. The functions of characterized PPR proteins include RNA processing, such as cleavage of RNA precursors and RNA editing. This discovery is consistent with the effects of *RF* genes on *CMS* genes, since in the presence of a restorer allele, transcripts of *CMS* ORFs fail to accumulate. One current hypothesis is that PPR proteins encoded by *Rf* alleles process transcripts produced by the *CMS* genes, thus restoring wild-type function to the affecting mitochondrial genes (❸; see Figure 17.16).

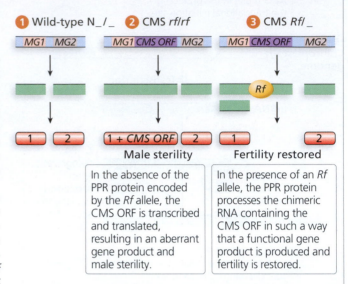

❶ Wild-type N_/_   ❷ CMS *rf/rf*   ❸ CMS *Rf/_*

Male sterility

In the absence of the PPR protein encoded by the *Rf* allele, the CMS ORF is transcribed and translated, resulting in an aberrant gene product and male sterility.

Fertility restored

In the presence of an *Rf* allele, the PPR protein processes the chimeric RNA containing the CMS ORF in such a way that a functional gene product is produced and fertility is restored.

CMS–RF systems have been harnessed to facilitate the production of hybrid seeds. The following double-cross hybrid scheme in maize utilizes four breeding lines as parents.

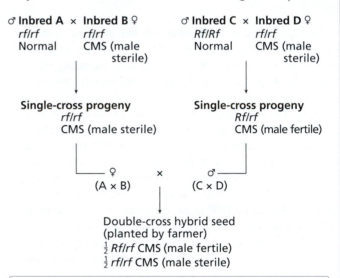

♂ Inbred A × Inbred B ♀
rf/rf   *rf/rf*
Normal   CMS (male sterile)

♂ Inbred C × Inbred D ♀
Rf/Rf   *rf/rf*
Normal   CMS (male sterile)

Single-cross progeny
rf/rf
CMS (male sterile)

Single-cross progeny
Rf/rf
CMS (male fertile)

♀   ×   ♂
(A × B)   (C × D)

Double-cross hybrid seed
(planted by farmer)
½ *Rf/rf* CMS (male fertile)
½ *rf/rf* CMS (male sterile)

The hybrid seed is ½ male fertile and ½ male sterile. When plants of both genotypes are planted together, pollen from the male fertile plants pollinate both kinds.

To produce each new generation of seeds for planting, breeders combine *CMS* and *RF* alleles so as to prevent female parents from self-fertilizing and to ensure that male parents have fertile pollen. In the first generation, two pairs of inbred parents are crossed, A × B and C × D. Both A and C have normal cytoplasm but differ at the *RF* locus: A is homozygous recessive (*rf/rf*), and C is homozygous dominant (*Rf/Rf*). In contrast, lines B and D are CMS and *rf/rf*. The progeny produced by A × B are CMS *rf/rf*, male sterile, and can be used as the female parents in the subsequent cross. The progeny produced by C × D are CMS *Rf/rf*, male fertile, and can be used as the male parents. The seeds that ultimately result have genomes derived from four different inbred lines and develop into larger, hardier plants due to hybrid vigor.

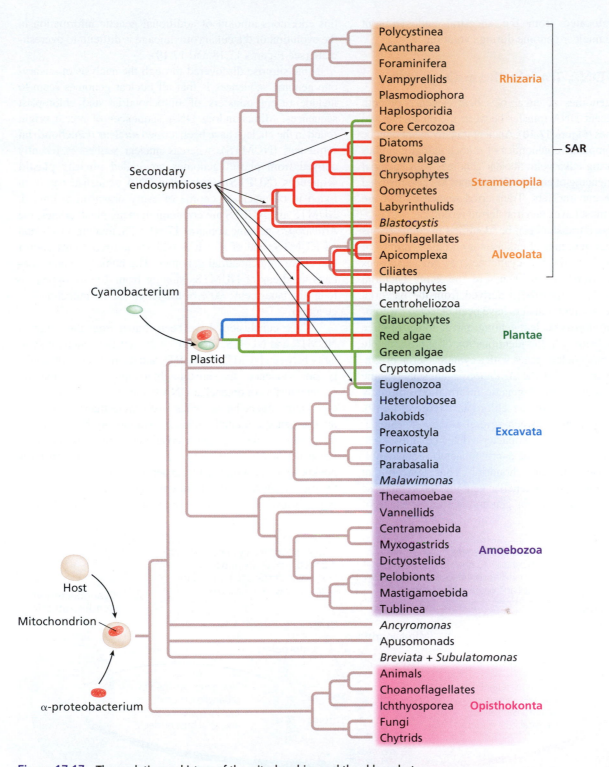

Figure 17.17 **The evolutionary history of the mitochondrion and the chloroplast.**

resulted in the horizontal transmission of chloroplasts among unrelated eukaryotic lineages.

Two fundamental questions arise when we consider the genomes of the organelles. First, given that mitochondrial and chloroplast genomes contain from 6 to 100 and from 20 to 200 genes, respectively, what happened to all the other genes of the ancestral symbiont? Second, given that the organelles contain many more organellar proteins than genes, what is the origin of the nuclear genes that encode so many organellar proteins? Are those nuclear genes derived from the ancestral symbiont genome, or did they evolve in the host genome? A possible answer was provided by the discovery that DNA is transferred from organellar genomes to nuclear genomes; this led to the hypothesis that genes have been relocated from the ancestral endosymbiont genome to the nuclear genome during evolution.

Continual DNA Transfer from Organelles

The nuclear genomes of eukaryotes bear evidence of both ancient and recent DNA transfer between the organellar and nuclear genomes (Figure 17.18). Ancient transfer events can be detected by comparative genomics of mitochondrial genomes and by comparing eukaryotic nuclear genomes with bacterial genomes. Sequencing of eukaryotic genomes has also revealed evidence of recent transfers. Transferred sequences that are highly similar must have been transferred recently.

Ancient gene transfers can be identified in comparisons between nuclear genomes of eukaryotes and the genomes of extant α-proteobacteria and cyanobacteria. Nuclear genes that are most similar to the genes of the living bacterial species are likely to have been derived from the bacterial endosymbiont. Ancient transfers have been detected by comparing the *Arabidopsis* nuclear genome and genomes of three cyanobacteria, leading to the identification of approximately 4300 *Arabidopsis* nuclear genes with a cyanobacterial origin. Thus, more than 10% of the *Arabidopsis* nuclear genome represents an acquisition of genetic information originally residing in the genome of the chloroplast (Figure 17.19). Similarly, comparisons between several eukaryotic nuclear genomes and those of α-proteobacteria detected at least 630 nuclear genes derived from the α-proteobacteria endosymbiont that gave rise to the mitochondrion. Thus, concomitant with the reduction in the organellar genomes is an increase in gene content in the nuclear genome. The importance of

this enormous amount of additional genetic information in the evolution of the eukaryotic lineage is difficult to overestimate (see Figures 17.18 and 17.19).

One surprise discovered through the analysis of eukaryotic genome sequences is that all nuclear genomes seem to include recent transfers of mitochondrial and chloroplast sequences. Mitochondrial DNA sequences of recent origin found in the nucleus have been termed **nuclear mitochondrial sequences (NUMTS)**, whereas nuclear sequences recently derived from plastid genomes are called **nuclear plastid sequences (NUPTS)**. Organellar DNA sequence has been found in the nuclear genome of every organism examined. NUMTS and NUPTS are common in many plant species; the *Arabidopsis* genome contains 17 NUPTS, totaling 11 kb, and 14 NUMTS, one of which is 620 kb and represents almost two entire mitochondrial genomes. The human genome contains hundreds of NUMTS, ranging from 106 to 14,654 bp long (the latter being 90% of the length of the mitochondrial genome).

Three conclusions have been drawn from the study of NUMTS and NUPTS. First, given the level of sequence similarity between NUMTS or NUPTS and the respective organelle genome sequences, they are thought to represent evolutionarily recent transfers of organellar DNA to the nuclear genome. Second, entire organellar genomes likely were transferred to the nuclear genome multiple times in evolutionary history. Third, the process is ongoing; DNA continues to move between the organelles and to the nucleus. Although the rate of transfer is not known in most organisms, experiments to directly measure the rate of DNA transfer from chloroplast to nuclear genome in plants revealed a new integration of chloroplast DNA in the

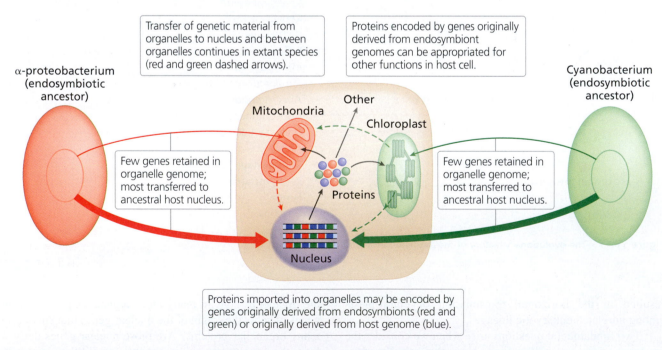

Figure 17.18   Transfer of endosymbiont genes to the nuclear genome and destinations of encoded protein products.

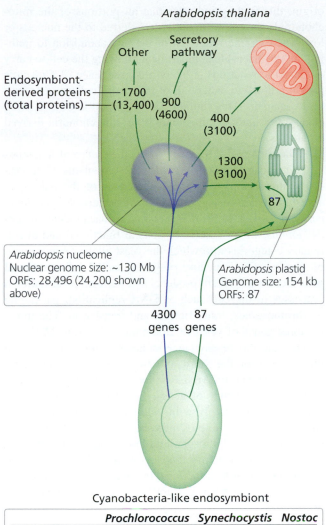

Arabidopsis thaliana

Endosymbiont-derived proteins (total proteins)

Arabidopsis nucleome
Nuclear genome size: ~130 Mb
ORFs: 28,496 (24,200 shown above)

Arabidopsis plastid
Genome size: 154 kb
ORFs: 87

4300 genes   87 genes

Cyanobacteria-like endosymbiont

	Prochlorococcus	*Synechocystis*	*Nostoc*
Genome size (Mb):	1.66	6.3	9.02
ORFs:	1694	3168	7281

Figure 17.19 Evolution of genes derived from the cyanobacteria-like endosymbiont.

Is an encoded protein of a gene originally derived from the cyanobacterium more likely to be targeted to the chloroplast or to elsewhere in the cell?

nuclear genome at a rate of 1 in 16,000 plants. This surprisingly high rate of DNA transfer between the organellar and nuclear genomes can account for the large numbers of evolutionarily recent insertions of organellar DNA (NUMTS and NUPTS) found in the nuclear genome of most organisms. Although the rate of transfer has not been directly measured in humans, it is likely that it is high enough for NUMTS polymorphisms to be present in the human population.

Although organellar genes are readily transferred into the nuclear genome, several events must occur for the transferred genes to be functional. Recall from Chapters 12 and 13 that the details of gene regulation differ between bacteria and eukaryotes. Since gene regulation in the organelles resembles that in bacteria, transferred genes must acquire sequences for proper transcriptional regulation in the nucleus. Researchers using an experimental system similar to the one for monitoring DNA transfer from chloroplast to nuclear genome in plants have demonstrated that transferred chloroplast genes can become functional nuclear genes at a frequency observable in the laboratory. In addition, as described in more detail below, the protein encoded by the transferred gene may be transported back to the organelle from which the gene was derived; or, alternatively, the protein may be directed to another cellular compartment. For the protein to be transported back to the organelle, an amino terminal signal sequence must be attached to it. Since signal sequences need only to have certain general structural features to function properly, the acquisition of functional signal sequences likely occurs at an appreciable frequency.

Encoding of Organellar Proteins

Organelles contain many more proteins than they encode in their genomes; this is an indication that most organellar proteins are encoded in the nuclear genome. For example, the yeast mitochondrion contains approximately 400 proteins, but only 16 proteins are encoded in its mitochondrial genome. The nucleus-encoded organellar proteins are translated in the cytoplasm and then imported into the organelles. These organellar proteins are targeted to their final location by signal sequences of 15 to 25 amino acids at the amino terminal end of the proteins. Different signal sequences label proteins for transport to different locations in organelles (such as the outer membrane, intermembrane space, inner membrane, matrix, and stroma and thylakoid membrane systems).

When the endosymbiotic theory of the origin of mitochondria and chloroplasts was first proposed, its framers predicted that proteins were always targeted to the cell compartment from which the genes encoding them were originally derived. In other words, if a protein was encoded by a nuclear gene that had originally been derived from the endosymbiont that gave rise to the mitochondrion, the protein would be targeted back to the mitochondrion. Contrary to expectations, however, the relationships between the endosymbiont origins of genes and the final destination of gene products are complex and difficult to predict. For example, in *Arabidopsis,* fewer than half the proteins identified as coming from the cyanobacterial endosymbiont are found to be targeted to the chloroplast (see Figure 17.19). Conversely, a number of proteins targeted to the chloroplast were not acquired from the cyanobacterial symbiont, but rather are descended from the original eukaryotic host genome. Similar observations have been made concerning the mitochondrion. Thus the proteins encoded by nuclear genes originally derived from endosymbiont genomes may be targeted to any location in the cell.

Although the diversity in the direction of protein transport was initially unexpected, perhaps consideration of the early stages of endosymbioses should have led scientists to expect it. When an endosymbiotic relationship was initially established, the genome of the ancestral mitochondrion would have been similar in size to that of its bacterial ancestors. If the rate of DNA transfer was similar to that measured today, the nuclear genome must have experienced a bombardment of DNA from the endosymbiont. Before the evolution of the mitochondrial protein-import machinery, proteins produced by genes transferred to the nuclear genome had to remain in the cytoplasm or be transported to the plasma membrane. Reduction in the endosymbiont genome could occur only after the evolution of systems able to import proteins into the endosymbiont. Such systems are composed of proteins encoded by genes originally derived from both the nuclear and endosymbiont genomes.

The Origin of the Eukaryotic Lineage

The tree of life is often depicted as having three major branches—the Bacteria, the Archaea, and the Eukarya—based on comparison of sequences of the rRNA genes (see Section 1.1). The extensive gene flow from bacterial endosymbionts to the nucleus, however, has resulted in the presence of significant numbers of "bacterial" genes in the nuclear genomes of eukaryotes. Given this situation, a simple tripartite view of life, in which three branches diverge from a single common ancestor, is overly simplistic. A fraction of the nuclear genome of every eukaryote is derived from bacterial endosymbionts, but where were all the remaining genes derived from? In other words, what was the original host of the α-proteobacterium that gave rise to the eukaryotes?

Two models have been proposed to answer this question. In one model, the original host is a cell described as having a nucleus but no mitochondria and as subsequently acquiring an α-proteobacterium as an endosymbiont. In this model, "eukaryotic" cells (cells having nuclei) existed before the endosymbiotic event, suggesting that such organisms lacking mitochondria might still exist. In the second model, the original host is a bacterial cell that acquires an α-proteobacterium as an endosymbiont; and subsequently, this host–endosymbiont system evolves other eukaryotic features, such as a nuclear membrane. If the latter model is correct, no intermediate eukaryotes lacking mitochondria should be found.

Two recent discoveries have contributed new fuel to this discussion. First, eukaryotic organisms that were originally thought to lack mitochondria, such as *Giardia intestinalis* (which causes diarrhea when it infects the human intestine), are now known to have mitochondria. In the case of *Giardia*, the mitochondria are reduced to double-membrane–bound structures called **mitosomes**. Mitosomes lack a genome, but proteins requiring an anaerobic environment to function are imported into them. Furthermore, the nuclear genome of *Giardia* harbors genes of mitochondrial

origin; this finding indicates that all portions of the mitochondrial genome were either transferred to the nucleus or lost. The extreme reduction of the mitochondrion to nothing but an anaerobic compartment allowing the cell to carry out specific reactions is likely a consequence of *Giardia*'s parasitic lifestyle, where all of its energy is derived from a host organism. This finding means that all known existing eukaryotes harbor mitochondria or mitochondria-derived organelles.

The second discovery concerns the nature of the genes in the nuclear genomes of eukaryotic organisms. Comparison of the complete genome sequences of the eukaryote *Saccharomyces cerevisiae* with two bacteria (*Escherichia coli* and *Synechocystis 6803*) and an archaea (*Methanococcus jannaschii*) revealed two general functional and evolutionary categories into which the yeast nuclear genes could be divided. One category of genes, called **informational genes**, encodes protein products that perform informational processes in the cell such as DNA replication, packaging of chromosomes, transcription, and translation. The informational genes of yeast resemble those found in *Methanococcus,* and this resemblance includes a similarity between the histones of the yeast and the histone-like chromatin proteins present in Archaea (see Sections 8.3 and 9.2). The second category of genes, called **operational genes**, encode proteins involved in cellular metabolic processes, such as amino acid biosynthesis, biosynthesis of cofactors, fatty acid and phospholipid biosynthesis, intermediary metabolism, energy metabolism, nucleotide biosynthesis, and some regulatory functions. In contrast to their informational genes, most yeast operational genes resemble those of Bacteria.

One scenario consistent with the apparent origins of informational and operational genes in yeast is that the original host cell of the α-proteobacterial endosymbiont was related to an archaeal cell (**Figure 17.20**). The original host genome would have contained both informational and operational genes, as would the α-proteobacterial endosymbiont. Over time, while both genomes retained their own informational genes, many endosymbiont operational genes were transferred to the nuclear genome and often replaced their host functional equivalents. Unlike the cases of the mitochondria and chloroplasts, where the endosymbionts can be traced to specific lineages of Bacteria, the putative archaeal host is unknown and may have been unrelated to any specific lineage of extant Archaea.

Secondary and Tertiary Endosymbioses

The melding together of genomes did not happen only during the endosymbioses that formed mitochondria and chloroplasts. **Secondary and even tertiary endosymbiotic events** have occurred between different lineages of eukaryotes, resulting in the dispersal of plastids into eukaryotic lineages that are distantly related (see Figure 17.17). In secondary and tertiary endosymbioses, typically, a

Figure 17.20 One hypothesis for the evolution of the eukaryotes.

What types of genes have we inherited from an ancestral archaeal cell?

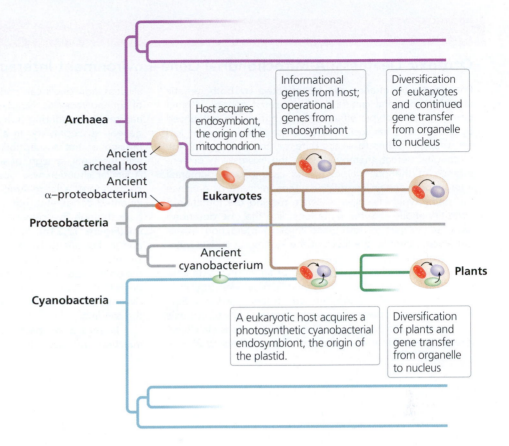

nonphotosynthetic eukaryote envelopes an algal cell and acquires a red or green algal endosymbiont. What happens to the nuclear genome of the secondary endosymbiont when one eukaryote envelops another eukaryote? Genes of the nuclear genome of the eukaryotic endosymbiont (the alga), whose products were targeted to the plastid, are translocated to the nucleus of the new, primary host in a process analogous to the movement of genes from the chloroplast genome to the primary endosymbiont host nuclear genome. Thus the nuclear genome of the algal endosymbiont, termed the **nucleomorph**, undergoes reduction to the extent that it encodes only some genes for products targeted to the plastid as well as some genes required for the maintenance of the nucleomorph genome. The plastid is serviced by three different genomes (nuclear, nucleomorph, and plastid), and the nuclear genome of photosynthetic secondary endosymbionts is a mixture of four genomes (mitochon- drial, chloroplast, and two nuclear genomes). Because secondary and tertiary endosymbioses have occurred many times during the evolution of eukaryotes (see Figure 17.17), the mixing and coevolution of genomes has been instrumental in shaping the evolution of several lineages of life.

The mixing and melding of genomes can sometimes result in biological anomalies. For example, the discovery of a reduced chloroplast (or apicoplast) in *Plasmodium falciparum*, the malarial parasite, came as quite a surprise because this is clearly not a photosynthetic organism.

Plasmodium resides within the phylum Apicomplexa, which would make it a descendant of an ancient secondary endosymbiosis involving a host eukaryote and an endosymbiotic chloroplast-containing red alga (see Figure 17.17). Is there a reason that *Plasmodium,* with its parasitic lifestyle, might have retained the apicoplast and its accompanying genome, albeit without any genes encoding proteins involved in photosynthesis?

One hypothesis explaining retention of the apicoplast in *Plasmodium* is based on differences in translation of organellar-encoded compared with nucleus-encoded genes. The initiator tRNA used in mitochondrial translation is a formylmethionyl-tRNA ($tRNA^{fMet}$), the same as used in bacteria. This special tRNA cannot be imported from the cytoplasm, since cytosolic translation in eukaryotes uses an initiator methionyl-tRNA that is not formylated. During the evolutionary history of *Plasmodium,* the gene encoding the enzyme that adds a formyl group to the methionyl-tRNA has been lost from the mitochondrial genome. Since the only methionyl-tRNA formyl transferase gene in *Plasmodium* is in the nuclear genome, it is thought that the protein product of this gene is transported to the apicoplast, and that $tRNA^{fMet}$ is produced in the apicoplast and then transported to the mitochondria. According to this hypothesis, the apicoplast may be maintained for the sole purpose of synthesizing $tRNA^{fMet}$ to be imported into the mitochondrion—a quirk of the evolutionary history of *Plasmodium.*

CASE STUDY

Ototoxic Deafness: A Mitochondrial Gene–Environment Interaction

Phenotypic penetrance can be affected by both genetic and environmental factors. In the case of genetic interactions, the phenotypic effects of a mutation are influenced by alleles at other loci. The gene products of other loci are thought either to exacerbate or compensate for the mutational defect, thereby altering the expressivity or penetrance of the phenotype. In the case of environmental interactions, certain conditions either mitigate or enhance the phenotypic effects, in essence making the mutation a conditional allele. Some mutations, like the one described here, are subject to both these kinds of interaction. In this particular example, the locus of the key mutation is a mitochondrial gene.

A rare complication of the use of aminoglycoside antibiotics, such as streptomycin, gentamicin, and kanamycin, is irreversible loss of hearing, termed ototoxic deafness. Several observations point to a genetic susceptibility to ototoxic deafness. Due to pervasive use of aminoglycosides in China, it was reported that in a district of Shanghai, nearly 25% of

all deaf individuals can trace their loss of hearing to the use of aminoglycosides. Nearly one-fourth of these patients also had relatives suffering from ototoxic deafness, suggesting a genetic susceptibility. In all 22 cases where genetic transmission of the susceptibility could be traced, inheritance was maternal, a sign of a mitochondrially inherited trait. A similar situation was observed for 26 families in Japan. Furthermore, a large Arab-Israeli pedigree with maternally inherited congenital (not ototoxic) deafness can be traced back through five generations to a common female ancestor (**Figure 17.21a**). In this case, the mitochondrial mutation is thought to be homoplasmic, since family members are either severely deaf or have normal hearing. However, the phenotype is not completely penetrant; this finding suggests that another mutation, likely to be an autosomal recessive nuclear mutation, contributes to the manifestation of the condition.

In studies on bacteria, aminoglycosides stabilize mismatched aminoacyl-tRNAs in the ribosome during translation;

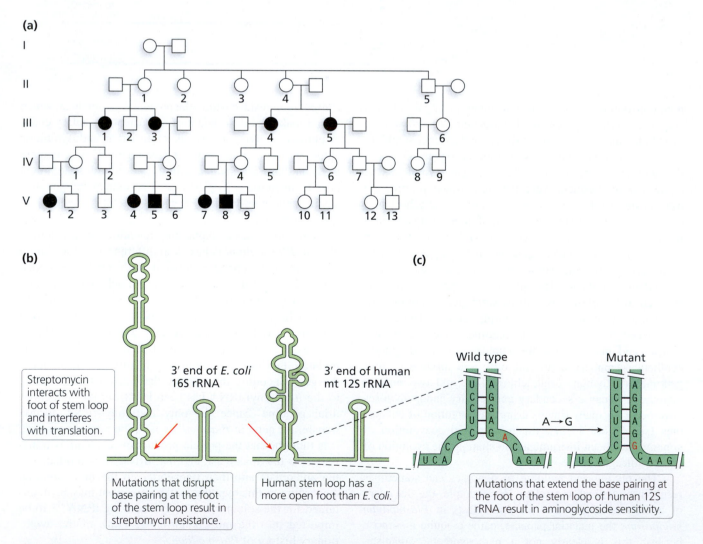

Figure 17.21 Genetic and environmental interactions in ototoxic deafness.

this finding explains their antibiotic effects. The presence of aminoglycosides causes a reduction in the fidelity of translation, leading to defective proteins. Aminoglycosides have been shown to interact directly both with ribosomal proteins and with the 16S rRNA of the 70S ribosome; and aminoglycoside-resistant bacteria have been shown to have point mutations in their 16S rRNA gene. Since the normal target of aminoglycosides is the bacterial ribosome, the likely target of aminoglycoside ototoxicity in humans is the evolutionarily related mitochondrial ribosomes, and perhaps specifically the 12S rRNA that is homologous to the 16S rRNA of bacteria.

Sequencing of the mitochondrial 12S rRNA gene in individuals with congenital deafness in the Arab-Israeli family and in other unrelated individuals with ototoxic deafness revealed that they shared a single A-to-G mutation in their 12S rRNA genes. The mutation lies at the foot of a stem loop conserved in bacteria, plants, and mammals. Studies on bacterial ribosomes have shown that this region of the 16S rRNA forms part of the aminoacyl site where mRNAs are decoded. Furthermore, aminoglycosides bind to this domain of the 16S rRNA, and bacterial mutants resistant to aminoglycosides map to this region of the 16S rRNA gene.

Thus, the cause of the aminoglycoside-induced deafness is a mutation in the mitochondrial 12S rRNA gene, but three intriguing questions remain. First, why is deafness the primary, and perhaps only, phenotypic defect? A characteristic of many mitochondrial diseases is pleiotropy due to a general loss of oxidative phosphorylation activity.

However, in these cases of maternally inherited deafness or susceptibility to aminoglycosides, no obvious pleiotropic phenotypes are associated with the deafness. Is the cochlea especially susceptible to a loss of mitochondrial function? Are the cochlear mitochondria especially sensitive to aminoglycosides? Second, what is the nature of the autosomal recessive mutation that acts to enhance the effect of the 12S rRNA mutation in the Arab-Israeli family? Could it be a nucleus-encoded ribosomal protein gene that interacts with the mitochondrial 12S rRNA? And third, if our mitochondrial ribosomes are evolutionarily related to bacterial ribosomes, why are humans able to utilize aminoglycosides as antibiotics in the first place?

Clues to the answer of the third question have come from comparative studies of mitochondrial ribosome function. The mutation causing deafness creates an extension of base pairing by one base in the stem loop of the mitochondrial 12S rRNA, in effect making its structure more closely resemble the structure of the aminoglycoside--binding site of the bacterial 16S rRNA (Figure 17.21b–c). Thus, in the 2 or so billion years since the separation of bacteria and mitochondria, the structure of the mitochondrial ribosome has changed just enough so that aminoglycosides do not normally interfere with the fidelity of translation in mitochondria; but mutations that result in a more bacteria-like ribosome structure bring back the ancient sensitivity to aminoglycosides. It is worth noting that—at least in this sense—translation in chloroplasts, which have diverged from bacteria for about 1.2 billion years, remains sensitive to aminoglycosides.

SUMMARY   Mastering Genetics   For activities, animations, and review quizzes, go to the Study Area.

17.1 Organellar Inheritance Transmits Genes Carried on Organellar Chromosomes

▌ Mitochondria and chloroplasts possess their own genomes, each encoding a small number of genes. The products of these genomes function within the respective organelle.

▌ Because many copies of organellar DNA occur in each cell, multiple genotypes may coexist in a single cell.

▌ Cells or organisms in which all genomic copies of an organellar gene have an identical sequence are said to be homoplasmic for that gene, whereas cells or organisms possessing multiple alleles for an organellar gene are called heteroplasmic.

▌ Replication of organellar genomes and organelle division are not directly coupled with the nuclear cell cycle.

▌ Replicative segregation of organelles can result in homoplasmic cells being derived from heteroplasmic cells.

▌ The proportion of mutant alleles in heteroplasmic cells influences the penetrance and expressivity of phenotypes.

17.2 Modes of Organellar Inheritance Depend on the Organism

▌ The transmission genetics of organellar genomes is often determined by the relative amounts of cytoplasm contributed by the parental gametes.

▌ Organelles are maternally inherited in mammals and many plant species, whereas in fungal species, mitochondria are often biparentally inherited. In some species, organellar inheritance is determined by alleles of a nuclear gene.

17.3 Mitochondria Are the Energy Factories of Eukaryotic Cells

▌ Mitochondria are the sites of energy production; the enzymes of oxidative phosphorylation are on the inner membrane.

▌ Mitochondrial mutations often have pleiotropic effects that reflect the role of mitochondria in energy production.

17.4 Chloroplasts Are the Sites of Photosynthesis

▌ Chloroplasts are the sites of photosynthesis, conducted by enzymatic reactions responsible for carbon fixation in the stroma and by photosystem complexes that convert light to chemical energy in the thylakoid membranes.

▌ Only a small fraction of the proteins present in a mitochondrion or chloroplast are encoded in the genome of the respective organelle; instead, most of the proteins are encoded in the nuclear genome and posttranslationally imported into the organelles.

17.5 The Endosymbiosis Theory Explains Mitochondrial and Chloroplast Evolution

▪ Both the mitochondrion and the chloroplast are evolutionarily derived from ancient endosymbioses in which a bacterium (of the phyla α-proteobacteria and cyanobacteria, respectively) was incorporated into a eukaryotic cell.

▪ The circular structure (in most organisms) and transcriptional and translational expression of mitochondrial and chloroplast genomes reflect their evolutionary origins as bacterial endosymbionts of eukaryotic cells.

▪ Many of the genes present in the ancestral endosymbiont have been transferred to the nuclear genome of the host cell and have contributed extensively to eukaryotic nuclear genome content.

▪ The process of DNA transfer from organellar genomes to the nuclear genome is ongoing, and recent transfers of organellar DNA into the nucleus can be detected in most, if not all, organisms.

▪ Genes transferred from the ancient endosymbiont genome to the host nuclear genome encode proteins that may be targeted to any compartment of the eukaryotic cell.

▪ Eukaryotic informational genes are related to archeal genes, thus suggesting that eukaryotes might be descended from an archaea-like cell that acquired a bacterial endosymbiont.

PREPARING FOR PROBLEM SOLVING

In addition to the list of problem-solving tips and suggestions given here, you can go to the Study Guide and Solutions Manual that accompanies this book for help at solving problems.

1. Know the meanings of homoplasmy and heteroplasmy and how these properties impinge upon expressivity and penetrance of organellar alleles.

2. Be familiar with how replicative segregation can result in homoplasmy from an initial state of heteroplasmy.

3. Recognize that the modes of organellar inheritance differ among eukaryotes.

4. Understand that the inheritance of mitochondria in mammals is maternal.

5. Know the general structure and contents of the organelle genomes.

6. Understand that organelles contain some proteins encoded in organelle genomes and other proteins encoded in nuclear genomes, and how this influences expressivity and penetrance of alleles of organellar and nuclear genes.

7. Recognize the origin of the organelles from ancestral bacterial endosymbionts.

8. Be aware of the continuing transfer of DNA between organelle genomes and the nuclear genome.

PROBLEMS

Mastering Genetics Visit for instructor-assigned tutorials and problems.

Chapter Concepts

For answers to selected even-numbered problems, see Appendix: Answers.

1. Reciprocal crosses of experimental animals or plants sometimes give different results in the F_1. What are two possible genetic explanations? How would you distinguish between these two possibilities (i.e., what crosses would you perform, and what would the results tell you)?

2. How are some of the characteristics of the organelles (the mitochondria and chloroplasts) explained by their origin as ancient bacterial endosymbionts?

3. The human mitochondrial genome encodes only 22 tRNAs, but at least 32 tRNAs are needed for cytoplasmic translation. How are all codons in mitochondrial transcripts accommodated by only 22 tRNAs? The *Plasmodium* mitochondrial genome does not encode any tRNAs; how are genes of the *Plasmodium* mitochondrial genome translated?

4. What is the evidence that transfer of DNA from the organelles to the nucleus continues to occur?

5. Draw a graph depicting the relative amounts of nuclear DNA present in the different stages of the cell cycle

(G_1, S, G_2, M). On the same graph, plot the amount of mitochondrial DNA present at each stage of the cell cycle.

6. What are the differences between the universal code and that found in the mitochondria of some species? Given that some changes (UGA $=$ stop $\rightarrow$ Trp) have occurred multiple independent times in evolution, can you think of any selective advantage to the mitochondrial code?

7. What is the evidence that the ancient mitochondrial and chloroplast endosymbionts are related to the α-proteobacteria and cyanobacteria, respectively?

8. Outline the steps required for a gene originally present in the endosymbiont genome to be transferred to the nuclear genome and be expressed, and for its product to be targeted back to the organelle of origin.

9. Consider the phylogenetic tree presented in Figure 17.17. How were the origins of secondary endosymbiosis in the brown algae determined?

Application and Integration

For answers to selected even-numbered problems, see Appendix: Answers.

10. You are a genetic counselor, and several members of the family whose pedigree for an inherited disorder is depicted in Genetic Analysis 17.2 consult with you about the probability that their progeny may be afflicted. What advice would you give individuals III-1, III-2, III-4, III-6, III-8, and III-9?

11. A mutation in *Arabidopsis immutans* results in the necrosis (death) of tissues in a mosaic configuration. Examination of the mitochondrial DNA detects deletions of various regions of the mitochondrial genome in the tissues that are necrotic. When *immutans* plants are crossed with wild-type plants, the F$_1$ are wild type, and the F$_2$ are wild type and *immutans* in a 3:1 ratio. Explain the inheritance of the *immutans* mutation and a possible origin of the mitochondrial DNA deletions.

12. What type or types of inheritance are consistent with the following pedigree?

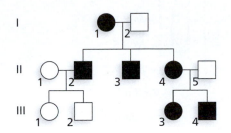

13. You have isolated (1) a streptomycin-resistant mutant (*str*^{R}) of *Chlamydomonas* that maps to the chloroplast genome and (2) a hygromycin-resistant mutant (*hyg*^{R}) of *Chlamydomonas* that maps to the mitochondrial genome. What types of progeny do you expect from the following reciprocal crosses?

$$mt^+ \ str^R \ hyg^S \times mt^- \ str^S \ hyg^R$$
$$mt^+ \ str^S \ hyg^R \times mt^- \ str^R \ hyg^S$$

14. You have isolated two *petite* mutants, *pet1* and *pet2*, in *Saccharomyces cerevisiae*. When *pet1* is mated with wild-type yeast, the haploid products following meiosis segregate 2:2 (wild type : *petite*). In contrast, when *pet2* is mated with wild type, all haploid products following meiosis are wild type. To what class of *petite* mutations does each of these *petite* mutants belong? What types of progeny do you expect from a *pet1* × *pet2* mating?

15. Consider this human pedigree for a vision defect.

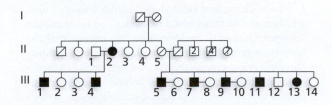

What is the most probable mode of inheritance of the disease? Identify any discrepancies between the pedigree and your proposed mode of transmission, and provide possible explanations for these exceptions.

16. A 50-year-old man has been diagnosed with MELAS syndrome (see Figure 17.6). His wife is phenotypically normal, and there is no history of MELAS syndrome in either of their families. The couple is concerned about whether their children will develop the disease. As a genetic counselor, what will you tell them? Would your answer change if it were the mother who exhibited disease symptoms rather than the father?

17. The first person in a family to exhibit Leber hereditary optic neuropathy (LHON) was II-3 in the pedigree shown below, and all of her children also exhibited the disease. Provide two possible explanations as to why II-3's mother (I-1) did not exhibit symptoms of LHON.

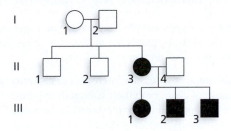

18. The following pedigree shows a family in which several individuals exhibit symptoms of the mitochondrial disease MERRF. Two siblings (II-2 and II-5) approach you to inquire about whether their children will also be afflicted with MERRF. What do you tell them?

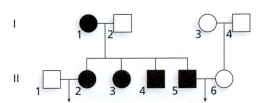

19. What is the most likely mode of inheritance for the trait depicted in the following human pedigree?

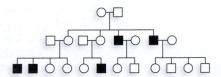

20. In 1918, the Russian Tsar Nicholas II was deposed, and he and his family were reportedly executed and buried in a shallow grave. During this chaotic time, rumors abounded that the youngest daughter, Anastasia, had escaped. In 1920, a woman in Germany claimed to be Anastasia. In 1979, remains were recovered for the tsar, his wife (the Tsarina Alexandra), and three of their children, but not Anastasia. How would you evaluate the claim of the woman in Germany?

21. The dodo bird (*Raphus cucullatus*) lived on the Mauritius Islands until the arrival of European sailors, who quickly

hunted the large, placid, flightless bird to extinction. Rapid morphological evolution such as often accompanies island isolation had caused the bird's huge size and obscured its physical resemblance to any near relatives. However, sequencing of mitochondrial DNA from dodo bones reveals that they were pigeons, closely related to the Nicobar pigeon from other islands in the Indian Ocean. Why was mitochondrial DNA suited to the study of this extinct species?

22. Cytoplasmic male sterility (CMS) in plants has been exploited to produce hybrid seeds (see Experimental Insight 17.1). Specific CMS alleles in the mitochondrial genome can be suppressed by specific dominant alleles in the nuclear genome, called *Restorer of fertility* alleles, *RF*. Consider the following cross:

    ♀ CMS 1*Rf1/Rf1 rf2/rf2* × ♂ CMS2 *rf1/rf1 Rf2/Rf2*

    What genotypes and phenotypes do you expect in the F_1? If some of the F_1 plants are male fertile, what genotypes and phenotypes do you expect in the F_2?

23. Wolves and coyotes can interbreed in captivity; and now, because of changes in their habitat distribution, they may have the opportunity to interbreed in the wild. To examine this possibility, mitochondrial DNA from wolf and coyote populations throughout North America—including habitats where the two species both reside—was analyzed, and a phylogenetic tree was constructed from the resulting data (see Section 1.4 for details on how this is accomplished). Sequence from a jackal was used as an outgroup and a sequence from a domestic dog was included, demonstrating wolves as the origin of domestic dogs.

    What do you conclude about the possibility that interspecific hybridization occurred between wolves and coyotes on the basis of this phylogenetic tree?

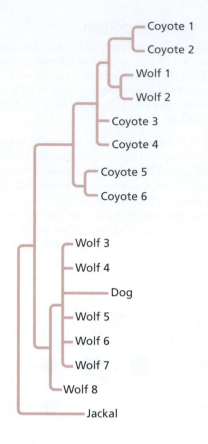

24. Considering the phylogenetic assignment of *Plasmodium falciparum*, the malarial parasite, to the phylum Apicomplexa (see Figure 17.17), what might you speculate as to whether the parasite is susceptible to aminoglycoside antibiotics?

Collaboration and Discussion

For answers to selected even-numbered problems, see Appendix: Answers.

25. *Elysia chlorotica* is a sea slug that acquires chloroplasts by consuming an algal food source, *Vaucheria litorea*. The ingested chloroplasts are sequestered in the sea slug's digestive epithelium, where they actively photosynthesize for months after ingestion. In the algae, the algal nuclear genome encodes more than 90% but not all of the proteins required for chloroplast metabolism. Thus it is suspected that the sea slug actively maintains ingested chloroplasts, supplying them with photosynthetic proteins encoded in the sea slug genome. How would you determine whether the sea slug has acquired photosynthetic genes by horizontal gene transfer from its algal food source? Discuss the steps required, and their plausibility, for heritable endosymbiosis to eventuate.

26. Most large protein complexes in mitochondria and chloroplasts are composed both of proteins encoded in the organelle genome and proteins encoded in the nuclear genome. What complexities does this introduce for gene

regulation (i.e., for ensuring that the appropriate relative numbers of the proteins in a complex are produced)?

27. As described in this chapter, mothers will pass on a mitochondrial defect to their offspring. In a type of gene therapy, one approach to circumvent this problem is to have two different maternal contributions, with the nucleus of the female with the defective mitochondria being placed in an enucleated egg derived from a female with normal mitochondria. After fertilization, the resulting offspring would have three parental sources of DNA—with nuclear DNA derived from a mother and a father, and mitochondrial DNA derived from another "mother." Recently, children with this genetic makeup have been born, but the elimination of defective mitochondria is not complete, with the amount of defective mitochondria derived from the defective mother ranging from 0 to 9%. Discuss potential complications resulting from such a mixture of genomes.

Developmental Genetics

18

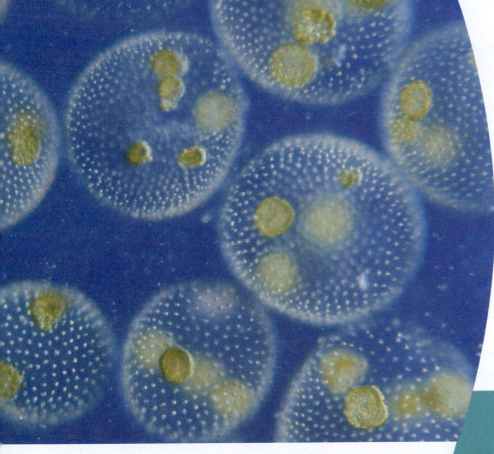

CHAPTER OUTLINE

18.1 Development Is the Building of a Multicellular Organism

18.2 *Drosophila* Development Is a Paradigm for Animal Development

18.3 Cellular Interactions Specify Cell Fate

18.4 "Evolution Behaves Like a Tinkerer"

18.5 Plants Represent an Independent Experiment in Multicellular Evolution

Multicellularity has evolved multiple times within the eukaryotes, as exemplified by *Volvox*, a chlorophyte green alga and member of a multicellular lineage independent of land plants and animals. In *Volvox*, the outer cells are somatic while the germ cells will be derived from the inner cells.

The development of a multicellular organism from a single fertilized egg cell is one of the wonders of evolution. Typically, the fertilized egg undergoes an initial mitotic division to produce two genetically identical daughter cells. Those two cells divide to produce four identical cells, which divide to produce eight cells, and so on. Yet, while all cells in the growing embryo continue to carry the same genetic information, many of them acquire different identities as the embryo develops different body parts, organs, and tissues. This development is a genetically programmed process, occurring in the same way in all members of a species. Different species exhibit both similarities and differences in development,

ESSENTIAL IDEAS

- Genes encoding transcription factors or signaling molecules direct the formation of specialized cell types.

- *Drosophila* embryos are subdivided into segments with unique identities by the sequential action of batteries of transcription factors.

- *Hox* genes specify the identity of body segments of *Drosophila* and are largely conserved throughout metazoans.

- Cells signal to either induce or inhibit neighboring cells from adopting particular developmental pathways.

- Morphological evolution can be the result of changes in gene expression patterns of a common genetic toolkit.

- Plant developmental genetics shares similarities with that of animals despite multicellularity evolving independently.

the former because of shared evolutionary ancestry and the latter because of species-specific adaptations.

Geneticists rely on defects in development to reveal the mechanisms of normal development. As early as 1790, the German scientist and philosopher Johann Wolfgang von Goethe recognized the potential of this approach:

> From our acquaintance with . . . abnormal metamorphosis, we are enabled to unveil the secrets that normal metamorphosis conceals from us, and to see distinctly what, from the regular course of development, we can only infer.

Even so, the connections between developmental abnormalities, gene mutations, and the mechanisms that control normal development could not be understood in any detail until scientists began to apply the basic principles of genetics to the study of development. This process began around 1900, when the young embryologist Thomas Hunt Morgan decided to shift his research to focus on the nascent field of genetics, using the fruit fly *Drosophila* as his experimental organism. Although Morgan never returned to the study of embryology, his students and his students' students blazed new trails by exploiting *Drosophila* genetics to illuminate many of the secrets of development in all metazoans (multicellular animals) and in plants as well.

In this chapter, we discuss the genetic processes that control development in complex multicellular organisms and the experimental approaches that led to their discovery.

18.1 Development Is the Building of a Multicellular Organism

An animal begins its life as a single cell, the zygote. All the cell types, each characterized by a specific gene expression pattern, of the adult animal ultimately are derived from the zygote. The key to understanding the molecular genetic basis of development is to understand how different patterns of gene expression are established and maintained as cells differentiate and specialize.

In 1915, Calvin Bridges (a student of Thomas Hunt Morgan) identified a *Drosophila* mutation in which the

small hind wings, the halteres, developed into structures resembling the forewings (**Figure 18.1a**). Mutations in which an apparently normal organ or body part develops in the wrong place are called **homeotic mutations** (from the Greek *homeos*, meaning "the same" or "similar"), and they have been central to the progress geneticists have made in understanding how complex organisms develop and evolve. Ed Lewis (a student of Morgan's student Alfred Sturtevant) later identified the *bithorax* complex of genes as being responsible for the homeotic mutation observed by Bridges. As we discuss in this chapter, mutations in *bithorax* genes change the developmental program of a portion of the fruit-fly body, resulting in the transformation of the halteres into a second set of forewings. Another example is the dominant *Antennapedia* mutation, in which relatively normal fly legs develop in the positions that should be occupied by the antennae (**Figure 18.1b**). To understand the cascades of events responsible for such developments, we must first examine the phenomenon of cell differentiation and pattern formation.

(a) In a *bithorax* mutation, halteres seen in wild-type *Drosophila* (left) develop instead into a second set of wings (right).

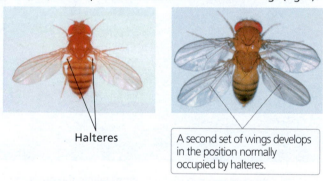

Halteres

A second set of wings develops in the position normally occupied by halteres.

(b) In an *Antennapedia* mutation, antennae in wild-type *Drosophila* (left) develop instead into legs (right).

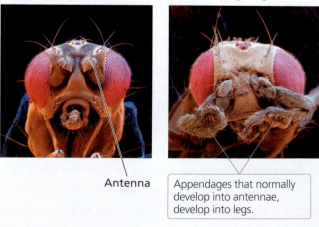

Antenna

Appendages that normally develop into antennae, develop into legs.

Figure 18.1 Inappropriate positions of organs and body structures in homeotic mutants.

Q What is the unique attribute of homeotic mutations?

Cell Differentiation

In an animal, fertilization of a haploid egg cell by a haploid sperm cell forms a single-celled diploid zygote, which undergoes several mitotic divisions to form a small cluster of embryonic cells that are genetically identical. These embryonic cells are **totipotent**, which means they have the potential to differentiate into any tissue or cell type the animal can produce. In vertebrates, totipotent cells of early embryos are called **embryonic stem cells**. In totipotent cells, all genes have the potential to be expressed given the appropriate cues. As development proceeds, however, cells become **differentiated**, taking on different morphologies and undertaking different physiological activities.

Differentiation is characterized by changes in patterns of gene expression that progressively limit which genes continue to be expressed by each cell type. At a certain stage in development, cells retain the potential to give rise to many different types of descendants, but not to all types—at this stage, the cells are said to be **pluripotent**. As development progresses further, however, most cells ultimately become specialized: These fully differentiated and specialized cells express only a subset of genes in the genome, and each cell type has its own characteristic pattern of gene expression. Thus development is a progressive process during which totipotent cells differentiate into specialized cell types through a series of genetically controlled steps that place ever more restrictive limits on their developmental potential.

Although most cells of adult animals are fully differentiated and locked into a specific cell fate, there are some exceptions. In our bodies, various types of pluripotent stem cells—such as muscle, epidermal, epithelial, and hematopoietic (blood) cells—retain the capacity to develop into a range of further-specialized cells to replenish cells that are lost.

Pattern Formation

How do genetically identical cells acquire different fates? Two mechanisms have been identified: Cells can inherit some definitive molecule that specifies cell fate, or the fate of cells can be determined by their interaction with neighboring cells through the action of signaling molecules. Inheritance of a fate-determining molecule depends on the identity of progenitor cells, whereas development through the influence of neighboring cells depends on the identity of those neighbors.

The term *pattern formation* describes the intricately interacting events that organize differentiating cells in the developing embryo to establish the three body-plan axes of many mature organisms: anterior–posterior, dorsal–ventral, and left–right (**Figure 18.2**). Cells have various ways of "knowing" their locations with regard to these axes. The combination of internal and external signals that a cell perceives during development provides information on the cell's location within an organism and its appropriate course of differentiation.

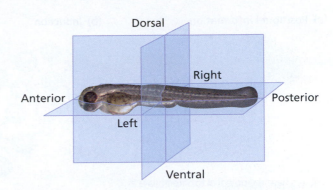

Figure 18.2 **The three embryonic axes of a zebrafish.**

To understand the role that the **positional information** represented by these signals plays in development, consider the French flag, which has a simple pattern of three vertical stripes in the order blue, white, and red, along a single (anterior–posterior) axis (**Figure 18.3a**). Although French flags may come in various sizes, the proportions of the stripes within each flag remain generally constant, dividing the flag into thirds. Imagine the entire flag to consist of cells descended from a single parent cell. How do daughter cells know whether they are to differentiate as blue, white, or red?

The cells could interpret their position by one or more of various mechanisms, but the simplest to envision is based on the concentration gradient of a molecule that is highly concentrated at one end of the embryonic flag and much less concentrated at the opposite end. The position of each cell on the flag's anterior–posterior axis is defined by the concentration of this molecule, in which threshold values define boundaries between discrete fates: Above a certain concentration, the result is blue cell identity; below this threshold concentration, white cells develop; and below an even lower threshold, red cells develop. Substances whose presence in different concentrations directs developmental fates are referred to as **morphogens**. If activation or repression of gene expression is dependent upon threshold concentrations of a morphogen (e.g., concentrations above which a gene is active and below which a gene is inactive), discrete boundaries of gene expression can be established.

Once a cell has acquired a specific identity, it may induce its neighbors to acquire a certain fate; this process is termed **induction**. A classic case of induction was first noted more than a century ago, when transplantation of cells from one region of a developing frog embryo to another region of a second embryo induced the surrounding cells to form a second body axis (**Figure 18.3b**). The region from which the transplanted cells were derived was called the **organizer** because the cells of that region possess the ability to organize cells in the surrounding tissue. Alternatively, a cell that acquires a specific fate may produce an inhibitory substance that prevents its neighbors from acquiring a certain fate, and this process is called **inhibition** (**Figure 18.3c**). Inhibition can be used to produce patterns of regularly spaced cells of a particular fate within a field of cells that would otherwise

(a) Positional information　　　**(b) Induction**　　　**(c) Inhibition**

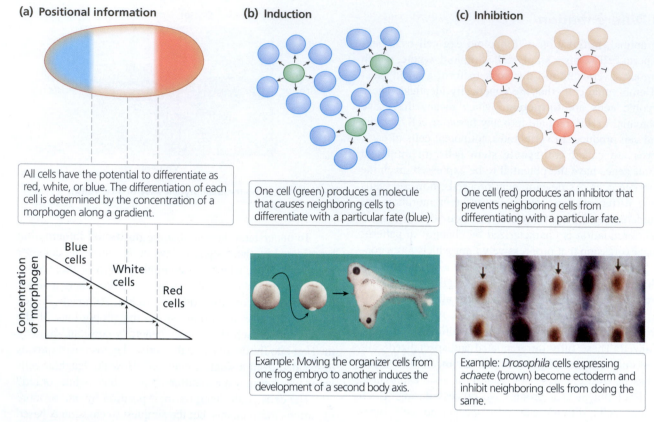

All cells have the potential to differentiate as red, white, or blue. The differentiation of each cell is determined by the concentration of a morphogen along a gradient.

One cell (green) produces a molecule that causes neighboring cells to differentiate with a particular fate (blue).

One cell (red) produces an inhibitor that prevents neighboring cells from differentiating with a particular fate.

Example: Moving the organizer cells from one frog embryo to another induces the development of a second body axis.

Example: *Drosophila* cells expressing *achaete* (brown) become ectoderm and inhibit neighboring cells from doing the same.

Figure 18.3 Mechanisms of differentiation.

all differentiate in the same manner, such as in the example of *Drosophila* shown in Figure 18.3c. Examples of tissues with regular spacing include many epidermal features, such as bristles, feathers, hairs, and scales.

The developmental histories of cells can affect how the cells respond to cues from their neighbors. For example, for a cell to be able to respond to an inductive or inhibitory signal from neighboring cells, it must express the appropriate receptor. In addition, cells able to respond to a signal may behave differently depending on what other factors are present in the cell. When a cell divides, the daughter cells usually inherit the same set of transcription factors and chromatin states that existed in the cell they were derived from (the importance of chromatin states is discussed in Section 18.2). However, occasional asymmetric cell divisions in which the two daughter cells inherit different cellular constituents and acquire different fates underlie developmental patterning events in some species.

Positional information, induction, inhibition, and asymmetric cell divisions are common processes directing cell differentiation and pattern formation in multicellular organisms. When employed sequentially and reiteratively during embryogenesis, these processes enable a single-celled zygote to develop into a complex organism having a multitude of cell types. Each cell division in the embryo brings about changes in the relative positional relationships between the cells, so new opportunities for cell–cell communication are constantly created. In keeping with the importance of positional information, induction, and inhibition in development, most genes identified as having prominent roles in developmental processes encode proteins that act as either transcription factors or signaling molecules.

18.2 *Drosophila* Development Is a Paradigm for Animal Development

Discoveries about the developmental processes of *Drosophila* have made it one of the best-understood animals on the planet. These insights have in turn profoundly influenced how geneticists perceive the development and evolution of all other animals, ourselves included. For their work in unraveling some of the mechanisms underlying pattern formation in *Drosophila*, Edward B. Lewis, Christiane Nüsslein-Volhard, and Eric Wieschaus were awarded the Nobel Prize in Physiology or Medicine in 1995.

One of the reasons that *Drosophila* is an ideal genetic experimental organism is its short, 9-day life cycle (**Figure 18.4a**). Embryogenesis spans the first 24 hours of *Drosophila* development, commencing with the deposition of a fertilized egg that immediately begins a rapid series of genetically controlled changes (**Figure 18.4b**). After embryogenesis, development progresses through three distinct larval stages, called instars. Each instar stage is marked

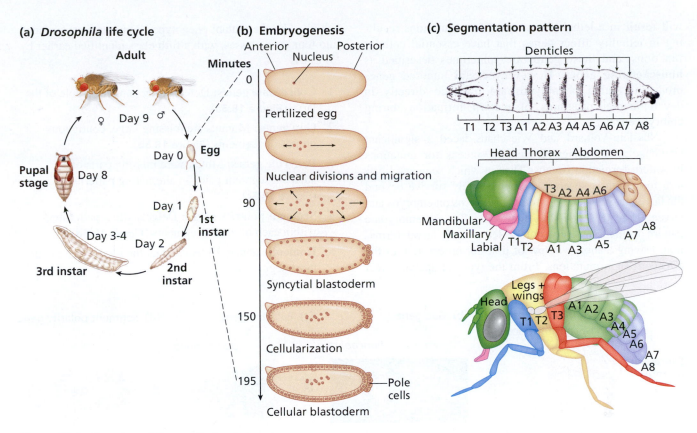

Figure 18.4 Overview of *Drosophila* development.

🔴 **At what time during *Drosophila* development do you expect genes directing the body plan to be active?**

by progressive development of tissues and structures that will form the adult fly. Following the third instar stage, the larva forms a pupa in which metamorphosis will take place. At the conclusion of pupation a fully formed adult fruit fly emerges, ready to begin the cycle anew.

The *Drosophila* egg has conspicuous anterior–posterior and dorsal–ventral polarities that are acquired during its production in the female fly. In contrast to early development in many other species, early embryonic development in *Drosophila* proceeds by nuclear division without division of cytoplasm. Rather than forming blastomeres, as in mammalian development, this process forms a **syncytium**, a multinucleate cell in which the nuclei are not separated by cell membranes (see Figure 18.4b). The fertilized egg undergoes nine mitotic nuclear divisions, after which the nuclei migrate to the periphery of the embryo. At this time, about 10 pole cells, from which the germ line will be derived, are set aside at the posterior end of the embryo. The somatic cells undergo another four rounds of mitotic divisions at the periphery, forming a **syncytial blastoderm** containing about 6000 nuclei. By about 3 hours after egg laying, cellularization of the syncytium occurs by the assembly of cell membranes that separate nuclei into individual cells, thus forming a **cellular blastoderm**.

During the syncytial blastoderm and cellularization stages, cells become progressively restricted in their developmental potential. This can be demonstrated experimentally

by transplanting cellular blastoderm cells from one embryo into another. Blastoderm cells implanted into an equivalent region of a host embryo are incorporated normally into host structures, but those transplanted into different regions will develop autonomously into tissues reflecting the original position of the cells in the donor embryo. Thus, at the cellular blastoderm stage, cells have already become committed to differentiate into particular tissues.

Drosophila is typical of insects in the segmentation pattern of its adult body. Eight abdominal and three thoracic segments are easily distinguished (**Figure 18.4c**). The head consists of at least three distinct developmental segments. The segments of the insect body are first visible during embryogenesis, where they are indicated by the pattern of denticles (small hooks for gripping during larval movement) on the ventral epidermis. The body plan established during embryogenesis determines the organization of tissues and organs in the adult fly.

The Developmental Toolkit of *Drosophila*

Large-scale genetic screens (see Section 14.1) were commenced by Christiane Nüsslein-Volhard, Eric Wieschaus, and others in the late 1970s and early 1980s to identify and describe the function of genes directing pattern formation in *Drosophila* embryos. It is estimated that mutations in about 5000 of the 14,000 genes in *Drosophila* will result in a lethal phenotype. Most mutations resulting in lethality affect genes that have essential cellular functions, and these genes are sometimes described as **housekeeping genes**. However, several hundred genes producing lethal phenotypes are involved directly in developmental programs of pattern formation during embryogenesis.

Nüsslein-Volhard and Wieschaus faced a significant challenge when designing genetic screens for mutations in pattern formation because flies in which segmental pattern formation is severely disrupted rarely survive beyond the larval stage. Their solution was to focus on embryos and larvae. They reasoned that mutations affecting embryonic pattern formation would not be lethal until larval formation, leaving a short window of time for observation of the effects of such mutations. From the types of spatial defect

exhibited by the mutant phenotypes, mutants were grouped into four gene classes, with a fifth class identified earlier by Ed Lewis:

1. **Coordinate genes:** Defects affect an entire pole of the larva (**Figure 18.5a**).

2. **Gap genes:** Mutants are missing large, contiguous groups of segments (**Figure 18.5b**).

3. **Pair-rule genes:** Mutants are missing parts of adjacent segment pairs, in alternating patterns (**Figure 18.5c**).

4. **Segment polarity genes:** Defects affect patterning within each of the 14 segments (**Figure 18.5d**).

5. **Homeotic genes:** Defects affect the identity of one or more segments.

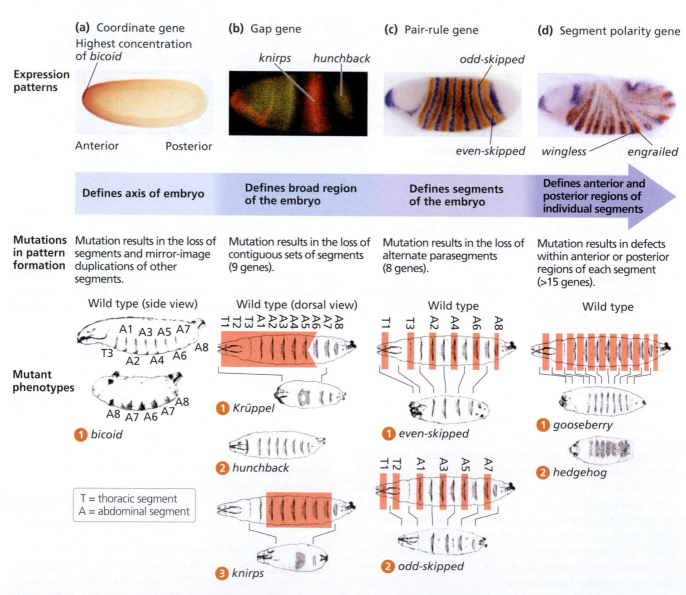

Figure 18.5 Mutations causing defects in pattern formation in *Drosophila*. A fifth class of mutations, homeotic gene mutations, is represented in Figure 18.10.

These five gene classes are expressed sequentially during embryogenesis: The coordinate genes act first, followed by gap genes, pair-rule genes, segment polarity genes, and finally homeotic genes. The cascade of gene expression subdivides the embryo in successive steps, first into broad regions and then into progressively smaller domains, and each of the 14 resulting segments acquires a specific identity. The patterns of mRNA and protein expression of each gene correspond, both in space and in time, to its mutant phenotype (see Figure 18.5). For example, expression of the gap gene *knirps* spans a contiguous embryonic domain that is destined to become abdominal segments. These abdominal segments are missing in *knirps* mutants, as is evident in the early larva (see Figure 18.5b).

Expression of the pair-rule genes follows that of gap genes and each is expressed in 7 stripes in the embryo. Curiously, the stripes of gene expression of some pair-rule genes do not correspond to the segments of the adult insect, but rather straddle the boundaries between segments, thus occupying the posterior part of one segment and the anterior part of its neighbor. The domains of gene expression controlled by these pair-rule genes are therefore called **parasegments**. In contrast, expression of the segment polarity genes occurs in 14 polar stripes (i.e., each stripe has anterior and posterior "poles") that do correspond to the segments of the embryo. The homeotic genes are the last to be expressed and affect broad domains of contiguous parasegments along the anterior–posterior axis. The anterior expression boundaries of the homeotic genes correspond to parasegment boundaries defined by the pair-rule genes. Thus, the sequential activation of different classes of genes during early development is reflected in the sequential subdivision of the organism, from a single-celled zygote into a segmented embryo.

When the expression pattern of a gene in a wild-type embryo corresponds precisely to the cell fates that are disrupted when the gene is mutated, the activity of the gene is said to be cell autonomous. A gene whose action is cell autonomous affects only the cells in which the gene is transcribed and expressed. Four of the five classes of genes act largely cell autonomously, an observation consistent with the identity of these genes as transcription factors. The exception is the segment polarity class of genes, which often encode signaling molecules that can act nonautonomously, that is, in cells other than where the gene is expressed. In the following sections, we examine how the embryo is successively subdivided by the activity of these sets of genes.

Maternal Effects on Pattern Formation

In animals, the mother often supplies critical gene products to the egg that subsequently direct embryo development. These genes are called **maternal effect genes**. Note that maternal effects are different from maternal inheritance (introduced in Chapter 17), in that maternal effects entail the maternal deposition of protein or mRNA in the

egg cell, whereas maternal inheritance refers to maternal transmission of genetic material (e.g., organelle genomes).

How can the maternal effect genes that influence development be identified in mutant screens, given that for these genes, the embryonic phenotype is determined by the genotype of the mother rather than that of the embryo? An answer becomes apparent when we compare the inheritance patterns observed with maternal effect genes against those observed with **zygotic genes**, genes that are active only in the zygote or embryo. For zygotic genes, *the genotype of the embryo determines the phenotype*. The following cross illustrates this principle for an autosomal recessive mutation (*m*):

Inheritance Pattern with Zygotic Genes

Parents	Offspring	Phenotype
m/+ × m/+	m/+, +/+	Normal (3)
	m/m	Mutant (1)

With maternal effect genes, where *the genotype of the mother determines the phenotype of the zygote*, the same cross as above, involving an autosomal recessive mutation (*m*), would give the following outcomes:

Inheritance Pattern with Maternal Effect Genes

Parents (female × male)	Offspring	Phenotype
m/+ × m/+	m/m, m/+, +/+	All normal
m/+ × m/m	m/m, m/+	All normal
m/m × +/+ or m/+ or m/m	m/m, m/+	All mutant

These divergent patterns allow discrimination between maternal effect genes and zygotic genes. Crosses can be performed to determine whether the genes are active maternally, zygotically, or both. When such crosses were performed to test the five classes of pattern formation mutants described above, the coordinate genes were found to be maternally active; their expression *in the mother* rather than in the embryo provides positional information to the egg. Most gap genes are active zygotically, but at least one, *hunchback*, also exhibits maternal activity. All pair-rule, segment polarity, and homeotic genes act strictly zygotically. These findings make sense given the developmental stage at which the different classes of gene are active and the observation that zygotic gene expression commences only in the syncytial blastoderm stage of embryogenesis.

Coordinate Gene Patterning of the Anterior–Posterior Axis

The genetic control of development is essentially a process of regulating gene expression in three-dimensional space over time. It is not surprising, then, that most of the early-acting genes establishing the anterior–posterior axis of *Drosophila* encode transcription factors. The interaction of transcription factors with cis-acting regulatory elements of target genes provides spatial control of gene expression.

This spatial control is coordinated over time by continual inputs from neighboring cells. In this section, we describe examples of the spatial and temporal regulation of gene expression that results in subdivision of a developing *Drosophila* embryo into its characteristic segments.

The coordinate gene *bicoid* plays a major role in the establishment of the anterior–posterior axis in *Drosophila*. Loss-of-function *bicoid* alleles result in a loss of anterior portions of the embryo; the anterior portions are replaced instead by a mirror-image duplication of posterior regions (**Figure 18.6a**). *Bicoid* mRNA is anchored to the anterior region of the egg during oogenesis in the mother (**Figure 18.6b**). After translation, the resulting protein (Bicoid) diffuses from its site of synthesis at the anterior pole of the embryo throughout the syncytial embryo, owing to the absence of cell membranes to impede protein diffusion. The diffusion results in a gradient of Bicoid in which the highest concentration is at the anterior end and very little Bicoid is detected beyond the middle of the embryo.

Cytoplasmic transplantation experiments elegantly demonstrate that Bicoid specifies anterior identity. Anterior cytoplasm extracted from a wild-type embryo and then injected into a *bicoid* mutant embryo causes anterior structures to develop at the site of injection (see Figure 18.6a, bottom panel). When the *bicoid* gene was cloned, similar experiments were carried out with purified *bicoid* mRNA, which produced the same result. These findings indicate that the concentration gradient of Bicoid provides positional information along the anterior–posterior axis of the embryo, presumably by differentially regulating several genes that respond to different concentrations of Bicoid. Among the known zygotic genes whose transcription is directly regulated by Bicoid is the gap gene *hunchback*.

Surprisingly, examination of the distribution of *hunchback* mRNA revealed that *hunchback* is also maternally expressed and that its maternal (mRNA) expression is uniform throughout the egg (**Figure 18.7a**). The hunchback protein (Hunchback), on the other hand, is found only at the anterior end of the early embryo, implying that posterior *hunchback* mRNA is not translated. This seeming contradiction was explained by the discovery of another maternally expressed coordinate gene, *nanos*. The posterior end of the embryo is patterned by *nanos*, whose protein forms a gradient with the highest concentration at the posterior end. Rather than encoding a transcription factor, *nanos* encodes a protein that represses translation of *hunchback* mRNA. Thus, Hunchback is restricted to the anterior end of the embryo by posterior translational repression of maternal *hunchback* mRNA. In addition, zygotic *hunchback* expression in the anterior end is transcriptionally activated by anteriorly localized Bicoid.

Patterning of the posterior end of the embryo is governed by similar interactions. In addition to acting as a transcription factor, Bicoid acts as a translational repressor of the maternally supplied *caudal* mRNA, which is uniformly distributed throughout the egg. Translational repression of *caudal* mRNA by the anterior gradient of Bicoid results in a posterior gradient of *caudal* protein (Caudal). The end result is an embryo with graded distributions of three transcription factors: Bicoid and Hunchback, in which the highest concentration is at the anterior end; and Caudal, in which the highest concentration is at the posterior end. The relative concentrations of these three proteins provide positional information along the length of the embryo, which is interpreted by the subsequently acting gap genes.

Domains of Gap Gene Expression

The broad gradients of maternally supplied coordinate gene products are transformed into domains of gap gene expression with discrete boundaries. This occurs through a combination of cooperative binding of transcription factors—similar to the activation of the lambda repressor described in Chapter 12—and cross-regulatory interactions among the gap genes themselves. To begin, let's

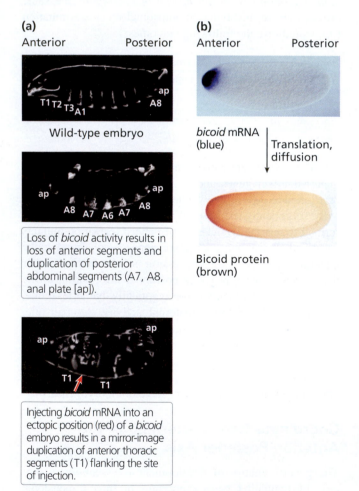

(a)

Anterior   Posterior

T1 T2 T3 A1   ap A8

Wild-type embryo

ap   ap A8 A7 A6 A7 A8

Loss of *bicoid* activity results in loss of anterior segments and duplication of posterior abdominal segments (A7, A8, anal plate [ap]).

ap   ap T1   T1

Injecting *bicoid* mRNA into an ectopic position (red) of a *bicoid* embryo results in a mirror-image duplication of anterior thoracic segments (T1) flanking the site of injection.

(b)

Anterior   Posterior

bicoid mRNA (blue) | Translation, diffusion

Bicoid protein (brown)

Figure 18.6 Maternal *bicoid* patterning of the embryo along the anterior–posterior axis.

Nanos protein is localized to the posterior terminus similar to the way that Bicoid is localized to the anterior end. Nanos acts as a translational repressor. Compare the actions of Nanos and Bicoid with that of inhibitors and inducers (defined in Figure 18.3).

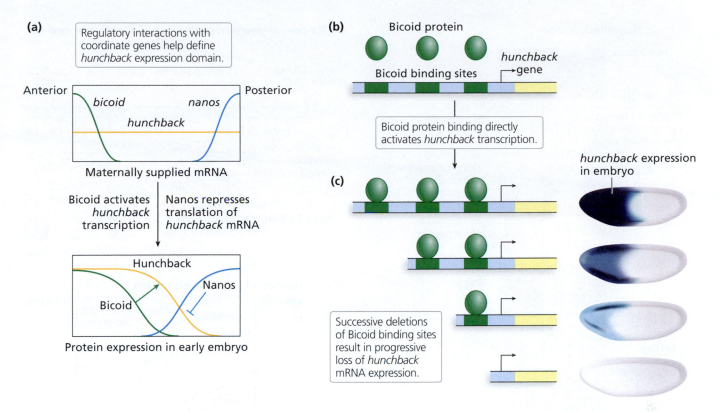

Figure 18.7 **Gap gene expression patterns are activated by coordinate genes.**

consider further how the gradual concentration gradient of Bicoid is translated into the more discrete pattern of *hunchback* mRNA expression.

As noted earlier, zygotic expression of the gap gene *hunchback* is confined to the anterior region of the embryo. Unlike Bicoid, which exhibits a gradual concentration gradient, the concentration of *hunchback* mRNA produced in the embryo declines precipitously at a particular point along the anterior–posterior axis. Transcription of *hunchback* is activated by the binding of Bicoid to cis-regulatory elements 5′ to the *hunchback* coding region (**Figure 18.7b**). In this location, there are multiple cis-acting sites to which Bicoid can bind, and these sites are bound in a cooperative manner, meaning that the binding of one Bicoid molecule to one site facilitates the binding of a second Bicoid molecule to a second nearby site, and so on. Mutation of the Bicoid binding sites alters the responsiveness of *hunchback* expression to Bicoid, and removal of all binding sites abolishes *hunchback* expression in the embryo (**Figure 18.7c**).

A threshold level of Bicoid must be present for *hunchback* expression to be activated. Consequently, *hunchback* expression occurs on one side of a threshold concentration with no expression on the other, and a sharp boundary is produced. In this manner, the gradual anterior concentration gradient of Bicoid is translated into a distinct anterior region of *hunchback* mRNA expression, which, after translation, produces a sharp gradient of Hunchback (see Figure 18.7a).

The gradient of hunchback protein is critical for the regulation of other gap genes, such as *Krüppel* (**Figure 18.8**), which is repressed by high levels of Hunchback but activated in the central region of the embryo where Bicoid levels are moderate. These interactions establish the anterior margin of *Krüppel* expression toward the posterior end of the Hunchback protein gradient. The posterior margin of *Krüppel* expression appears to be determined through negative regulation by other gap genes, *knirps* and *giant*. Similar regulatory interactions between other gap genes help establish the rest of the partially overlapping patterns of gap gene expression that subdivide the developing embryo into discrete domains.

Regulation of Pair-Rule Genes

From the domains of gap gene expression emerge narrower stripes of gene expression that represent the first manifestation of segmentation of the anterior–posterior body plan. Analysis of the regulation of the pair-rule gene *even-skipped* (*eve*) revealed that each stripe is established by independent enhancer modules of cis-acting regulatory sequences. Each enhancer module responds to specific combinations of gap genes (**Figure 18.9a**). Thus, the formation of stripes of gene expression is the result of combinatorial control of gene expression through multiple cis-acting regulatory elements of the pair-rule genes.

Stripe 2 of *eve* provides an example of modularity in gene regulation. Gene expression within stripe 2 is controlled

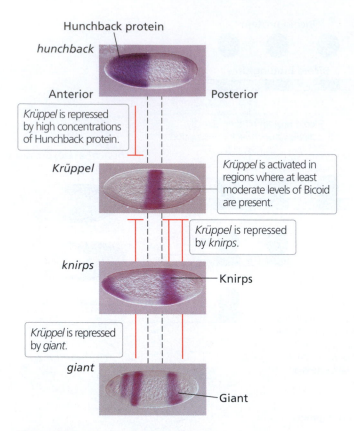

Hunchback protein

hunchback

Anterior   Posterior

Krüppel is repressed by high concentrations of Hunchback protein.

Krüppel

Krüppel is activated in regions where at least moderate levels of Bicoid are present.

Krüppel is repressed by *knirps*.

knirps

Knirps

Krüppel is repressed by *giant*.

giant

Giant

Figure 18.8 Cross-regulatory interactions among gap genes, defining their expression patterns.

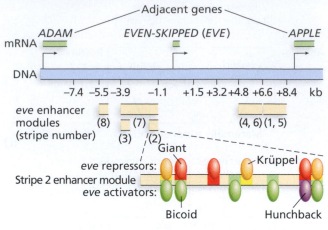

(a) The pair-rule gene *even-skipped* (*eve*) and its enhancer modules

Adjacent genes

ADAM   *EVEN-SKIPPED (EVE)*   *APPLE*

mRNA

DNA

−7.4 −5.5 −3.9   −1.1   +1.5 +3.2 +4.8 +6.6 +8.4   kb

eve enhancer modules (stripe number)

(8) (7) (3) (2)   (4, 6) (1, 5)

Giant   Krüppel

eve repressors:

Stripe 2 enhancer module

eve activators:

Bicoid   Hunchback

(b) Distribution of gap gene expression

Anterior   Posterior

hunchback   Position of 2nd stripe relative to gap gene expression
giant

Krüppel

bicoid

Gap expression

Parasegment   1   2   3   4   5   6

(c) Occupancy of regulatory sites on *eve* stripe 2 enhancer module in different parasegments

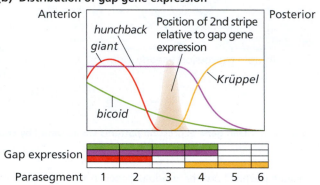

In parasegment 3 (*eve* stripe 2)

Bicoid   Hunchback

In parasegment 3, the concentration of the activators Bicoid and Hunchback is high, while the concentration of repressors Krüppel and Giant is low, causing activation of *eve* in stripe 2.

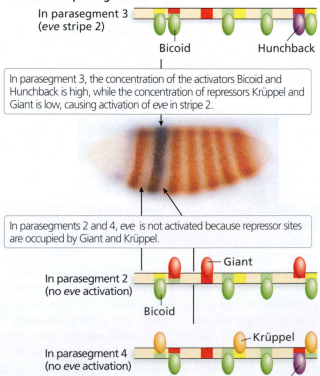

In parasegments 2 and 4, *eve* is not activated because repressor sites are occupied by Giant and Krüppel.

Giant

In parasegment 2 (no *eve* activation)

Bicoid

Krüppel

In parasegment 4 (no *eve* activation)

Hunchback

by a cis-regulatory element—the stripe 2 enhancer module—located about 1700 to 1000 bp upstream of the transcription initiation site of *eve* (see Figure 18.9a). When this regulatory element is isolated and used to drive a reporter gene (see Section 14.4) in transgenic *Drosophila* embryos, expression is observed only in stripe 2, indicating that these regulatory sequences are sufficient for stripe 2 expression. Detailed sequence analysis of this module identified binding sites for the gap proteins Hunchback, Krüppel, and Giant, as well as binding sites for Bicoid. Mutational analysis of different combinations of binding sites demonstrates that both Hunchback and Bicoid act as activators of *even-skipped* stripe 2 gene expression, whereas both Giant and Krüppel act as repressors.

Stripe 2 lies entirely within the *hunchback* expression domain of the embryo and is flanked on the anterior side by the *giant* expression domain and on the posterior side by the *Krüppel* expression domain (**Figure 18.9b**). It contains an intermediate level of Bicoid remaining from the maternally

Figure 18.9 Stripes of gene expression, established by combinatorial coordinate and gap gene activities.

Q Describe how the *eve* stripe 2 enhancer module activates expression exclusively in parasegment 3.

established gradient. Thus the position of *eve* stripe 2 along the anterior–posterior axis is a zone with a high concentration of Hunchback, low concentrations of Giant and Krüppel, and an intermediate concentration of Bicoid. Only in parasegment 3, which is the location of stripe 2, are both positive regulators present and both negative regulators absent (**Figure 18.9c**). This combination of gap and coordinate protein concentrations does not occur anywhere else along the axis of the embryo and uniquely defines the *eve* stripe 2 position. The integration of positive and negative regulators results in the precise limiting of *even-skipped* stripe 2 to a region only a few cells in width along the anterior–posterior axis. Similar combinatorial mechanisms are thought to control the expression patterns of all of the pair-rule and segment polarity genes.

The discovery that in multicellular organisms *the control of gene expression is modular* provided important insight into the evolution of organisms. Modularity of gene regulation allows changes in specific domains of expression without catastrophic disruption of global expression patterns.

Specification of Parasegments by *Hox* Genes

Having explored the mechanisms by which gap and pair-rule genes successively subdivide the *Drosophila* embryo into segments and parasegments, we can now consider how each segment acquires a unique identity through the action of the homeotic genes. Once again, the key discoveries were made through the study of mutations, pioneered by Edward B. Lewis starting in the 1950s.

As we saw at the beginning of the chapter, a remarkable aspect of homeotic mutant phenotypes is the development of relatively normal structures in inappropriate positions. Another general feature of homeotic mutations is that they cause identity transformations of serially repeated structures. Legs, for example, are appendages that are normally limited to the three thoracic segments in *Drosophila*, whereas antennae are appendages that normally develop only on the third cephalic (head) segment. In the case of *Antennapedia* mutants, however, a leg appears in a segment ordinarily reserved for an antenna (see Figure 18.1), suggesting that *Antennapedia* normally specifies the identity of one or more of the thoracic segments. Analyses of homeotic genes in *Drosophila* demonstrate that in fact they act in combination to specify the identity of each of the 14 body segments.

The homeotic genes of animals are also remarkable for being clustered in gene complexes. In *Drosophila* there are two homeotic clusters on the third chromosome: the *Antennapedia* **complex**, consisting of five genes, and the *bithorax* **complex**, consisting of three genes. In other organisms, the homeotic genes are usually in a single cluster. Amazingly, the order of the genes within the complexes reflects the positions along the anterior–posterior axis that are influenced by each gene (**Figure 18.10**).

The cloning of the homeotic genes revealed another surprise: All eight genes encode closely related proteins, suggesting that all members of the complex were derived from a common ancestor through a series of gene duplications. All of the genes share a conserved sequence of DNA of 180 nucleotides that was dubbed the **homeobox**, which encodes a 60–amino acid protein domain, termed the **homeodomain**, with a helix-turn-helix motif. Such motifs had previously been recognized in bacterial and phage transcription factors, such as the Lac repressor and the lambda repressor proteins. They function to bind cis-regulatory DNA sequences of target genes. Since the homeobox genes of the *Antennapedia* and *bithorax* complexes share both molecular and functional similarity as well as having a common evolutionary origin, they are known collectively as *Hox* **genes**.

The patterns of *Hox* gene expression correlate with the regions affected in the corresponding mutants. Each of the *Hox* genes has a well-defined anterior boundary of expression but in most cases a more diffuse boundary on the posterior end, resulting in overlapping domains of *Hox* gene expression. The anterior boundaries of *Hox* gene expression do not correspond to segmental boundaries but rather to boundaries of segment polarity gene expression. Thus, *Hox* gene expression is out of register with the groups of cells that give rise to segments in the adult fly and instead marks the boundaries of parasegments.

Because of the parasegmental pattern of *Hox* gene expression, mutations of those genes affect cellular identity in a parasegmental manner. Each parasegment of the embryo expresses a unique combination of *Hox* gene products, giving each parasegment a specific identity. The activation of *Hox* genes is controlled by the earlier-acting gap and pair-rule genes in a combinatorial manner similar to that described for the activation of pair-rule genes by the gap and coordinate genes. In the absence of all *Hox* gene activity, segments are formed, but they all differentiate into a "default" state that resembles a head segment. This outcome indicates that *Hox* genes are not required for the formation of the segments but rather for the specification of their identity.

The *Antennapedia* Complex The *Antennapedia* complex consists of five *Hox* genes—*labial, Deformed, Sex combs reduced, proboscipedia (Pb)*, and *Antennapedia*—that act in combination to specify the cephalic and thoracic parasegments (see Figure 18.10c). The original *Antennapedia* mutant (see Figure 18.1) was dominant and was found to be the result of a gain-of-function allele (see Section 4.1). The *Antennapedia* gene is normally expressed only in parasegments 4 and 5 (see Figure 18.10c), which give rise to thoracic segments that each produce a pair of legs. In flies carrying the dominant *Antennapedia* mutation, however,

(a) Adult body segments

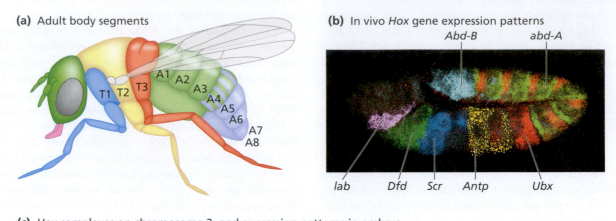

(b) In vivo *Hox* gene expression patterns

(c) *Hox* complexes on chromosome 3, and expression patterns in embryo

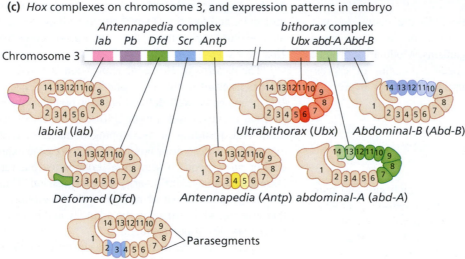

Figure 18.10 *Hox* genes of the *Antennapedia* and *bithorax* complexes.

Describe how the *Hox* gene products give each segment a unique identity.

Antennapedia is expressed ectopically—meaning it is expressed at an inappropriate time or place or both. One of the normal roles of *Antennapedia* expression in the thoracic segments is to promote the differentiation of thoracic appendages into legs. When expressed ectopically in the third head segment, *Antennapedia* inappropriately promotes differentiation of head appendages (antennae) into legs instead.

The *bithorax* Complex In contrast to *Antennapedia* mutations, which affect anterior body segments, mutations in the three genes of the *bithorax* complex—*Ultrabithorax*, *abdominal-A*, and *Abdominal-B*—affect more-posterior segments (**Figure 18.11a**). The *bithorax* complex genes are expressed in overlapping sets of thoracic and abdominal parasegments and act in combination to specify the identity of those parasegments. How do only three genes specify the identity of nine segments, one thoracic and eight abdominal? The three genes vary not only in their spatial patterns of expression but also

in expression levels between segments. Each has a sharp anterior border of expression and a more diffuse posterior boundary of expression. Thus, each segment exhibits a unique qualitative and quantitative pattern of *Hox* gene expression.

Loss of *Ultrabithorax* activity results in parasegments 5 and 6 having a combination of *Hox* gene products resembling that normally found in parasegment 4. This causes transformations of the identity of thoracic segment T3 and abdominal segment A1 into thoracic segment T2 (**Figure 18.11b**). Loss of the entire *bithorax* complex causes most abdominal segments to develop as T2, so each has legs as appendages (**Figure 18.11c**). This observation suggests that expression of *Antennapedia*, which promotes leg identity in appendages, extends posteriorly in such mutants and that genes of the *bithorax* complex normally repress posterior expression of *Antennapedia*. Such cross-regulatory interactions between *Hox* genes, whereby more posteriorly expressed *Hox* genes repress the expression of *Hox* genes normally expressed in more-anterior positions, is a common

(a) Wild type

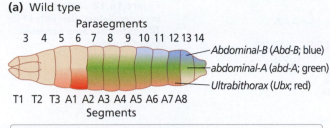

Parasegments
3 4 5 6 7 8 9 10 11 12 13 14

- Abdominal-B (*Abd-B*; blue)
- abdominal-A (*abd-A*; green)
- Ultrabithorax (*Ubx*; red)

T1 T2 T3 A1 A2 A3 A4 A5 A6 A7 A8
Segments

> Both *Ubx* and *abd-A* have a diffuse posterior boundary of expression due to negative regulatory interactions between genes.

(b) Loss of *Ubx*

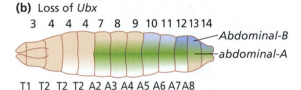

3 4 4 4 7 8 9 10 11 12 13 14

- Abdominal-B
- abdominal-A

T1 T2 T2 T2 A2 A3 A4 A5 A6 A7 A8

> T3 and A1 are incorrectly specified as T2 due to a failure to repress *Antennapedia* in these segments.

(c) Loss of all *bithorax* complex (*Ubx*, *abd-A*, and *Abd-B*)

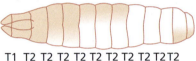

3 4 4 4 4 4 4 4 4 4 4 14

T1 T2 T2 T2 T2 T2 T2 T2 T2 T2 T2

> All segments posterior to T1 differentiate as T2 due to a failure to repress *Antennapedia* in all posterior segments.

(d) Loss of *abd-A* and *Abd-B*

3 4 5 6 6 6 6 6 6 6 6 14

- Ultrabithorax

T1 T2 T3 A1 A1 A1 A1 A1 A1 A1A1

> All abdominal segments differentiate as A1 due to failure of *abd-A* and *Abd-B* to repress *Ubx* expression in posterior segments.

(e) Loss of *Abd-B*

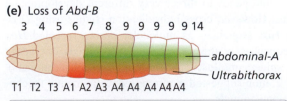

3 4 5 6 7 8 9 9 9 9 9 14

- abdominal-A
- Ultrabithorax

T1 T2 T3 A1 A2 A3 A4 A4 A4 A4A4

> *Ubx* and *abd-A* are both expressed more posteriorly due to loss of repression by *Abd-B*, leading to most posterior abdominal segments differentiating as A4.

Figure 18.11 **Cross-regulatory interactions between *bithorax* complex genes, specifying thoracic and abdominal segment fates.**

although not universal feature in the regulation of *Hox* genes (**Figure 18.11d–e**).

As you have probably noticed, there is no single *Hox* gene called *bithorax*; so what became of the original *bithorax (bx)* mutation that was isolated by Calvin Bridges? When Ed Lewis recognized that mutations such as *bithorax* could provide valuable insights into the genetic mechanisms of development, he began collecting mutations with similar but distinct phenotypic defects, some of which he called *postbithorax (pbx)*, *Contrabithorax*, *Ultrabithorax*, and *bithoraxoid (bxd)*. Each of these mutations mapped to a different position in the same chromosomal region, so that they were separable by recombination events, and double-mutant combinations could be constructed. At the time Lewis performed these studies, molecular cloning was unknown, and he assumed that each mutant he identified represented a different gene. When the *bithorax* complex was eventually cloned in 1983, however, many of the mutant phenotypes were found to result from mutations in different enhancer modules controlling the expression of a single coding region that is now called the *Ultrabithorax* gene (**Figure 18.12a**).

Mutations of the regulatory elements can be either recessive, if in an enhancer module that acts to positively regulate gene expression, or dominant, if in a silencer module that acts to negatively regulate gene expression. Whereas null loss-of-function alleles of *Ultrabithorax* result in embryo lethality, disruption of single enhancer modules results in milder defects. For example, recessive *Ultrabithorax*^bithorax mutations *(bx)* result in the transformation of the anterior part of T3 into T2, causing the anterior portion of the haltere to develop as a wing (**Figure 18.12b**). Conversely, recessive *Ultrabithorax*^postbithorax mutations *(pbx)* result in the transformation of the posterior region of T3 into T2 identity, and the posterior portion of the haltere develops as a wing. Only in the *Ultrabithorax*^bithorax *Ultrabithorax*^postbithorax double mutant is the identity of the entire T3 segment transformed into a T2 identity, causing a four-winged fly to develop (see Figure 18.1).

The cis-regulatory elements of *Ultrabithorax* span over 120 kb (see Figure 18.12a), and their modularity allows the evolution of changes in gene expression without catastrophic disruption of *Ultrabithorax* function, such as those caused by nonsense mutations within the coding region. Thus, *Ultrabithorax*^bithorax *Ultrabithorax*^postbithorax double mutants survive to adulthood because the remainder of the cis-regulatory elements controlling *Ultrabithorax* expression are intact. **Genetic Analysis 18.1** asks you to evaluate cross-regulatory interactions among *Hox* genes.

Downstream Targets of *Hox* Genes

Given that combinatorial action of the *Hox* genes specifies parasegment identity and that *Hox* genes encode transcription factors, it follows that the downstream target genes activated by the *Hox* genes must differ between segments. These *Hox* target genes have been called **realizator genes**, and their expression contributes to the characteristic

(a) *Ultrabithorax* gene

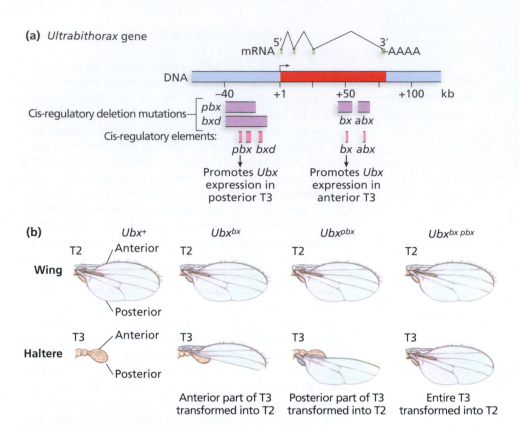

Figure 18.12 Mutations in cis-regulatory elements of *Ultrabithorax* cause homeotic transformations.

morphology of each segment. As an example, let's consider the formation of appendages on each segment.

Wild-type flies have antennae on the most-anterior head segment and have mandibles and maxillary and labial sense organs on other head segments. The three thoracic segments have legs; T2 and T3 also have wings and halteres, respectively. The eight abdominal segments lack appendages. Loss of all *Hox* activity is lethal to the embryo and causes all segments to resemble a head segment having antennae as appendages. This outcome indicates that all segments have the potential to form an appendage, and that expression of *Hox* genes can either specify the appendage identity or repress its formation.

The formation of an appendage is dependent on a gene called *Distal-less*. In wild-type *Drosophila, Distal-less* is expressed in the head and thoracic segments but not in any abdominal segments. This pattern suggests that the abdominal segment identity genes, *Ultrabithorax, abdominal-A,* and *Abdominal-B,* negatively regulate *Distal-less* expression in the abdominal segments. Loss of function of all *bithorax* complex genes results in ectopic *Distal-less* expression in all abdominal segments, along with a concomitant development of appendages (legs) on all abdominal segments. Conversely, if *Ultrabithorax* is ectopically expressed at high levels throughout the embryo, *Distal-less* is not activated in any segment and no appendages are formed. Thus, action of specific *bithorax* complex *Hox* proteins on *Distal-less* cis-regulatory sequences represses *Distal-less* gene expression in the abdominal segments. The identity of the appendages is determined by

the combinatorial activity of the *Hox* genes in conjunction with *Distal-less*. For example, the identity of the T1 leg is specified by *Distal-less* and *Sex combs reduced*, whereas the identity of the T2 leg is specified by *Distal-less* and *Antennapedia*.

Hox Genes throughout Metazoans

Soon after the discovery of *Hox* gene clusters in *Drosophila*, researchers began to inquire whether *Hox* genes are a peculiarity of *Drosophila* development, or whether they are found in a broader range of species. Many developmental biologists did not expect to find *Hox* genes in other animals, since there was no reason to expect that other animals would use the same genes to direct very different developmental programs. However, cross-hybridization studies using *Drosophila Hox* sequences as molecular probes revealed *Hox* gene sequences in the genomes of all animals, including insects, spiders, molluscs, and vertebrates (such as humans). This revelation suggested a common developmental mechanism among animals.

Subsequent experiments showed not only that most animals have clusters of *Hox* genes but also that they are arranged in a manner similar to that in *Drosophila* (**Figure 18.13**). Each cluster consists of genes corresponding to those in the *bithorax* and *Antennapedia* clusters of *Drosophila*, with some minor deletions and duplications. For example, as in *Drosophila*, the mouse *Hox* genes are expressed in an anterior-to-posterior pattern that corresponds to the chromosomal position of the genes within

PROBLEM Why do loss-of-function mutations in *bithorax* complex genes result in homeotic transformations of parasegments into identities that correspond to more-anterior parasegments, whereas gain-of-function mutations (see Section 4.1) tend to result in identities corresponding to more-posterior parasegments?

BREAK IT DOWN: The *bithorax* complex genes specify identity along the anterior–posterior axis of *Drosophila* (see p. 675).

BREAK IT DOWN: In a homeotic transformation, a normal body part is replaced by another body part normally found in another region of the body.

Solution Strategies	Solution Steps
Evaluate	
1. Identify the topic this problem addresses and the nature of the required answer.	1. The subject of this question is the effect of mutations in the *bithorax* complex on segment pattern formation. The answer requires descriptions of why loss-of-function mutations lead to segments that resemble more-anterior segments, whereas gain-of-function mutations lead to the formation of segments that resemble more-posterior segments.
2. Identify the critical information given in the problem.	2. The question suggests there is a key difference between the effects of loss-of-function mutations and gain-of-function mutations of the *bithorax* complex.
Deduce	
3. Review the general patterns of expression and segmental pattern formation resulting from the normal expression of homeotic genes. TIP: Use *Hox* genes as an example of a set of developmental genes.	3. Homeotic genes, such as the *Hox* genes, specify segment identity in a combinatorial manner through overlapping expression domains in parasegments. Each gene has a well-defined anterior boundary but a more diffuse posterior boundary. Cross-regulatory interactions refine *Hox* gene expression domains, with more-posterior genes repressing more anteriorly expressed genes.
4. Review the general pattern of expression and the normal segmental pattern formation of *bithorax* genes.	4. The *bithorax* complex consists of three genes, *Ubx*, *abd-A*, and *Abd-B*. *Ubx* is expressed in the anterior abdominal segments and posterior thoracic segments, *abd-A* is expressed in the middle abdominal segments, and *Abd-B* is expressed in the posterior abdominal segments. Segment identity is specified by the combination of *Hox* gene products and their levels of expression.
Solve	
5. Explain why loss-of-function mutations of *bithorax* genes lead parasegments to take on a more-anterior identity. TIP: Consider the cross-regulatory interactions of the *Hox* genes.	5. The loss of function of a posterior gene leads to both the absence of expression of the mutant gene and posterior expansion in the expression domains of more-anterior genes. For example, the posterior gene *Abd-B* acts to repress *abd-A* in the most-posterior segments. Loss-of-function mutations in *Abd-B* result in a posterior expansion of *abd-A* expression into more-posterior abdominal segments. The result is that both middle and posterior abdominal segments acquire an identity that is similar to that of the middle abdominal segments—a homeotic transformation to more-anterior identity.
6. Explain why gain-of-function mutations of *bithorax* genes lead parasegments to take on a more-posterior identity. TIP: Gain-of-function *Antennapedia* mutations cause legs (a posterior structure) to develop in the position normally occupied by antennae (an anterior structure).	6. Gain-of-function mutations cause gene expression at inappropriate times and locations. Gain-of-function alleles often, but not always, result in *Hox* gene expression in a more-anterior domain than in wild-type animals, thus resulting in homeotic transformations to a more-posterior identity.

For more practice, see Problems 6, 7, 21, and 24. Visit the Study Area to access study tools. **Mastering Genetics**

the *Hox* clusters. This pattern suggests that *Hox* genes also specify identity along the anterior–posterior axis of the mouse and, by extension, of mammals in general.

The conservation of *Hox* gene clusters among animals indicates that a common ancestor possessed a *Hox* gene cluster specifying pattern formation along its anterior–posterior axis. This cluster was duplicated during the evolution of the vertebrate genome, which has

four copies. The conservation of the *Hox* complexes for more than 500 million years suggests that the spatial colinearity of *Hox* genes along the chromosome with their expression along the body axis is essential for optimal functionality.

Mice embryos with loss-of-function alleles of *Hox* genes, constructed using gene-targeting techniques described in Section 15.2, exhibit defects in the identity of serially

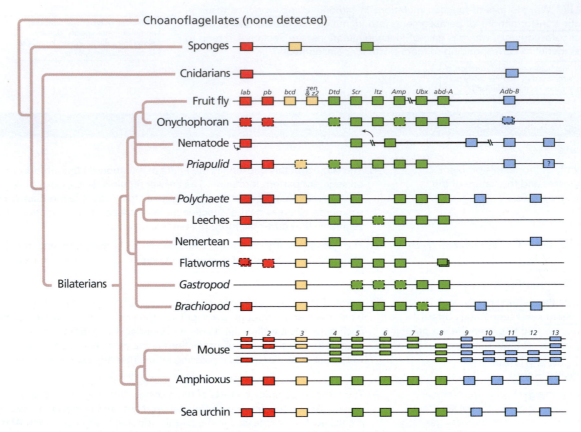

Figure 18.13   Occurrence and arrangement of *Hox* complexes in metazoans. *Hox* genes have not been detected in choanoflagellates, single-celled organisms that represent the sister clade to metazoans, but they are present in all metazoans. In the vertebrate lineage (exemplified by the mouse), the entire complex has been duplicated twice, resulting in four *Hox* complexes. Such events have produced duplicated genes that were later co-opted to new developmental functions.

repeated structures. For example, loss of *Hox* function results in a homeotic transformation of the lumbar and sacral vertebrae, which do not normally bear ribs, into structures resembling more-anterior thoracic vertebrae that do carry ribs (see Figure 14.1). These and additional *Hox* gene mutations suggest *Hox* genes direct the development of body plans in chordates as well as in annelids, arthropods, molluscs, nematodes, and other animals.

Studies of *Hox* complexes in other metazoans reveal that gene duplication took place before the divergence of bilaterian animals (animals that have bilateral symmetry). Thus, all bilaterian animals have essentially the same homeotic gene toolkit to pattern their anterior–posterior axis. This homology indicates that the differences between animals reflect how the toolkit is employed rather than differences in the component parts. Indeed, large-scale sequencing of cnidarian (jellyfish, sea anemone) genomes suggests that other components of the genetic toolkit are also largely shared by all metazoans. Given that all animals share fundamental developmental patterning processes and genes, much of what we learn from the study of model animals such as *Drosophila*, *Caenorhabditis elegans*, and mice

can be extended to other members of the animal kingdom, including ourselves.

Stabilization of Cellular Memory by Chromatin Architecture

The preceding sections describe how the basic body plan of *Drosophila* is established in early embryogenesis by the action of coordinate, gap, and segmentation genes and through spatially restricted patterns of *Hox* gene expression that specify segmental identity. The patterns of *Hox* gene expression are then faithfully propagated throughout the remainder of embryonic development. The proteins that activate *Hox* gene expression have an ephemeral pattern of expression; it disappears soon after *Hox* expression patterns are initiated. Thus, one challenge cells face during embryonic development is for specific lineages to maintain their identity as they proliferate.

Genetic screens for homeotic genes revealed that mutations at loci other than those encoding the *Hox* genes can also produce homeotic mutant phenotypes. In general, mutations at these other loci fall into two classes. The first class, exemplified by *trithorax* mutations, produces phenotypes reminiscent of multiple *Hox* loss-of-function mutations. In contrast, phenotypes of mutants of the second class, exemplified by *Polycomb* mutations, often resemble multiple gain-of-function alleles of *Hox* genes. At the molecular level, expression of multiple *Hox* genes is found to be ectopic in *Polycomb* mutants and reduced in *trithorax* mutants. Although *Hox* gene expression is established normally in both *Polycomb* and *trithorax* mutants, the expression either fails to be maintained (*trithorax* mutants) or is later activated in inappropriate locations (*Polycomb* mutants). Thus, rather than "remembering" what type of tissue they are destined to form, mutant *trithorax* and *Polycomb* cell lineages appear to "forget" their identity.

Recall the discussion in Section 13.2 of how Trithorax group (TrxG) and Polycomb group (PcG) protein complexes repress or activate, respectively, gene expression via chromatin modification. These proteins provide a type of epigenetic cellular memory that is propagated through cell divisions occurring long after the initial activators of *Hox* gene expression patterns have disappeared.

Study of *trithorax* and *Polycomb* mutants has helped clarify that the establishment of euchromatic or heterochromatic chromatin at specific developmental genes is a primary mechanism by which the potential fates of cells become restricted as development proceeds from totipotent zygote to differentiated cell types. The relative rigidity or plasticity of these different chromatin states is directly responsible for a cell's ability to express some genes and not express others, thus influencing the developmental potential of particular cell types.

18.3 Cellular Interactions Specify Cell Fate

The adult *C. elegans* contains only about 1000 cells, and its development provides a model of organogenesis. For example, the development of the *Caenorhabditis elegans* vulva demonstrates how inductive and inhibitory signals between cells direct the differentiation of distinct developmental fates in a group of pluripotent cells. John Sulston, Sydney Brenner, and Robert Horvitz shared the Nobel Prize in Physiology or Medicine in 2002 for their research on the genetic regulation of organ development and programmed cell death in *C. elegans*.

Inductive Signaling between Cells

Caenorhabditis elegans is a hermaphrodite nematode worm in which external genitalia, the vulva, forms a portal to the uterus through which eggs are laid. Early in their development, hermaphroditic worms produce sperm, which they store for later use. Eggs are subsequently produced in the gonads, fertilized with the stored sperm, and then extruded through the vulva. The vulva forms during the last larval stage, from six precursor cells called vulval precursor cells (VPCs); see **Figure 18.14a–b**. Three of these larval cells give

(a) Six cells, P3.p to P8.p, have potential to develop into vulva.

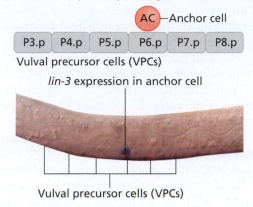

(b) The three cells closest to anchor cell—P5.p to P7.p—form the vulva; the other cells develop into hypodermis.

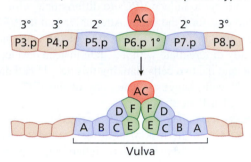

One cell has 1° identity and forms the central part; two flanking cells adopt 2° fate and form peripheral parts.

(c) Loss of the anchor cell results in loss of vulval development; all cells adopt hypodermal fate.

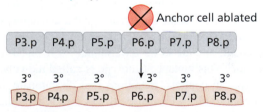

(d) Inductive signal from anchor cell induces vulval cell differentiation.

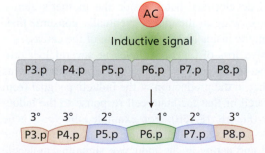

Figure 18.14   Inductive signaling during vulval development in *C. elegans*.

🔴 If the cell P6.p is ablated, will a 1° cell be specified, and if so, where?

rise to structures of the vulva itself: One is called the primary (1°) cell, and the other two are called secondary (2°) cells of the vulva. The other three cells differentiate into hypodermis and are called tertiary (3°) cells. The VPC closest to a specific gonadal cell called the anchor cell differentiates as the 1° cell and forms the central part of the vulva. The two cells flanking the 1° cell differentiate as the 2° cells and form the peripheral regions of the vulva. The 1° and 2° fates can be easily distinguished by their distinct cell-division patterns.

Initially, each of the six VPCs has the potential to differentiate along any of the pathways—1°, 2°, or 3°. This flexible cell-fate potential is demonstrated by laser-ablation experiments that destroy the anchor cell or one or more VPCs (**Figure 18.14c**). If the anchor cell is destroyed, no vulva will form, because all six VPCs differentiate with a 3° fate and become hypodermis. This suggests that the anchor cell must be present to induce VPCs to differentiate with 1° or 2° fates and thus form the vulva. Alternatively, if the VPC closest to the anchor cell is ablated, one of the cells that would normally differentiate with a 2° fate instead develops with a 1° fate and the two cells flanking this new 1° cell differentiate as 2° cells, suggesting that any of the VPCs can differentiate with a 1° or 2° fate.

What limits the number of VPCs destined to form the vulva to three? Given the loss of both the 1° and 2° fates when the anchor cell is removed, researchers hypothesized that the anchor cell might provide an **inductive signal** to induce vulval cell differentiation (**Figure 18.14d**). If this inductive signal is disseminated in a gradient, the cell closest to the anchor cell could acquire a different fate than cells that are more distant.

As predicted by the inductive interaction model, mutations that eliminate either the inductive signal or the ability of cells to respond to the inductive signal result in a loss of vulval development, and all VPCs differentiate as hypodermis (**Figure 18.15a**). This mutant phenotype is called the vulva-less phenotype. In contrast, mutations that disseminate the inductive signal to all VPCs cause all VPCs to differentiate into vulval cells, producing a multi-vulva phenotype. Multi-vulva mutants lay eggs similarly to normal worms; however, the fertilized eggs of vulva-less worms cannot be laid and instead develop and hatch inside the mother's uterus. Progeny developing in the uterus eventually consume their mother from the inside and then hatch out of the carcass.

Recessive loss-of-function alleles at several loci produce a vulva-less phenotype. These genes encode proteins that act either in the production of the inductive signal from the anchor cell or that facilitate cell response to the inductive signal (**Figure 18.15b**). For example, the *lin-3* gene encodes a small, secreted protein expressed only in the anchor cell and acting as the inductive signaling molecule (see Figure 18.14a and d). Mutations that result in a loss of active LIN-3 protein result in the loss of the inductive signal from the anchor cell. In contrast, the *let-23* and *let-60* genes are expressed in the VPCs and act as the receptor (LET-23) for the *lin-3*–encoded signal and as a signal transduction

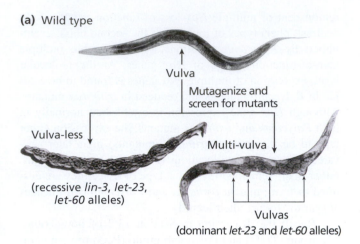

(a) Wild type

Vulva

Mutagenize and screen for mutants

Vulva-less

Multi-vulva

(recessive *lin-3*, *let-23*, *let-60* alleles)

Vulvas
(dominant *let-23* and *let-60* alleles)

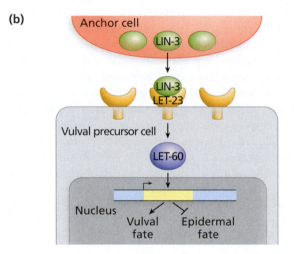

(b)

Anchor cell

LIN-3

LIN-3
LET-23

Vulval precursor cell

LET-60

Nucleus

Vulval fate   Epidermal fate

Figure 18.15 Genetic analysis of vulval development in *C. elegans*.

molecule (LET-60) that communicates the signal from the plasma membrane to the nucleus, where changes in gene expression are induced. The absence of a receptor for LIN-3, or the inability to transmit receipt of the signal, blocks the normal developmental fate of VPCs.

Epistatic analysis of developmental pathways, conducted by studying multiple mutant combinations, is used to identify groups of genes that interact to control a particular cellular process or pathway and to establish an order-of-function map for the genes in the pathway (see Section 4.3). Genetic analysis of developmental pathways can be more complicated than analysis of biochemical pathways because often there is no way of assaying intermediate steps in the developmental pathway. The analysis of double mutants and the availability of gain-of-function alleles can be crucial in these endeavors, as the studies of vulva-less and multi-vulva mutants in *C. elegans* show (**Figure 18.16**). In the case of recessive loss-of-function alleles of *lin-3*, *let-23*, and *let-60*, all single mutants have the same phenotype, suggesting all these genes might act in the same pathway (Figure 18.16b). However, all double-mutant loss-of-function combinations also exhibit a vulva-less

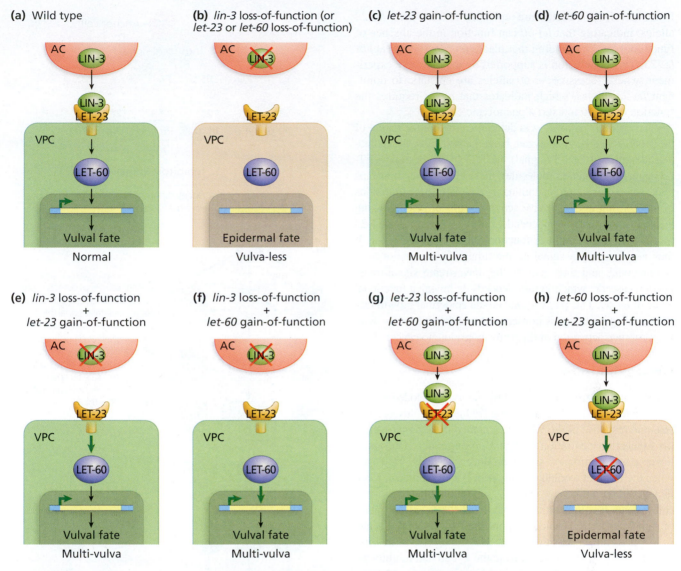

Figure 18.16 **Analysis of double-mutant phenotypes to find order of genes in developmental pathways.** (a) In wild-type worms, the vulva developmental pathway is active only in the presence of the signal (LIN-3). (b) In *lin-3* mutants, no signal is present, and worms develop with a vulva-less phenotype. (c) and (d) In either *let-23* or *let-60* gain-of-function alleles, the pathway is constitutively active, and worms develop with a multi-vulva phenotype. (e) and (f) Gain-of-function alleles of *let-23* and *let-60* are epistatic to loss-of-function *lin-3* alleles. The pathway is constitutively active regardless of whether the *lin-3* signal is present. (g) and (h) Gain-of-function alleles of *let-60* are epistatic to loss-of-function alleles of *let-23*. Conversely, loss-of-function alleles of *let-60* are epistatic to gain-of-function alleles of *let-23*. This places *let-60* downstream of *let-23*.

Q **Explain why gain-of-function alleles of either *let-23* or *let-60* are epistatic to loss-of-function alleles of *lin-3*.**

phenotype, which complicates the effort to discover the order of genes in the pathway.

As shown in Figure 18.15, genetic screens of *C. elegans* identified dominant multi-vulva mutations in which all VPCs differentiated as 1° or 2° cells. Two of the dominant mutations mapped to the same positions as *let-23* and *let-60*, suggesting that they might be gain-of-function alleles of these genes, and both dominant mutant alleles proved to be epistatic to (that is, to suppress or repress expression of) recessive

loss-of-function alleles of *lin-3* (i.e., the double mutants have a multi-vulva phenotype like the *let-23* and *let-60* gain-of-function single mutants), as outlined in Figure 18.16c–f. The double-mutant phenotype indicates that the gain-of-function alleles of either *let-23* or *let-60* do not require the function of *lin-3* to exert their phenotypic effects, thus placing both *let-23* and *let-60* downstream of *lin-3*.

Similar analysis enables the ordering of the *let-23* and *let-60* genes in the pathway (see Figure 18.16g–h).

Dominant *let-60* alleles are epistatic to recessive *let-23* alleles, indicating that *let-60* can function in the absence of functional *let-23*, a finding that places *let-60* downstream of *let-23*. This conclusion is supported by the converse experiment, where recessive *let-60* alleles are epistatic to dominant *let-23* alleles, which indicates that *let-23* requires the function of *let-60* to exert a phenotypic effect.

The genetic pathway was determined before the nature of the proteins had been analyzed. Now that we know the molecular identities of LIN-3 (signal), LET-23 (receptor), and LET-60 (signal transduction molecule), these epistatic relationships make sense. For example, dominant gain-of-function mutations of *let-60* result in constitutive activity of this protein, allowing it to transduce a signal independent of the state of the LET-23 receptor. Likewise, gain-of-function alleles of *let-23* act as if they are receiving a signal all the time, whether or not *lin-3* is functional, and thus activate the downstream signal-transduction cascade, which in turn depends on having a functional allele of *let-60*. This pathway, called the epidermal growth factor signaling pathway, is conserved throughout animals, with inappropriate activation of the pathway leading to cancer.

Lateral Inhibition

Given that they are both induced by the *lin-3*–encoded signal, how are the 1° and 2° fates specified? One possibility is a differential response of the VPCs to a graded *lin-3* signal, where the highest concentration of signal produces a 1° fate and a lower concentration of signal produces 2° cells. However, when the cell that would normally be a 1° cell is ablated, a cell that would normally have been a 2° cell differentiates into a 1° cell instead. It is thus unlikely that the absolute concentration of signal perceived is solely responsible for directing cell fate.

A possible explanation is that after reception of the *lin-3* signal, a second signal is sent from the 1° cell that inhibits the neighboring cells from becoming 1° cells (**Figure 18.17a**). This process is termed **lateral inhibition**, where an initial asymmetry is reinforced by signalling between adjacent cells (**Figure 18.17b**). All VPCs initially have the potential to express a lateral signal, encoded by the *lag-2* gene, and to express the receptor for the LAG-2 signal, encoded by the *lin-12* gene. The *lag-2* gene is activated in response to the LIN-3 signal, so it is expressed at higher levels in the 1° cell. Reception of LAG-2 results in down-regulation of the *lag-2* gene in the receiving cells and up-regulation of the gene for its receptor, LIN-12 (**Figure 18.17c**). This creates a feedback loop that reinforces the initial asymmetry between the 1° and 2° cells. Continued feedback between the signal and its perception amplifies the differences between the two cells, causing them to acquire distinct developmental fates.

Cell Death During Development

One of the striking observations made when Sulston, Brenner, and Horvitz tracked the fate of every cell during *C. elegans* development is that many cells are fated to die. Of the 1090 cells produced during the development

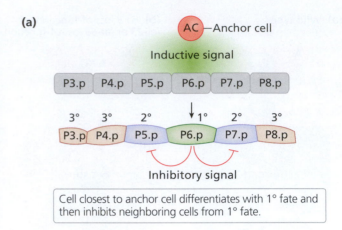

(a)

Cell closest to anchor cell differentiates with 1° fate and then inhibits neighboring cells from 1° fate.

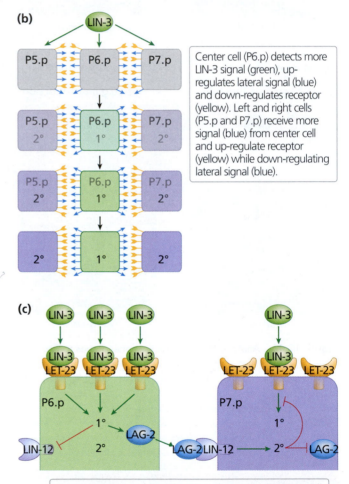

(b) Center cell (P6.p) detects more LIN-3 signal (green), up-regulates lateral signal (blue) and down-regulates receptor (yellow). Left and right cells (P5.p and P7.p) receive more signal (blue) from center cell and up-regulate receptor (yellow) while down-regulating lateral signal (blue).

(c) Strong activation of *lin-3/let-23* pathway promotes 1° cell fate, in turn activating the *lag-2/lin-12* pathway, which promotes a 2° cell fate in neighboring cells.

Figure 18.17   Lateral inhibition in *C. elegans* vulval differentiation.

of a hermaphrodite worm, 131 cells undergo a process called programmed cell death, or apoptosis (introduced in Sections 3.1 and 11.4).

Because the fate of every cell in *C. elegans* development is known, researchers have been able to identify mutants in which a cell fails to undergo apoptosis. Genetic analyses of such mutants have elucidated a genetic pathway that leads to cell death in response to a signaling molecule. This pathway is largely conserved across the animal kingdom (in humans, as well) and is a natural and important process that helps sculpt the development of tissues as well as maintain tissues in adult organisms. Indeed, it is estimated that 10^{11} cells are programmed to die every day in an adult human, many of them in epithelial tissues such as skin and intestine. Whereas loss-of-function mutants for genes in the apoptosis pathway are viable in *C. elegans*, loss-of-function mutations in homologous genes in mice result in embryo death, indicating that cell death is an essential part of life in mammals.

18.4 "Evolution Behaves Like a Tinkerer"

One of the major surprises emerging from genome sequence analysis of animals is that, within a factor of about 2, most animal genomes have very similar numbers of genes. The range is from about 12,000 to about 25,000. Thus relatively simple animals such as *Drosophila* have a genome containing about 14,000 genes, whereas the human genome contains about 25,000 genes. Even organisms such as jellyfish and sea anemones possess genomes with gene numbers largely similar to those of vertebrates.

Given this consistency of gene number, what is the biological explanation of how the presumed "complexity" of vertebrates is produced from a genetic toolkit that is similar to the one possessed by comparatively "simple" animals? The answer seems to lie in the relative complexity of gene regulation rather than the invention of new genes for additional developmental processes. This proposal suggests that existing genes are recruited for new roles by means of changes in their regulation, both in space and time. Biologist Francois Jacob summed up this view of evolution when he said, "Evolution behaves like a tinkerer. . . . [It] does not produce novelties from scratch. It works on what already exists, either transforming a system to give it new functions or combining several systems to produce a more elaborate one."

A common theme in the evolutionary history of all genes, and particularly those influencing development, is the **co-option** of genes and genetic modules to direct the patterning or growth of novel organs. In this section, we consider an example of the co-option of genes by evolutionary "tinkering" to form newly evolved structures: digits (fingers and toes) on tetrapod limb appendages such as hands and feet. The study of the evolution of development is often referred to as **evo-devo**.

Evolution through Co-option

Limb positioning in tetrapods (four-legged vertebrates) results in large measure from the expression of *Hox* genes that direct the anterior–posterior organization of the body.

Work on chickens and mice demonstrates that expression of *Hox* genes along the anterior–posterior body axis defines the position at which a limb will develop. The anterior limit of the expression domains of two *Hox* genes, *Hoxc8* and *Hoxc6*, demarcates the position of the forelimb, and the posterior limit of expression marks the position of the hindlimb (**Figure 18.18a**). The expression of these two genes specifies the thoracic region of vertebrates, which is characterized by the formation of ribs from the vertebral column.

Once limb positions are specified, cells of the mesenchyme (loosely connected sub-ectodermal cells) send a signal to the overlying ectodermal cells. This signal promotes changes within a narrow band of cells that then forms the apical ectodermal ridge (AER), whose primary function is to direct limb-bud outgrowth by responding to signals produced in a group of mesenchymal cells toward the posterior side of the limb bud called the **zone of polarizing activity** (**ZPA**; **Figure 18.18b**). The ZPA acts as an organizer that promotes digit formation at the distal ends of limb buds (that is, the ends farther from the center of the body) through the production of a morphogen, a small secreted signaling protein called Sonic hedgehog (Shh). The *Sonic hedgehog* (*Shh*) gene is orthologous to the *Drosophila* segment polarity gene *hedgehog*. *Sonic hedgehog* is expressed principally in the neural tube, where it helps organize the brain, eyes, and other structures through patterning of a group of cells known as the floor plate, and in developing limbs, where it directs the development of digits. The Case Study in this chapter discusses the consequences of different *Shh* mutations on mammalian development and morphology.

All extant tetrapods are characterized by five or fewer digits in each set, and each digit in the set has a unique identity. Tetrapod digits arise along the anterior–posterior axis of the limb bud. If you allow your arms to hang straight down, you will see that your thumb (digit 1) is in the anterior position on your hand, while your pinky (digit 5) is in the posterior position. *Sonic hedgehog* expressed in the ZPA plays an important role in initiating digit formation, and loss-of-function alleles of *Shh* result in a loss of digits 2–5; only digit 1 forms independently of *Shh* function. A second role of *Shh* in limb patterning is in the specification of digit identity. Experiments where a second ZPA is transplanted to an anterior position result in a mirror-image duplication of digits, suggesting that the ZPA instructs those digits closer to the ZPA to differentiate with posterior identity (see Figure 18.18b).

The *Hox* genes that play a conserved role in patterning the anterior–posterior axis in animals were considered candidates to be the genes acting downstream of *Shh* to specify the patterning events in digits. In mice (and by inference humans), five *Hox* genes are expressed in the limb bud at the time and place where the digits are developing: *Hoxd9*, *Hoxd10*, *Hoxd11*, *Hoxd12*, and *Hoxd13* (**Figure 18.18c**). These genes are also expressed in the posteriormost regions of the mouse embryo, where they contribute to patterning along the anterior–posterior body axis, and later in the

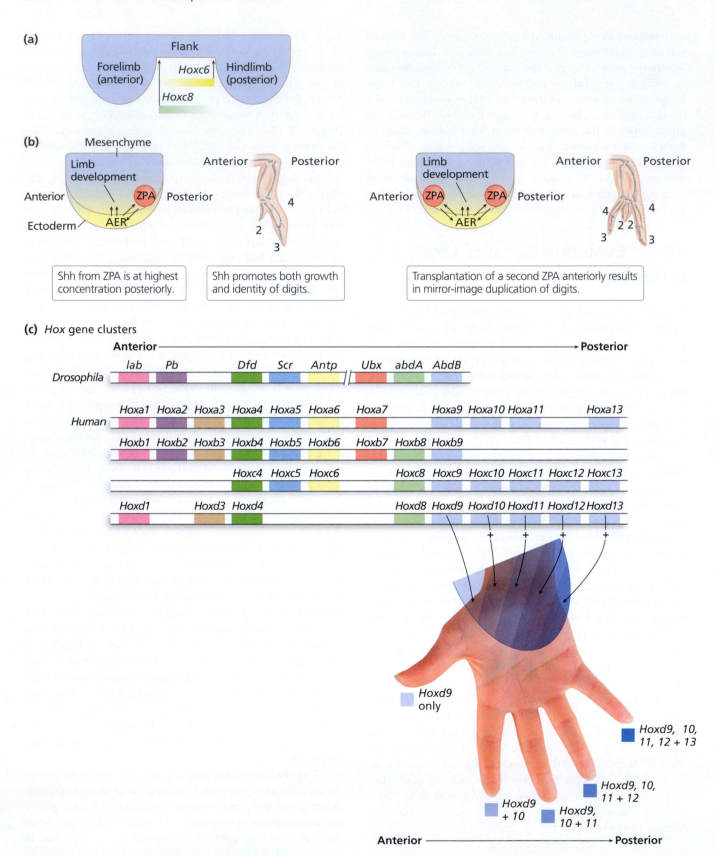

(a)

Flank

Forelimb (anterior)   *Hoxc6*   Hindlimb (posterior)

Hoxc8

(b)

Mesenchyme

Limb development

Anterior

Ectoderm

ZPA

AER

Posterior

Anterior   Posterior

4

2

3

Shh from ZPA is at highest concentration posteriorly.

Shh promotes both growth and identity of digits.

Limb development

Anterior

ZPA   ZPA

AER

Posterior

Anterior   Posterior

4   4

2 2

3   3

Transplantation of a second ZPA anteriorly results in mirror-image duplication of digits.

(c) *Hox* gene clusters

Anterior ————————————————————————→ **Posterior**

Drosophila   *lab* *Pb*   *Dfd* *Scr* *Antp*   *Ubx* *abdA* *AbdB*

Human   *Hoxa1 Hoxa2 Hoxa3 Hoxa4 Hoxa5 Hoxa6   Hoxa7   Hoxa9 Hoxa10 Hoxa11   Hoxa13*

Hoxb1 Hoxb2 Hoxb3 Hoxb4 Hoxb5 Hoxb6   Hoxb7 Hoxb8 Hoxb9

Hoxc4 Hoxc5 Hoxc6   Hoxc8 Hoxc9 Hoxc10 Hoxc11 Hoxc12 Hoxc13

Hoxd1   Hoxd3 Hoxd4   Hoxd8 Hoxd9 Hoxd10 Hoxd11 Hoxd12 Hoxd13

+   +   +   +

Hoxd9 only

Hoxd9, 10, 11, 12 + 13

Hoxd9, 10, 11 + 12

Hoxd9 + 10

Hoxd9, 10 + 11

Anterior ————————————————————————→ **Posterior**

Figure 18.18 **Limb-position and digit determination.**

developing nervous system. Despite the difference in position of hindlimb and forelimb along the body axis, the same five *Hox* genes are expressed in the developing digits of each limb. Their expression in the limb bud follows a precise temporal and spatial pattern and is dependent on *Shh* activity. The first gene to be expressed is *Hoxd9*, followed by *Hoxd10*, then *Hoxd11*, and so on through *Hoxd13*. Spatially, all genes share the same posterior boundary, but the anterior boundary of expression is different for each gene. Consequently, the five *Hoxd* genes subdivide the limb bud into five zones, each specified by a different combination of *Hoxd* gene expression. Analogous to patterning along the anterior–posterior axis, ectopic expression of different *Hoxd* genes within the developing limb bud results in transformations of digit identity. A similar combinatorial code of *Hox* gene expression also appears to specify the proximal–distal patterning of the limb buds themselves (e.g., upper arm, forearm, hand, digits).

Mutations that expand or increase *Shh* expression result in extra digits and have been documented in mice, chickens, dogs, cats, and humans. However, because identity is controlled by only five *Hox* genes, the extra digits always have a morphology closely resembling that of an adjacent digit, rather than having a unique identity (see Figure 4.13). Finally, it is worth noting that the separation of the human limb bud into individual digits requires programmed cell death (see Section 18.3) of the intervening cells—a process that has been lost in duck and bat limbs and has led to webbing in those animals.

These programs have been further modified during evolution in the secondary loss of legs in snakes and cetaceans. The loss of the front legs of snakes is due to an anterior shift in both *Hoxc6* and *Hoxc8* gene expression all the way to the base of the head. All vertebrae behind the snake head, except the first one, develop as thoracic vertebrae with ribs. In contrast, the convergent evolution of loss of hind legs in snakes and cetaceans is due to independent alterations in *Shh* activity in the developing hind limb bud.

Constraints on Co-option

The ancestral roles of *Hoxd* genes pertained to patterning along the anterior–posterior axis of the body. Therefore, the role of *Hoxd* genes in specifying digit identity represents a co-option of function of already existing genes. These same ancestral genes also acquired roles in the differentiation of the nervous system floor plate, whose presence in all vertebrates is an indication that it evolved before limbs during vertebrate evolution. Limbs developed later within the tetrapod lineage, and in the course of limb evolution, *Shh* was co-opted to pattern digits, structures that did not previously exist. By what process are genes co-opted for new functions during evolution?

In the case of limb evolution, genes of the *Hoxd* cluster could have come under control of limb-specific enhancer modules leading to expression of the *Hoxd* genes in developing limbs. As long as changes in regulation did not disrupt

Hoxd expression during anterior–posterior patterning of the body axis, the changes would not result in defects of this earlier process. The acquisition of gene expression in the developing limb could be thought of as a gain-of-function mutation. The modularity of enhancers and silencers facilitates evolution by co-option because individual enhancer modules are free to evolve independently. Thus the patterning of a novel tetrapod organ, the limb, involved the co-option of, or tinkering with, preexisting genetic programs that already had developmental roles elsewhere. As noted above, a major constraint on this type of evolutionary change is that the more ancestral functions of the gene must not be disrupted.

18.5 Plants Represent an Independent Experiment in Multicellular Evolution

Multicellularity has evolved independently many times in the history of life on Earth. The two lineages of multicellular organisms you are likely to be most familiar with are animals and land plants. Since the common ancestor of plants and animals was a single-celled organism, multicellularity evolved independently in each lineage.

Due to their independent origins, animals and plants differ in certain crucial aspects of their development. One difference is that germ-line cells in animals separate from somatic (body) cells much earlier in development than do the germ-line cells in land plants. Another difference is that animal cells are often motile during development, whereas plant cells are encased in a cell wall that essentially fixes them in the location at which they arise. Animals and land plants also differ with respect to when the basic form of the body plan takes shape. The animal body plan is established during embryogenesis, and subsequent development consists primarily of growth in size but without the addition of new organs. In contrast, throughout their lifetimes plants add new organs that are produced from pluripotent stem-cell populations. Finally, because plants often grow in a fixed location and are unable to migrate as many animals can, a plant must be able to alter its developmental program in response to changing environmental conditions throughout its lifetime. Thus, although identical twins in animals are nearly indistinguishable, genotypically identical plants may develop to look very different depending upon their growth environment. Despite these differences, developmental processes occurring in plants are remarkably similar to those in animals, especially in their reliance on the coordinated action of transcription factors and signaling molecules.

Development at Meristems

Plant development occurs at organized groups of pluripotent cells called **meristems**. The two functions of meristems are generation of organs and self-maintenance (to ensure that a pool of stem cells is always present). The above ground parts of a plant are produced by shoot meristems and the below ground parts by root meristems. The shoot meristem is divided into three functional domains—a peripheral zone from which leaves are formed, a rib zone from which part of the stem is derived, and a central zone that acts as a stem-cell reservoir to replenish cells lost to the developing leaves and stem (**Figure 18.19**). Meristems are generally indeterminate— that is, they can remain active for years, or in some cases the entire life of the plant. For example, the shoot meristem at the top of a pine tree can be active for centuries, continually producing leaves and side branches. Over time, the sizes of the central and peripheral domains remain remarkably constant. It is the continual production of new organs from meristems throughout the life of a plant that allows plants to adjust and adapt to changing local environmental conditions.

The identity of the meristem determines what types of organs are produced from its periphery. Early in the life of a flowering plant, leaves are produced from the flanks of the shoot meristem, and roots are produced from the root meristem. At the upper side of the attachment point of the leaf to the stem an axillary meristem is formed, from which a branch can arise. This reiterative formation of meristems that produce leaves that produce branches containing meristems forms the basis of most aboveground development of flowering plants.

In response to appropriate environmental conditions, the identity of meristems can change. For example, shoot meristems, which have been producing leaves, are converted in response to seasonal changes into reproductive meristems. A reproductive meristem may either develop directly into a flower meristem, or alternatively into an inflorescence meristem that produces flower meristems—an inflorescence being a group of flowers. In turn, flower meristems produce floral organs from their peripheral zones. Unlike the other meristems, flower meristems are determinate: no more stem cells are available after the flower meristem has produced a fixed number of organs.

Because each type of meristem is characterized by a specific pattern of gene expression, mutations in key genes can result in homeotic transformations of meristem types. We have all eaten one such mutant, cauliflower, in which meristems that would normally be specified as flowers behave instead as inflorescence meristems (see Figure 18.19, lower right). The genetic basis of this phenotype has been identified in *Arabidopsis* as loss-of-function alleles of two closely related paralogs, *APETALA1* and *CAULIFLOWER*, encoding transcription factors.

Combinatorial Homeotic Activity in Floral-Organ Identity

Several flowering plant species have been adopted as models for the study of genetics. For example, peas (*Pisum sativum*), with which Mendel performed his experiments, and maize (*Zea mays*), in which transposons were discovered, were introduced in earlier chapters. Due to its small size, short generation time, and fully sequenced genome,

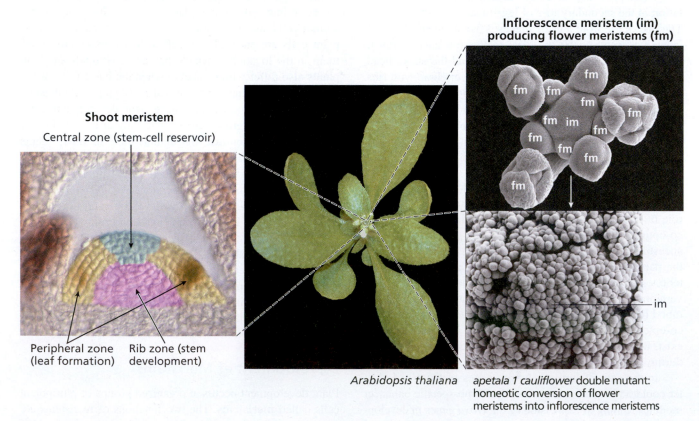

Inflorescence meristem (im) producing flower meristems (fm)

Shoot meristem

Central zone (stem-cell reservoir)

Peripheral zone (leaf formation)   Rib zone (stem development)

Arabidopsis thaliana

apetala 1 cauliflower double mutant: homeotic conversion of flower meristems into inflorescence meristems

Figure 18.19 Shoot meristems in plant growth.

the most widely used model plant is *Arabidopsis thaliana*. Since the 1980s, study of homeotic mutants in *Arabidopsis* and another plant species, *Antirrhinum* (snapdragon), has led to insights into the genetic basis of flower development and revealed developmental parallels with animals.

Arabidopsis flowers are composed of four concentric whorls of organs (**Figure 18.20**). The outermost whorl is occupied by sepals, organs that protect the flower bud during development. The second whorl is occupied by petals, which in many species attract pollinators. Stamens, the male organs that produce pollen, are located in the third whorl, and the female organs—carpels, containing the ovules—occupy the central whorl.

Homeotic Floral Mutants of *Arabidopsis* Recessive floral homeotic mutants of *Arabidopsis* fall into three classes, each having defects in two adjacent whorls (see Figure 18.20). One class, named the A class, exhibits homeotic transformations in the outer two whorls, where carpels develop in the positions normally occupied by sepals and stamens replace petals, so that the four floral whorls consist of carpels, stamens, stamens, and carpels (see Figure 18.20). A second class, the B-class mutants, exhibit homeotic transformations in the middle two whorls, where sepals replace petals and carpels replace stamens, so that the four whorls consist of sepals, sepals, carpels, and carpels. In C-class mutants, homeotic transformations in the third and fourth whorls result in flowers where petals develop in the positions normally occupied by stamens, and the cells that would normally give rise to the carpels behave as if they were another flower meristem that reiterates the developmental cycle. Similar mutants can be found in a number of ornamental plant species and are often referred to as "double flowers."

In *Arabidopsis*, A-class activity is promoted by two genes, *APETALA2* and *APETALA1*, B-class activity by the *APETALA3* and *PISTILLATA* genes, and C-class activity by the *AGAMOUS* gene. Double mutants either display an additive phenotype (e.g., *apetala3 agamous* flowers consisting of only sepals) or exhibit novel phenotypes (e.g., *apetala2 agamous* flowers with novel floral organs that do not exist in wild-type flowers). Additive double-mutant phenotypes suggest that the two genes do not interact, whereas nonadditive double-mutant phenotypes suggest that the two genes interact to influence a common developmental pathway. For example, in *apetala2 agamous* flowers, the first and fourth whorls have leaf-like carpels whereas the second and third whorls are occupied by organs with features of both petals and stamens. The *agamous* mutation has a phenotypic effect in the first and second whorls in an *apetala2* background (compare the identities of these whorls in an *apetala2* single mutant with a *apetala2 agamous* double mutant), an effect not observed in a wild-type background, where phenotypic defects of *agamous* are limited to the third and fourth whorls. This indicates that *AGAMOUS* is ectopically active in first and second whorls in *apetala2* mutants. Likewise, based on the double-mutant phenotype, *APETALA2* is active in the inner whorls of *agamous* mutants.

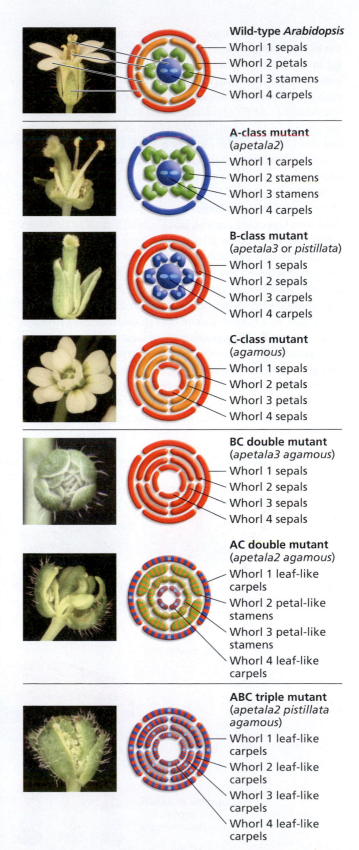

Wild-type *Arabidopsis*
Whorl 1 sepals
Whorl 2 petals
Whorl 3 stamens
Whorl 4 carpels

A-class mutant (*apetala2*)
Whorl 1 carpels
Whorl 2 stamens
Whorl 3 stamens
Whorl 4 carpels

B-class mutant (*apetala3* or *pistillata*)
Whorl 1 sepals
Whorl 2 sepals
Whorl 3 carpels
Whorl 4 carpels

C-class mutant (*agamous*)
Whorl 1 sepals
Whorl 2 petals
Whorl 3 petals
Whorl 4 sepals

BC double mutant (*apetala3 agamous*)
Whorl 1 sepals
Whorl 2 sepals
Whorl 3 sepals
Whorl 4 sepals

AC double mutant (*apetala2 agamous*)
Whorl 1 leaf-like carpels
Whorl 2 petal-like stamens
Whorl 3 petal-like stamens
Whorl 4 leaf-like carpels

ABC triple mutant (*apetala2 pistillata agamous*)
Whorl 1 leaf-like carpels
Whorl 2 leaf-like carpels
Whorl 3 leaf-like carpels
Whorl 4 leaf-like carpels

Figure 18.20 Floral homeotic mutations in *Arabidopsis*.

On the basis of single and multiple mutant phenotypes, a model was formulated in which the identity of organs developing in any whorl is determined by the combination of homeotic genes active in that whorl (**Figure 18.21**). It was presumed that each class of gene is active in the whorls seen to be in the respective mutants: *APETALA2* and *APETALA1* in the outer two whorls, *APETALA3* and *PISTILLATA* in the middle two whorls, and *AGAMOUS* in the inner two whorls. Thus, each whorl is characterized by a different combination of homeotic gene activity that specifies floral organ identity. The A-class activity by itself in the first whorl specifies sepals, A-class + B-class in the second whorl specifies petals, B-class + C-class in the third whorl specifies stamens, and C-class by itself in the fourth whorl specifies carpels. To account for the mutant phenotypes (specifically the *apetala2 agamous* mutant described above), a second postulate of the model is that the A-class and C-class activities are mutually antagonistic, so that in an A-class mutant background, C-class activity is found in all four whorls; and conversely, in a C-class mutant background, A-class activity is in all four whorls. The specification of identity by combinations of homeotic gene activities and cross-regulatory interactions between the floral homeotic genes is reminiscent of specification of segmental identity in *Drosophila* by *Hox* genes.

The model successfully predicts the phenotypes of multiple mutants. For example, in a double mutant in which both B-class and C-class activities are absent, only A-class genes are expressed in all four whorls, and a flower with only sepals develops (see Figure 18.20). In ABC triple mutants, in which all floral-organ–identity gene activity is compromised, leaf-like organs are found in all whorls. These observations suggest that since floral organs are evolutionarily derived from leaves, one role of the floral homeotic genes is to modify a leaf into a specialized floral organ.

Homeotic MADS Box Transcription Factors Many floral homeotic genes encode closely related transcription factors, similar to the situation with animal homeotic genes. However, rather than encoding homeobox genes, the floral homeotic genes encode **MADS box** genes, named after the DNA-binding domain of the transcription factors. The name MADS box is derived from four members of the gene family: *MCM1* of *Saccharomyces cerevisiae*, *AGAMOUS* of *Arabidopsis*, *DEFICIENS* of *Antirrhinum*, and *SRF* of humans. All of the B- and C-class genes, as well as *APETALA1*, encode MADS boxes. Consistent with the model described above, the B-class genes are expressed in whorls two and three, and the C-class gene, *AGAMOUS*, is expressed in the third and fourth whorls (see Figure 18.21).

Subsequent studies have shown that the ABC classes of MADS box proteins interact with another class of MADS

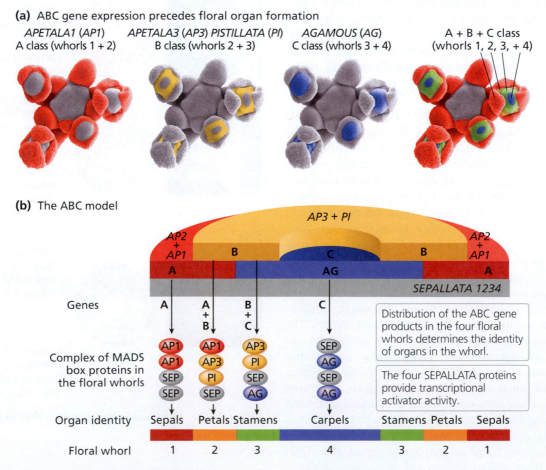

(a) ABC gene expression precedes floral organ formation

APETALA1 (AP1) A class (whorls 1 + 2)	*APETALA3 (AP3) PISTILLATA (PI)* B class (whorls 2 + 3)	*AGAMOUS (AG)* C class (whorls 3 + 4)	A + B + C class (whorls 1, 2, 3, + 4)

(b) The ABC model

Figure 18.21 **The ABC model of flower development.**

PROBLEM You are interested in the development of the body plan of kelp, a common brown alga found along many coastlines. Would reverse or forward genetics approaches be more suited to identifying the genes required for early kelp development?

BREAK IT DOWN: Review Figure 17.17 to find the relationship between brown algae and the other organisms you have been studying.

BREAK IT DOWN: In a "forward genetics" approach, no prior knowledge of gene identity is required, while a "reverse genetic" approach starts with known gene sequences.

Solution Strategies	Solution Steps
Evaluate	
1. Identify the topic this problem addresses and the nature of the required answer.	1. This problem concerns the investigation of genes determining development of kelp. Devising an answer requires evaluating the relative potential of reverse genetic analysis versus forward genetic analysis (see Sections 14.1 and 14.3).
2. Identify the critical information given in the problem.	2. Kelp is identified as brown algae, a form of life distinct from land plants and animals.
Deduce	
3. Determine if looking for gene homology (a reverse genetic approach) has a high probability of successfully identifying developmental genes in kelp.	3. Examination of Figure 16.12 indicates that kelp is only distantly related to either land plants or animals. Therefore, searching for brown algal genes based on the sequences of plant or animal developmental genes is something of a fishing expedition (i.e., holds little promise of success).
Solve	
4. Determine whether the use of mutagenesis (a forward genetics approach) is likely to help identify kelp developmental genes.	4. A good approach to finding developmental genes is to perform a mutagenesis experiment that will identify mutants in which pattern formation is perturbed. Mutagenesis can potentially affect any gene; thus, the forward genetics approach is not biased or restricted to genes that share homology with genes in other species. Mutants displaying abnormalities of wild-type pattern formation are likely to carry mutations of pattern-forming genes.

TIP: Was the common ancestor of animals, plants, and kelp unicellular or multicellular? Review Figure 16.12.

PITFALL: Distantly related organisms are likely to have evolved substantially since they last shared a common ancestor, and the extent of gene homology decreases as evolutionary distance between species increases.

TIP: How were genes that regulate development in *Drosophila* originally identified?

For more practice, see Problems 17, 19, 22, 23, and 26. Visit the Study Area to access study tools. **Mastering Genetics**

---

box protein encoded by the *SEPALLATA* (*SEP*) genes (see Chapter 14 Case Study). The SEP proteins together with the A-, B-, and C-class proteins form higher-order complexes that regulate transcription (see Figure 18.21). The SEP proteins provide a transcriptional activation activity to the complexes, an activity that the B and C proteins lack. Conversely, the A, B, and C proteins provide specificity to the complexes, an activity the SEP proteins lack. When A-, B-, or C-class genes are ectopically expressed throughout the flower meristem, they cause homeotic transformations of floral organ identity. For example, if B-class genes are ectopically expressed throughout the flower, the result is a flower with organ identities of petal, petal, stamen, stamen, from the first to the fourth whorls. In contrast, ectopic expression of the A-, B-, and C-class genes alone is not sufficient to convert the leaves of the *Arabidopsis* plant into floral organs. However, if the *SEP* genes are ectopically expressed in addition to, for example, the A and B genes, the combination is sufficient to convert leaves into petals. In this manner, the identities of leaves and floral organs are interconvertible by the absence or presence of the expression of the floral homeotic genes, consistent with floral organs evolving by modification of an ancestral leaf.

Studies of B- and C-class genes from flowering plants and gymnosperms (e.g., conifers) suggest that for all seed plants, C-class genes alone promote female reproductive development and that B + C gene activity promotes male reproductive development. However, unlike the *Hox* genes, which appear to have evolved at the base of the animal lineage and which control patterning in all known animals, the B- and C-class genes are unknown in earlier-diverging lineages of land plants, such as ferns, lycophytes, and bryophytes, whose reproductive structures differ substantially in morphology and development and whose leaf-like organs evolved independently.

We have seen that the specification of serially repeated structures in both *Drosophila* and *Arabidopsis* is controlled in a similar manner via the combinatorial action of closely related transcription factors. Although the mechanism of developmental patterning in plants and animals is similar, the genes involved in development in the two kingdoms are not related; this is consistent with the independent evolution of multicellularity in plants and animals.

Genetic Analysis 18.2 asks you to design an experimental strategy to genetically dissect development in another group of multicellular eukaryotes.

CASE STUDY

Cyclopia and Polydactyly—Different *Shh* Mutations with Distinctive Phenotypes

Sonic hedgehog (*Shh*), introduced in Section 18.4, is an evolutionarily conserved gene that performs multiple related but distinct roles in developing tissues of animals. The gene's best-understood developmental roles, stemming from its expression in limb buds and in the neural tube, pertain to digit formation and to the development of the floor plate. The floor plate divides the brain into hemispheres and is required for midline separation of other anatomical features, including separating developing eye tissue into right and left eyes. Given the central role of *Shh* in development, it stands to reason that *Shh* mutations profoundly affect normal development and morphology. Here we briefly examine two abnormal conditions that are caused by changes in *Shh* activity: holoprosencephaly/cyclopia and polydactyly.

HOLOPROSENCEPHALY/CYCLOPIA Holoprosencephaly (HPE) is a genetically heterogeneous abnormality, meaning that mutations in different genes can cause the disorder. One form of holoprosencephaly, HPE3, is caused by *Shh* mutations. HPE3 is a clinically variable disorder that produces many different morphological abnormalities in patients. The most subtle phenotypic defect is a slight loss of midline separation, resulting in a single central incisor. More severe defects include characteristic brain abnormalities; abnormalities of the mid-face, such as the formation of a proboscis-like nose; or possibly, in the most extreme cases, cyclopia, the presence of a single large mass of eye tissue rather than two separate eyes.

Numerous *Shh* mutations that cause HPE3 affect the coding region of the gene and result in the production of

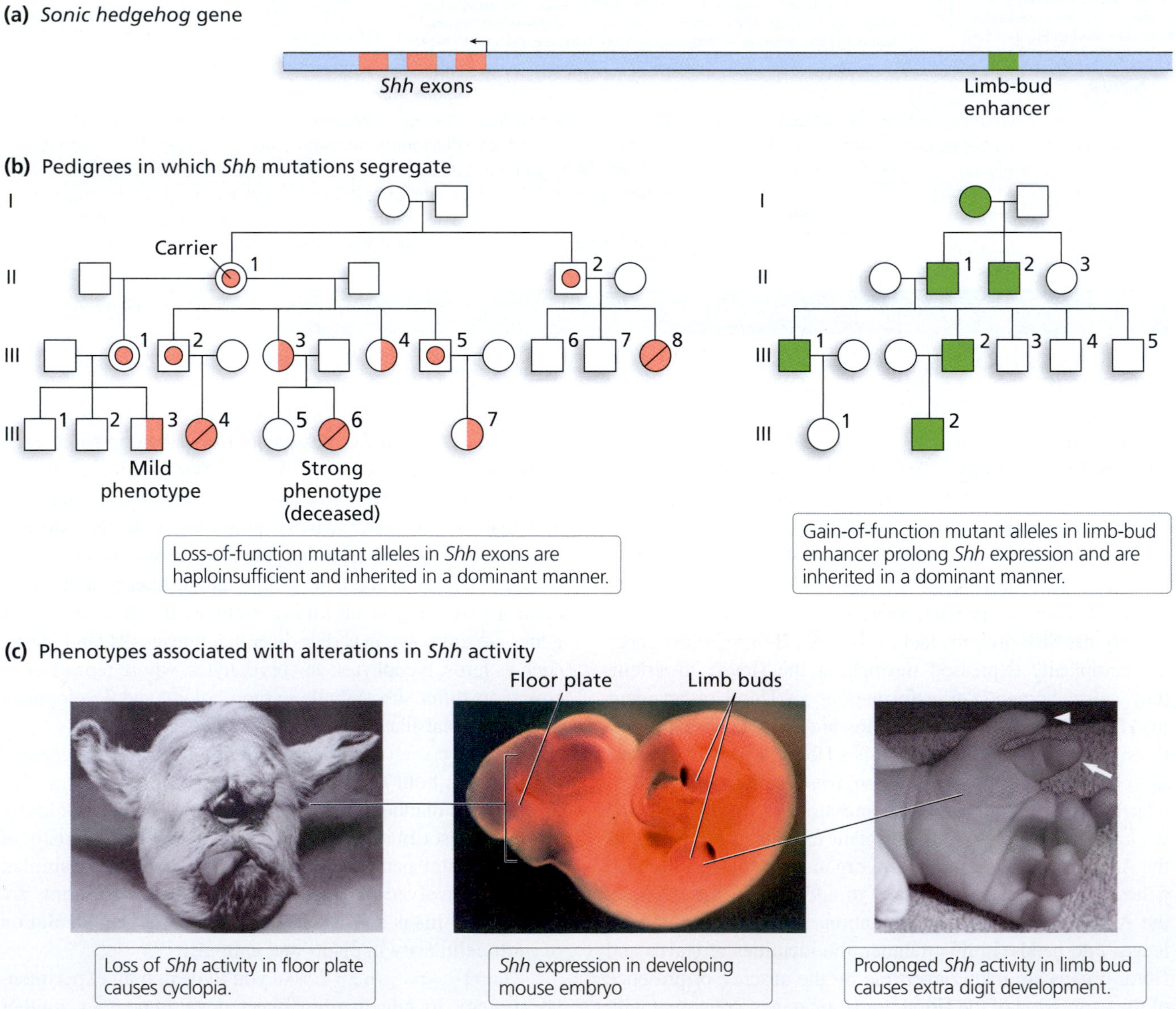

(a) *Sonic hedgehog* gene

Shh exons

Limb-bud enhancer

(b) Pedigrees in which *Shh* mutations segregate

Carrier

Mild phenotype

Strong phenotype (deceased)

Loss-of-function mutant alleles in *Shh* exons are haploinsufficient and inherited in a dominant manner.

Gain-of-function mutant alleles in limb-bud enhancer prolong *Shh* expression and are inherited in a dominant manner.

(c) Phenotypes associated with alterations in *Shh* activity

Floor plate   Limb buds

Loss of *Shh* activity in floor plate causes cyclopia.

Shh expression in developing mouse embryo

Prolonged *Shh* activity in limb bud causes extra digit development.

Figure 18.22 Effects of alterations in Shh morphogen activity in the floor plate and the limb bud.

a severely defective or nonfunctional protein product, leading to a failure to form the floor plate and thus to form brain hemispheres. To date, there are no specific genotype–phenotype correlations that tie specific *Shh* mutations to more severe or less severe manifestations of HPE3 or cyclopia. Although the HPE3 mutations in Shh are missense, nonsense, and frameshift loss-of-function alleles, familial cases of HPE3 are inherited in an autosomal dominant manner, indicating that the *Shh* mutations are haploinsufficient: The presence of a single copy of a wild-type allele is not sufficient for normal activity. Nevertheless, pedigrees exhibit variation in both penetrance and expressivity, most likely because other genes involved in brain and mid-face formation (i.e., the other genes that cause the HPE phenotype) influence the extent of morphological abnormality (**Figure 18.22a–b**). Thus, as with most genetic disorders that have been characterized in humans, both penetrance and expressivity of abnormal phenotypes are modified significantly by genetic background.

During the 1950s, an epidemic of cyclopia was reported among sheep in the western United States (**Figure 18.22c**). The compound cyclopamine, found in the plant *Veratrum californicum*, was implicated as an environmental cause of the abnormalities. Evidence indicated that ingestion of *V. californicum* during gestation caused the production of lambs with cyclopia. In 2002, Philip Beachy and colleagues looked at the mechanism by which cyclopamine caused cyclopia and discovered that the compound binds to the *Shh* receptor expressed in cells in the floor plate and blocks their response to Shh protein. This study illustrates that the action of normal proteins can be inhibited under certain environmental circumstances to produce effects similar to those seen with gene mutation. When an environmental condition induces a phenotype similar to that caused by mutation, the environmental condition is said to induce a phenocopy of the mutant phenotype.

POLYDACTYLY If *Shh* expression is eliminated from the developing limb bud by loss-of-function mutations inactivating the Shh protein, limb patterning is perturbed and digits do not form. However, if *Shh* expression is altered by mutation in the cis-regulatory region of the gene, changes in the Shh protein concentration gradient can result in polydactyly, the presence of extra digits (see Figure 18.22c). The extra digits develop because Shh protein is present in high concentration in parts of the limb bud where it is not normally found. Polydactyly in humans (discussed in Section 4.2) is an autosomal dominant disorder. Its inheritance is dominant because the ectopic expression resulting from the mutation is a gain of function. The enhancer element responsible for appropriate Shh expression in the developing limb buds was identified using a phylogenetic footprinting approach (see Figure 16.17).

SUMMARY   Mastering Genetics   For activities, animations, and review quizzes, go to the Study Area.

18.1 Development Is the Building of a Multicellular Organism

- Multicellularity has evolved independently multiple times.
- The development of a multicellular organism from a fertilized egg cell entails the formation of specialized cell types, driven by differential expression of genes.
- As animal development proceeds, cells become progressively restricted in their potential developmental fates, changing from totipotent to pluripotent to differentiated.
- Morphogens can provide positional information that is converted into differential gene expression.
- Signaling between neighboring cells can induce or inhibit developmental pathways. Genes controlling developmental processes often encode transcription factors or molecules involved in signaling between cells.

18.2 *Drosophila* Development Is a Paradigm for Animal Development

- Genetic screens of *Drosophila* identified sets of successively acting genes directing pattern formation during embryonic development.
- The *Drosophila* embryo is successively subdivided into segments, each with a unique identity, by the sequential action of batteries of transcription factors.
- Genes whose products are supplied to the egg by the mother and act to guide the development of the embryo are called maternal effect genes. The genotype of the mother, rather than that of the embryo, dictates the embryonic phenotype for the traits these genes determine.
- Gap genes are regulated by maternal effect genes and subdivide the *Drosophila* embryo into several broad regions. Pair-rule genes are regulated by both maternal effect and gap genes, and they subdivide the embryo into parasegments.
- Homeotic genes known as the *Hox* genes act in combination to specify the parasegments of *Drosophila*. *Hox* genes are largely conserved throughout the metazoan kingdom.
- Downstream targets of the *Hox* genes contribute to the morphogenesis of body segments.
- *Hox* gene expression patterns are maintained by regulation at the level of chromatin, providing a cellular memory of gene expression propagated through mitoses.

18.3 Cellular Interactions Specify Cell Fate

- In *C. elegans*, an inductive signal from the anchor cell determines vulval cell fates, and lateral inhibition refines cell specification in the developing vulva.
- Programmed cell death, or apoptosis, is a normal aspect of development in animals. It is required for sculpting the body plan during embryogenesis and maintaining tissues postembryonically.

18.4 "Evolution Behaves Like a Tinkerer"

- Most animals possess the same types of genes; therefore, the differences between animals are largely due to differences in how genes are deployed during development.

■ Genes can be co-opted to direct the development of new organs and tissues, often through changes in gene expression patterns. For example, the evolution of limbs and digits in tetrapods occurred through changes in *Hox* and *Sonic hedgehog* gene expression.

18.5 Plants Represent an Independent Experiment in Multicellular Evolution

■ Despite differences in cellular behavior between plants and animals, the genetic control of development in plants has many similarities to that of animals.

■ Plants continue to add organs throughout their life span due to the action of meristems, which are groups of pluripotent stem cells.

■ Combinatorial action of homeotic genes specifies the identity of floral organs in flowering plants; the homeotic genes in plants encode MADS box transcription factors, analogous to the transcription factors encoded by the homeobox in animals.

PREPARING FOR PROBLEM SOLVING

In addition to the list of problem-solving tips and suggestions given here, you can go to the Study Guide and Solutions Manual that accompanies this book for help at solving problems.

1. Understand how cell identity can be specified in multicellular organisms via the processes of pattern formation, induction, and inhibition.

2. Be familiar with the hierarchy of gene activity that leads to the *Drosophila* embryo being more and more finely subdivided.

3. Understand the different inheritance patterns for maternal effect versus zygotic genes.

4. Be familiar with how the homeotic genes, acting alone and in combination, specify segmental identity.

5. Review the mechanisms (induction and lateral inhibition) by which cell fate is specified during vulval development in *C. elegans*.

6. Understand that old genes may be co-opted to perform new functions in the course of evolution.

7. Understand that plants, animals, fungi, and brown algae have all evolved multicellularity independently from single-celled ancestors.

8. Be prepared to compare and contrast the specification of segmental identity in *Drosophila* with the specification of floral organ identity in *Arabidopsis*.

PROBLEMS

Mastering Genetics Visit for instructor-assigned tutorials and problems.

Chapter Concepts

For answers to selected even-numbered problems, see Appendix: Answers.

1. Explain why many developmental genes encode either transcription factors or signaling molecules.

2. Bird beaks develop from an embryonic group of cells called neural crest cells that are part of the neural tube that gives rise to the spinal column and related structures. Amazingly, neural crest cells can be surgically transplanted from one embryo to another, even between embryos of different species. When quail neural crest cells were transplanted into duck embryos, the beak of the host embryo developed into a shape similar to that found in quails, creating the "quck." Duck cells were recruited in addition to the quail cells to form part of the quck beak. Conversely, when duck neural crest cells were transplanted into quail embryos, the beak of the embryo resembled that of a duck, creating a "duail," and quail cells were recruited to form part of the beak. What do these experiments tell you about the autonomy or nonautonomy of the transplanted and host cells during beak development?

3. How is positional information provided along the anterior–posterior axis in *Drosophila*? What are the functions of *bicoid* and *nanos*?

4. Early development in *Drosophila* is atypical in that pattern formation takes place in a syncytial blastoderm, allowing free diffusion of transcription factors between nuclei. In many other animal species, the fertilized egg is divided by cellular cleavages into a larger and larger number of smaller and smaller cells.

   a. What constraints does the formation of a syncytial blastoderm impose on the mechanisms of pattern formation?

   b. How must the model that describes *Drosophila* development be modified for describing other animal species whose early development is not syncytial?

5. Consider the *even-skipped* regulatory sequences in Figure 18.9.

   a. How are the sharp boundaries of expression of *eve* stripe 2 formed?

   b. Consider the binding sites for gap proteins and Bicoid in the stripe 2 enhancer module. What sites are occupied in parasegments 2, 3, and 4, and how does this result in expression or no expression?

c. Explain what you expect to see happen to *even-skipped* stripe 2 if it is expressed in a *Krüppel* mutant background. A *hunchback* mutant background? A *giant* mutant background? A *bicoid* mutant background?

6. What is the difference between a parasegment and segment in *Drosophila* development? Why do developmental biologists think of parasegments as the subdivisions that are produced during development of flies?

7. Why do loss-of-function mutations in *Hox* genes usually result in embryo lethality, whereas gain-of-function mutants can be viable? Why are flies homozygous for the recessive loss-of-function alleles *Ultrabithorax^bithorax* and *Ultrabithorax^postbithorax* viable?

8. Compare and contrast the specification of segmental identity in *Drosophila* with that of floral organ specification in *Arabidopsis*. What is the same in this process, and what is different?

9. Actinomycin D is a drug that inhibits the activity of RNA polymerase II. In the presence of actinomycin D, early development in many vertebrate species, such as frogs, can proceed past the formation of a blastula, a hollow ball of cells that forms after early cleavage divisions; but development ceases before gastrulation (the stage at which cell layers are established). What does this tell you about maternal versus zygotic gene activity in early frog development?

10. Ablation of the anchor cell in wild-type *C. elegans* results in a vulva-less phenotype.
    a. What phenotype is to be expected if the anchor cell is ablated in a *let-23* loss-of-function mutant?
    b. What about if the anchor cell is ablated in a *let-23* gain-of-function mutant?

11. In gain-of-function *let-23* and *let-60 C. elegans* mutants, all of the vulval precursor cells differentiate with 1° or 2° fates. Do you expect adjacent cells to differentiate with 1° fates or with 2° fates? Explain.

12. In mammals, identical twins arise when an embryo derived from a single fertilized egg splits into two independent embryos, producing two genetically identical individuals.
    a. What limits might there be, from a developmental genetic viewpoint, as to when this can occur?
    b. The converse phenotype, fusion of two genetically distinct embryos into a single individual, is also known. What are the genetic implications of such an event?

Application and Integration

For answers to selected even-numbered problems, see Appendix: Answers.

13. The *bicoid* gene is a coordinate, maternal effect gene.
    a. A female *Drosophila* heterozygous for a loss-of-function *bicoid* allele is mated to a male that is heterozygous for the same allele. What are the phenotypes of their progeny?
    b. A female that is homozygous for a loss-of-function *bicoid* allele is mated to a wild-type male. What are the phenotypes of their progeny?
    c. If loss of *bicoid* function in the egg leads to lethality during embryogenesis, how are females homozygous for *bicoid* produced? What is the phenotype of a male homozygous for *bicoid* loss-of-function alleles?

14. Given that maternal Bicoid activates the expression of *hunchback* (see Figure 18.7), what would be the consequence of adding extra copies of the *bicoid* gene by transgenic means to a wild-type female with two copies, thus creating a female fly with three or four copies of the *bicoid* gene? How would *hunchback* expression be altered? What about the expression of other gap genes and pair-rule genes?

15. What phenotypes do you expect in flies homozygous for loss-of-function mutations in the following genes: *Krüppel, odd-skipped, hedgehog,* and *Ultrabithorax*?

16. The pair-rule gene *fushi tarazu* is expressed in the seven even-numbered parasegments during *Drosophila* embryogenesis. In contrast, the segment polarity gene *engrailed* is expressed in the anterior part of each of the 14 parasegments. Since both genes are active at similar times and places during development, it is possible that the expression of one gene is required for the expression of the other. This can be tested by examining expression of the genes in a mutant background—for example, looking at *fushi tarazu* expression in an *engrailed* mutant background, and vice versa.
    a. Given the hierarchy of gene action during *Drosophila* embryogenesis, what might you predict to be the result of these experiments?
    b. Based on your prediction, can you predict the phenotype of the *fushi tarazu* and *engrailed* double mutant?

17. In contrast to *Drosophila*, some insects (e.g., centipedes) have legs on almost every segment posterior to the head. Based on your knowledge of *Drosophila*, propose a genetic explanation for this phenotype, and describe the expected expression patterns of genes of the *Antennapedia* and *bithorax* complexes.

18. The bristles that develop from the epidermis in *Drosophila* are evenly spaced, so that two bristles never occur immediately adjacent to each other. How might this pattern be established during development?

19. You are traveling in the Netherlands and overhear a tulip breeder describe a puzzling event. Tulips normally have two outer whorls of brightly colored petal-like organs, a third whorl of stamens, and an inner (fourth) whorl of carpels. However, the breeder found a recessive mutant in his field in which the outer two whorls were green and sepal-like, whereas the third and fourth whorls both contained carpels. What can you speculate about the nature of the gene that was mutated?

20. A powerful approach to identifying genes of a developmental pathway is to screen for mutations that suppress or enhance the phenotype of interest. This approach was

undertaken to elucidate the genetic pathway controlling *C. elegans* vulval development.

a. A *lin-3* loss-of-function mutant with a vulva-less phenotype was mutagenized. Based on your knowledge of the genetic pathway, what types of mutations will suppress the vulva-less phenotype?

b. In a complementary experiment, a gain-of-function *let-23* mutant with a multi-vulva phenotype was also mutagenized. What types of mutations will suppress the multi-vulva phenotype?

21. The *Hoxd9–13* genes are thought to specify digit identity (see Figure 18.18).

a. What would be the consequence of ectopically expressing *Hoxd10* throughout the developing mouse limb bud? What about *Hoxd11*? What about both *Hoxd10* and *Hoxd11*?

b. You wish to examine the effect of loss-of-function alleles in developing limbs. How would you construct a mouse in which the function of *Hoxd9–13* is retained during anterior–posterior embryonic patterning but is absent from developing limbs?

22. Three-spined stickleback fish live in lakes formed when the last ice age ended 10,000 to 15,000 years ago. In lakes where the sticklebacks are prey for larger fish, they develop 35 bony plates along their body as armor. In contrast, sticklebacks in lakes where there are no predators develop only a few or no bony plates.

a. In crosses between fish of the two different morphologies, the lack of bony armor segregates as a recessive trait that maps to the *ectodermal dysplasin (Eda)* gene. Comparisons between the *Eda*-coding regions of the armored and nonarmored fish revealed no differences. How can you explain this result?

b. Loss-of-function mutations in the coding region of the homologous gene in humans result in loss of hair, teeth, and sweat glands, as in the toothless men of Sind (India). What does this suggest about hair, teeth, and sweat glands in humans?

23. The flowering jungle plant *Lacandonia schismatica*, discovered in southern Mexico, has a unique floral structure. Petal-like organs are in the outer whorls surrounding a number of carpels, and stamens are in the center of the flower. Closely related species are dioecious; female plants bear flowers that resemble those of *Lacandonia*, but without the central stamens. What type of mutation could have resulted in the evolution of *Lacandonia* flowers?

24. Homeotic genes are thought to regulate each other.

a. What aspect of the phenotype of *apetala2 agamous* double mutants indicates that these two genes act antagonistically?

b. Are similar interactions observed between *Hox* genes?

25. Dipterans (two-winged insects) are thought to have evolved from a four-winged ancestor that had wings on both T2 and T3 thoracic segments, as in extant butterflies and dragonflies. Describe an evolutionary scenario for the evolution of dipterans from four-winged ancestors. What types of mutations could lead to a butterfly developing with only two wings?

26. Basidiomycota is a monophyletic group of fungi that includes most of the common mushrooms. You are interested in the development of the body plan of mushrooms. How would you identify the genes required for patterning during mushroom development?

Collaboration and Discussion

For answers to selected even-numbered problems, see Appendix: Answers.

27. *Zea mays* (maize, or corn) was originally domesticated in central Mexico at least 7000 years ago from an endemic grass called teosinte. Teosinte is generally unbranched, has male and female flowers on the same branch, and has few kernels per "cob," each encased in a hard, leaf-like organ called a glume. In contrast, maize is highly branched, with a male inflorescence (tassel) on its central branch and female inflorescences (cobs) on axillary branches. In addition, maize cobs have many rows of kernels and soft glumes. George Beadle crossed cultivated maize and wild teosinte, which resulted in fully fertile F_1 plants. When the F_1 plants were self-fertilized, about 1 plant in every 1000 of the F_2 progeny resembled either a modern maize plant or a wild teosinte plant. What did Beadle conclude about whether the different architectures of maize and teosinte were caused by changes with a small effect in many genes or changes with a large effect in just a few genes?

28. In *C. elegans* there are two sexes: hermaphrodite and male. Sex is determined by the ratio of X chromosomes to haploid sets of autosomes (X/A). An X/A ratio of 1.0 produces a hermaphrodite (XX), and an X/A ratio of 0.5 results in a male (XO). In the 1970s, Jonathan Hodgkin and Sydney

Brenner carried out genetic screens to identify mutations in three genes that result in either XX males (*tra-1*, *tra-2*) or XO hermaphrodites (*her-1*). Double-mutant strains were constructed to assess for epistatic interactions between the genes (see table). Propose a genetic model of how the *her* and *tra* genes control sex determination.

Genotype[a]	XX Phenotype	XO Phenotype
Wild-type	Hermaphrodite	Male
tra-1^{rec}	Male	Male
tra-2^{rec}	Male	Male
her-1^{rec}	Hermaphrodite	Hermaphrodite
tra-1^{dom}/+	Hermaphrodite	Hermaphrodite
tra-^{rec}1 tra-2^{rec}	Male	Male
tra-1^{rec} her-1^{rec}	Male	Male
tra-2^{rec} her-1^{rec}	Male	Male
tra-2^{rec} tra-1^{dom}/+	Hermaphrodite	Hermaphrodite

[a]*rec* = recessive mutation; *dom* = dominant mutation.

29. In *Drosophila*, recessive mutations in the *fruitless* gene (*fru*) result in males courting other males; and recessive mutations in the *Antennapedia* gene (*Ant⁻*) lead to defects in the body plan, specifically in the thoracic region of the body, where mutants fail to develop legs. The two genes map 15 cM apart on chromosome 3. You have isolated a new dominant Ant^d mutant allele that you induced by treating your flies with X-rays. Your new mutant has legs developing instead of antennae on the head of the fly. You cross your newly induced dominant Ant^d mutant (a pure-breeding line) with a homozygous recessive *fru* mutant (which is homozygous wild type at the Ant^+ locus), as diagrammed below:

$$\frac{Ant^d fru^+}{Ant^d fru^+} \times \frac{Ant^+ fru}{Ant^+ fru} \rightarrow F_1 \frac{Ant^d fru^+}{Ant^+ fru}$$

a. What phenotypes, and in what proportions, do you expect in the F₂ obtained by interbreeding F₁ animals?

b. Your cross results in the following phenotypic proportions:

Legs on head, normal courting behavior	75
Normal head, abnormal courting behavior	25
Legs on head, abnormal courting behavior	0
Normal head, normal courting behavior	0

Provide a genetic explanation for these results and describe a test for your hypothesis.

c. Provide a molecular explanation for the reason your new Ant^d mutant is dominant and for its novel phenotype.

19

Genetic Analysis of Quantitative Traits

CHAPTER OUTLINE

19.1 Quantitative Traits Display Continuous Phenotype Variation

19.2 Quantitative Trait Analysis Is Statistical

19.3 Heritability Measures the Genetic Component of Phenotypic Variation

19.4 Quantitative Trait Loci Are the Genes That Contribute to Quantitative Traits

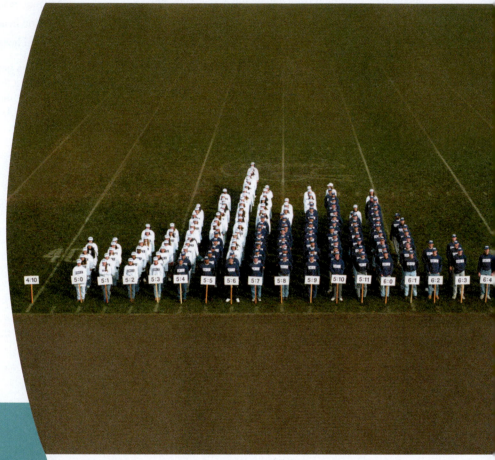

A human histogram depicting the distribution of heights of 138 faculty members and students of the University of Connecticut. The women are in white shirts and the men are in blue shirts.

ESSENTIAL IDEAS

▮ Quantitative traits are influenced by multiple genes and may also be influenced by the environment. They are continuously distributed along a phenotypic scale. Some quantitative traits are separated into distinct phenotypes by a threshold.

▮ The phenotypic distributions of quantitative traits are described by statistical measures that also estimate the genetic and environmental contributions to phenotype.

▮ The extent to which genetic variation contributes to phenotype variability can be estimated for quantitative traits and provides an indication of how traits may respond to artificial selection.

▮ The genes that influence quantitative traits are identified and mapped using genetic crosses and molecular and statistical techniques.

E xplaining the connection between phenotypes and genotypes is simplest when the phenotypic variation in a trait is decided by variation in a single gene. The segregation of alleles of a single gene determining whether peas are round or wrinkled, as in Mendel's studies, is a classic example. Other genes are not involved, and there is no evidence of gene interaction (i.e., epistasis) or of interaction between the gene and specific environmental factors.

In reality, however, such direct correlations between phenotypes and genotypes are not common. Many traits display variation resulting from epistatic gene interactions (see Section 4.3). In addition, numerous traits, known as **polygenic traits,** result from the influence of multiple genes. The genes contributing to polygenic traits generally assort independently to produce a large number of genotypes and multiple phenotypes. The inheritance of polygenic traits is identified as **polygenic inheritance.** Further complicating the imperfect correlations between genotypes and phenotypes in polygenic inheritance is the possibility that environmental factors or circumstances during development can interact with one or more of the genes to shape the phenotype. Thus both genetic variation and nongenetic variation can contribute to the phenotypic variation of certain traits, which are therefore identified as **multifactorial traits.**

Many multifactorial traits have phenotypes that are best described in *quantitative* rather than *qualitative* terms, that is, with the aid of numbers rather than descriptive adjectives. Qualitative phenotypes often fall into discrete categories that may correspond to specific genotypes and that are distinctly different from one another. "Round seeds" versus "wrinkled seeds" or "blood type A" versus "blood type B" are examples of qualitative phenotypic differences. In contrast, quantitative phenotypic variation usually takes the form of continuous variation along a phenotypic scale, and the traits are frequently described using units of measure. For example, one might use kilograms to measure quantitative variation in the weight of cattle or centimeters to measure quantitative variation in the length of ears of corn. Traits of this kind are often identified as **quantitative traits.** Note, however, that this term is also used for traits that are nonnumeric but vary over a phenotypic range, as with a range of color phenotypes (e.g., from black through shades of gray to white).

The genetic study and analysis of quantitative traits is the focus of the field of inquiry known as **quantitative genetics.** In this chapter, we explore how quantitative genetics examines the hereditary variation of polygenic and multifactorial traits. In the process, we address some of the ways geneticists attempt to disentangle the genetic and environmental influences on trait variation and discuss genetic approaches to interpreting the relative effects of those factors on quantitative trait phenotypes.

19.1 Quantitative Traits Display Continuous Phenotype Variation

For most of the traits we discuss in earlier chapters, phenotypic variation is controlled by allelic variation at single genes. The phenotypes of these single-gene traits commonly display **discontinuous variation**, meaning differences that allow organisms to be assigned to discrete, sharply distinguishable phenotypic categories. The discontinuous patterns of variation lead to the specification of consistent phenotype ratios, such as a 3:1 ratio among the F_2 progeny of self-fertilized F_1 organisms. Even when two genes take part in epistatic interactions that affect phenotypic expression, the phenotypes are discrete and occur in predictable ratios (see Section 4.3).

In contrast, polygenic and multifactorial traits usually display **continuous variation**, which is phenotypic variation distributed across a range of values in an uninterrupted continuum. This section explores the genetic factors contributing to traits displaying continuous variation.

Genetic Potential

Human adult height is an example of a multifactorial trait that varies continuously along a scale of measurement usually marked off in centimeters or inches. This continuous variation is demonstrated in the chapter-opening photo, in which 138 University of Connecticut students and faculty are arranged according to height. The height distribution of this sample, divided into 1-inch increments, ranges from 60 inches (5 feet) to 77 inches (6 feet, 5 inches). The length of each line of individuals behind the height markers represents the frequency of each incremental category, and the sweatshirt and hat color identifies the wearer's sex (white for women and blue for men). Examining the overall distribution, you can see that it is actually composed of two different distributions, one for each sex, and you can also see that the distribution is uneven.

Adult height is influenced by multiple genes. For example, in a 2011 study by Matthew Lanktree and many colleagues, analysis of human genomic variation combined with statistical methods suggested that more than 60 genes may influence adult height. Although the actual number of genes influencing human height continues to be investigated, your own personal experiences most likely agree with the data from population studies, telling you that taller parents tend to have taller children and shorter parents tend to have shorter children.

In addition to this genetic influence, however, environmental and developmental factors can have a significant effect. If your genetics class is typical of most, a survey of your classmates would likely find that many of the men are taller than their fathers and grandfathers and that many of the women are taller than their mothers and grandmothers.

These differences are due almost exclusively to improved prenatal and childhood health and nutrition and only minimally to changes in the population genetic makeup influencing adult height. Longitudinal studies confirm that much of the world's population is getting taller. During the 20th century, the height of the average American woman increased from approximately 5 feet, 2 inches in 1900 to almost 5 feet, 5 inches in 2000. An even more dramatic increase in average adult height can be observed by walking through the doors of houses and other structures built a few centuries ago. Most modern-day visitors have to stoop to enter! Such observations lead to the clear conclusion that adult height is a multifactorial trait.

To understand the role of genetics in a trait like adult height, you might think of parents as transmitting to their children a "genetic potential" for reaching a certain maximum adult height; the genetic potential will be attained if the child grows and develops under ideal conditions. Not all of the children of a particular pair of parents will have the same genetic potential, since segregation and independent assortment of the contributing genes can produce many different genotypes. These processes produce offspring with different genotypes conveying genetic potential for a range of heights, including heights that are greater or lesser than those of their parents. On average, however, progeny genetic potential for height will be at approximately the midpoint of the two parents' genetic potential. The phenotypic outcome (actual adult height) is subject to various influences on the height potential of the genotype, including prenatal and maternal health and childhood health and nutrition, as the following discussions illustrate.

Major Gene Effects

The continuous phenotypic variation of polygenic traits results from the effects of multiple genes that may each exert about the same amount of influence or may exert different amounts of influence on the phenotype. One example of a polygenic trait with a wide range of phenotypes determined by genes with different levels of influence on the phenotype is eye color in humans. Contrary to popular misconception, eye color is a polygenic trait that is influenced by up to 15 genes. Two principal factors affect eye color: (1) the amount of the pigment called melanin deposited in the iris and (2) the turbidity of the viscous stroma of the iris, which can also contain melanin. Individuals with the darkest eye colors (black and dark brown) have irises and stroma containing the most melanin, whereas those with the lightest eye colors (blue and light green) have irises and stroma containing the least amount of melanin. Melanin is also responsible for skin pigmentation. Populations with darker eye colors tend to have darker skin tones as well, and conversely, populations with higher rates of light eye colors tend to have lighter skin tones.

Two genes having strong effects on human eye color are *OCA2* and *HERC2*. Because of their predominating effects,

these two genes are identified as **major genes**. *OCA2* has several alleles that greatly influence eye color and skin tone. One variant of the gene produces an autosomal recessive form of albinism called oculocutaneous albinism type 2. This form of albinism features very lightly pigmented eyes and skin. The gene derives its name from this condition. Other alleles of *OCA2* reduce the amount of melanin pigment production to a lesser extent. These alleles are strongly associated with blue and green eye colors. Along with light eye colors, the joint effects of *OCA2* alleles that produce small amounts of melanin include freckling, moles, and light hair color. The *HERC2* gene regulates the expression of *OCA2*; thus, alleles of *HERC2* that down-regulate *OCA2* expression are associated with blue and green eye colors. A dozen or more additional genes have minor effects on eye color. These are classified as **modifier genes**.

Additive Gene Effects

Polygenic traits for which no individual gene or genes exert major gene effects have a continuous phenotypic distribution that results from incremental contributions by multiple genes. Genes contributing to phenotypic variation in this way are known as **additive genes**. The alleles of each additive gene can be assigned their own quantitative values that indicate the contribution to the trait. In the absence of environmental influence, phenotypes can sometimes be predicted by adding the values of the alleles together. For certain traits, each of the additive genes has an approximately equal effect on the phenotype, or at least a level of effect that does not differ substantially from that of the other genes. For other traits the influence of each gene is distinguishable.

Grasping the notion of additive genes requires a different way of thinking about genotypes and phenotypes than we have discussed previously. Since traits controlled by additive genes have a phenotype that is the sum of allelic contributions across multiple genes, it is possible for more than one genotype to correspond to certain phenotypes. Segregation and independent assortment of alleles of additive genes produces the various genotypes, but the phenotype corresponding to each is based on the sum of the values of the alleles at all the contributing loci.

In the early 1900s, coinciding with the verification and expansion of the then recently rediscovered hereditary principles of Mendel, geneticists began to explore the hypothesis that the segregation of alleles of multiple genes played a role in phenotypic variation of particular traits. Known as the **multiple-gene hypothesis**, the proposal was that alleles of each of the contributing genes obeyed the principles of segregation and independent assortment and had an additive effect in the production of phenotypic variation.

The multiple-gene hypothesis was the foundation of quantitative genetics, and the plant geneticist Hermann Nilsson-Ehle was one of the first to use the hypothesis in his 1909 description of genetic control of kernel color in wheat. **Figure 19.1** illustrates one of Nilsson-Ehle's genetic models,

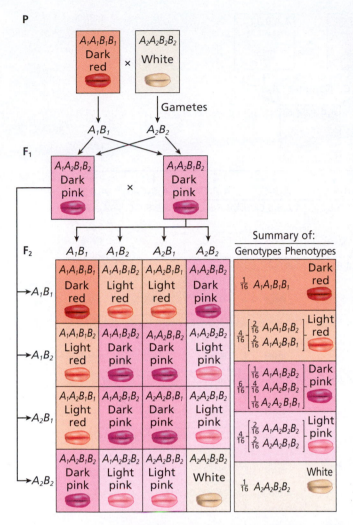

Figure 19.1   Polygenic inheritance of wheat kernel color controlled by two additive genes. Each number 1 allele (either A_1 or B_1) adds a unit of color, but number 2 alleles (A_2 or B_2) add no units of color. Pure-breeding parents (one dark red, one white) produce dihybrid F_1 with dark pink kernel color. Five phenotype classes are predicted among F_2 progeny in a ratio determined by the total number of A_1 plus B_1 alleles in the genotype.

Figure 19.1 shows a cross between pure-breeding dark red and pure-breeding white plants. The cross produces F_1 plants that are dihybrid ($A_1A_2B_1B_2$) and have dark pink kernel color as a consequence of carrying just two number 1 alleles. Crossing the F_1 plants produces an F_2 generation with five different kernel colors, each dependent on the total number of number 1 alleles in the genotype. For these two loci, genotypes can have a maximum of four number 1 alleles and a minimum of zero number 1 alleles. The five different totals of number 1 alleles produce the five different phenotypes in the F_2 generation, in proportions determined by independent assortment. Among the F_2, 1/16 carry four number 1 alleles and produce dark red kernels like the parental plant, 4/16 carry three number 1 alleles and have light red kernels, 6/16 have two number 1 alleles and have dark pink kernels, 4/16 carry a single number 1 allele and have light pink kernels, and the final 1/16 have no number 1 alleles and have white kernels like the parental plant.

As the number of additive genes contributing to a phenotypic trait increases, the number of phenotype categories also increases (see Pascal's triangle, Figure 2.14, and the associated discussion in Section 2.4). **Figure 19.2** illustrates an additive genetic model in which wheat kernel color is determined by three genes. In this example, genes A, B, and C each have two alleles whose additive effect is computed in the same way as for the two-gene system of Figure 19.1: Phenotype categories are determined by the number of 1 alleles contained in a genotype. A cross of pure-breeding dark red and pure-breeding white parental plants produces an F_1 of an intermediate (dark pink) color as a result of its trihybrid genotype ($A_1A_2B_1B_2C_1C_2$). Independent assortment produces an F_2 that falls into seven phenotypic categories that are determined by genotypes that have a maximum of six number 1 alleles and a minimum of zero number 1 alleles.

Continuous Phenotypic Variation from Multiple Additive Genes

The more phenotypes that occur along a limited scale of phenotype measurement, the narrower is the slice of the distribution each category occupies and the less obvious the demarcation between categories may become. **Figure 19.3** shows five histograms illustrating the distribution of F_2 phenotypes produced by different numbers of additive genes having two alleles each. As in the preceding examples, each number 1 allele adds a unit of color to the phenotype, but number 2 alleles do not. Notice that as the number of phenotype classes increases, the classes are more tightly packed, blending into a continuous phenotypic distribution in Figure 19.3e.

In a diploid organism, the number of distinct phenotype categories for a polygenic trait produced by the segregation of additive alleles of a given number of genes (n) is calculated as $2n + 1$. For example, for three additive

describing the determination of wheat kernel color by additive alleles of two genes. In this model, only genetic effects on phenotype are being considered. The model predicts that kernel color spans a spectrum from dark red to white. Gene A and gene B each have two alleles. Alleles A_1 and B_1 are equivalent to one another, each adding an equal unit of color to the phenotype. Alleles A_2 and B_2 are also equivalent, neither adding any units of color to the phenotype. Under the additive genetic model, the more "number 1" alleles, either A_1 or B_1, the genotype contains, the darker the color of wheat kernels. Conversely, the fewer number 1 alleles (or the more "number 2" alleles) there are in the genotype, the lighter the kernel color. The deepest red color (dark red) is present when four number 1 alleles are present ($A_1A_1B_1B_1$). Conversely, white kernels are produced when no copies of number 1 alleles are in the genotype ($A_2A_2B_2B_2$).

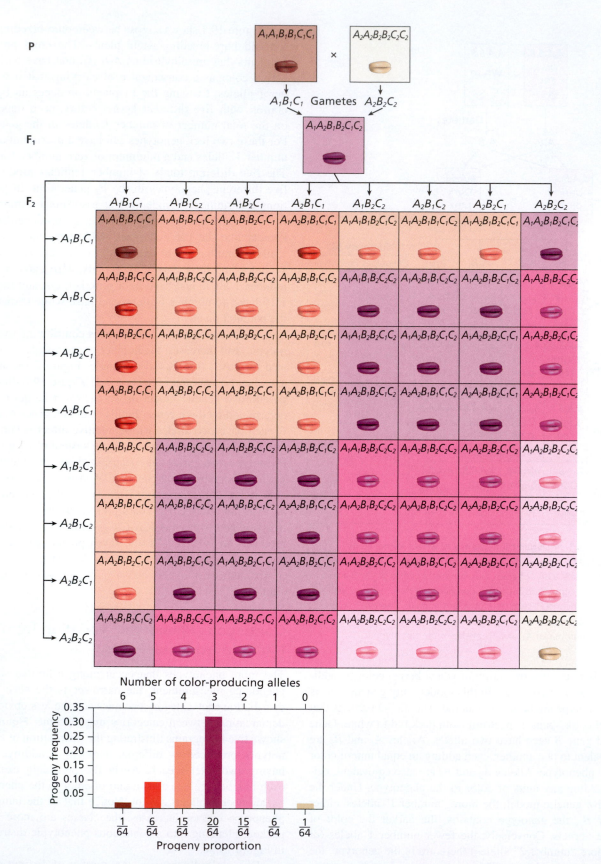

Figure 19.2 **A three-gene additive model for wheat kernel color.** Color is determined by total number of 1 alleles (A_1, B_1, and C_1) in the genotype. The F_2 have seven phenotypic classes in proportions generated by independent assortment at three loci.

Explain how additivity generates a continuous phenotypic distribution.

(a) One locus: $A_1A_2 \times A_1A_2$

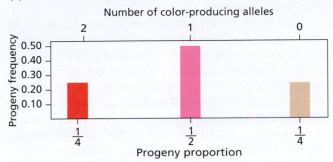

(b) Two loci: $A_1A_2B_1B_2 \times A_1A_2B_1B_2$

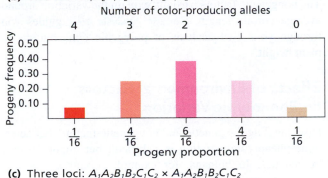

(c) Three loci: $A_1A_2B_1B_2C_1C_2 \times A_1A_2B_1B_2C_1C_2$

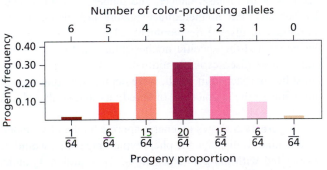

(d) Four loci: $A_1A_2B_1B_2C_1C_2D_1D_2 \times A_1A_2B_1B_2C_1C_2D_1D_2$

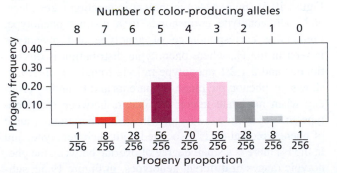

(e) Five loci: $A_1A_2B_1B_2C_1C_2D_1D_2E_1E_2 \times A_1A_2B_1B_2C_1C_2D_1D_2E_1E_2$

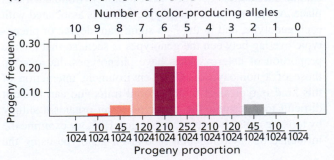

Figure 19.3 Phenotype distributions with additive genes. The parents producing progeny in each example are heterozygous for each gene. The color-contributing alleles are designated as 1 for each gene. The number of F_2 phenotype categories increases with the number of additive genes.

Q **If a trait was produced by the action of six additive genes, how many phenotype categories would there be?**

genes contributing to a polygenic trait, $n = 3$, and the number of distinct phenotypic categories is $2(3) + 1 = 7$. The expected frequencies of the most extreme phenotypes are (4^n). **Table 19.1** lists the numbers of phenotypic categories for different numbers of contributing genes and gives the frequency of the most extreme phenotypes in each distribution. If more than two alleles occur for the contributing genes, the number of phenotypes can increase.

Allele Segregation in Quantitative Trait Production

In 1916, plant geneticist Edward East undertook a comprehensive examination of the multiple-gene hypothesis by testing its ability to explain patterns of inherited variation that he produced in the length of the corolla (the petal-producing part of the flower) in *Nicotiana longiflora*. In this long-flower species of tobacco, the corolla is a tube-shaped structure whose length can be measured and compared with corollas in other plants.

East began his experiments with pure-breeding parental lines, one having a short corolla approximately 40 millimeters (mm) long and the other producing a long corolla of approximately 90 mm (**Figure 19.4**). Note that there is a small amount of variation in corolla length in each pure-breeding line, suggesting that despite attempts to produce pure-breeding lines, gene–gene interaction,

Table 19.1	The Effect of Multiple Contributing Genes on Phenotypic Variation	
Number of Genes	Number of Phenotype Categories	Frequency of Most Extreme Phenotypes
1	3	1/4
2	5	1/16
3	7	1/64
4	9	1/256
5	11	1/1024
6	13	1/4096
7	15	1/16,384
8	17	1/65,536
9	19	1/262,144
10	21	1/1,048,576

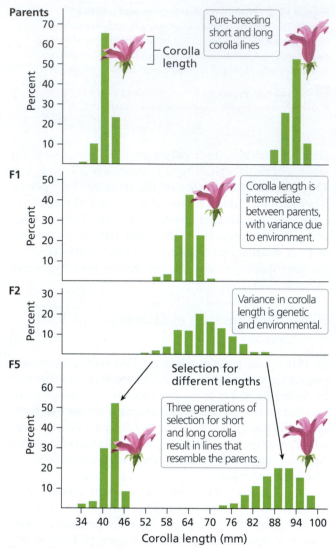

Figure 19.4 Corolla length in tobacco. Edward East determined that alleles of multiple genes control genetic variance in corolla length of tobacco (*Nicotiana longiflora*).

corolla lengths approximating those found in the original pure-breeding parents.

East reached two general conclusions based on his observations. Both conclusions are consistent with the models of continuous phenotypic variation of quantitative traits we have discussed. First, he concluded that corolla length in *Nicotiana longiflora,* particularly in the F_2, results from the segregation of alleles of multiple genes. Second, East concluded that the phenotypic expression of each genotype is influenced by nongenetic factors, that is, genes interacting with environmental factors to blur the direct correspondence between a given genotype and a specific phenotype. The nongenetic factors partially explain the variation around average corolla length. Genetic Analysis 19.1 guides you through your own analysis of polygenic contributions to plant height.

Effects of Environmental Factors on Phenotypic Variation

Disentangling the genetic and nongenetic factors that determine phenotypic variation is a difficult but important task in genetics. In humans, for example, common diseases such as heart disease, cancer, and diabetes are influenced by heredity, but nonhereditary factors are also critically important in disease development. Identifying the particular genes and the specific nonhereditary factors contributing to these diseases is the ultimate goal of research, but it must be approached in small, incremental steps that include modeling of the interactions of hereditary and nonhereditary factors.

Figure 19.5 shows a general approach taken by models of this kind. It displays the phenotypic ranges that would be associated with the genotypes A_1A_1, A_1A_2, and A_2A_2 under different assumptions of gene–environment interaction. In Figure 19.5a, no gene–environment interaction takes place, and each genotype corresponds to a distinct phenotype. Predictable correspondence of genotype and phenotype is seen in the F_2, where phenotypic distribution is discontinuous and a 1:2:1 phenotype ratio is found. Figure 19.5b shows the phenotypic ranges of parents and F_1 and F_2 progeny when moderate interaction occurs between the genotype and environmental factors. In each generation, a range of phenotypic values is associated with each genotype, and in the F_2, there is a small degree of overlap between the phenotypic ranges of different genotypes. In Figure 19.5c, substantial interaction between genes and environment takes place. A wide range of phenotypic values is associated with each genotype, and in the F_2 a significant degree of phenotypic overlap between the genotypes is seen, so that a large proportion of heterozygotes have phenotypes that overlap those of a homozygote. Gene–environment interaction of this kind is typical of multifactorial traits and can make it difficult to determine the genotype of an organism simply by looking at its phenotype. In Section 19.2, we examine the influence of environmental factors on genotype using the

environmental effects, or multifactorial effects produce some variability. The F_1 progeny of this cross had an average corolla length of about 65 mm, approximately midway between the parental averages. These "mid-parental" values are an indication of strong genetic control of corolla length. Once again, there is some variability around the average corolla length value, but none of the F_1 have corolla lengths that are near the parental values.

East allowed F_1 plants to self-fertilize to produce about 450 F_2, among which he observed a wider distribution of corolla length than in the F_1, although the average length was about the same as that of the F_1. None of the F_2 East produced had corolla lengths equal to those of the pure-breeding parental lines. Then, over three additional generations beginning with F_2, East selectively bred plants to produce a line having a short corolla and a line having a long corolla, achieving new collections of plants with

PROBLEM Dr. Ara B. Dopsis, a famous plant geneticist, develops several pure-breeding lines of daffodils. Under ideal growth conditions, line A plants are the tallest and grow to a height of 48 centimeters (cm), whereas line B plants are the shortest and grow to 12 cm. Dr. Dopsis devises a genetic model with three additive genes that contribute equally to explain polygenic inheritance of plant height. He assumes that line A has the genotype $A_1A_1B_1B_1C_1C_1$ and that line B has the genotype $A_2A_2B_2B_2C_2C_2$. In answering the following questions, assume that genotype alone determines plant height under ideal growth conditions.

> **BREAK IT DOWN:** Pure-breeding plants in line A and line B are homozygous for 1 and 2 alleles, respectively. Seven progeny categories will produce continuous variation in height (p. 699 and Figure 19.3c).

a. If these two pure-breeding parental plants are crossed, what will be the genotype and height of the F_1 progeny plants?

b. If F_2 are produced, what plant heights are expected and at what frequencies?

> **BREAK IT DOWN:** Three additive genes have a total of six alleles that make approximately equal contributions to continuous variation in plant height (p. 699).

Solution Strategies	Solution Steps
Evaluate	
1. Identify the topic this problem addresses and the nature of the required answer.	1. This problem concerns assessment of a three-gene additive model for plant height. The model is to be applied to crosses of pure-breeding parental plants of different heights to predict the frequencies of genotypes and heights in the F_1 and F_2 progeny.
2. Identify the critical information given in the problem.	2. The genotypes of the pure-breeding parents are given. In applying the polygenic additive model, we are to assume that genotype alone determines variation in plant height.
Deduce	
3. Deduce the contribution of each allele of the additive genes to height in line A. *TIP: Assume that each allele makes an equal contribution in this additive genetic model.*	3. The 48-cm height of line A plants is determined by six alleles of additive genes. Each 1 allele in the line A genotype contributes 48 cm/6 = 8 cm to plant height.
4. Deduce the contribution of each allele of the additive genes to height in line B.	4. Six alleles also contribute equally to the 12-cm height of line B plants. Each 2 allele in the line B genotype contributes 12 cm/6 = 2 cm to plant height.
5. Deduce the gametes produced by each pure-breeding line. *TIP: The laws of segregation and independent assortment apply to genes controlling polygenic traits.*	5. Line 1 has the genotype $A_1A_1B_1B_1C_1C_1$ and produces gametes with the genotype $A_1B_1C_1$. Line 2 has the genotype $A_2A_2B_2B_2C_2C_2$ and produces the gamete genotype $A_2B_2C_2$.
Solve	**Answer a**
6. Determine the genotype and height of F_1 plants.	6. F_1 progeny of these pure-breeding parental plants will have the genotype $A_1A_2B_1B_2C_1C_2$. Based on the contribution of each 1 and 2 allele, the predicted F_1 plant height is [(3)(8 cm)] + [(3)(2 cm)] = 30 cm.
	Answer b
7. Determine the frequency and height of each category of F_2 plants. *TIP: Either use Pascal's triangle (Figure 2.14) or determine the probability of genotypes containing different numbers of 1 and 2 alleles.* *PITFALL: Remember that for most categories there are multiple genotypes with the same total number of 1 and 2 alleles.*	7. The expected F_2 progeny are

Number of Alleles		Frequency	Height (cm)
1	2		
0	6	1/64	12
1	5	6/64	18
2	4	15/64	24
3	3	20/64	30
4	2	15/64	36
5	1	6/64	42
6	0	1/64	48

For more practice, see Problems 10 and 22.   Visit the Study Area to access study tools.

Mastering Genetics

Figure 19.5 **The effect of gene–environment interaction.** The phenotype determined by a single gene with codominant alleles can be modified by the action of environmental factors.

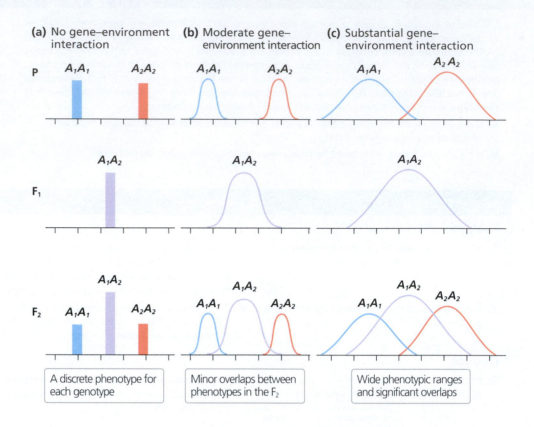

(a) No gene–environment interaction

(b) Moderate gene–environment interaction

(c) Substantial gene–environment interaction

A discrete phenotype for each genotype

Minor overlaps between phenotypes in the F₂

Wide phenotypic ranges and significant overlaps

term *environmental variance*. In that section, we employ a quantitative approach to determining how much of the variance in phenotype is due to environmental factors.

Threshold Traits

Most polygenic and multifactorial traits exhibit a continuous phenotypic distribution, but certain of these traits, while having an underlying continuous distribution, can nevertheless be divided into distinct categories. Such traits are often called **threshold traits**. Traits of this kind are especially important in medical contexts, where individuals are often classified (not always with great clarity) as falling into one of two clinical categories—"unaffected" (or "normal") and "affected" (or "abnormal")—to distinguish individuals who have an abnormality from those that do not. Traits such as cleft lip (the failure of the upper lip to fully close), cleft palate (the failure of the hard palate in the mouth to fully close), and congenital hip dysplasia (the misalignment of the upper leg bone ball with its socket on the hip) are examples of human traits in this category.

For human threshold traits, the vast majority of the population will have phenotypes on the unaffected side of the threshold and will display the normal phenotype. A small proportion of the population, however, will be situated on the affected side of the threshold and have the abnormal phenotype. Cases that lie at the borderline between the two categories can be problematic to diagnose.

The genetic hypothesis explaining threshold traits proposes that such traits are polygenic or multifactorial, so that

underlying the categorization of "affected" and "unaffected" phenotypes is a continuous phenotypic distribution. Some of the alleles contributing to the continuous distribution each carry a certain level of **genetic liability**—a term conveying the idea that certain alleles can push the phenotype toward the "affected" end of the continuous distribution. Each person's risk of having the affected phenotype is the result of the individual's genotype—or of the individual's genotype along with nongenetic influences, in cases of multifactorial phenotypes. Different genotypes may confer different amounts of genetic liability, making some individuals more likely to cross the threshold and display an affected phenotype. **Figure 19.6** shows a continuous distribution of genetic

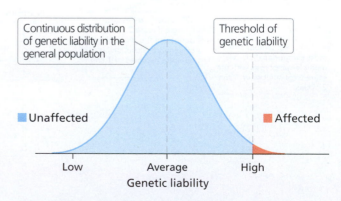

Continuous distribution of genetic liability in the general population

Threshold of genetic liability

■ Unaffected

■ Affected

Low   Average   High
Genetic liability

Figure 19.6 **Threshold traits.** A theoretical continuous phenotypic distribution and a threshold of genetic liability for a threshold trait.

liability for a population and the designation of a threshold that separates unaffected from affected individuals in the population. The portion of the population to the left of the **threshold of genetic liability**, by far the majority, are identified as unaffected or normal, and the small group to the right of the threshold are classified as affected or abnormal.

Models used to simulate these concepts generally assume that alleles of the genes affecting the trait are distributed as described by Mendel's law of independent assortment and that the threshold of liability that marks the transition from unaffected to affected is crossed when a sufficient number of "liability alleles" are present in the genotype. For example, **Figure 19.7** depicts a hypothetical three-gene model in which alleles are designated as either

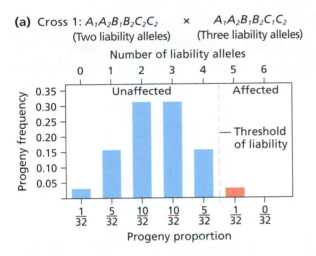

(a) Cross 1: $A_1A_2B_1B_2C_2C_2$ × $A_1A_2B_1B_2C_1C_2$
(Two liability alleles)   (Three liability alleles)

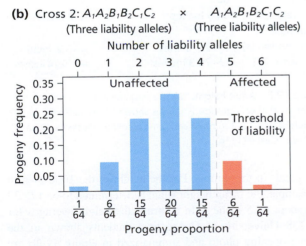

(b) Cross 2: $A_1A_2B_1B_2C_1C_2$ × $A_1A_2B_1B_2C_1C_2$
(Three liability alleles)   (Three liability alleles)

Figure 19.7   A polygenic model for a threshold trait. Any allele designated as 1 confers genetic liability, any allele designated as 2 confers no liability, and the 1 alleles are additive. **(a)** In Cross 1, the couple has a 1/32 chance of producing an affected child. **(b)** In Cross 2, the couple has a 7/64 chance of producing an affected child.

Q Explain why the siblings of an affected child of either of the couples illustrated are at greater risk of having the condition than the siblings of unaffected children from the general population.

1 or 2 at each locus. The genetic liability increases with a greater number of 1 alleles. In this model, the threshold of liability is passed when at least five 1 alleles are present. Because independent assortment drives the distribution of alleles from parents to offspring, a greater number of 1 alleles in parental genotypes increases the proportion of progeny that will cross the threshold of liability and display an affected phenotype. The model can compare the risks of having a child affected by a threshold trait for parents carrying different numbers of liability alleles. Notice that the overall shape of the phenotypic distribution is reminiscent of the kind of continuous distribution expected for polygenic traits. The difference here is that one end of the continuous distribution crosses the phenotypic threshold into the affected category.

Cross 1, in Figure 19.7a, is between a parent with two 1 alleles and a parent with three 1 alleles. Both parents have the unaffected (normal) phenotype. Among the progeny of this cross, 1/32 (3%) are expected to carry five 1 alleles, but none can carry six 1 alleles. Thus, 1/32 is the chance that a child of this cross will have the affected phenotype. Figure 19.7b shows Cross 2, with parents that each carry three liability alleles. Neither of these parents is affected, but because together they carry more liability alleles than the parents in Cross 1 (six liability alleles versus five liability alleles), independent assortment predicts that among their offspring 7/64 (11%) will have genotypes that contain five or more 1 alleles and will have the affected phenotype. Notice that like the phenotypic distribution depicted in Figure 19.7a, this distribution is continuous, with one end of the distribution crossing the threshold into the affected category.

The parental genotypes in Cross 2 lead to an almost fourfold increased risk (3% versus 11%) of producing an affected offspring compared with Cross 1. This difference is analogous to the difference we might see between different families in a population. Overall, a mating in the general population has a low risk of producing a child with a threshold trait. Different families may have different risks, however, and a mating of parents that both come from families with a history of the trait will be most likely to produce children who also have the trait. This kind of modeling also supports the observation that if neither of the parents is affected but they have a child that is affected, there is an elevated risk of the affected phenotype recurring in a subsequent child. It also supports an observation concerning **first-degree relatives**, individuals such as siblings and parents and children who share 50% of their genes. The observation is that if a person is affected by a polygenic or threshold trait, his or her first-degree relatives are more likely than an average person in the population to be affected by the trait or condition. This elevated risk is due to the sharing of genetic liability within families.

The influence of environmental and developmental factors on phenotypes of threshold traits is an important additional component contributing to the probability of expressing a particular trait. These factors can play a role in determining whether individuals whose genetic liability places them near the threshold of liability express the affected phenotype or not. Gene–gene interactions such as epistasis (see Section 4.3) can also contribute to phenotype outcomes of threshold traits.

19.2 Quantitative Trait Analysis Is Statistical

The statistical methods applied today to the study of quantitative traits are a direct extension of contributions made nearly a century ago by statistician and evolutionary biologist Sir Ronald Fisher. In 1918, Fisher used statistical analysis to show that quantitative traits result from the segregation of alleles of multiple genes displaying an additive effect. Fisher also showed that interactions between genes (i.e., epistasis) can be detected by these methods. In addition, he explored the role of gene–environment interaction and concluded that environmental factors contribute to continuous variation by blurring the lines between phenotypic classes. The tools and approaches described here and pioneered by Fisher allow scientists to identify genetic influences on phenotypes in terms of quantitative measurement rather than qualitative appearance.

Statistical Description of Phenotypic Variation

The first step in quantifying the phenotypic variation of a trait in a population is to construct a **frequency distribution** of values of the trait on a quantitative scale.

A frequency distribution shows what proportion of the population exhibits each measured value of the trait or falls into each category defined for the trait. **Figure 19.8a** provides an example, showing the number and frequency of each designated height category in a sample of 1000 college-aged males.

Since the individuals in this study were not selected for any attribute related to height, they are considered a random sample of college-aged males. Random samples are used in quantitative trait analysis for two reasons. First, it is often impossible or impractical to collect data on every individual in a population; and second, random samples can be just as accurate in the statistical sense as "samples" consisting of whole populations. As an analogy, about 10 milliliters of blood—approximately two-tenths of 1% of a person's total blood volume—is drawn for most routine blood tests. The amount taken is not large enough to cause physiological problems, but it is representative enough to provide dependable information concerning a person's health status.

After the frequency distribution is constructed, the first piece of information to be calculated is the average, or **mean**, value ($\bar{x}$) of the distribution. This is calculated by summing all the values in the sample and dividing by the total number of

(a) Number and frequency of heights in 3-cm intervals

Height (cm)	Number	Frequency (%)
155–157	4	0.4
158–160	8	0.8
161–163	26	2.6
164–166	53	5.3
167–169	89	8.9
170–172	146	14.6
173–175	188	18.8
176–178	181	18.1
179–181	125	12.5
182–184	92	9.2
185–187	60	6.0
188–190	22	2.2
191–193	4	0.4
194–196	1	0.1
197–199	1	0.1
	1000	100

(b) Number of females and males of each height

Female		Male	
Height (in)	Number	Height (in)	Number
60	5	64	2
61	5	65	5
62	7	66	2
63	7	67	6
64	9	68	7
65	9	69	7
66	12	70	9
67	6	71	6
68	3	72	10
69	2	73	7
70	1	74	2
71	1	75	3
72	1	76	1
		77	3

Total	68		70
Average ($\bar{x}$)	64.5 inches	70.2 inches	
Standard deviation (s)	+/– 2.7 inches	+/– 3.2 inches	
Variance (s^2)	+/– 7.29 inches	+/– 10.24 inches	

Figure 19.8 **Adult height.** **(a)** The frequency distribution of height in 1000 college-aged males is shown in tabular form. **(b)** Height data for 138 male and female college students. Data from W.E. Castle (1916)

individuals in the sample. For the height of the 1000 men in this sample, the mean height value is determined to be 175.33 cm (about 68.5 inches). In contrast, the height averages for the 138 University of Connecticut students shown in the chapter-opening photo and summarized in **Figure 19.8b** are 64.5 inches for the women and 70.2 inches for the men. Both of these values are very close to the current U.S. population averages. The increase of 1.7 inches in average male height is likely an example of the influence of improved nutrition and child and maternal health on adult height.

Frequency distributions vary depending on several factors, including the sample size and the number of classification categories for the trait. When graphed, the distinct frequency distributions dictated by different data sets can have different shapes, as is seen for the three distributions depicted in **Figure 19.9.** As a consequence of such differences in distributions, it is necessary to provide a statistical description of the shape of the frequency distribution when comparing trait values. For example, it is important to report the **mode**, or **modal value**, that is, the most common value in a distribution. For the height data shown in Figure 19.8a, the mode is the 173–175 cm category, containing 188 individual values. Each distribution also possesses a middle value, known as the **median**, or **median value**. In the height distribution, you can think of the median value as entry number 500 (in order of increasing height) of the 1000 entries in the distribution. This median value also resides in the 173–175 cm category.

Data in the real world are usually skewed—that is, unevenly distributed on either side of the mean, as Figure 19.8a and the chapter-opening photo both illustrate. Therefore, to describe the frequency distribution, we must

also have ways of measuring (and thus describing) the nature of the distribution around the mean. Two forms of measurement are commonly used.

The first, called the **variance (s^2)**, is a numerical measure of the spread of the distribution around the mean. This measure interprets how much variation exists among individuals in the sample. The variance value depends on the relationship between the width of the distribution and the number of observations in the sample. It will be small if all the observations are close to the mean, and it will be large if the observations are widely spread around the mean (see Figure 19.9). The variance is determined by summing the squares of the difference between each individual value and the sample mean and dividing that sum by the number of degrees of freedom (df) in the sample. The number of degrees of freedom is equal to the number of independent variables. Squaring the differences between individual values and the sample mean prevents positive and negative differences from canceling each other out. This is why the variance is expressed as squared units:

$$s^2 = \sum (x_i - \bar{x})^2 / \mathrm{df}$$

In our example of variation in a quantitative phenotype, the variance is described as **phenotypic variance (V_P)**. Figure 19.8a reports the measured values for height in centimeters, so the variance would be expressed in centimeters squared.

The second measure that describes the distribution of data is the **standard deviation (s)**, a value expressing deviation from the mean in the same units as the scale of measurement for the sample. The standard deviation (s) is calculated as $\sqrt{s^2}$. In our sample of the heights of 1000 college-aged males, $V_P = s^2 = 43.30 \ \mathrm{cm}^2$, and the standard deviation is $s = 6.58 \ \mathrm{cm}$. In a recent sample of 138 college students enrolled in a genetics course, the standard deviations and variances for height of the 68 females and 70 males are reported in inches as 64.5 +/− 2.7 inches for females and 70.2 +/− 3.2 inches for males (see Figure 19.8b).

Partitioning Phenotypic Variance

A key part of analyzing quantitative trait variation is quantifying the effect of factors thought to contribute to phenotypic variance, V_P. Quantitative phenotypes are the joint product of genes, environment, and gene interactions; consequently, phenotypic variance can be partitioned among those influences. As a first step, the phenotypic variance can be divided into two principal components: *genetic variance* (V_G) and *environmental variance* (V_E). Under this assumption, phenotypic variance can be expressed as genetic variance plus environmental variance: $V_P = V_G + V_E$.

In this expression, **genetic variance (V_G)** is the proportion of phenotypic variance that is due to differences among genotypes. In highly inbred populations in which all individuals are homozygous for alleles controlling a quantitative phenotype, $V_G = 0$. Such populations are found only

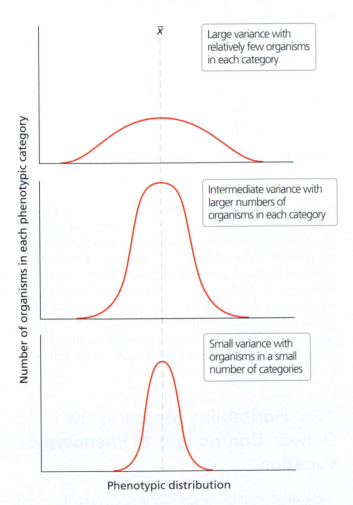

Figure 19.9 Distributions and variance. The shape of curves depicting variance is changed by the sample size and the number of outcome classes. Variance around the average is correspondingly large, intermediate, and small.

🔵 **How do you think the number of phenotypic categories might be related to the variance?**

after strictly controlled laboratory inbreeding, however; they are rarely found in nature, due to the ubiquitous presence of genetic variation in natural populations. Genetic variation in natural populations generates individuals with different genotypes for quantitative traits and leads to phenotypic variability that is directly attributable to the genetic variability.

Environmental variance (V_E) is the portion of phenotypic variance that is due to variability of the environments inhabited by individual members of a population. Differences in sun exposure, in water and nutrient content of the soil, and in exposure to pests are examples of environmental variables that influence V_E in plants. Carefully controlled laboratory experiments can sometimes control all of the environmental variables and produce a situation in which V_E approximates zero. In nature, however, such circumstances rarely occur. Individual members of natural populations are almost certain to experience variability in the environmental conditions they encounter.

Some differences may be systematic and predictable. For example, members of a plant population growing below a natural spring will experience wetter growth conditions than plants living above the spring. Other environmental variables are sporadic or unpredictable. For example, a dry year might reduce the flow of water from a natural spring and affect the plants living below the spring more severely than those living above it.

Let's use an example to illustrate the dissection of V_G and V_E as components of V_P. Suppose that two different pure-breeding parental lines are established. Each line is genetically uniform, with $V_G = 0$; therefore, $V_P = V_E$ (**Figure 19.10a**). The pure-breeding lines are crossed to produce F_1 progeny that are genetically uniform. In the F_1, $V_G = 0$ because there is no genetic variation among the individuals, and $V_P = V_E$ (**Figure 19.10b**). Production of F_2, however, leads to genotypic variation and thus to the production of phenotypic variation that results from a combination of genetic variance and environmental variance (**Figure 19.10c**). Among the F_2, $V_P = V_E + V_G$. Since V_E has been determined for the parents and the F_1, genetic variance can be calculated by subtracting environmental variance from the phenotypic variance among the F_2. In other words, $V_G = V_P - V_E$. **Genetic Analysis 19.2** provides practice in determining environmental and genetic variance.

Partitioning Genetic Variance

Each allelic difference affecting a quantitative trait contributes to genetic variance in a population, but not necessarily each in the same way. Indeed, it can be difficult to measure the specific effect of each allelic variant. Nevertheless, genetic variance can theoretically be partitioned into three different *kinds* of allelic effects. **Additive variance** (V_A) derives from the additive effects of all alleles contributing to a trait. Additive variance is the result of incomplete dominance of alleles at a locus, which causes heterozygotes to have a phenotype intermediate between the homozygous

(a) Parental lines

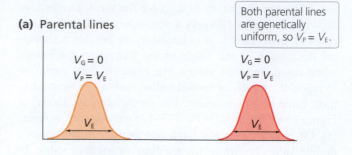

(b) F_1 progeny

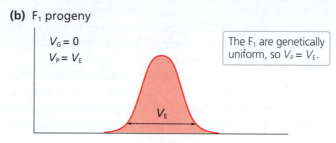

(c) F_2 progeny

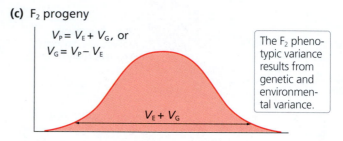

FIGURE 19.10   Sources of phenotypic variance.

phenotypes. **Dominance variance** (V_D) is variance resulting from dominance relationships in which alleles of a heterozygote produce a phenotype that is not exactly intermediate between those of homozygotes (i.e., the nonadditive effects of alleles of contributing genes). Lastly, **interactive variance** (V_I) derives from epistatic interactions between the alleles of different genes that influence a quantitative phenotype. Collectively these three components unite to produce the genetic variance in a model summarized by $V_G = V_A + V_D + V_I$. We use these values in the following section to discuss *heritability*.

19.3 Heritability Measures the Genetic Component of Phenotypic Variation

One goal of quantitative genetics is to estimate the extent to which genetic variation influences the phenotypic variation seen in a trait. This is a challenging task under many circumstances and particularly so when a trait is determined by a combination of genetic variation, environmental variation, and gene–environment interaction. The concept of trait

PROBLEM Two pure-breeding lines of tomatoes, P_1 and P_2, producing fruit with different average weights, are crossed. The means and variances of their F_1 and F_2 progeny are shown in the table to the right.

a. What is the environmental variance (V_E) for this trait?

b. What is the genetic variance (V_G) determined from the F_2?

Line	Average Fruit Weight (g)	V_P
P_1	6.5	$1.6\ g^2$
P_2	14.2	$3.5\ g^2$
F_1	10.2	$2.2\ g^2$
F_2	9.8	$4.0\ g^2$

BREAK IT DOWN: Phenotypic variance equals genetic variance plus environmental variance. The three values can be manipulated to isolate and quantify one value at a time (p. 708).

Solution Strategies	Solution Steps
Evaluate	
1. Identify the topic this problem addresses and the nature of the required answer.	1. This problem concerns the determination of environmental variance and genetic variance for the tomato plant data given.
2. Identify the critical information given in the problem.	2. Fruit weight and phenotypic variance are given for the two pure-breeding parental lines and for the F_1 and F_2 progeny.
Deduce	
3. Describe the relationship between V_P, V_G, and V_E.	3. $V_P = V_G + V_E$
4. Identify the variance values that contribute to V_P in each line and generation. TIP: For organisms that are genetically identical, $V_P = V_E$.	4. Each of the pure-breeding parental lines (P_1 and P_2) and the F_1 progeny are genetically uniform. As a consequence, all phenotypic variance is due to environmental variance, and genetic variance makes no contribution. The F_2 contains genotypic variety, so both V_G and V_E contribute to V_P.
Solve	**Answer a**
5. Determine VE for this trait.	5. In the genetically uniform P_1, P_2, and F_1, $V_G = 0$, and in each line $V_P = V_E$. The average environmental variance among these three lines is calculated as $(1.6 + 3.5 + 2.2)/3 = 2.43$ grams.
	Answer b
6. Determine V_G for this trait.	6. V_G is calculated by rearranging the expression in step 3 to $V_G = V_P - V_E$. The genetic variance for these data is $V_G = 4.0 - 2.43 = 1.57$ grams.

For more practice, see Problems 4, 12, and 14.   Visit the Study Area to access study tools.   **Mastering** Genetics

---

heritability was developed to help measure the proportion of phenotypic variation that is due to genetic variation.

Heritability differs from trait to trait, and it can change for the same trait measured in different environments or under different conditions. Heritability is an important measure of the potential responsiveness of a trait to natural selection or artificial selection. It is of special interest to evolutionary biologists and to plant and animal breeders, who use it to assess the potential impact of selection on traits of agricultural or economic importance.

A high heritability value indicates that most of the observed phenotypic variation is due to genetic variation. Such a finding implies that the trait can be strongly influenced by natural selection or by artificial selection programs focused on changing the frequency of a phenotype in a population. Conversely, a low heritability value indicates that little of the observed phenotypic variation is due to inherited genetic variation, but that most of it is due to influences of the environment, so the expression of the trait in a population is not effectively changed by selection processes. Two widely used measures of heritability assess different components of the contribution of genetic variation to phenotypic variation. **Broad sense heritability (H^2)** estimates the proportion of phenotypic variation that is due to total genetic variation. This form of heritability is defined by the equality $H^2 = V_G/V_P$. **Narrow sense heritability (h^2)** estimates the proportion of phenotypic variation that is due to additive genetic variation. Narrow sense heritability is defined by the equality $h^2 = V_A/V_P$. Both measures of heritability are expressed as proportions that range in magnitude from 0.0 to 1.0. In all cases, greater heritability values indicate a larger role for genetic variation in phenotypic variation.

Heritability is easily misunderstood. An erroneous understanding can lead to the mistaken idea that genetic variation makes a much larger contribution to phenotypic variation than the data actually support. Heritability is difficult to apply to humans except under limited circumstances (described later in the discussion of twin studies), but it can be used for other organisms. The following attributes of heritability are central to its meaning:

1. Heritability is a measure of the degree to which *genetic differences* contribute to *phenotypic variation* of a trait. In other words, heritability is high when much of the phenotypic variation is produced by genetic variation and little is contributed by environmental variation. Heritability *is not* an indication of the mechanism by which genes control a trait, nor is it a measure of how much of a trait is produced by gene action.

2. Heritability values are accurate only for the environment and population in which they are measured. Heritability values measured in one population cannot be transferred to another population, because both genetic and environmental factors may differ between populations.

3. Heritability for a given trait in a population can change if environmental factors change, and changes in the proportions of genotypes in a population can alter the effect of environmental factors on phenotypic variation, thus changing heritability.

4. High heritability does not mean that a trait is not influenced by environmental factors. Traits with high heritability can be very responsive to environmental changes.

Broad Sense Heritability

We have seen that genetic variance (V_G) is a composite value that derives its magnitude from additive, dominance, and interaction variance. Unfortunately, genetic variance is not always easy to partition into these separate components. Fortunately, broad sense heritability ($H^2 = V_G/V_P$) can be used as a general measure of the magnitude of genetic influence over phenotypic variation of a trait, when V_G cannot be partitioned.

In a 1988 study of the genetics and evolution of cave fish (*Astyanax fasciatus*), Horst Wilkens used broad sense heritability analysis to describe the genetic contribution to the evolution of the organism's eye tissue. Some populations of this species live in completely dark underground cave streams in eastern Mexico and have a dramatically reduced amount of eye tissue in comparison with closely related fish living aboveground. In these populations, the eye tissue appears to be undergoing rapid evolutionary change. The eyes in sighted fish of this species are approximately 0.7 cm in diameter. In comparison, blind cave fish have less than 0.2 cm of eye tissue diameter.

Wilkens crossed sighted cave fish with blind cave fish, measured eye tissue mean and variance in the F_1,

and then produced F_2 fish and measured their eye tissue as well. Since the F_1 fish were nearly genetically uniform, the variance in the amount of eye tissue was due entirely to the environment. In these F_1, V_E was 0.057 cm^2. Among the F_2, phenotypic variance (V_P) was 0.563 cm^2 and was the result of both genetic and environmental variance ($V_G + V_E$). Broad sense heritability is derived by determining V_G and dividing it by phenotypic variation. In this case,

$$V_G = V_P - V_E = 0.563 - 0.057 = 0.506$$
$$H^2 = V_G/V_P = 0.506/0.563 = 0.899$$

This broad sense heritability of approximately 0.90 means that approximately 90% of the phenotypic variation in eye size between these populations of cave fish is due to genetic variation.

Twin Studies

Heritability can be quantified when both mating and environmental factors can be controlled. However, when mating and environmental variation are not among the controlled experimental parameters, heritability is far more difficult—some would say impossible—to measure accurately. This limitation applies to attempts to measure the heritability of traits in humans. Fortunately, studies of phenotypic variation in human twins can offer insights into broad sense heritability of human traits.

Identical twins, also known as monozygotic (MZ) twins, are produced by a single fertilization event that is followed by a splitting of the fertilized embryo into two zygotes. MZ twins share all of their alleles. Theoretically, broad sense heritability can be determined by assuming that phenotypic variance between them is fully attributable to environmental variance. Under this assumption, in MZ twin pairs, $V_P = V_E$.

Fraternal twins, on the other hand, are dizygotic (DZ), produced by two independent fertilization events that take place at the same time. DZ twins are siblings that are born at the same time, but they are no more closely related than siblings born at different times. Like all full siblings, DZ twins have an average of 50% of their alleles in common. To control for differences between the sexes, only DZ twins of the same sex are used in twin studies. Phenotypic variance between DZ twins is the sum of environmental variance plus one-half of the genetic variance (the 50% of alleles not shared by the average DZ twin pair): In DZ twin pairs, $V_P = V_E + 1/2V_G$. On the basis of these general formulas for calculation of H^2, broad sense heritability can be estimated for human traits by methods we do not discuss here (Table 19.2).

Studies of traits in human twins usually compare MZ twins with same-sex DZ twins to make heritability estimates

Table 19.2	Selected Broad Sense Heritability (H^2) Values from Human Twin Studies	
Trait	**Heritability (H^2), %**	
Biological Traits		
Total fingerprint ridge count	90	
Height	85	
Maximum heart rate	85	
Club foot	80	
Amino acid excretion	70	
Weight	60	
Total serum cholesterol	60	
Blood pressure	60	
Body mass index (BMI)	50	
Longevity	29	
Behavioral Traits		
Verbal ability	65	
Sociability index	65	
Temperament index	60	
Spelling aptitude	50	
Memory	50	
Mathematical aptitude	30	

Because of the difficulties and the potential sources of error in making heritability estimates based on twin studies, the values in Table 19.2 are more likely to be too high than too low.

The study of identical twins reared together versus those reared apart is an alternative approach to estimating the influence of genes on phenotypic variation. Such studies measure the **concordance,** the percentage of twin pairs in which both members of the pair have the same phenotype for a trait, versus the **discordance,** the percentage in which the twins of a pair have dissimilar phenotypes for a trait. Concordance and discordance frequencies give a general picture of the overall influence of genes on phenotypes. If phenotypic variation for a trait is 100% genetic, MZ twins should always be concordant for their phenotypes, whether reared together or apart. In this case, concordance would be 100%. DZ twins share an average of 50% of their genes in common and would have concordance of about 50% for a trait whose variation is completely genetic. When phenotypic variation of a trait is due entirely to nongenetic factors, on the other hand, concordance among MZ and DZ twins will be approximately equal.

For the intermediate situation in which phenotypic variation of a trait is determined to a significant extent by genetic variation, concordance among MZ twin pairs will be high, and it will be substantially greater than for DZ twins. Because MZ twins share not only genes but also a common environment, a high concordance value alone does not necessarily indicate strong genetic influence. Even so, measuring a substantial difference in concordance rates between MZ and DZ twins is consistent with the possibility of strong genetic influence on a trait.

Table 19.3, showing MZ and DZ twin concordance values for some common medical and behavioral conditions, offers an opportunity for interpretation of the role genetics may play in the production of the conditions listed. A comparison of the MZ and DZ concordance values for medical conditions such as cleft lip and club foot indicates a prominent role for genetics. In each of these conditions, the concordance of MZ twins is several-fold greater than DZ concordance. On the other hand, heart attack concordance values show little evidence of genetic influence. Similarly, values for handedness, although highly concordant in all twins, show no difference between MZ versus DZ twin pairs, suggesting strong environmental or learning influence.

Behavioral conditions present a much greater challenge in that both their diagnosis and genetic investigation is more complex. Data aggregated from multiple studies indicate a moderate level of genetic influence on the development of bipolar disorder and schizophrenia. Numerous studies have examined the genome in an attempt to identify specific gene variants that are strongly associated with the development of these conditions. Multiple family studies have identified numerous candidate genes that may be involved in generating the conditions in families, but none of the candidates have shown the same level of significance in larger population-based studies. Autism spectrum disorders (ASD) are

more accurate. Even so, heritability studies of human twins are prone to several sources of error that lead to inaccurately high values. Following are the most common sources of error:

1. *Stronger shared maternal effects in identical twins than in fraternal twins.* These effects include the sharing of embryonic membranes and other aspects of the uterine environment that lead to more similar developmental conditions for identical twins than for fraternal twins.

2. *Greater similarity of treatment of identical twins than of fraternal twins.* Parents, other adults, and peers have a tendency to treat identical twins more equally than they treat fraternal twins of the same sex. This gives identical twins a similar social and behavioral environmental experience, whereas fraternal twins more often are treated differently.

3. *Greater similarity of interactions between genes and environmental factors in identical twins than in fraternal twins.* Identical twins have the same genotype and are affected in similar, if not identical, ways by environmental factors. On the other hand, fraternal twins have genetic differences that can be influenced differently by environmental factors. This may result in greater variance between fraternal twins than between identical twins.

Table 19.3	Concordance Values for Common Medical and Behavioral Conditions in Humans	
Trait	**Percent Concordance**	
	MZ Twins	**DZ Twins**
Medical Conditions with Likely Genetic Influence		
Cleft lip	40	4
Club foot	30	2
Congenital hip dislocation	35	3
Epilepsy	60	20
Multiple sclerosis	30	6
Pyloric stenosis	25	3
Rheumatoid arthritis	35	6
Medical Conditions Unlikely to Have Strong Genetic Influence		
Handedness (left and right)	79	77
Heart attack (both sexes)	37	20
Behavioral Conditions with Likely Genetic Influence		
Bipolar disorder[a]	40–60	8–10
Schizophrenia[b]	35–75	10–28
Autism spectrum disorder[c,d]	60–82	10–25

[a] Smoller, J. W., and C. T. Finn. 2003. *Am. J. Med. Genet.* 123C: 48.
[b] Sullivan, P. F., et al. 2003. *Arch. Gen. Psychiatry* 60:1187.
[c] Hallmayer, J., et al. 2011. *Arch. Gen. Psychiatry* 68:1095.
[d] Folstein, S., and M. Rutter. 1977. *J. Child. Psychol. Psychiatry* 18:297.

Table 19.4	Selected Narrow Sense Heritability (h^2) Values for Animals and Plants	
Organism	**Trait**	**Heritability (h^2)**
Cattle	Body weight	0.65
	Milk production	0.40
Corn	Plant height	0.70
	Ear length	0.55
	Ear diameter	0.14
Horse	Racing speed	0.60
	Trotting speed	0.40
Pig	Back-fat thickness	0.70
	Weight gain	0.40
	Litter size	0.05
Poultry	Body weight (8 weeks)	0.50
	Egg production	0.20

particularly challenging to study, due to the diversity of the conditions categorized as ASD and the complex genetic picture they present. Concordance values suggest that genes play a part in ASD, but as with studies of bipolar disorder and schizophrenia, none of the numerous candidate genes that have been suggested have been identified as causal in large population-based studies. The Case Study in this chapter explores the genetics of ASD in more detail.

Narrow Sense Heritability and Artificial Selection

Narrow sense heritability ($h^2 = V_A/V_P$) estimates the proportion of phenotypic variation that is due to additive genetic variance (V_A), variance resulting from the alleles of additive genes. These estimates are particularly useful in agriculture, where they predict the potential responsiveness of a trait in an animal or plant to artificial selection imposed through selective breeding programs or controlled growth conditions. High narrow sense heritability values are correlated with a greater degree of response to selection than low values, because additive genetic variance is responsive to selection.

Table 19.4 gives examples of h^2 values, covering a broad spectrum of magnitude, for several characteristics of plants and animals. Since higher h^2 values have the strongest correlation with selection response, biologists predict that traits such as body weight in cattle, back-fat thickness in pigs, and plant height in corn will be most amenable to change through artificial selection schemes. On the other hand, litter size in pigs, egg production in poultry, and ear diameter in corn have low h^2 values and will be less responsive to selection.

Estimating the potential response to selection for a trait begins with calculation of a value known as the **selection differential (S)**, which measures the difference between the population mean value for a trait and the mean trait value for the mating portion of a population. Suppose, for example, that a goal of an artificial selection experiment is to increase plant height. Choosing taller-than-average plants to mate will be an effective way to increase the height of progeny if h^2 is high. If the population average height is 37.5 cm and the average height of plants selected for mating is 42 cm, then $S = 42$ cm $- 37.5$ cm $= 4.5$ cm.

The potential **response to selection (R)** depends on the extent to which the difference between the mating trait mean value and the population mean value can be passed on to progeny. This probability is estimated using the formula $R = S(h^2)$. For this plant height example, let's use the value for corn plant height, $h^2 = 0.70$ (see Table 19.4). The estimated response to selection would be $R = (4.5$ cm$)(0.70) = 3.15$ cm. Under stable growth conditions, the progeny plants could be expected to have a height equal to the population average plus the value of R, or 37.5 cm $+ 3.15$ cm $= 40.65$ cm. Narrow sense heritability can be measured by rearranging the terms in the response-to-selection equation to $h^2 = R/S$. For the plant-height example, $h^2 = 3.15$ cm$/4.5$ cm $= 0.70$.

Estimates of heritability have important practical applications for plant and animal breeders, and for evolutionary biologists. Whether traits are subjected to artificial selection by breeders or to natural selection, the extent to which the mean value of a trait changes in a population depends on its heritability. Breeders and evolutionary biologists predict substantial change in trait mean values (i.e., large values for R) when heritability is high, but little or no change in trait mean values when heritability is low. In other words, traits evolve when a substantial proportion of the phenotypic variation is due to genetic variation.

Figure 19.11a shows three examples in which the selection differentials are the same but the response to

selection differs as a result of different degrees of heritability. This comparison illustrates that selection response is expected to be maximal when heritability is $h^2 = 1.0$. Selection response is substantially less when heritability is $h^2 = 0.2$, and there is no selection response when heritability is $h^2 = 0$. Figure 19.11b shows selection operating over many generations in three different modes that have different effects on phenotypic means and variances. In the mode known as **directional selection**, the mean phenotypic value is shifted in one direction because one extreme of the phenotype distribution is favored. This narrows the phenotypic range and reduces phenotypic variance. In contrast, selection favoring an intermediate phenotype over extreme phenotypes results in **stabilizing selection** that reduces the phenotypic variance without shifting the mean value. **Disruptive selection** occurs when both extreme phenotypes are favored over intermediate phenotypes. The result is an increase in the phenotypic variance and, potentially, a phenotypic split within the population. These modes can operate in both artificial selection and natural selection.

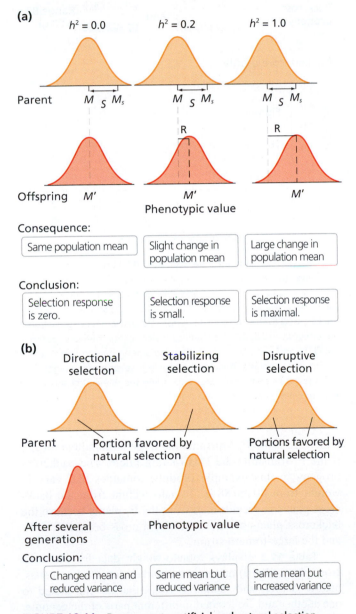

FIGURE 19.11 **Responses to artificial and natural selection.** (a) Response to artificial selection after one generation depends on h^2. M is mean phenotype in parental generation; M_S is the mean phenotype selected for mating; M' is the mean phenotype of offspring after selection; selection differential is $S = M_S - M$. (b) Three modes of artificial or natural selection produce different results after several generations.

19.4 Quantitative Trait Loci Are the Genes That Contribute to Quantitative Traits

The genes that contribute to the variation in a quantitative trait are collectively called **quantitative trait loci (QTLs)**. Individually, a gene that contributes to a quantitative trait is referred to as a **quantitative trait locus**. QTLs were initially of interest in agricultural plants such as tomatoes and corn, where they influence important attributes such as fruit sweetness, acidity, and color. The analysis of QTLs has expanded greatly in recent decades and been used to study many distinct traits in plants and animals, including humans.

In one way, QTLs are no different from other genes we discuss. For example, they often produce polypeptides that operate in metabolic pathways to produce compounds that give flavor or color to fruit. Identifying QTLs by experimental analysis is different from identifying other genes that control phenotypic variation, however, because many genes are influencing the trait, and the presence or absence of any one allele does not correlate well with distinct phenotypes. Specialized statistical methods have been developed to detect and map QTLs. This process is called **QTL mapping**, and it involves the identification of chromosome regions that are likely to contain QTLs.

The general process of QTL mapping is similar to the methods used to determine genetic linkage between genes. A chromosome region likely to contain a QTL is identified by the frequent co-occurrence of a specific genetic marker such as a single nucleotide polymorphism (SNP) in organisms with a particular phenotype.

The inherited DNA sequence variation of a SNP is usually not the molecular basis of the QTL. Instead, the SNP is usually genetically linked to the QTL. The connection between the genetic marker and the phenotype implies that a QTL exists near the genome location encoding the genetic marker.

QTL Mapping Strategies

Contemporary QTL mapping uses DNA markers that have known chromosome locations to assist with the mapping and identification of genes. SNPs are particularly useful in these analyses.

Multiple approaches can be taken in QTL mapping experiments. At its core, however, QTL mapping is a statistical process that seeks to identify regions of genomes containing genetic markers that are linked to QTLs. The statistical analysis for QTLs is closely related to the statistical analysis of genetic linkage using logarithm of the odds (lod) score analysis (see Section 5.5). QTL analysis can lead to identification of the potential *chromosome location* of a QTL influencing phenotypic variation of a quantitative trait, but by itself it does not identify the molecular basis of action of the QTL. Other genetic methods are available for molecular description of QTL action.

QTL mapping uses the parents and progeny produced by controlled crosses as the sources of DNA for genetic marker identification and as the source of data for the quantitative trait of interest. If, for example, a researcher wants to identify QTLs that influence large fruit size in tomatoes, he or she will cross two parental lines of tomatoes that differ in fruit size. The F$_1$ progeny of this cross could then be used to produce F$_2$ progeny or, as we illustrate here, the F$_1$ could be used in a backcross to one of the parental lines. Genetic markers will be determined in the original parental lines and in the backcross progeny. Tomato sizes produced by backcross progeny will be weighed and the results compared with genetic markers in the individual plants.

Figure 19.12a illustrates the structure of a backcross experiment designed to collect genetic marker and tomato-weight data for QTL mapping analysis. One parental tomato strain producing large fruit that averages 100 grams (g) contains an allele of a genetic marker that is identified by the letter *L*. There are actually many markers linked to QTLs in the line, and for each marker gene tested, the large-tomato strain will have two copies of the large-strain marker allele, designated *LL*. Similarly, a small-tomato–producing strain, with an average tomato weight of 10 g, is characterized for the same genetic marker, and the locus tested in the small-strain genotype is designated *SS*. The F$_1$ progeny of the large × small cross is heterozygous for the marker locus and is designated *LS*. These plants in this example are shown to produce tomatoes that weigh 60 g. The backcross is made to the large-tomato strain, and the marker genotype will be

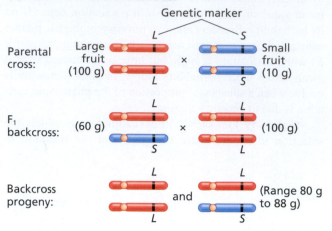

(a) Parental cross and backcross

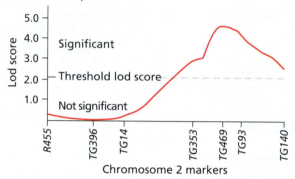

(b) Lod score profile

FIGURE 19.12 **Quantitative trait locus (QTL) detection and mapping. (a)** Parental tomato plants producing large fruit (and homozygous for *L marker alleles*) or small fruit (and homozygous for *S marker alleles*) are crossed to produce F$_1$ (*LS*). The F$_1$ are then backcrossed to the large-fruit line to yield backcross progeny that are either *LL* or *LS*. **(b)** The significance of linkage between potential QTLs and genetic markers is tested among backcross progeny by lod score analysis. A lod score profile assessing fruit-weight QTLs reveals significant scores exceeding the threshold value on tomato chromosome 2.

either *LL*, if the F$_1$ transmits the large-strain allele, or *LS*, if the F$_1$ transmits the small-strain allele. The backcross progeny in this example produce tomatoes that vary in weight from 80 to 88 g. Tomato weight from the backcross plants is greater than from the F$_1$ plants because the backcross plants are the result of a cross between the F$_1$ and the large-tomato strain.

Table 19.5 displays tomato-weight data for 10 backcross plants (1–10) and genetic marker data for two genes, marker A (M_A) and marker B (M_B), that are not linked to one another and are located in different parts of the genome. In an actual QTL backcross experiment, several hundred backcross plants might be examined, and each plant might be genotyped for dozens of genetic markers that ideally would be spaced about every 5 to 10 centimorgans (cM) in the genome. This number of genetic markers and their close

Table 19.5	QTL Analysis of Tomato Weight in Backcross Progeny		
Backcross Plant	Average Fruit Weight (g)	Genotype	
		Marker M_A	Marker M_B
1	86	LS	LL
2	82	LL	LS
3	85	LL	LL
4	88	LL	LL
5	81	LS	LS
6	83	LS	LS
7	84	LL	LL
8	80	LL	LS
9	84	LS	LS
10	87	LS	LL
Total average weight	84		
LL average weight		83.8	86.0
LS average weight		84.2	82.0

proximity maximize the chance of identifying the location of QTLs detected by the analysis.

In Table 19.5, the average weight of tomatoes from backcross plants is 84 g. Average tomato weight is compared for *LL* plants versus *LS* plants for each marker. There is almost no difference in average weight for M_A (*LL* = 83.8 g versus *LS* = 84.2 g), but for M_B, *LL* plants produce tomatoes that are 4 g heavier on average than are the tomatoes from *LS* plants (*LL* = 86.0 g versus *LS* = 82.0 g). These data may indicate that a QTL influencing tomato weight is located near M_B. Conversely, there is no evidence to indicate that a QTL is located near M_A.

To determine the statistical significance of this kind of information provided for genetic markers and tomato weight, a lod score is calculated. In this case, the lod score is based on odds ratios dividing the probability of the data if a QTL is linked to the marker by the probability of the data if there is no QTL linked to the marker. The odds ratios for the backcross plants are added together, and the log (the *log* of the *odd*s) is taken to yield the lod score. Like the analysis of lod scores for genetic linkage, there is a threshold value for significance of the score (see Section 5.5). If the lod score for a genetic marker is greater than the threshold value, the lod score indicates a statistically significant probability that a QTL is linked to the marker.

In **Figure 19.12b**, a lod score profile for several genetic markers located on chromosome 2 of tomato reveals significant evidence indicating genetic linkage to a QTL. Beginning at the marker designated *TG353* and spanning to the right through marker *TG140*, the lod score

values are greater than the threshold value and give statistically significant evidence favoring linkage between these genetic markers and a QTL. On the other hand, the lod scores falling below the threshold value in the figure give no statistical evidence of linkage to a QTL. For chromosome 2 in tomato, lod scores for genetic markers to the left of *TG353* are less than the threshold lod score value.

Andrew Paterson and his colleagues published a 1988 study mapping 15 QTLs in the tomato genome that influence fruit weight, fruit acidity, and the amount of soluble solids in the fruit. Each trait has agricultural importance, and together they determine the quality and yield of tomato paste from the fruit. Paterson's study used 70 DNA markers spaced an average of 20 cM apart throughout the tomato genome. Collectively, these markers span about 95% of the 12 chromosomes that constitute the tomato genome.

The parental plants were two closely related and interfertile species: a domestic tomato (*Solanum esculentum*) and a wild South American green-fruited tomato (*Solanum chmielewskii*). The F$_1$ hybrids were backcrossed to *S. esculentum*, producing 237 backcross progeny plants for analysis. All backcross plants were grown under identical conditions to minimize the influence of environmental factors on the traits of interest. Individual fruits from backcross plants were assayed for fruit weight (grams), soluble solids content (percentage), and acidity (pH). Lod score analysis was used to test whether genes influencing any of the three traits exhibited genetic linkage to genome markers. Significant lod score values traced six genes influencing fruit weight, five influencing acidity, and four influencing soluble solids content to regions of nine chromosomes in the tomato genome. The regions of tomato chromosomes 6 and 7 containing QTLs influencing the three traits are shown in **Figure 19.13**.

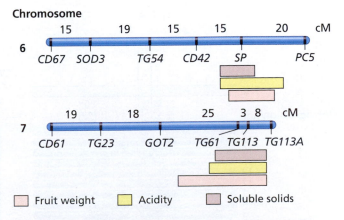

FIGURE 19.13 QTL mapping in domestic tomato. Multiple QTLs influencing fruit weight, fruit acidity, and percentage of soluble solids of tomatoes are shown on chromosome 6 and chromosome 7. Many other QTLs populate the rest of the genome. Distances between genes are in cM (centimorgans).

Identification of QTL Genes

Since QTL mapping identifies the location of genes influencing quantitative traits but not the genes themselves, additional genetic analysis is required to identify the genes. To acquire information leading to gene identity, researchers use **near isogenic lines (NILs)**, also called **introgression lines (ILs)**. These are lines of organisms derived from backcross progeny produced as described earlier. Different backcross progeny are self-fertilized over many generations to form highly inbred lines that are nearly isogenic, meaning they are genetically identical at almost all genes. The lines differ from one another, however, as a result of different crossovers that occurred during the backcrossing and that introduced different alleles near the site of a QTL. The introduced

differences are called introgressions, thus giving these lines their name.

Figure 19.14a illustrates six introgression lines (IL1 to IL6) descended from a cross between two original parental lines, one a domesticated species and the other a wild species. The chromosome colors illustrate crossovers that produce differences between the introgression lines. Crossover locations are identified by analysis of genetic markers, and each introgression line is characterized for a trait phenotype. In the figure, the bars to the right of each line indicate the percentage difference between the phenotype of the IL and the domesticated parental species. Two potential QTL regions, QTL-A and QTL-B, contain variations of the crossover segments. The greatest positive percentage difference relative to the domesticated species phenotype occurs in IL2 and IL3

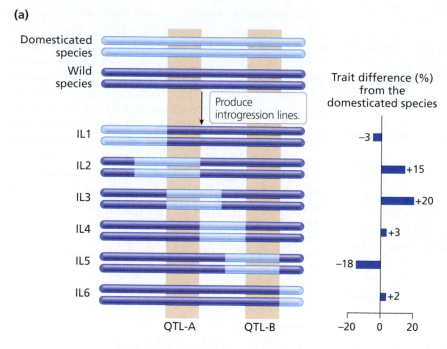

(a)

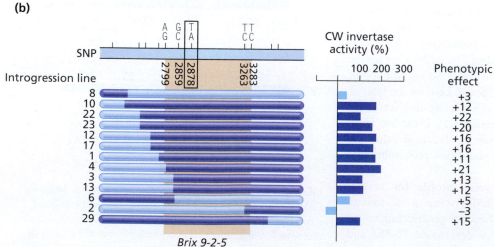

(b)

FIGURE 19.14 QTL analysis in introgression lines. (a) Six introgression lines (IL1 to IL6) formed by mating between a domesticated species and a wild species have different patterns of recombination in the region of two QTLs. The difference in trait expression between the trait in the domesticated species and each IL is given as a percentage. **(b)** Analysis of *Brix 9-2-5* in 13 introgression lines identifies SNPs that alter CW invertase activity. The SNP at position 2878 has a substantial influence on CW invertase function.

that carry crossover chromosomes containing domesticated DNA in the vicinity of QTL-A and wild-species DNA near QTL-B.

To identify the genes responsible for QTL variation, "candidate genes," genes that are potentially responsible for the observed variation, must be identified and investigated. Genes in the QTL-A and QTL-B regions are located by examining DNA sequences, and sequence variants in candidate genes among introgression lines are identified. The sequence differences detected are studied to determine if they correlate with phenotypic variation.

Figure 19.14b illustrates a portion the results of experimental analysis of tomato introgression lines by Eyal Fridman and colleagues in 2004 designed to identify genes contributing to Brix value in tomato. The Brix value of fruit refers to the total soluble solids content, of which sugars and acids are the primary constituents. Fridman and colleagues created a large number of ILs from an initial cross between the domesticated tomato species (*Solanum lycopersicum*) and a wild relative (*Solanum pennellii*).

The parental species and each of the ILs were assessed for Brix value, and a QTL found to have a high Brix value, *Brix 9-2-5,* was intensively studied. DNA sequencing of the 484 nucleotides (positions 2799 to 3283) in *Brix 9-2-5* revealed the five SNP variants shown in the figure. The *Brix 9-2-5* QTL corresponds to a segment of the tomato *LIN5* gene that produces the cell wall enzyme invertase (CW invertase). In the figure, the positions of SNPs are shown relative to 13 ILs that carry recombination in or near *Brix 9-2-5*. The bar to the right of each IL indicates its percentage difference in CW invertase activity relative to *S. lycopersicum*. The results show that when the *S. pennellii* sequence is present, CW invertase activity is significantly greater than in *S. lycopersicum*. The data shown, along with additional data not shown, indicated that the SNP at position 2878 (boxed) was strongly correlated with increased CW invertase activity. DNA and protein sequence analysis revealed that this SNP produced an amino acid difference that altered CW invertase activity.

Genome-Wide Association Studies

The widespread availability of genome sequencing information has opened a new avenue to the identification of QTLs in numerous species, including humans. As described in Section 5.5, the method known as **genome-wide association studies (GWAS)** seeks to tie the presence of a DNA marker to a QTL influencing a specific phenotype. Recall that in GWAS studies the inherited genetic marker variant and the phenotype are related by "association," which means organisms that carry a particular variant are more likely to have a certain phenotype than are organisms that carry a different variant. The assessment of association is quantitative; that is, it expresses the percentage of organisms with a genetic marker that also display a certain phenotype versus the percentage that have the phenotype but not the genetic marker.

One advantage of GWAS over other QTL mapping approaches is that GWAS can scan the entire genome for QTLs by statistically testing for marker variants that are associated with phenotypic variation. Positive statistical results indicating association identify chromosome regions that can be more closely inspected for genes that influence the trait. A second advantage of GWAS is that organisms in random mating populations can be analyzed. Rather than requiring controlled crosses and the formation of introgression lines, GWAS uses "cases," or organisms with a particular phenotype, and compares them with "controls" that lack the particular phenotype to assess the association between QTL markers and a phenotype.

This case–control approach identifies the SNP genotypes in all the individuals with, for example, a genetic disease (the cases) as well as in healthy controls. The frequency of each SNP allele in the cases is compared with the allele frequency in the controls. When the allele frequency in the case group is greater than the frequency in the control group, the odds ratio is greater than 1.0. Statistics applied to the odds ratio determine the *P* value of each odds ratio. Significant association between a SNP and a disease is found when the *P* value is less than the cutoff value. The results of each SNP examination are plotted as in the following description of a GWAS analysis of Crohn's disease.

Discussion on pages 173–174 and associated with Figure 5.17 describes the use of GWAS analysis to identify genome regions that may contain genes influencing the development of selected human disorders. An example of the human hereditary condition known as Crohn's disease (CD) investigated by GWAS is displayed in Figure 5.17. CD is an intestinal disorder that is influenced by inherited variation. No single gene with a major effect is known for CD, but GWAS analysis identified nine genome regions having significant associations with CD. Any or all of them may contain genes whose variants play a functional role in the development of CD.

To verify the possibility of genetic influence identified by GWAS analysis, it is necessary to find the gene or genes involved. This requires close examination of each identified region. For CD, the chromosome region 16q.2.1 revealed a highly significant association, and Yasunori Ogura and colleagues dissected this region, ultimately identifying a gene known as *CARD15* (caspase recruitment domain, member 15) as a candidate for a gene influencing susceptibility to CD.

CARD15 encodes 12 exons that direct the production of a 1040–amino acid protein. The protein is involved in recognizing bacterial proteins and stimulating an immune response. Ogura and colleagues sequenced the exons and introns of *CARD15* in 12 CD patients from different families having multiple cases of CD. They performed the same gene sequencing on four healthy control individuals as well. The study identified an identical C–G base pair insertion at nucleotide 3020 of exon 11 in three of the 12 CD patients. The insertion, designated *3020insC*, induces a frameshift mutation that generates a premature stop codon, shortening the mutant protein by 1007 amino acids.

Ogura and colleagues developed an allele-specific polymerase chain reaction (PCR) assay for *3020insC* and tested 101 CD patients whose parents were heterozygous for the wild-type allele and the *3020insC* allele. Of the 101 CD patients, 68 were homozygous for *3020insC* (**Figure 19.15**). Biochemical analysis shows mutant protein from the gene has only a small fraction of the activity of the wild-type protein. The diminished capacity of the mutant protein reduces the sensitivity of the immune system to the microbial invader. It may be that this allows bacteria to bypass the first line of immune system defenses, leading to a large inflammatory immune response—a primary feature of CD—when other immune system proteins recognize the presence of bacteria. Since the identification of *3020insC*, two additional mutations of *CARD15* have been found to increase the risk of CD. All three mutations appear to be null alleles, meaning there is no functional protein product produced. It is suspected that the absence of this protein leads to an increased inflammatory response as seen in CD.

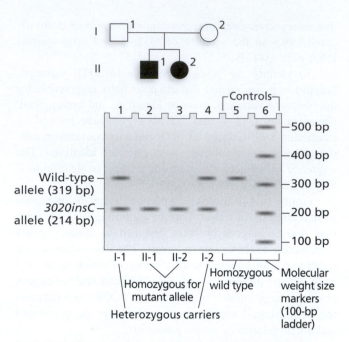

FIGURE 19.15 Detection of *3020insC* in *CARD15* in a family with Crohn's disease. Gel electrophoresis of PCR products from four members of a family are shown in lanes 1 through 4. A wild-type control is in lane 5, and molecular weight size markers are in lane 6.

🅠 Draw the band pattern for a child of this couple who does not have Crohn's disease. Offer a genetic reason to explain why this person does not experience the condition.

CASE STUDY

The Genetics of Autism Spectrum Disorders

Autism spectrum disorders (ASD) are a large group of neurodevelopmental impairments affecting language, social cognition, and mental flexibility in humans. ASD generally has its onset by the age of 3, and most cases are diagnosed in young children. When autism was first described, in the early 1940s, it was thought to be a single, severe condition of social and language dysfunction that primarily affects boys. This unitary definition has expanded in the ensuing decades, and now neurobiologists and psychiatric specialists recognize ASD to be a large collection of conditions rather than only one. In addition, ASD is now known to have a biological basis, and it is no longer classified as a psychiatric condition. A number of hypotheses have been proposed regarding its causation, and over recent decades, evidence of significant genetic influence in ASD has mounted.

The first strong evidence of a genetic basis for ASD came in 1977 when Susan Folstein and Michael Rutter published research that examined concordance for ASD in MZ and DZ twin pairs. Their finding of 82% concordance for cognitive disabilities associated with ASD in MZ twin pairs versus 10% in DZ twin pairs led to the conclusion that genetic variation plays a major role in ASD.

These findings have been supported in numerous follow-on studies. In addition to providing support for the overall concordance results identified by Folstein and Rutter, the follow-on studies have identified two additional features

of ASD that point to a role for genetic influence. First, studies have found that the first-degree relatives of children with ASD are much more likely to develop ASD than the population average. (Recall that first-degree relatives, e.g., full siblings, share 50% of their DNA and have the closest genetic relationships in families; see the discussion in Section 19.1 and Figure 19.7.) Second, the studies have identified several genetic syndromes in which ASD can be one component of the syndrome. One example is fragile X syndrome. Recall from Section 11.2 and Table 11.2 that fragile X syndrome is caused by a large DNA triplet repeat expansion mutation affecting the *FMR1* gene. The gene normally has between 6 and about 50 repeats of a CGG triplet repeat. Fragile X syndrome occurs in males who have a large expansion containing more than 200 of the CGG repeats in *FMR1*.

Fragile X syndrome symptoms include physical abnormalities and mental impairment. The link to ASD is detected in males and females who carry abnormal X chromosomes with CGG triplet expansions between 50 and 200 copies. These are not as large as the expansions of full-mutation X chromosomes that cause fragile X syndrome. There is evidence that the function of *FMR1* is altered but not inactivated by these smaller expansions. The role they play in generating ASD-like symptoms is a subject of active investigation.

The search for gene mutations and variants that may be responsible for large numbers of ASD cases has not produced results. However, it has led to the identification of dozens of genes whose mutations play a role in a small percentage (at most 2% or so) of cases of ASD. Frequently, these are mutations classified as copy number variants (CNVs)—submicroscopic chromosome duplication or deletion mutations that usually affect just a few kilobases of DNA. Collectively, the identified CNVs are associated with approximately 10% of all ASD cases. The CNVs that are implicated are scattered throughout the genome. They and other variants associated with ASD appear to affect many different molecular processes, including cell adhesion, synaptic structure and function, pre-mRNA processing and splicing, and protein production.

The picture of ASD that has emerged over the past two decades is one of disruption to complex brain circuitry in which many different developmental and communication pathways must be functional for optimal performance. In other words, the complexities of brain function that lead to "normal" language, social skills, and mental flexibility can potentially be disrupted by the mutation of any one of hundreds of different genes. Sections 4.2 and 4.3 describe the concept of genes operating in pathways to produce certain phenotypic features. Those sections also describe pleiotropy between genes (situations in which mutation of one gene can affect multiple, usually distinct, attributes of the individual; see Figure 4.16) and epistasis (situations

in which mutation of one gene modifies or prevents the expression of another gene or genes; see Foundation Figure 4.21). We can think of the many gene variants and mutations associated with ASD as being part of large, complex pathways, and of these genes often having pleiotropic or epistatic effects. Many distinct pathways and features must, and usually do, develop normally to generate language and social skills classified as falling within the "normal" range. Mutations can alter these pathways in manners that disable social ability, language function, or mental flexibility to the extent that a child suffers an identifiable abnormality.

Research into the genetic and biological foundations of ASD is active and ongoing. Examples of the directions in which the study of ASD is moving include genome sequencing to identify any genetic similarities among groups of ASD patients with similar manifestations of the condition, examination of how mutations affect synaptic and cellular circuits that are disrupted in ASD, studies of potential epigenetic contributions to ASD, and the search for the mutational basis and categorization of different subtypes of ASD. ASD is a complex and diverse set of conditions with many distinct causes. It is a goal of neuroscience and neurogenetics that the next decade or two provide a much clearer picture of the causes and development of ASD, along with effective methods of treatment.

SUMMARY
Mastering Genetics For activities, animations, and review quizzes, go to the Study Area.

19.1 Quantitative Traits Display Continuous Phenotype Variation

- Quantitative phenotypic traits are polygenic and are described by scales of measure that can be assigned values having a quantitative basis.

- The phenotypes of multifactorial traits result from polygenic inheritance and the influence of environmental factors.

- Most quantitative traits have a continuous phenotypic distribution. Those influenced by larger numbers of genes are more likely to display continuous variation. Discontinuous variation in phenotype is a frequent feature of threshold traits.

- Threshold traits are explained by additive alleles and have a threshold of liability that separates one phenotypic category (unaffected) from another (affected). The threshold of liability is crossed when a sufficient number of additive alleles accumulate in the genotype.

19.2 Quantitative Trait Analysis Is Statistical

- Quantitative traits are analyzed using statistical methods that evaluate the mean, median, mode, and variance of quantitative trait phenotype distribution.

- The frequency distribution for the phenotype range is described by the variance or the standard deviation in sample values. In the case of quantitative trait phenotypes, the phenotypic variance (V_P) is a useful measure of the sample distribution.

- The phenotypic variance of a trait is the sum of genetic variance (V_G) and environmental variance (V_E).

- Genetic variance is partitioned into additive variance (V_A), dominance variance (V_D), and interactive variance (V_I), the latter resulting from the epistatic interaction of genes determining a phenotype.

19.3 Heritability Measures the Genetic Component of Phenotypic Variation

- Heritability is a measure of the extent to which genetic variation contributes to total phenotypic variation.

- Broad sense heritability (H^2) measures the ratio of genetic variance to phenotypic variance (V_G/V_P). One method of applying broad sense heritability analysis to humans is through twin studies that give a general estimate of heritability.

- Narrow sense heritability (h^2) measures the contribution of additive genetic variance to phenotypic variance (V_A/V_P).

- Narrow sense heritability is used to predict the selection response (R) of a trait to artificial selection or to natural selection.

19.4 Quantitative Trait Loci Are the Genes That Contribute to Quantitative Traits

- QTL mapping is used to determine the location of potential QTLs in genomes.

- QTL mapping uses methods that closely resemble recombination mapping, such as controlled crosses and analysis of recombinant chromosomes.

■ Specific genes influencing quantitative trait phenotypes are identified and their variation characterized through QTL candidate locus analysis.

■ Genome-wide association studies (GWAS) scan the entire genome of organisms in randomly mating populations for statistical evidence of QTLs.

PREPARING FOR PROBLEM SOLVING

In addition to the list of problem-solving tips and suggestions given here, you can go to the Study Guide and Solutions Manual that accompanies this book for help at solving problems.

1. Be able to analyze the results of crosses involving polygenic traits and to predict the possible outcomes of crosses.

2. Understand the concepts pertaining to multifactorial traits, their inheritance, and their expression.

3. Be prepared to define and explain threshold traits and to describe their relationship to polygenic or multifactorial traits.

4. Understand the definitions and concepts pertaining to broad sense heritability and narrow sense heritability.

5. Be prepared to describe the concept of heritability and the use of concordance in twin studies for assessing it in humans.

6. Be prepared to calculate the mean, standard deviation, variance, and heritability of quantitative traits.

7. Be prepared to assess the results of artificial selection experiments.

PROBLEMS

Mastering Genetics Visit for instructor-assigned tutorials and problems.

Chapter Concepts

For answers to selected even-numbered problems, see Appendix: Answers.

1. Which of the following traits would you expect to be inherited as quantitative traits?
   a. body weight in chickens
   b. growth rate in sheep
   c. milk production in cattle
   d. fruit weight in tomatoes
   e. coat color in dogs

2. For the traits listed in the previous problem, which do you think are likely to be multifactorial traits, with phenotypes that are influenced by genes and environment? Identify two environmental factors that might play a role in phenotypic variation of the traits you identified.

3. Compare and contrast broad sense heritability and narrow sense heritability, giving an example of each measurement and identifying how the measurement is used.

4. In a cross of two pure-breeding lines of tomatoes producing different fruit sizes, the variance in grams (g) of fruit weight in the F_1 is 2.25 g, and the variance among the F_2 is 5.40 g. Determine the genetic and environmental variance (V_G and V_E) for the trait and the broad sense heritability of the trait.

5. Describe the difference between continuous phenotypic variation and discontinuous variation. Explain how polygenic inheritance could be the basis of a trait showing continuous phenotypic variation. Explain how polygenic inheritance can be the basis of a threshold trait.

6. Calculate the mean, variance, and standard deviation for a sample of turkeys weighed at 8 weeks of age that have the following weights in ounces: 161, 172, 155, 173, 149, 177, 156, 174, 158, 162, 171, 181.

7. Provide a definition and an example for each of the following terms:
   a. additive genes
   b. concordance of twin pairs
   c. multifactorial inheritance
   d. polygenic inheritance
   e. quantitative trait locus
   f. threshold trait

8. What is a random sample, and why can a random sample be used to represent a population?

9. Why is heritability an important phenomenon in plant and animal agriculture?

Application and Integration

For answers to selected even-numbered problems, see Appendix: Answers.

10. Three pairs of genes with two alleles each (A_1 and A_2, B_1 and B_2, and C_1 and C_2) control the height of a plant. The alleles of these genes have an additive relationship: each copy of alleles A_1, B_1, and C_1 contributes 6 cm to plant height, and each copy of alleles A_2, B_2, and C_2 contributes 3 cm.
    a. What are the expected heights of plants with each of the homozygous genotypes $A_1A_1B_1B_1C_1C_1$ and $A_2A_2B_2B_2C_2C_2$?
    b. What height is expected in the F_1 progeny of a cross between $A_1A_1B_1B_1C_1C_1$ and $A_2A_2B_2B_2C_2C_2$?
    c. What is the expected height of a plant with the genotype $A_1A_2B_2B_2C_1C_2$?
    d. Identify all possible genotypes for plants with an expected height of 33 cm.
    e. Identify the number of different genotypes that are possible with these three genes.

f. Identify the number of different phenotypes (expected plant heights) that are possible with these three genes.

11. In selective breeding experiments, it is frequently observed that the strains respond to artificial selection for many generations, with the selected phenotype changing in the desired direction. Often, however, the response to artificial selection reaches a plateau after many generations, and the phenotype no longer changes as it did in past generations.

   a. What is the genetic explanation for the plateau phenomenon?

   b. Once a plateau has been reached, is the heritability of the trait very high or is it very low? Explain.

12. Two inbred lines of sunflowers (P_1 and P_2) produce different total weights of seeds per flower head. The mean weight of seeds (grams) and the variance of seed weights in different generations are as follows.

Generation	Mean Weight/Head (g)	Variance
P_1	105	3.0
P_2	135	3.8
F_1	122	3.5
F_2	125	7.4

   a. Use the information above to determine V_G, V_E, and V_P for this trait.

   b. Determine H^2 for this trait.

13 What is a quantitative trait locus (QTL)? Suppose you wanted to search for QTLs influencing fruit size in tomatoes. Describe the general structure of a QTL experiment, including the kind of tomato strains you would use, how molecular markers should be distributed in the genome, how the genetic marker alleles should differ between the two strains, and how you would use the F_1 progeny in a subsequent cross to obtain information about the possible location(s) of QTLs of interest.

14. In *Nicotiana*, two inbred strains produce long (P_L) and short (P_S) corollas. These lines are crossed to produce F_1, and the F_1 are crossed to produce F_2 plants in which corolla length and variance are measured. The following table summarizes mean and variance of corolla length in each generation. Calculate H^2 for corolla length in *Nicotiana*.

Generation	Mean Corolla Length (mm)	Variance
P_L	85.75	4.21
P_S	43.15	2.89
F_1	62.26	3.62
F_2	67.37	38.10

15. Suppose the length of maize ears has narrow sense heritability (h^2) of 0.70. A population produces ears that have an average length of 28 cm, and from this population a breeder selects a plant producing 34-cm ears to cross by self-fertilization. Predict the selection differential (S) and the response to selection (R) for this cross.

16. In a line of cherry tomatoes, the average fruit weight is 16 g. A plant producing tomatoes with an average weight of 12 g is used in one self-fertilization cross to produce a line of smaller tomatoes, and a plant producing tomatoes of 24 g is used in a second cross to produce larger tomatoes.

   a. What is the selection differential (S) for fruit weight in each cross?

   b. If narrow sense heritability (h^2) for this trait is 0.80, what are the expected responses to selection (R) for fruit weight in the crosses?

17. Two pure-breeding wheat strains, one producing dark red kernels and the other producing white kernels, are crossed to produce F_1 with pink kernel color. When an F_1 plant is self-fertilized and its seed collected and planted, the resulting F_2 consist of 160 plants with kernel colors as shown in the following table.

Kernel Color	Number
White	9
Dark red	12
Red	39
Light pink	41
Pink	59

   a. Based on the F_2 progeny, how many genes are involved in kernel color determination?

   b. How many additive alleles are required to explain the five phenotypes seen in the F_2?

   c. Using clearly defined allele symbols of your choice, give genotypes for the parental strains and the F_1. Describe the genotypes that produce the different phenotypes in the F_2.

   d. If an F_1 plant is crossed to a dark red plant, what are the expected progeny phenotypes and what is the expected proportion of each phenotype?

18. In studies of human MZ and DZ twin pairs of the same sex who are reared together, the following concordance values are identified for various traits. Based on the values shown, describe the relative importance of genes versus the influence of environmental factors for each trait.

Trait	Concordance	
	MZ	DZ
Blood type	100	65
Chicken pox	89	87
Manic depression	67	13
Schizophrenia	72	12
Diabetes	62	15
Cleft lip	51	6
Club foot	40	4

19. During a visit with your grandparents, they comment on how tall you are compared with them. You tell them that in your genetics class, you learned that height in humans

has high heritability, although environmental factors also influence adult height. You correctly explain the meaning of heritability, and your grandfather asks, "How can height be highly heritable and still be influenced by the environment?" What explanation do you give your grandfather?

20. An association of racehorse owners is seeking a new genetic strategy to improve the running speed of their horses. Traditional breeding of fast male and female horses has proven expensive and time-consuming, and the breeders are interested in an approach using quantitative trait loci as a basis for selecting breeding pairs of horses. Write a brief synopsis (~50 words) of QTL mapping to explain how genes influencing running speed might be identified in horses.

21. Applied to the study of the human genome, a goal of GWAS is to locate chromosome regions that are likely to contain genes influencing the risk of disease. Specific genes can be identified in these regions, and particular mutant alleles that increase disease risk can be sequenced. To date, the identification of alleles that increase disease risk has occasionally led to a new therapeutic strategy, but more often the identification of disease alleles is the only outcome.

    a. From a physician's point of view, what is the value of being able to identify alleles that increase the risk of a particular disease?
    b. What is the value of being able to identify alleles that increase disease risk for a person who is currently free of the disease but who is at risk of developing the disease due to its presence in the family?
    c. What personal or ethical issues arising from GWAS might be of concern to physicians or to those who might carry an allele that increases disease risk?

22. Suppose a polygenic system for producing color in kernels of a grain is controlled by three additive genes, G, M, and T. There are two alleles of each gene, G_1 and G_2, M_1 and M_2, and T_1 and T_2. The phenotypic effects of the three genotypes of the G gene are $G_1G_1 = 6$ units of color, $G_1G_2 = 3$ units of color, and $G_2G_2 = 1$ unit of color. The phenotypic effects for genes M and T are similar, giving the phenotype of a plant with the genotype $G_1G_1M_1M_1T_1T_1$ a total of 18 units of color and a plant with the genotype $G_2G_2M_2M_2T_2T_2$ a total of 3 units of color.

    a. How many units of color are found in trihybrid plants?
    b. Two trihybrid plants are mated. What is the expected proportion of progeny plants displaying 9 units of color? Explain your answer.
    c. Suppose that instead of an additive genetic system, kernel-color determination in this organism is a threshold system. The appearance of color in kernels requires nine or more units of color; otherwise, kernels have no color and appear white. In other words, plants whose phenotypes contain eight or fewer units of color are white. Based on the threshold model, what proportion of the F_2 progeny produced by the trihybrid cross in part (b) will be white? Explain your answer.
    d. Assuming the threshold model applies to this kernel-color system, what proportion of the progeny of the cross $G_1G_2M_1M_2T_2T_2 \times G_1G_2M_1M_2T_1T_2$ do you expect to display colored kernels?

23. New Zealand lamb breeders measure the following variance values for their herd.

Trait	V_P	V_G	V_A
Body mass (kg)	42.4	20.5	7.4
Body fat (%)	38.9	16.2	5.7
Body length (cm)	51.6	26.4	8.1

    a. Calculate the broad sense heritability (H^2) and the narrow sense heritability (h^2) for each trait in this lamb herd.
    b. How would you characterize the potential response to selection (R) for each trait?

24. Cattle breeders would like to improve the protein content and butterfat content of milk produced by a herd of cows. Narrow sense heritability values are 0.60 for protein content and 0.80 for butterfat content. The average percentages of these traits in the herd and the percentages of the traits in cows selected for breeding are as follows.

Trait	Herd Average	Selected Cows
Protein content	20.2%	22.7%
Butterfat content	6.5%	7.4%

    a. Determine the selection differential (S) for each trait in this herd.
    b. Which trait is likely to be the most responsive to artificial selection applied by the cattle breeders through selection of cows for mating?

25. In human gestational development, abnormalities of the closure of the lower part of the midface can result in cleft lip, if the lip alone is affected by the closure defect, or in cleft lip and palate (the roof of the mouth), if the closure defect is more extensive. Cleft lip and cleft lip with cleft palate are multifactorial disorders that are threshold traits. A family with a history of either condition has a significantly increased chance of a recurrence of midface cleft disorder in comparison with families without such a history. However, the recurrence risk of a midface cleft disorder is higher in families with a history of cleft lip with cleft palate than in families with a history of cleft lip alone.

    a. Suppose a friend of yours who has not taken genetics asks you to explain these observations. Construct a genetic explanation for the increased recurrence risk of midface clefting in families that have a history of cleft disorders versus families without a history of such disorders.
    b. Construct a similar explanation of why the recurrence risk of a cleft disorder is higher in families with a history of cleft lip with cleft palate than in families with a history of cleft lip alone.

26. The children of couples in which one partner has blood type O (genotype *ii*) and the other partner has blood type AB (genotype $I^A I^B$) are studied.

    a. What is the expected concordance rate for blood type of MZ twins in this study? Explain your answer.
    b. What is the expected concordance rate for blood type of DZ twins in this study? Explain why this answer is different from the answer to part (a).

27. Answer the following in regard to multifactorial traits in human twins.

    a. If the trait is substantially influenced by genes, would you expect the concordance rate to be higher in MZ twins or higher in DZ twins? Explain your reasoning.
    b. If the trait is produced with little contribution from genetic variation, what would you expect to see if you compared the concordance rates of MZ twins versus DZ twins? Explain your reasoning.

Collaboration and Discussion

For answers to selected even-numbered problems, see Appendix: Answers.

28. Suppose the mature height of a plant is a multifactorial trait under the control of five independently assorting genes, designated *A, B, C, D,* and *E,* and five environmental factors. There are two alleles of each gene (A_1, A_2, etc.). Each allele with a subscript 1 (i.e., A_1, etc.) contributes 5 cm to potential plant height, and each allele with a 2 subscript (i.e., A_2, etc.) contributes 10 cm to potential plant height. In other words, a genotype containing only 1 alleles ($A_1 A_1 B_1 B_1 C_1 C_1 D_1 D_1 E_1 E_1$) would have a potential height of $[(10)(5)] = 50$ cm, and a genotype with only 2 alleles ($A_2 A_2 B_2 B_2 C_2 C_2 D_2 D_2 E_2 E_2$) would have a potential height of $[(10)(10)] = 100$ cm.

    The five environmental factors are (1) amount of water, (2) amount of sunlight, (3) soil drainage, (4) nutrient content of soil, and (5) temperature. Each environmental factor can vary from optimal to poor. If all factors are optimal, assume that full potential height is attained. However, if one or more of the environmental factors is less than optimal, then height is reduced. The state of each environmental factor has an effect on growth. In this exercise, we'll assume that the growth is affected according to the following scale:

Environmental Factor State	Height Lost
Optimal (O)	0 cm lost
Good (G)	4 cm lost
Fair (F)	8 cm lost
Marginal (M)	12 cm lost
Poor (P)	16 cm lost

Thus, for example, if one environmental factor is optimal, two are good, one is fair, and one is marginal, the loss of potential height is $(0 + 4 + 4 + 8 + 12) = 28$ cm. If the loss of height potential is greater than the height potential of the plant, the plant does not survive.

    a. Calculate the potential height, based on inherited alleles, and the attained height, based on growth in the environmental circumstances given, for the three plants (a, b, and c) in the accompanying table.
    b. How many 1 and 2 alleles must be present to give a height potential of 80 cm?

    c. List two genotypes that have a height potential of 80 cm.
    d. If two plants that each have a height potential of 75 cm are crossed, what proportion of the progeny will have a height potential of 80 cm? (Hint: See Figure 19.3e for assistance making this determination.)

		Environmental Factor States				
Genotype		1	2	3	4	5
a. $A_1 A_2 B_1 B_2 C_2$ $C_2 D_1 D_2 E_1 E_2$		G	F	O	G	M
b. $A_1 A_2 B_1 B_2 C_2$ $C_2 D_1 D_2 E_1 E_2$		F	M	G	G	F
c. $A_1 A_1 B_1 B_2 C_1$ $C_2 D_1 D_2 E_1 E_2$		O	G	G	G	G

29. A three-gene system of additive genes (*A, B,* and *C*) controls plant height. Each gene has two alleles (*A* and *a, B* and *b,* and *C* and *c*). There is dominance among the alleles of each gene, with alleles *A, B,* and *C* dominant over *a, b,* and *c*. Under this scheme, the dominant genotype for a gene contributes 10 cm to height potential, and the recessive genotype contributes 4 cm.

    a. What is the height potential of a plant that is homozygous for all three dominant alleles?
    b. What is the height potential of a plant that is homozygous for all three recessive alleles?
    c. What is the height potential of the F_1 progeny of the homozygous plants identified in (a) and (b) of this problem?
    d. What are the phenotypes and proportions of each phenotype among the F_2?

30. Congenital dislocation of the hip is a threshold condition in which the head of the femur (the femoral head) is out of its normal position relative to the bones that will form the socket of the hip (the acetabulum). This misplacement can lead to potentially serious orthopedic problems later in life if the condition is not treated in infancy. Numerous studies have shown that (a) brothers and sisters of infants born with congenital hip dislocation are more likely to develop the condition

than are the siblings of those without the condition. These studies also find that (b) more female infants than male infants have the trait, and (c) if the affected child is a girl, the risk to her siblings is lower than if the affected infant is a boy. Explain the meaning of the three observations (a, b, and c) in the context of proposing a threshold model that explains these observations.

31. A total of 20 men and 20 women volunteer to participate in a statistics project. The height and weight of each subject are given in the table.

    a. Draw one histogram for height of the subjects and a separate histogram for weight. Use different colors for men and women so that you can visually compare the distributions by sex and plot weights in 10-lb intervals (i.e., 90–99 lb, 100–109 lb, 110–119 lb, etc.).

    b. Calculate the mean, variance, and standard deviation for height and weight in men and women.

    c. Compare the numerical values with the visual distribution of heights and weights you drew in the histograms and describe whether you think your visual impression matches the numerical values.

Subject	Men		Women	
	Height (in)	Weight (lb)	Height (in)	Weight (lb)
1	65	136	60	95
2	66	146	61	103
3	67	141	62	110
4	67	148	62	109
5	68	147	62	118
6	68	166	63	137
7	69	165	63	152
8	69	173	64	134
9	69	159	64	127
10	70	188	64	166
11	70	183	65	129
12	70	179	65	130
13	70	190	66	148
14	71	169	66	152
15	71	186	67	155
16	71	190	67	149
17	72	206	68	157
18	72	210	68	138
19	73	238	69	162
20	74	267	70	169

Population Genetics and Evolution at the Population, Species, and Molecular Levels

20

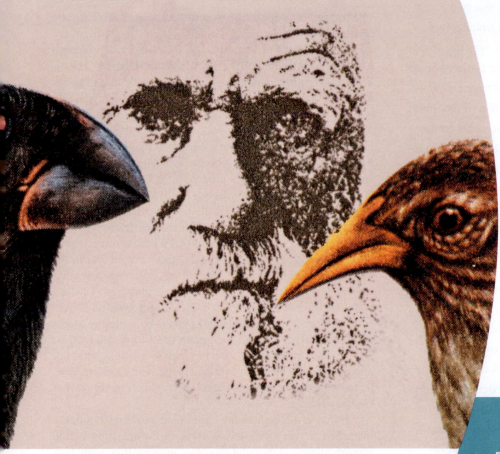

CHAPTER OUTLINE

20.1 The Hardy–Weinberg Equilibrium Describes the Relationship of Allele and Genotype Frequencies in Populations

20.2 Natural Selection Operates through Differential Reproductive Fitness within a Population

20.3 Mutation Diversifies Gene Pools

20.4 Gene Flow Occurs by the Movement of Organisms and Genes between Populations

20.5 Genetic Drift Causes Allele Frequency Change by Sampling Error

20.6 Inbreeding Alters Genotype Frequencies but Not Allele Frequencies

20.7 New Species Evolve by Reproductive Isolation

20.8 Molecular Evolution Changes Genes and Genomes through Time

Charles Darwin (1809–1882) studied the morphology and adaptation of finches on islands of the Galápagos and Cocos chains in formulating his theory of evolution by natural selection. The molecular genetics underlying the evolution of the two predominant beak shapes in finches—pointed for insect eating and blunt for seed crushing—have recently been described. The two shapes are shown along with an image of Darwin on this United Kingdom stamp commemorating the 100th anniversary of his death.

I n 1970, Theodosius Dobzhansky, one of the most influential geneticists of the 20th century, wrote,

> Nothing in biology makes sense except in the light of evolution.

Dobzhansky and the other architects of the *modern synthesis of evolution* (see Section 1.5) identified evolution and evolutionary analysis as central organizing principles of biology, necessary for understanding modern forms of life and their origins. Evolution shaped the living world we see today,

ESSENTIAL IDEAS

- The Hardy–Weinberg equilibrium predicts frequencies of genotypes in populations.
- The impact of natural selection on allele frequencies can be estimated.
- The effect of mutations on allele frequencies can be quantified.
- The effects of gene flow on allele frequencies in populations can be calculated.
- Chance events can lead to changes in allele frequency.
- Inbreeding is a pattern of nonrandom mating that can alter genotype frequencies.
- Species and higher taxonomic groups evolve in genetic isolation.
- Molecular genetic evolution parallels speciation and higher-level diversification.

just as it shaped life in the past, and will continue to shape it into the future. All four of the evolutionary processes described in Section 1.5—natural selection, mutation, migration (gene flow), and genetic drift—play a role in shaping the evolution of genes, proteins, populations, and species.

The modern synthesis focused on uniting two elements of evolutionary biology. One was the large-scale evolutionary change linked to speciation and to the divergence of taxonomic groups above the species level. The second element consisted of what was known about Mendelian inheritance and the connection between inherited molecular variation (i.e., variation of DNA and protein sequences) and evolutionary change. Through this unification, the modern synthesis has given rise to a simple definition of evolution: the change in allele frequencies in populations over time. Much of the discussion in this chapter centers on that definition of evolution.

The impact of the evolutionary processes on populations has been a focus of population biologists, evolutionary biologists, and mathematicians since the beginning of the 20th century, several decades before DNA was identified as the hereditary molecule and its structure became known. The central predictions that were made more than a century ago about populations on the basis of evolutionary principles have been proven correct time and again in countless experiments and observations in natural and experimental populations. In this chapter, we focus on the connection between the evolution of populations and evolution at the molecular level, that is, the evolution of genes, genomes, and proteins. We begin our discussion with the application of evolutionary principles to populations that forms the foundation of the field of **population genetics**. We then discuss the operation of each of the evolutionary processes, using examples that largely focus on humans. The causes of speciation are then explored, and we conclude the chapter with a discussion of molecular evolution.

20.1 The Hardy–Weinberg Equilibrium Describes the Relationship of Allele and Genotype Frequencies in Populations

The origin of population genetics can be traced to the earliest years of the 1900s, shortly after the rediscovery of Mendel's laws of heredity, and to a time when George Udny Yule, William Castle, Karl Pearson, Godfrey Hardy, Wilhelm Weinberg, and others first debated the fate of genes in populations. In 1902, the inheritance of brachydactyly (OMIM 112500), an autosomal dominant condition characterized by shortening of fingers and toes, was described in humans as a trait paralleling a Mendelian pattern of heredity. In contemplating this observation, Yule proposed that since three-quarters of the progeny of a cross of heterozygous parents with brachydactyly will also display shortened digits, the frequency of the dominant allele might be expected to increase over time. William Castle thought Yule was wrong, and in 1903 he offered, as a partial refutation of Yule's contention, a mathematical demonstration that in the absence of natural selection, genotype frequencies remain stable in populations. Karl Pearson supported Castle's position by showing that if two alleles of a gene had equal frequency in a population, there would be a single, stable equilibrium frequency for their genotypes. Reginald Punnett (of Punnett square fame) also thought Yule was wrong, but unable to formulate a mathematical argument to refute Yule, he took the problem to his friend and regular cricket partner Godfrey Hardy.

Hardy, a mathematician rather than a biologist, quickly identified a "very simple" solution to the question of the fate of alleles in populations. He showed that with random mating and in the absence of evolutionary change in a population, the allele frequencies result in a stable equilibrium frequency. Hardy also showed that, at equilibrium, allele frequencies are stable and that genotypes occur in predictable frequencies derived directly from allele frequencies. In 1908, Hardy penned a letter to the editors of *Science* magazine that began with these self-effacing words:

> I am reluctant to intrude in a discussion concerning matters of which I have no expert knowledge, and I should have expected the very simple point which I wish to make to have been familiar to biologists. However, some remarks of Mr. Udny Yule, to which Mr. R. C. Punnett has called my attention, suggest it may be worth making.

In his letter, Hardy demonstrated that Yule was wrong. Dominant alleles *do not* increase in frequency over time. His letter laid out the concept that has become known as the **Hardy–Weinberg (H-W) equilibrium**. The name recognizes Hardy's explanation of allele and genotype frequencies in populations as well as an independent explanation of the same principle by Wilhelm Weinberg (a German physician) that was also published in 1908. The H-W equilibrium is a cornerstone of population genetics and was the first of many developments in evolutionary genetics that culminated in the modern synthesis. Hardy may have been reluctant to intrude into matters of biology, but biologists for more than 100 years have been glad he did!

Populations and Gene Pools

A **population** is a group of interbreeding organisms. The collection of genes and alleles found in the members of a population is known as a **gene pool**. The gene pool is the source of genetic information from which the next generation is produced. Each population member carries a portion of the gene pool in its genome, but typically, the amount of genetic variation in a gene pool is greater than the variation carried by individual members of the population. The pattern of mating between individuals and the effect of evolutionary processes on alleles determine (1) how alleles are dispersed into genotypes and (2) their frequencies in successive generations.

The H-W equilibrium serves as a model demonstrating that the frequencies of alleles and genotypes in a theoretical population of infinite size that practices random mating does not experience evolutionary change. In other words, allele frequencies do not change over time if there is no evolution. The H-W equilibrium predicts that allele frequencies will be stable from generation to generation, that the frequencies of genotypes are predictable from their constituent allele frequencies, and that genotype frequencies too will remain the same in successive generations.

In nature, however, no real population meets all the criteria assumed by the H-W equilibrium. For example, all populations are finite in size and are subject to genetic drift as a consequence (an evolutionary mechanism we encounter in Section 20.5). In addition, natural selection, migration, and mutation each exert their influences on a population. Despite these circumstances, most populations adhere closely enough to the assumptions of the H-W equilibrium that alleles are distributed into genotypes in the proportions it predicts. The H-W equilibrium has proven to be a dependable arithmetic tool for assessing population genetic structure and detecting evolutionary change and nonrandom mating, and it is applied in numerous ways to the analysis of autosomal and X-linked genes in populations.

The Hardy–Weinberg Equilibrium

The predictions of the H-W equilibrium can be modeled for any number of alleles of an autosomal or an X-linked gene. The simplest model, however, is for two alleles of an autosomal gene, here designated A_1 and A_2, and this is the model we will focus on for most of our discussion. The assumptions and predictions of the H-W equilibrium are given

Table 20.1	The Hardy–Weinberg Equilibrium

Assumptions

1. Population size is infinite.
2. Random mating occurs in the population, allowing genotype frequencies to be predicted by allele frequencies.
3. Natural selection does not operate.
4. Migration (gene flow) does not introduce new alleles.
5. Mutation does not introduce new alleles.
6. Genetic drift does not occur.

Predictions

1. Allele frequencies remain stable over time.
2. Allele distribution into genotypes is predictable.
3. Stable equilibrium frequencies of alleles and genotypes are maintained.
4. Evolutionary and nonrandom mating effects are predictable.

in **Table 20.1**. The assumptions of the H-W equilibrium can be thought of simply as meaning that the population is infinitely large, experiences no evolution, and contains members that mate at random. As stated previously, these assumptions are not met by real populations, but reality is often close enough to the theory to allow accurate predictions to be made based on the H-W equilibrium. For the general case of two alleles of an autosomal gene, the alleles are given frequencies of $f(A_1) = p$ and $f(A_2) = q$, with the frequencies equal in males and females. Since A_1 and A_2 are the only alleles that occur at this gene, the sum of their frequencies is $p + q = 1.0$. Rearrangements of this equality allow the frequency of one allele to be used to determine the frequency of the other allele; thus, $p = 1 - q$ and $q = 1 - p$.

Allelic segregation governs the relationship between allele frequencies and genotype frequencies in populations. For the two alleles in our example, there are three genotypes: A_1A_1, A_1A_2, and A_2A_2. The genotype frequencies are computed using a binomial expansion $[(p + q)^2]$, where the two $(p + q)$ expressions represent male and female contributions to mating. Alternatively, a representation of random mating in the population that resembles a Punnett square can be used. Both methods make the same genotype frequency predictions of $f(A_1A_1) = p^2, f(A_1A_2) = 2pq$, and $f(A_2A_2) = q^2$ (**Figure 20.1**). The summation of these three genotype frequencies equals unity: $p^2 + 2pq + q^2 = 1.0$.

We can demonstrate the application of the H-W equilibrium by assigning frequencies to each allele in a hypothetical population. Say that in a certain population, $f(A_1) = p = 0.6$ and $f(A_2) = q = 0.4$. As required, the sum of the two allele frequencies is $0.6 + 0.4 = 1.0$. Therefore, in this hypothetical population example, 60 percent of gametes carry A_1 and 40 percent carry A_2 (**Figure 20.2**). If the population is in H-W equilibrium, probability predicts that an A_1-containing

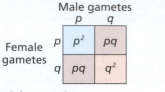

Binomial expansion
$(p + q)(p + q) = p^2 + pq + pq + q^2 = p^2 + 2pq + q^2 = 1$

Figure 20.1   The Hardy–Weinberg equilibrium for autosomal genes. The Punnett square method and the binomial expansion of alleles with frequencies p and q predict genotype frequencies under assumptions of the Hardy–Weinberg equilibrium.

◉ **The diagram is reminiscent of a Punnett square, but it represents mating in a population rather than between two organisms. In one or two sentences, describe what the diagram is showing.**

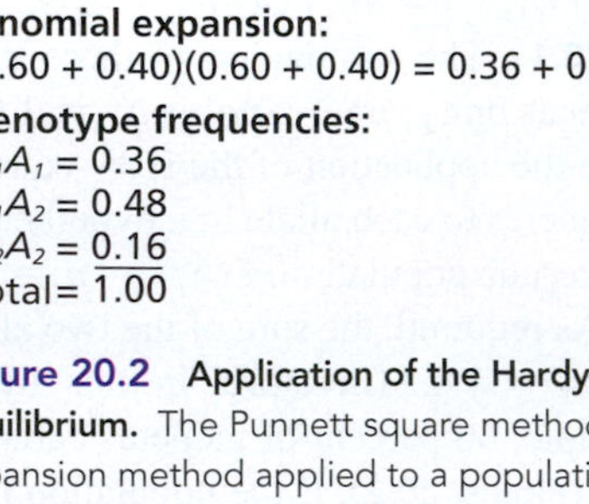

gamete from a male and an A_1-containing female gamete will unite to produce A_1A_1 progeny with a frequency of $(0.6)(0.6) = 0.36$. Similarly, the production of A_2A_2 progeny, from the union of two A_2-containing gametes, has a frequency of $(0.4)(0.4) = 0.16$. Heterozygous progeny are produced in two ways, with a combined frequency predicted as $(0.6)(0.4) + (0.6)(0.4) = 0.48$. The sum of frequencies of the three genotypes is $(0.36) + (0.48) + (0.16) = 1.00$. The binomial expansion method of calculating the genotype frequencies in progeny makes identical predictions.

In this example we see one of the predictions of the H-W equilibrium: Random mating for one generation produces genotype frequencies that can be predicted from allele frequencies. For any frequencies of p and q between 0.0 and 1.0, an expected equilibrium distribution of genotype frequencies can be derived (**Figure 20.3**). Notice that as the frequency of

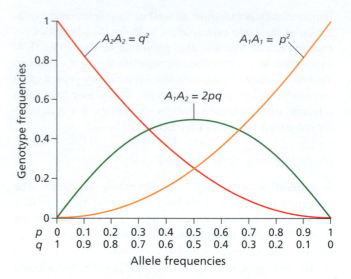

Figure 20.3   The Hardy–Weinberg equilibrium for two autosomal alleles. Each curve shows the frequency of the genotype for the indicated frequencies of the alleles p and q.

◉ **Assuming a gene has two alleles that are in H-W equilibrium frequencies, a) what are the allele frequencies if $A_1A_1 = 0.81$? b) What are the allele frequencies if $A_1A_2 = 0.42$?**

p decreases and q increases, the proportions of genotypes shift, altering the frequency of each homozygous class and the frequency of heterozygotes in the population. Heterozygous frequency has a maximum of 0.50 (50 percent), when the frequencies are $p = q = 0.50$.

This example also allows us to observe the second prediction of the H-W equilibrium: With random mating and no evolution, allele frequencies do not change from one generation to the next. We see this if we count the alleles in progeny genotypes, recognizing that *all* of the alleles in A_1A_1 are alleles of a single type, and all the alleles in A_2A_2 progeny are alleles of the other type. The A_1A_1 progeny are 36 percent of the new generation, and A_2A_2 are 16 percent. Among the 48 percent of the progeny that are heterozygotes, exactly *one-half* of the alleles are A_1 and *one-half* are A_2. Consequently, the frequency of A_1 among the progeny is 36 percent plus 24 percent, or 60 percent of the alleles carried by progeny, which is the same frequency that was seen in the parental generation. The A_2 frequency is 16 percent plus 24 percent, or 40 percent of the progeny-generation alleles, also the same as the frequency found in the parental generation. Expressed as p and q, the frequency of A_1 in the progeny generation is $f(A_1) = p^2 + pq$, and the frequency of A_2 is $f(A_2) = q^2 + pq$.

The observations that random mating leads to predictable genotype frequencies and that allele frequencies are stable from one generation to the next can be portrayed in a mating-table format that shows the consequence of reproduction under the assumptions of the H-W equilibrium (**Table 20.2**). In the mating-table analysis, parental genotypes unite to reproduce at proportions predicted by their frequency. If parents have the same genotype, there is no

Male gametes

	A_1 0.60	A_2 0.40
Female gametes A_1 0.60	A_1A_1 0.36	A_1A_2 0.24
A_2 0.40	A_1A_2 0.24	A_2A_2 0.16

Binomial expansion:
$(0.60 + 0.40)(0.60 + 0.40) = 0.36 + 0.24 + 0.24 + 0.16 = 1.00$

Genotype frequencies:
$A_1A_1 = 0.36$
$A_1A_2 = 0.48$
$A_2A_2 = 0.16$
Total $= 1.00$

Figure 20.2   Application of the Hardy–Weinberg equilibrium. The Punnett square method and the binomial expansion method applied to a population in which $f(A_1) = 0.60$ and $f(A_2) = 0.40$.

Table 20.2	Hardy–Weinberg Mating Table for Two Alleles of an Autosomal Gene			
Mating	**Mating Frequency**	**Progeny Genotypes**		
		A_1A_1	A_1A_2	A_2A_2
$A_1A_1 \times A_1A_1$	$(p^2)(p^2) = p^4$	p^4	—	—
$A_1A_1 \times A_1A_2$	$2[(p^2)(2pq)] = 4p^3q$	$2p^3q$	$2p^3q$	—
$A_1A_1 \times A_2A_2$	$2[(p^2)(q^2)] = 2p^2q^2$	—	$2p^2q^2$	—
$A_1A_2 \times A_1A_2$	$(2pq)(2pq) = 4p^2q^2$	p^2q^2	$2p^2q^2$	p^2q^2
$A_1A_2 \times A_2A_2$	$2[(2pq)(q^2)] = 4pq^3$	—	$2pq^3$	$2pq^3$
$A_2A_2 \times A_2A_2$	$(q^2)(q^2) = q^4$	—	—	q^4
Total	1.0	p^2	$2pq$	q^2

Among the progeny, a common term is factored out of each summation to produce the frequency of each genotype:

$$A_1A_1 = p^4 + 2p^3q + p^2q^2 = p^2 1 p^2 + 2pq + q^2 2 = p^2$$

$$A_1A_2 = 2p^3q + 2p^2q^2 + 2p^2q^2 + 2pq^3 = 2pq 1 p^2 + pq + pq + q^2 2 = 2pq$$

$$A_2A_2 = p^2q^2 + 2pq^3 + q^4 = q^2(p^2 + 2pq + q^2) = q^2$$

The sum of progeny genotype frequencies is $p^2 + 2pq + q^2 = 1.0$.

reciprocal mating to account for, but if different genotypes occur in the parents, the reciprocal matings must be taken into account. The progeny of each mating are predicted according to Mendelian principles. The frequency or fraction of offspring with each genotype is summed once the table is filled. The term that is the sum of each genotype frequency can be simplified to show that offspring are produced in the genotype proportions p^2, $2pq$, and q^2, just as they occur in the parents. This analysis is compelling evidence that in the presence of random mating and the absence of evolutionary change, the allele frequencies in populations are stable over time.

In populations that meet the assumptions of the H-W equilibrium, a single generation of random mating will "reset" the genotype frequencies in the population into the predicted proportions p^2, $2pq$, and q^2. Moreover, if a population meets the assumptions but *is not* initially in H-W equilibrium, we can predict what the consequence of one generation of random mating will be. As an example, **Figure 20.4** illustrates the effect of uniting two previously separate populations with different frequencies of A_1 and A_2 to form a new population. Each of the contributing populations originally contained 500 individuals, and the new population contains 1000 individuals. Immediately after forming the new population, the genotypes *are not* in Hardy–Weinberg proportions. One generation of mating in the new population under Hardy–Weinberg assumptions, however, produces genotype frequencies in the next generation that *are* in H-W equilibrium. The new population has new allele frequencies as a result of the mixing of the two populations.

Determining Autosomal Allele Frequencies in Populations

Allele frequencies and genotype frequencies are commonly used measures of the genetic structure of populations. Comparison of these frequencies between populations can identify relationships and diversification of populations, and documentation of allele frequency change over time is evidence of population evolution.

Allele frequencies in populations can be estimated by two methods, the gene-counting method and the square root method. The gene-counting method does not require any assumptions about the population; it only requires that all genotypes can be identified. It can be used whether or not one knows or can assume the population is in H-W equilibrium. For the square root method, on the other hand, one must know or must assume that the population is in H-W equilibrium. The square root method is often used when the trait of interest is the result of a recessive homozygous genotype and where the heterozygous and homozygous dominant genotypes result in identical phenotypes.

The gene-counting method can be accomplished in either of two ways: by calculating the proportions of genotypes or by directly counting the number of alleles from the genotypes themselves. We describe these two "gene-counting" approaches separately for convenience, but they are really the same. The choice is dictated by the type of genotype or phenotype information available and the composition of the population or of the sample data.

Figure 20.4 One generation of random mating produces Hardy–Weinberg equilibrium frequencies for genotypes of autosomal genes.

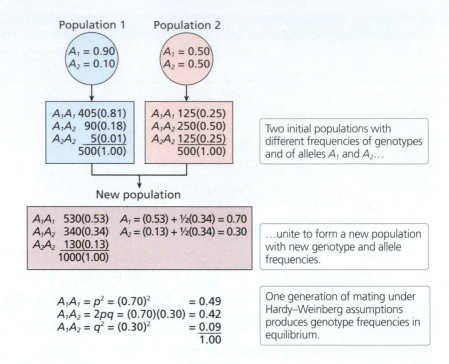

The Genotype Proportion Method

The first approach to gene counting is called the **genotype proportion method**. This approach calculates allele frequencies (f) as already demonstrated in one of the examples above, by adding the frequency of the homozygotes for the allele and the frequency of one-half of the heterozygotes carrying the allele. For instance, suppose that a population has the following composition: $B_1B_1 = 0.64$, $B_1B_2 = 0.32$, $B_2B_2 = 0.04$. Applying the genotype proportion method, the frequency of B_1 is the sum of the frequency of B_1B_1 plus one-half the frequency of B_1B_2 heterozygotes. In this case, $f(B_1) = p = (0.64) + [(0.5)(0.32)] = 0.80$. Similarly, for B_2, the allele frequency is calculated by adding the frequency of B_2B_2 and one-half the frequency of B_1B_2, or $f(B_2) = q = (0.04) + [(0.5)(0.32)] = 0.20$. For this example, notice that $p + q = 0.80 + 0.20 = 1.0$.

The Allele-Counting Method

The second approach to the gene-counting method is called the **allele-counting method**. As an example of the allele-counting method, consider the human MN blood group system, a codominant system produced by two alleles, M and N. Both alleles are present in all human populations and produce three blood group phenotypes: type M, type MN, and type N. Each blood group has a corresponding genotype. Individuals with blood type M or blood type N have homozygous genotypes MM and NN, respectively, and the blood type MN is produced by the MN genotype. MN blood group testing of 1482 members of a Japanese population produced the following results:

Blood group	M	MN	N	
Number	406	744	332	= 1482

The allele frequency calculation recognizes that each of the 1482 people in the sample carries two alleles of the gene and that there are $(2)(1482) = 2964$ alleles represented in the sample. The frequency of each allele is determined by counting the two alleles of that type from each homozygote and the single allele of that type from each heterozygote and dividing the result by the total alleles in the sample. The allele frequencies are therefore $f(M) = [(2)(406) + (744)]/2964 = 0.525$ and $f(N) = [(2)(332) + (744)]/2964 = 0.475$.

The Square Root Method

The alternative approach for allele frequency determination in populations is the **square root method**. It is used only when the gene has two alleles, one dominant and one recessive; the condition or trait of interest is recessive; and the investigator knows or can assume that the population is in H-W equilibrium. In the human autosomal recessive disorder cystic fibrosis, for example, one allele (*cf*) is recessive and therefore is evident only in the homozygous genotype. When the recessive allele is in a heterozygous genotype, it is "hidden" by the dominant allele (*CF*). In a circumstance like this, the dominant phenotype consists of two genotypes, *CFCF* and *CFcf*. In contrast, the recessive phenotype is produced only by the homozygous recessive genotype *cfcf*. The correspondence of the recessive phenotype and homozygous genotype allows use of Hardy–Weinberg principles to estimate the frequency of the recessive allele by taking the square root of the recessive homozygous genotype frequency. In the U.S. population, the frequency of cystic fibrosis among newborn infants is approximately 1 in 2000. Where $f(CF) = p$ and $f(cf) = q$, $f(cfcf) = q^2 = 0.0005$. The frequency of q is thus estimated as the square root of 0.0005, or $f(q) = 0.022$; that is, about 2.2 percent.

With $f(cf)$ determined, the frequency of CF is estimated as $f(CF) = p = 1 - q = 1.0 - 0.022 = 0.978$. Then, according to the Hardy–Weinberg principle, the population frequency of carriers is $f(CFcf) = 2pq = 2(0.978)(0.022) = 0.043$. In other words, approximately 4.3 percent of the population, or about 1 in 23 people, carry a recessive mutant allele for cystic fibrosis. The frequency of carriers of cystic fibrosis is of practical importance for determining the chance that a person could pass the allele on to his or her progeny. Estimates like this can be particularly valuable in genetic counseling situations, where it is desirable to know the probability that a person who has a dominant phenotype might be a heterozygous carrier of a recessive allele. Genetic Analysis 20.1 provides more practice in calculating allele frequencies and applying the H-W equilibrium.

The Hardy–Weinberg Equilibrium for More than Two Alleles

Having examined the application of the H-W equilibrium to genes with two alleles, we can now consider the more complex case of a gene that has more than two alleles. We shall limit our discussion to three alleles, whose frequencies are represented by the variables p, q, and r, where $p + q + r = 1.0$, and where the trinomial expansion $(p + q + r)^2$ represents random mating and predicts the distribution of alleles in genotypes. Assuming that the population is in H-W equilibrium, the frequencies of the six resulting genotypes are predicted to be as listed in Table 20.3a, and the sum of

genotype frequencies resulting from the trinomial expansion is $(p + q + r)^2 = p^2 + 2pq + q^2 + 2pr + r^2 + 2qr = 1.0$.

The human ABO blood group system provides an opportunity for applying the H-W equilibrium to a gene with three alleles (see Section 4.1). Recall that among the three alleles producing ABO blood types (I^A, I^B, and i) I^A and I^B exhibit dominance over i but are codominant to one another. These allelic relationships result in four blood types from the six genotypes (see Figure 4.3). Using $f(I^A) = p, f(I^B) = q$, and $f(i) = r$, along with data reporting the frequencies of each blood type in a population as type O = 46%, type A = 37%, type B = 13%, and type AB = 4%, we can estimate the frequency of each allele by applying a version of the square root method. Table 20.3b shows the calculations of the genotype frequencies from allele frequencies. They are derived as follows:

Step 1. Blood type O is found with recessive homozygous genotypes, and the frequency of the blood type is $r^2 = 0.46$. The square root of $0.46 = r$; thus, the allele frequency is $f(i) = r = 0.68$.

Step 2. The combined frequency of blood types A and O is $p^2 + 2pr + r^2 = (p + r)^2$, so $f(I^A) = p$ is estimated by the square root of the combined frequency of A plus the frequency of O minus r. The calculation is $f(I^A) = p = \sqrt{[0.37 + 0.46]} - r = 0.91 - 0.68 = 0.23$.

Step 3. Having estimated p and r, we can solve for q by $q = 1 - (p + r) = 1 - (0.23 + 0.68) = 0.09$.

The Chi-Square Test of Hardy–Weinberg Predictions

Strictly speaking, the assumptions of the H-W equilibrium are unattainable in real populations. From a statistical perspective, however, what matters is whether the observed genotype frequencies in populations deviate *significantly* from the predictions of the H-W equilibrium. The chi-square test is used when it is not known whether or not the population is in H-W equilibrium. Chi-square analysis tests the hypothesis that H-W equilibrium exists in the population by comparing observed and expected results. If there is no significant deviation between observed and expected values, the hypothesis of H-W equilibrium in the population is not rejected. If, on the other hand, the test reveals a significant deviation, the hypothesis of H-W equilibrium in the population is rejected.

If chi square analysis finds that a population does not deviate significantly from H-W equilibrium predictions, the population is assumed to be exhibiting random mating and not to be experiencing significant evolutionary change in the current generation. If, instead, chi-square analysis detects a significant deviation from H-W equilibrium expectations, the cause can be investigated. The reasons can differ, but for human populations the sources of

Table 20.3	Hardy–Weinberg Equilibrium Genotype Frequencies for Three Alleles of a Gene

(a) Genotype prediction for three alleles

Genotype	Genotype Frequency
A_1A_1	p^2
A_1A_2	$2pq$
A_1A_3	$2pr$
A_2A_2	q^2
A_2A_3	$2qr$
A_3A_3	r^2

(b) Hardy–Weinberg analysis of ABO blood group data

Genotype	Genotype Frequency[a]	Blood Type
I^AI^A	$p^2 = (0.23)^2 = 0.053$	A
I^Ai	$2pr = 2[(0.23)(0.68)] = 0.314$	A
I^BI^B	$q^2 = (0.09)^2 = 0.008$	B
I^Bi	$2qr = 2[(0.09)(0.68)] = 0.122$	B
I^AI^B	$2pq = 2[(0.23)(0.09)] = 0.041$	AB
ii	$r^2 = (0.68)^2 = 0.462$	O

[a] Where $f(A_1) = p$; $f(A_2) = q$; $f(A_3) = r$; and $p + q + r = 1.0$

PROBLEM A worldwide survey of genetic variation in human populations reported the autosomal codominant MN blood group types in a sample of 1029 Chinese from Hong Kong. The sample contained 342 people with blood type M, 500 with blood type MN, and 187 with blood type N.

a. Determine the frequencies of both alleles (*M* and *N*) using the genotype proportion method and the allele-counting method.

b. Determine the expected genotype frequencies and the number of individuals with each genotype under assumptions of the H-W equilibrium.

> **BREAK IT DOWN:** Since we know the number of individuals with each genotype for this codominant trait in a sample of 1029 individuals, the 2058 alleles can each be enumerated (p. 730).

Solution Strategies	Solution Steps
Evaluate	
1. Identify the topic this problem addresses and the nature of the required answer.	1. This problem addresses the determination of allele frequencies from population data and the determination of expected genotype frequencies under assumptions of the H-W equilibrium.
2. Identify the critical information given in the problem.	2. The number of individuals with each blood type is given, and the blood type is identified as an autosomal codominant trait.
Deduce	
3. Determine the genotype corresponding to each blood group.	3. For this autosomal codominant trait, blood type M individuals have the genotype *MM*, those with blood type N are *NN*, and MN individuals are *MN*.
4. Calculate the frequency of each blood type in the sample.	4. Blood type M is 342/1029 = 0.332, MN is 500/1029 = 0.486, and N is 187/1029 = 0.186.

> **TIP:** The frequency of each genotype is the number of people with the genotype over the total sample size.

Solve	Answer a
5. Calculate allele frequencies using the genotype proportion method.	5. The frequencies are $$f(M) = (0.332) + [(0.5)(0.486)] = 0.575 \text{ and}$$ $$f(N) = (0.186) + [(0.5)(0.486)] = 0.425$$
6. Calculate the allele frequencies by the allele-counting method	6. For the sample of 1029 people, there are 2058 alleles. The allele frequencies are $$f(M) = [(2)(342)] + (500)/2058 = 0.575 \text{ and}$$ $$f(N) = [(2)(187)] + (500)/2058 = 0.425$$

> **TIP:** If the allele frequencies are calculated correctly, their sum will be 1.0.

	Answer b
7. Determine the expected genotype frequencies and the number of individuals with each genotype under Hardy–Weinberg assumptions.	7. The expected genotype frequencies are $$MM = (0.575)^2 = 0.33; (0.33)(1029) = 339.57$$ $$MN = 2[(0.575)(0.425)] = 0.49; (0.49)(1029) = 504.21 \text{ and}$$ $$NN = (0.425)^2 = 0.18; (0.18)(1029) = 185.22$$

> **TIP:** Assume $f(M) = p$ and $f(N) = q$, and expand the binomial equation $(p + q)^2 = p^2 + 2pq + q^2$.

For more practice, see Problems 17, 18, 21, and 25.   Visit the Study Area to access study tools.   **Mastering Genetics**

significant deviation are most often either small population size, substantial migration in or out of the population, or nonrandom mating. We discuss these effects in following sections.

The H-W equilibrium has application beyond the mere examination of populations. Some of the most interesting applications are seen in forensic genetics—for instance in crime scene analysis of DNA or in paternity assessment. Application Chapter E: Forensic Genetics explores these applications.

20.2 Natural Selection Operates through Differential Reproductive Fitness within a Population

Application of the H-W equilibrium to idealized populations reveals that allele frequencies, along with the frequencies of genotypes, are maintained when the population mates at random and in the absence of the action of evolutionary mechanisms. But what happens to allele frequencies when evolution does occur? The simple answer is that allele frequencies change, and along with them genotype frequencies are altered. The evolutionary impact can be quantified by determining the change in allele frequencies. An implicit component of the description of evolution as change in allele frequencies in a population over time is the presence of inherited genetic diversity. If there is no genetic diversity, there can be no evolution.

In this section, we look at the effects of different mechanisms of natural selection on allele frequencies and H-W equilibrium. In later sections, we examine how the other evolutionary processes—mutation, migration (gene flow), and genetic drift—affect allele frequencies and H-W equilibrium in populations (see Section 1.5).

Differential Reproductive Fitness and Relative Fitness

Natural selection results from the differential reproductive success of organisms in the population. Organisms that leave more offspring distribute more copies of their alleles to the next generation, and this increases the frequency of the alleles that those most successful reproducers pass on. Natural selection usually operates as a result of differences in anatomical, physiological, behavioral, or other traits passed to progeny by the more successful reproducers and not present in organisms that are less successful at reproduction. The most successful individuals may survive to reproductive age at higher rates than other population members, they may reproduce at higher rates, or both. This phenomenon is called **differential reproductive fitness**, and it is a central feature of natural selection. The consequence of differential reproductive fitness is that more of some alleles than others are passed to the next generation, and this imbalance changes allele frequencies in the population over time. On this basis, natural selection is sometimes said to "favor the most fit" organisms in the population, meaning those with the highest reproductive fitness among the organisms in the population.

Reproductive fitness is not an idealized concept or value. It is a real consequence of inherited variation operated on by natural selection, causing the most fit among a generation of organisms to produce more offspring. A common way to measure the intensity of natural selection is to determine the impact of differential reproduction on the next generation. This involves use of the **relative fitness (w)** of organisms, a value that quantifies the reproductive success of other genotypes relative to the most favored genotype. Since this is a relative comparison, organisms with the greatest reproductive success have a relative fitness of $w = 1.0$.

The genotypes that reproduce less successfully than the most favored genotype have a relative fitness of less than $w = 1.0$. These less fit genotypes have their relative fitness reduced by a proportion called the **selection coefficient (s)**. The selection coefficient identifies the proportionate difference between the fitnesses of organisms with different traits.

For example, if an organism not having the favored trait reproduces 80 percent as well as the organism with the trait, the selection coefficient is $s = 0.2$, and the relative fitness of the organism is expressed as $w = 1 - s$, or $1 - 0.2 = 0.8$. If other organisms experience yet a different level of relative fitness, a second selection coefficient, designated t, is used. Where an organism with one genotype is most fit and organisms with either of two other genotypes experience reduced fitness, the relative fitness values for the two less fit genotypes are expressed as $w = 1 - s$ and $w = 1 - t$.

Directional Natural Selection

In the pattern of natural selection called **directional natural selection (directional selection**, for short), the favored phenotype has a homozygous genotype. Organisms with this phenotype have higher relative fitness than other phenotypes in the population. Natural selection favoring one homozygous genotype produces a directional change in allele frequencies that increases the favored allele frequency and decreases others.

In the directional selection example that follows, assume alleles B_1 and B_2 are codominant. The codominant relationship of these alleles will result in one genotype that occurs in organisms with the highest relative fitness and in reduced fitness in organisms with the other genotypes. In this example, the allele frequencies are $f(B_1) = 0.6$ and $f(B_2) = 0.4$, there are 1000 members of the population, the favored phenotype has a relative fitness of $w = 1.0$, and the other phenotypes have different relative fitness values of $w = 0.80$ and $w = 0.40$. The genetic profile of the population, therefore, is as follows:

Genotype	B_1B_1	B_1B_2	B_2B_2
Frequency	0.36	0.48	0.16
Number	360	480	160
Relative fitness (w)	1.0	0.80	0.40

As this table shows, the B_1B_1 organisms have the highest relative fitness ($w = 1.0$). In comparison, B_1B_2 organisms have $s = 0.20$ and $w = 1 - s = 0.80$, and organisms with the B_2B_2 genotype have a selection coefficient of $t = 0.60$ and a relative fitness of $w = 1 - t = 0.40$.

Given this profile as a starting point, the impact of natural selection on the population is computed in two steps. First, assuming natural selection has its effect before organisms reach reproductive age, the surviving number of organisms of each genotype is calculated by multiplying the original number of each genotype by the relative fitness value of the genotype. In this case the numbers of survivors of each genotype are $B_1B_1 = (1.0)(360) = 360$, $B_1B_2 = (0.80)(480) = 384$, and $B_2B_2 = (0.40)(160) = 64$. In this hypothetical population, 808 organisms of the original 1000 remain after natural selection.

The second step is determination of the allele frequencies after natural selection and of the genotype frequencies in the next generation. In this case, the frequencies are most readily calculated using the allele-counting method, since we can identify the genotype of each survivor. There are a total of 1616 alleles in the 808 survivors, and the allele frequencies after natural selection are $f(B_1) = [(2)(360) + (384)]/1616 = 1104/1616 = 0.683$, and $f(B_2) = [(2)(64) + (384)]/(2)(808) = 512/1616 = 0.317$. If we assume that random mating takes place among the survivors and that no other evolutionary mechanism other than natural selection is operating, the genotype frequencies in the next generation are $f(B_1B_1) = (0.683)^2 = 0.467, f(B_1B_2) = 2(0.683)(0.317) = 0.433$, and $f(B_2B_2) = (0.317)^2 = 0.100$.

The changes in allele frequencies are symbolized by the Greek delta (Δ) and found by taking the absolute value of the difference between the original allele frequency and the new allele frequency. For this example in which B_1 has increased and B_2 has decreased, the values are, $\Delta B_1 = 0.683 - 0.60 = 0.083$, and $\Delta B_2 = 0.317 - 0.40 = 0.083$. If this pattern of natural selection continues for enough generations, the frequency of the B_1 allele will eventually become fixed at $f(B_1) = 1.0$, and the frequency of B_2 will be eliminated, so that its final frequency will be $f(B_2) = 0.0$. Once an allele frequency is either fixed ($f = 1.0$) or eliminated ($f = 0.0$), natural selection can no longer change the frequency. Population allele frequencies of 0.0 or 1.0 can, however, be changed by migration and mutation. **Figure 20.5** illustrates that

directional selection favoring B_1 increases the frequency of that allele at a pace determined by the intensity of natural selection.

The concept of relative fitness values can be applied to populations in several ways. **Table 20.4** illustrates a case of natural selection against a homozygous recessive genotype. In this case, frequencies of $f(B) = 0.50$ and $f(b) = 0.50$ are subjected to natural selection against bb, where $w_{bb} = 0.0$ and $w_{Bb} = w_{BB} = 1.0$. No bb individuals survive to reproductive age, thus removing 25 percent of the population. When the relative genotype frequencies are determined using their new proportions in the surviving reproductive population, $f(B)$ and $f(b)$ are calculated to be $f(B) = 0.667$ and $f(b) = 0.333$. Among the progeny in generation 1, genotype frequencies are $f(BB) = 0.445$, $f(Bb) = 0.444$, and $f(bb) = 0.111$.

Directional natural selection against the homozygous recessive genotype causes the frequency of the dominant allele to increase and the frequency of the recessive allele to decrease. Eventually, the recessive allele may be eliminated from the population gene pool. The recessive allele is not eliminated quickly, however, and its frequency changes slowly, especially as the allele gets less frequent. The slow pace of evolutionary change at low allele frequencies is due to the smaller number of recessive homozygotes in the population.

Numerous directional selection experiments, taking place over the last several decades of research, demonstrate support for the theoretical predictions for populations under directional selection. A 1981 study by Douglas Cavener and Michael Clegg examined four subpopulations of *Drosophila melanogaster* for 50 generations to test the effectiveness of artificial directional selection at increasing the frequency of the allele Adh^F of the *alcohol dehydrogenase (Adh)* gene. The enzyme product of Adh^F breaks ethanol down rapidly. An original population with an Adh^F frequency of 0.38 was

(a)

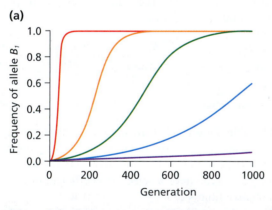

(b)

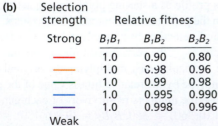

Figure 20.5 The consequences of the intensity of natural selection on allele frequency. (a) The curves illustrate the relationship between the rate of change in $f(B_1)$ and the intensity of natural selection. **(b)** Relative fitness values for natural selection of different intensities.

Table 20.4	A Model of Directional Selection against a Recessive Lethal Allele		
	Genotype		
	BB	**Bb**	**bb**
Frequency	0.25	0.50	0.25
Relative fitness (w)	1.0	1.0	0.0
Survivors after selection (total, 0.75)	0.25	0.50	0.00
Relative genotype frequencies	0.25/0.75 = 0.333	0.50/0.75 = 0.667	0.00

Estimated allele frequencies after natural selection:
$$f(B) = (0.333) + (0.5)(0.667) = 0.667$$
$$f(b) = (0) + (0.5)(0.667) = 0.333$$

Estimated genotype frequencies after reproduction:
$$f(BB) = (0.667)^2 = 0.445$$
$$f(Bb) = 2(0.667)(0.333) = 0.444$$
$$f(bb) = (0.333)^2 = 0.111$$

divided into four subpopulations of equal size. Two subpopulations reared on ethanol-rich food (population 1 and population 2) showed progressive increases in the frequency of Adh^F over 50 generations (**Figure 20.6**). In contrast, control populations (control 1 and control 2), which were reared on food without ethanol, showed an overall upward (control 1) and downward (control 2) drift of Adh^F frequency.

A similar effect is seen in the action of strong directional natural selection in human populations. Two independent reports published in 2010, one by Xin Yi and colleagues and the other by Tatum Simonson and colleagues, describe the rapid evolutionary changes that have occurred in the last 5000 years in native Tibetans who have adapted to low oxygen conditions in the high-altitude environment of the Himalayan mountains. Strong directional natural selection has operated in favor of certain alleles of multiple genes that increase oxygen utilization and improve oxygen transport and metabolism.

Natural Selection Favoring Heterozygotes

A pattern of natural selection that can produce and maintain genetic diversity in populations is seen when the heterozygous genotype is favored. The consequence of natural selection favoring the heterozygote is a **balanced polymorphism**, in which alleles reach stable equilibrium frequencies that are maintained in a steady state, balancing the selective pressures favoring the maintenance of a mutant allele when it occurs in a heterozygote but acting against it when it occurs in a homozygous genotype.

Table 20.5 depicts a natural selection scheme favoring heterozygotes. In this example, the relative fitness values are based on the heterozygous genotype (Cc) being 1.0, the relative fitness of CC being 0.80, and the fitness of cc being 0.20,

Table 20.5	A Model of Natural Selection Favoring the Heterozygous Genotype		
	Genotype		
	CC	**Cc**	**cc**
Frequency	0.25	0.50	0.25
Relative fitness	0.65	1.0	0.20
Survivors after selection (total = 0.7125)	0.1625	0.50	0.05
Relative genotype frequencies	0.1625/ 0.7125 = 0.228	0.50/ 0.7125 = 0.702	0.05/ 0.7125 = 0.070

New allele frequencies after natural selection:
$$f(C) = 0.579$$
$$f(c) = 0.421$$

Genotype frequencies after reproduction:
$$f(CC) = (0.579)^2 = 0.335$$
$$f(Cc) = 2[(0.579)(0.421)] = 0.448$$
$$f(cc) = (0.421)^2 = 0.177$$

indicating that few homozygotes with the cc genotype survive to reproductive age. The example assumes that the allele frequencies are initially equal—that is, $f(C) = f(c) = 0.50$ in generation 0. One generation of natural selection changes the allele frequencies to $f(C) = 0.579$ and $f(c) = 0.421$. The table shows calculations illustrating the action of natural selection in the production of generation 1.

Natural selection operating in favor of heterozygotes will eventually lead to a balanced polymorphism. (We explore another example of this pattern of natural selection in the Case Study at the end of the chapter.) Once attained, the equilibrium frequencies of the alleles will be maintained in a balanced polymorphism as long as natural selection remains steady. Population geneticists can predict the stable equilibrium frequencies of alleles in a balanced polymorphism using the relative intensity of natural selection against the homozygous genotypes. Using the variables s and t to represent the natural selection coefficients operating against the homozygous genotypes in the preceding example, the relative fitness of CC is $1 - s$ and the relative fitness of cc is $1 - t$. Solving for the values of s and t,

$$s = 1.0 - 0.65 = 0.35 \text{ and}$$
$$t = 1.0 - 0.20 = 0.80$$

The stable equilibrium values for p and q, designated p_E and q_E, in the balanced polymorphism are calculated as ratios of selection coefficients operating against the homozygous genotypes. In this example, the equilibrium p_E and q_E values are

$$p_E = t/(s + t) = 0.80/(0.35 + 0.80) = 0.696 \text{ and}$$
$$q_E = s/(s + t) = 0.35/(0.35 + 0.80) = 0.304$$

Genetic Analysis 20.2 examines a case of natural selection involving variant chromosomes, and calculation of their equilibrium frequencies, in a population of fruit flies.

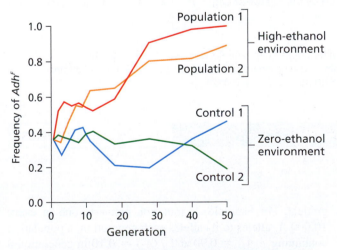

Figure 20.6 Directional artificial selection favoring the Adh^F allele in experimental *Drosophila* populations. The Adh^F allele increases in frequency in both of the experimental populations exposed to an ethanol-rich environment. Allele frequencies in the two control populations (no natural selection) drift up and down over the generations, ending up higher (control 1) and lower (control 2) than their starting frequencies.

PROBLEM In a *Drosophila* species, a naturally occurring autosomal inversion is found in two forms, Arrowhead (AR) and Standard (ST). Flies of this species can be homozygous for either chromosome form (AR/AR or ST/ST), or they can be heterozygous (AR/ST). In the 1970s, researchers determined that the relative fitness values for the three genotypes differed with respect to the fruit flies' ability to resist the now banned insecticide DDT. The relative fitness values are listed in the table to the right.

Genotype	Relative Fitness
AR/AR	0.65
AR/ST	1.00
ST/ST	0.50

a. Describe the pattern of natural selection operating on these chromosomes, and make a statement about the eventual fate of the two chromosome forms in this species.

b. Use the information provided to determine the equilibrium frequencies of AR and ST.

BREAK IT DOWN: The pattern of natural selection is determined by the relative fitness values that assign a fitness of 1.0 to the most fit genotype and lesser relative fitness values to the other genotypes (p. 733).

BREAK IT DOWN: Natural selection can eliminate an allele (frequency 0.0), fix an allele (frequency 1.0), or establish equilibrium frequencies for two or more alleles, depending on the pattern of natural selection (p. 734).

Solution Strategies	Solution Steps
Evaluate	
1. Identify the topic of this problem and the nature of the required answer.	1. This problem is about the effects of natural selection on the frequencies of two chromosome forms, AR and ST. The answer requires an explanation of the pattern of natural selection and a calculation to determine the ultimate frequencies of the chromosome forms.
2. Identify the critical information given in the problem.	2. The relative fitness values are given, and these can be used to determine the final frequencies of AR and ST.
Deduce	
3. Examine the relative fitness values for each genotype, and calculate the selection coefficients (s and t) against each genotype. TIP: Subtract the relative fitness of a genotype from 1.0 to determine the selection coefficients s and t.	3. The relative fitness value for the heterozygous genotype is 1.0, and the relative fitnesses of the homozygous genotypes are lower. The selection coefficient s operating against AR/AR is $1.0 - 0.65 = 0.35$. The selection coefficient t operating against ST/ST is $1.0 - 0.50 = 0.50$.
4. Consider how the relative fitness values can be used to calculate the final frequencies of AR and ST.	4. A ratio of relative fitness values operating against each homozygous genotype can be used to calculate the equilibrium frequency of each of the chromosome forms, with $p_E = t/(s + t)$ and $q_E = s/(s + t)$.
Solve	Answer a
5. Describe the natural selection pattern operating on these genotypes.	5. This is an example of heterozygous advantage, and both chromosome forms are expected to remain in the population at equilibrium values determined by the relative strength of natural selection against each form.
	Answer b
6. Determine the equilibrium frequencies of each chromosome form. PITFALL: Double-check your arithmetic by making sure that the sum of the equilibrium frequencies you calculate is 1.0.	6. If the equilibrium frequency of AR is p_E and of ST is q_E, the equilibrium frequencies are $p_E = 0.50/(0.35 + 0.50) = 0.588$ and $q_E = 0.35/(0.35 + 0.50) = 0.412$.

For additional practice see Problems 4, 11, and 24. Visit the Study Area to access study tools. **Mastering** Genetics

20.3 Mutation Diversifies Gene Pools

Mutation is the ultimate source of all new genetic variation in populations, and the genetic variation it generates is an indispensable component of evolution. By itself, however, gene mutation is a very slow evolutionary process because its effect on allele frequencies in populations is small and gradual. For example, if mutation converts one in every 10,000 A_1 alleles to A_2 alleles each generation, a population containing $f(A_1) = 0.90$ and $f(A_2) = 0.10$ in generation 0 will have frequencies $f(A_1) = 0.81$ and $f(A_2) = 0.19$ after 1000 generations, assuming no effects from the other evolutionary processes.

An additional reason that mutation alone is a slow evolutionary process has to do with the two directions in which mutation can affect any given allele. The **forward mutation** rate (μ) pertains to mutations that create a new A_2 allele by mutation of A_1, whereas the **reverse mutation rate** (v), also known as the **reversion rate**, pertains to mutation of alleles in the opposite direction, A_2 to A_1. Forward and reverse mutation can create a balanced equilibrium, given a sufficient number of generations and the absence of other evolutionary processes.

Quantifying the Effects of Mutation on Allele Frequencies

In the absence of other evolutionary effects, the consequences of forward and reverse mutation (reversion) for allele frequencies in a population can be quantified. If $f(A_1) = p$ and $f(A_2) = q$, the effect of forward mutation on $f(A_1)$ is described by the value μp, and the effect of reversion on $f(A_2) = vq$. These two expressions identify, respectively, the rate at which A_2 alleles are created from A_1 by forward mutation and the rate at which A_2 alleles are reverted to A_1. In each generation, the change in the frequency of A_2 is quantified by the expression Δq ("delta q") that is calculated as $\Delta q = \mu p - vq$. Over an infinite number of generations in a theoretical population where μ and v are constant and no other evolutionary processes are operating, allele frequency equilibrium is established.

The equilibrium frequencies of alleles subject only to mutation and reversion are a ratio of the frequencies of the respective events. Since the equilibrium frequencies are purely a function of the ratios of the rates at which new copies of an allele are added and removed from the population gene pool, they are calculated as $p_E = v/(\mu + v)$ and $q_E = \mu/(\mu + v)$. In a theoretical population where $f(A_1) = 0.99, f(A_2) = 0.01, \mu = 2 \times 10^{-6}$, and $v = 3 \times 10^{-8}$, Δq is expressed as $\Delta q = [(2 \times 10^{-6})(0.99) - (3 10^{-8})(0.01)] = 1.9810^{-6}$. This small change gradually increases $f(A_2)$ and decreases $f(A_1)$, leading eventually to equilibrium allele frequencies. When equilibrium is achieved by the interaction of forward and reverse mutation rates in this population, the allele frequencies will be

$$p_E = 3 \times 10^{-8}/(2 \times 10^{-6} + 3 \times 10^{-8}) = 0.015 \text{ and}$$
$$q_E = 2 \times 10^{-6}/(2 \times 10^{-6} + 3 \times 10^{-8}) = 0.985$$

These are stable allele frequencies that, once achieved, will be maintained as long as the forward and reverse mutation rates stay the same and no other evolutionary process intervenes.

Mutation–Selection Balance

Unlike the theoretical population just described, mutations in the real world are commonly subject to natural selection. In cases where the deleterious mutation is recessive, the mutant allele is masked by the wild-type dominant allele in heterozygous genotypes. Recessive mutant alleles are subjected to natural selection only when they occur in the homozygous recessive genotype. This results in the persistence of recessive mutant alleles in most populations at a frequency somewhat greater than the mutation frequency.

Under these circumstances, the frequency of mutant alleles in a population is a balance of the intensity of natural selection against the mutant and the frequency of mutation of the gene. This expression is called the **mutation–selection balance**, and it determines the equilibrium frequency of the mutant allele (q_E) by considering the rate of elimination of deleterious alleles by natural selection (s) and the rate at which new mutant alleles are generated (μ).

Consider the following situation for a recessive lethal mutation.

Genotype	A_1A_1	A_1A_2	A_2A_2
Relative fitness	1	1	$1 - s$

Here, the equilibrium frequency of the recessive allele (q_E) is calculated as the balance between selection against a recessive genotype (s) and the rate of mutation (μ):

$$q_E = \sqrt{\mu/s}$$

This expression predicts that when selection against the recessive genotype is complete (i.e., $s = 1.0$), the equilibrium frequency of the mutant allele is approximately the square root of the mutation rate. When the selection coefficient is less than 1.0, the equilibrium frequency is greater than the square root of the mutation frequency.

In the case of complete selection against a lethal dominant mutant allele B_2, the relative fitness values of the genotypes are as follows.

Genotype	B_1B_1	B_1B_2	B_2B_2
Relative fitness	1	$1 - s$	$1 - s$

In this case, $q_E = \mu$. In other words, when $s = 1.0$ against a lethal dominant mutation, the equilibrium frequency of the mutant allele is equal to the mutation frequency.

Numerous examples of mutation–selection balance have been investigated in organisms, including humans. Several studies of human hereditary disease alleles reveal that recessive mutant alleles are maintained in populations at frequencies predicted by calculating the mutation–selection balance.

20.4 Gene Flow Occurs by the Movement of Organisms and Genes between Populations

In evolutionary terms, **gene flow**, also known as migration, refers to the movement of alleles into and out of populations. It can bring novel alleles into a population, it can increase the frequency of alleles already present in a population, or it can remove alleles from a population. These events can potentially have the immediate effect of changing allele frequencies in a population. Gene flow brought about by the addition of new organisms to an existing population generates a new population, identified as an **admixed population**, consisting of members from the two formerly distinct populations. In more familiar terms, you can think of gene flow as the consequence of the migration of organisms into a new population or the emigration of organisms out of a population. These organisms carry their genes with them as they move, creating a flow of genes into or out of a population.

Effects of Gene Flow

Gene flow has two principal effects on populations. First, in the short run, gene flow can cause the admixed population to have a different frequency of alleles, particularly if the starting allele frequencies in one of the participating populations differ from those in the other and if the number of immigrants constitutes a large proportion of the admixed population. Second, in the long run, gene flow acts to equalize frequencies of alleles between populations that remain in genetic contact by the exchange of population members back and forth between the populations. This exchange can also slow genetic divergence of populations and block speciation. Let's look at how both of these effects are explained.

The change in allele frequencies produced in an admixed population by gene flow from population 1 into population 2 can be described by the **island model** of migration that depicts a one-way process of gene flow, that is, from a mainland population to an island population. In the example illustrated in **Figure 20.7a**, gene flow changes allele frequencies by reducing $f(A_1)$ on the island from 1.0 to 0.60 and increasing $f(A_2)$ from 0.0 to 0.40. In this example, gene flow has produced an almost instantaneous evolutionary change (**Figure 20.7b**). The admixed population has allele frequencies of $f(A_1) = 0.60$ and $f(A_2) = 0.40$, but the genotypes are not in H-W equilibrium immediately following migration. A single generation of random mating, however, will bring the genotype frequencies into ratios consistent with the H-W equilibrium: $A_1A_1 = 0.36, A_1A_2 = 0.48,$ and $A_2A_2 = 0.16$.

The impact of gene flow on allele frequencies in an admixed population is expressed by a formula that calculates p_N, the new value of p, as the weighted average of the allele frequency among island residents and mainland immigrants. The expression uses p_I and p_C to represent $f(A_1)$ in the original island and mainland populations, respectively. The formula identifies the fraction of individuals or alleles from the mainland population as m, and the fraction contributed by island residents as $1 - m$. The value of p_N as a result of gene flow is $p_N = (1 - m)(p_I) + (m)(p_C)$. Applying this formula to our example in Figure 20.7, we find $p_N(0.20)(1.0) + (0.80)(0.50) = 0.60$.

Examples of gene flow abound in animals and plants. For example, bees can facilitate gene flow between plant

(a) The island model of migration

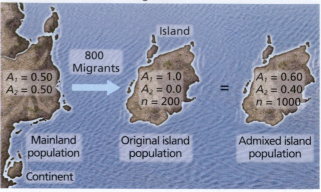

(b) Consequence of migration

Island population	A_1A_1	A_1A_2	A_2A_2	Allele frequencies in admixed population
Original (n = 200)	200	0	0	$f(A_1) = 0.60$ $f(A_2) = 0.40$
Admixed (n = 1000)	400	400	200	
Genotype frequencies in admixed population	0.36	0.48	0.16	

Figure 20.7 **The island model of migration.**

populations by collecting pollen from plants in one population of plants and depositing it on flowers in a different population. Gene flow can also occur through the action of the organisms themselves. As an example, the escape of farm-raised salmon from their ocean pen can lead to their reproducing with wild salmon.

Examples of gene flow in humans exist as well, but one example, harking back to events that affect the composition of the present-day human genome, is of particular note. The Neanderthals were an archaic human lineage that was distributed across Europe and large parts of Asia from about 400,000 to approximately 30,000 years ago. A second archaic human lineage, the Denisovans, also inhabited parts of Europe and Asia. Beginning about 70,000 to 80,000 years ago, a new human lineage—the lineage that would displace Neanderthals and Denisovans and give rise to all contemporary human populations—migrated out of Africa and into Europe and Asia. Evidence from the sequencing of ancient Neanderthal DNA, ancient Denisovan DNA, and modern human genomes reveals that the genomes of many present-day humans contain small amounts of DNA that originated in Neanderthals or Denisovans. On average this DNA, a consequence of gene flow from Neanderthals and Denisovans, makes up approximately 2 to 4% of the genome in a living human. Application Chapter D: Human Evolutionary Genetics discusses more details of this analysis.

Allele Frequency Equilibrium and Equalization

We have just seen that gene flow can produce rapid evolutionary change in the allele frequencies of populations. In the short term, the effect of gene flow is determined by the change in the frequency of p in the new gene pool of the island population. This value, Δp_I, is the difference in allele frequency before and after migration, and is defined as $\Delta p_I = p_N - p_I$. Substituting the formula for p_N and simplifying gives $\Delta p_I = [(1 - m)(p_I) + (m)(p_C)] - p_I = m(p_C - p_I)$. Allele frequency equilibrium occurs when $\Delta p_I = 0$; thus, at equilibrium, $m(p_C - p_I) = 0$, indicating that p remains constant either when there is no migration ($m = 0$) or when p in the island gene pool equals the allele frequency in the mainland gene pool ($p_I = p_C$).

Population and evolutionary biologists use this reasoning to conclude that gene flow has a homogenizing, or equalizing, effect on allele frequencies among participating populations. By this mechanism, gene flow maintains genetic contact between populations and can thus prevent evolutionary divergence of populations. In broader evolutionary terms, gene flow hinders the establishment of the reproductive isolation that is an important component of evolutionary divergence between populations and of potential speciation.

20.5 Genetic Drift Causes Allele Frequency Change by Sampling Error

The term **genetic drift** refers to chance fluctuations of allele frequencies that result from "sampling error," a statistical term signifying that a small sample taken from a larger population is not likely to contain all alleles in exactly the same frequencies as in the larger population. Genetic drift affects all populations, but it is especially prominent in small populations in which a small number of gametes unite to produce each subsequent generation.

To appreciate the cause and consequences of genetic drift, picture a gene pool with alleles at frequencies $f(A_1) = f(A_2) = 0.50$ from which two separate samples are drawn. In sample one, 20 alleles are drawn at random, whereas in the second sample, 1000 alleles are drawn. These two separate draws represent the alleles that, in the two respective cases, unite to form the next generation. In the first sample, containing 20 alleles, each allele represents 5 percent (one allele out of 20) of the total for the next generation, whereas in the 1000-allele sample, each allele only represents 1/1000 of the alleles in the next generation. Any deviation from exactly 10 A_1 alleles and 10 A_2 alleles in the first sample will substantially change allele frequencies in

the next generation. If, for example, the draw of 20 alleles contains 12 A_1 alleles and 8 A_2 alleles, the allele frequencies in the next generation will be $f(A_1) = 12/20 = 0.60$ and $f(A_2) = 8/20 = 0.40$. A change of such magnitude can easily occur by chance in the small sample, but it is very unlikely to occur in the larger sample of 1000 alleles.

Sampling errors of the kind described for the first sample can randomly raise or lower the frequency of an allele in a small population each generation. Once the allele frequencies are changed, the next generation, when it reproduces, has the new allele frequencies as a starting point. Over multiple generations, the frequency of an allele in a small population will randomly fluctuate, or "drift," sometimes increasing and sometimes decreasing, due to nothing more than the chance deviations in small random samples.

Allele frequency changes due to genetic drift are random. In the absence of any other evolutionary influence, and given a sufficient number of generations, allele frequencies will drift until, ultimately, one allele reaches fixation at a frequency of 1.0 and all other alleles are eliminated. **Figure 20.8** illustrates four different simulations of genetic drift of an allele in experimental populations and shows how the result of genetic drift for 30 generations can vary among populations that are initially identical. Each experimental population begins with 20 organisms and maintains that number throughout the 30 generations. The initial starting frequency of the allele is 0.50 in each population, so there is no frequency bias that favors or disfavors the allele at the beginning of the simulations.

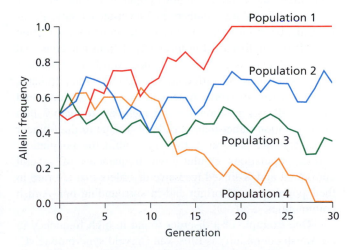

Figure 20.8 Genetic drift of an allele frequency. Four simulated populations each start with a frequency of 0.50 for a hypothetical allele whose frequency fluctuates randomly in each population over 30 generations. The allele eventually becomes fixed in population 1, is eliminated in population 4, and is still present in populations 2 and 3 at distinct frequencies.

⊙ Based on the results shown, write a general description of the impact of genetic drift on allele frequencies in a population.

The Founder Effect

As was stated previously, genetic drift affects all populations but is most pronounced in small populations. Small population size provides the conditions under which sampling errors can produce significant genetic drift of allele frequency. Two kinds of special cases of genetic drift stem from events that affect either the establishment of a new population or the survival of a population that has experienced a dramatic reduction in its membership.

The first special case of genetic drift is called the **founder effect**. It occurs when a new, small population branches off from a larger population. Since the founders of the new population are drawn from a larger original population, and the number of founders is small, the allele frequencies carried by the founders may be higher or lower than those in the original population, and some alleles may be missing altogether. These changes are due to sampling error. The founder effect can create new populations having allele frequencies that differ substantially from those found in the original population.

Small human populations whose origins can be traced to religious, social, political, or other distinctions are often established by a small number of individuals and contain few members of reproductive age. Often, the founders consist of several families. Since the family members are related and share alleles, allele frequencies among the founders likely will differ from allele frequencies in the larger population from which the founders emigrate.

One consequence of founder effect and genetic drift can be high frequencies of autosomal recessive disorders in the new population that are rare in the original population. The Old Order Amish are a religious population established by about 200 founding members in Lancaster County, Pennsylvania, between 1720 and 1770. The founding population came from English and European populations and consisted of several extended families. Other Amish communities were established by different founders in Ohio, Indiana, and elsewhere in North America. These populations tend to be small, yet it is common for members to mate within the population rather than outside of it. Due to the founder effect and the preference to mate within the population, Amish populations exhibit high frequencies of several autosomal and X-linked recessive disorders that are rare in their populations of origin and in surrounding non-Amish communities.

One example of a disorder found in high frequency in an Amish community is Ellis–van Creveld syndrome (EvC; OMIM 225500), an autosomal recessive disorder that produces short stature accompanied by short forearms and short lower legs and by the frequent appearance of extra digits on hands or feet. In a survey of nearly 8000 Old Order Amish in Lancaster County completed several years ago, 43 cases of EvC were identified. We can estimate the frequency of the allele producing EvC in the population by taking the square root of the frequency of the recessive trait in the

population. The calculation is $q = \sqrt{43/8000} = 0.073$, or about 7.3 percent. Among other Amish populations, and in the general (non-Amish) population, the frequency of this recessive allele is $q < 0.001$.

The genealogical history of the Old Order Amish community in Lancaster County, Pennsylvania, reveals that all families with EvC trace their genealogies to Mr. and Mrs. Samuel King, who immigrated to Lancaster County in 1744. At the time, there were about 400 people in the Lancaster County population, and the evidence suggests that both Mr. King and Mrs. King were carriers of the recessive mutant allele for EvC. This information establishes the initial frequency of the mutant allele in the founding population at approximately $f(q) = 2/800 = 0.0025$, more than twice the frequency in the population of origin. Genetic drift and the tendency for the Amish to mate within the Lancaster County community subsequently contributed to the rise in the frequency of the allele in the population.

Genetic Bottlenecks

A second special case of genetic drift is the **genetic bottleneck**. A genetic bottleneck occurs when a relatively large population is substantially reduced in number by a catastrophic event independent of natural selection. The survivors of the bottleneck—a small sample of the original population—are likely to have a very low level of genetic diversity due to the loss of alleles from the gene pool. They are likely to carry alleles in frequencies that differ radically from those in the original population (**Figure 20.9**). In the statistical sense, founder effect and genetic bottlenecks are equivalent. Indeed, the founder effect is essentially one version of a genetic bottleneck. Both establish a new breeding population from a small subset of the ancestral population.

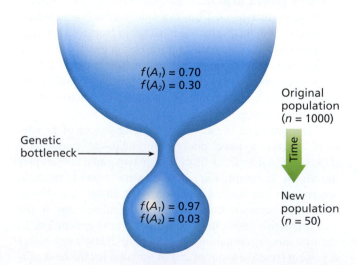

Figure 20.9 A genetic bottleneck. Catastrophic population reduction not due to natural selection can restrict or eliminate the alleles that pass through the bottleneck and alter allele frequencies in the surviving population.

The loss of genetic diversity from a genetic bottleneck can be quantified in two ways: first, by determining the percentage of polymorphic loci in the population, and second, by determining the percentage of loci that are heterozygous in an average individual.

Genetic bottlenecks can affect single populations, or they can affect an entire species. An example of the latter case would be a near-extinction event such as the one that affected the northern elephant seal (*Mirounga angustirostris*). This animal was historically distributed along the western coast of North America, in numbers that exceeded 150,000 in the mid-1800s. Extensive hunting devastated the rookeries where young elephant seals were raised, and by 1884 fewer than 100 elephant seals remained. Some biologists have estimated that the surviving population may have been as small as 20 individuals. The entire remaining population bred at an isolated rookery on Guadalupe Island, about 200 miles off the western shore of Baja California. Elephant seal protection measures put in place by the U.S. and Mexican governments in the early 1900s led to population growth and the reestablishment of additional rookeries. Today, the northern elephant seal remains a protected species that has returned to its historic population size of approximately 150,000 individuals.

In 1974, Robert Selander and his colleagues collected blood samples from 159 northern elephant seals from five populations and examined 24 blood protein and enzyme genes for evidence of genetic variation. All 24 genes were monomorphic, and the single allele of each gene was identical in all five populations! About 20 years later, A. Rus Hoelzel and colleagues expanded the genetic survey of northern elephant seals to include 43 genes in 61 individuals from the five populations. They also found no genetic variation. Additionally, Hoelzel and colleagues examined variation of mitochondrial DNA in northern elephant seals and found a low level of sequence variation in two distinctive mitochondrial DNA haplotypes that had frequencies of 0.725 and 0.275. The extremely limited genetic variation in northern elephant seals is wholly consistent with the historical genetic bottleneck that left very little genetic variation in the surviving population members.

20.6 Inbreeding Alters Genotype Frequencies but Not Allele Frequencies

Descriptions of population genetic structure based on the Hardy–Weinberg principle assume random mating within the population. If this assumption is not met, however—if mating in the population is nonrandom—the distribution of alleles into genotypes occurs in frequencies inconsistent with the chance predictions of the H-W equilibrium.

Inbreeding, mating between related individuals, is a form of nonrandom mating that alters the distribution of alleles into genotypes.

The Coefficient of Inbreeding

Inbreeding, also known as **consanguineous mating** (consanguineous means "with blood"), is mating between related individuals who share a greater proportion of alleles with one another than with random members of a population. The principal genetic consequences of inbreeding are an increase in the frequency of homozygous genotypes in a population and a decrease in the frequency of heterozygous genotypes relative to the frequencies expected from random matings. The likelihood of homozygosity is increased because related organisms share alleles and are thus more likely to produce homozygotes, especially when the alleles involved are rare in the general population. Inbreeding *does not* change allele frequencies. Instead, it systematically redistributes alleles into genotypes in a manner that increases homozygosity and reduces heterozygosity relative to the frequencies expected under H-W equilibrium.

Inbreeding is a normal reproductive process for self-fertilizing plants and for some animals that reproduce by self-fertilization. The effect of self-fertilization on genotype proportions is shown in **Table 20.6**, where a heterozygous organism self-fertilizes and produces genotypes in generation 1 in a 1:2:1 ratio. Self-fertilization of generation 1 individuals produces a generation 2 that has an overall increase in the frequency of both homozygous genotypes and a decrease of one-half in the frequency of the heterozygous genotype. The decrease in heterozygous frequency of one-half occurs each generation. By generation 4, a little more than 6 percent of the progeny are heterozygous, and more than 93 percent are homozygous. Note, however, that the allele frequencies of A_1 and A_2 remain unchanged at $f(A_1) = f(A_2) = 0.50$ in each generation.

Among sexually reproducing organisms, the effect of inbreeding is similar, but it takes place over a larger number of generations since the proportion of organisms in a population participating in consanguineous matings is generally low. The population geneticist Sewall Wright investigated

Table 20.6	Consequences of Self-Fertilization for Genotype Frequencies		

P: A_1A_2 (self-fertilization)

	Genotype		
Progeny Generation	A_1A_1	A_1A_2	A_2A_2
1	0.250	0.500	0.250
2	0.375	0.250	0.375
3	0.437	0.125	0.437
4	0.468	0.063	0.468

the consequences of inbreeding in sexually reproducing populations and devised the **coefficient of inbreeding (F)** as an arithmetic measure of the probability of homozygosity for an allele obtained in identical copies from an ancestor. The coefficient of inbreeding quantifies the probability that two alleles in a homozygous individual are **identical by descent (IBD)**, having descended from the same copy of the allele carried by a common ancestor of the inbred individual. A common ancestor is an ancestor shared by two inbreeding organisms, and potentially the source of identical alleles that could be carried by the inbreeding organisms. If inbreeding takes place, all genes in the genome are susceptible to the same inbreeding effects. Thus F can also be used to estimate the proportion of loci that will be homozygous IBD.

The quantification of F as a measure of the likelihood that a particular allele is IBD is most readily accomplished through pedigree analysis. The three key elements for determining F from pedigrees are (1) the number of alleles of a gene carried by common ancestors, (2) the number of transmission events required to produce a genotype that is homozygous IBD, and (3) the probability of transmission for each event linking the allele in a common ancestor to the inbred individual. **Figures 20.10a** and **20.10b** show a mating between half-siblings having the same mother (I-2) as the common ancestor. The general solution for F is $(1/2)^n$, where $1/2$ is the probability of transmission of an allele and n is the number of transmission events required to produce identity by descent. In this example, either allele A_1 or A_2 of the mother could be transmitted to both II-1 and II-2 and then to their offspring III-1, so the general solution for F is $(1/2)^n + (1/2)^n$. The arrows in the figure show the four transmission steps that are required for either allele to end up in III-1 IBD. Each required transmission event has a probability of 50 percent. Thus, the probability that either allele is found in III-1 in a homozygous IBD genotype is $(1/2)^4 = 1/16$. For this case, the inbreeding coefficient is the probability that *any* allele of a locus is homozygous IBD; thus, for each gene, $F = (1/2)^4 + (1/2)^4 = 1/8$. Notice that the arrows in the figure indicating transmission of alleles from I-2 to III-3 trace the two sides of a loop. This visual representation indicates the movement of the allele from generation to generation. If this loop were incomplete, identity by descent could not occur.

Figure 20.10c shows a first-cousin mating in a pedigree in which alleles from either I-1 or I-2 could make their way to IV-1. Here there are four alleles, any of which could be IBD in IV-1. Each allele must complete six transmission steps (indicated by arrows in the figure) to be identical by descent in IV-1, and the transmission probability for each step is $1/2$. For each allele carried by I-1 and each allele carried by I-2, the probability the allele is IBD in IV-1 is $(1/2)^6 = 1/64$. For this pedigree, there are four alleles for each gene, two per common ancestor, and F is determined

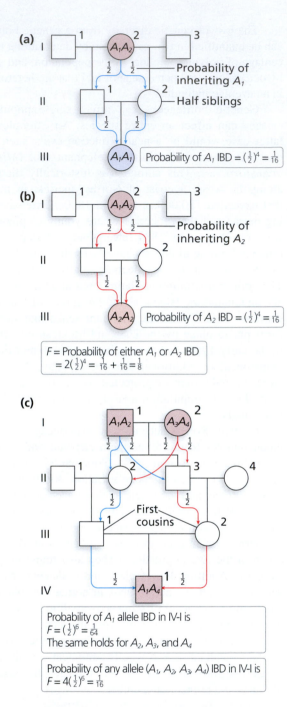

Figure 20.10   **Calculation of the inbreeding coefficient (F).**
(a) The probability of A_1 IBD equals the likelihood of four transmission events, each with a probability of 1/2. **(b)** The probability of A_2 IBD also requires four transmission events, each with a probability of 1/2. The likelihood of either allele IBD is $F = 2(1/2)^4$. **(c)** With two common ancestors, there are four alleles $(A_1, A_2, A_3,$ and $A_4)$ that can be IBD. For this first-cousin mating, the probability for each allele IBD is the same: $F = (1/2)^6$. For all shared alleles combined, $F = 4(1/2)^6 = 1/16$.

🅠 Draw a new version of the pedigree in part (c), with a single common ancestor in generation I and an inbred organism in generation IV. What is the inbreeding coefficient (F) of the inbred organism in generation IV?

by adding the probability of the four complete loops (one for each allele) that could link an allele in a common ancestor to an inbred homozygous IBD descendant. In this case, $F = (1/2)^6 + (1/2)^6 + (1/2)^6 + (1/2)^6 = 1/16$. The value can also be determined as $F = 4(1/2)^6 = 1/16$. Genetic Analysis 20.3 demonstrates another computation of an inbreeding coefficient.

First-cousin mating is a form of inbreeding that is relatively common in many human societies and is common in mammals in general. It can have negative genetic outcomes in the form of infants with recessive conditions due to homozygosity for recessive alleles that are very rare in a population (i.e., $q = 0.005$ or less). In such cases there can be a 20- to 30-fold increase in the likelihood that a first-cousin mating will produce a child with a recessive phenotype compared with the risk by random mating. However, when the recessive allele frequency is as common as $q = 0.01$, for example, the chance of producing a recessive homozygote from a first-cousin mating is only a few times more likely than the chance of producing a recessive homozygote by random mating. The effect disappears as the frequency of q in the population increases further.

Inbreeding Depression

The genetic consequences of inbreeding for populations are an increase in the frequency of homozygous genotypes and a decrease in the frequency of heterozygous genotypes. One immediate impact of these consequences is seen when small, captive populations of organisms are bred to perpetuate a nearly extinct species. The increased frequency of homozygosity can lead to a phenomenon known as **inbreeding depression**, the reduction in fitness of inbred organisms, often as a result of the reduced level of genetic heterozygosity. The reduced fitness associated with inbreeding depression can be due either to an increase in the proportion of deleterious homozygous genotypes or to the higher fitness of heterozygotes.

Inbreeding and inbreeding depression have real-world consequences for the planet's biodiversity and for efforts to preserve nearly extinct species. One of several strategies adopted by biological scientists and others interested in preserving nearly extinct species is the design of captive breeding programs. These programs are part of **conservation genetics**, a branch of population genetics that designs, conducts, and monitors captive breeding programs with the intent of maintaining vanishing populations. One of the principal areas of concern for managers of captive breeding programs is the magnitude of inbreeding coefficients and the danger of inbreeding depression for the captive breeding populations. Captive breeding program managers attempt to avoid the negative consequences of inbreeding depression by designing mating strategies that include as little inbreeding as possible.

The magnitude of inbreeding depression depends on the organism. Among plants that naturally reproduce by self-fertilization, the inbreeding depression is small. Many bird species also experience only relatively minor inbreeding depression. This lack of negative consequence has been particularly beneficial in captive breeding programs that have bred bird species such as the California condor and then reintroduced the birds into their natural environment.

In contrast to birds and plants, however, mammals experience severe inbreeding depression. The scientific literature contains about 20 reports on inbreeding and inbreeding depression from captive mammal breeding programs. The reports outline that inbreeding depression is a serious issue, resulting in reduced reproductive success of captive animals, reduced litter size, decreased longevity, and reduced survival of infant and juvenile animals. To maximize the chances of success in captive breeding programs for mammals, matings are carefully managed to avoid mating inbred animals when possible and to minimize F by using just one inbred animal in a mating when the use of an inbred animal is necessary or cannot be avoided.

20.7 New Species Evolve by Reproductive Isolation

Our discussion to this point has focused on microevolution, that is, evolution operating at the population level. In this section, we broaden our perspective to examine evolution at the species level and above.

The most widely used definition of a species, and the definition we use for purposes of this discussion, is the **biological species concept (BSC)**. It was developed in 1942 by the biologist Ernst Mayr, who also made important contributions to the modern synthesis of evolution (see Section 1.5). Mayr stated that from a biological perspective a species could be described as a group of organisms capable of interbreeding with one another but isolated from members of other species. By this definition, the alleles carried by a species stay within the confines of the species and are not exchanged with other species. This definition presents some problems for application in the real world. One problem is that the BSC cannot be used when one is dealing with fossilized remains or extinct species. A second problem is the difficulty in some cases of discovering whether or not two organisms are capable of reproducing. Third, the BSC cannot be applied to organisms that do not engage in sexual reproduction. And, finally, the assumption of the BSC is violated by organisms capable of interspecies hybridization. A well-known example is the mating of a male donkey ($2n = 62$) and a female horse ($2n = 64$) to produce the infertile hybrid known as a mule. The mule gets 31 chromosomes from the donkey parent and 32 chromosomes from the horse parent for a total of 63 chromosomes. Mules are

PROBLEM The pedigree shown here depicts crosses performed as part of an antelope captive-breeding program. Use the pedigree information to calculate the coefficient of inbreeding (*F*) for the mating of IV-1 and III-3 that produces the animal identified as V-1.

> **BREAK IT DOWN:** Each allele transmission probability is 1/2. Individual V-1 has two common ancestors, either of whom could be the source of an allele that is IBD (p. 742).

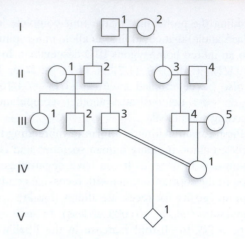

Solution Strategies	Solution Steps
Evaluate	
1. Identify the topic of this problem and the nature of the required answer.	1. This problem concerns determination of the coefficient of inbreeding (*F*) for a specific mating.
2. Identify the critical information given in the problem.	2. The pedigree depicting the common ancestry of the related animals is given.
Deduce	
3. Count the number of transmission events that must occur for an allele to be identical by descent (IBD) in V-1.	3. Counting from a common ancestor to individual V-1, there are seven transmission steps required to produce an allele that is IBD.
4. Identify the transmission probability for each step of transmission.	4. For an autosomal allele, the transmission probability is 1/2.
5. Identify the total number of alleles of an autosomal gene in the common ancestors of V-1.	5. There are two common ancestors (I-1 and I-2) for the inbred individual (V-1). There are two alleles per gene in each common ancestor, for a total of four alleles at each locus.
Solve	
6. Calculate the coefficient of inbreeding for this pedigree.	6. The coefficient of inbreeding is $F = 4(1/2)^7 = 1/32$.

For more practice, see Problems 33–36.

Visit the Study Area to access study tools.   **Mastering Genetics**

---

infertile due to their odd number of chromosomes that cannot properly segregate to form gametes (see Section 10.3).

Given the potential difficulties of applying the BSC, alternatives have been developed. One alternative is the **morphospecies concept**, which defines species based exclusively on morphology. A second alternative is the **phylogenetic species concept**, which defines a species as the smallest recognizable group with a unique evolutionary history.

Processes of Speciation

Charles Darwin was the first to describe the concept that existing species evolve from preexisting species. In his famous 1859 book, *On the Origin of Species by Means of Natural Selection*, he laid out two guiding principles of species formation that are still considered fundamental aspects of macroevolution. First, Darwin proposed that hereditary variation is present in all species and controls the phenotypic variability in each species. Second, Darwin proposed that natural selection allows species members with favored phenotypic attributes to survive and reproduce in greater numbers than species members with other phenotypes. Darwin described his model combining these principles as "the theory of descent with modification through variation and natural selection." In other words, Darwin viewed inherited variation and the operation of natural selection as the elements essential to the transformation of one species into another.

Innumerable biological investigations in the last 150 years have verified and elaborated upon Darwin's original proposals as well as quantifying the effects and the interplay of each of the four evolutionary processes (natural selection, mutation, migration, and genetic drift) on speciation.

The clear picture of speciation that emerges from these studies is that the evolutionary lineages leading from ancestral organisms to descendant forms are almost never simple, straight lines of descent. Instead, the evolutionary history of modern species is filled with side branches that died out because a species, once developed, could not adapt to new environments or was displaced by competing species. It can be tempting to look backward into the evolutionary past and identify a linear step-by-step procession leading to modern species, but this perspective minimizes the occurrence of adaptive changes that led to evolutionary "dead ends." More important, the backward-looking approach ignores a major reality of evolution: Evolutionary history is far more like a multibranched bush rather than like a tree with a long, straight branches connecting past and present.

The evolutionary history of modern horses and their living relatives, zebras and donkeys (all three being members of the genus *Equus*), is an example of the typical complexity of evolutionary history (**Figure 20.11**). One can trace a lineage leading more or less directly from *Hyracotherium* in the early Eocene (about 54 million years ago) to modern *Equus*, but this would ignore the many other branches of the evolutionary tree that did not produce modern-day organisms.

The evolutionary tree leading to the modern species of *Equus* illustrates the complex patterns of relationships that can occur as new species evolve. The figure illustrates a phylogenetic tree that is inferred from the physical characteristics identified in fossil remains. In identifying the evolution of horses, characteristics of the skull, teeth, and hoof are particularly important in determining which ancestral

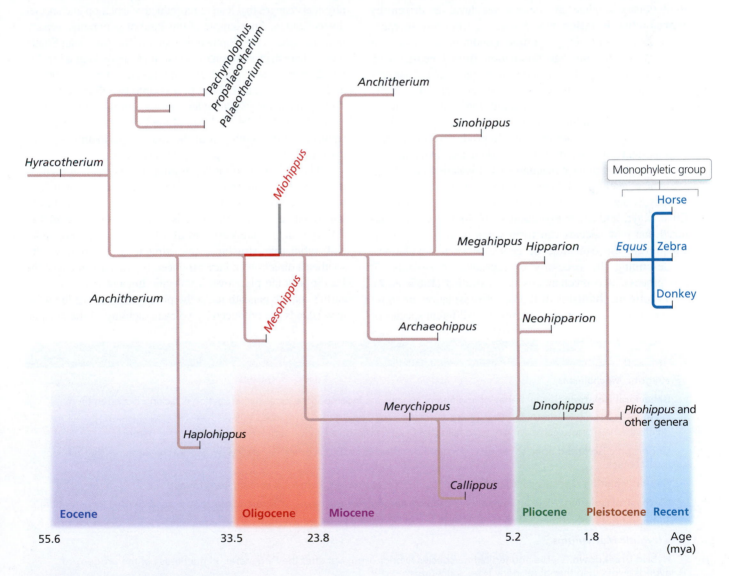

Figure 20.11 Evolution of the genus *Equus*. This multibranched evolutionary tree includes the monophyletic group that includes the modern species of the genus *Equus* and shows a few of the nearly 200 branches of the phylogeny descending from *Hyracotherium*.

traits present in an ancestor correlate with derived traits present in a descendant. The modern species of the genus *Equus* form a monophyletic group of the modern species and their common ancestor.

DNA sequences can also be used to determine phylogenetic relationships. Recall from the Case Study in Chapter 1 (pp. 24–26), that the relationship of an extinct relative of the zebra called the quagga was determined by collecting DNA from preserved quagga hides and comparing it to DNA from zebra species. Whether phylogenies are constructed using morphologic traits or DNA sequence, they share two essential features: (1) inherited variation controlling critical phenotypic variation and (2) morphology and genome content evolve through evolutionary processes.

Reproductive Isolation and Speciation

Evolutionary change at the species level is driven by **reproductive isolation** that can result from any morphological, behavioral, or geographic condition or set of conditions that prevents one population from breeding with others. Reproductively isolated populations adapt separately to their particular circumstances, and divergence is a likely consequence. In each environment, differential reproductive success driven by natural selection allows the better-adapted organisms to leave more progeny. Reproductive isolation is an important component for both cladogenesis and anagenesis, although the precise mechanisms of isolation may differ.

The concept of cladogenesis and reproductive isolation of species derives from work by Theodosius Dobzhansky, Ernst Mayr, and other evolutionary biologists who recognized that new species can form when reproductive barriers prevent the exchange of genes between populations. In describing the necessity of reproductive isolation in this process, two mechanisms are identified (**Table 20.7**). **Prezygotic mechanisms** of reproductive isolation are those that prevent mating between members of different species or prevent the formation of a zygote following interspecies mating. On the other hand, **postzygotic mechanisms** of reproductive isolation result in the failure of a fertilized zygote to survive, or result in sterile offspring of an interspecies mating. These mechanisms of reproductive and genetic isolation lead to allopatric speciation or sympatric speciation.

Allopatric Speciation In **allopatric speciation**, populations are separated by a physical barrier. New species can develop in separate geographic locations as a consequence of their reproductive isolation. Two principal mechanisms create the separations that lead to reproductive isolation: (1) physical separation of a segment of a large population by a physical barrier that prevents gene flow and (2) colonization of new territory (**Figure 20.12**). Geographic events such as the advance of a glacier, the emergence of a mountain range, change in flow pattern of a river, or erosion of a canyon are typical of the kinds of physical changes that lead to reproductive isolation and species diversification. An example of this kind of geographic separation and species development is found in the American Southwest, where the formation of the Grand Canyon beginning 5 to 6 million years ago split an ancestral species of ground squirrel and led to its eventual diversification into two distinct species. Today, *Ammospermophilus leucurus* is a gray-colored ground squirrel found on the north rim of the Grand Canyon, whereas squirrels on the south rim of the canyon are members of the chestnut-colored *Ammospermophilus harrisii*.

The colonization model of allopatric speciation predicts that new species diversify following colonization of new habitats. The diversification of *Drosophila* species on the Hawaiian Islands is a case study of this mechanism (**Figure 20.13**). The Hawaiian Islands are part of a long chain of landmasses and submarine structures that stretch in a northwest-to-southeast direction and are produced by the movement of the Pacific tectonic plate over a volcanic hotspot that lies in the earth's mantle beneath it. As the plate slides toward the west, new islands are produced by volcanic activity of the hotspot.

Table 20.7	Mechanisms of Reproductive Isolation

Prezygotic Mechanisms

Behavioral isolation: Sexual behavior in different species are incompatible, or sexual attraction is lacking between them.

Gametic isolation: Mating takes place between different species, but the gametes fail to unite with one another due to differences in gamete compatibility or to failure of male gametes to survive until fertilization of female gametes.

Geographic isolation: Species reside in separate geographic locations or are separated by geographic features that prevent their contact.

Habitat isolation: Species inhabit different ecosystems that prevent them from coming into contact.

Mechanical isolation: Male and female genitalia or reproductive structures of different species are anatomically incompatible.

Temporal isolation: Timing of reproductive ability or receptivity in different species is incompatible.

Postzygotic Mechanisms

Hybrid breakdown: Viable and fertile interspecies hybrids form, but after the F_1 generation the fitness of the progeny of hybrids is less than that of progeny from nonhybrids.

Hybrid inviability: The fertilized zygote of an interspecies mating fails to survive gestation.

Hybrid sterility: Interspecies hybrids are viable but infertile.

(a) Population bifurcation by a barrier to reproduction

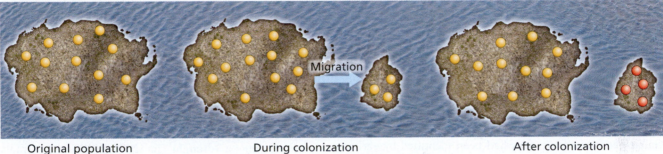

Original population   During bifurcation   Separate populations after bifurcation

(b) Colonization of new territory by migration

Original population   During colonization   After colonization

Figure 20.12 Processes leading to allopatric speciation.

The oldest of the islands are Nihau and Kauai to the northwest; the youngest island is Hawaii, which is still growing by volcanic eruptions of Mauna Loa and Kilauea.

In 2005, James Bonacum and his colleagues examined genetic and morphologic data in numerous Hawaiian *Drosophila* species to test the allopatric speciation model. They found that the most closely related species occur on adjacent islands and that the phylogenetic pattern of species formation corresponds to the pattern of emergence of islands. These results provide support and documentation for the model of allopatric speciation by colonization.

Sympatric Speciation   In **sympatric speciation**, populations share a single habitat but are isolated by genetic, behavioral, seasonal, or ecosystem-based mechanisms that prevent gene flow. Species that diverge while occupying the same geographic area are sympatric species.

One clear example of sympatric speciation occurs in plant species that diversify from one another through the development of polyploidy. Mating between a polyploid species and one that is not polyploid can result in reduced fertility of hybrid individuals. Section 10.3 discusses the development of polyploidy through nondisjunction and highlights the evolution of the modern bread wheat species (*Triticum aestivum*)

from a wild diploid grass to its contemporary allohexaploid form (see Figure 10.12). Animals that develop nocturnal or diurnal patterns of activity that make them more likely to encounter only those other members of the population that are active at the same time are another example of potential sympatric speciation. Similarly, changes in the seasonality of reproduction can limit organisms to the ability to reproduce only during certain times of the year. Organisms living in the same geographic area that do not have the same reproductive seasonality will be unable to mate.

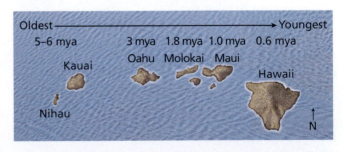

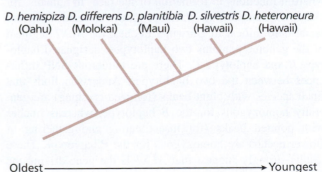

Figure 20.13 **Phylogenetic relationships among Hawaiian *Drosophila* species.** Evolutionary evidence supports the colonization of younger islands and the formation of new species following migration from older islands.

🔘 **Describe how the evolution of Hawaiian *Drosophila* is an example of allopatric speciation.**

The Molecular Genetics of Evolution in Darwin's Finches

As the Hawaiian Islands study of *Drosophila* clearly illustrates, the examination of living organisms can reveal enlightening details of evolutionary relationships. Another example comes from long-term studies of Darwin's finches in the Galápagos Island chain and the nearby Cocos Islands. Multiple studies, including recent analysis of the genomes, have provided insight into the relationships between the various Galápagos finch species and offer powerful support for contemporary concepts of evolution and speciation.

In 2015, a group of researchers led by Leif Andersson completed the genomic sequencing of 120 finches from the Galápagos Islands and the Cocos Islands. Earlier taxonomic analysis of the birds' morphology had identified 14 finch species on the Galápagos Islands, and an additional species on the Cocos Islands. In contrast, phylogenetic analysis based on the genome sequences obtained by Andersson's group identified a total of 17 species on the Galápagos, three more than had been identified by earlier methodologies.

The genome sequence data revealed three significant features of the evolution of Galápagos finches. First, Darwin's finches have a long evolutionary history that is distinct from the history of other finches. This observation is in line with Darwin's original contention that the Galápagos finches were an isolated population that diversified and speciated in place. Second, there is substantial evidence of gene flow between the Galápagos finch species, as well as multiple examples of hybrid populations generated by mating between closely related species. These results comport with the modern view of species evolution as a gradual and sometimes fitful process, with natural selection driving diversification and gene flow slowing it through exchanges of genes among populations.

The third finding from the finch genome analysis is the identification of the probable genetic basis of beak shape, the phenotypic characteristic thought to be at the heart of Galápagos finch speciation (see the chapter opener image). Andersson's genome sequence data identify a 240-kb region of the finch genome that includes the *ALX1* gene, which produces a transcription factor protein. *ALX1* is found in many vertebrate genomes, including mammals and fish, where it functions in formation of the face. In humans, for example, mutations of *ALX1* are known to result in severe facial deformities. In Darwin's finches, the *ALX1* segment of the genome contains two haplotypes, designated haplotype *B* and haplotype *P*. There are numerous SNP differences between the two haplotypes. Andersson finds that finch species with blunt beaks (for seed crushing) are generally homozygous for the *B* haplotype, whereas finches with pointed beaks (for insect eating and gathering of flower nectar) are homozygous for the *P* haplotype. These results strongly suggest that *ALX1* is the gene driving the diversification of beak shape in Darwin's finches. The *B* and *P* haplotypes are also found to correlate with beak shape in hybrid finch populations that contain birds with different beak shapes.

The genome sequencing also reveals pertinent details about a second region, that which includes the *HGMA2* gene. The protein product of *HGMA2* associates with chromatin and appears to bind to it as part of a complex that activates transcription of several other genes. *HGMA2* alleles *HGMA2*S* and *HGMA2*L* are associated with variation in beak size in finches, with large-beaked birds usually having the *LL* genotype and small-beaked birds the *SS* genotype.

The *HGMA2* genotype variation and its relation to beak size dovetails nicely with data gathered since the early 1980s by Peter and Rosemary Grant. In studying the finches on the Galápagos Island of Daphne Major, the Grants have followed the population through four periods of drought that have altered the vegetation pattern—for example, greatly reducing the availability of seeds that are the preferred food source of large-beaked finches.

Following a drought in 2004–2005, the Grants reported a major shift in beak size in the finch population on Daphne Major. They observed that finches with large beaks survived poorly while finches with smaller beaks survived in much larger numbers. The Grants proposed that the effects of the drought on the availability of seeds had exerted natural selection pressure against birds with large beaks and in favor of birds with small beaks. Andersson examined *HGMA2* genotypes in 37 survivors and 34 deceased birds from the 2004–2005 Daphne Major drought and found that many more *SS* birds than *LL* birds survived the drought. The frequency of the *S* allele was 61% among survivors versus 37% among deceased birds. This translates to a selection coefficient against *LL* of approximately $s = 0.59$. The results led the Andersson group to conclude that there was a relationship between *HGMA2* and the fitness of finches based on their beak size. More generally, the data illustrate that Andersson and colleagues' two genes, *ALX1* and *HGMA2*, are involved in the adaptation of Darwin's finches to the Galápagos Islands and in the evolution of beak shape in the diverse finch species of the islands.

20.8 Molecular Evolution Changes Genes and Genomes through Time

The heritable variation that provides the raw material of evolution begins at the molecular level, with alterations in DNA sequence and proteins. These molecular changes are part and parcel of the evolutionary process and they can be examined at several levels, from the evolution of individual genes and gene families to the evolution of entire genomes. In this final section, we examine the molecular evolutionary analysis of the vertebrate steroid receptor (SR) family and discuss the evolutionary process that has generated multiple new molecular functions from an ancestral gene of limited function. Application Chapter D: Human Evolutionary Genetics, which follows this chapter contains another example of molecular genetic evolution, that of the human genome, with its evidence of the introgression of Neanderthal DNA through human–Neanderthal interbreeding.

Vertebrate Steroid Receptor Evolution

Evolutionary theory predicts that novel molecular functions are acquired as a consequence of the action of natural selection on favorable mutations. In the case of complex systems with multiple active elements, however, the challenge for evolutionary biology is to identify how new protein functions arise when all the components of the complex are not initially present. The evolution of vertebrate steroid receptors (SRs) illustrates one way in which this has occurred. Dissection of this process shows how an ancestral receptor with a single original function underwent duplication and diversification to produce new genes and proteins with the ability to bind new compounds. The basic scenario of duplication of the ancestral gene followed by diversification of function is one commonly encountered in evolutionary biology.

Contemporary vertebrates possess several closely related genes that are responsible for producing SR proteins. Functionally, SR proteins are a family of proteins that have the capability of binding a ligand (a smaller molecule—in this case, a hormone). Hormone binding changes the SR protein conformation so as to initiate the transcription of particular genes. In this way, the hormones act as signaling molecules that work through SRs to initiate transcription. The contemporary vertebrate SR protein family includes two estrogen receptors (ERα and ERβ) and one receptor each for androgens (AR), progesterones (PR), mineralocorticoids (MR), and glucocorticoids (GR).

The SR proteins have highly conserved DNA-binding domains (DBDs) that recognize specific DNA sequences called response elements in the promoter regions of specific target genes. Hormone binding to the ligand-binding domains (LBDs) triggers conformational change of the proteins into their transcription-activating forms that are capable of binding to response elements. Activated ER proteins recognize the response element sequence AGGTCA; the other activated SR proteins (AR, PR, MR, and GR) recognize the response element sequence AGAACA. Differences in response element recognition enable the vertebrate SR proteins to mediate hormone-induced transcription of a range of different genes. SR proteins that are closely related to the vertebrate SRs have been found in mollusks, annelids, and the invertebrate cephalochordates. How did this closely related yet diversified family of proteins evolve?

Novel Functions from the Ancestral Steroid Receptor

The first step in tracing the evolutionary pathway of SR protein diversification is to identify the clades to which contemporary SRs belong. Based on their sequences, two major SR clades have been identified. One contains the ERs, and the other contains the other SR proteins (ARs, PRs, MRs, and GRs; **Figure 20.14**). The SR proteins of all organisms have the capacity to bind estrogen as a ligand. This is one of several clues indicating that the ancestral SR protein, called *AncSR1*, was an estrogen-binding protein. The strong sequence similarities among the other SR genes and proteins indicate that the diversification of SRs began when *AncSR1* underwent a gene-duplication event. This gave rise to the two major SR protein clades. In the ER clade, the proteins diversified to produce estrogen-binding capability in mollusks, annelids, and cephalochordates. Later gene-duplication events in this clade gave rise to the vertebrate ERα and ERβ proteins. In the clade of the other SRs, the original duplication of *AncSR1* was followed by additional gene duplication and diversification to produce the four new vertebrate SR proteins (see Section 16.3 for additional discussion of genome duplication).

Ancestral Gene and Protein Reconstruction Phylogenetic reconstruction based on comparisons of gene and protein sequence similarities is one way to identify the probable evolutionary history and function of the ancestral SR protein. Over more than a decade of such analysis, Joseph Thornton and his colleagues have developed several lines of evidence to demonstrate that *AncSR1* was an ER, and they have deciphered the process that led to the evolution of new SR functions in vertebrates. Part of Thornton's identification of *AncSR1* function is based on statistical analysis of the phylogenetic information to identify the

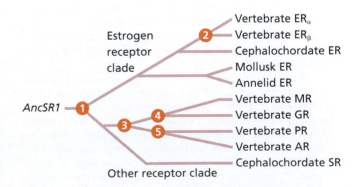

Figure 20.14 Evolution of the vertebrate SR gene family.
Multiple duplications of the ancestral estrogen receptor gene *AncSR1* were followed by diversification to produce two vertebrate estrogen receptors (ERs) and other ERs. Other vertebrate steroid receptors (MR, GR, PR, and AR) evolved to use intermediates in the estrogen biosynthetic pathway as ligands.

 Speculate about the role gene duplication may have played in the evolution of vertebrate steroid receptors.

most likely nucleotide at each location in the ancestral gene. The researchers used these data to recreate multiple versions of the inferred ancestral protein by placing a synthesized DNA copy of each putative ancestral gene into an expression system capable of transcription and translation. Each recreated version of *AncSR1* produced slightly different results, but all versions functioned as estrogen receptors.

The Evolution of Novelty Results by Thornton and others show that the inferred *AncSR1* sequence is highly similar to vertebrate ERs in both its LBD and DBD domains. This provides additional evidence that the function of *AncSR1* was estrogen binding and indicates that the ancestral protein most likely recognized an AGGTCA-containing response element as do contemporary ERs. The subsequent diversification of the SR protein occurred with a switch of the DBD to recognize AGAACA response-element sequences and with changes in the LBDs to facilitate binding of the new ligands. Research indicates that just two nucleotide base pair changes are required to switch DBD recognition from one response element sequence to the other.

Changing the LBDs to recognize new hormone ligands may seem to be a more complex evolutionary problem than switching DBD recognition. In reality, however, this may

be a simple and common occurrence. Estrogen is the end product of a multistep biochemical pathway that begins with cholesterol and has progesterone, corticosteroids, and testosterone as intermediates (**Figure 20.15**). The emergence of diverse SR proteins able to bind new ligand targets is an example of an evolutionary mechanism in which the ancestral molecule recognized the end product of a multistep biosynthetic pathway, estrogen in this case, and duplication and subsequent diversification eventually produced proteins that recognize and interact with intermediate compounds in the same pathway. Computer simulation studies have found that changing just two to four amino acids in the LBD of a modern human ER is sufficient to change its LBD to one binding progesterone or testosterone. Derived copies of *AncSR1* may have undergone similar changes in ligand recognition by equally simple alterations.

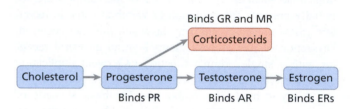

Figure 20.15 The estrogen biosynthesis pathway.

Sickle Cell Disease Evolution and Natural Selection in Humans

Dozens of variant alleles of hemoglobin genes produce one form or another of hereditary anemia, a condition characterized by a chronic abnormally low level of red blood cells. According to the World Health Organization, hereditary anemias are the most common of all human genetic diseases, occurring in an estimated 250 to 300 million people around the world. Most of the globin-gene mutations causing hereditary anemia are rare, but a few are found in high frequency in certain populations.

Recall from Table 9.2 and its associated discussion that the red blood cell protein hemoglobin is a heterotetrameric protein composed of two different globin proteins—two polypeptides are products of the α-globin gene and two are products of the β-globin gene. The specific allelic variants we focus on here are alleles of the β-globin gene. At this gene, the wild-type allele is designated β^A. In certain populations, one of the variant alleles, β^S, β^E, or β^C can be found at polymorphic frequencies (population frequencies of 1% or more). Each of these variant alleles is caused by a single base pair substitution that generates a missense mutation. Recall from Section 11.1 and Figure 11.2 that a missense mutation is characterized by the substitution of one amino acid in the mutant protein. Homozygosity for any of these three variants (i.e., genotypes $\beta^S\beta^S$, $\beta^E\beta^E$, or $\beta^C\beta^C$) produces a form of hereditary anemia. The hereditary anemia in individuals with the $\beta^S\beta^S$ genotype is called **sickle cell disease (SCD)**. It

is a very serious and potentially fatal condition. The other hereditary anemias are also serious diseases, although they are not often fatal.

Given the seriousness of these hereditary anemias, one might think that natural selection would act against the mutant alleles and reduce their frequencies to very low levels. Thus you may be wondering why each of the variant alleles occurs at polymorphic frequencies. The β^S allele occurs in frequencies as high as 15% in several indigenous populations of Africa, the Middle East, and the Indian subcontinent; the β^E allele occurs at frequencies exceeding 10% in some populations of Southeast Asia and the Pacific Islands; and the β^C allele occurs at frequencies of 10% or more in certain West African populations.

The origin and maintenance of β^S, β^C, and β^E has been studied for more than 50 years, and researchers have firmly established that the infectious disease malaria is the agent driving natural selection. Malaria is a potentially fatal infectious disease caused by the protozoan *Plasmodium falciparum*. This protozoan is carried by the mosquito vector *Anopheles gambiae*, which transfers the protozoan to animals, including humans, when it bites them. The malarial parasite matures in red blood cells of its host.

In populations where malaria is endemic (present throughout the year), heterozygous individuals, with genotypes $\beta^A\beta^S$, $\beta^A\beta^E$, or $\beta^A\beta^C$, have higher reproductive fitness than individuals with other genotypes. This is because of the reduced incidence and lessened severity of malarial infections in heterozygous individuals as compared with individuals in the same populations who are $\beta^A\beta^A$. In other words, heterozygous advantage is the natural selection mechanism at work in populations experiencing endemic malaria where one of these variant alleles is present. The result of this pattern of natural selection has been the establishment of balanced polymorphisms that maintain the mutant allele at polymorphic frequencies in numerous populations (see Section 20.2).

The physiological basis for the heterozygous advantage in this example is that heterozygosity shortens the life span of the average red blood cell by about one-third. This shortened red blood cell life span disrupts development of the mature parasite, leading to a reduction in disease incidence and severity. The consequence is higher reproductive fitness of heterozygous individuals compared with $\beta^A\beta^A$ individuals, who suffer more malaria, and compared with homozygous mutant individuals, who suffer hereditary anemia.

Figure 20.16 shows a map of the distribution of endemic malaria and maps of the frequency distribution of the β^S and β^E alleles. Notice two things about these maps. First, there is strong overlap between the distribution of malaria and the distribution of the mutant β-globin alleles. Second, the β^S allele has a wide geographic distribution, appearing in African populations and in populations around the Mediterranean, in the Middle East, and on the Indian subcontinent. Molecular genetic evidence demonstrates that the mutations in these diverse geographic areas derive from independent events. In other words, the β^S allele arose independently multiple times. Examination of the haplotypes of the chromosomes carrying the β^S allele in each geographic area reveals that the mutant alleles belong to distinctly different chromosome haplotypes. This situation could only have come about through independent mutational events. That the mutant allele is at polymorphic frequencies in these distinct populations means that balanced polymorphism has been established in each population through heterozygous advantage. This is just one of several examples offering evidence of the ongoing action of natural selection in human populations.

(a)

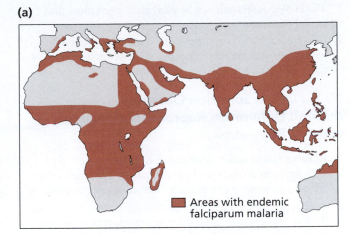

Areas with endemic falciparum malaria

(b)

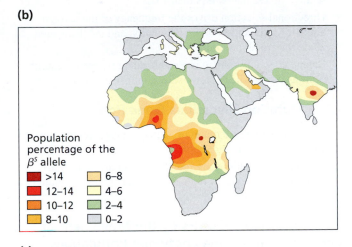

Population percentage of the β^S allele

>14	6–8
12–14	4–6
10–12	2–4
8–10	0–2

(c)

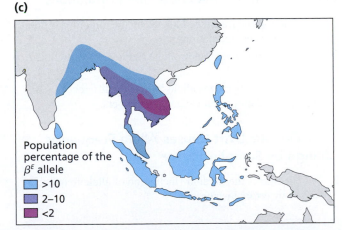

Population percentage of the β^E allele

>10
2–10
<2

Figure 20.16   The distribution of malaria and of the hemoglobin variants β^S and β^E. (a) Regions of the world where malaria is endemic are shown. **(b)** The frequency distribution of the β^S allele in Africa, Southern Europe, the Middle East, and the Indian subcontinent. **(c)** The frequency distribution of the β^E allele in Southeast Asia and the Pacific Islands.

SUMMARY   Mastering Genetics   For activities, animations, and review quizzes, go to the Study Area.

20.1 The Hardy–Weinberg Equilibrium Describes the Relationship of Allele and Genotype Frequencies in Populations

▌ A population is a group of interbreeding organisms that share a collection of genes known as a gene pool.

▌ If there are two alleles at a locus, with frequencies represented by p and q, the sum of allele frequencies $p + q = 1.0$.

▌ The H-W equilibrium predicts that two alleles will be distributed into genotypes of frequencies p^2, $2pq$, and q^2. The sum of genotype frequencies $p^2 + 2pq + q^2 = 1.0$.

▌ The H-W equilibrium assumes that the members of a population mate at random and that the population is not altered by any of the four evolutionary processes.

▌ Allele frequencies in populations can be determined by the genotype proportion method, allele counting, or the square root method.

- The H-W equilibrium can be used even when more than two alleles occur for a gene.
- Chi-square analysis compares the number of observed genotypes with the number expected under assumptions of the H-W equilibrium.

20.2 Natural Selection Operates through Differential Reproductive Fitness within a Population

- Relative fitness is the comparative capacity of individuals with different phenotypes to make genetic contributions to the next generation due to the influence of natural selection.
- A selection coefficient is the percentage decrease in reproductive success experienced by an organism possessing a relative fitness that is less than 1.0.
- Directional selection drives the frequency of the favored allele toward fixation in the population and the disfavored allele toward elimination.
- Balanced polymorphism is a stable allele frequency equilibrium resulting when natural selection favors heterozygotes.

20.3 Mutation Diversifies Gene Pools

- Forward and reverse mutation slowly change the frequencies of alleles in populations.
- Deleterious mutations are removed by natural selection, striking an equilibrium frequency by balancing mutation and selection rates.

20.4 Gene Flow Occurs by the Movement of Organisms and Genes between Populations

- Gene flow is the transfer of alleles by the migration of individuals between populations.
- Gene flow can produce new allele frequencies in admixed populations.
- Gene flow homogenizes allele frequency differences among populations that exchange members.

20.5 Genetic Drift Causes Allele Frequency Change by Sampling Error

- Genetic drift is the random fluctuation of allele frequencies caused by errors in sampling.

- Genetic drift leads ultimately to allele fixation and elimination, but small populations are particularly susceptible to its effects.
- Founder effect is a special form of genetic drift that occurs when a small number of individuals from a larger population establish a new, small population.
- A genetic bottleneck is a random and substantial reduction in population size that significantly changes allele frequencies among survivors.

20.6 Inbreeding Alters Genotype Frequencies but Not Allele Frequencies

- Inbreeding is nonrandom mating based on genotype that occurs between relatives who are more closely related to one another than to a random member of the population.
- The coefficient of inbreeding (F) is the probability that an allele is homozygous identical by descent in an inbred individual.
- Inbreeding increases the frequency of homozygosity and decreases heterozygosity.
- Inbreeding depression often develops in inbred populations due to the cumulative effects of numerous homozygous loci.

20.7 New Species Evolve by Reproductive Isolation

- New species emerge in reproductive isolation through adaptive change in response to conditions.
- Prezygotic reproductive isolation prevents mating between individuals in different populations. Postzygotic reproductive isolation reduces the ability of individuals from different populations to produce living and fertile offspring when they mate.
- In allopatric speciation, new species develop as a result of the physical separation of populations into different geographic areas.
- Sympatric speciation results from genetic differences that prevent reproduction among organisms that occupy the same habitat.

20.8 Molecular Evolution Changes Genes and Genomes through Time

- The evolution of gene families often occurs by one or more duplications of an ancestral gene followed by diversification of sequence and function of the new gene copies.

PREPARING FOR PROBLEM SOLVING

In addition to the list of problem-solving tips and suggestions given here, you can go to the Study Guide and Solutions Manual that accompanies this book for help at solving problems.

1. Be prepared to use population data to calculate the allele, genotype, and phenotype frequencies expected under the assumptions of the H-W equilibrium.

2. Be prepared to define and explain the terminology of population genetics and of evolutionary genetics.

3. Be prepared to calculate allele and genotype frequencies produced in populations as a consequence of the action of natural selection or gene flow.

4. Be prepared to describe the impact of mutation and genetic drift on populations.

5. Be prepared to use pedigrees to analyze inbreeding and to calculate inbreeding coefficients.

Chapter Concepts

For answers to selected even-numbered problems, see Appendix: Answers.

1. Compare and contrast the terms in each of the following pairs:
   a. population and gene pool
   b. random mating and inbreeding
   c. natural selection and genetic drift
   d. a polymorphic trait and a polymorphic gene
   e. founder effect and genetic bottleneck

2. In a population, what is the consequence of inbreeding? Does inbreeding change allele frequencies? What is the effect of inbreeding with regard to rare recessive alleles in a population?

3. Identify and describe the evolutionary forces that can cause allele frequencies to change from one generation to the next.

4. Describe how natural selection can produce balanced polymorphism of allele frequencies through selection that favors heterozygotes.

5. Thinking creatively about evolutionary mechanisms, identify at least two schemes that could generate allelic polymorphism in a population. Do not include the processes described in the answer to Problem 4.

6. Genetic drift, an evolutionary process affecting all populations, can have a significant effect in small populations, even though its effect is negligible in large populations. Explain why this is the case.

7. Over the course of many generations in a small population, what effect does random genetic drift have on allele frequencies?

8. Catastrophic events such as loss of habitat, famine, or overhunting can push species to the brink of extinction and result in a genetic bottleneck. What happens to allele frequencies in a species that experiences a near-extinction event, and what is expected to happen to allele frequencies if the species recovers from near extinction?

9. George Udny Yule was wrong in suggesting that an autosomal dominant trait like brachydactyly will increase in frequency in populations. Explain why Yule was incorrect.

10. The ability to taste the bitter compound phenylthiocarbamide (PTC) is an autosomal dominant trait. The inability to taste PTC is a recessive condition. In a sample of 500 people, 360 have the ability to taste PTC and 140 do not. Calculate the frequency of
    a. the recessive allele
    b. the dominant allele
    c. each genotype

11. Figure 20.6 illustrates the effect of an ethanol-rich and an ethanol-free environment on the frequency of the *Drosophila Adh^F* allele in four populations in a 50-generation laboratory experiment. Population 1 and population 2 were reared for 50 generations in a high-ethanol environment, while control 1 and control 2 populations were reared for 50 generations in a zero-ethanol environment. Describe the effect of each environment on the populations, and state any conclusions you can reach about the role of any of the evolutionary processes in producing these effects.

12. Biologists have proposed that the use of antibiotics to treat human infectious disease has played a role in the evolution of widespread antibiotic resistance in several bacterial species, including *Staphylococcus aureus* and the bacteria causing gonorrhea, tuberculosis, and other infectious diseases. Explain how the evolutionary mechanisms mutation and natural selection may have contributed to the development of antibiotic resistance.

13. Two populations of deer, one of them large and living in a mainland forest and the other small and inhabiting a forest on an island, regularly exchange members who migrate across a land bridge that connects the island to the mainland.
    a. If you compared the allele frequencies in the two populations, what would you expect to find?
    b. An earthquake destroys the bridge between the island and the mainland, making migration impossible for the deer. What do you expect will happen to allele frequencies in the two populations over the following 10 generations?
    c. In which population do you expect to see the greatest allele frequency change? Why?

14. Directional selection presents an apparent paradox. By favoring one allele and disfavoring others, directional selection can lead to fixation (a frequency of 1.0) of the favored allele, after which there is no genetic variation at the locus, and its evolution stops. Explain why directional selection no longer operates in populations after the favored allele reaches fixation.

15. What is inbreeding depression? Why is inbreeding depression a serious concern for animal biologists involved in species-conservation breeding programs?

16. Certain animal species, such as the black-footed ferret, are nearly extinct and currently exist only in captive populations. Other species, such as the panda, are also threatened but exist in the wild thanks to intensive captive-breeding programs. What strategies would you suggest in the case of black-footed ferrets and in the case of pandas to monitor and minimize inbreeding depression?

Application and Integration

For answers to selected even-numbered problems, see Appendix: Answers.

17. Genetic Analysis 20.1 predicts the number of individuals expected to have the blood group genotypes *MM, MN,* and *NN.* Perform a chi-square analysis using the number of people observed and expected in each blood-type category, and state whether the sample is in H-W equilibrium (see pages 50 and 51 for the chi-square formula and table).

18. In a population of rabbits, $f(C_1) = 0.70$ and $f(C_2) = 0.30$. The alleles exhibit an incomplete dominance relationship in which C_1C_1 produces black rabbits, C_1C_2 tan-colored rabbits, and C_2C_2 rabbits with white fur. If the assumptions of the Hardy–Weinberg principle apply to the rabbit population, what are the expected frequencies of black, tan, and white rabbits?

19. Sickle cell disease (SCD) is found in numerous populations whose ancestral homes are in the malaria belt of Africa and Asia. SCD is an autosomal recessive disorder that results from homozygosity for a mutant β-globin gene allele. Data on one affected population indicates that approximately 8 in 100 newborn infants have SCD.
    a. What are the frequencies of the wild-type (β^A) and mutant (β^S) alleles in this population?
    b. What is the frequency of carriers of SCD in the population?

20. Epidemiologic data on the population in the previous problem reveal that before the application of modern medical treatment, natural selection played a major role in shaping the frequencies of alleles. Heterozygous individuals have the highest relative fitness, and in comparison with heterozygotes, those who are $\beta^A\beta^A$ have a relative fitness of 82 percent, but only about 32 percent of those with SCD survived to reproduce. What are the estimated equilibrium frequencies of β^A and β^S in this population?

21. The frequency of tasters and nontasters of PTC (see Problem 10) varies among populations. In population A, 64 percent of people are tasters (an autosomal dominant trait) and 36 percent are nontasters. In population B, tasters are 75 percent and nontasters 25 percent. In population C, tasters are 91 percent and nontasters are 9 percent.
    a. Calculate the frequency of the dominant (*T*) allele for PTC tasting and the recessive (*t*) allele for nontasting in each population.
    b. Assuming that Hardy–Weinberg conditions apply, determine the genotype frequencies in each population.

22. Tay–Sachs disease is an autosomal recessive neurological disorder that is fatal in infancy. Despite its invariably lethal effect, Tay–Sachs disease occurs at very high frequency in some Central and Eastern European (Ashkenazi) Jewish populations. In certain Ashkenazi populations, 1 in 750 infants has Tay–Sachs disease. Population biologists believe the high frequency is a consequence of genetic bottlenecks caused by pogroms (genocide) that have reduced

the population multiple times in the past several hundred years.
    a. What is a genetic bottleneck?
    b. Explain how a genetic bottleneck and its aftermath could result in a population that carries a lethal allele in high frequency.
    c. In the population described, what is the frequency of the recessive allele that produces Tay–Sachs disease?
    d. Assuming mating occurs at random in this population, what is the probability a couple are both carriers of Tay–Sachs disease?

23. Cystic fibrosis (CF) is the most common autosomal recessive disorder in certain Caucasian populations. In some populations, approximately 1 in 2000 children have CF. Determine the frequency of CF carriers in this population.

24. In the mouse, *Mus musculus,* survival in agricultural fields that are regularly sprayed with a herbicide is determined by the genotype for a detoxification enzyme encoded by a gene with two alleles, *F* and *S*. The relative fitness values for the genotypes are

Genotype	Relative fitness
FF	0.72
FS	1.00
SS	0.45

    a. Why will this pattern of natural selection result in a stable equilibrium of frequencies of *F* and *S*?
    b. Calculate the equilibrium frequencies of the alleles.

25. In a population of flowers growing in a meadow, C_1 and C_2 are autosomal codominant alleles that control flower color. The alleles are polymorphic in the population, with $f(C_1) = 0.80$ and $f(C_2) = 0.20$. Flowers that are C_1C_1 are yellow, orange flowers are C_1C_2, and C_2C_2 flowers are red. A storm blows a new species of hungry insects into the meadow, and they begin to eat yellow and orange flowers but not red flowers. The predation exerts strong natural selection on the flower population, resulting in relative fitness values of $C_1C_1 = 0.30$, $C_1C_2 = 0.60$, and $C_2C_2 = 1.0$.
    a. Assuming the population begins in H-W equilibrium, what are the allele frequencies after one generation of natural selection?
    b. Assuming random mating takes place among survivors, what are the genotype frequencies in the second generation?
    c. If predation continues, what are the allele frequencies when the second generation mates?
    d. What are the equilibrium frequencies of C_1 and C_2 if predation continues?

26. Assume that the flower population described in the previous problem undergoes a different pattern of predation. Flower color determination and the starting

frequencies of C_1 and C_2 are as described above, but the new insects attack yellow and red flowers, not orange flowers. As a result of the predation pattern, the relative fitness values are $C_1C_1 = 0.40$, $C_1C_2 = 1.0$, and $C_2C_2 = 0.80$.

a. What are the allele frequencies after one generation of natural selection?

b. What are the genotype frequencies among the progeny of predation survivors?

c. What are the equilibrium allele frequencies in the predation environment?

27. ABO blood type is examined in a Taiwanese population, and allele frequencies are determined. In the population, $f(I^A) = 0.30$, $f(I^B) = 0.15$, and $f(i) = 0.55$. Assuming Hardy–Weinberg conditions apply, what are the frequencies of genotypes, and what are the blood group frequencies in this population?

28. A total of 1000 members of a Central American population are typed for the ABO blood group. In the sample, 421 have blood type A, 168 have blood type B, 336 have blood type O, and 75 have blood type AB. Use this information to determine the frequency of ABO blood group alleles in the sample.

29. A sample of 500 field mice contains 225 individuals that are D_1D_1, 175 that are D_1D_2, and 100 that are D_2D_2.

a. What are the frequencies of D_1 and D_2 in this sample?

b. Is this population in H-W equilibrium? Use the chi-square test to justify your answer.

c. Is inbreeding a possible genetic explanation for the observed distribution of genotypes? Why or why not?

30. In humans the presence of chin and cheek dimples is dominant to the absence of dimples, and the ability to taste the compound PTC is dominant to the inability to taste the compound. Both traits are autosomal, and they are unlinked. The frequencies of alleles for dimples are $D = 0.62$ and $d = 0.38$. For tasting, the allele frequencies are $T = 0.76$ and $t = 0.24$.

a. Determine the frequency of genotypes for each gene and the frequency of each phenotype.

b. What are the expected frequencies of the four possible phenotype combinations: dimpled tasters, undimpled tasters, dimpled nontasters, and undimpled nontasters?

31. Albinism, an autosomal recessive trait characterized by an absence of skin pigmentation, is found in 1 in 4000 people in populations at equilibrium. Brachydactyly, an autosomal dominant trait producing shortened fingers and toes, is found in 1 in 6000 people in populations at equilibrium. For each of these traits, calculate the frequency of

a. the recessive allele at the locus

b. the dominant allele at the locus

c. heterozygotes in the population

d. For albinism only, what is the frequency of mating between heterozygotes?

32. The frequency of an autosomal recessive condition is 0.001 (1 in 1000) in a population.

a. What is the frequency of the mutant allele?

b. What is the frequency of carriers of the mutant allele?

c. Assuming individuals mate at random, what is the chance that two heterozygous individuals will mate?

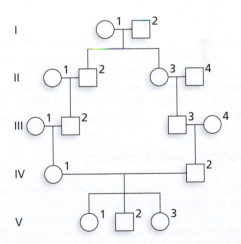

33. Evaluate the following pedigree, and answer the questions below for individual IV-1.

a. Is IV-1 an inbred individual? If so, who is/are the common ancestor(s)?

b. What is F for this individual?

34. Evaluate the following pedigree, and answer the questions below.

a. Which individual(s) in this family is/are inbred?

b. Who is/are the common ancestor(s) of the inbred individual(s)?

c. Calculate F for any inbred members of this family.

35. The following is a partial pedigree of the British royal family. The family contains several inbred individuals and a number of inbreeding pathways. Carefully evaluate the pedigree, and identify the pathways and common ancestors that produce inbred individuals A (Alice in generation IV), B (George VI in generation VI), and C (Charles in generation VIII).

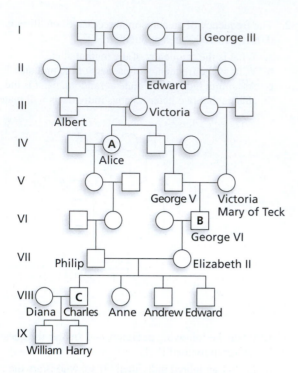

Although this research found several *MC1R* alleles in African populations, *MC1R* alleles that decrease the production of eumelanin were rare. In contrast, several alleles decreasing eumelanin production were found in European populations. How can these results be explained by natural selection?

38. Achromatopsia is a rare autosomal recessive form of complete color blindness that affects about 1 in 20,000 people in most populations. People with this disorder see only in black and white and have extreme sensitivity to light and poor visual acuity. On Pingelap Island, one of a cluster of coral atoll islands in the Federated States of Micronesia, approximately 10 percent of the 3000 indigenous Pingelapese inhabitants have achromatopsia.

    Achromatopsia was first recorded on Pingelap in the mid-1800s, about four generations after a typhoon devastated Pingelap and reduced the island population to about 20 people. All Pingelapese with achromatopsia trace their ancestry to one male who was one of the 20 typhoon survivors. Provide a genetic explanation for the origin of achromatopsia on Pingelap, and explain the most likely evolutionary model for the high frequency there of achromatopsia.

36. Draw a separate hypothetical pedigree identifying the inbred individuals and the inbreeding pathways for each of the following inbreeding coefficients:

    a. $F = 4(1/2)^6$
    b. $F = 2(1/2)^5$
    c. $F = 4(1/2)^8$
    d. $F = 2(1/2)^7$

37. The human melanocortin 1 receptor gene (*MC1R*) plays a major role in producing eumelanin, a black-brown pigment that helps determine hair color and skin color. Jonathan Rees and several colleagues (J. L. Rees et al., *Am. J. Human Genet.* 66(2000): 1351–1361) studied multiple *MC1R* alleles in African and European populations.

39. New allopolyploid plant species can arise by hybridization between two species. If hybridization occurs between a diploid plant species with $2n = 14$ and a second diploid species with $2n = 22$, the new allopolyploid would have 36 chromosomes.

    a. Is it likely that sexual reproduction between the allopolyploid species and either of its diploid ancestors would yield fertile progeny? Why or why not?
    b. What type of isolation mechanism is most likely to prevent hybridization between the allopolyploid and the diploid species?
    c. What pattern of speciation is illustrated by the development of the allopolyploid species?

Collaboration and Discussion

For answers to selected even-numbered problems, see Appendix: Answers.

The problems in this section are best done in small groups of three to six people, if possible. These exercises use a large (12- to 16-ounce) bag of M&M's candies or a similar generic candy. The idea for these exercises was inspired by a 2002 paper titled "Teaching evolutionary mechanisms: Genetic drift and M&M's," by Professor Nancy Staub of Gonzaga University (Staub, N. L. 2002. *BioScience*, 52:373–377). We thank Professor Staub for permission to borrow her approach.

40. Divide the contents of a large bag of different colored candies randomly and approximately equally among the members of the group. Do not pick specific candy colors, but simply empty the contents of the bag onto a table and quickly divide the pile. If you are doing this exercise by yourself, divide the contents of the bag into five piles.

    a. Have each person count the number of candies of each color in his or her pile and calculate the frequency of each color in the pile.
    b. Tabulate the total number of candies of each color in the original bag by combining the numbers from each

    person. Use these numbers to determine the frequency of each color in the original bag.
    c. Have each person compare the frequencies of each color in his or her pile with the frequencies in the original bag. Describe any differences in frequency between the pile and the original bag.
    d. Identify what phenomenon explains the observed differences. What evolutionary mechanism do the observations emulate?

41. Put all the candies used in Problem 40 into a single mound and then divide them into four equal piles, this time being sure that the frequency of each color is the same in each pile. Label two of these piles "male" and the other two "female." Half of the group will take one male and one female pile, and the other half of the group will take the other two piles. Each half of the group will carry out its own experiments:

    a. Blindly draw one candy from the male pile and one candy from the female pile. Record the colors of the two candies as though they were a genotype. Put the candies back into their respective piles.

b. Repeat this activity 24 more times, recording the "genotype" each time.

c. Determine the frequency of each candy color in the total of 25 draws (a total of 50 candies) and compare these frequencies with the original frequencies of the colors in the pile.

d. Explain any observed differences in frequencies in terms of the evolutionary mechanism the results best emulate.

42. Put all the candies used in Problem 41 back into a single mound and then divide them into two piles, being sure that the frequencies of each color are the same in each pile. Make a note of the starting frequency of each color. Label one pile "male" and the other pile "female."

a. Have one person blindly draw one candy from the male pile and one candy from the female pile. Record the colors as though they were genotypes.

b. If *both* colors drawn are *yellow*, eat the candies! If the two colors are any other combination, including yellow with any other color, put the candies back into their respective piles.

c. Repeat this process of blindly drawing one male and one female candy 12 to 15 times for each person in the group.

d. When all selection rounds have been completed, combine the two piles and determine the frequency of each color.

e. Compare the starting frequency of each color with the frequency after drawing. Describe the observed differences and identify the evolutionary mechanism this exercise best emulates.

43. There are usually five or more colors of candy in each bag. Sort the candies by color, and if your bag has more than four colors, eat the least frequent color or colors. Once that is done, calculate the frequencies of the four remaining colors. Assume these frequencies represent four alleles of a gene, and use the description of the H-W equilibrium for more than two alleles for assistance (Section 20.1).

a. Using a different one of the following variables for each color frequency, write out the expected results of a quadrinomial expansion of the expression $(p + q + r + t)^2$.

b. Use this expansion to calculate the expected frequency of each possible genotype produced in a randomly mating population.

Human Evolutionary Genetics

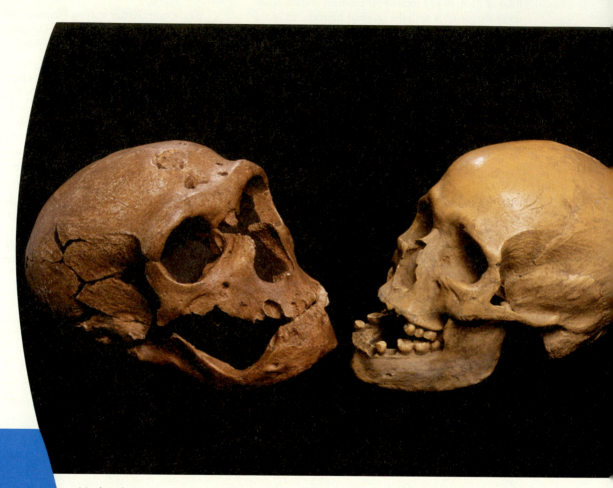

Modern humans, represented by the skull of *Homo sapiens sapiens* at the right, evolved from a branch of the human phylogenetic tree that also gave rise to Neandertals, represented by the skull of *Homo sapiens neanderthalensis* at the left. Neandertals lived in Europe and Asia until about 30,000 years ago, and recent research comparing the modern human and Neandertal genomes finds telltale evidence of interbreeding between the lineages.

Modern humans and their early ancestors—collectively, an evolutionary group known as hominins—evolved in Africa and moved out of Africa to Europe, Asia, and beyond in an undetermined number of successive migrations that began nearly 2 million years ago. The original migrants were most likely the common ancestors of *Homo erectus* and other hominins. Later migrants included the Neandertals, who coexisted with modern humans in Europe and western Asia. The most recent migrants out of Africa, about 60,000 to 80,000 years ago, were ourselves—anatomically modern humans who constitute all of the world's populations today.

Archaeological work over the past century laid the foundation for understanding this more "recent" human history, pointing to an origin in Africa for modern humans, with a subsequent migration to other regions of the world. However, the fragmentary nature of the fossil record left many questions unanswered. For example, how many separate migrations out of Africa contributed to modern humans? Did modern humans interbreed with hominins from earlier migrations out of Africa? If so, what is the imprint of those hominins in the genomes of modern humans? Can genomes from ancient modern humans inform us about past migrations and admixing of populations? Can they tell us about cultural developments? For example, is the spread of farming due to the exchange of ideas or the displacement of populations? Although modern humans likely evolved in a subtropical climate, we now occupy almost every ecological niche of the planet. Is climatic adaptation reflected in our genetics? Finally, how have we changed the genomes of plants and animals during domestication?

Although the stories to be told are far from complete, analyses comparing genome sequences from extant modern humans with the sequences obtained from remains of archaic hominins are providing unprecedented insight into who we are as a species.

Prior to the late 1990s, only fossil evidence was available on which to model hominin evolution. Two principal hypotheses, the multiregional (MRE) hypothesis and the recent African origin (RAO) hypothesis, emerged to explain the evolution of modern humans from our fossilized ancestors (**Figure D.1**). The models agreed that the genus *Homo* evolved in Africa and that multiple waves of early hominins migrated out of Africa to populate Europe and Asia. The MRE hypothesis proposed that local development of modern humans occurred in several locales at about the same time. Under this model, all humans share a deep, common origin but have been distributed in many global locations for a very long time and have diversified locally to produce the populations we observe today. In contrast, the RAO hypothesis proposed that anatomically modern humans migrated out of Africa in a single wave about 80,000 to 100,000 years ago, supplanting the descendants of earlier hominin migrations they encountered and establishing modern-day human populations.

As we shall see, recent genetic and genomic data strongly support the RAO model of modern human evolution, but with a twist. Since the late 1990s, increasingly efficient methods have been developed to isolate and sequence DNA derived from fossilized bones. First demonstrated on bones from Neandertals in 1997, these methods have now produced extensive "archaic" genomic DNA sequences for multiple hominins that are now extinct. The analyses of these sequences lend support to the RAO hypothesis, but they also provide evidence that encounters took place between modern humans and archaic hominins, with various consequences for the modern human genome.

D.1 Genome Sequences Reveal Extent of Human Genetic Diversity

The Human Genome Sequencing Project, completed in the early 2000s, was a significant milestone in biology that has paved the way for an unprecedented wave of new information about the composition, evolution, and genetic diversity of the human genome. As expected based on previous study of evolutionary relationships, genome sequencing has shown many human genes to be directly related to genes of our primate and mammalian relatives. The advances in our understanding of these evolutionary relationships and of our human genetic diversity are enabling us to address two especially intriguing questions: (1) To what extent does genomic sequence vary from one person to another? and (2) What does it mean to be human in the genomic sense? The rest of this chapter outlines the answers that are beginning to emerge.

As described in Chapter 16, the first "draft" of the human genome was actually two draft sequences from two different projects, one funded by the government and the other by Celera Corporation. The DNA sequenced in the publicly funded human genome project was isolated from sperm cells of a number of anonymous male donors and from white blood cells of anonymous female donors. Thus, multiple alleles for a given site were sometimes revealed in the data from this project. In contrast, the DNA sequenced by Celera was isolated from a single individual, company founder J. Craig Venter; therefore, the maximum number of alleles that could be detected for any autosomal gene in that DNA was two.

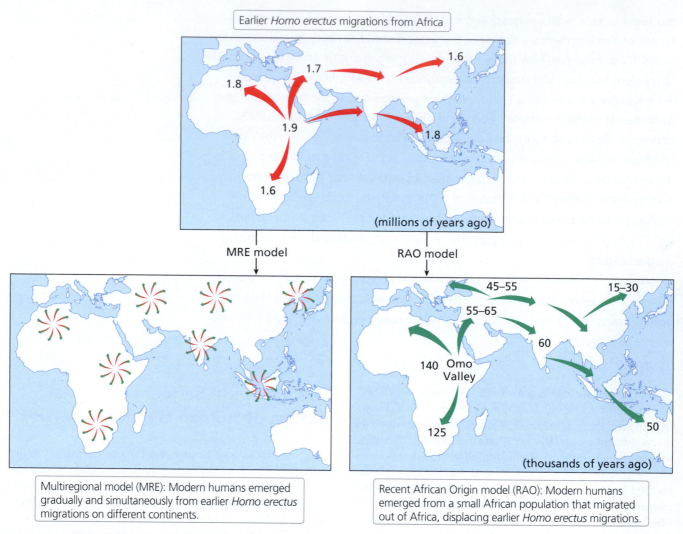

Figure D.1   MRE and RAO models of hominin migration. Genomic evidence indicates multiple migrations with replacement of archaic hominins by modern humans accompanied by interbreeding.

How would the pattern of fossil hominin remains differ under the MRE and RAO scenarios?

By the end of 2015, entire genome sequences for thousands of individuals were available, representing much human diversity from every inhabited continent. These included the genome of !Gubi, a Khoisan indigenous hunter-gatherer from the Kalahari Desert; and Archbishop Desmond Tutu, a South African of Bantu descent. Through the Human Genome Diversity Project, begun at Stanford University in the early 1990s, the sequencing of genomic DNA from a broad spectrum of humans around the world has identified millions of polymorphisms distinguishing individuals and populations. The genomes of ancient modern humans, including Inuk, a paleo-Eskimo from Greenland represented by 4000-year-old permafrost-preserved hair, and dozens of Europeans dating to as far back as 24,000 years, have also been sequenced. Comparisons of these modern human genomes with those of our extinct hominin cousins the Neandertals and Denisovans, as well as those of living great apes, have illuminated our recent evolutionary past.

SNP Variation in Humans

Recall from Chapter 16 that genetic variation takes different forms, ranging from variations in the identity of a single nucleotide, or single nucleotide polymorphisms (SNPs), to larger-scale structural differences, including copy number variants (CNVs; see Figure 16.6). A sampling of SNP variation between two randomly chosen humans reveals differences at about 1 in 1000 bases in DNA sequence, or approximately 3 million base pairs (bp) in the 3×10^9 bp human genome. Variation is greatest in African genomes, consistent with Africa being the place where our species originated. However, it is important to note that genetic diversity between populations is a small fraction of the diversity found within our species.

Differentiation between populations is often expressed as the fraction of the species' global diversity that is due to allele frequency differences between populations; this measure is called the fixation index and abbreviated F_{ST}. An F_{ST} of 0 would mean that allele frequencies are the same between two populations, whereas an F_{ST} of 1 would mean that the two populations have differed fixedly in all alleles. Obviously, neither of these extremes exists in reality. Fixation index values vary from 0.05 to 0.25 between major geographic human populations—that is, between 5 and 25% of the genetic diversity between two of these populations will be attributable to differences in alleles that are unique to a population. For example, the mean F_{ST} between Asians and Europeans is about 0.05, whereas that between African hunter-gatherers and Europeans can be as high as 0.25.

Frequencies of specific alleles also vary enormously. So-called rare alleles are those found at frequencies less than or equal to 1% in the population, with common alleles being more frequent. Alleles may also be referred to as "private alleles," although the meaning of this term varies with context—a SNP might be private to an individual or a family, or to a population. Studies analyzing genome sequences of parents and their offspring indicate that SNP variation accumulates due to mutation at the rate of about 30 to 50 new SNPs in each individual's germ cells in each generation, providing a continuous source of new, often private, alleles. In contrast, most nonprivate alleles are not unique to a population, but rather are shared, often at different frequencies in different populations.

A study of 525,910 SNPs in 29 populations found that 81% of SNPs were cosmopolitan, occurring on all continents, whereas only 1.66% were regionally specific. The latter were seen mostly in Africa. This distribution of alleles indicates that, as a species, the various human populations did not evolve in isolation but rather maintained connections and extensive gene flow. However, although most genetic variation can be found within populations, the fact that F_{ST} values are not 0 indicates that human populations possess some geographic structure. Indeed, genotyping a large enough number of SNPs in a genome can reliably predict its geographic region of origin, often to within a few hundred kilometers or even less.

Variation in CNVs

Between individuals, the number of base pair differences due to CNVs is more than 100 times higher than that due to SNPs. Although the full extent of CNVs is not known, a survey of 2500 individuals revealed substantial variation. On average, individuals had more than 500 kilobase (kb) of CNVs, and although most CNVs were small, 65–80% had a CNV larger than 100 kb, 5–10% had a CNV larger than 500 kb, and 1–2% had a CNV larger than 1 Mb. Only the largest of these CNVs would have been detected by karyotype analysis. Most of the larger CNVs were rare, present in less than 1% of the population. Whether or not these rare CNVs are associated with genetic disease is an active area of investigation. As with SNP variation, the genomes of African donors possessed much greater diversity than those of non-Africans. Studies analyzing genome sequences of parents and their offspring indicate that 8–25 kb of CNV variation accumulates due to mutation in each individual's germ cells in each generation.

One surprising finding from the sequencing of large numbers of individual genomes is the prevalence of deleterious mutations in all of our genomes. In a survey of European and African American populations, each genome carried hundreds of alleles predicted to be missense mutations, of which dozens are homozygous. Of the hundreds of missense alleles, dozens were classified by the Human Gene Mutation Database (HGMD) as disease-causing mutations, and these alleles were occasionally homozygous. Thus, most, if not all, individuals carry potential disease-causing mutations in their genomes. The consequence of these missense alleles is largely unknown, but it is possible that epistatic interactions with other genes may mitigate the phenotypic effects of disease-causing alleles. Nonetheless, these observations underscore the uncertainty inherent in predicting phenotype from genotype, and the need for greater understanding to close this gap in our current knowledge.

D.2 Diversity of Extant Humans Suggests an African Origin

The first genetic evidence for an African origin of modern humans came from analysis of mitochondrial DNA polymorphisms. Mitochondrial DNA sequences are particularly suited for deciphering the genealogical history and evolutionary relationships of mammalian species. First, since mitochondria are strictly maternally inherited in mammals, they undergo no recombination of alleles as occurs in the nuclear genome. Second, some noncoding regions of mitochondrial genomes evolve quickly, with the result that many differences in mitochondrial DNA sequence are present even in closely related populations. This is especially true for mammals, where the rate of mutation in the mitochondrial genome is about 10 times that in the nuclear genome, reflecting lower levels of DNA mutation repair in mitochondria versus repair of nuclear DNA. Since there is little selective pressure to maintain a specific sequence in noncoding regions, mutations in these regions accumulate at a relatively steady rate.

Once a mitochondrial mutation becomes homoplasmic in the germ cells of an individual female, the mutation is transmitted to all her progeny. Therefore, maternal lineages can be traced by following the mutational changes back in time. The mitochondrial DNA sequences in the present population reflect the maternal genealogy of the population as a whole, and construction of a phylogenetic tree based on these sequences should allow the identification of the common ancestor(s) of the species.

Mitochondrial Eve

Analyses of mitochondrial DNA variation in human populations provided our first view of our early human ancestors' journey out of Africa. The regions around the Great Rift Valley of East Africa have been home to humans and our hominin ancestors for at least 4 million years. Based on the fossil record, dispersals from Africa have also been a regular feature throughout hominin evolution.

As described in the chapter introduction, genetic studies have supported a model of human evolution called the RAO model (for *recent African origin*), which proposes that modern humans evolved from a small African population that migrated out of Africa, displacing other hominin species. The RAO model postulates that modern humans arose approximately 120,000 to 200,000 years ago, whereas a competing model, the MRE model (for *multiregional*), posits a much older age for our species—up to 2 million years ago. The RAO model suggests genetic diversity should be greatest in Africa, since humans would have diversified there before migrating outward. In the RAO scenario, the genetic diversity outside of Africa would be a subset of that found in Africa and so would reflect the subpopulation of humans who migrated from Africa.

Allan Wilson and colleagues used the mitochondrial genome to analyze genetic diversity in modern humans (**Figure D.2**). Their phylogenetic analysis of mtDNA sequences from individuals representative of distinct geographic regions leads to two major conclusions: First, Africans are genetically more diverse than humans from other continents (see the right half of Figure D.2); and second, the genetic diversity of non-Africans is a subset of that found in Africans. In addition, comparison of human sequences with those of chimpanzees allowed the researchers to estimate when the divergence of modern humans occurred. This is calculated by first working out the rate of sequence evolution in terms of base pair changes per million years. The researchers divided the number of sequence differences between humans and chimpanzees by 5 to 7 million years (the divergence time of the two species) and then calculated the minimum divergence time of humans by applying the rate of sequence evolution to the two most divergent human sequences. Such calculations led to the estimate that modern humans first appeared about 200,000 years ago. Several subsequent studies of mtDNA diversity have supported these initial findings, and have estimated the common ancestor of extant humans to have lived 172,000 years ago and the separation of African and non-African mtDNA lineages to have originated 50,000 years ago.

The patterns of mitochondrial DNA variation suggest that modern humans evolved in Africa and subsequently migrated around the world, largely displacing other hominid populations. The mtDNA of all humans living today is descended from a female or group of females living in East Africa 120,000 to 200,000 years ago. The carrier of this ancestral mtDNA has been called our "mitochondrial Eve."

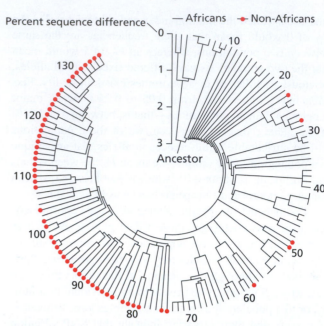

Figure D.2 **Human evolution.** This genealogical tree of modern humans based on phylogenetic analyses of mitochondrial restriction fragment length polymorphisms (RFLPs) strongly supports the RAO model. The population affinities of the mtDNA types are as follows (lineages are identified by the numbers around the outside of the tree): Western Pygmies (1, 2, 37–48); Eastern Pygmies (4–6, 30–32, 65–73); !Kung (7–22); African Americans (3, 27, 33, 35, 36, 59, 63, 100); Yorubans (24–26, 29, 51, 57, 60, 63, 77, 78,103, 106, 107); Australian (49); Herero (34, 52–56, 105, 127); Asians (23, 28, 58, 74, 75, 84–88, 90–93, 95, 98, 112, 113, 121–124, 126, 128); Papua New Guineans (50, 79–82, 97, 108–110, 125, 129–135); Hadza (61, 62, 64, 83); Naron (76); and Europeans (89, 94, 96, 99, 101, 102, 104, 111, 114–120).

❯ How does the phylogenetic pattern support an African origin for modern humans?

Y Chromosome Phylogeny

Analyses of Y chromosome sequence variation provide a convenient complement to mtDNA analyses, as the Y chromosome is strictly paternally inherited and, outside the pseudoautosomal regions, it does not recombine with other chromosomes. The size of the Y chromosome, 23 Mb, provides ample sequence diversity, especially since the chromosome is gene poor, with only a few dozen genes present in the male-specific euchromatin. In particular, Y chromosome short tandem repeats (Y-STR) have been useful, as they are estimated to mutate rapidly, as much as 0.1% per Y-STR per generation. As with the mtDNA analyses, African and non-African Y chromosome lineages are recognizable. Consistent with the RAO model, more diversity is present within African Y chromosome sequences than non-African sequences.

Since in humans inheritance of mtDNA and the Y chromosome is strictly maternal and paternal, respectively, their haplotypes can be used to trace migration patterns following marriage. For example, about 70% of human societies are patrilocal, meaning that following marriage, the couple make their home near the male's birthplace rather than the female's. Other societies may be matrilocal. In patrilocal societies, the geographical distribution of Y chromosome haplotypes is predicted to increase, whereas in matrilocal societies the mtDNA haplotypes are predicted to spread geographically. Studies on mtDNA and Y chromosome haplotypes in matrilocal and patrilocal societies have confirmed these hypotheses.

Due to the high mutation rates of the Y-STRs, a study analyzing a set of 10–20 Y-STR loci in a small population of males showed most of them to possess a unique pattern. This makes the Y-STR polymorphisms useful for forensic or paternity assessments. Occasionally, however, a population possesses clusters of very similar Y chromosome Y-STR haplotypes, implying a rapid expansion in that population of a particular Y chromosome lineage. One such case was found in a survey of 2123 Asian males, where greater than 90% of haplotypes were rare but one cluster of closely related haplotypes had a frequency of 8%. This cluster was geographically widespread, from the Pacific to the Caspian Sea, with its highest frequency occurring in Mongolia. It has been suggested that the expansion of this lineage may have been due to Ghengis Khan and his descendants, whose empire was centered in Mongolia. Similar clusters have also been hypothesized to be associated with the establishment of the Qing dynasty in 16th century China, where rulers had many concubines, and to the Uí Néill royal family in medieval Ireland. The ties to historical figures are hypothetical at present, but access to relevant ancient DNA samples could confirm or refute the links.

Autosomal Loci

With the advent of new sequencing technologies, thousands of human genome sequences have been generated, providing an unprecedented view of our genetic diversity. An analysis of 1327 microsatellite and insertion/deletion (indel) markers in 185 populations (121 African, 4 African American, and 60 non-African) demonstrated that autosomal genetic diversity is greater in African populatons compared with non-African populations (**Figure D.3**). Similarly, in the previously described study of 525,910 SNPs in a worldwide sample of 29 populations, analysis revealed that African populations had the highest frequency of unique alleles and that non-Africans harbored only a subset of the diversity present within Africa—a distribution consistent with the theory arguing for a recent migration of humans out of Africa. Another study examining the distribution of 650,000 SNPs found that mean heterozygosity decreased as distance from Addis Ababa (Ethiopia) increased (**Figure D.4**). These data all strongly suggest an African origin for our species, but do not distinguish between a southern or eastern origin within the continent.

Within Africa, genetic diversity, including the number of private alleles, is highest in hunter-gatherer populations of southern and eastern Africa—specifically, Khoisan speakers (whose languages include click sounds) and Pygmies. For example, SNP differences between two Namibian Khoisan individuals (1.2 per kb) are greater than differences between European and Asian individuals (1.0 per kb). Analysis of several related hunter-gatherer populations in sub-Saharan Africa, including the Hadza and Sandawe of Tanzania and click-speaking ‡Khomani Bushmen of southern Africa, revealed the lowest levels of linkage disequilibrium (see Section 5.5) and highest population differentiation of any population in Africa, pointing to a southern African origin for modern humans. Not only are these hunter-gatherer tribes highly differentiated from other African populations, they are also highly differentiated from one another, indicating that they form distinct isolated populations that have been separated from one another for thousands of years. This provides genetic evidence that the Khoisan have continuously occupied southern Africa for up to 40,000 years.

As noted above, genetic diversity of non-Africans is largely a subset of diversity found among Africans. Since only a subset of humans migrated from Africa, the alleles they carried were only a subset of the alleles present in Africa at the time. As human populations traveled further from their ancestral homeland, subsequent splittings of migrant groups would experience successive reductions in genetic diversity—a pattern referred to as a serial founder effect. Interestingly, the diversity of phonemes, the basic units of sound in speech, also decreases with distance from the Khoisan speakers in central and southern Africa, a distribution also hypothesized to reflect a serial founder effect.

D.3 Comparisons between Great Apes Identify Human-Specific Traits

Although analysis and comparisons are made among modern human genomes for insight into what makes us individuals, biologists and geneticists look to our closest primate relatives and to our recently extinct human relatives to understand what makes us human.

Revelations of Great Ape Genomes

The genomes of all of the extant great apes (**Figure D.5**) have been sequenced, allowing comparisons of both chromosome and gene evolution. Differences can be found at the levels of chromosome architecture, gene content, and SNP diversity. One characteristic of humans relative to all other primates is our comparatively reduced individual genetic diversity, despite our population size being vastly larger than those of the great apes. Whereas F_{ST} levels vary between 0.05 and 0.25 for human populations (see above), the F_{ST} values for chimps (0.32) and gorillas (0.38) are both higher, and global

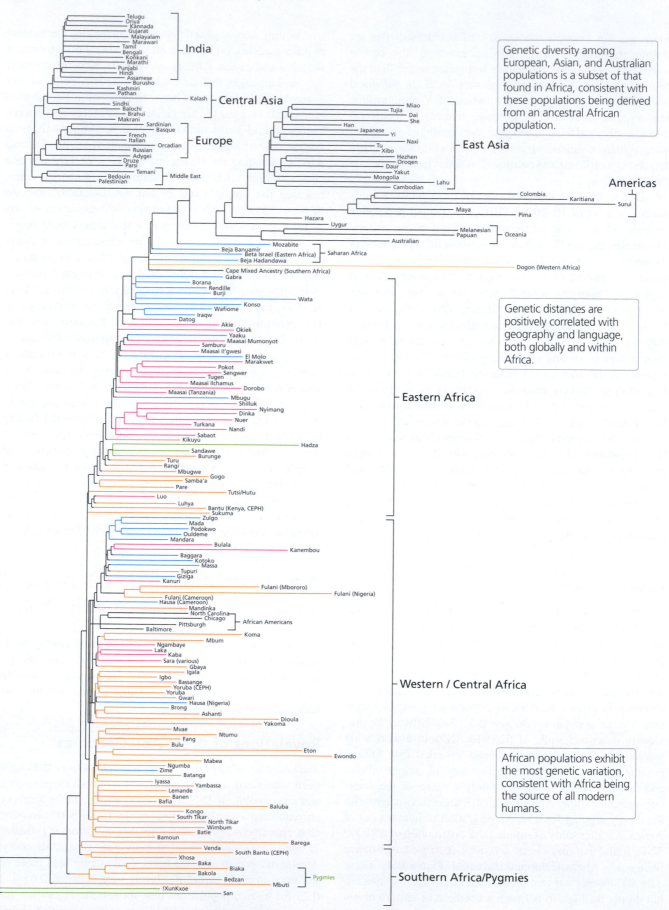

Genetic diversity among European, Asian, and Australian populations is a subset of that found in Africa, consistent with these populations being derived from an ancestral African population.

Genetic distances are positively correlated with geography and language, both globally and within Africa.

African populations exhibit the most genetic variation, consistent with Africa being the source of all modern humans.

Figure D.3 **Cladogram showing genetic distances and relationships between human populations.** This phylogenetic tree is based on 1327 polymorphic markers, 848 repetitive sequence variants, 476 indels, and 3 SNPs.

How does recent admixture confound identification of past population divergences?

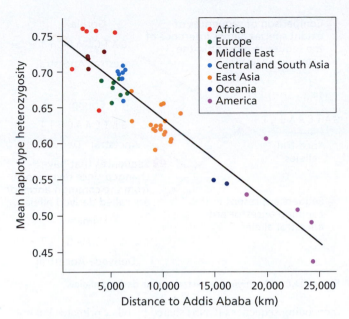

Figure D.4 Decrease in mean haplotype heterozygosity as distance from Addis Ababa increases.

🔴 **Explain how diversity might be lost over geographic distance.**

genetic diversity of orangutans is estimated to be twice that of humans. This spectrum of genetic diversity is interpreted as being a consequence of our recent population expansion, with gene flow and admixture (see Section 20.4) having a greater impact than geographic isolation and differentiation.

Genomic comparisons among the various species of great apes and old world monkeys (the nearest relatives of the great apes), reveal changes in gene content related to interactions with the environment. For example, the common ancestor of old world monkeys and great apes had trichromatic vision due to a tandem duplication of the long-wavelength opsin gene on the X chromosome. In contrast, because the old world monkeys and great apes rely less on their sense of smell than this ancestor did, and than most other mammals do, they have consequently experienced a loss of genes encoding olfactory receptors—with many of those genes becoming pseudogenes. This form of change is particularly pronounced in humans, where slightly more than half of our olfactory receptor genes have become nonfunctional.

Comparing the Human and Chimpanzee Genomes

Humans and chimpanzees last shared a common ancestor about 6 million years ago. Both lineages have diverged since that time. Many phenotypic and behavioral differences between humans and chimpanzees are obvious, but what about genetic differences? Genetic and genomic analysis indicates that about 5% of each genome is lineage-specific, that is, found in one lineage exclusively but not in the other. Stated another way, the genomes of humans and chimpanzees are about 95% identical.

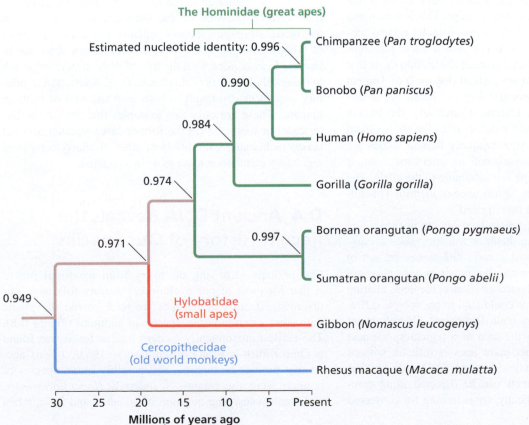

Figure D.5 Phylogenetic relationships among apes and monkeys.

There are about 35 million SNPs differentiating the human and chimpanzee genomes, or roughly 10 times the number that differentiate one human from another (the vast majority being in noncoding regions). This corresponds to a frequency of 1.23% in nucleotide differences between the human and chimp genomes. Of these differences, 86% are fixed between species—meaning they are differences in which humans are homozygous for one allele and chimps are homozygous for another. In addition, there are about 5 million indels accounting for a further portion of the difference. When orthologous proteins are compared, 29% of human and chimpanzee proteins are seen to have identical amino acid sequences, and the average protein differs by about two amino acids between the two lineages.

Beyond these differences are gains and losses of genes in each lineage, such as the olfactory receptor genes mentioned previously. Complete genome tabulations show that the number of genes differs by several hundred. A gene loss specific to the human lineage is *MYH16*, which encodes a myosin heavy chain expressed in the mandible in other apes, perhaps reflecting the gracile phenotype of humans relative to other great apes. Other losses include several genes involved in sialic acid biology. Sialic acid has a role in cell–cell communication, and one conjecture is that the genes were lost through positive selection owing to pathogens binding to sialic acids at the cell surface.

How can biologists determine which changes were functionally important in the evolution of humans as they diversified from their shared common ancestor with the chimpanzee? The first step is to identify those changes that occurred exclusively in the human lineage. This is done using the genome sequence of a third, more distantly related species, such as *Gorilla*, for comparisons that allow researchers to separate human and chimpanzee alleles into those that are ancestral and those that are derived (**Figure D.6**). Human alleles are considered *ancestral* if they are shared by humans and gorillas but differ in chimps. Conversely, the human allele is considered *derived* if it differs from the allele shared by chimps and gorillas. After uniquely human alleles are identified, they can be investigated to determine what, if any, difference in phenotype is attributable to the allele. The functional and evolutionary significance of identified phenotypic variation can then be investigated.

Given that protein sequences between chimpanzees and humans are often indistinguishable, it was speculated as early as the 1970s that the causal genetic differences are not in the coding regions of the genes, but rather in how genes are regulated. Mutations in enhancer or silencer elements altering expression levels or patterns could lead to phenotypic differences without creating large-scale disruptions of development and physiology. Detecting the gain of a regulatory element in humans relative to other great apes is difficult without performing functional studies. In contrast, human-specific losses of regulatory elements can be detected using comparative genomics—specifically, by searching for conserved

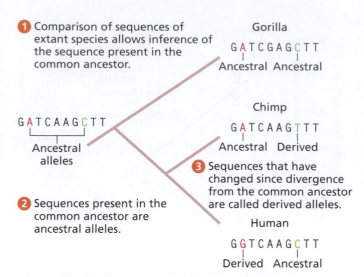

Figure D.6 Identifying ancestral versus derived alleles.

noncoding sequences (CNS) shared by other primates but not present in humans (**Figure D.7**; see also Figure 16.17).

In a systematic screen of CNSs found throughout mammals but lost in humans, 510 potential regulatory sequences were identified. One of these may regulate the tumor suppressor gene *GADD45G*. Because loss-of-function alleles of this gene result in expansion of growth of specific brain regions, it was speculated that in humans the loss of a positive regulatory sequence driving expression of this gene could have led to more extensive growth of regions of the brain relative to that in other mammals. Another example of a loss of regulation is the loss of an enhancer sequence that drives expression of the androgen receptor gene in the facial vibrissae (sensory whiskers) and penile spines of other mammals. The loss of this regulatory sequence in humans is associated with the loss of these structures, much to the relief of readers of this book. Thus, deletion of regulatory sequences can result in both gain and loss of traits in humans. These are only two examples that are (in the latter case) or might be (in the former case) relevant to what makes us human. A multitude of other, similarly conserved regulatory elements remain to be investigated.

D.4 Ancient DNA Reveals the Recent History of Our Species

One perhaps surprising discovery from the fossil record is that for most of our evolutionary history following our divergence from chimpanzees we have shared the planet with other, often multiple, species of hominins (**Figure D.8**). The earliest anatomically modern human fossil was found at Omo Kibish in Ethiopia and dates to 195,000 years ago. At that time at least three, and possibly more, species of hominin were also extant—Neandertals, *Homo floresiensis*, and Denisovans. The question of whether, and if so, when

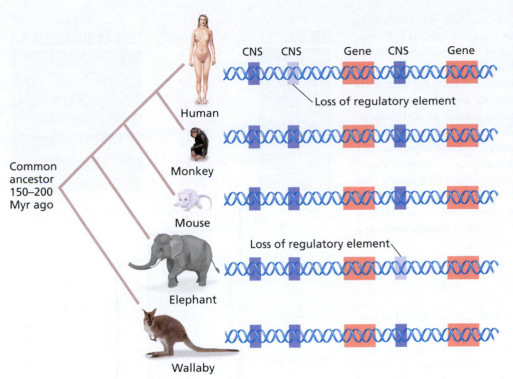

Figure D.7 Identification of conserved noncoding sequences (CNS) lost in specific lineages. Dark blue boxes represent CNS conserved throughout mammals and light blue boxes indicate CNS lost during the evolution of specific lineages, e.g., elephant or human.

🔵 **How can we determine whether a CNS has been lost rather than never acquired?**

and where, we interbred with our hominin cousins has fascinated anthropologists.

In addition to approaches that identify important human alleles by comparing our genome with those of our living relatives, developments within the past decade now allow comparisons of our genome with high-quality genome sequences from ancient remains (see Chapter 1 Case Study). Genomics has undergone amazingly rapid development

of methods and applications in recent years, and genome experts such as Svante Pääbo have used new methods to decipher the genomes of so-called archaic hominins. The archaic genomes are derived from DNA isolated from bone fragments that are 30,000 or more years old. Using highly specialized techniques, Pääbo and his colleagues have assembled genomic sequence data on two archaic hominins that rival the genome data for modern humans in depth and

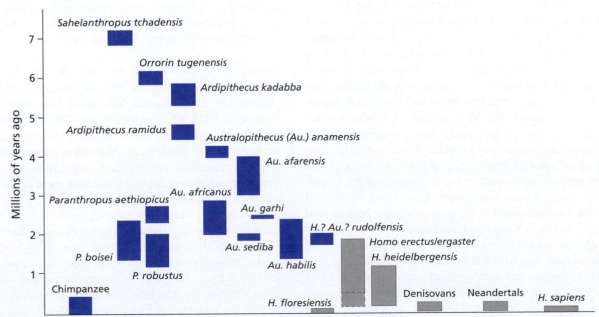

Figure D.8 **Fossil hominins.** The hominin fossil record reveals potential human ancestors. The length of the bars represents the approximate temporal existence of the taxa. Blue represents taxa found only in Africa; grey represents taxa found in Africa and elsewhere or only outside Africa.

accuracy of genome coverage. One archaic genome is from Neandertals, a hominin that was widely dispersed in Europe and Asia from 400,000 years ago or more until about 30,000 years ago (Figure D.8). The second archaic genome is from Denisovans, a more recently identified hominin named for Denisova cave in Siberia, where its bones were first discovered. Denisovans were closely related to and contemporaneous with Neandertals. Both these hominins diverged from the lineage leading to modern humans approximately 500,000 years ago, and both lineages, or a common ancestor, migrated out of Africa and into the Middle East and Eurasia, where their descendants lived until about 30,000 years ago. Modern humans stayed in Africa until about 75,000 to 85,000 years ago, when they migrated to Eurasia and coexisted with Neandertals and Denisovans.

Neandertals

Because modern humans and Neandertals cohabited in Eurasia for millennia, scientists have looked for indications of whether interbreeding occurred between the lineages. Although the mtDNA sequence of Neandertals is distinct from that of modern humans and provided no evidence of interbreeding, comparisons of nuclear genome sequences revealed that up to about 4% of the modern human genome is of Neandertal origin. Introgression (incorporation through hybridization) of Neandertal DNA into the modern human genome is found in all non-Africans assayed, but not in sub-Saharan African genomes, indicating that interbreeding took place following the migration of modern humans out of Africa. Additional analysis of high-quality Neandertal genomic sequence has determined that whereas the average modern non-African human carries a few percentages of Neandertal DNA in the genome, it is not the same DNA in each person. The current estimate is that 30% of the Neandertal genome is present today if all modern human genomes are considered collectively (**Figure D.9**). Thus, as modern humans left Africa, they interbred with Neandertals during at least one episode, perhaps in the Middle East prior to the divergence of Europeans and East Asian human populations (**Figure D.10**). More recently, it was shown that East Asians have proportionally more Neandertal DNA than Europeans, suggesting a more complex model of interbreeding between the hominins, perhaps involving at least a second episode subsequent to the divergence of Europeans and East Asian human populations. In addition, Neandertal DNA has been identified in the genomes of the Maasai who currently reside in Kenya and Tanzania, but this introgression appears to have been recent, possibly a consequence of migration back into Africa in the past few thousand years.

This analysis has also revealed that Neandertal DNA is unevenly distributed in the human genome. For example, there is virtually no Neandertal DNA on the X chromosome. Each autosome, on the other hand, carries Neandertal DNA, with the precise distribution differing among human populations (Figure D.9). The absence of Neandertal DNA from

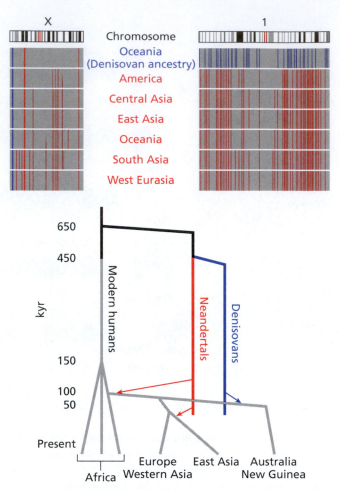

Figure D.9   The distribution of Neandertal and Denisovan DNA in the modern human genome. The X chromosome and a representative autosome, chromosome 1, are shown. Red indicates regions in which the likelihood of Neandertal sequence is greater than zero; blue indicates the same for Denisovan sequence. The relationships between humans and other hominins and the proposed interbreeding are depicted in the lower panel.

the human X chromosome may indicate that the descendants of human–Neandertal hybrids bearing Neandertal X chromosome DNA became less fertile over time and the Neandertal DNA was eventually lost. This may have been particularly the case for males, whose X chromosome genes are present in a single copy. Without a second copy of a gene to compensate, the less-fit X-linked Neandertal alleles were selected against, so that eventually most of them were lost from the human X chromosome.

Whatever the fate of Neandertal genes on the X chromosome may have been, what is known about the functions of genes for which Neandertal alleles do occur at high frequency in the human genome? Genome-wide association analyses (see Section 5.5) have uncovered Neandertal alleles for genes affecting the skin, hair, and nail protein keratin in about 60% of the genomes of Europeans and East Asians. Keratin thickens and toughens the skin, giving it elasticity and protection against water, heat, cold, and pathogens. The researchers speculate that the additional protection afforded to the

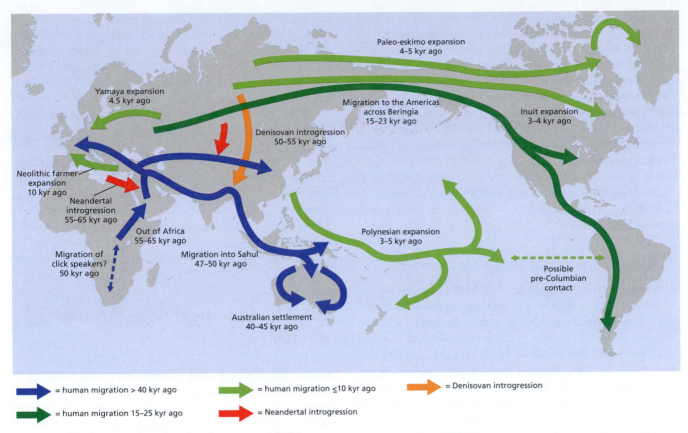

Figure D.10   The migration of modern humans out of Africa.

skin was advantageous in the colder and wetter climates of Europe and Asia. A Neandertal gene that affects the size of the optic disc in the eye has also been identified. However, the most common Neandertal haplotypes involve genes related to immune system functions. As humans entered new environments, they were exposed to new pathogens. Perhaps Neandertals, who had been exposed to the pathogenic environment for hundreds of thousands of years prior to the arrival of humans, were a source of adaptive alleles.

Although some Neandertal alleles may have helped humans emigrating from Africa adapt to their new, colder habitats, other Neandertal alleles may have increased their vulnerability to certain human disorders. Neandertal genes that make humans more susceptible to Crohn's disease, lupus, and type 2 diabetes, and even a gene influencing potential addiction to smoking (nicotine addiction), have been identified. Researchers speculate that these alleles did not harm Neandertals and that, until very recently, they did not harm the humans who carried the Neandertal alleles. It may be that prior to the last century or so, the average human life span was not long enough for the ill effects of these alleles to manifest themselves, or perhaps those alleles provided some as yet unidentified advantage in a hunter-gatherer life history.

The ultimate fate of the Neandertals has been the subject of much discussion, with one extreme possibility being that modern humans drove the Neandertals to extinction, either violently or by outcompeting them for resources. However,

the presence of 30% of the Neandertal genome residing within that of modern humans has suggested another possible fate at the other extreme. Since the estimated Neandertal population size was small compared with that of the humans who were migrating from Africa, it may be that the Neandertals largely admixed with the humans and were subsumed into the expanding human population, leaving within the human genome a legacy in the form of a collection of adaptive alleles that facilitated the further spread of humans around the world.

Denisovans

Similar questions are being asked about the second archaic genome, from the Denisovans, who are only known to us by a few finger bone fragments and some teeth. Based on nuclear DNA comparisons, Denisovans are thought to have been more closely related to Neandertals than either was to humans, diverging from Neandertals perhaps 400,000 years ago. Remarkably, genome sequences of four Denisovan individuals from a single location have genetic diversity comparable with that seen in Neandertals from all across Eurasia and from periods spanning tens of thousands of years. Comparisons of the sequence of the Denisovan genome with those of modern humans suggest that up to about 5% of the genomes of Melanesians, Papuans, and Aboriginals was derived from Denisovans, implying interbreeding between modern humans migrating eastward out of Africa toward Australia (Figure D.10). Closer inspection of the genomes of East Asians and Native Americans indicates a low level of Denisovan ancestry that may be derived from the ancestral modern human population colonizing Papua and Australia, or perhaps a separate admixture event. As with the Neandertals, some Denisovan alleles that have been retained are involved in immune system functions. In another case of ancient hominin alleles being potentially adaptive, Tibetan populations living at high altitudes harbor a Denisovan allele of the *EPAS1* gene, which encodes a transcription factor induced under hypoxic conditions and thought to provide an advantage in high-altitude environments with lower oxygen levels.

Finding Genes That Make Us Human

Now that genome sequences for both Neandertals and Denisovans are available, we can begin to ask what alleles have been derived specifically within the modern human lineage. Initially there was much interest in *FOXP2*, a gene associated with our ability to speak and use language and for which the human version harbors two functionally relevant amino acid changes relative to the version seen in other great apes. However, both archaic hominins have the same changes as found in modern humans, hinting that Neandertals and Denisovans may have possessed language capabilities similar to those of modern humans. A study designed to identify alleles for which archaic hominins possess the ancestral variant (found in great apes) and for which modern humans are fixed for a derived nonsynonymous amino acid change identified only 90 loci. At one locus, *AHR*, the nonsynonymous change is in the ligand-binding domain of an aryl hydrocarbon receptor, a protein that senses polycyclic aromatic hydrocarbons and induces expression of genes encoding enzymes that break down cyclic hydrocarbons, often into toxic or carcinogenic products. The ancestral version of *AHR* is 150–1000 times more sensitive in inducing expression of cyclic hydrocarbon metabolic enzymes than is the derived human allele. Why might such an allele have been selected in modern humans? One idea is that the derived human allele might make us less sensitive to some smoke-derived toxins than other hominins were, lending support to a theory proposing that the invention of cooking contributed to the success of early humans.

Several questions regarding the evolution of the modern human genome remain to be answered. For example, was there any other ancient human lineage that contributed to the makeup of the human genome? Indeed, analyses of the genomes of sub-Saharan Africans suggest ancient admixture with additional hominins for which there is no known fossil record, perhaps due to the tropical climate in central Africa. Also, if modern humans were around for 200,000 or more years, why did it take them so long to walk out of Africa, given that a land bridge to Eurasia existed? An answer to

this puzzle is beginning to emerge based on sequences of Neandertal mtDNA, which provide evidence that an early out-of-Africa migration of ancestors of modern humans may have interbred with Neandertals, but not Denisovans, at least 270,000 years ago. This suggests that the lineage leading to modern humans likely ventured outside of Africa, just as the ancestral Neandertal and Denisovan populations did before them.

The holy grails of researchers seeking ancient DNA from additional hominin species are genomes from *Homo erectus* and *Homo floresiensis*, as these could illuminate, respectively, the more distant past and more recent interactions of our species. There is much to be added to the story of what in our genetic and evolutionary history makes us human, and undoubtedly some surprises will be revealed, as researchers study the evolution of the human genome.

D.5 Human Migrations Around the Globe

Just as analyses of ancient genomes have illuminated early hominin migration patterns, similar analyses of more recent genomes have provided insight into the migration patterns of modern humans out of Africa and their colonization of other continents. The patterns emerging from studies of genomes typical of Europe and Australia, for example, present contrasting patterns of settlement and in the case of Europe highlight how human demographics change when farmers replace hunter-gatherer populations.

Europe

One question that has occupied scientists for a long time is whether farming and agricultural practices spread through populations via information exchange from one population to another or via a migration of populations in space and time. Analyses of both modern and ancient genomes have helped resolve this question with respect to the peopling of Europe.

Present-day Europeans have a genetic constitution primarily composed of lineages from three separate migrations into Europe (Figure D.10). The genetic contribution to present-day Europeans from the first modern humans that migrated into Europe (about 45,000 thousand years ago) appears limited, but DNA sequences dated to 37,000 years ago, in the Upper Paleolithic, already contain some major genetic components found in Europe today. The population of these hunter-gatherers passed through a population bottleneck (see Section 20.5) during the Last Glacial Maximum (LGM; 26,500–19,000 years ago) as they were displaced into refugia by the advance of ice from the north. Following the LGM, the hunter-gatherers repopulated the European continent, and the population may have remained relatively uniform for many millennia. Interestingly, the genomes of several hunter-gatherers revealed that they had dark skin and hair but blue or light-colored eyes.

The transition from a hunter-gatherer lifestyle to one incorporating agriculture is a major event in the history of any human population, and it is one that has occurred independently in different populations around the world. In western Eurasia this transition, called the Neolithic transition, took place approximately 11,000–12,000 years ago in the Fertile Crescent, from where it spread to Anatolia and then into Europe, arriving in Scandinavia and the British Isles about 6000 years ago. The movement of farming into Europe was driven by farmers from Anatolia, who expanded into Europe via two routes, along the Danube River and along the Mediterranean coast. Based on genome sequences from Neolithic farmers, the preexisting hunter-gatherer population and the migrating farmers did not remain genetically isolated from one another, but rather mixed.

Thus, farming and agricultural practices spread through Europe as a result of both a displacing population from Anatolia and an incorporation by that population of the original hunter-gatherer population. The hunter-gatherer lifestyle was gradually replaced, and their genes became admixed with those of the influx of farmers. Today there is a gradient across Europe of genetic evidence from the two groups—southern Europeans have a greater contribution from the Anatolian farmers, whereas northern Europeans retain a greater contribution from the original hunter-gatherers. However, given the larger population sizes of agricultural societies, the Anatolian farmers contributed a greater fraction to modern genomes in most regions. Of interest is the observation that the people that now live in Anatolia do not have any genetic signature of the Neolithic farmers that emigrated from there to Europe, suggesting that this population was also displaced by subsequent migrations and highlighting the importance of ancient DNA to untangle past human movements.

The third genetic component of modern Europeans came from the migration of the Yamnaya herders from the Pontic–Caspian steppe in present-day Russia about 4500 years ago. The Yamnaya, in turn, are at least in part descended from a population that lived in northeastern Eurasia, a conclusion based on the genome sequence from 24,000-year-old remains of a Siberian boy, whose genetic affinities include both modern Europeans and Native Americans. As with the Anatolian farmers, the migration of the Yamnaya, who were pastoralists with horses, displaced and incorporated preexisting hunter-gatherer populations across northern Europe. The Yamnaya were light-skinned and brown-eyed, and it is thought that they are the source of one of the alleles for light skin in modern-day Europe, although infrequent alleles for these features already existed in some northern hunter-gatherers (see below). Surprisingly, although the Yamnaya were herders, they were unable to digest raw milk as adults, and thus were not the source for alleles conferring this ability (discussed further below).

Australia

In contrast to Europe, only a single ancient human migration was responsible for the initial colonization of Sahul, the continent consisting of what is now Australia, Tasmania, and New Guinea, which formed a single land mass for much of the past 100,000 years. Multiple studies in 2016 support the idea that Sahul was first settled 47,000–55,000 years ago by a single population migrating from the Indonesian archipelago (Figure D.10). Thus, Australians were the first people to migrate across an open expanse of ocean while losing sight of land. As with Europeans, Australians admixed with Neandertals, and in addition admixed with Denisovans at a slightly later date. Both admixtures occurred prior to their migration to Sahul.

A study that analyzed the genomes of 25 Highland Papuans and 83 Pama–Nyungan-speaking Aboriginal Australians from throughout the Australian continent indicates that the populations in New Guinea and Australia split about 37,000 years ago, long before the land masses were separated by water about 8000 years ago. Additional details come from a second study in which 111 mtDNA sequences were derived from hair samples collected from throughout the continent in the mid-20th century and analyzed with the consent of living descendants of the donors. It finds that the initial single Australian population spread rapidly around the perimeter of the continent, following both east and west coasts and arriving in southern Australia by 45,000 to 49,000 years ago, while the inland regions were colonized at least 42,000 years ago (Figure D.10). However, perhaps because the formation of the central deserts acted as a migration barrier, present-day populations in eastern and western Australia have been separated for as much as 31,000 years—a time frame similar to that for the separation of modern day Siberians and Native Americans!

This scenario is supported by the distribution of mtDNA haplotypes, which provide evidence for the continuous presence of specific populations in distinct geographic locations dating back to the original settlement of the continent, despite significant climatic, cultural, artistic, and technological changes (e.g., the LGM and the intensification of the El Niño/Southern Oscillation 2000–4000 years ago) occurring during the period in question. About 6000 years ago, migrations from northeastern Australia southwest into the interior brought some gene flow and a change in language. Variation between populations is greater for mtDNA than for the Y chromosome, reflecting more male than female migration, possibly due to the complex marriage and postmarital residence traditions among Pama–Nyungan-speaking Australians. In inland populations, adaptation to the harsh climate of the central desert, with its cold winter nights, is reflected in alleles of genes associated with the thyroid system that facilitate adaptation to desert cold and with serum urate levels that regulate dehydration. Although more is to be learned from studying non-Pama–Nyungan-speaking populations largely inhabiting northwest Australia, the striking differences between the ancient histories of Europe and Australia shed some light on certain Aboriginal Australian traditions. The Aboriginal connection to "country"—a deep kin-group–based affinity for the land in which they were born, which is reinforced by song lines and dreaming narratives based on the Australian landscape—appears to be rooted in tens of thousands of years of residence.

D.6 Genetic Evidence for Adaptation to New Environments

As humans migrated out of Africa they encountered a wide range of different climates, food sources, and pathogens. A number of polymorphic alleles have arisen in modern humans in the past 80,000 years that are associated with changes in diet or adaptation to pathogens or the environment. The alleles persisting in human populations today reflect their recent evolutionary history. Some of the polymorphic alleles may still be adaptive in the modern world, whereas others may be relics of past environments and may be maladaptive in some present-day environments. An example of the former is β-globin alleles that confer a level of resistance to malaria when in the heterozygous state but that have severe consequences when homozygous. The genetics of such alleles is explored more fully in Chapter 20. Here, we examine in more detail alleles affecting three other traits: the ability to digest lactose, skin color, and adaptation to living at high altitude.

How are adaptive alleles that are under selection identified? One approach is to ask whether a particular haplotype is overrepresented in a population. Under neutral selection, recombination will result in a shuffling of different alleles within a haplotype. However, under natural selection, there is a reduction in variation at the locus under selection, with the frequency of the beneficial allele potentially rising to fixation (see Section 20.5). This reduction or elimination of polymorphism at a locus under selection is referred to as a **selective sweep** (**Figure D.11a**), and it is explained as follows. Evolutionary theory predicts that if a particular SNP is favored, its frequency will increase, but so too will the frequency of alleles that are linked to the favored SNP; natural selection directly favors a specific allele and indirectly favors the alleles of genes closely linked to it. Initially, this leads to linkage disequilibrium (LD) in which the favored allele and the alleles closely linked to it occur together on chromosomes significantly more often than expected by chance (see Section 5.5 for a discussion).

The name for this phenomenon is **genetic hitchhiking**, because the alleles of genes that happen to be closely linked on the same chromosome as the favored allele are taken along for the evolutionary ride, leading to distinctive haplotypes on those chromosomes, at least temporarily. Over time, homologous recombination will break up the haplotype and randomize the combinations of alleles among the linked genes. In other words, recombination gradually eliminates LD and restores linkage equilibrium.

Lactose Tolerance

Lactose is a carbohydrate component of mammalian breast milk. All humans have the ability to break it down at birth, but like most other mammals, a majority of individuals lose that ability rapidly after weaning. Lactose digestion in newborns is made possible by production of the enzyme lactase-phlorizin hydrolase, commonly known as "lactase," encoded by the *LCT* gene on chromosome 2. Lactase is functionally equivalent to β-galactosidase, the bacterial enzyme for cleaving lactose that we discussed in Section 12.2.

Individuals who lose the ability to digest lactose after weaning are often identified as "lactose intolerant," whereas those who digest lactose into adulthood are termed "lactase persistent." Approximately one-third of humans exhibit lactase persistence, with the frequency varying greatly between populations, from as low as 5% to as high as nearly 100%. Lactase persistence is common in individuals of European ancestry descended from populations of pastoralists. The evolution of lactase persistence in these populations is associated with the domestication of cattle 7500 to 9000 years ago and with the availability of milk and other dairy products that provided a readily accessible source of protein. Lactase-persistent individuals have the evolutionary advantage, in the pastoral environment, of being able to exploit that protein source. Recent analyses of the genomes of ancient Eurasians suggest that the allele conferring lactase persistence in modern Europeans may have been brought into Europe by the Yamnaya, but its frequency rose due to selection only about 4000 years ago, postdating the domestication of cattle and consistent with the idea that the allele increased in frequency due to selection related to diet.

Lactase persistence is not limited to Europeans, however, and a 2007 study by Sarah Tishkoff and colleagues studied the evolution of lactase persistence in pastoral African populations in Tanzania, Kenya, and the Sudan to determine if lactase persistence in Europeans and Africans has the same genetic basis or is the result of different mutations and a separate evolutionary history. The study determined that European and African lactase persistence is produced by different mutations of the *LCT* gene, and furthermore, that different African populations harbor different alleles. In addition, Middle Eastern populations of Bedouin camel and goat herders possess a fifth lactase persistence haplotype. A SNP in the upstream regulatory region of *LCT* is responsible for lactase persistence in Europeans (**Figure D.11b**). This SNP is a bp substitution that substitutes a cytosine with a thymine at nucleotide position −13910, located approximately 14 kb upstream from the *LCT* transcription start site and residing within an intron of the adjacent *MCM6* gene. The SNP is designated C/T−13910, and it occurs in nearly 100% of Europeans with lactase persistence; this SNP is

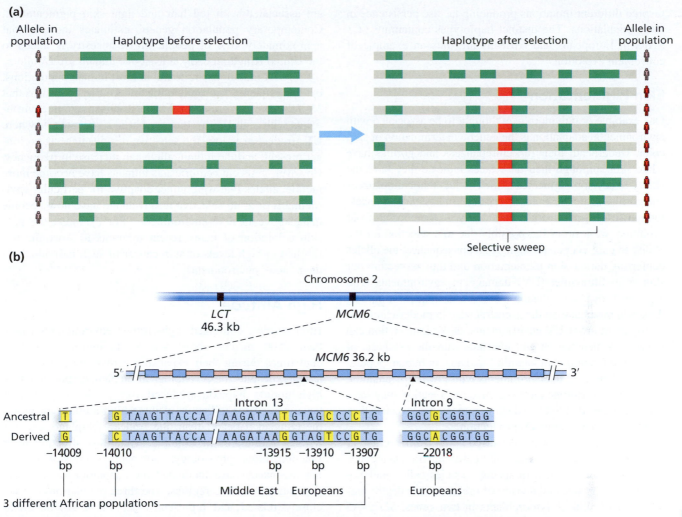

Figure D.11 **Adaptive alleles in modern humans. (a)** Selective sweeps result in a reduction in polymorphism surrounding the locus of selection. **(b)** Lactose tolerance has evolved independently in Europeans and Africans and in the Middle East. Each of the SNPs conferring lactase persistence is located in an intron of a gene adjacent to the LCT gene.

Is the favored haplotype expected to expand or contract over evolutionary time?

in strong linkage disequilibrium with a second SNP, G/A-22018, suggesting they may act together. The C/T-13910 SNP creates a new binding site for the transcription factor Oct-1, and thus leads to an alternative molecular pathway for *LCT* expression.

The C/T-13910 SNP is widespread among lactase-persistent individuals in Eurasia. In contrast, the C/T-13910 allele is not found in Africans with lactase persistence. Instead, four other SNPs also located in the upstream *LCT* regulatory region are detected: T/G-14009, G/C-14010, T/G-13915, and C/G-13907 are each associated with lactase persistence in Africans, with the T/G-13915 allele being frequent in the Middle East as well. The G/C-14010 SNP is prevalent among East and South African pastoralists, whereas the T/G-14009 and C/G-13907 alleles are common among the Beja people of Sudan. At least two of the SNPs, T/G-13915, and C/G-13907, affect Oct-1 binding,

suggesting a similar molecular mode of action as the C/T-13910 allele. Given the molecular genetic data identifying distinct SNPs associated with lactase persistence in pastoral Europeans and Africans, a logical hypothesis is that natural selection favored different mutations producing lactase persistence in these populations. In this case, the evolution of a new binding site for a transcription factor leads to persistence of *LCT* expression that would otherwise disappear with age.

Natural selection favors the most fit organism in a given environment, and on occasion, mutant alleles that are identical or nearly identical can be independently generated and can be similarly favored in separate populations. When this occurs, the mutant traits evolve independently in each population, a phenomenon known as **convergent evolution**. Given the molecular genetic data identifying distinct SNPs associated with lactase persistence in pastoral Europeans and Africans, a logical hypothesis is that natural selection favored different mutations producing lactase persistence in these populations. The distinct haplotypes containing *LCT* SNPs in Europeans and Africans are thus an example of convergent evolution.

Skin Pigmentation

One example of polymorphism thought to be associated with environmental adaptation is the genetic determination of skin color. Underneath their fur, chimpanzees and gorillas have white skin, although their dark faces indicate they have the ability to develop pigmented skin. The fact that chimpanzees and gorillas share these characteristics implies that our ancestors possessed similar traits and ability. In the course of our evolution, we lost our fur, possibly due to a selection for the ability to cool via perspiration. As a consequence, the alleles conferring darker skin pigmentation and thus protecting our skin from ultraviolet (UV) damage in environments with high levels of UV irradiation increased in frequency, making dark skin pigmentation the ancestral state in modern humans. However, in lower UV environments, dark pigmentation can reduce UV penetration and interfere with the synthesis of the essential compound vitamin D_3. Thus, in human populations that migrated to environments with low UV irradiation, particularly in Europe and Asia, natural selection may have favored alleles that lightened skin pigmentation because they promoted easier vitamin D_3 production.

Our skin pigmentation is caused by melanin, a granular substance produced in specialized cells called melanocytes. Melanin is concentrated in special vesicles called melanosomes, and the size and density of melanosomes determines the color of skin. Polymorphisms in two genes, *SLC24A5* and *SLC45A2*, encoding transporters involved in melanin biosynthesis contribute to the light skin pigmentation in Europeans. The derived allele of *SLC24A5* is almost fixed in European populations and is associated with pale skin, whereas the ancestral allele is found in Africa, Australia, East Asia, and the Americas. That East Asians, who have light skin, harbor the ancestral allele suggests that light skin has evolved independently multiple times among modern humans. As the derived *SLC24A5* allele is almost fixed in Anatolian Neolithic farmers, it is thought that its widespread occurrence in Europe is due to the migration of Neolithic farmers. In contrast, the derived *SLC45A2* allele conferring light skin pigmentation that is almost fixed in present-day Europeans is not found at high frequencies in ancient Eurasian genomes. In this case the derived allele likely made its way to Europe via the Yamnaya, in which the derived allele has been found, and then due to subsequent selection its frequency rose to near fixation later.

Another allele of interest in this regard is a mutation of the melanocortin-1 receptor (*MC1R*) gene that is particularly common in northern Europe. The melanocortin-1 receptor binds to the α-melanocyte stimulating hormone, subsequently signaling melanocytes to produce mature malanosomes. Specific mutant alleles of *MC1R* are associated with red hair and light skin pigmentation. Contemporary population genetic estimates indicate that approximately 40% of people whose ancestry is traced to the United Kingdom carry at least one mutant *MC1R* allele.

MC1R mutations are found in most human populations, but the frequency is usually quite low. One hypothesis is that *MC1R* mutations are at a selective disadvantage in environments with high UV irradiation; but in environments where UV irradiation is low, the selective disadvantage is no longer present, and the mutant allele can increase in frequency. However, in recent centuries, as humans have become more mobile, alleles that were either adaptive for particular environments or at no selective disadvantage have now become maladaptive in new environments. For example, the pale skin coloration of many recent migrants to Australia has resulted in high levels of skin cancer of such individuals in their "new" environment.

High Altitude

Humans have colonized high-altitude environments (more than 2500 meters above sea level) multiple independent times during their expansion across the globe. Most notably, despite the physiological challenges presented by high-altitude hypoxia (reduced oxygen levels), humans have resided for millennia at three high-altitude locations: the Qinghai–Tibet Plateau, the Andean Altiplano, and the Semien Mountains in Ethiopia. Mutations affecting heart function, blood physiology, and maternal physiology during pregnancy have facilitated the adaptation of the local populations to these regions. The three populations are not closely related and represent independent colonizations, allowing comparisons that reveal examples of both distinct and converging evolutionary events in genetic adaptation to high-altitude hypoxia.

Genome-wide association studies in each of the three populations have identified candidate genes, many of which are in the hypoxia-inducible factor (HIF) pathway. Not surprisingly, given the independent adaptations by the different populations, alleles in both common and distinct HIF pathway and non-HIF pathway genes were identified. In both the Tibetan and Ethiopian populations, alleles at the *EPAS1* locus were identified as contributing to hypoxia adaptation, but the alleles in the two populations were different. Moreover, *EPAS1* alleles were not identified in the Andean populations. One locus identified in all three populations was *EGLN1*, which regulates the HIF transcriptional response via hydroxylation of HIF-1α, a transcription factor mediating cellular oxygen homeostasis and activated by hypoxia. In Tibetan populations, two nonsynonymous mutations, D4E and C127S, reduce binding between EGLN1 protein and an accessory protein that mediates its interaction with HIF-1α. Thus, it was proposed that this is a loss-of-function allele that results in reduced down-regulation of the HIF pathway, overcoming hypoxic stress by keeping the HIF pathway activated. Although the *EGLN1* locus was identified in both of the other populations as well, the alleles in those populations differ from that of the Tibetans, and their mode of action is unknown.

D.7 Domestication of Plants and Animals: Maize

Fly over any arable region of the Earth and you will see that the most conspicuous, and in many ways destructive, change that humans have wrought upon the environment is agriculture, made possible by the domestication of plant and animal species. About 15,000 years ago, dogs were domesticated from ancestral wolves, presaging a momentous change in lifestyle for many human populations. By 10,000 years ago, with the domestication of several plant and animal species, pastoral and farming societies emerged from previous hunter-gatherer populations. Remarkably, domestication of different plant and animal species occurred independently in several regions of the globe, where local indigenous plants and animals were exploited and managed. Goats, sheep, barley, chickpeas, and beans were first domesticated throughout the Fertile Crescent about 10,000 years ago, followed by turkeys, llamas, maize, tomatoes, and peppers in two centers of domestication in Central and South America a few thousand years later. Other centers of domestication occurred independently in South and East Asia, Africa, and New Guinea.

With respect to genetics, domestication results in a population bottleneck, as only a subset of a population of a species contributes to the domesticated variety. In addition, selection for specific traits, such as nondispersing seed in plants or tameness in animals, results in selective sweeps at loci controlling those traits. During the early stages of domestication, admixing with local wild progenitors likely occurred. Charles Darwin noted the remarkable phenotypic variation selected by animal breeders, and pointed to human-mediated artificial selection to support his ideas regarding evolution, natural selection, and the origins of domestic animals.

As described in detail below for maize, genetic and genomic analyses of domesticated species in comparison with their wild relatives have provided insight into the alleles that contribute to agronomically important traits. In addition, experimental approaches to breeding tameness in silver foxes and rats have led to the identification of quantitative trait loci including genes for neurotransmitters, suggesting that changes in gene expression regulating brain chemistry underlie the behavioral changes that adapt animals to domestication.

At the turn of the 20th century, there were multiple theories for the origin of maize, given the many aspects in which it differs significantly from any of its alleged wild ancestors (Table D.1; Figure D.12). The phenotypes that distinguish domesticated maize were likely selected by early

Maize (*Z. mays ssp. mays*)	Teosinte (*Z. mays ssp. parviglumis*)
Short lateral branches	Long lateral branches
Lateral branches tipped by ears (female)	Lateral branches tipped by tassels (male)
Short, soft glumes	Long, hard glumes
Ears 4-ranked (or more)	Ears 2-ranked
Ears nonshattering	Ears shattering
Cupules with 2 spikelets	Cupules with 1 spikelet

Table D.1 Major phenotypic differences between maize and teosinte

Mesoamerican farmers as being desirable traits for cultivation, though not necessarily adaptive in the wild. For example, the lack of ear-shattering in the domestic plant facilitates harvesting of the crop but would be disadvantageous in a wild species whose seed needs to be dispersed. Alleles conferring nondispersing seeds have been independently selected in nearly all crop species. Likewise, the differences in plant architecture between maize and its wild relatives allow maize plants to be grown more densely in fields.

Classic experiments by George Beadle, of one gene–one enzyme fame (Section 4.3), firmly established the grass teosinte as the wild progenitor of maize. To understand the inheritance of morphological traits, Beadle crossed a primitive "landrace" maize (domesticated but similar to maize that existed prior to modern breeding) with wild teosinte and examined 50,000 F_2 progeny. He observed that in about 1 in 500 F_2 plants, the phenotype was nearly identical to that of teosinte, whereas about 1 in 500 F_2 plants had a phenotype similar to the maize parental line. From these numbers he deduced that alleles at four to five major genes could explain the genetic basis for the differences in morphology between maize and teosinte.

Toward the end of the 20th century, John Doebley and his colleagues set out to identify the molecular basis for the difference between teosinte and maize. A survey of genomic

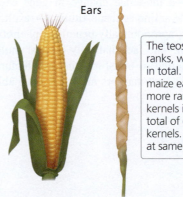

Ears

The teosinte ear has two ranks, with 6–10 kernels in total. The modern maize ear contains 16 or more ranks, with more kernels in each rank and a total of close to 1000 kernels. (Ears not drawn at same scale.)

Figure D.12 Phenotypes of maize and teosinte.

regions encoding typical neutral genes (that is, genes not under domestication selection) suggests that maize retains about 70% of the nucleotide diversity observed in teosinte, indicating a modest population bottleneck associated with the domestication event. Quantitative trait locus (QTL) mapping (see Section 19.4) facilitated identification of the genomic regions for several of the domestication traits, two of which—plant architecture and glume architecture—we examine here.

The difference in plant architecture, with teosinte having long lateral branches tipped by tassels (male inflorescences) in contrast to maize having short lateral branches with ears at their tips, is largely controlled by alleles at a single locus called *teosinte branched1* (*tb1*). The *tb1* gene encodes a transcription factor that represses the outgrowth of lateral branches. The derived maize allele encodes the same protein, but its expression is about twice the level as that of the teosinte allele. Introgression of the maize *tb1* allele into teosinte can confer a maize-like architecture to the teosinte plants, and vice versa. The maize *tb1* allele is the same in all domesticated varieties, with evidence of a selective sweep at the locus: only 2% of the diversity found in teosinte is present in the 5′ upstream region of the *tb1* coding sequence.

Another trait under selection is glume architecture; the teosinte glume (a modified leaf) is hard and covers the kernels, whereas the maize glume is short and soft, allowing easy access to the kernels. The hardness of the teosinte glume makes its seeds similar to the hardness of popcorn, leading to speculation that this may have been one of the earliest forms of maize eaten. Again, this difference in phenotype is largely determined by alleles at a single locus, *teosinte glume architecture1* (*tga1*). The difference between the ancestral teosinte allele and the derived maize allele is a single base pair mutation in a gene encoding a transcription factor, resulting in an amino acid substitution (leucine in place of asparagine at position 6). This single amino acid change is thought to endow the transcription factor with a strong repressor activity, leading directly or indirectly to a loss of development of the glume.

Thus, during the domestication of maize, two semidominant mutations—a moderate change in gene expression levels and a single amino acid substitution—resulted in dramatically different, agronomically beneficial phenotypes in the cultivated plant. The fact that only modest molecular changes were required to transform the architecture of this plant suggests that early farmers may have been able to assemble the basic suite of traits found in modern maize in a short span of time.

D.8 The Future

The recent evolutionary past of our species is written in the distribution of polymorphic alleles in our genome sequences and reflects a combination of serial founder effects and locally restricted new mutations. These polymorphisms, whose distributions have accumulated over the past 150,000 years, make it possible to pinpoint the geographic origin of anyone by the person's genomic sequence alone. However, since the Renaissance, and especially in the past 50 years, the accelerating mobility of man has resulted in increasing admixture of populations. This can be seen by the placement of African Americans in Figure D.3, in a position intermediate between peoples indigenous to West Africa and peoples indigenous to Europe—two groups of whom African Americans are an admixture. With continued elevated rates of migration and admixture, phenotypic and genotypic differences between populations are expected to decrease, and if our species ever reaches panmixis (random mating), all traces of historical movements will be erased from our genomes.

Can we predict the role of natural selection on the human genome in the future? Many of the adaptive alleles that have been selected for in our past may not have selective advantage in present-day societies (for example, lactase persistence) or may even present a disadvantage (for example, pale skin color for recent migrants to subtropical or tropical environments). However, because people in most developed societies typically live well beyond the age of reproduction, these alleles, previously adaptive, but now neutral or only mildly problematic, will likely undergo genetic drift in future populations. In contrast, one environmental factor imposing selection will likely be with us for as long as our species exists—infectious disease. Although the diseases of the future may be different from those that are scourges today or from those (such as malaria) that have been powerful influences in shaping our present genomes, infectious diseases will likely continue to be a significant influence on our genomes in the future. It is an interesting intellectual exercise to consider what other types of alleles might be selected for in the future of our species given that the mutation rate will not diminish over time.

For answers to selected even-numbered problems, see Appendix: Answers.

1. Why might mitochondrial, Y chromosome, and autosomal DNA provide different perspectives on our evolutionary past—for example, with respect to our relationship with Neandertals?

2. What insights have analyses of human mitochondrial DNA provided into our recent evolutionary past?

3. What lines of evidence support the hypothesis that modern humans evolved in Africa and then subsequently migrated throughout the globe?

4. Discuss how both gains and losses of regulatory elements may lead to human-specific traits.

5. How do copy number variants arise? Do they account for more polymorphism than SNPs within the human population?

6. Consider possible societal and ethical dilemmas that might arise if we currently shared the planet with another hominin.

7. Carl Linnaeus, the 18th century botanist who laid the foundation for the modern system of taxonomic nomenclature, placed chimpanzees and humans in the same genus. Discuss the merits of this classification.

8. Describe how selection at a locus can result in a loss of polymorphism surrounding the locus.

9. How can ancient DNA provide insight into past migrations that analyses of extant human genomes fail to uncover?

10. Denisovans are known from bones found in Denisova Cave in the Altai Mountains in Siberia, but traces of their DNA are found in Australians and Melanesians, whose ancestors likely migrated across Asia much farther to the south. How can these geographic differences be reconciled?

11. In Island Melanesia and Polynesia, most mtDNA haplotypes are of Asian ancestry, whereas Y chromosome haplotypes are predominantly New Guinean. Provide a hypothesis for this sex-biased distribution.

12. A 9-bp deletion in the mitochondrial genome between the gene for cytochrome oxidase subunit II and the gene for tRNA^{Lys} is a common polymorphism among Polynesians and also in a population of Taiwanese natives. The frequency of the polymorphism varies between populations: the highest frequency is seen in the Maoris of New Zealand (98%), lower levels are seen in eastern Polynesia (80%) and western Polynesia (89%), and the lowest level is seen in the Taiwanese population. What do these frequencies tell us about the settlement of the Pacific by the ancestors of the present-day Polynesians?

13. When the human genome is examined, the chromosomes appear to have undergone only minimal rearrangement in the 100 million years since the last common ancestor of eutherian mammals. However, when individual humans are examined or when the human genome is compared with that of chimpanzees, a large number of small indels and SNPs can be detected. How are these observations reconciled?

14. The mtDNA sequence of Neandertals is more similar to that of modern humans than to that of Denisovans. However, analyses of nuclear DNA clearly indicate that Neandertals and Denisovans share a more recent common ancestor than either of these hominins shares with modern humans. Propose a hypothesis to resolve the discrepancy between the mtDNA and the nuclear genome.

15. If you were to compare your genome sequence with that of your parents, how would it differ? If you were to compare your genome sequence with another student's in the class, how would it differ? What additional difference might you see if your genome was compared with that of a sub-Saharan African, or if you are of sub-Saharan African descent, with that of a non-African?

Forensic Genetics

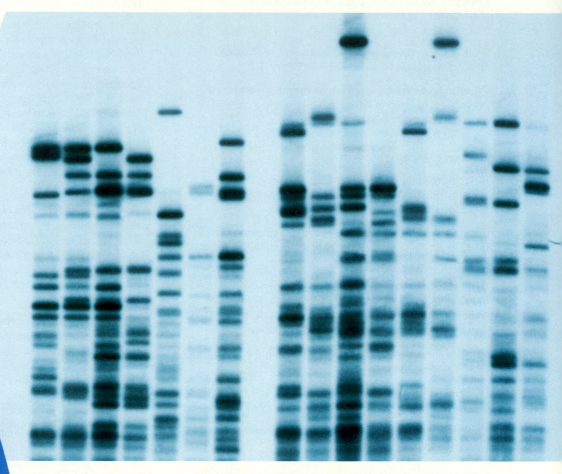

PCR-based analysis of short tandem repeats (STRs) provides the basis for forensic genetic analysis, paternity testing, and individual genetic assessment.

In late 1983 a 15-year-old young woman named Lynda Mann was raped and murdered in the English village of Narborough in Leicestershire. No suspects were identified and the case remained unsolved. In mid-1986, a similar rape and murder of a 17-year-old young woman named Dawn Ashworth occurred in the nearby village of Enderby. Shortly after Ashworth's rape and murder, a 17-year-old young man named Richard Buckland, who had been spotted near the location of that murder, was taken into custody. Under intense questioning, Buckland repeatedly confessed and retracted his confession to the Ashworth murder. He did not confess to Mann's murder. The Leicestershire police were convinced Buckland was responsible for both crimes but needed more evidence to bring murder charges against him.

To obtain more information, a Leicestershire police investigator contacted Alec Jeffreys, a professor of genetics at the University of Leicester. The inspector asked Jeffreys if he knew of any way to compare the sperm samples from the two murder cases to see if they came from the same man. Jeffreys said he did, and if samples were provided, he thought he could also match the sperm to the man who produced it, using a new method of DNA analysis. Jeffreys had discovered this new method quite by accident while investigating the inheritance of diseases in families. Jeffreys's accidental discovery would quickly evolve into the worldwide standard for the analysis of crime scene DNA.

Jeffreys used his method to determine that the sperm samples for the Mann and Ashworth cases came from the same man. He then tested DNA from Buckland and found that Buckland *was not* the source of the sperm. The police made Jeffreys test the Buckland sample three times, convinced he must be wrong. After the third test, they had to admit that although they once thought Buckland was responsible for the murders, they now had clear evidence that he was not. Buckland became the first person exonerated of rape and murder based on DNA analysis.

In early 1987, with no suspects in either case, Leicestershire police turned to a new strategy—the voluntary mass screening of all men aged 17 to 34 years from Narborough, Enderby, and the nearby village of Littlethorpe. More than 98% of men in the villages complied with the request, but after the screening of 5511 men, there were no matches to the sperm samples.

In August 1987 came a break in the case. Someone reported to Leicestershire police an overheard conversation between two colleagues. One colleague was boasting to the other that he had given a DNA sample to investigators for a friend of his named Colin Pitchfork. Pitchfork had told the man he had already given a sample for another friend and couldn't contribute under both his real name and a false name. The man said Pitchfork doctored his own passport, substituting the man's picture for Pitchfork's, and had driven the man, who was now posing as Pitchfork, to the clinic to have his blood sample collected. Following a police investigation of these suspicious circumstances, Pitchfork and the imposter were both arrested in August 1987, and Pitchfork's DNA was collected. It was a match to the sperm samples from the Mann and Ashworth cases. Pitchfork confessed to the crimes, and in January 1988 Pitchfork became the first person convicted of murder using DNA analysis. He continues to serve a life sentence in Britain for the two rapes and murders.

Each of us, with the exception of monozygotic multiple births, has a unique genome. This genetic uniqueness has practical applications in individual identification through the identification of genotypes of DNA marker genes. The techniques used for this identification are commonly known as **DNA fingerprinting, DNA profiling, forensic genetics,** or **forensic genetic analysis.** By any name you prefer, they have come a long way since Sir Alec Jeffreys's initial version was used to exonerate Buckland and to convict Pitchfork. The contemporary methods generate individual genetic profiles using laboratory analyses of carefully selected genetic markers and then evaluate them statistically according to the Hardy–Weinberg equilibrium (H-W equilibrium). The calculated result informs investigators of the frequency of a person's genotypes and the probability that the person is the source of a specific DNA sample.

Today, this methodology is used for three primary kinds of forensic analysis, which we discuss in the first portion of this chapter: the analysis of crime scene DNA, DNA analysis for paternity testing, and examination of DNA for the individual identification of remains. The second portion of the chapter addresses three direct-to-consumer uses of DNA analysis. Two of the applications are closely related: the analysis of DNA for genealogical purposes (identification of relatives) and DNA analysis to determine genetic ancestry (geographic origin of one's ancestors). These kinds of analysis are conducted by a number of companies, such as Ancestry.com. The third direct-to-consumer application is the use of DNA for genetic health risk assessment. These kinds of assessments are performed at this time by the company 23andMe.

E.1 CODIS and Forensic Genetic Analysis

The genetic markers used in forensic genetic analysis are short tandem repeats (STRs) that contain different numbers of copies of short, repeating DNA sequences. The repeat sequences of STRs are very similar to those of variable number tandem repeats (VNTRs; see Figure 5.13a), except that STR repeats are less than 10 base pairs (bp) long, whereas VNTRs contain repeats that are longer than 10 bp each. Like VNTRs, the inheritance of STRs follows a codominant pattern (see Figure 5.13b and Figure 7.27c).

The STRs used in forensic genetic analysis are examined by first using the polymerase chain reaction (PCR) to amplify target DNA segments that contain an STR gene. Recall from Figures 7.27a and 7.27b, and the accompanying discussion, that the DNA fragments generated by PCR for alleles of a gene that differ by the number of DNA sequence repeats are of different lengths. The differences in the lengths of PCR-amplified DNA are multiples of the number of base pairs in each sequence repeat. For example, if one allele (A_8) contains 8 repeats of a repetitive 4-bp STR sequence and another allele of the gene (A_{12}) contains 12 repeats of the same sequence, the difference in the lengths of the PCR fragments for the alleles will be (4 repeats)(4 bp/repeat) = 16 bp. If the gene happens to have alleles with consecutive numbers of repeats (i.e., alleles with 5 repeats, 6 repeats, 7 repeats, and so on), the respective PCR fragments from each allele will differ from the preceding and following one by 4 bp each. Each allele generates a PCR-amplified DNA fragment of a distinctive length.

CODIS History and Markers

The contemporary forensic genetic analysis that has grown out of Jeffreys's original analysis of the Leicestershire cases is an example of international scientific cooperation. Laboratories in the United States, Canada, Europe, Africa, Asia, and elsewhere have contributed to the identification of STR genetic markers that have the right characteristics for forensic genetic analysis. These efforts include the assembly of detailed population genetic analyses that provide the number of alleles and the frequencies of each allele in populations around the world.

In 1990, the United States Federal Bureau of Investigation (FBI) began a process of extensive analysis that culminated in the selection of 13 independently assorting human STR markers to form the core of the FBI's *Combined DNA Index System* (CODIS) and that also determined the number and frequencies of alleles for those markers in most human populations. In 1994, federal legislation known as the DNA Identification Act led the FBI to establish the National DNA Index System (NDIS) that uses CODIS genetic markers as a basis for comparison of DNA information. Local agencies can submit samples to the FBI for analysis; or as an alternative, the methods used for CODIS-based analysis are made available to local law enforcement agencies and municipalities that often conduct their own genetic analysis. The NDIS allows the sharing of genetic identification information between states and between local, national, and international law enforcement agencies. Today, nearly 200 law enforcement agencies in the United States participate in NDIS. Internationally, almost 100 law enforcement agencies in 50 different countries use the CODIS markers and CODIS DNA identification software for their forensic genetic analyses. Beginning on January 1, 2017, seven new STR markers were added to the CODIS list, bringing the total to 20 STR markers (Table E.1). The additional markers were identified through international research and investigation. Adoption of the seven new markers into CODIS followed their use and adoption by multiple European law enforcement agencies.

A CODIS marker must meet four critical criteria. First, a CODIS STR must have a known chromosome location, and its location must ensure that the STR assorts independently of all other CODIS markers. This condition contributes importantly to the calculation of individual identity that we discuss below. Most CODIS STRs are located in noncoding regions of the genome, meaning that they are not part of an expressed gene. These noncoding STRs are designated by gene labels reading "*D*S****." The "*D*" indicates that the STR is encoded in DNA, the number following *D* is the chromosome on which the STR is located, and the "*S*" indicates that the repetitive sequence of the STR is a "single" repetitive sequence, meaning that the STR is found just once in the genome. The final numbers either are part of a consecutive count of genetic markers on the particular chromosome or are a reference to the position of the STR on the chromosome. Notice that five CODIS markers have designations that are all letters or are letters and a number. These STRs are parts of intron sequences of expressed genes. Because they are located in intron sequences, the variation in repeat number of these STRs does not affect the polypeptide product of the genes.

The second criterion for CODIS STR markers is that they must have multiple alleles in all populations examined.

Table E.1	The 20 CODIS Core Loci[a]	
Locus	Location	Sequence
STRs in noncoding sequences		
D1S1656	1q42.1	$(GATA)_n$
D2S441	2p14	$(TCTA)_n$
D2S1338	2q35	$(GGAA)_n$
D3S1358	3p21.31	$(TCTG/TCTA)_n$
D5S818	5q23.2	$(AGAT)_n$
D7S820	7q21.11	$(GATA)_n$
D8S1179	8q24.13	$(TCTA/TCTG)_n$
D10S1248	10q26.3	$(GGAA)_n$
D12S391	12p12	$(AGAT/AGAC)_n$
D13S317	13q31.1	$(TATC)_n$
D16S539	16q24.1	$(GATA)_n$
D18S51	18q21.33	$(AGAA)_n$
D19S433	19q12	$(AGAT/AGAC)_n$
D21S11	21q21.1	$(TCTA/TCTG)_n$
D22S1045	22q13.3	$(TAA)_n$
STRs in introns of expressed genes		
CSF1PO[b]	5q33.1	$(TAGA)_n$
FGA[c]	4q31.3	$(CTTT)_n$
TH01[d]	11p15.5	$(TCAT)_n$
TPOX[e]	2p25.3	$(GAAT)_n$
vWA[f]	12p13.31	$(TCTG/TCTA)_n$

[a] As of January 1, 2017.
[b] 6th intron of the *c-fms* protooncogene.
[c] 3rd intron of the fibrinogen alpha chain gene.
[d] 1st intron of the tyrosine hydroxylase gene.
[e] 10th intron of the thyroid peroxidase gene.
[f] 40th intron of the von Willebrand factor gene.

Table E.2	Examples of Allele Frequencies for Three STR Markers Used in CODIS				
D3S1358		*vWA*		*FGA*	
Allele[a]	Frequency	Allele	Frequency	Allele	Frequency
12	0.015	12	0.015	18	0.017
13	0.015	14	0.131	19	0.061
14	0.134	15	0.119	20	0.125
15	0.270	16	0.186	21	0.180
16	0.227	17	0.257	22	0.209
17	0.162	18	0.189	23	0.131
18	0.162	19	0.088	24	0.146
19	0.015	20	0.015	25	0.094
				26	0.018
				27	0.019

[a] Identified by number of repeats.

In addition, beginning with the collection and initial handling of DNA samples, the entire process is controlled under strict evidentiary rules, and once a sample reaches the laboratory it is handled by specially trained laboratory technicians. Exacting handling and processing are essential, as the results of analysis must be among the most reproducible and reliable in all of science, to guarantee accuracy and fairness. Because the reliability of the laboratory procedures and results themselves are so high, the most common legal challenges to forensic genetic analysis of DNA concern the potential mishandling or mislabeling of samples before they arrive at the laboratory.

The final criterion for CODIS STRs is that their PCR products must distinguish alleles from one another clearly enough for automated PCR amplification and gel electrophoresis to reliably identify each allele. Experience has shown that a difference of 4 bp is adequate to ensure consistently accurate analysis. All but one of the 20 CODIS alleles are 4-bp repeat sequences. Notice from Table E.1 that most CODIS STRs are simple tetranucleotide repeats; that is, the same 4-bp sequence, is repeated multiple times. A few contain complex tetranucleotide repeats that are a mixture of two different 4-bp sequences repeated multiple times. All of the amplified DNA fragments are small, and the results are reliably repeatable. The fragment lengths for the CODIS gene producing the smallest PCR fragments are between approximately 110 and 150 bp. The gene producing the largest fragments generates a size range between about 310 and 350 bp.

Electrophoretic Analysis

The analysis of PCR-amplified STR fragments is carried out by a form of gel electrophoresis known as capillary gel electrophoresis. The term derives from the fact that the

None of the alleles can be more frequent in a population than about 20 to 25%. A typical CODIS STR will have 8 to 16 alleles that each have population frequencies between 1 or 2% on the low end and 20 or 25% on the high end. Table E.2 gives the population allele frequencies for three CODIS markers. Notice that the total of all allele frequencies for each of the markers is 1.00. Allele profiles of this kind mean that for each CODIS STR, a high proportion of the population is heterozygous. For most CODIS markers, the proportion of heterozygotes is around 80%. This high percentage of heterozygosity increases the effectiveness of individual genetic identification.

Third, the STR markers selected for CODIS must carry alleles that can be consistently, reliably, and accurately amplified by PCR and analyzed in highly automated laboratory settings in specially equipped laboratories. The high level of automation minimizes the risk of contaminating the DNA samples, and ensures that the results are highly reproducible.

electrophoresis gel is poured into a narrow glass tube about the size of a small drinking straw. Electrical current applied to the capillary gel separates the amplified DNA fragments as described in Section 1.4. The smaller fragments migrate more rapidly in the capillary gel and the larger fragments migrate more slowly. The PCR-amplified fragments are labeled with a fluorescent compound that allows their detection using laser light. As migrating fluorescent-labeled DNA fragments pass the laser light, their fluorescent compounds are excited by the light, and a photoreceptor records their emission. The length of each fragment and the number of fragments are recorded for each STR.

Figure E.1 illustrates example results obtained from the electrophoretic analysis of the 13 original CODIS markers. For each gene, one peak indicates a homozygous genotype and two peaks indicate a heterozygous genotype. For example, the sample shown is homozygous for *D8S1179* and for *D21S11*, and it is heterozygous for *FGA*, *D7S820*, and *CSF1PO*. Overall, this sample is homozygous for five genes and heterozygous for the other eight genes. The horizontal axis indicates the fragment length. Near each peak in the figure is a number indicating the number of repeats in each DNA fragment. These numbers are used to designate the different alleles for each STR. In this instance, the sample is homozygous *12/12* for *D8S1179*, homozygous *15/15* for *D21S11*, heterozygous *18/20* for *FGA*, and so on through the 13 STR genes.

Forensic Analysis Using CODIS

The statistical power of CODIS-based identification rests on the H-W equilibrium and the product rule of probability for independently assorting genes. The STR allele frequencies are determined for each population, and the population-specific frequencies are used to predict population genotype frequencies. Table E.2 lists example frequencies of alleles for three STR loci, *D3S1358*, *vWA*, and *FGA*. Using these frequencies and H-W equilibrium, we can determine the probability that a person selected at random from the example population has a specific genotype (see Example Analysis E.1).

In criminal cases where the DNA of a suspect is compared with a sample from a crime scene, the genotypes for as many of the CODIS markers as possible are compared to discover whether any mismatches are present. The principle at work in these comparisons is the principle of *exclusion*, meaning that if just one of the STR markers analyzed fails to match between a suspect and the crime scene or reference sample, the suspect is excluded as the source of the crime scene or reference DNA. The logic of the exclusion principle is rooted in scientific investigation and hypothesis testing. In scientific investigations, experimental data that do not match the predicted outcome can be used to *reject* a hypothesis. In those cases where the data do *not* reject the hypothesis, scientists say they have *failed to reject* the hypothesis (see Section 2.5). A similar practice is followed in forensic analyses. However, rather than speaking in terms of "rejecting" and "failing

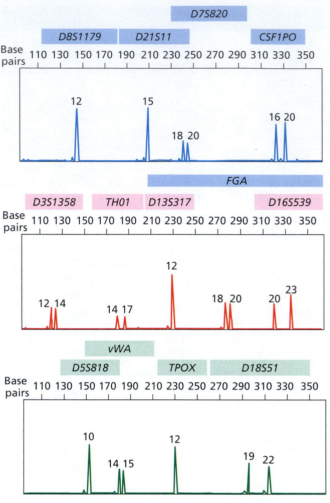

Figure E.1   An example of DNA profile results for the 13 original CODIS STRs. Homozygous STRs have one peak and heterozygous STRs have two peaks. Alleles are determined by the migration of DNA fragments along the base pair scale.

to reject" a hypothesis, forensic genetic investigators speak of "excluding" and "failing to exclude" a suspect as the source of a DNA sample.

These methods for laboratory and computational analysis of CODIS STR markers have been used in countless criminal and paternity cases since the mid-1990s. By itself, however, DNA evidence is rarely sufficient to demonstrate beyond a reasonable doubt that a particular person is responsible for a crime. Additional corroborating evidence, such as evidence placing the suspect at or near the crime scene at the time the crime occurred, is required. Nevertheless, DNA analysis is a powerful piece of evidence both for excluding individuals and for identifying individuals as the source of a certain DNA sample.

Example Analysis E.1 For this example, let's assume that the person in question is heterozygous for the 17 and 19 alleles of *D3S1358* (that is, has the *17/19* genotype), homozygous for the 14 alleles at *vWA* (that is, has the *14/14* genotype), and is heterozygous *20/25* for *FGA*. What we want to find out is, how frequently does this genotype occur?

To calculate the genotype frequency, we use arithmetic similar to the formula for calculating the H-W equilibrium. In this case, the frequency of *17/19* heterozygosity of *D3S1358* is $f(17/19) = 2[(0.162)(0.015)] = 0.0049$ (or 0.4%). The homozygous *14/14* frequency for *vWA* is $f(14/14) = (0.134)(0.134) = 0.018$ (or 1.8%). The genotype frequency for *FGA 20/25* heterozygosity is $f(20/25) = 2[(0.125)(0.094)] = 0.0235$ (or 2.35%). Based on independent assortment of the three markers, the joint probability of the three-gene genotype is the product of the genotype frequencies for each gene. The joint probability of the genotype is therefore $(0.0049)(0.0180)(0.0235) = 2.0 \times 10^{-6}$. This value indicates that approximately two people per million are expected to have this genotype.

From this analysis, it can be seen why it is not always necessary to use all 20 CODIS markers to obtain a statistically strong forensic genetic identification. When more CODIS markers are used, however, they are capable, in essence, of uniquely identifying every person in the world. Stated another way, the theoretical probability of a random match of two unrelated people for the 13 CODIS markers is on the order of 10^{-25} to 10^{-30}.

Example Analysis E.2 **Figure E.2** shows a hypothetical forensic genetic analysis of the genes *D3S1358, vWA,* and *FGA* from five samples: a crime scene sample, a sample from the crime victim, and samples from three suspects. (The DNA of the victim is analyzed to identify the genotype so that it can be eliminated from consideration in analysis of the crime scene.) The DNA samples are PCR amplified, and the resulting DNA fragments are separated by gel electrophoresis (see Section 1.4 to review gel electrophoresis and Section 7.5 to review PCR). Mismatches between the crime scene sample and Suspects 1 and 3 are evident from mismatches of the DNA-fragment patterns. These two individuals are excluded as sources of the crime scene sample. On the other hand, Suspect 2 is not excluded on the basis of analysis of the band patterns for these three genes. In a case like this, it is likely that the DNA of Suspect 2 would then be analyzed for additional CODIS markers, if more of the person's DNA is available. However, the frequency of a genotype match involving these three STR markers alone—genes *FGA, vWA,* and *D3S1358*—can be determined as was done in Example Analysis E.1. Thus, if Suspect 2 has the genotype described in Example Analysis E.1, investigators would estimate that there are approximately two people per million in the population who possess the genotype found in Suspect 2 and in the crime scene DNA sample.

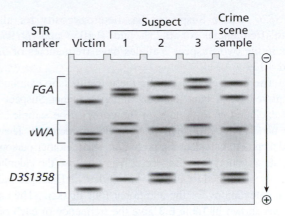

Figure E.2   STR marker comparison. Three suspect samples, a victim sample, and a crime scene sample are compared for three STRs to determine whether a suspect profile matches the crime scene profile. Suspects 1 and 3 are excluded based on mismatches, but Suspect 2 is not excluded.

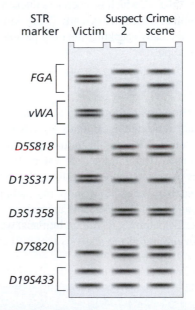

Figure E.3   Expanded STR marker comparison for seven markers. Suspect 2 is not excluded by analysis of additional STRs. The probability of a match is calculated using population frequencies of STR alleles.

Example Analysis E.3 In most instances, numerous CODIS STRs are used in an analysis. Let us therefore expand the analysis of three CODIS markers we performed in the first example into an example using seven CODIS markers. **Figure E.3** shows hypothetical electrophoretic results from PCR amplification of seven CODIS markers for Suspect 2, the victim, and the crime scene DNA from Example Analysis E.2. Three of the CODIS markers are *FGA, vWA,* and *D3S1358* from that example. The added markers are *D5S818,* where Suspect 2 is heterozygous for alleles with frequencies of 0.112 and 0.081; *D13S317,* where Suspect 2 is homozygous for an allele with a frequency of 0.095;

D7S820, where Suspect 2 has heterozygosity for alleles with frequencies of 0.231 and 0.105; and *D19S443,* where the two Suspect 2 alleles have frequencies of 0.082 and 0.131.

The first step in assessing these results is to examine the amplified DNA band patterns and notice that Suspect 2 is not excluded as the source of the crime scene sample, since the band patterns of the two samples are identical. The second step is to calculate the probability that another person has the same genotype as Suspect 2. Here we use the calculation already performed for three of the markers in Example 1 along with calculations for the additional four markers. The calculations shown in Table E.3 give the frequency of each of the genotypes carried by Suspect 2 and the joint probability for the seven genotypes combined. (The joint probability is the product of the seven individual genotype frequencies since the seven genes assort independently.) On the basis of these seven, as opposed to the earlier three, independently assorting CODIS markers, the joint probability of the Suspect 2 genotype is 3.52×10^{-13}, which is much less than one in 1 trillion. Given the number of people currently living on Earth, Suspect 2 may be, statistically speaking, the only person on the planet with this genotype!

Paternity Testing

The identification of paternity can be made in humans and other sexually reproducing animals by DNA analysis. The same approach that is used in human paternity determination can be used in the context of veterinary medicine, or for purposes of selective breeding, to ascertain the paternity of animals such as racehorses, show or champion dogs and cats, cattle, and other domesticated animals.

To describe paternity testing in humans, we will assume that at the beginning of the analysis there is certainty about the identity of the mother and the child. As you might imagine, there are situations in which this relationship is not certain, as in cases of the abandonment of an infant for example. In these cases it is readily possible to match a child to its mother by methods similar to those described here.

Recall from discussion in Section 3.2 that a child will have received exactly one-half of his or her genes from the mother; therefore, genetic testing will reveal that one-half of the genetic markers in the child match those of the mother. Genetic markers that are not maternal in origin must have come from the father. These are designated either "paternal markers" or "nonmaternal markers." To conclusively identify paternity, *every* nonmaternal marker carried by a child *must be* carried by the father. Analogous to crime scene genetic analysis, exclusion of a man as the father of a child is based on the presence in the child of a nonmaternal marker that the man does not carry. On the other hand, if all the nonmaternal markers in a child are carried in the putative father's genome, a probability calculation can be made to determine the likelihood that another man carries the same alleles contributed as the nonmaternal markers.

Example Analysis E.4 Table E.4 lists hypothetical DNA marker results for the 13 original CODIS STR markers

Table E.3	Calculation of Joint Probability of a Genotype Based on Seven CODIS STR Markers	
Marker	**Genotype Frequency**	
From Example Analysis E.2:		
D3S1358	2[(0.162)(0.015)] =	0.0049
vWA	$(0.134)^2 =$	0.0180
FGA	2[(0.125)(0.094)] =	0.0235
From Example Analysis E.3:		
D5S818	2[(0.112)(0.081)] =	0.0181
D13S317	$(0.095)^2 =$	0.0090
D7S820	2[(0.231)(0.105)] =	0.0485
D19S443	2[(0.082)(0.131)] =	0.0215

The joint probability of the genotype is the product of the individual genotype frequencies: (0.0049)(0.0180)(0.0235)(0.0181)(0.0090)(0.0485)(0.0215) = 3.52×10^{-13}.

Table E.4	Data for a Hypothetical Paternity Test Using 13 CODIS Genes				
Gene	**M**	**C**	**F1**	**F2**	**F3**
CSF1PO	10, 11	10, 12	11, 12	11, 12	10, 12
FGA	23, 24	20, 23	20, 24	18, 23	20, 24
THO1	8, 8	7, 8	7, 8	7, 8	7, 8
TPOX	9, 11	11, 11	10, 11	11, 11	9, 10
vWA	18, 18	17, 18	17,18	18, 18	17, 17
D3S1358	16, 17	16, 16	16, 16	16, 17	16, 17
D5S818	10, 10	10, 10	10, 16	10, 17	16, 17
D7S820	12, 12	10, 12	10, 12	10, 11	10, 14
D8S1179	12, 14	14, 14	12, 14	11, 16	13, 13
D13S317	12, 12	12, 13	11, 13	12, 13	11, 11
D16S539	10, 12	12, 14	14, 14	11, 15	12, 13
D18S51	15, 15	15, 15	15, 15	15, 16	16, 16
D21S11	29, 30	28, 30	28, 29	29, 30	30, 30
Paternity index (PI) and combined paternity index (CPI) calculation for five genes:					
FGA	PI = 0.5/0.125 = 4.00				
vWA	PI = 0.5/0.257 = 1.95				
D3S1358	PI = 1.0/0.227 = 4.40				
CSF1PO	PI = 0.5/0.361 = 1.39				
D16S539	PI = 1.0/0.232 = 4.31				
CPI = (4.00)(1.95)(4.40)(1.39)(4.31) = 205.60.					

for a mother (M), her child (C), and three putative fathers, F1, F2, and F3. Based on a gene-by-gene assessment of the nonmaternal alleles, F1 matches for all 13 genes. On the other hand, F2 does not match the nonmaternal allele for five genes (*FGA, vWA, D8S1179,* and *D16S539,* and *D21S11*), and F3 does not match for seven genes (*TOPX, D5S818, D8S1179, D13S317, D16S539, D18S51,* and *D21S11*). On this basis, both F2 and F3 are excluded as the father of the child. F1 is not excluded as the father of the child. For purposes of paternity identification, however, the critical question is what is the probability F1 is the actual father?

This is determined by a two-stage calculation. First, a **Paternity Index (PI)** is calculated for each gene tested. A PI is determined as x/y, where x is the probability that the nonmaternal allele comes from the putative father and y is the probability the allele comes from another male in the population. A PI value for a gene will be greater than 1.0 if it is more likely the nonmaternal allele came from the putative father than from a random male in the population. PI will be less than 1.0 if a random male is more likely than the putative father to have contributed the nonmaternal allele, and PI will be exactly 1.0 if there is no information on the contribution of the nonmaternal allele. Once a PI value is determined for each gene, the individual PI values are multiplied (because the genes assort independently), and their product is the **Combined Paternity Index (CPI)**. A CPI greater than 100 indicates a 99% or higher probability that the man is the father of the child.

Table E.4 shows the calculation of PI for five of the thirteen CODIS genes and the CPI produced for the five PI values. These PI calculations were performed as follows. F1 is heterozygous (*20, 23*) for *FGA*. His probability of transmitting the nonmaternal allele (FGA_{20}) is 0.5. The frequency of the FGA_{20} in the population is 0.125 (see Table E.2); thus the PI is $0.5/0.125 = 4.0$ for *FGA*. Similarly, the PI calculation for the nonmaternal vWA_{17} allele is $PI = 0.5/0.257 = 1.95$. The PI for the nonmaternal $D3S1358_{16}$ allele has a numerator of 1.0 since F1 is homozygous (*16/16*) for this gene and can only transmit a $D3S1358_{16}$ allele. For this gene, $PI = 1.0/0.227 = 4.40$. A frequency of 0.361 for the $CSF1PO_{12}$ allele and a population frequency of 0.232 for the $D16S539_{12}$ allele are used to calculate the PI values for both of those genes. The five PI values are then multiplied to give a product of 205.60, well above the CPI = 100 threshold. This CPI result based on five genes indicates with greater than 99% certainty that F1 is the father of the child.

Individual Identification

Several unfortunate kinds of circumstances necessitate the individual identification of people or their remains, and DNA is the material of choice for making these determinations. The analysis is done by matching alleles of DNA collected from the unidentified person or remains to either a reference DNA sample collected from a known source or by obtaining partial DNA matches to someone thought to be a close relative, such as a parent or sibling. In cases where a reference DNA sample is available, an allele-for-allele match can be expected if the identification is correct. In cases where close relatives are used to determine partial DNA matches, each parent will share one-half of his or her DNA with a child in a manner similar to what is seen in paternity testing. When siblings are used for partial DNA matches, it is expected that full siblings, with the same mother and father, will share, on average, about 50% of their alleles.

Remains Identified following the 9-11 Attack

On September 11, 2001, the Twin Towers in New York City were destroyed in coordinated terrorists attacks and 2753 people were killed. Some of the bodies of the deceased were recovered and identified, but most were not. Unidentified remains generally consisted of partial remains for which there was no possible identification method other than DNA testing. In total, almost 22,000 human samples were collected. Of these, more than 14,000 samples were bones or teeth, the most difficult tissues from which to extract DNA for analysis.

To accomplish DNA testing and identification of the recovered samples, family members were asked to submit personal objects from the victims that might contain DNA. A toothbrush, for example, could contain epithelial cells from inside the mouth from which DNA could be extracted; a hair brush or comb could contain hair roots that are a source of DNA. DNA collected in this way was analyzed, and the allelic data was stored for later comparison with recovered remains.

There are three types of chromosomes that can serve as sources of DNA for these analyses. Autosomes are the most common DNA source, but genetic markers on the Y chromosome can be used when the victim is male. In these cases, either a reference sample from the victim or DNA from the victim's father or sons will contain the same Y chromosome DNA, since the Y chromosome is transmitted from fathers to sons (see Section 3.5). The third DNA source is mitochondria, which are transmitted from mothers to their children (see Section 17.1). The mother of a victim will share mitochondrial DNA with the victim. If the victim was a mother, her children will carry the same mitochondrial DNA she carried.

Matching of DNA data from the analysis of partial remains to stored autosomal, Y chromosome, or mitochondrial DNA data has been attempted. As of late 2016, 15 years after the event, DNA identification had been made for 1637 of the 2753 victims of the attack. The identity of approximately 40% of the victims remains to be confirmed by DNA analysis, although the effort continues.

Identification of the Disappeared in Argentina

In 1976 a military coup led to the removal of the lawfully elected president of Argentina. In the 8 years that followed, the military dictatorship carried out a "dirty war" on its political opponents. This war consisted of kidnapping as many as 30,000 people, many of them university students, and killing many of them. A large number simply disappeared and were presumed killed by the military. In 1977, a brave group of about a dozen women whose children had disappeared formed a group known as the Madres de Plaza de Mayo (Mothers of May Square, a Buenos Aires landmark) to raise awareness of the loss of their children. The Madres gave rise to another group, the Abuelas de Plaza de Mayo (Grandmothers of May Square). Together, these groups brought international attention to the military's dirty war and helped initiate the search for their missing children and grandchildren.

In 1984, the American geneticist Mary-Claire King, whom we discuss in Experimental Insight 5.1 in connection with her work identifying the breast cancer susceptibility gene BRCA1, began to work with the Madres and the Abuelas in an effort to use DNA analysis to identify the remains of the missing. King was successful in identifying many of those who had disappeared. Her methods were similar to those that would be used several years later to identify remains of those killed in the attack on the Twin Towers.

At the urging of the Abuelas, however, King also took on an even more challenging task. The military dictatorship had abducted a number of pregnant young women or mothers with young infants. As many as 500 babies may either have been abducted with their mothers or have been born while their mothers were in detention. Most of the young women were later executed, but many of their babies survived. A large number of the babies of executed women were suspected to have been illegally adopted by military families. King realized that she might be able to identify these children and connect them to their biological families through mitochondrial DNA. Mitochondria are maternally transmitted, so mothers and their children have the same mitochondria. King reasoned that the Abuelas passed mitochondrial DNA to their daughters, who in turn passed it to their children. She correctly surmised that grandmothers and grandchildren would match for mitochondrial DNA variants, and that women who illegally adopted the babies would not match their adopted child's mitochondrial DNA. King collected donated mitochondrial DNA from the Abuelas and from suspected illegally adopted children and made comparisons of mitochondrial DNA variation. King's efforts were a success and have resulted in the identification of more than 100 illegally adopted children.

E.2 DNA Analysis for Genealogy, Genetic Ancestry, and Genetic Health Risk Assessment

Direct-to-consumer DNA testing is a relatively new commercial enterprise that seeks to provide general information to customers concerning their genealogical relationships, their individual genetic ancestry, and, to a limited extent, their personal genetic risk for certain diseases or conditions. Several different companies have entered this market, conducting DNA testing through DNA chip–based assessment of hundreds of thousands of single nucleotide polymorphisms (SNPs). The results represent a genome-wide genetic profile of each subscriber-contributed sample (see Section 16.4 for a discussion of SNP analysis using DNA chips). The DNA used for SNP analysis is usually collected from epithelial cells present in saliva. After paying a fee, subscribers receive a saliva collection tube that they fill with their own saliva and return to the company for SNP analysis. The full analysis generally takes 4 to 6 weeks, and the results can identify potential genealogical relationships and probable geographic areas of ancestral origin (genetic ancestry). As of this writing, one company also can provide some genetic health risk assessment.

The number of SNP markers screened by different companies varies, as does the accuracy and interpretation of the results. The most comprehensive of the DNA chips used to amass SNP data screens more than 730,000 SNPs, about 24,000 of which are located on the X chromosome or the Y chromosome. Separate analysis can examine mitochondrial DNA for sequence variants. A great deal of computational biology goes into converting the SNP data into forms that can be used to provide personalized genetic information. We will not address many of the computational details here, but we will discuss in a broad way how the assessments are performed and the conclusions and inferences that can be drawn from them.

Assessing Genealogical Relationships

A genealogical relationship is a genetic connection between related individuals as a result of shared ancestry. These relationships are identified by shared alleles. The process of sharing alleles is identified as identity by descent (IBD). This is the same term used to describe alleles found in inbred organisms whose parents share one or more relatives (see Section 20.6). Both the allele sharing of inbreeding and allele sharing in a genealogical context reflect a genetic connection between individuals. The connection comes about in the same way—having one or more ancestors in common.

The SNPs screened from each submitted DNA sample are used to identify haplotypes, or regions of shared alleles, on chromosome segments. Computer algorithms make comparisons between chromosome segments of individuals to identify these haplotypes, which span multiple SNPs along segments measured in centiMorgans (cM). (Recall this unit for measuring distance along a chromosome from our discussion of recombination in Section 5.2, where we use the formula of 1 cM equaling 1% recombination.) For statistical reasons related to the significance of haplotype sharing, haplotype regions indicating IBD in two individuals must usually be 7 cM or more in length. A chromosome region of this length is likely to encompass at least a few million base pairs. This means that sharing a few SNP alleles by chance is not sufficient to indicate a genetic relationship between two individuals. Instead, much longer shared haplotype regions are required to produce a statistically valid conclusion that two individuals are related by common ancestry.

The number of shared haplotype segments and the total length of those segments (i.e., the total number of centiMorgans) can indicate the degree of closeness of the relationship between individuals. In these comparisons, parents and children will appear as the closest relatives since they share 50% of their alleles. This level of shared genes indicates **first-degree relationships**. Siblings as well as grandparents and grandchildren share 25% of their genes and are connected by **second-degree relationships**. **Third-degree relationships** are between individuals who share 12.5% of their genes. Examples of your third-degree relatives are your uncles and aunts or your first cousins. The assortment of chromosomes during meiosis is one of the principal drivers of the decreased level of shared haplotypes with more distant relationships. Homologous recombination is the other driver of haplotype diversification. Recombination reshuffles chromosomes to break up large haplotype regions.

As the degree of relationship is reduced, so is the average centiMorgan length of shared haplotypes. Recall from Section 5.4 that there are about 3300 cM in the human genome. This means that a parent is expected to share 1650 cM (50% of the genome) with each of his or her children. Second-degree relatives will share approximately 800 cM, third-degree relatives approximately 400 cM or so, and so on. As a consequence of recombination, the shared haplotype regions tend to get smaller as individuals become more distantly related, but even fairly distant relatives such as fourth cousins (6.25% of genes shared) or fifth cousins (3.12% of genes shared) can establish the likely authenticity of a genetic relationship if they share haplotype segments of 7 cM or more.

Assessing Genetic Ancestry

Most of us are curious about our ancestors. We would like to know who they were, and we would like to know their stories. Sometimes this information can be obtained from genealogical and historical records, but often there are no records going back more than a few generations. For people trying to trace their family tree beyond grandparents or great-grandparents, the question often becomes, "Where did my ancestors come from?" This question is answerable using population-based haplotype analysis.

Companies engaging in the determination of genetic ancestry attempt to identify the most likely geographic areas of the subscriber's ancestral origin. This is accomplished by comparing the SNP data for the subscriber against a series of reference genomes representing different geographic areas. The most active company in this arena has collected and analyzed DNA samples from several thousand people who can each trace their origins to a single geographic region. These genomes are used as the reference samples with which individual subscriber samples are compared to estimate likely ancestral origins. Ancestry.com, the company with the largest collection of reference samples, identifies 26 different geographic regions of origin. Among these are nine populations from Africa, eight populations in Europe, three Asian populations, two populations each from Great Britain and the Pacific islands, and one population each representing Native Americans and individuals from the Indian subcontinent.

The data on reference populations consist of multiple haplotypes, but whereas the individuals contributing to each reference population have a single ancestral region of origin, most of us do not. The vast majority of people submitting DNA for genetic ancestry assessment are from admixed populations. In other words, their genomes are composed of a mixture of haplotypes and haplotype segments that originated in different reference populations. The genetic ancestry results produced for a subscriber with an admixed background might identify, for example, that the subscriber's genetic ancestry is 40% Great Britain, 35% Iberian Peninsula, 10% northern European, 8% eastern European, 4% Native American, and 3% African. These percentages are determined by complex computational biology that surveys each SNP to identify the most likely reference population of origin.

For example, if a SNP contains the nucleotides A/A, the reference populations most likely to have contributed adenines at this SNP location can be estimated. Suppose that for this SNP the eastern European reference population is 80% A and 20% G, the Iberian reference population is 90% A and 10% G, the Irish population is 50% A and 50% G, and an Asian population is 10% A and 90% G. It is most likely that the eastern European and Iberian populations are the populations of origin for this SNP. Similar estimates are made hundreds of thousands of times as SNPs comprising haplotypes are compared between a subscriber's DNA and the reference populations. The final percentages of ancestral origin are the accumulation of the most likely results across the genome. Put another way, genetic ancestry is the most likely estimate of the proportion of one's genome that originated in each geographic region. These assignments are susceptible to inaccuracy due to genetic overlaps between reference populations that are near one another and may have experienced gene flow in the past. There is, for example, occasional misassignment of genetic ancestry between Great Britain and Western Europe, between other European populations, and between some African populations.

There is a 27th and a 28th reference genome to consider as well—the Neandertal genome. As Application Chapter D makes clear, large numbers of people alive today have small proportions of genomic sequence that evolved in Neandertals or in Denisovans. For example, mating between Neanderthals and the early humans who gave rise to modern-day populations introduced Neandertal DNA into the contemporary human genome. Surviving Neandertal DNA has its own unique haplotype patterns. These can be identified and their percentage of the total genome determined by the same computations that are used to identify the reference populations of origin for other genome sequences.

Genetic Health Risk Assessment

The third category of direct-to-consumer assessment available at this time is genetic health risk assessment. These assessments estimate the risk that a person might develop specific diseases or conditions relative to the chance that an average member of the population will develop the same condition. These are based on the inheritance of specific SNPs or alleles that are associated with (but do not cause) the diseases or conditions of interest. The estimates are often expressed in terms of susceptible individuals having *n* times the risk of disease compared with a nonsusceptible person.

The last section of Application Chapter B contains a discussion of direct-to-consumer tests and uses the term *association* in describing the inheritance of SNP alleles whose presence is statistically connected to a greater or lesser likelihood of the presence of a disease or condition. The concept of association is also discussed in Sections 5.5 and 19.4, in the context of genome-wide association studies (GWAS). As a reminder, association between a SNP and a disease or condition does not imply causation, and inheriting an associated SNP *does not* determine whether or not an individual will develop a disease. Instead, the association is a statistical statement about the co-occurrence of certain SNP alleles with a disease phenotype. SNP allele *A* is associated with condition *C* if people who have *C* also carry *A* significantly more often than would be predicted by chance. The chance probability is determined by the frequencies of *A* and *C* in the population. For example, if allele *A* has a population frequency of 30% but occurs in 75% of people with condition *C*, statistical testing will reveal that the allele *A* is associated with condition *C*.

The important point to understand is that genetic health risk assessment is probabilistic rather than predictive. It can only indicate higher or lower likelihoods of certain conditions occurring. The presence of a particular SNP variant does not mean an individual will develop a specific disease and condition, and the absence of the variant doesn't guarantee that a person will not develop the disease or condition. The reason these assessments are not predictive of disease is that the diseases and conditions are multifactorial. Genetic variants may influence the onset of a disease, but environmental factors, including age, lifestyle, diet, and exposure to agents in the surroundings, are also at work in the disease development process (see Section 19.1 for a discussion of multifactorial conditions).

Let's look at a couple of examples of direct-to-consumer genetic health risk assessment. In April 2017, the company 23andMe received approval from the United States Food and Drug Administration (FDA) to make genetic health risk estimates available to subscribers for 10 diseases and conditions. Application Chapter B described how inherited SNP variation is associated with the condition alpha-1 antitrypsin deficiency. Here we look at two other conditions, late-onset Alzheimer disease and celiac disease.

Late-Onset Alzheimer Disease

Late-onset Alzheimer disease (AD) is the most common form of the disease, which is a condition marked by cognitive deficits, personality changes, confusion, loss of short-term memory, and other difficulties tied to memory and cognition. The cause of AD is not known, and diagnosis in living persons is difficult because the telltale indicator of the condition is a buildup of β-amyloid protein in the brain, discoverable only in an autopsy. It is thought that β-amyloid protein forms clusters that interfere with and are toxic to neurons, but a causative mechanism is not established.

Research dating from the early 1990s identified what is to date the leading genetic risk factor for AD. Apolipoprotein E (ApoE) is the principal cholesterol-transporting protein in the brain. The gene for this protein *(APOE)* came to the attention of AD researchers when they extracted ApoE from brain and spinal fluid and realized that it was encoded by a gene on chromosome 19, where previous studies had detected a gene influencing AD onset. The *APOE* gene has three allelic variants—*APOE2, APOE3,* and *APOE4. APOE3* is the most common allele in populations, averaging a frequency of about 78%. *APOE2* has an average population frequency of 8%, and *APOE4* an average frequency of 14%. Studies in several populations have identified that having one or two copies of *APOE4* in one's genome is a significant risk factor for AD. A heterozygous genotype such as *APOE2/APOE4* or *APOE3/APOE4* produces about a three- to fourfold increased lifetime risk of AD, and being homozygous *APOE4/APOE4* generates a lifetime AD risk that is about 12-fold greater than for a person without a copy of *APOE4*. The 23andMe genetic heath risk assessment screens the *APOE* gene and identifies the alleles a person carries.

To correctly interpret the *APOE* genotype and AD risk, four things are important to remember. First, *APOE* does not cause AD, and it is not known if *APOE4* plays any direct role in disease causation. Second, several other biological and medical factors, including total blood cholesterol level and high blood pressure, are known to influence AD risk. Third, many people who carry one or two copies of *APOE4 will never* develop AD. And, lastly, many people who do not carry any copies of *APOE4 will* develop AD.

Celiac Disease

Our second example of a direct-to-consumer health risk assessment is for celiac disease (CD), a digestive condition caused by a severe sensitivity to the grain protein gluten. Gluten is the main protein component of wheat, barley, oats, and rye. CD is a serious disease marked by severe intestinal distress and bloating. It causes inflammation of the mucosal lining of the intestines and can lead to deficient absorption of nutrients. The symptoms of CD are brought on by the immune system; the root cause of the condition is an abnormal immune response to gluten.

Genes of the human leucocyte antigen (HLA) system are encoded in a region of about 3 million base pairs on chromosome 6p21. These genes produce antigens that form the major histocompatibility complex. There are two major classes of HLA genes. HLA class I genes are *HLA-A*, *HLA-B*, and *HLA-C*. HLA class II also includes three genes, *HLA-DP*, *HLA-DQ*, and *HLA-DR*. These six genes are highly diverse, producing dozens of different antigens that help the immune system identify cells as "self." The antigens are also important in the immune system response to infection, and they are the primary antigens involved in tissue matching for organ transplantation.

Certain of the HLA antigens are associated with autoimmune diseases. These are diseases arising as a result of the immune system incorrectly or overactively attacking and destroying or disabling specific cells in the body. Well-characterized autoimmune diseases include insulin-dependent diabetes, rheumatoid arthritis, systemic lupus erythematosus, and CD. In insulin-dependent diabetes, for example, the immune system overreaction leads to the death of insulin-producing islet cells in the pancreas; and in rheumatoid arthritis, immune system overreaction generates excessive inflammation in joints that leads to destruction of cartilage and bone.

Two specific antigens of the *HLA-DQ* gene are closely tied to CD risk. Surveys detect the allele *HLA-DQ2* in nearly 80% of patients with CD; the allele *HLA-DQ8* is detected in approximately 8% of CD patients; and both alleles together are detected in nearly 11% of CD patients. Overall, either *HLA-DQ2* or *HLA-DQ8* or both are present in about 98% of CD patients.

This does not mean that these immune system alleles cause CD. Approximately 56% of the CD–free general population have *HLA-DQ2*, *HLA-DQ8*, or both. This means that many people with one or both of these alleles will never develop CD. In addition, CD is a multifactorial disease, to which environmental factors and genes outside the HLA system make contributions. The strong association of *HLA-DQ2* and *HLA-DQ8* with CD has led some people to suggest that having one or more of these alleles is necessary but not sufficient to produce CD. In any case, the presence of either or both alleles is thought to exert a strong influence on cellular reaction to gluten that triggers cells of the immune system to attack intestinal cells, inducing an aggressive inflammatory response that may lead to the disease. This scenario parallels those of other autoimmune conditions where specific HLA antigens are thought to play prominent roles in immune system overreaction to environmental stimuli.

One Side of the Equation

The genetic health risk assessments provided by 23andMe are purely advisory in nature. The associations between the inherited variants in a subscriber's DNA and specific diseases do not predict disease, they merely indicate the possibility of an increased risk of disease.

The genetic health risk assessment is only one side— the genetic side—of the equation. No information about lifestyle, behavior, related medical conditions, or environmental factors that might affect disease risk is taken into account in making a genetic health risk assessment. Even so, the information can be useful, encouraging greater awareness of disease symptoms and more active monitoring of potential symptoms earlier in life than a person might otherwise exercise. But a result indicating an increased risk must not be misinterpreted as certainty that the disease will occur, since large numbers of people with the same inherited risk factors will never develop the disease.

PROBLEMS

Mastering Genetics Visit for instructor-assigned tutorials and problems.

For answers to selected even-numbered problems, see Appendix: Answers.

1. What is CODIS? Describe the four most important features of genetic markers used in this system.

2. Compare and contrast the terms *paternity index* (PI) and *combined paternity index* (CPI). How does each contribute to paternity determination?

3. What is the exclusion principle? How is it used in forensic genetic analysis and in paternity determination?

4. What is the statistical principle underlying genetic health risk assessment? Why are these assessments not predictive of disease occurrence?

5. Explain the meaning of "identity by descent" in the context of identifying genealogical relationship between individuals. In these analyses, why are segments of chromosomes (haplotypes) rather than individual STRs used to identify genetic relationships?

6. A victim of murder is found to have scrapings containing skin cells under several of her fingernails. Genetic analysis confirms that the DNA isolated from these cells came from the same individual and does not match the DNA of the victim. The results shown below are for six CODIS STR markers from the crime scene DNA (from under the victim's fingernails and presumed to be the murderer's), and from three suspects (A, B, and C) who have been detained for questioning about the murder.

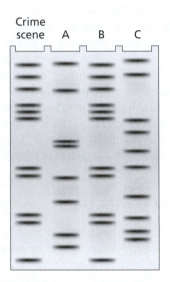

Crime
scene   A   B   C

a. Do the STR results exclude any of the three suspects? Explain.
b. Is there a failure to exclude any of the suspects? Explain.

7. The results shown are from a DNA test for four genes used in a paternity identification case. DNA for the mother (M) and her child (C) are shown along with DNA from two possible fathers, F1 and F2.

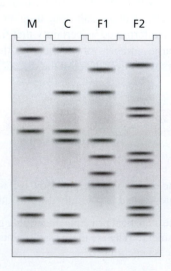

M   C   F1   F2

a. In the "C" column, label the DNA bands contributed by the mother with "M" and the DNA bands contributed by the father with "F."
b. Based on the exclusion principle, is either man excluded as the possible father? Explain.
c. What can you conclude based on the DNA results available?

8. Figure E.1 illustrates the results of an electrophoretic analysis of 13 CODIS STR markers on a DNA sample and identifies the alleles for each gene. Table E.2 lists the frequencies for alleles of three of the STRs shown in the figure. Use this information to calculate the frequency of the genotype for STR genes *FGA, vWA,* and *D3S1358* given in Figure E.1.

9. Additional STR allele frequency information can be added to improve the analysis in Problem 8. The frequency of $D8S1179_{12} = 0.12$. The frequency of $D16S539_{18} = 0.08$ and of $D16S539_{20} = 0.21$. Lastly, $D18S51_{19} = 0.13$ and $D18S51_{20} = 0.10$. Combine the allele frequency information for these three STR genes with the information used in Problem 8 to calculate the frequency of the genotype for six of the STR genes.

10. The frequencies of the four alleles contributed to the child by possible father F1 in Problem 7 are 0.18, 0.23, 0.13, and 0.14.
    a. Calculate the combined paternity index (CPI) for the four genes in this analysis.
    b. Make a statement about the possible paternity of F1 based on this analysis.

11. In an inheritance case, a man has died leaving his estate to be divided equally between "his wife and his offspring." His wife (M) has an adult daughter (D), and they argue that they should split the estate equally. As a young couple, however, the man and his wife had a son that they gave up for adoption. Two men have appeared, each claiming to be the son of the couple and therefore entitled to a one-third share of the estate. The accompanying illustration shows the results of DNA analysis for five genes for the mother (M), her daughter (D), and the two claimants (S1 and S2).

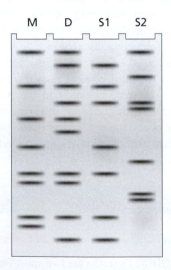

M   D   S1   S2

a. How many nonmaternal DNA bands are shared by D and S1? By D and S2?
b. Do the DNA results suggest that either man is likely to be the son of the man and his wife? Explain.

12. Three independently assorting STR markers (*A*, *B*, and *C*) are used to assess the paternity of a colt recently born to a quarter horse mare. Blood samples are drawn from the mare, her colt, and three possible male sires (S$_1$, S$_2$, and S$_3$). DNA at each marker locus is amplified by PCR, and a DNA electrophoresis gel is run for each marker. Amplified DNA bands are visualized in each gel by ethidium bromide staining. Gel results are shown below for each marker.

Marker *A*

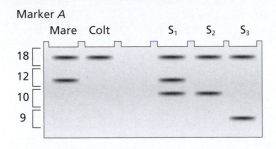

Marker *B*

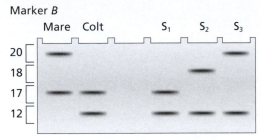

Marker *C*

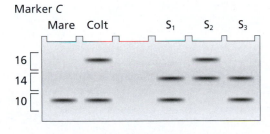

a. Evaluate the data and determine if any of the potential sires can be excluded. Explain the basis of exclusion, if any, in each case.

b. Calculate the PI and CPI based on these STR markers, using the following population frequencies: $A_{12} = 0.12$, $A_{10} = 0.18$; $B_{18} = 0.08$, $B_{12} = 0.17$; $C_{16} = 0.11$, $C_{14} = 0.20$.

13. Look over the 10 diseases approved for genetic health risk assessment listed in Application Chapter B. Select one disease other than the three discussed in Application Chapter B or in this chapter (alpha-1 antitrypsin deficiency, late-onset Alzheimer disease, and celiac disease) or another of the diseases of your choice. Do a brief Internet search to find and download (1) one article for a nonscientific audience identifying the gene or genes whose alleles are associated with occurrence of the disease and (2) one scientific paper that provides data supporting the association of specific alleles of the gene or genes with the disease. Write a short summary combining the information contained in the two papers.

References and Additional Reading

Chapter 1 The Molecular Basis of Heredity, Variation, and Evolution

Chargaff, E. 1951. Structure and function of nucleic acids as cell constituents. *Fed. Proc.* 10: 654–59.

Dronamraju, K. 1992. Profiles in genetics: Archibald E. Garrod. *Am. J. Hum. Genet.* 51: 216–19.

Dunn, L. C. 1965. *A Short History of Genetics.* New York: McGraw-Hill.

Garrod, A. E. 1902. The incidence of alkaptonuria: A study in chemical -individuality. *Lancet* ii: 1616–20.

———. 1909. *Inborn Errors of Metabolism.* London: Frowde, Hodder and Stoughton.

Green, R.E. et al. 2010. A draft sequence of the Neandertal genome. Science, 328:710–722.

Higuchi, R. et al. 1984. DNA sequences from the quagga, an extinct member of the horse family. Nature, 312:282–284

Judson, H. F. 1978. *The Eighth Day of Creation: Makers of the Revolution in Biology.* Woodbury, NY: Cold Spring Harbor Press.

Lander, E. S., and R. A. Weinberg. 2000. Genomics: Journey to the center of -biology. *Science* 287: 1777–82.

Meyer, M., M. Kircher, M-T. Gansauge, et al. 2012. A high-coverage genome -sequence from an archaic Denisovan individual. *Science* 338: 222–26.

Neel, J. V. 1949. The inheritance of sickle cell anemia. *Science* 110: 64–66.

Pääbo, S. 2014. Neanderthal Man: In Search of Lost Genomes. Basic Books, New York.

Pauling, L., et al. 1949. Sickle cell anemia, a molecular disease. *Science* 110: 543–48.

Ridley, M. 1999. *Genome: The Autobiography of a Species in 23 Chapters.* New York: Perennial.

Slon, V. et al. 2017. Neandertal and Denisovan DNA from Pleistocene sediments. Science, 356:605–608.

Sturtevant, A. H. 1965. *A History of Genetics.* New York: Harper and Row.

Vernot, B., and J. M. Akey. 2014. Resurrecting surviving Neandertal lineages from modern human genomes. *Science* 343: 1017–21.

Wacey, D., M. R. Kilburn, M. Saunders, et al. 2011. Microfossils of sulphur–metabolizing cells in 3.4 billion year old rocks of Western Australia. *Nature Genetics* 4: 698–702.

Watson, J. D. 1968. *The Double Helix.* New York: Atheneum.

Watson, J. D., and F. H. C. Crick. 1953. Genetical implications of the structure of deoxyribonucleic acid. *Nature* 171: 964–69.

———. 1953. Molecular structure of nucleic acids: A structure for deoxyribose -nucleic acid. *Nature* 171: 737–38.

Chapter 2 Transmission Genetics

Armstead, I. I., et al. 2007. Cross-species identification of Mendel's *I* locus. *Science* 315: 73.

Aubry, S., J. Mani, and S. Hörtensteiner. 2008. Stay-green protein, defective in Mendel's green cotyledon mutant, acts independently and upstream of pheophorbide *a* oxidase in the chlorophyll catabolic pathway. *Plant Mol. Biol.* 67: 243–56.

Bateson, W. 1913. *Mendel's Principles of Heredity.* Cambridge: Cambridge University Press.

Bennett, R. L., et al. 1995. Recommendations for standardized human pedigree nomenclature. *Am. J. Hum. Genet.* 56: 745–52.

Bhattacharyya, M., C. Martin, and A. Smith. 1993. The importance of starch -biosynthesis in the wrinkled shape character of peas studied by Mendel. *Plant Mol. Biol.* 22: 525–31.

Bhattacharyya, M., et al. 1990. The wrinkled-seed character of pea described by Mendel is caused by a transposon-like insertion in a gene coding starch-branching enzyme. *Cell* 60: 115–22.

Detlefsen, J. A. 1918. Fluctuations of sampling in a Mendelian population. *Genetics* 3: 599–607.

Fisher, R. A. 1936. Has Mendel's work been rediscovered? *Ann. Science* 1: 115–37.

Goss, J. 1822. On the variation in the colour of peas. Trans. Horticult. Soc. London, I:234–237.

Hartl, D., and V. Orel. 1992. What did Gregor Mendel think he discovered? *Genetics* 131: 245–53.

Hellens, R. P., et al. 2010. Identification of Mendel's white flower character. *PLoS ONE* 5: 1–7.

Henig, R. M. 2001. *A Monk in the Garden: The Lost and Found Genius of Gregor Mendel, the Father of Genetics.* New York: Houghton-Mifflin.

Knight, T.A. 1823. Some remarks on the supposed influence of the pollen, in cross breeding, upon the colour of seed coats of plants, and the qualities of fruits. Trans. Horticult. Soc. London, V:377–380.

Lester, D. R., et al. 1997. Mendel's stem length gene (*Le*) encodes a gibberellin 3 β-hydroxylase. *Plant Cell* 9: 1435–43.

Martin, D. N., W. M. Proebsting, and P. Hedden. 1997. Mendel's dwarfing gene: cDNAs from the *Le* alleles and function of the expressed proteins. *Proc. Natl. Acad. Sci. USA* 94: 8907–11.

Mendel, G. (1866) 1966. Experiments in plant hybridization. In *The Origins of Genetics: A Mendel Source Book*, edited by C. Stern and E. Sherwood. Translated. San Francisco: W. H. Freeman.

Olby, R. C. 1985. *Origins of Mendelism.* London: Constable.

Orel, V. 1996. *Gregor Mendel: The First Geneticist.* Oxford: Oxford University Press.

Peters, J. (ed.). 1959. *Classic Papers in Genetics.* Englewood Cliffs NJ: Prentice-Hall.

Reid, J. B., and J. J. Ross. 2011. Mendel's genes: Toward a full molecular characterization. *Genetics* 189: 3–10.

Stern, C., and E. Sherwood (eds.). 1966. *The Origins of Genetics: A Mendel Source Book.* San Francisco: W. H. Freeman.

Stubbe, H. 1972. *History of Genetics: From Prehistoric Times to the Rediscovery of Mendel's Laws.* Cambridge, MA: MIT Press.

Tschermak-Seysenegg, E. 1951. The rediscovery of Mendel's work. *J. Hered.* 42: 162–72.

Welling, F. 1991. Historical study: Johann Gregor Mendel 1822–1884. *Am. J. Med. Genet.* 40: 1–25.

White, O. E. 1917. Studies of inheritance in *Pisum.* II. The present state of -knowledge of heredity and variation in peas. *Proc. Am. Phil. Soc.* 56: 487–88.

Chapter 3 Cell Division and Chromosome Heredity

Barr, M. L. 1960. Sexual dimorphism in interphase nuclei. *Am. J. Hum. Genet.* 12: 118–27.

Bridges, C. B. 1916. Nondisjunction as proof of the chromosome theory of -heredity. *Genetics* 1: 1–52 and 107–63.

Craig, J. M., W. C. Earnshaw, and P. Vagnarelli. 1999. Mammalian centromeres: DNA sequence, protein composition, and role in cell cycle progression. *Exp. Cell. Res.* 246: 249–62.

Gonzalez, A. N., et al. 2008. A shared enhancer controls a temporal switch -between promoters during Drosophila primary sex determination. *Proc. Natl. Acad. Sci. USA* 105: 18436–41.

Gould, K. L., and P. Nurse. 1989. Tyrosine phosphorylation of the fission yeast cdc2+ protein kinase regulates entry into mitosis. *Nature* 342: 39–45.

Hartwell, L. H. 1991. Twenty-five years of cell cycle genetics. *Genetics* 129: 975–80.

Hartwell, L. H., et al. 1974. Genetic control of cell division cycle in yeast. *Science* 183: 46–51.

Hartwell, L. H., J. Culotti, and B. J. Reid. 1970. Genetic control of cell division in yeast. I. Detection of mutants. *Proc. Natl. Acad. Sci. USA* 66: 352–59.

Hartwell, L. H., and M. W. Unger. 1977. Unequal division in *Saccharomyces -cerevisiae* and its implications for the control of cell division. *J. Biol. Chem.* 75: 422–35.

Hodgkin, J. 1989. *Drosophila* sex determination: Cascade of regulated splicing. *Cell* 56: 905–6.

Hunt, D. M., et al. 1995. The chemistry of John Dalton's color blindness. *Science* 267: 984–88.

Hunt, T., and M. W. Kirschner. 1993. Cell manipulation. *Current Opinions in Cell Biol.* 5: 163–65.

Jegalian, K. and B.T. Jahn. 2001. Why the Y is so weird. Sci. Am., February:56–61.

Johnson, R. T., and P. N. Rao. 1970. Mammalian cell fusion: Induction of premature chromosome condensation in interphase nuclei. *Nature* 226: 717–22.

Koopman, P., et al. 1991. Male development of chromosomally female mice -transgenic for *Sry. Nature* 351: 117–21.

Lahn, B.T. and D. Page. 1999. Four evolutionary strata of the human X chromosome. Science, 286:964–967.

Lyon, M. F. 1962. Sex chromatin and gene action in the mammalian X-chromosome. *Am. J. Hum. Genet.* 14: 135–48.

Masui, Y., and C. L. Markert. 1971. Cytoplasmic control of nuclear behavior -during meiotic maturation of frog oocytes. *J. Exp. Zool.* 177: 129–45.

Morgan, T. H. 1910. Sex-limited inheritance in *Drosophila*. *Science* 32: 120–22.

Murray, A. W., and M. W. Kirschner. 1989. Cyclin synthesis drives the early -embryonic cell cycle. *Nature* 339: 275–80.

Nathans, J., D. Thomas, and D. S. Hogness. 1986. Molecular genetics of human color vision: The genes encoding blue, green, and red pigments. *Science* 232: 193–202.

Nathans, J., et al. 1986. Molecular genetics of inherited variation in human color vision. *Science* 232: 203–10.

Page, D. C., A. de la Chapelle, and J. Weissenbach. 1985. Chromosome Y-specific DNA in human XX males. *Nature* 315: 224–26.

Page, D. C., et al. 1987. The sex-determining region of the Y chromosome encodes a finger protein. *Cell* 51: 1091–1104.

Rao, P. N., and R. T. Johnson. 1970. Mammalian cell fusion studies on the regulation of DNA synthesis and mitosis. *Nature* 225: 159–64.

Salz, H. K., and J. W. Erickson. 2010. Sex determination in *Drosophila*: The view from the top. *Fly* 4: 60–70.

Stevens, N. M. 1905. Studies in spermatogenesis with especial reference to the "accessory chromosome." Washington, DC: Carnegie Institute of Washington, Publication No. 36.

Willard, H. F. 1996. X chromosome inactivation, *XIST*, and pursuit of the X-inactivation center. *Cell* 86: 5–7.

Wilson, E. B. 1895. *An Atlas of the Fertilization and Karyokinesis of the Ovum*. New York: Columbia University Press.

Chapter 4 Gene Interaction

Beadle, G. W., and E. L. Tatum. 1941. Genetic control of biochemical reactions in *Neurospora*. *Proc. Natl. Acad. Sci. USA* 27: 499–506.

Bultman, S. J., E. J. Michaud, and R. P. Woychik. 1992. Molecular characterization of the mouse *agouti* locus. *Cell* 71: 1195–1204.

Duhl, D. M. J., et al. 1994. Pleiotropic effects of the mouse *lethal yellow* (A^Y) -mutation explained by detection of a maternally expressed gene and the -simultaneous production of *agouti* fusion RNAs. *Development* 120: 1695–1708.

Flatt, T., M-P. Tu, and M. Tatar. 2005. Hormonal pleiotropy and the juvenile hormone regulation of *Drosophila* development and life history. *BioEssays* 27: 999–1010.

Garrod, A. E. 1902. The incidence of alkaptonuria: A study in chemical -individuality. *Lancet* 2: 1616–20.

———. (1909) 1963. *Inborn Errors of Metabolism*. London: Oxford University Press.

Garrod, S. C. 1989. Family influences on A. E. Garrod's thinking. *J. Inherit. Metabol. Dis.* 12: 2–8.

Jackson, I. J. 1994. Molecular and developmental genetics of mouse coat color. *Ann Rev. Genet.* 28: 189–217.

Landsteiner, K., and P. Levine. 1927. Further observations on individual differences of blood group. *Proc. Soc. Exp. Biol. Med.* 24: 941–42.

Michaud, E. J., et al. 1994. A molecular model for the genetic and phenotypic characteristics of the mouse lethal yellow (Ay) mutation. *Proc. Natl. Acad. Sci. USA* 91: 2562–66.

Phillips, P. C. 1998. The language of gene interaction. *Genetics* 149: 1167–71.

Race, R. R., and R. Sanger. 1975. *Blood Groups in Man*. 6th ed. Cambridge: Oxford University Press.

Sandstedt, S. A., and P. K. Tucker. 2004. Evolutionary strata on the mouse X chromosome correspond to strata on the human X chromosome. *Genome Res.* 14: 267–72.

Siracusa, L. D. 1994. The *agouti* gene: Turned on to yellow. *Trends Genet.* 10: 423–28.

Srb, A. M., and N. H. Horowitz. 1944. The ornithine cycle in *Neurospora* and its genetic control. *J. Biol. Chem.* 154: 129–39.

Yamamoto, F., et al. 1990. Molecular genetic basis of the histo-blood group ABO system. *Nature* 345: 229–33.

Chapter 5 Genetic Linkage and Mapping in Eukaryotes

Bateson, W., E. R. Saunders, and R. C. Punnett. 1905. Experimental studies in the physiology of heredity. *Rep. Evol. Committee Royal Soc.* II: 1–55, 80–99.

Baudat. F. et al. 2010. PRDM9 is a major determinant of meiotic recombination hotspots in humans and mice. Science, 327:836–840.

Bregger, T. 1918. Linkage in maize: The *C* aleurone factor and waxy endosperm. *Am. Nat.* 52: 57–61.

Bridges, C. B., and T. M. Olbrycht. 1926. The multiple stock "Xple" and its use. *Genetics* 11: 41–56.

Coop, G. and M. Prezworski. 2007. An evolutionary view of human recombination. Nature Rev. Genet., 8:23–34.

Creighton, H. B., and B. McClintock. 1931. A correlation of cytological and genetic crossing over in *Zea mays*. *Proc. Natl. Acad. Sci. USA* 17: 492–97.

Green, M. M., and K. C. Green. 1949. Crossing-over between alleles at the Lozenge locus in *Drosophila melanogaster*. *Proc. Natl. Acad. Sci. USA* 35: 596–91.

Gusella, J. F., et al. 1983. A polymorphic DNA marker genetically linked to Huntington's disease. *Nature* 306: 234–38.

Hall, J. M., et al. 1990. Linkage of early-onset familial breast cancer to chromosome 17q21. *Science* 250: 1684–89.

———. 1992. Closing in on a breast cancer gene on chromosome 17q. *Am. J. Hum. Genet.* 50: 1235–42.

Houlahan, M. B., G. W. Beadle, and H. G. Calhoun. 1949. Linkage studies with biochemical mutants of *Neurospora crassa*. *Genetics* 34: 493–507.

Huntington's Disease Collaborative Research Group (58 authors). 1993. A novel gene containing a trinucleotide repeat that is expanded and unstable on Huntington's disease chromosomes. *Cell* 72: 971–83.

Ikeda, Y., et al. 2006. Spectrin mutations cause spinocerebellar ataxia type 5. *Nat. Genet.* 38: 184–90.

Janssens, F. A. 1909. La theorie de la chiasmatypie. *La Cellule* 25: 389–411.

Knudson, A. G. Jr. 1971. Mutation and cancer: Statistical study of retinoblastoma. *Proc. Natl. Acad. Sci. USA* 68: 820–23.

Lindegren, C. C. 1933. The genetics of *Neurospora*. III. Pure-bred stocks and crossing over in *N. crassa*. *Bull. Torrey Bot. Club* 60: 133–54.

Mancera, E. et al. 2008. High-resolution mapping of meiotic crossovers and noncrossovers in yeast. Nature, 454:479–486.

Morgan, T. H. 1910. Sex-limited inheritance in *Drosophila*. *Science* 32: 120–22.

———. 1910. The method of inheritance of two sex-limited characters in the same animal. *Proc. Soc. Exp. Biol. Med.* 8: 17.

———. 1911. An attempt to analyze the constitution of the chromosomes on the basis of sex-limited inheritance in *Drosophila*. *J. Exp. Zool.* 11: 365–414.

———. 1911. Random segregation versus coupling in Mendelian inheritance. *Science* 34: 384.

Morgan, T. H., et al. 1915. *The Mechanism of Mendelian Heredity*. New York: Henry Holt.

Morton, N. E. 1955. Sequential tests for the detection of linkage. *Am. J. Hum. Genet.* 7: 277–318.

Paigen, K. and P. Petkov. 2010. Mammalian recombination hotspots: properties, control and evolution. Nature Rev. Genet., 11:221–233.

Singh, N.D. et al. 2013. Fine-scale heterogeneity in crossover rate in the *garnet-scalloped* region of the *Drosophila melanogaster* X chromosome. Genetics, 194:375–387

Stern, C. 1931. Zytologisch-genetische untersuchungen als beweise fur die Morgansche theorie des fakorenaustauchs. *Biol. Zentrabl.* 51: 547–87.

Stern, C., and D. Doan. 1936. A cytogenetic demonstration of crossing-over -between X- and Y-chromosomes in the male of *Drosophila melanogaster*. *Proc. Natl. Acad. Sci. USA* 22: 649–54.

Strachan, T., and A. P. Read. 2004. *Human Molecular Genetics*. 3rd ed. London and New York: Garland Science.

Sturtevant, A. H. 1913. The linear arrangement of six sex-linked factors in *Drosophila* as shown by their mode of association. *J. Exp. Zool.* 14: 43–59.

Weber, J. L., et al. 1993. Evidence for human meiotic recombination - interference obtained through construction of a short tandem repeat -polymorphism -linkage map of chromosome 19. *Am. J. Hum. Genet.* 53: 1079–95.

Wexler, Alice. 1995. *Mapping Fate: A Memoir of Family, Risk, and Genetic Research*. New York: Times Books, Random House.

Chapter 6 Gene Analysis and Mapping in Bacteria and Bacteriophages

Bachmann, B. J. 1990. Linkage map of *Escherichia coli* K-12, Edition 8. *Microbiol. Rev.* 54: 130–97.

Benzer, S. 1959. On the topology of the genetic fine structure. *Proc. Natl. Acad. Sci. USA* 45: 1607–20.

———. 1961. On the topology of the genetic fine structure. *Proc. Natl. Acad. Sci. USA* 47: 403–16.

Blattner, F. R., G. Plunkett III, and C. A. Bloch. 1997. The complete genome -sequence of *Escherichia coli* K-12. *Science* 277: 1453–62.

Curtiss, R. 1969. Bacterial conjugation. *Ann. Rev. Microbiol.* 23: 69–123.

Davies, J. and D. Davies. 2010. The origin and evolution of antibiotic resistance. Microbiol. and Molec. Biol. Rev., 74:417–433.

Davis, B. D. 1950. Nonfiltrability of the agents of recombination. *J. Bacteriol.* 60: 507–8.

Hayes, W. 1953. Observations on a transmissible agent determining sexual -differentiation in Bact. Coli. *J. Gen. Microbiol.* 8: 72–88.

Hotchkiss, R. D., and M. Gabor. 1970. Bacterial transformation with special -reference to recombination processes. *Ann. Rev. Genet.* 4: 193–224.

Lederberg, J. 1986. Forty years of genetic recombination in bacteria: A fortieth -anniversary reminiscence. *Genetics* 28: 491–511.

Lederberg, J., and E. L. Tatum. 1946. Gene recombination in *Escherichia coli. Nature* 158: 558–59.

Nakamura, Y., T. Itoh, H. Matsuda, and T. Gojobori. 2004. Biased biological - functions of horizontally transferred genes in prokaryotic genomes. *Nature Genet.* 36: 760–66.

Robinson, K. M., K. B. Sieber, and J. C. Dunning Hotopp. 2013. A review of -bacterial-animal lateral gene transfer may inform our understanding of -diseases like cancer. *PLOS Genetics* 9: 1–6.

Stent, G. S. 1963. *Molecular Biology of Bacterial Viruses*. San Francisco: W. H. Freeman.

Susman, M. 1970. General bacterial genetics. *Ann. Rev. Genet.* 4: 135–76.

Wollman, E. L., F. Jacob, and W. Hayes. 1962. Conjugation and genetic -recombination in *E. coli* K-12. *Cold Spring Harbor Symp. Quant. Biol.* 21: 141–62.

Yanofsky, C., and E. S. Lennox. 1959. Transduction and recombination study of linkage relationships among the genes controlling tryptophan synthesis in *Escherichia coli. Virology* 8: 425–47.

Zinder, N. D. 1958. Transduction in bacteria. *Sci. Am.* 199: 38–46.

Zinder, N. D., and J. L. Lederberg. 1952. Genetic exchange in *Salmonella. J. Bacteriol.* 64: 679–99.

Application Chapter A Human Hereditary Disease and Genetic Counseling

Dolan, S.M. 2009. Prenatal genetic testing. *Ann. Pediatrics*, 38:426–430.

Garrod, A. E. 1902. The incidence of alkaptonuria: A study in chemical individuality. Lancet, vol ii: 1616–1632.

MacLeod, E.L. and D. M. Nei. 2010. Nutritional management of phenylketonuria. *Ann. Nestle Eng.*, 68: 58–69.

Schneider, K. 2011. Counseling About Cancer. *John Wiley and Sons*. New York, NY.

Stern, A. M. 2012. Telling Genes: The Story of Genetic Counseling in America. *Johns Hopkins Univ. Press, Baltimore*, MD.

Williams, R.A. et al. 2008. Phenylketonuria: An inborn error of phenylalanine metabolism. *Clin. Biochem. Rev.*, 29:31–41.

Websites for information on genetic counseling;

American Board of Genetic Counseling (U.S.) http://www.abgc.net

National Society of Genetics Counselors (U.S.) http://www.nsgc.org

Canadian Association of Genetic Counsellors (Canada) http://www.cagc-accg.ca

Association of Genetic Nurses and Counsellors (U.K.) http://www.agnc.org.uk

Chinese Board of Genetic Counselors (China) http://www.cbgc.org.cn/en

Websites for information on genetic testing:

The Genetic Alliance – An international organization of health professionals, consumers, health companies and non-profit organizations dedicated to improving the lives of people with genetic conditions (http://www.geneticalliance.org)

Recommended Uniform Screening Panel – Information on the panel of genetic tests mandated on newborn infants (http://www.hrsa.gov/advisorycommitees/mchba)

Newborn genetic testing – http://www.kidshealth.org

Genetic testing and counseling in Europe (http://www.eurogentest.org)

On-line Mendelian Index in Man (OMIM) – http://www.ncbi.nlm.nih.gov/omim

Chapter 7 DNA Structure and Replication

Avery, O. T., C. M. Macleod, and M. McCarty. 1944. Studies on the chemical nature of the substance inducing transformation of pneumococcal types: Induction of transformation by a desoxyribonucleic acid fraction isolated from pneumococcus type III. *J. Exp. Med.* 79: 137–58.

Barry, E. R., and S. D. Bell. 2006. DNA replication in Archaea. *Microbiol. Molec. Biol. Rev.* 70: 876–87.

Blackburn, E. H. 1991. Structure and function of telomeres. *Nature* 350: 569–73.

Blackwood, J. K., N. J. Rzechorzek, A. S. Abrams, et al. 2011. Structural and functional insights into DNA-end processing by the archaeal HerA helicase-NurR nuclease complex. *Nuc. Acids Res.* 39: 1–14.

Cairns, J. 1963. The bacterial chromosome and its manner of replication as seen by autoradiography. *J. Mol. Biol.* 6: 208–13.

De Lange, T. 2004. T-loops and the origin of telomers. Nature Rev. Molec. Cell. Biol., 5:323–329.

DeLucia, P., and J. Cairns. 1969. Isolation of an *E. coli* strain with a mutation -affecting DNA polymerase. *Nature* 224: 1164–66.

Franklin, R. E. and R. G. Gosling. 1953. Molecular configuration in sodium thymonucleate. nature, 171:740–741.

Garrett, R. A. and H-P. Klenk (eds.) 2007. *Archaea: Evolution, Physiology, and Molecular Biology*. Malden, MA: Blackwell Publishing.

Georgescu, R. E., et al. 2007. Structure of a sliding clamp on DNA. *Cell* 132: 43–54.

Gordon, L.B. et al. 2012. Progeria: Translational insights from cell biology. J. Cell. Biol., 199:9–13.

Greider, C. W., and E. H. Blackburn. 1987. The telomere terminal transferase of *Tetrahymena* is a ribonucleoprotein enzyme with two kinds of primer specificity. *Cell* 51: 887–98.

Griffith, F. 1928. The significance of pneumococcal types. *J. Hyg.* 27: 113–59.

Hanahan, D., and R. Weinberg. 2000. The hallmarks of cancer. *Cell* 100: 57–70.

Harley, C. B., A. B. Futcher, and C. W. Greider. 1990. Telomeres shorten during ageing of human fibroblasts. *Nature* 345: 458–60.

Hayflick, L., and P. S. Moorhead. 1961. The serial cultivation of human diploid cell strains. *Exp. Cell. Res.* 25: 585–621.

Heather, J. M. and B. Chain. 2016. The sequence of sequencers: The history of DNA sequencing. Genomics, 107: 1–8

Hershey, A. D., and M. Chase. 1952. Independent function of viral protein and nucleic acid in growth of bacteriophage. *J. Genet. Phys.* 36: 39–56.

Huberman, J. A., and A. D. Riggs. 1968. On the mechanism of DNA replication in mammalian chromosomes. *J. Mol. Biol.* 32: 327–41.

Huberman, J. A., and A. Tsai. 1973. Direction of DNA replication in mammalian cells. *J. Mol. Biol.* 75: 5–12.

Huntington's Disease Collaborative Research Group. 1993. A novel gene containing a trinucleotide repeat that is expanded and unstable on Huntington's -disease chromosomes. *Cell* 72: 971–83.

Kornberg, A. 1960. Biological synthesis of DNA. *Science* 131: 1503–8.

Lemon, K. P., and A. D. Grossman. 2000. Movement of replicating DNA through a stationary replisome. *Mol. Cell* 6: 1321–30.

Leonard, A.C. and M. Méchali. 2013. DNA replication origins. Cold Spring Harbor Perspect. Biol., 5: 1–17.

Margulies, M., et al. 2005. Genome sequencing in microfabricated high-density picolitrereactors. *Nature* 437: 376–80.

Meselson, M., and F. W. Stahl. 1958. The replication of DNA in *Escherichia coli. Proc. Natl. Acad. Sci. USA* 44: 671–82.

Navarro, C.L. et al. 2006. Molecular bases of progeroid syndromes. Human Molec. Genet., 15 Spec. No. 2:R151–161.

O'Donnel, M., and J. Kuriyan. 2006. Clamp loaders and replication initiation. *Curr. Opin. Struct. Biol.* 16: 405–15.

Ogawa, T., and R. Okazaki. 1980. Discontinuous DNA replication. *Ann. Rev. Biochem.* 49: 421–57.

Rodriguez, R. L., M. S. Dalbey, and C. I. Davern. 1973. Autoradiographic evidence for bidirectional DNA replication in *Escherichia coli. J. Molec. Biol.* 74: 599–604.

Spies, M., I. Amitani, R. J. Baskin, and S. C. Kowalczykowski. 2007. RecBCD enzyme switches lead motor subunits in response to chi recognition. *Cell* 131: 694–705.

Steitz, T. A. 1998. A mechanism for all polymerases. *Nature* 391: 231–32.

———. 2006. Visualizing polynucleotide polymerase machines at work. *EMBO J.* 25: 3458–68.

Vulliamy, T. et al. 2004. Disease anticipation is associated with progressive telomere shortening in families with dyskeratosis congenita due to mutations in *TERC*. Nature Genet., 5:447–449.

Wilkins, M.H.F. et al. 1953. Molecular structure of deoxypentose nucleic acids. Nature, 171:738–740.

Chapter 8 Molecular Biology of Transcription and RNA Processing

Berget, S. M., C. Moore, and P. Sharp. 1977. Spliced segments at the 5′ terminus of adenovirus 2 late mRNA. *Proc. Natl. Acad. Sci. USA* 74: 3171–75.

Bogenhagen, D. F., S. Sakonju, and D. D. Brown. 1980. A control region in the center of the 5S RNA gene directs specific initiation of transcription: II. the 3′ border of the region. *Cell* 19: 27–35.

Brenner, S., F. Jacob, and M. Meselson. 1961. An unstable intermediate -carrying information from genes to ribosomes for protein synthesis. *Nature* 190: 575–80.

Cech, T. 1987. The chemistry of self-splicing RNA and RNA enzymes. *Science* 236: 1532–39.

Chambon, P. 1981. Split genes. *Sci. Am.* 244: 60–71.

Cramer, P., et al. 2000. Architecture of RNA polymerase II and implications for the transcription mechanism. *Science* 288: 640–49.

Darnell, J. E. 1983. The processing of RNA. *Sci. Am.* 249: 90–100.

De Carlo, S., S-C. Lin, D. J. Taatjes, and A. Hoenger. 2010. Molecular basis of -transcription initiation in archaea. *Transcription* 1: 103–11.

Dugaiczyk, A., et al. 1978. The natural ovalbumin gene contains seven intervening sequences. *Nature* 274: 328–33.

Hamkalo, B. 1985. Visualizing transcription in chromosomes. *Trends. Genet.* 1: 255–60.

Kersanach, R., et al. 1994. Five identical intron positions in ancient duplicated genes of eubacterial origin. *Nature* 367: 387–89.

Kim, M., et al. 2006. Distinct pathways for snoRNA and mRNA termination. *Mol. Cell* 24: 723–34.

Lees-Miller, J. P., L. O. Goodwin, and D. M. Helfman. 1990. Three novel brain tropomyosin isoforms are expressed from the rat α-tropomyosin gene through the use of alternative promoters and alternative RNA processing. *Mol. Cell. Biol.* 10: 1729–42.

Logsdon, J. M. Jr., et al. 1995. Seven newly discovered intron positions in the triose-phosphate isomerase gene: Evidence for the intron-late theory. *Proc. Natl. Acad. Sci. USA* 92: 8507–11.

Maniatis, T., S. Goodbourn, and J. A. Fischer. 1987. Regulation of inducible and tissue-specific gene expression. *Science* 236: 1237–45.

Maniatis, T., and R. Reed 2002. An extensive network of coupling among gene expression machines. *Nature* 416: 499–506.

Myers, R. M., K. Tilly, and T. Maniatis. 1986. Fine structure genetic analysis of the β-globin promoter. *Science* 232: 613–18.

Peng, N., Y. X. Liang, and Q. She. 2011. Archaeal promoter architecture and mechanism of gene activation. *Biochem. Soc Trans.* 39: 99–103.

Pribnow, D. 1975. Nucleotide sequence of an RNA binding site at an early T7 -promoter. *Proc. Natl. Acad. Sci. USA* 72: 784–88.

Reed, R. 2003. Coupling transcription, splicing, and mRNA export. *Curr. Opin. Cell Biol.* 15: 326–31.

Reed, R., and T. Maniatis. 1985. Intron sequences involved in lariat formation -during pre-mRNA splicing. *Cell* 41: 95–105.

Sakonju, S., D. F. Bogenhagen, and D. D. Brown. 1980. A control region in the center of the 5S RNA gene directs specific initiation of transcription: I. the 5′ border of the region. *Cell* 19: 13–25.

Sharp, P. 1994. Nobel Lecture: Split genes and RNA splicing. *Cell* 77: 805–15.

Sudhof, T. C., et al. 1985. Cassette of eight exons shared by genes for LDL and EGF precursors. *Science* 228: 893–95.

Tilghman, S., et al. 1978. The intervening sequence of a mouse beta-globin gene is traced to the 15S beta-globin mRNA precursor. *Proc. Natl. Acad. Sci. USA* 75: 1309–13.

Tocchini-Valentini, G., P. Fruscoloni, and G. P. Tocchini-Valentini. 2011. Evolution of introns in the archaeal world. *Proc. Nat. Acad. Sci. USA* 108: 4782–87.

Chapter 9 The Molecular Biology of Translation

Blobel, G., and B. Dobberstein. 1975. Transfer of proteins across membranes. I. Presence of proteolytically processed and unprocessed nascent immunoglobulin light chains on membrane-bound ribosomes of murine myeloma. *J. Cell. Biol.* 67: 835–51.

Brenner, S., F. Jacob, and M. Meselson. 1969. An unstable intermediate carrying information from genes to ribosomes for protein synthesis. *Nature* 190: 576–81.

Carrell, R. W., and D. A. Lomas. 2002. Alpha-1 antitrypsin deficiency—a model conformational disease. *N. Engl. J. Med.*, 346: 45–53.

Cech, T. R. 2000. The ribosome is a ribozyme. *Science* 289: 878–79.

Chapeville, F. F., et al. 1962. On the role of soluble ribonucleic acid in coding for nucleic acids. *Proc. Natl. Acad. Sci. USA* 48: 1086–92.

Crick, F. 1966. Codon-anticodon pairing: The wobble hypothesis. *J. Mol. Biol.* 19: 548–55.

Crick, F., et al. 1961. General nature of the genetic code for proteins. *Nature* 192: 1227–32.

Fox, T. D. 1987. Natural variation in the genetic code. *Ann. Rev. Genet.* 21: 67–91.

Johnson, A. W., E. Lund, and J. Dahlberg. 2002. Nuclear export of ribosomal -subunits. *Trends Biochem. Sci.* 27: 850–57.

Kaltschmidt, E. and H.G. Wittmann. 1970. Ribosomal proteins, XII. Number of proteins in small and large ribosomal subunits in *Escherichia coli* as determined by two-dimensional gel electrophoresis.

Khorana, H. G., et al. 1967. Polynucleotide synthesis and the genetic code. *Cold Spring Harbor Symp.* 31: 39–49.

Kloc, M., N. R. Zearfoss, and L. D. Etkin. 2002. Mechanisms of subcellular mRNA localization. *Cell* 108: 533–44.

Kozak, M. 1978. How do eukaryotic ribosomes select initiation regions in mRNA? *Cell* 15: 1109–23.

———. 1987. An analysis of 5′-noncoding sequences from 699 vertebrate -messenger RNAs. *Nuc. Acid Res.* 15: 8125–48.

Nirenberg, M. W., and P. Leder. 1964. RNA code words and protein synthesis. I. The effects of trinucleotides upon the binding of sRNA to ribosomes. *Science* 145: 1399–1407.

Nirenberg, M. W., and J. H. Matthaei. 1961. The dependence of cell-free protein synthesis in *E. coli* upon naturally occurring or synthetic polyribosome *Proc. Natl. Acad. Sci. USA* 47: 1588–1602.

Patil, C., and P. Walter. 2001. Intracellular signaling from the endoplasmic reticulum to the nucleus: The unfolding protein response in yeast and mammals. *Curr. Opin. Cell Biol.* 13: 349–55.

Sachs, A. B., P. Sarnow, and M. W. Hentz. 1997. Starting at the beginning, middle, and end: Translation initiation in eukaryotes. *Cell* 89: 831–38.

Saito, K., K. Kobayashi, M. Wada, I. Kikuno, et al. 2010. Omnipotent role of -archaeal elongation factor 1 alpha (EF1α) in translation elongation and termination, and quality control of protein synthesis. *Proc. Natl. Acad. Sci. USA* 107: 19242–47.

Shine, J., and L. Dalgarno. 1974. The 3′-terminal sequence of *Escherichia coli* 16S ribosomal RNA: Complementary to nonsense triplet and ribosome binding sites. *Proc. Natl. Acad. Sci. USA* 71: 1342–46.

Tsugita, A., et al. 1962. Demonstration of the messenger role of viral RNA. *Proc. Natl. Acad. Sci. USA* 48: 846–53.

Watson, J. D. 1963. Involvement of RNA in the synthesis of proteins. *Science* 140: 17–26.

Zheng, N., and L. M. Gierasch. 1996. Signal sequences: The same yet different. *Cell* 86: 849–52.

Application Chapter B Human Genetic Screening

Boue, A. et al. 1985. The cytogenetics of fetal wastage. *Adv. Hum. Genet.*, 14: 1–57.

Caskey, C. 1993. Presymptomatic diagnosis: A step toward genetic health care. *Science*, 262:48–49.

Green, J.E. et al. 1988. Chorionic villus sampling: Experience with an initial 940 cases. *Obstet. Gynecol.*, 71:208–212.

Huntington's Disease Collaborative Group. 1993. A novel gene containing a trinucleotide repeat that is expanded and unstable in Huntington's disease chromosomes. *Cell*, 72:971–983.

Huntington's Disease News. Genetic testing: Does Kristen Powers have her mom's fatal gene? http://www.newshd.net/journals/1544.

Jacobs, P. A. and T. J. Hassold. 1995. The origins of numerical chromosome abnormalities. *Adv. Genet.*, 33: 101–133.

Fiddler, M. 2014. Fetal cell based prenatal diagnosis: Perspectives on the present and future. *J. Clin. Med.*, 3:972–985.

Kinney, L. Stanford freshman to release documentary on dealing with family history of Huntington's. http://www.stanforddaily.com/2013/02/13.

Lloyd, J. Genetic testing and disease: Would you want to know? http://usatoday30.usatoday.com/news/health/story/2012-04-09.

Marshall, E. 1996. The genome program's conscience. *Science*, 274:488–490.

Philip, J. et al. 1994. Prenatal aneuploidy detection in interphase cells by fluorescence in situ hybridization (FISH). *Prenatal Diag.*, 14: 1203–1215.

Shiefa, S. et al. 2013. First trimester maternal serum screening using biochemical markers PAPP-A and free β-hCG for Down syndrome, Patau symdrome, and Edward syndrome. *Indian J. Clin. Biochem.*, 28:3–12.

Wald, N. J. et al. 1988. Maternal serum screening for Down's syndrome in early pregnancy. *British Med. J.*, 297:883–887.

Wapner, R. J. and L. Jackson. 1988. Chorionic villus sampling. *Clin. Obstet. Gynecol.*, 31:328–344.

Chapter 10 Eukaryotic Chromosome Abnormalities and Molecular Organization

Bendich, A. J., and K. Drlica. 2000. Prokaryotic and eukaryotic chromosomes: What's the difference? *BioEssays* 22: 481–86.

Blakeslee, A. F. 1934. New jimson weeds from old chromosomes. *J. Hered.* 25: 80–108.

Carbon, J. 1984. Yeast centromeres: Structure and function. *Cell* 37: 352–53.

Clarke, L. 1990. Centromeres of budding and fission yeasts. *Trends Genet.* 6: 150–54.

Cremer, T., and C. Cremer. 2001. Chromosome territories, nuclear architecture and gene regulation in mammalian cells. *Nat. Rev. Genet.* 2: 292–301.

Cross, I., and J. Wolstenholme. 2001. An introduction to human chromosomes and their analysis. In *Human Cytogenetics: Constitutional Analysis* (3rd ed.), edited by D. E. Rooney. Oxford: Oxford University Press.

Deal, R. B., J. Henikoff, and S. Henikoff. 2010. Genome-wide kinetics of -nucleosome turnover determined by metabolic labeling of histones. *Science* 328: 1161–64.

DeLange, R. J., et al. 1969. Calf and pea histone IV. III. Complete amino acid sequence of pea seedling histone IV; comparison with the homologous calf thymus histone. *J. Biol. Chem.* 244: 5669–79.

Duan, Z., et al. 2010. A three-dimensional model of the yeast genome. *Nature* 465: 363–67.

Federoff, N. V. 1993. Barbara McClintock (June 16, 1902–September 2, 1992). *Genetics* 136: 1–10.

Feldman, M., and E. R. Sears. 1981. The wild gene resources of wheat. *Sci. Am.* 244: 102–12.

Gardner, R. J. M., and G. R. Sutherland. 2004. *Chromosome Abnormalities and Genetic Counseling.* 3rd ed. Oxford: Oxford University Press.

Gersh, et al. 1995. Evidence for a distinct region causing a catlike cry in -patients with 5p deletions. *Am. J. Hum. Genet.* 56: 1404–10.

Hassold, T. J., and D. Chiu. 1985. Maternal age-specific rates of numerical -chromosome abnormalities with special reference to trisomy. *Hum. Genet.* 70: 11–17.

Hassold, T. J., and P. Hunt. 2001. To err (meiotically) is human: The genesis of -human aneuploidy. *Nat. Rev. Genet.* 2: 280–91.

Hassold, T. J., and P. A. Jacobs. 1984. Trisomy in man. *Annu. Rev. Genet.* 18: 69–97.

Hayes, J. J., and J. C. Hansen. 2001. Nucleosomes and the chromatin fiber. *Curr. Opin. Genet. Dev.* 11: 124–29.

Heikanen, M., L. Peltonen, and A. Palotie. 1996. Visual mapping with high resolution FISH. *Trends Genet.* 12: 379–84.

Hook, E. B., and A. Linsjo. 1978. Down syndrome by single year maternal age interval in a Swedish study: Comparison with results from a New York study. *Am. J. Hum. Genet.* 30: 19–27.

Hunt, P. A., and T. J. Hassold. 2008. Human female meiosis: What makes a good egg go bad? *Trends Genet.* 24: 86–93.

Kaiser, P. 1984. Pericentric inversions: Problems and significance for clinical g-enetics. *Hum. Genet.* 68: 1–47.

Luger, K., et al. 1997. Crystal structure of the nucleosome core particle at 2.8 Å resolution. *Nature* 389: 251–60.

Luger, K., and T. J. Richmond. 1998. DNA binding within the nucleosome core. *Curr. Opin. Struct. Biol.* 8: 33–40.

———. 1998. The histone tails of the nucleosome. *Curr. Opin. Genet. Dev.* 8: 140–46.

Madan, K. 1995. Paracentric inversions: A review. *Hum Genet.* 96: 503–15.

McClintock, B. 1939. The behavior in successive nuclear divisions of a chromosome broken at meiosis. *Proc. Natl. Acad. Sci. USA* 25: 406–16.

———. 1951. Chromosome organization and genic expression. *Cold Spring Harbor Symp. Quant. Biol.* 16: 13–47.

Nelson, D. L., and R. A. Gibbs. 2004. The critical region in trisomy 21. *Science* 306: 619–21.

Page, S. L., and R. S. Hawley. 2003. Chromosome choreography: The meiotic -ballet. *Science* 301: 785–89.

Patterson, D., and A. Costa. 2005. Down syndrome and genetics—A case of linked histories. *Nat. Rev. Genet.* 6: 137–45.

Thanbichler, M., and L. Shapiro. 2006. Chromosome organization and segregation in bacteria. *J. Struct. Biol.* 156: 292–303.

Thanbichler, M., S. C. Wang, and L. Shapiro. 2005. The bacterial nucleoid: A highly organized and dynamic structure. *J. Cell. Biochem.* 96: 506–21.

Trask, B. J. 2002. Human chromosomes: 46 chromosomes, 46 years and counting. *Nat. Rev. Genet.* 3: 769–78.

Warburton, D. 2005. Biological aging and the etiology of aneuploidy. *Cytogenet. Genome Res.* 111: 266–72.

Woodcock, C. L., and S. Dimitrov. 2001. Higher-order structure of chromatin and chromosomes. *Curr. Opin. Genet. Dev.* 11: 130–35.

Yunis, J. J. 1982. The origin of man: A chromosomal pictorial legacy. *Science* 215: 1525–30.

Chapter 11 Gene Mutation, DNA Repair, and Homologous Recombination

Bzymek, M., et al. 2010. Double Holliday junctions are intermediates of DNA break repair. *Nature* 464: 937–41.

Cox, M. M. 2001. Recombinational DNA repair of damaged replication forks in *Escherichia coli*: Ques. *Ann Rev. Genet.* 35: 53–82.

De Laat, W. L., N. G. Jaspers, and J. H. Hoeijmakers. 1999. Molecular mechanism of excision nucleotide repair. *Genes Dev.* 13: 768–85.

Deininger, P. L., and M. A. Batzer. 1999. Alu repeats and human disease. *Molec. Genet. Metabol.* 67: 183–93.

Drucker, R., and E. Whitelaw. 2004. Retrotransposon-derived elements in the mammalian genome: A potential source of disease. *J. Inherit. Metabol. Dis.* 27: 319–30.

Eichler, E. E., and D. Sankoff. 2003. Structural dynamics of eukaryotic chromosome evolution. *Science* 301: 793–97.

Grindley, N. D. F., and R. R. Reed. 1985. Transpositional recombination in -prokaryotes. *Annu. Rev. Biochem.* 54: 863–96.

Kazazian, H.H. et al. 1988. Hemophilia A resulting from de novo insertion of *L1* sequences represents a novel mechanism for mutation in man. Nature, 332: 164–166.

Kowalczykowski, S. C. 2000. Initiation of genetic recombination and -recombination-dependent replication. *Trends Biochem. Sci.* 25: 156–64.

Kunkel, T. A., and D. A. Erie. 2005. DNA mismatch repair. *Annu. Rev. Biochem.* 76: 681–710.

Lusetti, S. L., and M. M. Cox. 2002. The bacterial RecA protein and the recombinational DNA repair of stalled replication forks. *Annu. Rev. Biochem.* 71: 71–100.

Lynch, M. 2010. Evolution of mutation rate. *Trends Genet.* 26: 345–52.

McCann, J., and B. N. Ames. 1978. The *Salmonella*/microsome mutagenicity test: Predictive value for animal carcinogenicity. In *Advances in Modern Technology* (Vol. 5: Mutagenesis), edited by W. G. Flamm and M. A. Mehlman. Washington, DC: Hemisphere Publishing.

Medstrand, P., et al. 2005. Impact of transposable elements on the evolution of mammalian gene regulation. *Cytogenet. Genome Res.* 110: 342–52.

Miki, Y. 1998. Retrotransposal integration of mobile genetic elements in human disease. *J. Hum. Genet.* 43: 77–84.

O'Hare, K. 1985. The mechanism and control of *P* element transposition in *Drosophila*. *Trends Genet.* 1: 250–54.

Ossowski, S., et al. 2010. The rate and molecular spectrum of spontaneous -mutations in *Arabidopsis thaliana*. *Science* 327: 92–94.

Sekiguchi, J. M., and D. O. Freguson. 2006. DNA double-strand break repair: A relentless hunt uncovers new prey. *Cell* 124: 260–62.

Szostak, J. W., et al. 1983. The double-strand break repair model for recombination. *Cell* 33: 25–35.

Walsh, T., M. K. Lee, S. Casadei, A. M. Thornton, et al. 2010. Detection of -inherited mutations for breast and ovarian cancer using genomic capture and -massively parallel sequencing. *Proc. Nat. Acad. Sci. USA* 107: 12629–33.

Walsh, T., S. Casadei, M. K. Lee, C. C. Pennil, et al. 2011. Mutations in 12 genes for inherited ovarian, fallopian tube, and peritoneal carcinoma identified by massively parallel sequencing. *Proc. Nat. Acad. Sci. USA* 108: 18032–37.

Chapter 12 Regulation of Gene Expression in Bacteria and Bacteriophage

Bell, S. D. 2005. Archaeal transcription regulation—variation on a bacterial theme? *Trends Microbiol.* 13: 262–65.

Bertrand, K., and C. Yanofsky. 1976. Regulation of transcription termination in the leader region of the tryptophan operon of *Escherichia coli*. *J. Mol. Biol.* 103: 339–49.

Bocobza, S. et al. 2007. Riboswitch-dependent gene regulation and it evolution in the plant kingdom. Genes Dev., 21:2874–2879.

Cheah, M.T. et al. 2007. Control of alternative RNA splicing and gene expression by eukaryotic riboswitches. Nature, 447:497–500.

Dickson, R. C., et al. 1975. Genetic regulation: The *Lac* control region. *Science* 187: 27–33.

Fisher, R. F., et al. 1985. Analysis of the requirements for transcription pausing in the tryptophan operon. *J. Mol. Biol.* 182: 397–409.

Fried, M. G. 1996. DNA looping and *Lac* repressor–CAP interaction. *Science* 274: 1930.

Jacob, F., and J. Monod. 1961. Genetic regulatory mechanisms in the synthesis of proteins. *J. Mol. Biol.* 3: 318–56.

Lee, D., and R. Schleif. 1989. In vivo loops in *araCBAD*: Size limits and helical -repeats. *Proc. Natl. Acad. Sci. USA* 86: 476–80.

Lewis, M., et al. 1996. Crystal structure of the lactose operon repressor and its complexes with DNA and inducer. *Science* 271: 1247–54.

Matthews, K. S. 1996. The whole lactose repressor. *Science* 271: 1245–46.

Nudler, E. and A.S. Mironov. 2004. The riboswitch control of bacterial metabolism. Trends in genetics, 29: 11–17.

Pardee, A. B., F. Jacob, and J. Monod. 1959. The genetic control and cytoplasmic expression of inducibility in the synthesis of β-galactosidase by *E. coli*. *J. Mol. Biol.* 1: 165–78.

Ptashne, M. 2005. *A Genetic Switch: Phage Lambda Revisited*. 3rd ed. Cold Spring Harbor, NY: Cold Spring Harbor Laboratory Press.

Ptashne, M., and A. Gann. 2002. *Genes and Signals*. Cold Spring Harbor, NY: Cold Spring Harbor Laboratory Press.

Schlief, R. 2000. Regulation of the L-arabinose operon of *Escherichia coli*. *Trends Genet.* 16: 559–66.

———. 2003. AraC protein: A love-hate relationship. *BioEssays* 25: 274–82.

Schultz, S. C., G. C. Shields, and T. A. Steitz. 1991. Crystal structure of a -CAP-DNA complex: The DNA is bent 90°. *Science* 253: 1001–7.

Tijan, R. 1995. Molecular machines that control genes. *Sci. Am.* 272: 55–61.

Tucker, B.J. and R.R. Breaker. 2005. Riboswitches as versatile gene control elements. Curr. Opin. Struct. Biol., 15:342–348.

Ullman, A. 2003. *Origins of Molecular Biology: A Tribute to Jacques Monod*. rev. ed. Washington, DC: ASM Press.

Chapter 13 Regulation of Gene Expression in Eukaryotes

Augui, S., et al. 2011. Regulation of X-chromosome inactivation by the X-inactivation centre. *Nat. Rev. Genet.* 12: 429–42.

Ambrose, V., and X. Chen. 2007. The regulation of genes and genomes by small RNAs. *Development* 134: 1635–41.

Black, D. L. 2000. Protein diversity from alternative splicing: A challenge for -bioinformatics and postgenomic biology. *Cell* 103: 367–70.

Cairns, B. R. 2009. The logic of chromatin architecture and remodeling at -promoters. *Nature* 461: 193–98.

Dillon, N., and P. Sabbattini. 2000. Functional gene expression domains: Defining the functional unit of eukaryotic gene regulation. *BioEssays* 22: 657–65.

Fedoriw, A. M., et al. 2004. Transgenic RNAi reveals essential function of CTCF in H19 gene imprinting. *Science* 303: 238–40.

Filion, G. J., et al. 2010. Systematic protein location mapping reveals five principal chromatin types in *Drosophila* cells. *Cell* 143: 212–24.

Flintoft, L. 2010. Complex diseases: Adding epigenetics to the mix. *Nat. Rev. Genet.* 11: 94–95.

Fuda, N. J., M. Behfar Ardehali, and J. T. Lis. 2009. Defining mechanisms that regulate RNA polymerase II transcription *in vivo*. *Nature* 461: 186–92.

Gregory, P. D., K. Wagner, and W. Hurz. 2001. Histone acetylation and chromatin remodeling. *Exp. Cell Res.* 265: 195–202.

Grewal, S. I. S., and S. Jia. 2008. Heterochromatin revisited. *Nat. Rev. Genet.* 8: 35–46.

Guttman, M. et al. 2011. lincRNAs act in the circuitry controlling pluripotentcy and differentiation. *Nature* 477: 295–300.

Hassan, A. H., et al. 2001. Promoter targeting of chromatin-modifying complexes. *Frontiers in Bioscience* 6: 1054–64.

Horn, P. J., and C. L. Peterson. 2002. Chromatin higher order folding: Wrapping up transcription. *Science* 297: 1824–27.

Jenuwein, T., and C. D. Allis. 2001. Translating the histone code. *Science* 293: 1074–80.

Kappeler, L., and M. J. Meaney. 2010. Epigenetics and parental effects. *BioEssays* 32: 818–27.

Kucharski, R., et al. 2008. Nutritional control of reproductive status in honeybees via DNA methylation. *Science* 319: 1827–30.

Lawrence, P. A. 1992. *How to Make a Fly*. London: Blackwell Scientific.

Lusser, A., and J. T. Kadonaga. 2003. Chromatin remodeling by ATP-dependent molecular machines. *BioEssays* 25: 1192–1200.

MacRae, I. J., et al. 2006. Structural basis for double-stranded RNA processing by Dicer. *Science* 311: 195–98.

Margueron, R., and D. Reinberg. 2010. Chromatin structure and the inheritance of epigenetic information. *Nat. Rev. Genet.* 11: 285–96.

Meister, G., and T. Tuschl. 2004. Mechanisms of gene silencing by double-stranded RNA. *Nature* 431: 343–49.

Moore, M. J. 2005. From birth to death: The complex lives of eukaryotic mRNAs. *Science* 309: 1514–18.

Piunti, A., and Shilatifard, A. (2016). Epigenetic balance of gene expression by Polycomb and COMPASS families. Science *352*.

Roudier, F., et al. 2011. Integrative epigenomic mapping defines four main chromatin states in *Arabidopsis*. *EMBO J.* 30: 1928–38, doi:10.1038/emboj.2011.103.

Schwarz, Y. B., and Pirrotta, V. 2007. Polycomb silencing mechanisms and the management of genomic programs. *Nat. Rev. Genet.* 8: 9–22.

Siomi, H., and M. C. Siomi. 2007. Expanding RNA physiology: MicroRNAs in -unicellular organisms. *Genes Dev.* 21: 1153–56.

Small, S., et al. 1991. Transcriptional regulation of a pair-rule gene in *Drosophila*. *Genes Develop.* 5: 827–39.

Small, S., A. Blair, and M. Levine. 1992. Regulation of *even-skipped* stripe-2 in the *Drosophila* embryo. *EMBO J.* 11: 4047–57.

Sudarsanam, P., and F. Winston. 2000. The SWI/SNF family of nucleosome-remodeling complexes and transcriptional control. *Trends Genet.* 16: 345–51.

Turner, B. M. 2000. Histone acetylation and the epigenetic code. *BioEssays* 22: 836–45.

Van Steensel, B. 2011. Chromatin: Constructing the big picture. *EMBO J.* 30: 1885–95, doi:10.1038/emboj.2011.135.

Visel, A., E. M. Rubin, and L. A. Pennacchio. 2009. Genomic views of distant-acting enhancers. *Nature* 461: 199–205.

Wang, H., et al. 2004. Using atomic force microscopy to study nucleosome remodeling on individual nucleosomal arrays in situ. *Biophys. J.* 87: 1964–71.

Weake, V. M., and J. L. Workman. 2010. Inducible gene expression: diverse regulatory mechanisms. *Nat. Rev. Genet.* 11: 426–37.

Zaret, K.S., and Carroll, J.S. (2011). Pioneer transcription factors: establishing competence for gene expression. Gene Dev *25*, 2227–2241.

Chapter 14 Analysis of Gene Function by Forward Genetics and Reverse Genetics

Austin, C. P., et al. 2004. The knockout mouse project. *Nat. Genet.* 36: 921–24.

Bellen, H. J., et al. 1989. P-element-mediated enhancer detection—A versatile method to study development in *Drosophila*. *Genes & Development* 3: 1288–300.

Boone, C., H. Bussey, and B. J. Andrews. 2007. Exploring genetic interactions and networks with yeast. *Nat. Rev. Genet.* 8: 437–49.

Doudna, J.A., and Charpentier, E. (2014). The new frontier of genome engineering with CRISPR-Cas9. Science *346*, 1077–+.

Echeverri, C. J., and N. Perrimon. 2006. High-throughput RNAi screening in -cultured cells: A user's guide. *Nat. Rev. Genet.* 7: 373–84.

Forsburg, S. L. 2001. The art and design of genetic screens: Yeast. *Nat. Rev. Genet.* 2: 659–68.

Gantz, V.M., and Bier, E. (2015). The mutagenic chain reaction: A method for converting heterozygous to homozygous mutations. Science *348*, 442–444.

Halder, G., P. Callaerts, and W. J. Gehring. 1995. Induction of ectopic eyes by -targeted expression of the eyeless gene in *Drosophila*. *Science* 267: 1788–92.

Hannon, G. J. 2002. RNA interference. *Nature* 418: 244–51.

Hartwell, L. H., et al. 1973. Genetic control of the cell division cycle in yeast: V. genetic analysis of *cdc* mutants. *Genetics* 74: 267–86.

Jiang, F.G., and Doudna, J.A. (2017). CRISPR-Cas9 Structures and Mechanisms. Annu Rev Biophys *46*, 505–529.

Kile, B. T., and D. J. Hilton. 2005. The art and design of genetic screens: Mouse. *Nat. Rev. Genet.* 6: 557–67.

Komor, A.C., Badran, A.H., and Liu, D.R. (2017). CRISPR-Based Technologies for the Manipulation of Eukaryotic Genomes. Cell *168*, 20–36.

Marraffini, L.A., and Sontheimer, E.J. (2010). CRISPR interference: RNA-directed adaptive immunity in bacteria and archaea. Nat Rev Genet *11*, 181–190.

McCallum, C. M., et al. 2000. Targeting induced local lesions in genomes (TILLING) for plant functional genomics. *Plant Physiol.* 123: 439–42.

Mojica, F.J.M., and Montoliu, L. (2016). On the Origin of CRISPR-Cas Technology: From Prokaryotes to Mammals. Trends Microbiol *24*, 811–820.

Page, D. R., and U. Grossniklaus. 2002. The art and design of genetic screens: *Arabidopsis thaliana*. *Nat. Rev. Genet.* 3: 124–36.

Pelaz, S., et al. 2000. B and C floral organ identity functions require *SEPALLATA* MADS-box genes. *Nature* 405: 200–203.

Shuman, H. A., and T. J. Silhavy. 2003. The art and design of genetic screens: *Escherichia coli*. *Nat. Rev. Genet.* 4: 419–31.

St Johnston, D. 2002. The art and design of genetic screens: *Drosophila melanogaster*. *Nat. Rev. Genet.* 3: 176–88.

Sturtevant, A. H. 1955. A highly specific complementary lethal system in *Drosophila melanogaster*. *Genetics* 40: 118–23.

Thomas, J. H. 1993. Thinking about genetic redundancy. *Trends Genet.* 9: 395–399.

Application Chapter C The Genetics of Cancer

Brennan, C. W. et al. 2013. The somatic genomic landscape of glioblastoma. *Cell*, 155:462–477.

Calabrese, P. et al. 2004. Colorectal pretumor progression before and after loss of DNA mismatch repair. *Am. J. Pathol.*, 164: 1447–1453.

Grady, D. 2017. F.D.A. approves first gene-altering leukemia treatment, costing $475,000. https://www.nytimes.com/2017/08/30/health.

Hanahan, D. and R. A. Weinberg. 2000. The hallmarks of cancer. *Cell*, 100:57–70

Hanahan, D. and R. A. Weinberg. 2011. The hallmarks of cancer: the next generation. *Cell*, 144:646–674.

Kaiser, J. 2017. Modified T cells that attack leukemia become first gene therapy approved in the United States. *Science*, DOI:10,1126/science.aap8293.

Kamiyama, H. et al. 2012. DNA methylation in normal colon tissue predicts predisposition to multiple cancers. *Oncogene*, 31:5029–5037.

Kandoth, C. et al. 2013. Mutational landscape and significance across 12 major cancer types. *Nature*, 502:333–339.

Mavaddat, N. et al. 2013. Cancer risks for *BRCA1* and *BRCA2* mutation carriers: Results from prospective analysis of EMBRACE. *J. Natl. Cancer Inst.*, 105:812–822.

Stahl, M. et al. 2016. Epigenetics of cancer: A hematological perspective. PLoS Genetics, DOI:10.1371/journal.pgen.1006193.

Waddell, N. et al. 2014. Whole genomes redefine the mutational landscape of pancreatic cancer. *Nature*, 518:495–501.

Walther, A. et al. 2009. Genetic prognostic and predictive markers in colorectal cancer. *Nature Rev. Cancer*, 9:489–499.

Chapter 15 Recombinant DNA Technology and Its Applications

Barrangou, R., and Doudna, J.A. (2016). Applications of CRISPR technologies in research and beyond. Nat Biotechnol *34*, 933–941.

Berg, P., et al. 1974. Potential biohazards of recombinant DNA molecules. *Proc. Natl. Acad. Sci. USA* 71: 2593–94.

———. 1975. Summary Statement of the Asilomar Conference on recombinant DNA molecules. *Proc. Natl. Acad. Sci. USA* 72: 1981–84.

Berg, P., and Singer, M. A. 1995. The recombinant DNA controversy: Twenty years later. *Proc. Natl. Acad. Sci. USA* 92: 9011–13.

Champer, J., Buchman, A., and Akbari, O.S. (2016). Cheating evolution: engineering gene drives to manipulate the fate of wild populations. Nat Rev Genet *17*, 146–159.

Chilton, M. D., et al. 1977. Stable incorporation of plasmid DNA into higher plant cells: The molecular basis of crown gall tumorigenesis. *Cell* 11: 263–71.

Cohen, S. A., et al. 1973. Construction of biologically functional plasmids in vitro. *Proc. Natl. Acad. Sci. USA* 70: 3240–44.

Danna, K., and D. Nathans. 1971. Specific cleavage of simian virus 40 DNA by restriction endonuclease of *Hemophilus influenzae. Proc. Natl. Acad. Sci. USA* 68: 2913–17.

Dever, D.P., Bak, R.O., Reinisch, A., Camarena, J., Washington, G., Nicolas, C.E., Pavel-Dinu, M., Saxena, N., Wilkens, A.B., Mantri, S., et al. (2016). CRISPR/Cas9 beta-globin gene targeting in human haematopoietic stem cells. Nature *539*, 384–389.

DiCarlo, J.E., Chavez, A., Dietz, S.L., Esvelt, K.M., and Church, G.M. (2015). Safeguarding CRISPR-Cas9 gene drives in yeast. Nat Biotechnol *33*, 1250–+.

Goeddel, D. V., et al. 1979. Expression in *Escherichia coli* of chemically synthesized genes for human insulin. *Proc. Natl. Acad. Sci.* 76: 106–10.

Grunstein, M., and D. S. Hogness. 1975. Colony hybridization—Method for isolation of cloned DNAs that contain a specific gene. *Proc. Natl. Acad. Sci. USA* 72: 3961–65.

Hanna, J., et al. 2007. Treatment of sickle cell anemia mouse model with iPS cells generated from autologous skin. *Science* 318: 1920–23.

Hershfie, V., et al. 1974. Plasmid ColE1 as a molecular vehicle for cloning and -amplification of DNA. *Proc. Natl. Acad. Sci. USA* 71: 3455–59.

Kelley, T. J. Jr., and H. O. Smith. 1970. A restriction enzyme from *Hemophilus influenzae*. II. Base sequence of the recognition site. *J. Molec. Biol.* 51: 393–409.

Kimmelman, J. 2008. Science and society: The ethics of human gene transfer. *Nat. Rev. Genet.* 9: 239–44.

Kyndt, T., Quispe, D., Zhai, H., Jarret, R., Ghislain, M., Liu, Q.C., Gheysen, G., and Kreuze, J.F. (2015). The genome of cultivated sweet potato contains Agrobacterium T-DNAs with expressed genes: An example of a naturally transgenic food crop. P Natl Acad Sci USA *112*, 5844–5849.

Linn, S., and W. Arber. 1968. Host specificity of DNA produced by *Escherichia coli*. X. In vitro restriction of phage fd replicative form. *Proc. Natl. Acad. Sci. USA* 59: 1300–6.

Long, C.Z., Amoasii, L., Mireault, A.A., McAnally, J.R., Li, H., Sanchez-Ortiz, E., Bhattacharyya, S., Shelton, J.M., Bassel-Duby, R., and Olson, E.N. (2016). Postnatal genome editing partially restores dystrophin expression in a mouse model of muscular dystrophy. Science *351*, 400–403.

Martin, V. J. J., et al. 2003. Engineering a mevalonate pathway in *Escherichia coli* for production of terpenoids. *Nat. Biotechnol.* 21: 796–802.

Rubin, G. M., and A. C. Spradling. 1982. Genetic-transformation of *Drosophila* with transposable element vectors. *Science* 218: 348–53.

Sambrook, J., E. F. Fitch, and T. Maniatis. 1989. *Molecular Cloning: A Laboratory Manual.* 2nd ed. Cold Spring Harbor, NY: Cold Spring Harbor Press.

Smith, H. O., and K. W. Wilcox. 1970. A restriction enzyme from *Hemophilus -influenzae*. I. Purification and general properties. *J. Molec. Biol.*, 51: 379–91.

Thomas, K. R., and M. R. Capecchi. 1987. Site-directed mutagenesis by gene -targeting in mouse embryo-derived stem-cells. *Cell* 51: 503–12.

Waehler, R., S. J. Russell, and D. T. Curiel. 2007. Engineering targeted viral vectors for gene therapy. *Nat. Rev. Genet.* 8: 573–87.

Wilmut, I., et al. 1997. Viable offspring derived from fetal and adult mammalian cells. *Nature* 385: 810–13.

Wofenbarger, L. L., and P. R. Phifer. 2000. The ecological risks and benefits of -genetically engineered plants. *Science* 290: 2088–93.

Ye, X., et al. 2000. Engineering the provitamin A (β-carotene) biosynthetic -pathway into (carotenoid-free) rice endosperm. *Science* 287: 303–5.

Chapter 16 Genomics: Genetics from a Whole-Genome Perspective

Adams, M. D., et al. 2000. The genome sequence of *Drosophila melanogaster. Science* 287: 2185–95.

The *Arabidopsis* Genome Initiative. 2000. Analysis of the genome sequence of the flowering plant *Arabidopsis thaliana. Nature* 408: 796–814.

Blattner, F. R., et al. 1997. The complete genome sequence of *Escherichia coli* K-12. *Science* 277: 1453–61.

Boffelli, D., M. A. Nobrega, and E. M. Rubin. 2004. Comparative genomics at the vertebrate extremes. *Nat. Rev. Genet.* 5: 456–65.

Boone, C., H. Bussey, and B. J. Andrews. 2007. Exploring genetic interactions and networks with yeast. *Nat. Rev. Genet.* 8: 437–49.

Brune, A. 2007. Woodworker's digest. *Nature* 450: 487–88.

Chu, S., et al. 1998. The transcriptional program of sporulation in budding yeast. *Science* 282: 699–705.

DeRisi, J. L., V. R. Iyer, and P. O. Brown. 1997. Exploring the metabolic and -genetic control of gene expression on a genomic scale. *Science* 278: 680–86.

Feuk, L., A. R. Carson, and S. W. Scherer. 2006. Structural variation in the human genome. *Nat. Rev. Genet.* 7: 85–97.

Fleischmann, R. D., et al. 1995. Whole genome random sequencing and assembly of *Haemophilus influenzae* Rd. *Science* 269: 496–512.

Giaever, G., et al. 2002. Functional profiling of the *Saccharomyces cerevisiae* -genome. *Nature* 418: 387–91.

Geib, S. M., et al. 2008. Lignin degradation in wood-feeding insects. *Proc. Natl. Acad. Sci. USA* 105: 12932–37.

Girirajan, S. et al. 2011. Human copy number variation and complex genetic -disease. *Annu. Rev. Genet.* 45: 203–26.

Goffeau, A., et al. 1996. Life with 6000 genes. *Science* 274: 562–67.

Gonzalez, A. et al. 2011. Our microbial selves: what ecology can teach us. *EMBO Reports* 12: 775–84.

Grice, E. A., and A. Sgre, J. A. 2011. The skin microbiome. *Nature Reviews Microbiology* 9: 244–53.

Hattori, M., et al. 2000. The DNA sequence of human chromosome 21. *Nature* 405: 311–19.

Hui, L., and D. W. Bianchi. 2013. Recent advances in the prenatal interrogation of the human fetal genome. *Trends Genet.* 29: 84–91.

International Human Genome Sequencing Consortium. 2001. Initial sequencing and analysis of the human genome. *Nature* 409: 860–921.

Keeling, P. J., et al. 2005. The tree of eukaryotes. *Trends Ecol. and Evol.* 12: 670–76.

Kellis, M., et al. 2003. Sequencing and comparison of yeast species to identify genes and regulatory elements. *Nature* 423: 241–54.

Knight, R., Callewaert, C., Marotz, C., Hyde, E.R., Debelius, J.W., McDonald, D., and Sogin, M.L. (2017). The Microbiome and Human Biology. Annual Review of Genomics and Human Genetics *18*, 3.1–3.22.

Kobayashi, K., et al. 2003. Essential *Bacillus subtilis* genes. *Proc. Natl. Acad. Sci. USA* 100: 4678–83.

Lindblad-Toh, K., et al. 2005. Genome sequence, comparative analysis and -haplotype structure of the domestic dog. *Nature* 438: 803–19.

Long, M., et al. 2003. The origin of new genes: Glimpses from the young and old. *Nat. Rev. Genet.* 4, 865–75.

Mazurkiewicz, P., et al. 2006. Signature-tagged mutagenesis: Barcoding mutants for genome-wide screens. *Nat. Rev. Genet.* 7: 929–39.

Mouse Genome Sequencing Consortium. 2002. Initial sequencing and comparative analysis of the mouse genome. *Nature* 420: 520–62.

Poinar, H. N., et al. 2006. Metagenomics to paleogenomics: Large-scale sequencing of mammoth DNA. *Science* 311: 392–94.

Tautz, D., and Domazet-Lošo, T. (2011). The evolutionary origin of orphan genes. Nat Rev Genet *12*, 692–702.

Turnbaugh, P. J., et al. 2007. The Human Microbiome Project. *Nature* 449: 804–10.

Uetz, P., et al. 2000. A comprehensive analysis of protein-protein interactions in *Saccharomyces cerevisiae. Nature* 403: 623–27.

Van De Peer, Y., Mizrachi, E., and Marchal, K. (2017). The evolutionary significance of polyploidy. Nat Rev Genet *18*, 411–424.

Venter, J. C., et al. 2001. The sequence of the human genome. *Science* 291: 1304–51.

———. 2004. Environmental genome shotgun sequencing of the Sargasso Sea. *Science* 304: 66–74.

Warnecke, F., et al. 2007. Metagenomic and functional analysis of hindgut -microbiota of a wood-feeding higher termite. *Nature* 450: 560–69.

Warren, W. C., et al. 2008. Genome analysis of the platypus reveals unique -signatures of evolution. *Nature* 453: 175–84.

Wienberg, J. 2004. The evolution of eutherian chromosomes. *Curr. Opinion in Gen. Devel.* 14: 657–66.

Chapter 17 Organelle Inheritance and the Evolution of Organelle Genomes

Brown, J. R. 2003. Ancient horizontal gene transfer. *Nat. Rev. Genet.* 4: 121–32.

Burger, G., M. W. Gray, and B. F. Lang. 2003. Mitochondrial genomes: Anything goes. *Trends Genet.* 19: 709–16.

Chase, C. D. 2007. Cytoplasmic male sterility: A window to the world of plant mitochondrial-nuclear interactions. *Trends Genet.* 23: 81–90.

Chen, X. J., and R. A. Butow. 2005. The organization and inheritance of the -mitochondrial genome. *Nat. Rev. Genet.* 6: 815–25.

Embley, T. M., and W. Martin. 2006. Eukaryotic evolution, changes and -challenges. *Nature* 440: 623–30.

Finlayson, C. 2005. Biogeography and evolution of the genus *Homo. Trends Ecol. Evol.* 20: 457–63.

Garrigan, D., and M. F. Hammer. 2006. Reconstructing human origins in the -genomic era. *Nat. Rev. Genet.* 7: 669–80.

Gilson, P. R., et al. 2006. Complete nucleotide sequence of the chlorarachniophyte nucleomorph: Nature's smallest nucleus. *Proc. Natl. Acad. Sci. USA* 103: 9566–71.

Huang, C. Y., M. A. Ayliffe, and J. N. Timmis. 2003. Direct measurement of the transfer rate of chloroplast DNA into the nucleus. *Nature* 422: 72–76.

Kotera, E., M. Tasaka, and T. Shikanai. 2005. A pentatricopeptide repeat protein is essential for RNA editing in chloroplast. *Nature* 433: 326–30.

Lang, B. F., et al. 1997. An ancestral mitochondrial DNA resembling a eubacterial genome in miniature. *Nature* 387: 493–97.

Lehman, N., et al. 1991. Introgression of coyote mitochondrial DNA into -sympatric North American gray wolf populations. *Evolution* 45: 104–19.

Leister, D. 2003. Chloroplast research in the genomic age. *Trends Genet.* 19: 47–56.

Martin, W. 2002. Evolutionary analysis of *Arabidopsis*, cyanobacterial, and chloroplast genomes reveals plastid phylogeny and thousands of cyanobacterial genes in the nucleus. *Proc. Natl. Acad. Sci. USA* 99: 12246–51.

Oda, K., et al. 1992. Gene organization deduced from the complete sequence of liverwort *Marchantia polymorpha* mitochondrial DNA. *J. Mol. Biol.* 223: 1–7.

Prezant, T. R., et al. 1993. Mitochondrial ribosomal RNA mutation associated with both antibiotic-induced and non-syndromic deafness. *Nat. Genet.* 4: 289–94.

Rivera, M. C., et al. 1998. Genomic evidence for two functionally distinct gene classes. *Proc. Natl. Acad. Sci. USA* 95: 6239–44.

Stegemann, S., and R. Bock. 2006. Experimental reconstruction of functional gene transfer from the tobacco plastid genome to the nucleus. *Plant Cell* 18: 2869–78.

Taylor, R. W., and D. M. Turnbull 2005. Mitochondrial DNA mutations in human disease. *Nat. Rev. Genet.* 6: 389–402.

Timmis, J. N., et al. 2004. Endosymbiotic gene transfer: Organelle genomes forge eukaryotic chromosomes. *Nat. Rev. Genet.* 5: 123–35.

Trifunovic, A., et al. 2004. Premature ageing in mice expressing defective -mitochondrial DNA polymerase. *Nature* 429: 417–23.

Wallace, D. C., et al. 1988. Mitochondrial DNA mutation associated with Leber's hereditary optic neuropathy. *Science* 242: 1427–30.

Ward, T. J., et al. 1999. Identification of domestic cattle hybrids in wild cattle and bison species: A general approach using mtDNA markers and the parametric bootstrap. *Animal Conservation* 2: 51–57.

Chapter 18 Developmental Genetics

Bender, W., et al. 1983. Molecular-genetics of the bithorax complex in *Drosophila melanogaster*. *Science* 221: 23–29.

Binns, W., L. F. James, and J. L. Shupe. 1964. Toxicosis of *Veratrum californicum* in ewes and its relationship to a congenital deformity in lambs. *Ann. N.Y. Acad. Sci.* 111: 571–76.

Bowman, J. L., D. R. Smyth, and E. M. Meyerowitz. 1991. Genetic interactions among floral homeotic genes of *Arabidopsis*. *Development* 112: 1–20.

Chen, J. K., et al. 2002. Inhibition of hedgehog signaling by direct binding of -cyclopamine to smoothened. *Genes Dev.* 16: 2743–48.

Coen, E. S., and Meyerowitz, E. M. 1991. The war of the whorls: Genetic interactions controlling flower development. *Nature* 353: 31–37.

De Robertis, E. M., and H. Kuroda. 2004. Dorsal-ventral patterning and neural -induction in *Xenopus* embryos. *Annu. Rev. Cell Dev. Biol.* 20: 285–308.

de Rosa, R., et al. 1999. Hox genes in brachiopods and priapulids and protostome evolution. *Nature* 399: 772–76.

Driever, W., and C. Nusslein-Volhard. 1988. The Bicoid protein determines position in the *Drosophila* embryo in a concentration-dependent manner. *Cell* 54: 95–104.

Driever, W., V. Siegel, and C. Nusslein-Volhard. 1990. Autonomous determination of anterior structures in the early *Drosophila* embryo by the Bicoid -morphogen. *Development* 109: 811–20.

Horvitz, H. R. 2003. Worms, life and death. *Bioscience Reports* 23: 239–69.

Lemons, D., and W. McGinnis. 2006. Genomic evolution of Hox gene clusters. *Science* 313: 1918–22.

Lettice, L. A., et al. 2002. Disruption of a long range *cis*-acting regulator for *Shh* causes preaxial polydactyly. *Proc. Natl. Acad. Sci. USA* 99: 7548–53.

Lewis, E. B. 1978. Gene complex controlling segmentation in *Drosophila*. *Nature* 276: 565–70.

Nanni, L., et al. 1999. The mutational spectrum of the *sonic hedgehog* gene in holoproencephaly: *Shh* mutations cause a significant proportion of autosomal dominant holoproencephaly. *Hum. Mol. Genet.* 8: 2479–88.

Nusslein-Volhard, C., and Wieschaus, E. 1980. Mutations affecting segment -number and polarity in *Drosophila*. *Nature* 287: 795–801.

Shubin, N., C. Tabin, and S. Carroll. 1997. Fossils, genes, and the evolution of -animal limbs. *Nature* 388: 639–48.

———. 2009. Deep homology and the origins of evolutionary novelty. *Nature* 457: 818–23.

Small, S., A. Blair, and M. Levine. 1992. Regulation of *even-skipped* stripe-2 in the *Drosophila* embryo. *EMBO J.* 11: 4047–57.

Sternberg, P. W., and M. Han. 1998. Genetics of RAS signaling in *C. elegans*. *Trends Genet.* 14: 466–72.

Chapter 19 Genetic Analysis of Quantitative Traits

Castle, W. 1916. *Genetics and Eugenics*. Cambridge, MA: Harvard University Press.

deVicente, M. C., and S. D. Tanksley. 1993. QTL analysis of transgressive -segregation in an interspecific tomato cross. *Genetics* 134: 585–96.

Dudley, J. W. 1977. 76 generations of selection for oil and protein percentage in maize. In *Proc. Internat. Conf. on Quant. Gene.*, edited by E. Pollack, O. Kempthorne, and T. Bailey. Ames: Iowa State University Press.

East, E. M. 1910. A Mendelian interpretation of variation that is apparently -continuous. *Am. Nat.* 44: 65–82.

———. 1916. Studies on size inheritance in *Nicotiana*. *Genetics* 1: 161–76.

Fridman, E., et al. 2004. Zooming in on a quantitative trait for tomato yield using interspecific introgressions. *Science* 305: 1786–89.

Geschwind, D.H. 2011. Genetics of autism spectrum disorders. Trends Cog. Sci., 15:409–416.

Hallmayer, J. et al. 2011. Genetic heritability and shared environmental factors among twin pairs with autism. Arch. Gen. Psychiatry, 68: 1095–1102.

Lanktree, M. B., et al. 2011. Meta-analysis of dense gene centric association studies reveals common and uncommon variants associated with height. *Am. J. Hum. Genet.* 88: 6–18.

Laurie, C. C., et al. 2004. The genetic architecture of response to long-term selection for oil concentration in the maize kernel. *Genetics* 168: 2141–55.

Moose, S. D., J. W. Dudley, and T. R. Rocheford. 2004. Maize selection passes the century mark: A unique resource for 21st century genomics. *Trends Plant Sci.* 7: 358–64.

Nilsson-Ehle, H. 1909. Kreuzengsunter-su-chungen an hafer und weizen. *Lunds Univ. Aarskrift, N.F. Atd.*, Ser. 2, 5: 1–122.

Ogura, Y., et al. 2001. A frameshift mutation in *NOD2* associated with susceptibility to Crohn's disease. *Nature* 411: 603–6.

Smoller, J.W. and C. T. Finn. 2003. Family, twin, and adoption studies of bipolar disorder. Am. J. Med. Genet. part C (Semin. Med. Genet.), 123C:48–58.

Sullivan, P.F. et al. 2003. Schizophrenia as a complex trait. Arch. Gen. Psychiatry, 60: 1187–1192.

Tanksley, S. D. 2004. The genetic, developmental, and molecular bases of fruit size and shape variation in tomato. *Plant Cell* 16: S181–89.

Weedon, M. N., et al. 2008. Genome-wide association analysis identifies 20 loci that influence human height. *Nat. Genet.* 40: 575–83.

Wellcome Trust Case Control Consortium. 2007. Genome wide association study of 14,000 cases of seven common diseases and 3,000 shared controls. *Nature* 447: 661–78.

Chapter 20 Population Genetics and Evolution at the Population, Species, and Molecular Levels

Abzhanov, A., M. Protas, B. R. Grant, et al. 2004. *Bmp4* and morphological -variation in beaks in Darwin's finches. *Science* 305: 1462–65.

Cavalli-Sforza, L. L., and W. F. Bodmer. 1971. *The Genetics of Human Populations*. San Francisco: W. H. Freeman and Co.

Cavener, D. R., and M. T. Clegg. 1981. Multigenic response to ethanol in *Drosophila melanogaster*. *Evolution* 35: 1–10.

Crow, J. F. 1986. *Basic Concepts in Population, Quantitative, and Evolutionary Genetics*. New York: W. H. Freeman.

Diamond, J. M., and J. I. Rotter. 1987. Observing the founder effect in human -evolution. *Nature* 329: 105–6.

Dobzhansky, T. 1970. *Genetics of the Evolutionary Process*. New York: Columbia University Press.

Eick, G., and J. W. Thornton. 2011. Evolution of steroid receptors from an -estrogen-sensitive ancestral receptor. *Molec. and Cell. Endocrin.* 334: 31–38.

Elena, S. F., V. S. Cooper, and R. E. Lenski. 1996. Punctuated evolution caused by selection of rare beneficial mutations. *Science* 272: 1802–4.

Freeman, S., and J. C. Herron. 2001. *Evolutionary Analysis*. Upper Saddle River, NJ: Prentice Hall.

Grant, P. R., and B. R. Grant. 2006. Evolution of character displacement in Darwin's finches. *Science* 313: 224–26.

———. 2009. The secondary contact phase of allopatric speciation in Darwin's finches. *Proc. Nat. Acad. Sci. USA* 106: 20141–48.

Green, R. E., et al. 2010. A draft sequence of the Neandertal genome. *Science* 328: 710–22.

Hardy, G. H. 1908. Mendelian proportions in a mixed population. *Science* 28: 49–50.

Lamichhaney, S. et al. 2015. Evolution of Darwin's and their beaks revealed by genome sequence. Nature, 518:371–375

Lamichhaney, S. et al. 2016. A beak size locus in Darwin's finches facilitated character displacement during a drought. Science, 352:470–473.

McKusick, V. A. 2000. Ellis-van Crevald syndrome and the Amish. *Nature Genet.* 24: 203–4.

National Institute of Standards (NIST). "Overview of STR Fact Sheets." Last -updated May 20, 2011. www.cstl.nist.gov/strbase/str_fact.htm.

———. "Material Measurement Laboratory." Last updated May 25, 2011. www.cstl.nist.gov/strbase/fbicore.htm.

Ralls, K., K, Brugger, and J. Ballou. 1979. Inbreeding and juvenile mortality in small populations of ungulates. *Science* 206: 1101–3.

Simonson, T. S., et al. 2010. Genetic evidence for high-altitude adaptation in Tibet. *Science* 329: 72–75.

Slatkin, M. 1987. Gene flow and the geographic structure of natural populations. *Science* 236: 787–92.

Smith, J. M. 1989. *Evolutionary Genetics*. New York: Oxford University Press.

Staub, N.L. Teaching evolutionary mechanisms: Genetic drift and M&M's. BioScience, 52:373–377.

Thornton, J. W. 2001. Evolution of vertebrate steroid receptors from an -ancestral estrogen receptor by ligand exploitation and serial genome expansions. *Proc. Nat. Acad. Sci. USA* 98: 5671–76.

Tishkoff, S. A., F. A. Reed, A. Ranciaro, et al. 2007. Convergent adaptation of -human lactase persistence in Africa and Europe. *Nature Genet.* 39: 31–40.

Vernot, B., and J. M. Akey. 2014. Resurrecting surviving Neandertal lineages from modern human genomes. *Science* 343: 1017–21.

Weinberg, W. 1908. Ueber den nachweis der vererbung beim menschen. *Jahreshefte des Vereins für Vaterländische Naturkunde in Württemburg* 64: 368–82. English translation in Boyer, S. H. 1963. *Papers on Human Genetics*. Englewood Cliffs, NJ: Prentice Hall.

Yi, X., et al. 2010. Sequencing of 50 human exomes reveals adaptation to high -altitude. *Science* 329: 75–78.

Yule, G. U. 1902. Mendel's laws and their probable relations to intra-racial -heredity. *New Phytologist* 1: 193–207.

Application Chapter D Human Evolutionary Genetics

Barbujani, G., Ghirotto, S., and Tassi, F. (2013). Nine things to remember about human genome diversity. Tissue Antigens 82, 155–164.

Beadle, G.W. (1939). Teosinte and the origin of maize. J Hered 30, 245–247.

Bigham, A.W. (2016). Genetics of human origin and evolution: high-altitude adaptations. Curr Opin Genet Dev 41, 8–13.

Campbell, M.C., and Tishkoff, S.A. (2010). The Evolution of Human Genetic and Phenotypic Variation in Africa. Curr Biol 20, R166–R173.

Cann, R. L., M. Stoneking, and A. C. Wilson. 1987. Mitochondrial DNA and -human evolution. *Nature* 325: 31–36.

Cavalli-Sforza, L. L. 2005. The Human Genome Diversity Project: Past, present, and future. *Nat. Rev. Genet.* 6: 333–40.

The Chimpanzee Sequencing and Analysis Consortium. 2005. Initial sequence of the chimpanzee genome and comparison with the human genome. *Nature* 437: 69–87.

Doebley, J. (2004). The genetics of maize evolution. Annu Rev Genet 38, 37–59.

Fan, S.H., Hansen, M.E.B., Lo, Y., and Tishkoff, S.A. (2016). Going global by adapting local: A review of recent human adaptation. Science 354, 54–59.

Fu, Q.M., Posth, C., Hajdinjak, M., Petr, M., Mallick, S., Fernandes, D., Furtwangler, A., Haak, W., Meyer, M., Mittnik, A., et al. (2016). The genetic history of Ice Age Europe. Nature 534, 200–+.

Green, R. E., et al. 2010. A draft sequence of the Neanderthal genome. *Science* 328: 710–22.

Henn, B.M., Gignoux, C.R., Jobin, M., Granka, J.M., Macpherson, J.M., Kidd, J.M., Rodriguez-Botigue, L., Ramachandran, S., Hon, L., Brisbin, A., et al. (2011). Hunter-gatherer genomic diversity suggests a southern African origin for modern humans. P Natl Acad Sci USA 108, 5154–5162.

Hubbard, T.D., Murray, I.A., Bisson, W.H., Sullivan, A.P., Sebastian, A., Perry, G.H., Jablonski, N.G., and Perdew, G.H. (2016). Divergent Ah Receptor Ligand Selectivity during Hominin Evolution. Mol Biol Evol 33, 2648–2658.

Huerta-Sanchez, E., Jin, X., Asan, Bianba, Z., Peter, B.M., Vinckenbosch, N., Liang, Y., Yi, X., He, M.Z., Somel, M., *et al.* (2014). Altitude adaptation in Tibetans caused by introgression of Denisovan-like DNA. Nature 512, 194–+.

Jakobsson, M., Scholz, S.W., Scheet, P., Gibbs, J.R., VanLiere, J.M., Fung, H.C., Szpiech, Z.A., Degnan, J.H., Wang, K., Guerreiro, R., et al. (2008). Genotype, haplotype and copy-number variation in worldwide human populations. Nature 451, 998–1003.

Lachance, J., Vernot, B., Elbers, C.C., Ferwerda, B., Froment, A., Bodo, J.M., Lema, G., Fu, W.Q., Nyambo, T.B., Rebbeck, T.R., et al. (2012). Evolutionary History and Adaptation from High-Coverage Whole-Genome Sequences of Diverse African Hunter-Gatherers. Cell 150, 457–469.

Lazaridis, I., Nadel, D., Rollefson, G., Merrett, D.C., Rohland, N., Mallick, S., Fernandes, D., Novak, M., Gamarra, B., Sirak, K., et al. (2016). Genomic insights into the origin of farming in the ancient Near East. Nature 536, 419–+.

Lazaridis, I., Patterson, N., Mittnik, A., Renaud, G., Mallick, S., Kirsanow, K., Sudmant, P.H., Schraiber, J.G., Castellano, S., Lipson, M., et al. (2014). Ancient human genomes suggest three ancestral populations for present-day Europeans. Nature 513, 409–+.

Malaspinas, A.S., Westaway, M.C., Muller, C., Sousa, V.C., Lao, O., Alves, I., Bergstrom, A., Athanasiadis, G., Cheng, J.Y., Crawford, J.E., et al. (2016). A genomic history of Aboriginal Australia. Nature 538, 207–+.

Mallick, S., Li, H., Lipson, M., Mathieson, I., Gymrek, M., Racimo, F., Zhao, M.Y., Chennagiri, N., Nordenfelt, S., Tandon, A., et al. (2016). The Simons Genome Diversity Project: 300 genomes from 142 diverse populations. Nature 538, 201–+.

Nielsen, R., Akey, J.M., Jakobsson, M., Pritchard, J.K., Tishkoff, S., and Willerslev, E. (2017). Tracing the peopling of the world through genomics. Nature 541, 302–310.

Pagani, L., Lawson, D.J., Jagoda, E., Morseburg, A., Eriksson, A., Mitt, M., Clemente, F., Hudjashov, G., DeGiorgio, M., Saag, L., et al. (2016). Genomic analyses inform on migration events during the peopling of Eurasia. Nature 538, 238–+.

Pickrell, J.K., and Reich, D. (2014). Toward a new history and geography of human genes informed by ancient DNA. Trends Genet 30, 377–389.

Poznik, G.D., Xue, Y.L., Mendez, F.L., Willems, T.F., Massaia, A., Sayres, M.A.W., Ayub, Q., McCarthy, S.A., Narechania, A., Kashin, S., et al. (2016). Punctuated bursts in human male demography inferred from 1,244 worldwide Y-chromosome sequences. Nat Genet 48, 593–+.

Sankararaman, S., Mallick, S., Patterson, N., and Reich, D. (2016). The Combined Landscape of Denisovan and Neanderthal Ancestry in Present-Day Humans. Curr Biol 26, 1241–1247.

Ségurel, L., and Bon, C. (2017). On the Evolution of Lactase Persistence in Humans. Annual Review of Genomics and Human Genetics 18, 8.1–8.23.

Simonti, C.N., Vernot, B., Bastarache, L., Bottinger, E., Carrell, D.S., Chisholm, R.L., Crosslin, D.R., Hebbring, S.J., Jarvik, G.P., Kullo, I.J., et al. (2016). The phenotypic legacy of admixture between modern humans and Neandertals. Science 351, 737–741.

Tishkoff, S.A., Reed, F.A., Friedlaender, F.R., Ehret, C., Ranciaro, A., Froment, A., Hirbo, J.B., Awomoyi, A.A., Bodo, J.M., Doumbo, O., et al. (2009). The Genetic Structure and History of Africans and African Americans. Science 324, 1035–1044.

Tobler, R., Rohrlach, A., Soubrier, J., Bover, P., Llamas, B., Tuke, J., Bean, N., Abdullah-Highfold, A., Agius, S., O'Donoghue, A., et al. (2017). Aboriginal mitogenomes reveal 50,000 years of regionalism in Australia. Nature 544, 180–+.

Xue, Y.L., Chen, Y., Ayub, Q., Huang, N., Ball, E.V., Mort, M., Phillips, A.D., Shaw, K., Stenson, P.D., Cooper, D.N., et al. (2012). Deleterious- and Disease-Allele Prevalence in Healthy Individuals: Insights from Current Predictions, Mutation Databases, and Population-Scale Resequencing. Am J Hum Genet 91, 1022–1032.

Application Chapter E Forensic Genetics

Ball, C.A. et al. 2013. Ethnicity estimate white paper. AncestryDNA.com

Birney, E. 2016. Epigenome-wide association studies and the interpretation of disease-omics. *PloS Genetics*, DOI:10.1371/journal .pgen.1006105.

Brettell, T. A. et al. 2009. Forensic science. Analytical Chem., 81:4695–4711.

Budowle, B. et al. 2001. CODIS STR loci data for 41 sample populations. *J. Forensic Sci.*, 46:453–489.

Baur, M. P, et al. 1986. No fallacies in the formulation of the paternity index. *Am. J. Hum. Genet.*, 39:528–536.

Cecilio, L. and M. W. Bonatto. 2015. The prevalence of HLA DQ2 and DQ8 in patients with celiac disease, in family and in general population. *ABCD arq. Bras. Cir. Dig.* 28: 183–185.

Cifuentes, L. O. et al. 2006. Probability of exclusion in paternity testing: time to reassess. *J. Forensic Sci.*, 51:349–350.

Cobain, I. 2016. Killer breakthrough – the day DNA evidence first nailed a murderer. https://www.theguardian.com/uk-news/2016/jun/07.

Federal Bureau of Investigation. Combined DNA index system (CODIS). https://www.fbi.gov/services/laboratory/biometric-analysis/codis.

Gill, P. et al. 2005. Forensic applications of DNA "fingerprints". *Nature*, 318:577–579.

Green, P. H. and C. Cellier. 2007. Celiac disease. *N. Engl. J. Med.*, 357: 1731–1743.

Jobling, M. A. and P. Gill. 2004. Encoded evidence: DNA in forensic analysis. *Nature Rev. Genet.*, 5:739–750.

Masunaga, S. 2017, What the new, FDA-approved 23andMe genetic health risk reports can, and can't tell you. http://www.latimes.com/business/la-fi-23andme-reports-20170414.

Spinney, L. 2014. The forgetting gene. *Nature*, 510:26–28.

Appendix: Answers

Chapter 1

2. Protein, not DNA, was the focus of efforts to understand heredity before this discovery. Only after this discovery was serious attention turned to understanding DNA structure and function. Whereas the complexity of protein structure confounded thinking about mechanisms of inheritance, DNA structure provided profound insight into the mechanism of heredity, suggesting a simple, elegant mechanism for duplication (inheritance), change (mutation and evolution), and phenotype specification (coding). The finding that DNA is universal facilitated rapid progress because study results from all organisms were now directly related. This also fostered the development of recombinant DNA technologies in bacteria and bacteriophage, which led to the explosion of biological information that excites and confounds us today.

4. Evolution states that all life descended from a common ancestor, which passed its genes and the mechanisms by which those genes were used to its descendants. These mechanisms would include the structure of nucleotides, the structure of DNA, the enzymes that replicate and read DNA, the enzymes that translate mRNA into amino acid sequences, and many more. Any change to one of these components would be harmful, slowing or preventing reproduction, and would be removed by natural selection (mountains of experimental evidence demonstrate that mutations in genes encoding basic genetic machinery are lethal). Thus, once established as the genetic material, DNA would be maintained as the genetic material by natural selection and therefore would be expected to be found as the genetic material in all existing organisms.

6. *Genotype* refers to the genetic makeup of a cell or organism, whereas *phenotype* refers to observable characteristics of the cell or organism, such as appearance, physiology, and behavior. The genotype of an organism is part of what determines the phenotype of the organism; however, environment also plays a role in the organism's phenotype. The genotype is heritable, and, therefore, its contribution to phenotype will be inherited. The aspects of phenotype that are due to environment are not heritable.

8. The modern synthesis of evolution is the reconciliation of Darwin's evolutionary theory with the findings of modern genetics. Darwin's theory proposed that all evolution was adaptive. Genetic studies on mutation and genetic recombination initially argued against the importance of natural selection as an agent for change because mutation and recombination were nonadaptive. The modern synthesis stated that evolution is due to the combined action of adaptive and nonadaptive evolutionary forces. In particular, the modern synthesis explained how mutation and recombination could provide the raw material (new genotypes and phenotypes) on which natural selection acts.

10a. *Transcription* is the synthesis of RNA by RNA polymerase. The RNA is complementary to the strand of DNA that was used as the template for transcription.

10b. An *allele* is a specific form of a gene or genetic locus.

10c. The *central dogma of biology* originally stated that genetic information flows from DNA to RNA (by transcription) and from RNA to protein (by translation). A point of emphasis of this dogma was that information does not flow in the reverse direction and has been modified to account for reverse transcription.

10d. *Translation* is the synthesis of a polypeptide using the information in an mRNA. *Translation* and *protein synthesis* are synonyms.

10e. *DNA replication* is the process by which DNA is copied by DNA polymerase.

10f. A *gene* is a segment of DNA that contains all the information necessary for its proper transcription, including the promoter, transcribed region, and termination signals.

10g. A *chromosome* is a heritable molecule composed of DNA and protein that typically contains genes.

10h. The term *antiparallel* refers to the orientation of the two strands of nucleic acid in a double-stranded nucleic acid (RNA or DNA). Each end of the double-stranded nucleic acid will contain the 5′ end of one strand and the 3′ end of the other.

10i. *Phenotype* refers to the observable characteristics of an organism, which include morphology, physiology, and molecular composition. The phenotype of an organism is a product of the interaction between its genotype and its environment.

10j. *Complementary base pair* refers to the two nucleotides on opposite, antiparallel strands of a double-stranded nucleic acid, which are hydrogen bonded to each other. One nucleotide contains a purine base that makes hydrogen bond to the pyrimidine base that is part of the other nucleotide.

10k. *Nucleic acid strand polarity* refers to the orientation of the nucleotides along a single strand of nucleic acid. One end of the strand terminates at the 3′ hydroxyl group of a ribose (or deoxyribose) sugar, whereas the other strand terminates at the 5′ phosphate group on the sugar. These are commonly referred to as the 3′ and 5′ ends of the strand.

10l. *Genotype* refers to the genetic makeup of an organism. The genotype can refer either to the organism's entire genetic makeup or to the genetic information at only one or a few loci.

10m. *Natural selection* is the process by which populations and species evolve and diverge through differential rates of survival and reproduction of members that are due to their inherited differences.

10n. *Mutation* is the process that generates new genetic variety through change to existing alleles.

10o. *Modern synthesis of evolution* is the term applied to the reconciliation of modern genetic analysis with Darwin's theory of evolution by natural selection.

12. The template DNA strand is complementary and antiparallel to the RNA transcript. The coding DNA strand is parallel and identical to the mRNA transcript, except that thymidine is located in the DNA strand where uridine is located in RNA.

16. The 5′ end is a phosphate group. The 3′ end is a hydroxyl group. A phosphodiester bond is a covalent bond that joins nucleotides in a strand of nucleic acid.

18. The central dogma is a description of the flow of genetic information. The flow is unidirectional, from DNA to RNA to protein. The process by which information flows from DNA to RNA is called transcription. Transcription is the synthesis of RNA by RNA polymerase. The RNA is complementary to the strand of DNA that was used as the template for transcription. The flow of information from RNA to protein is called translation. Translation is the synthesis of a polypeptide using the information in an mRNA.

20a. The mRNA sequence is 5′-UUCCAUGUC-3′.

20b. The amino acid sequence is Phe-His-Val.

22a. Six clades

22b. A backbone (They are all vertebrates.)

22c. The characteristics that are shared by primates and mammals are (1) backbone, (2) four legs, and (3) fur and milk. The characteristic that distinguishes primates from other mammals is opposable thumbs.

26. The samples are (1) double-stranded DNA, (2) single-stranded RNA, (3) double-stranded RNA, and (4) single-stranded DNA.

28. Mammals

Chapter 2

2. The genotype ratio will be 1/2 *BB* and 1/2 *BB*. The phenotype will be all B.

8a. False. The expected *phenotype* ratio is 9/16 : 3/16 : 3/16 : 1/16, assuming simple dominance and independent assortment of genetic loci (*AaBb* × *AaBb*). There are nine different genotypes, and the genotype ratio is 1/16 (*AABB*) : 2/16 (*AABb*) : 1/16 (*AAbb*) : 2/16 (*AaBB*) : 4/16 (*AaBb*) : 2/16 (*Aabb*) : 1/16 (*aaBB*) : 2/16 (*aaBb*) : 1/16 (*aabb*).

8b. True

8c. True

8d. False. The law of *independent assortment* is of primary importance in predicting the outcome of dihybrid and trihybrid crosses. The law of segregation is also necessary but not sufficient.

8e. False. Reciprocal crosses that produce identical results indicate that the traits being studied are autosomal.

8f. False. The law of segregation predicts that she will produce two gamete genotypes with respect to her albinism gene at equal frequency.

8g. True

8h(1). True

8h(2). False. There will be 1/16 *AABB*, 1/16 *AAbb*, 1/16 *aaBB*, and 1/16 *aabb*. All four genotypes will be true-breeding; therefore, 1/4 of the progeny will be true-breeding.

8h(3). False. Being "heterozygous at one or both loci" excludes only the progeny that are homozygous at both loci. In part (b) of this question, it was calculated that 1/4 will be homozygous at both loci; therefore, 3/4 will be heterozygous at one or both loci (2/16 *AABB*, 2/16 *AaBB*, 4/16 *AaBb*, 2/16 *Aabb*, and 2/16 *aaBB*).

10a. Mottled is the dominant phenotype.

10b. The results are consistent with autosomal inheritance.

10c. 1/2 of the F_2 of both crosses are expected to be homozygous, and 1/2 are expected to be heterozygous.

10d. One cross would be a test cross, and the other would be a backcross. The test cross would be the mottled F_2 to a true-breeding leopard individual. The backcross would be the mottled F_2 to one of its parents (both are heterozygotes).

12a. The mode of fur color inheritance in these crosses is likely to be a single gene with two alleles controlling fur color, and black will be dominant to brown.

12b. Assign the letter *B* for the black allele and *b* for the brown allele. The brown male must be *bb*. The black female in the first cross must be *Bb*. The black female in the second cross must be *BB*.

14a. The results suggest that the inheritances of color and fin shape are each due to segregation of two alleles at a single gene.

14b. The results indicate that gold is dominant to black and that split fin is dominant to single fin.

14c. The chi-square value for color is 0.061, which corresponds to a *P* value between 0.7 and 0.9. The chi-square value for fin shape is 0.05, which corresponds to a *P* value between 0.7 and 0.9. Neither *P* value is less than 0.05, which indicates that the hypothesis of one gene with two alleles for color and fin shape cannot be rejected.

16b. Of the F_2 progeny, 3/4 will have yellow seeds, 1/4 will have green seeds, 3/4 will have round seeds, and 1/4 will have wrinkled seeds.

16c. 9/16 yellow, round; 3/16 yellow, wrinkled; 3/16 green, round; 1/16 green, wrinkled

20. The χ^2 value is 0.591. There is one degree of freedom (df = 1), therefore the *P* value is greater than 0.05 and the hypothesis cannot be rejected.

22a. 0.132

22b. 0.178

22c. 0.822

24a. 0.422

24b. 0.0313

24c. 0.4219

24d. 0.0469

26. 1800 full wings and gray bodies, 600 full wings and ebony bodies, 600 vestigial wings and gray bodies, 200 vestigial wings and ebony bodies

28a. Tall and white are the dominant traits, whereas short and blue are recessive.

28b. The expected phenotypic distribution in the F_2 is 9/16 tall, white; 3/16 tall, blue; 3/16 short, white; and 1/16 short, blue.

28c. The hypothesis being tested in this experiment is that the two pea plant varieties differ at two independently assorting genetic loci, and two alleles show simple dominance at each locus.

28d. The chi-square value is 0.78, which corresponds to a *P* value between 0.9 and 0.7, indicating that the hypothesis cannot be rejected (the results are consistent with the hypothesis).

30a. 9/16

30b. 3/8

30c. 3/4

32. 0.988

34. The probability of five unaffected children is 0.237, of four unaffected and one affected is 0.396, of three unaffected and two affected is 0.264, of two unaffected and three affected is 0.0879, of one unaffected and four affected is 0.0146, and of all five affected is 0.000977.

36 *Experiment One:* (1) Cross the true-breeding short, brown-furred and long, white-furred guinea pigs to create an F_1 population; (2) test that they are dihybrids by crossing male F_1 with female F_1 to produce F_2 guinea pigs; (3) cross both sets of pure-breeding parents to create 24 F_1 progeny and intercross all the F_1 (12 crosses) to produce 144 F_2; (4) compare observed phenotypic distribution with expected results. *Experiment Two:* (1) Cross the F_1 with their long, white-furred parent to produce backcrossed guinea pigs; (2) cross two of the F_1 males with their long, white-haired mother, thus producing 24 progeny; and (3) cross the long, white-haired male guinea pig with all of the short, brown-haired female F_1, which would produce 144 progeny.

38. Cross the parents to produce (*FfRrTt*) trihybrids, and self-fertilize the F_1 to create an F_2 population that will include all possible phenotypes and genotypes. Among the F_2, 3/64 will produce yellow, pear-shaped tomatoes and have axial flowers (*ffrr*). To determine which of these plants are *TT*, self-fertilize them and identify the plants that breed true for axial flower position.

40a. All four adults are heterozygous carriers of alkaptonuria (*Aa*).

40b. 1/1500

40c. 1/4

40d. 3/4

40e. The probability that one of their children with alkaptonuria will have a child with alkaptonuria is dependent on the genotype of their child's mate. If their child's mate has no family history of alkaptonuria, then the probability is about 1/500. If their child's mate has a close relative with the disorder, then the probability increases dramatically. For example, if their child's mate's grandmother had alkaptonuria, then the probability increases to 1/4.

44. The genotypic ratios will be 4/9 *FFpp*, 4/9 *Ffpp*, and 1/9 *ffpp*. The phenotypic ratio will be 8/9 feathered legs and single comb, and 1/9 no leg feathers and single comb.

Chapter 3

2a. 48 chromosomes

2b. 48 chromosomes

2c. 24 chromosomes (23 autosomes and 1 sex chromosome)

2d. 48 chromosomes

2e. 48 chromosomes

2f. 48 chromosomes

4. Cohesion opposes the pulling forces attempting to separate sister chromatids until all pairs of sister chromatids are attached to microtubules from opposite poles of the spindle (i.e., bipolar attachment). Premature, as well as delayed, sister chromatid separation can cause sister chromatids to partition together instead of separating during anaphase and can lead to errors in chromosome segregation. Sister chromatid cohesion is due to cohesin, a protein complex that binds to sister chromatids and attaches them to each other. When all pairs of sister chromatids are under the tension generated by bipolar attachment and sister chromatid cohesion, the protease separase is activated. Separase cleaves a component of cohesin, which simultaneously ends cohesion on all pairs of sister chromatids and allows sister chromatids to be pulled toward opposite poles of the spindle.

8. Anaphase II

10. A normal human female nucleus contains one Barr body, whereas a normal male nucleus contains no Barr bodies.

12a. *Dd*

12b. 50%

12c. There is no chance that her daughter will have OTD, but there is a 1/2 or 50% chance that her daughter will be a carrier for OTD.

12d. *dY*

12e. 1/2 of the daughters and 1/2 of the sons will have OTD.

14a. The male parent was M^+Y and P^+p^- and the female was M^+m^- and P^+p^-.

14b. Among the females with purple eyes, half are M^+m^- and p^-p^- and half are M^+M^+ and p^-p^-. Males with purple eyes and miniature wings are m-Y and p^-p^-.

16. The unusual number of Barr bodies seen in the rare male and female infants is the result of nondisjunction during meiosis, which creates abnormal gametes containing an additional X chromosome or lacking an X chromosome.

18. In female carriers that show symptoms of an X-linked recessive trait, X-inactivation must have occurred such that wild-type gene expression was insufficient for normal development. The symptoms are less severe in these symptomatic female carriers because they express some level of the wild-type allele.

22. For cross A, all males are barred-feathered, 1/2 of the females are barred-feathered and 1/2 are nonbarred. For cross B, 1/2 males are barred, 1/2 males are nonbarred, 1/2 females are barred, and 1/2 are nonbarred.

24a. The reciprocal crosses produced different results, which is diagnostic for sex-linked traits.

24b. The female is the heterogametic sex (ZW), whereas males are homogametic (ZZ). Black spot is dominant, and nonspotted is recessive. Using Z-linked alleles designated *B* for black-spot and *b* for nonspotted, the parents of cross I are *Bb* male and *b*W female. Their progeny are 1/4 black-spot males (*Bb*), 1/4 nonspotted males (*bb*), 1/4 black-spot females (*B*W), and 1/4 nonspotted females (*b*W). For cross II, the parents are a *bb* male and a *B*W female. Their progeny are approximately 1/2 *Bb* males and 1/2 *b*W females.

26. Rare sex-reversed males carry an altered X chromosome that contains a fragment of the Y chromosome including the *SRY* gene. Thus, they develop male sex characteristics yet lack a Y chromosome. Rare sex-reversed females carry an altered Y chromosome the lacks the *SRY* gene. Thus, they develop female sex characteristics even though they have a Y chromosome.

28a. Female is *ECec; Vv* and the male is *ecY; Vv*.

28b. The parents are *ECec; Vv Ee* female and *ECY; Vv Ee* male.

28c. The parents are *ECec; Vv ee* female and *ecY; Vv Ee* male.

30. The results suggest recessive inheritance because the mother in the first mating is not affected but has affected children. The results differ from those predicted for autosomal recessive inheritance because the second mating yields all males with one phenotype and all females with the other.

Chapter 4

2. Epistasis and pleiotropy can be distinguished by inheritance patterns in pedigrees or from crosses. If the inheritance pattern of one phenotype indicates that more than one gene is segregating, then epistasis is occurring. If

two or more phenotypes are inherited together in a pattern, then pleiotropy is occurring.

4a. The bacteria in the 12 colonies that grew on minimal medium are prototrophs, whereas those in the 3 colonies that could not grow on minimal medium were auxotrophs.

4b. The bacteria in the three colonies that could not grow on minimal medium but could grow on minimal medium plus serine are serine-requiring auxotrophs. They carry mutations in one or more genes required for the biosynthesis of serine.

4c. Mutant 1 carries a mutation in the gene coding for a component of enzyme C, mutant 2 carries a mutation in the gene coding for a component of enzyme A, and mutant 3 carries a mutation in the gene coding for enzyme B.

6. Child b's parents must be 1. Child a's parents could be 1 or 3; however, since child b's parents are 1, child a's parents must be 3. Child c's parents could be 3 or 4; however, since child a's parents are 3, child c's parents must be 4. Child d's parents could be 2, 3, or 4; however, since child a's parents are 3 and child c's parents are 4, child d's parents must be 2.

10a. At the B locus, one parent was *Bb* and the other was *bb*. At the D locus, one parent was *Dd* and the other was *dd*.

10b. One parent was *BbDd* (brown) and the other was *bbDd* (yellow).

10c. At the B locus, one parent was *BB* and the other parent could have had any genotype (*BB, Bb,* or *bb*). At the D locus, one parent was *Dd* and the other was *dd*.

12a. One parent was *BBDdCc* and the other was *DdCc*. Any genotype is possible at the B locus.

12b. The parents were *BbddCc* × *bbddCc*.

12c. Both parents were *BbDdCc*.

12d. The parents were both *Bb* at the *B* locus. Between the two parents, there was a *DD* and a *CC* locus, but these need not have been in the same parent. The other *D* and *C* loci could have any genotype.

14. The F_2 will be 1/4 red, 1/2 pink, and 1/4 ivory.

16. 2/3 short stature and short limbs and 1/3 normal stature and limbs

18a. Pure-breeding red petunias are *aaBB*.

18b. Pure-breeding blue petunias are *AAbb*.

18c. The phenotypic distribution in the F_2 will be 9/16 purple, 3/16 red, 3/16 blue, and 1/16 white.

20a. Yes, there is evidence for variable expressivity in this pedigree. Variable expressivity indicates that individuals with the same mutant genotype vary in severity of mutant phenotype. In this pedigree, some affected individuals have two thumbs affected whereas others have only one thumb affected.

20b. Yes, there is evidence of incomplete penetrance. Incomplete penetrance indicates that not all individuals with a mutant genotype show the mutant phenotype. In this pedigree, IV-4 and IV-5 are affected children of unaffected parents, therefore at least one of their parents has the mutant allele but not a mutant phenotype.

22a. Genetic heterogeneity

22b. There are five complementation groups: Group 1 is defined by mutations 1, 3, and 7; Group 2 is defined by mutations 4 and 8; Group 3 is defined by mutations 5, 6, and 10 and Group 4 is defined by mutation 2. Mutation 9 fails to complement any of the other mutants and may represent complementation group 5.

24a. The parental strains are *AAbb* and *aaBB*.

24b. The phenotypic distribution will be 9/16 blue (*A_B_*), 6/16 purple (*A_bb + aaB_*), and 1/16 red (*aabb*).

24c. The progeny of the backcross of the F_1 to the *AAbb* parent will be 1/2 blue (*AABb* and *AaBb*) and 1/2 purple (*AAbb* and *Aabb*) progeny. The progeny of the backcross of the F_1 to the *aaBB* parent will be 1/2 blue (*AaBB* and *AaBb*) and 1/2 purple (*aaBB* and *aaBb*).

26a. The results of these crosses indicate that two genes control squash fruit color. $Y_1 \times G_1$ produces all yellow F_1, which produce 3/4 yellow and 1/4 green F_2. Green is recessive and the 3:1 ratio suggests segregation of alleles of a single gene. $Y_2 \times G_1$ produces all green F_1, which produces 3/4 green and 1/4 yellow. Here, yellow is recessive and the 3:1 ratio suggests segregation of alleles at a single gene. $Y_1 \times Y_2$ produces all yellow F_1, which produces 13/16 yellow and 3/16 green. The sixteenths in the F_2 suggests that alleles at two genes are segregating and that the two genes segregating in the first two crosses are different.

26b. In cross I, Y_1 is *AABB*, and G_1 is *aaBB*. Their yellow F_1 progeny are *AaBB*, and their F_2 are 3/4 yellow (*A_BB*) and 1/4 green (*aaBB*). In cross II, Y_2 is *aabb*, G_1 is *aaBB*, their green F_1 are *aaBb*, and their F_2 are 3/4 green (*aaB_*) and 1/4 yellow (*aabb*). The F_1 of $Y_1 \times Y_2$ resulting from cross III are *AaBb* and their F_2 are 9/16 yellow (*A_B_*), 3/16 yellow (*A_bb*), 3/16 green (*aaB_*), and 1/16 yellow (*aabb*).

26c. The progeny will be 1/2 yellow (*AaBB* and *AaBb*) and 1/2 green (*aaBB* and *aaBb*).

28a. All the mutants are temperature-sensitive mutants, carrying a mutant allele of a gene required for normal growth at 37°C. The typical mechanistic explanation of this is that the gene is required for growth at all temperatures, and the mutant allele is functional at 25°C but not 37°C (an alternative explanation is that the gene is required only at 37°C). This explains the five mutants that cannot grow at 37°C. For the two mutants that grow slowly at 37°C, the alleles probably retain partial function at 37°C.

28b. This study identifies three complementation groups: Group 1 is defined by A, D and F, Group 2 is defined by B and G, and Group 3 is defined by C and E.

30a. The chi-square value is

$$\frac{(22 - 25)^2}{25} + \frac{(23 - 25)^2}{25} + \frac{(55 - 50)^2}{50} = 1.02.$$ There are three phenotypic classes; therefore, this calculation has two degrees of freedom. A chi-square value of 1.02 with 2 df gives a P value between 0.5 and 0.7; therefore, the results are consistent with a 1:2:1 hypothesis, and that hypothesis cannot be rejected.

30b. The chi-square value is

$$\frac{(22 - 18.75)^2}{18.75} + \frac{(55 - 56)^2}{55} + \frac{(23 - 25)^2}{25} = 0.75.$$ There are three phenotypic classes; this calculation has two degrees of freedom. A chi-square value of 0.75 with 2 df gives a P value between 0.5 and 0.7; therefore, the results are consistent with a 9:4:3 hypothesis, and that hypothesis cannot be rejected.

30c. Neither hypothesis can be rejected based on the chi-square analysis.

30d. Self-fertilize all the purple progeny and determine the proportion that breed true. If 1:2:1 is correct, all purple plants will breed true. If 9:4:3 is correct, then 2/3 of the purple plants will not breed true (i.e., they will produce some whites).

32. Strains 1 and 2 are homozygous for mutations in the same gene, *A*, that causes albinism. Strain 3 is homozygous for a mutation in a different gene, *B*, which causes albinism. Strains 1 and 2 are *aaBB*, as are the F_1 and F_2 of cross A. Strain 3 is *AAbb*. The F_1 of cross B and cross C are *AaBb*. The F_2 of cross B and cross C are 9/16 *A_B_* (pigmented), 3/16 *A_bb* (albino), 3/16 *aaB_* (albino), and 1/16 *aabb* (albino).

Chapter 5

2a. Parental: 41% *DR*, 41% *dr*; recombinant: 9% *Dr*, 9% *dR*

2b. Parental: 41% *Dr*, 41% *dR*; recombinant: 9% *DR*, 9% *dr*

4. *E* and *H* are not genetically linked, because a single crossover in every meiosis results in production of equal proportions of *EH*, *Eh*, *eH*, and *eh* gametes. *EH* and *eh* are parental gametes, whereas *Eh* and *eH* are recombinant gametes. The percentage of parental gametes is the same as the percentage of recombinant gametes, which is 50%.

6a. Yes, the *y* and *w* genes are expected to show linkage because they are less than 50 map units (m.u.) apart.

6b. Yes, *y* is expected to assort independently of *f* because *y* and *f* are more than 50 m.u. apart. The same applies to *w* and *f*.

6c. There will be 24.625% of each of the following progeny types: gray with red eyes and forked bristles, gray with red eyes and normal bristles,

yellow with white eyes and forked bristles, and yellow with white eyes and normal bristles. There will be 0.375% of each of the following types: gray with white eyes and forked bristles, gray with white eyes and normal bristles, yellow with red eyes and forked bristles, and yellow with red eyes and normal bristles.

6d. The female is heterozygous at *y*, *w*, and *f*, and the male is hemizygous recessive. Consider the linked *y* and *w* loci first. The *y* and *w* genes are 1.5 m.u. apart, so the females will make 0.4925 of each parental gamete type, which are y^+w^+ and y^-w^-. They will make 0.0075 of each recombinant gamete type, which are y^+w^- and y^-w^+. The *f* gene is unlinked to *y* and *w*, so its alleles assort independently of *y* and *w*; 0.50 of each y^-w^- genotype receives an f^+ allele and 0.50 receives an *f* allele. The fraction of $y^+w^+f^+$ is $0.4925 \times 0.5 = 0.24625$. The same is true for y^+w^+f, $y^-w^-f^+$, and y^-w^-f. The fraction of $y^+w^-f^+$ is $0.0075 \times 0.50 = 0.00375$. The same is true for $y^+w^-f^-$, $y^-w^+f^+$, and $y^-w^+f^-$.

8a. See figure.

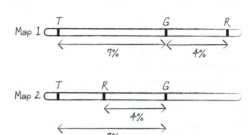

8b. A trihybrid organism with dominant alleles on one chromosome and recessive alleles on the homologous chromosome (*GRT/grt*) could be test crossed to a pure-breeding recessive (*grt/grt*). The number of test-cross progeny in each outcome category can be used to determine which genetic map is correct.

10. Syntenic genes that are separated by 50 map units or more will assort independently because there will be one or more crossovers between them per meiosis.

12a. To measure distance between *Y* and *Lz*, cross a *yll/y^+l^+* female to a *yl/Y* male. The progeny should be 36% (360/1000) yellow lozenge, 36% (360/1000) gray normal eyes, 14% (140/1000) yellow normal eyes, and 14% gray lozenge eyes. To measure the distance between *Lz* and *F*, cross an *lfl^+f^+* female to an *lf/Y* male. The progeny will be 34% (340/1000) lozenge forked bristles, 34% (340/1000) normal eyes and normal bristles, 16% (160/1000) normal eyes with forked bristles, and 16% (160/1000) with lozenge eyes and normal bristles.

12b. No cross can demonstrate genetic linkage between genes *Y* and *F* because the recombination frequency between genes *Y* and *Lz* plus that between *Lz* and *F* is greater than 50%; therefore, the percent recombination between *Y* and *F* in any cross will be 50%.

12c. Syntenic genes (genes on the same chromosome) that are separated by more than 50 map units do not display genetic linkage and, therefore, assort independently.

14a. Nail–patella syndrome (NPS) is a dominant trait.

14b. Yes, NPS appears to segregate with blood type A in this pedigree, indicating genetic linkage between these traits.

14c. I-1 is I^On/I^On, I-2 is I^AN/I^On, II-2 is I^On/I^On, II-4 is I^AN/I^On, II-6 is I^AN/I^On, II-7 is I^On/I^On, and II-9 is I^AN/I^On.

14d. III-6 is I^ON/I^On and III-8 is I^On/I^On. Even though III-6 and III-8 are both *O* blood type, III-6 has NPS because he inherited the recombinant chromosome, I^ON, from his mother, whereas III-8 inherited the nonrecombinant I^On from her mother.

14e. The genotypes of III-11 and III-12 cannot be unambiguously determined because they have type A blood and both of their parents are I^AI^O. Thus, either or both could be I^AI^A or I^AI^O. For this reason, it is not clear whether III-11 and III-12 are parental-type or recombinant-type progeny.

16a. The order is *G T L*.

16b. The recombination frequencies are 0.139 between G and T, 0.088 between T and L, and 0.214 between G and L.

16c. The recombination frequency for G and L is less than for G and T plus T and L because the double-crossover progeny do not appear to be recombinant for G and L and, therefore, are not counted.

16d. The interference value (I) is 0.49.

16e. The meaning of $I = 0.49$ is that only half of the expected number of double-crossover progeny were observed. This indicates that a meiotic cell undergoing a crossover between G and T is about half as likely to also have a crossover occur between T and L. Similarly, a crossover between T and L reduces the likelihood of a crossover between G and T.

18a. Yes, the data provides strong support for linkage between Rh and elliptocytosis because the maximum lod score supporting linkage is above 3 (it's about 5.5 for linkage at a θ value just over 0.1).

18b. The maximum lod score is about 5.5 for linkage at a θ value just over 0.1.

18c. The results support linkage at θ values from just under 0.05 to about 0.30.

22. The chi-square value is 168.3. For 3 degrees of freedom, this corresponds to a P value of less than 0.001.

24a. The pure-breeding brown-eyed fly line is ccd^+d^+, the pure-breeding short-bristled line is c^+c^+dd, and the F_1 is cc^+dd^+.

24b. The cross should be a test cross of the F_1 dihybrid. The test-cross strain would be $ccdd$. The test cross will yield four progeny categories whose phenotypes will be determined by the dominant or recessive alleles contributed by the F_1 dihybrid.

24c. The progeny will be 36% cd^+, 36% c^+d, 14% cd, and 14% c^+d^+.

24d. The progeny will be 25% cd^+, 25% c^+d, 25% cd, and 25% c^+d^+.

28a. I-1 is either $N1/n2$ or $N2/n1$. I-2 is $n2/n2$. II-1 is $N1/n2$. II-2 is $n2/n2$. III-1 is $N1/n2$. III-2 is $N1/n2$. III-3 is $n2/n2$. III-4 is $N1/n2$. III-5 is $n2/n2$. III-6 is $N2/n2$. III-7 is $N1/n2$. III-8 is $n2/n2$.

28b. III-6 is a recombinant. Her genotype indicates that the marker allele 2 is on the same chromosome as the $NF1$ allele, unlike the allele arrangement in her mother (II-1).

28c. 1/8

30a. The gene order is scute, echinus, crossveinless. The allelic phase in the trihybrid is $+\ e\ +\ /\ s\ +\ c$.

30b. The recombination frequency between scute and echinus is 0.067. The recombination frequency between echinus and crossveinless is 0.095. The recombination frequency between scute and crossveinless is 0.162.

30c. There are no discrepancies across this genetic interval.

30d. The chi-square value is 38,555, which corresponds to a P value well below 0.01, which indicates that the results of this experiment are not due to independent assortment.

32a. The chi-square values for both sets of data correspond to P values well below 0.01 and therefore indicate that the results significantly deviate from expectation based on independent assortment. This supports linkage of the colorless and waxy genes.

32b. The recombination frequency from cross 1 was 0.27, and the recombination frequency from cross 2 was 0.24.

32c. Yes, both sets of data are compatible with the hypothesis of genetic linkage, although the recombination frequencies of the two sets differed slightly.

32d. The recombination frequency using combined data is 0.27

Chapter 6

2. Link 1: Transfer of an entire F^+ plasmid from an F^+ cell to an F^- cell converts an F^- cell to an F^+ cell. Link 2: Integration of the F plasmid into the host chromosome converts an F^+ cell to an Hfr cell. Link 3: Precise excision of the F plasmid from the chromosome of an Hfr cell converts an Hfr cell to an F^+ cell. Link 4: Excision of the F plasmid plus some host DNA from the chromosome of an Hfr cell converts an Hfr cell into an F' cell.

4. All three mechanisms can involve homologous recombination of the transferred DNA into the recipient chromosome. In all three mechanisms, if the DNA entering the cell is linear or does not contain an origin of replication, then recombination of the DNA into the recipient cell chromosome or episome is required for the DNA to be stably maintained. If the DNA entering the recipient is circular and contains sequences required for replication and maintenance, then recombination into the recipient cell chromosome or an episome is not required.

These three mechanisms differ in how DNA is transferred from one cell to another. Only conjugation requires genetic information for transfer in the donor cell (F plasmid DNA) and physical contact between the donor and recipient cell. Transduction is characterized by infection of the donor cell by a bacteriophage. On the other hand, transformation does not require particular genes in the donor or the help of a phage: DNA is released from the "donor" cell due to cell lysis and enters the "recipient" cell via DNA transporters.

6. Lysis of an infected bacterial host cell, and the release of progeny phage particles, is the end result of the lytic cycle of bacteriophage. Lysogeny involves the integration of the phage chromosome (known as a prophage once integrated) by site-specific recombination into a specific site (DNA sequence) in the bacterial chromosome. Once integrated, the prophage can replicate along with the rest of the bacterial chromosome until conditions induce excision of the prophage and resumption of the lytic cycle.

8. A *prophage* is a bacteriophage genome that is part of the host cell chromosome. It is formed by integration of a bacteriophage chromosome into the host cell chromosome by site-specific recombination.

10. In genetic complementation, bacterial lysis occurs because the two viruses have mutations in different genes. This is analogous to complementation analysis in eukaryotes. In recombination, bacterial lysis occurs because, although the viruses have mutations in the same gene, rare homologous recombination events produce recombinant wild-type viruses. Complementation and recombination can be differentiated by the frequency of bacterial lysis after simultaneous infection with two mutant viruses: lysis is frequent in the case of complementation (many plaques are formed), whereas it is rare in the case of recombination.

20a. Selection for met^+ was done on minimal medium containing glucose and phenylalanine. The met^+ transductants were assayed for cotransduction of phe^+ using minimal medium containing glucose. The met^+ transductants were assayed for cotransduction of ara^+ using minimal medium containing arabinose. Selection of phe^+ transductants was done on minimal medium containing glucose and methionine. The phe^+ transductants were assayed for cotransduction of met^+ on minimal medium containing glucose. The phe^+ transductants were assayed for cotransduction of ara^+ on minimal medium containing arabinose. The met^+ phe^+ transductants were selected on minimal medium containing glucose. The met^+ phe^+ transductants were assayed for cotransduction of ara^+ on minimal medium containing arabinose. The ara^+ transductants were selected on minimal medium containing arabinose, phenylalanine, and methionine. The ara^+ transductants were assayed for cotransduction of met^+ on minimal medium containing arabinose and phenylalanine. The ara^+ transductants were assayed for cotransduction of phe^+ on minimal medium containing arabinose and methionine.

20b. The gene order is *phe-ara-met* or *met-ara-phe*.

22a. Four genes

22b. Mutations 1, 5, and 8 are in one gene. Mutation 2 is in a second gene. Mutations 3 and 7 are in a third gene. Mutations 4 and 6 are in a fourth gene.

22c. Complementation resulted in the formation of many plaques on each plate (the lysis of many different bacteria) due to coinfection by bacteriophage with mutations in different genes. The vast majority of these phage are mutants that cannot by themselves infect and lyse bacteria. Recombination between mutations in the same gene results in rare plaques (very few bacteria lyse); however, all the virus particles produced are wild type and can infect and lyse bacteria.

22d. Mutation 9 is a deletion that inactivates two genes. It overlaps mutations 1 and 7 but not mutation 3, 5, or 8.

22e. Mutation 10 is a deletion mutation that inactivates two genes. It overlaps mutations 4 and 8 but not mutation 1, 5, 6, or 9.

22f. The mutation order is 3, 7, 1, 5, 8, 4, 6, and 2.

Application Chapter A

2a. The affected gene in Tay–Sachs disease is referred to as HEXA, which stands for the hexoseaminidase A gene, and it is located on chromosome 15, at 15q23.

2b. Tay–Sachs disease is most frequently found in infants of Ashkenazi Jewish ancestry. The frequency of carriers in North American Jews is about 1/45 or 2.2%.

2c. The affected gene in cystic fibrosis is referred to as CFTR, which stands for the cystic fibrosis transmembrane regulator, and it is located on chromosome 7, at 7q31.2.

2d. The most common mutation in the CFTR gene is called ΔF508, which is a deletion of the 508th codon in the CFTR coding sequence, which removes a single phenylalanine amino acid from the CFTR protein.

4. J.B. and S.B. each have a 2/3 conditional probability of being carriers. If J.B. and S.B. are both heterozygous carriers, then the probability that their first son or daughter will have galactosemia is 1/4. The joint probability that the first child of J.B. and S.B. will have galactosemia is $\frac{2}{3} \times \frac{2}{3} \times \frac{1}{4} = \frac{4}{36} = \frac{1}{9}$.

Chapter 7

2. The key results were those showing that enzymes that destroyed RNA and protein did not destroy the transforming principle, whereas enzymes that destroyed DNA did. The transforming principle was considered to be genetic material. The most reasonable interpretation of those results was that DNA was the only essential component of the transforming principle, and therefore, the genetic material.

4. Hershey and Chase prepared T2 particles whose protein was labeled with the radioactive sulfur, S^{35}, and whose DNA was labeled with radioactive phosphorous, P^{32}. They used the labeled T2 to infect bacteria and then separated the infected bacteria from the empty phage shells (phage ghosts) using a blender. They found that essentially all the P^{32}-labeled T2 DNA but little to none of the S^{35}-labeled T2 protein was in the infected bacterial cells. Since T2 genetic material must be inside the infected cells to direct new virus particle synthesis, these results pointed to DNA as the genetic material of phage T2.

6. The chemical bonds that form base pairs in double-stranded DNA are weak, noncovalent bonds called hydrogen bonds. Hydrogen bonds involve two atoms sharing a hydrogen nucleus, and the distance between the atoms sharing the hydrogen nucleus is critical for hydrogen bonds to form. The bases in the two complementary antiparallel DNA strands are aligned such that each of the atoms that share hydrogen nuclei (N and O or N and N) in each base are positioned next to each other at a distance that allows all possible hydrogen bonds to form. The bases in the complementary but parallel strands are not aligned in this manner; therefore, the atoms that could form hydrogen bonds do not align and are not close enough together to allow hydrogen bonding between all possible and necessary chemical groups.

8a. Phosphodiester bonds

8b. Hydrogen bonds

8c. There are 12 phosphodiester bonds in the molecule.

8d. There are 17 hydrogen bonds in the DNA molecule.

10. DNA polymerase III determines which free nucleotide triphosphate is complementary to the base being copied. DNA polymerase III catalyzes phosphodiester bond formation between the α-phosphate of the incoming nucleotide triphosphate and the 3′ hydroxyl group of the last nucleotide added to the strand.

12. RNA is synthesized and serves as a primer for elongation by DNA polymerase.

14a. DNA polymerase I is required to remove the RNA primer and fill in the gap with DNA. DNA polymerase III is responsible for the bulk of synthesis of DNA on the leading and lagging strands.

14b. The absence of DNA pol I will not prevent the bulk of DNA replication but will result in newly replicated DNA containing small segments of RNA and nicks at the junctions of polymerase III synthesized DNA and the 5′ end of the RNA primers.

14c. An *E. coli* mutant without a functional DNA polymerase III will be unable to replicate its DNA because it lacks the enzyme responsible for the bulk of DNA synthesis during replication.

16a. True

16b. False

16c. True

16d. False

16e. True

18. Helicase, SSB, primase, DNA pol III, DNA pol I, ligase

20. Recall the Meselson-Stahl experiment and consider how the results excluded the alternatives to the semiconservative model for DNA replication. Meselson and Stahl initially cultured *E. coli* in medium containing only N15 (heavy nitrogen) until all cells contained only N15/N15 DNA. They then cultured the N15/N15 *E. coli* in normal medium (N14) and collected samples after one, two, and three rounds of DNA replication. The results showed that before transfer to N14 medium, only N15/N15 DNA was present. After one round of replication in N14 medium, all of the DNA was N15/N14; after two rounds of replication, half the DNA was N15/N14 and half was N14/N14; and after the third round of replication, 1/4 of the DNA was N15/N14 and 3/4 was N14/N14. The conservative model predicted that the original N15/N15 DNA would remain throughout, and therefore the results ruled out the conservative model after one round of replication. The dispersive model predicted that after each round of replication there would be only one form of DNA, which would become less and less dense. Although this model was not ruled out after one round of replication, the persistence of the N15/N14 DNA and the presence of two classes of DNA (N15/N14 and N14/N14) after rounds two and three ruled out the dispersive model.

22. Cells were incubated in medium containing 3H-thymine for a short period of time (a "pulse") and then transferred to medium containing an excess of unlabeled thymine (the "chase"). The cells were then collected and their DNA was prepared for electron microscopy, which can detect replication structures in DNA, and for autoradiography, which reveals the location of 3H-thymine incorporation into DNA. The results showed DNA replication bubbles that contained regions of label on both ends of the bubble. Since bidirectional replication produces a replication bubble with DNA synthesis occurring at both ends, whereas unidirectional replication results in a replication bubble with DNA synthesis occurring at one end, these results excluded unidirectional DNA replication and supported bidirectional replication.

24. DNA helicases unwind dsDNA during DNA replication and repair. Bloom syndrome is characterized by chromosome instability and an increased rate of cancer. Chromosome instability is evident when chromosomes are lost from cells, typically because of a failure during mitosis. Mitosis fails to occur properly if chromosomes are not completely replicated. Cancer is a disease caused by accumulation of somatic mutations, which will accumulate at an elevated rate if DNA repair by DNA replication is defective. Based on the information provided, it is reasonable to speculate that lack of the DNA helicase encoded by the Bloom syndrome gene results in incomplete replication during S phase and during repair of DNA damage. Failure to completely replicate chromosomes could result in a failure to pass chromosomes on to progeny cells during mitosis, which would result in chromosome instability. Failure to repair DNA damage would also lead to an increased rate of somatic mutation, which would lead to cancer.

26a. Telomeric DNA is composed of a repetitive, short DNA sequence. In many organisms, the repeated sequence is 5′-TTAGGG-3′ or a variant thereof.

26b. Telomerase uses a segment of its RNA as the template to add multiple copies of a simple sequence to the 3′ end of each strand of DNA on a linear chromosome. This strand, which corresponds to the template for lagging strand synthesis, is copied by the normal mechanism of lagging strand synthesis after it is extended by telomerase.

26c. Telomeres are thought to provide two functions, one in chromosome replication and the other in chromosome protection. Telomeres provide a mechanism for replication of the ends of linear chromosomes. Without telomeres, lagging strand synthesis would fail to extend to the chromosome ends, leaving a gap at each end after each round of replication. This would shorten the chromosome and, after many rounds of replication, would result in loss of important DNA sequences (genes). Telomeres are repetitive DNA, which prevents loss of important DNA sequences if shortening occurs. Telomeres are also the binding site for telomerase, which extends the lagging strand template to compensate for sequences lost during incomplete lagging strand synthesis. Telomeres also provide a protective "cap" on the ends of linear chromosomes; this cap distinguishes normal chromosome ends from ends generated by double-stranded chromosome breaks (DNA damage). Without telomeric DNA and the proteins that bind telomeric DNA, the ends of chromosomes are recognized as broken chromosomes and are fused together by DNA repair enzymes. Such breakage can create chromosome end-to-end fusions, which then create dicentric chromosomes that can be broken during the next cell division, creating new breaks and new fusions in an endless cycle known as the bridge-break-fusion cycle.

26d. Telomerase is required to ensure complete the replication of chromosome ends (telomeres), ensuring that every cell division produces two daughter cells with complete chromosomes. In the absence of telomerase, chromosomes shorten with every cell division, eventually resulting in loss of telomeres and nearby genes. Germ-line cells divide many times; therefore, they require telomerase. Somatic cells are capable of a limited number of cell divisions (some are unable to divide at all); therefore, they do not require telomerase. It is also thought that the lack of telomerase in somatic cells helps prevent indefinite cell division because loss of telomeres activates DNA damage responses that stop cell division and lead to cell death. This response would help protect the organism from the spread of cancerous cells.

28a. The reaction would have equal concentrations of deoxycytidine triphosphate, deoxythymidine triphosphate, and deoxyguanidine triphosphate. It would also have a mixture of deoxyadenosine triphosphate and dideoxyadenosine triphosphate.

28b. Dideoxysequencing uses DNA synthesis to generate labeled DNA fragments of different lengths, which are then resolved by gel electrophoresis or column chromatography. To visualize the products of DNA synthesis in traditional dideoxysequencing, relatively high levels of template were necessary. The use of PCR allows detectable levels of DNA synthesis from much lower levels of template DNA.

28c. Dideoxynucleotides contain a hydrogen group instead of a hydroxyl group on their 3′ carbon. When a dideoxynucleotide is incorporated into a growing DNA strand, there is no 3′ hydroxyl group present to allow phosphodiester bond formation with the next nucleotide to be added; therefore, no additional nucleotides are added to this DNA strand, and thus synthesis of this strand is terminated.

32. Approximately 7500 origins of replication. Five minutes = 300 seconds. Working bidirectionally, each origin generates (300 sec.)(40 nt.)(2) = 24,000 nucleotides per second, requiring $1.8 \times 10^8 / 2.4 \times 10^4 = 0.75 \times 10^4$ origins.

Chapter 8

2. The three major modifications of mRNA are 5′ capping, intron splicing, and 3′ polyadenylation. The process of 5′ capping involves addition of a guanosine monophosphate by guanylyl transferase to the 5′ end of a pre-mRNA via a 5′-to-5′ triphosphate linkage and the subsequent methylation of the guanine and sometimes additional nucleotides on the pre-mRNA. Intron splicing involves the removal of introns from the pre-mRNA and the joining of adjacent exons by the spliceosome. The process of 3′ polyadenylation involves the cleavage of the pre-mRNA downstream of the polyadenylation sequence by cleavage factors and addition of 20 to 200 adenine nucleotides by polyadenylate polymerase.

6. DNA and RNA polymerases are similar in that both (1) catalyze phosphodiester bond formation to polymerize nucleotides into nucleic acids, (2) polymerize in a 5′-to-3′ direction, and (3) are dependent on a DNA

sequence template. DNA and RNA polymerases differ in that (1) RNA polymerase can initiate strand synthesis whereas DNA polymerase can only extend an existing strand, (2) most DNA polymerases can proofread using a 3′-to-5′ exonuclease activity whereas RNA polymerases cannot, and (3) DNA polymerases use deoxyribonuclotide triphosphates as substrates whereas RNA polymerases use ribonucleotide triphosphates as substrates.

8. The primary transcripts of bacterial and eukaryotic genes differ in that bacterial transcripts often contain more than one coding sequence (they are polycistronic) whereas eukaryotic transcripts do not. Polycistronic mRNAs allow for coordinate regulation of production of several proteins by controlling initiation of transcription of only one gene. Eukaryotes accomplish this by coordinate regulation of transcription of multiple genes by gene-specific transcription factors. Prokaryotic and eukaryotic primary transcripts differ in that eukaryotic transcripts are extensively modified before translation whereas prokaryotic transcripts are not. The modification of eukaryotic transcripts includes 5′ capping and 3′ polyadenylation, which generate structures that are critical for regulation of the initiation of translation and for controlling the half-life of the mRNA. Mechanisms controlling translation initiation and mRNA half-life in bacteria do not involve these structures. The modification of eukaryotic transcripts also includes intron splicing, which is required for generating the complete open reading frame used in translation and allows for the generation of multiple, different (but related) mRNAs from a single primary transcript. This last mechanism increases the number of different proteins that are coded by a genome without increasing the number of genes present.

10. Recall that enhancers are DNA sequences that increase the level (rate) of transcription of genes in a position- and orientation-independent manner. Enhancers are binding sites for transcription factors that stimulate transcription of one or more genes. Since the expression of the transcription factors is often specific to the cell type or tissue, enhancers often provide for a mechanism to stimulate transcription of genes in a manner specific to the cell type or tissue. Possible rationales for the lack of enhancers in bacteria include (1) the lack of differentiated cell types in most bacteria; (2) little to no intergenic space on bacterial chromosomes, which makes long-range-acting enhancer sequences unnecessary; and (3) bacterial operons make coordinate regulation of protein synthesis by enhancers unnecessary.

18. The bands in lanes 2 and 4 have migrated the most rapidly; therefore, they correspond to naked DNA molecules. Lanes 1, 3, and 5 have migrated more slowly than naked DNA; therefore, they are DNA + protein complexes. Lane 1 showed slightly higher mobility than lane 5, which showed higher mobility than lane 3. Higher mobility indicates less protein is bound to the DNA. Conditions c and d should result in naked DNA because c contains DNA only, and d contains DNA plus RNA pol II, which cannot bind to DNA in the absence of general transcription factors. Therefore, c and d correspond to lanes 2 and 4 (either lane is equally possible for either condition). Condition e contains the lowest number of transcription factors, followed by condition a, and condition b has the most transcription factors. Thus, lane 1 corresponds to condition e, lane 5 corresponds to condition a, and lane 3 corresponds to condition b.

20a. The organism transcribes as a wild type.

20b. The organism transcribes slowly (i.e., is leaky).

20c. The organism does not transcribe genes.

20d. Temperature-sensitive mutant

22a. Since this mutation is in an intron but causes a defect in β-globin, it must affect splicing efficiency. The mutation replaces A with U, changing the 3′ splice site sequence AG to UG. This change is likely to affect the efficiency with which the spliceosome recognizes the end of intron 2 and leads to either inclusion of intron 2 in the mRNA—which results in an insertion or premature termination—or causes a change in the location of the 3′ splice junction, which leads to an insertion, deletion, or frameshift mutation.

22b. This problem requires you to consider the structure of genes and identify important DNA sequences that are not part of exons. Nonexon-located mutations that could prevent gene function include mutations in the promoter or terminator sequences as well as in enhancer or silencer sequences. Mutations in the promoter would diminish or prevent transcription, which would reduce or eliminate the mRNA. Mutations in the terminator could prevent or alter termination, which would elongate the mRNA. Mutations in an enhancer would diminish transcription, which would reduce mRNA abundance. Mutations in the silencer would enhance transcription, which would increase mRNA abundance.

24a. First, the eukaryotic promoter is unlikely to be recognized by bacterial RNA polymerase holoenzyme. Second, the introns will not be removed from the pre-mRNA, which will result in production of an abnormal protein. Third, sequences required for efficient translation initiation in bacteria are not present.

24b. First, I would make a cDNA copy of the gene. The cDNA is a DNA copy of the mRNA sequence, which lacks introns. Second, I would place the cDNA sequence downstream of a known bacterial promoter, which will ensure that the gene is transcribed. Third, I would modify the coding sequence upstream of the ATG start codon to contain a Shine–Dalgarno sequence, which is important for proper initiation of translation. Fourth, I would place an intrinsic or rho-dependent termination sequence downstream of the cDNA to ensure efficient transcription termination.

26a. The DNA-only and DNA + protein lanes differ in that bands are missing from the DNA + protein lanes. This result indicates that the proteins are bound to the DNA in a 200 base pair region about 80 base pairs in from one end. Since the proteins are transcription factors and RNA polymerase, which bind to promoters, it is reasonable to conclude that the DNA fragment contains a promoter sequence.

26b. 200 base pairs

26c. One reasonable experiment would be to clone this DNA sequence upstream of the coding sequence for a protein whose expression is easy to assay and then introduce that chimeric construct into cells and assay for protein expression. If the result is negative, then the orientation of the fragment should be inverted to check that it was not inserted backward in the first attempt. Also, a known, control promoter should be used to confirm that the protein-coding sequence is correct and that the protein can be detected in the cells used.

Chapter 9

2a. Nirenberg and Matthaei developed an in vitro translation system that contained everything necessary for translation except for amino acids and mRNAs. Synthetic RNA composed of only U (poly-U) was added to 20 separate reactions, each containing a different radioactive amino acid as well as the other 19 nonradioactive amino acids. Only the reaction with radioactive phenylalanine produced radioactive protein. Since the RNA sequence poly-U contains only UUU codons, then UUU codes for phenylalanine.

2b. Only reaction with radioactive proline produces radioactive protein. Since poly-C contains only CCC codons, CCC codes for proline.

2c. One type of polypeptide composed of alternating Arg and Glu amino acids was produced.

2d. No detectable polypeptides would be produced.

4. First, preinitiation complex formation: the small ribosomal subunit and IF3 bind to the mRNA, the AUG start codon is identified by 16S rRNA base pairing with the Shine–Dalgarno sequence, and the AUG codon is in the ribosomal P site. Second, formation of the 30S preinitiation complex: fMet−tRNA^{fMEt} bound to IF2–GTP binds to start codon in the P site, and IF1 binds. Third, formation of the 70S initiation complex: 50S ribosomal subunit binds; IF2 cleaves GTP to GDP + phosphate; and IF1, IF2–GDP, and IF3 leave the complex.

6. tRNAs that are charged with different amino acids have unique structural features that allow them to interact with their cognate aminoacyl tRNA synthetases. Unique features include the anticodon sequence as well as sequences and base modifications in the T-arm and D-arm.

8a. 5′-CUA-3′ and 5′-CUG-3′

8b. 5′-UUU-3′

8c. 5′-GAG-3′

8d. 5′-CAU-3′

8e. 5′-AUC-3′ and 5′-AUU-3′

10. See table.

	Bacterial Ribosome	Eukaryotic Ribosome
Similarities		
Composition	RNA and protein	RNA and protein
Number of subunits	two (small and large)	two (small and large)
tRNA binding sites	three (E, P, and A)	three (E, P, and A)
Differences		
Number and size of rRNAs	three (16S, 23S, and 5S)	four (18S, 28S, 5.8S, 5S)
Size of subunits	30S and 50S	40S and 60S
Numbers of proteins	21 in the small subunit and 34 in the large subunit	34 in the small subunit and 49 in the large subunit

12a. The errors in the diagram are (1) ribosome is moving in the wrong direction along mRNA, (2) mRNA contains T's, (3) amino terminal amino acid of the peptide is incorrect, (4) ribosomal subunit sizes are incorrect, (5) anticodon sequence of the tRNA in P site is incorrect, and (6) amino acids on tRNAs in P and A sites are incorrect.

14. 31

16. See table.

DNA	Non-template (5′ to 3′)	AAC	ATA	TGT	GAA	<u>GGC</u>	GAG	AA<u>T</u>	GAA	CGA
	Template (3′ to 5′)	TTG	TAT	ACA	CTT	CCG	CTC	TTA	CTT	GCT
RNA	mRNA (5′ to 3′)	AAC	AUA	UGU	GAA	GGC	GAG	AAU	GAA	CGA
	tRNA (3′ to 5′)	UUG	UAU	ACA	CUU	CCG	CUC	UUA	CUU	GCU
Amino acid abbreviations	3-letter	Asn	Ile	Cys	Glu	Gly	Glu	Asn	Glu	Arg
	1-letter	N	I	C	E	G	E	N	E	R

22. Soon after initiation of translation of an mRNA coding for a secretory protein, the amino terminus of the secretory protein is synthesized and is exposed on the surface of the ribosome. The amino terminus contains the signal sequence that marks this protein for cotranslational translocation into the endoplasmic reticulum (ER). The signal receptor particle (SRP) binds to the signal sequence and the ribosome and halts further translation. The SRP/ribosome/mRNA complex binds to the ER membrane—SRP binds to its receptor, and the ribosome binds to a protein translocation channel. SRP is released, translation resumes, and the growing polypeptide is extruded through the channel into the lumen of the ER. There, the signal sequence is cleaved by signal peptidase and the protein is glycosylated, folded with the help of chaperones, and packaged into transport vesicles destined for the Golgi apparatus. The carbohydrate on the protein is modified as the protein passes through the compartments of the Golgi, and the protein is packaged into vesicles destined for transport to the plasma membrane. Fusion of the transport vesicle membrane with the plasma membrane releases the secretory protein into the extracellular fluid.

24a. 5′-UGUGUGUGUGUGUGUG ...-3′

24b. Cys-Val-Cys-Val-Cys-Val-Cys-Val ...

24c. The experiment resulted in production of a polypeptide composed of alternating Val and Cys amino acids, which is what was predicted for a nonoverlapping triplet code.

24d. Two polypeptides, each composed of a single type of amino acid, would be produced if the code had been a doublet, nonoverlapping code.

24e. Translation of the RNA using an overlapping doublet or triplet code gives the same result—a single type of polypeptide with two alternating types of amino acids. This result does not differ from that predicted based on a nonoverlapping three-letter code but does differ from that predicted for a nonoverlapping two-letter code.

26. 438

32a. The start and stop codon are in bold print. 5′-CAPCCAA-GCGUUACAUGUAUGGAGAGAAUGAAACUGAGGCUUGCCACGUUU GUUAAGCACCUAUGCUACCGAAAAAAAAAAAAAAAAAAAAA-AAA-3′

32b. Met-Tyr-Gly-Glu-Asn-Glu-Thr-Glu-Ala-Cys-His-Val-Cys (MYGENETEACHVC)

34. The consensus sequence is CCCGCCGCCACCAUGG. Also see table.

Position	12	11	10	9	8	7	6	5	4	3	2	1	[start]4
Percent A	23	26	25	23	19	23	17	18	25	61	27	15	[AUG] 23
Percent C	35	35	35	26	39	37	19	39	53	2	49	55	[AUG] 16
Percent G	23	21	22	33	23	20	44	23	15	36	13	21	[AUG] 46
Percent T	19	18	18	18	19	20	20	20	7	1	11	9	[AUG] 15
Consensus	C	C	C	G	C	C	G	C	C	A	C	C	AUGG

36. GCCACCAUGG

Application Chapter B

2a. A low methionine diet reduces the levels of homocysteine accumulation, reducing or eliminating the physiological defects that lead to homocystinuria.

2b. Accumulation of high homocysteine levels at any stage of life result in physiological abnormalities; therefore, individuals unable to metabolize methionine must maintain a low methionine diet throughout their lives.

4. Community-based genetic screening programs recruit members of targeted populations to undergo carrier screening. The purpose of these programs is to identify individuals who are heterozygous carriers of recessive genetic disorders so that they can add that knowledge to their considerations as part of their family planning. These programs focus on populations that have a relatively high frequency of specific mutant alleles that underlie recessive disorders. One reason to target specific subpopulations rather than encourage genetic screening of everyone at random is to optimize the benefit-to-risk ratio of carrier screening: knowledge of an individual's genetic makeup has serious personal, ethical, legal, and societal implications that have not yet been thoroughly debated by professionals or effectively communicated to the general public.

8. Arguments for why community-based genetic screening should remain voluntary include concerns over the potential emotional, social, and financial impact that genetic information can have on individuals and communities. Arguments for why community-based genetic screening should become mandatory include the concerns over the financial and emotional costs to society that are imposed by individuals that have debilitating genetic conditions.

10. Two individuals who are heterozygous for a fatal condition that is not on the RUSP list should consider several factors as they make decisions about having children. One factor is the details of the condition, the effectiveness of existing medical treatments, how they feel about having a child who lives with the disorder, and whether they are financially capable of dealing with the costs associated with caring for an individuals with that condition.

12a. Many different mutant alleles of the gene *GBA* have been identified. L44P is a common mutation that results in substitution of the amino acid leucine at position 44 with the amino acid proline. The L44P mutation has been shown to cause retention of acid-β-glucosidase in the ER, which prevents its transport to the lysosome. The N370S mutation (asparagine at position 370 changed to serine) is the most common allele in the Ashkenazi Jewish population. The N370S mutation inactivates the enzymatic activity of the enzyme. Individuals with Gaucher disease who are homozygous for L44P or N370S or who are L44P/N370S heterozygotes have been identified.

12b. There does not appear to be a direct relationship between the severity of Gaucher disease and specific mutant alleles: the same mutations can be found in individuals diagnosed with type I, II, or III forms of Gaucher. It is thought that the severity of the disorder relates to the degree to which the cells of the individual are deficient in acid-β-glucosidase in the lysosome, and therefore it may be that specific combinations of mutant *GBA* alleles or other genetic and environmental factors influence the severity and time of onset of Gaucher disease.

14a. Sickle cell anemia is an autosomal recessive condition that is found in about 1 out of every 1000 births in non-Hispanic black populations in the United States and at a significantly lower frequency in populations that are of non-African and non-Mediterranean origin.

14b. Sickle cell anemia is due to one of two mutations in the adult beta globin gene (HBB). One is E6V (Glu6Val), and one is E6K (Glu6Lys).

14c. Sickle cell mutations cause hemoglobin proteins composed of sickle cell beta globin to polymerize at low oxygen partial pressures. Polymerization of hemoglobin creates sickled red blood cells, which shortens the half-life of red blood cells and leads to anemia. The abnormal red blood cells can block narrow blood vessels, occluding the passage of blood to organs and peripheral tissues, leading to organ failure. Spleen function is typically lost in individuals with sickle cell anemia.

14d–f. Most treatments for sickle cell anemia are designed to anticipate symptoms, reduce the severity of complications, and alleviate pain. Newborns are typically prescribed oral penicillin to prevent infections; this can continue to age 5 or beyond. Routine exams for blood, solid tissue, and organ function are recommended throughout life to promote early intervention when complications arise. Episodes of acute pain can be treated with over-the-counter nonsteroidal anti-inflammatory medicine. Hydroxyurea may also be prescribed in response to acute pain because it induces expression of fetal beta globin, which can partially replace the defective adult beta globin, and it has been found to be effective at alleviating the symptoms of sickle cell disease. Severe episodes require at least a visit to the emergency room for pain management and may require blood transfusions. Hematopoietic stem cell transplantation (HSCT) is the only cure for sickle cell anemia, but it is difficult to find an appropriate donor and this procedure is risky in adults. If HSCT is successful, then no further treatment is necessary.

Chapter 10

2. Approximately $2.9 \times 10^9/(146 + 50) = 1.48 \times 10^7$ nucleosomes.

4. Recall that the G-banding pattern of light and dark bands of chromosomes is characteristic for each chromosome. These distinctive band patterns allow a cytologist to unambiguously identify each chromosome in a human karyotype. This pattern allowed for the development of cytogenetics, which is the genetic analysis of an individual that is performed by microscopy. Genetic abnormalities associated with alterations in chromosome number or structure can be detected by cytogenetic analysis, allowing for the rapid diagnosis of some genetic diseases.

6. The diploid will have 18 bivalents whereas the triploid will have a combination of trivalents, bivalents, and monovalents.

8. If the *haploid* number is 4, then (a) a *diloid* species would have two copies of each chromosome, for a total of 8 chromosomes; (b) a *pentaploid* species would have five copies of each chromosome, for a total of 20 chromosomes; (c) an *octaploid* species would have eight copies of each chromosome, for a total of 32 chromosomes; (d) a *trisomic* species would have two copies of three chromosomes and three copies of the fourth chromosome, for a total of 9 chromosomes; (e) a *triploid* species would have three copies of each chromosome, for a total of 12 chromosomes; (f) a *monosomic* species would have two copies of three chromosomes and one copy of the fourth, for a total of 7 chromosomes; (g) a *tetraploid* species would have four copies of each chromosome, for a total of 16 chromosomes; (h) a *hexaploid* species would have six copies of each chromosome, for a total of 24 chromosomes.

10a. There will be two green spots and two red spots in cells from a female.

10b. There will be two green spots and one red spot in cells from a male.

14a. The hybrid will have 24 + 6 = 30 chromosomes.

14b. The hybrid will be infertile.

14c. The hybrid will have 60 chromosomes.

14d. The phenotype of an allopolyploid cannot be predicted. The combination of genes from the two genomes results in tens of thousands of genetic interactions that have never been seen before. To predict the phenotype of the allopolyploid, it would be necessary to predict the outcome of all of these genetic interactions, and this is not yet possible.

16a. The chromosome is submetacentric because the centromere is neither directly in the middle nor at an end.

16b. No; the centromeric region is constitutive heterochromatin, as are both telomeres.

16c. Telomeric regions of chromosomes generally lack genes because these chromosomal regions are heterochromatic and therefore inhibit gene expression. Thus, any gene located at telomeres would be silenced unless something altered telomeric heterochromatin structure.

16d. The amylase gene would be expected to be found in a euchromatic region of a chromosome.

18. The nucleosome spacing in species A is 200 base pairs (bp), whereas the spacing in species B is 400 bp.

20. Tetraploids produce diploid gametes, and diploids produce haploid gametes; therefore, a hybrid of the tetraploid and diploid will be a triploid. The triploid will have either bivalents plus monovalents or all trivalents during synapsis in meiosis I. It will produce unbalanced, nonviable gametes and thus will be seedless.

22a. Neither line is expected to be fertile, because the hexaploidy line contributes three of each of its eight different homologous chromosomes to the experimental varieties. These chromosomes will form trivalents or bivalents plus a monovalent during synapsis in meiosis I, thus preventing the formation of balanced gametes.

22b. The hexaploid line contributed 24 chromosomes to both experimental varieties.

22c. The tetraploid line contributed 16 chromosomes to experimental variety 1 and 32 chromosomes to experimental variety 2.

24a. The boy with Down syndrome must have three copies of at least part of chromosome 21. Since he has only 46 chromosomes, one of his chromosomes must contain two copies of chromosome 21 information. Since his sisters are phenotypically normal but have 45 chromosomes, they must have a chromosome that contains all the information from two chromosomes. This is reminiscent of a Robertsonian translocation involving chromosomes 14 and 21. This could explain why the boy has Down syndrome; he would have one normal chromosome 14, two normal copies of 21, and one 14:21 Robertsonian translocation.

24b. Since both parents are phenotypically normal, the parent carrying the 14:21 chromosome must have only one copy of chromosomes 14 and 21 and, therefore, only 45 total chromosomes. One parent is expected to have a normal karyotype and the other is expected to have 45 chromosomes; one 14, one 21, and one 14:21.

24c. A fusion of two acrocentric chromosomes is called a Robertsonian translocation.

26a. The results show that 1 hour is required for the majority of DNase I-sensitive sites to be cut under these conditions.

26b. The majority of human DNA in this sample is packaged in a chromatin structure that contains nucleosomes and is accessible to DNase I. A portion of the DNA in this sample is packaged in a higher order structure that is resistant to DNase I treatment.

Chapter 11

2. Nitrous acid causes the deamination of adenine, creating hyoxanthine. Hypoxanthine pairs with C; therefore, nitrous acid causes an A:T to G:C transition mutation. BU (5-bromodeoxyruidine) is incorporated into DNA in place of T or C. Since 5 BrdU can pair like T or C, it can cause A:T to G:C transitions.

4. A synonymous mutation converts one codon into a different codon that codes for the same amino acid (for example, AAG to AAA). A missense mutation converts one codon that codes for one amino acid into a different codon that codes for a different amino acid (for example, AAG to AAC). A nonsense mutation converts a codon that codes for an amino acid into a stop codon (for example, AAG to TAG).

6a. UV causes aberrant structures called photoproducts to form. The most common is the covalent bonding of adjacent thymines in one strand of DNA: these are called thymine dimers.

6b. Thymine dimers are not recognized by standard DNA polymerase as adjacent thymine containing nucleotides and therefore often not accurately replicated.

6c. One DNA repair mechanism that removes thymine dimers is photoreactive repair, which uses the enzyme photolyase to cleave the bonds holding thymine dimers together. Photolyase, which requires visible light, directly reverses the damage caused by UV. Another DNA repair mechanism that removes thymine dimers is the nucleotide excision repair (NER) pathway.

8. Nucleotide substitutions can result in silent, missense, or nonsense mutations. Silent mutations do not change the amino acid sequence of the protein and therefore have no effect on protein function. Missense mutations change one amino acid in a protein and the effect of this change depends on the importance of the amino acid that was replaced and the functional similarity (or lack thereof) of the R-group on the substituted amino to that of the wild-type amino acid.

10. Recessive mutations are typically loss-of-function mutations because the wild-type gene sequences have been selected during evolution for optimum function; therefore, any change (mutation) to that sequence is likely to replace a nucleotide maintained by natural selection with one that reduces the function of the gene. Forward mutations include all mutations in a gene that convert it from wild type to mutant, whereas reverse mutations are only those that precisely reverse a specific mutation to wild type. Thus, the number of possible nucleotide changes corresponding to a forward mutation is much greater than those that reverse a given mutation, making forward mutations far more frequent than reversion.

12. Insertion of a *Ds* element into the maize *C* gene inactivates the *C* gene and results in yellow kernels. If the activator of *Ds* transposition, called *Ac*, is present, then occasionally a *Ds* element is activated to precisely excise out of the *C* gene. This restores that *C* gene to wild-type function and causing all kernel cells that descend from that cell to be purple. The excision of *Ds* from the *C* gene occurs randomly on a cell-by-cell basis, which leads to a mostly yellow kernel (*Ds* gene remaining in the *C* gene) but with random, purple spots (cells in which *Ds* was induced to excise by *Ac*).

16. *E. coli recA* mutants are unable to use homologous recombination to repair their DNA by the SOS pathway. The *RecA* protein is required for strand exchange, which is a critical step in repair pathway, which uses the DNA sequence on a homologous DNA molecule to repair damaged DNA.

18. Flanking direct repeats are created at the site of transposon insertion. First, a staggered double-stranded DNA cut is made at the site of insertion, leaving complementary single-stranded sequences. The transposon is inserted at the site of the cut and the single-stranded DNA gaps are filled in by DNA polymerase. The single-stranded DNA sequence is now repeated on either side of the inserted transposon. See Figure 11.25.

20a. The mutation is a frameshift mutation (insertion or deletion).

20b. TCT/G-TAC-ATA-TGC-GAG-ACA-AGN

22a. The mouse (*Mus musculus*) is a widely used model organism for genetic analysis of mammalian development and physiology, specifically in relation to human disease, because many of these processes in mice and humans are evolutionarily conserved and because researchers can perform experimental manipulations using mice that are not possible when studying humans or even nonhuman primates.

22b. Although the mouse (*Mus musculus*) is a mammal, there are many developmental, behavioral, and physiological differences between mice and humans. In addition, not every human gene has a homolog in the mouse genome. Therefore, in cases where the physiology or genetics of mice and humans differ, mutations in a mouse homolog to a human disease gene may not provide useful information on the human disease process.

24. Mutational hotspots are genes or DNA sequences mutate at a higher rate than the average. Genes that are significantly larger than average have a higher than average mutation rate (examples include the human dystrophin (Dys) and neurofibromatosis (NF1) genes. The cytosine of CpG dinucleotide DNA sequences are also hotspots of mutation because C is often methylated at position 5 (creating 5-methylcytosine), and spontaneous deamination of 5-methylcytosine (which is common), creates thymine, which is not repaired efficiently and lead to C:G to T:A mutations.

26. Mismatch repair corrects DNA replication mistakes by removing the incorrect nucleotide of a mismatched base pair and then re-replicating that part of the DNA molecule. The incorrect nucleotide of a mismatched base pair is on the newly synthesized, daughter DNA strand and the correct nucleotide is on the parental, template DNA strand. If the identification of new versus template strands was not possible, then the nucleotide removed from the mismatched base pair would be random, causing mutation instead of repair half of the time. The template strand is identified in bacteria as the strand that contains methylated nucleotides.

28a. The results indicate that the test compound treated with the S9 extract was mutagenic whereas the test compound along was not. This indicates that the sample contains a chemical that can be converted into a mutagen by an activity in the S9 extract.

28b. The S9 extract is thought to simulate enzymatic activities present in our liver, therefore the results indicate a potential that something in the test compound could be converted into a mutagen when ingested. Therefore, the test compound should be considered a potential mutagen.

30a. Mutant 1 is a missense mutant, mutant 2 is a nonsense mutant, and mutants 3 and 4 are both frameshift mutants.

30b. The wild-type mRNA sequence is ACN CAC UCU GGA UUG AAG GCN.

30c. Mutant 1 is a G to T transversion, mutant 2 is a G to T transversion, mutant 3 is a deletion of the fourth nucleotide in the sequence, and mutant 4 is an insertion of either a G or an A after the fifth nucleotide of the sequence.

34a. Mistakes during DNA replication create mismatched based pairs. The mismatch repair pathway will repair the abnormal DNA created by mistakes during DNA replication.

34b. Heavily damaged bacterial DNA induces the SOS repair system. SOS repair allows for error-prone repair to prevent cell death due to high levels of DNA damage.

34c. Thymine dimers are repaired by two pathways: nucleotide excision repair (NER) and photoreactive repair.

34d. In cells that have completed DNA synthesis, double-stranded DNA breaks are repaired by homologous recombination in bacteria and archaea, and primarily by synthesis-dependent strand annealing (SDSA) in eukaryotes, although nonhomologous end-joining (NHEJ) and homologous recombination may also be used by eukaryotic cells.

34e. In eukaryotic cells that suffer a double-stranded DNA break in G1 phase, nonhomologous end-joining (NHEJ) is the primary pathway for repair.

34f. Conversion of cytosine to uracil by deamination creates G:U base pairs in DNA. Uracil is removed from DNA by the base excision repair (BER) pathway.

Chapter 12

2a. A DNA sequence that binds a regulatory protein, such as the *lac* operator sequence.

2b. A regulatory protein that binds DNA, such as the *lac* repressor protein.

2c. A compound that induces or activates transcription, such as lactose.

2d. A compound that interacts with another protein or compound to form an active repressor, such as the *trp* corepressor.

2e. A DNA sequence that binds RNA polymerase and regulates transcription, such as the *lac* promoter.

2f. A process of transcription regulation through which the binding of regulatory proteins to DNA activates transcription, such as the CAP binding site of the *lac* promoter.

2g. A process by which the stereochemistry of a protein is altered to change its interaction capabilities, such as the *lac* repressor protein.

2h. A process of transcriptional regulation through which binding of regulatory proteins to DNA blocks transcription, such as *lac* repressor protein binding to *lac O*.

2i. A mechanism of transcriptional regulation in which transcription level is modified (attenuated) to meet environmental requirements, such as *trp* operon attenuation.

4a. *Similarities:* Both have promoter and operator regulatory sequences. *Differences:* Inducible operons bind repressor protein to block transcription and may use positive control to help activate transcription. Inducible operons require an inducer substance to activate transcription. Repressible operons use a corepressor plus the pathway end product to repress transcription. Repressible operons often utilize attenuation.

4b. *Similarities:* Both types of regulatory systems utilize allostery in regulating transcription. *Differences:* The mechanism and consequences of allostery differ. In *lac* operon regulation, the repressor protein binds the operator, but allosteric change caused by allolactose prevents binding. In *trp* operon regulation, the corepressor protein cannot bind the operator until its allosteric shape is changed by binding to tryptophan.

4c. *Similarities:* Both types of operons contain multiple genes that share a single promoter and a single operator sequence. *Differences:* Repressible operons often use attenuation and contain a transcribed leader sequence that participates in determining structural gene transcription. This mechanism is not found in inducible operons.

6. Attenuation does not involve allosteric changes. Attenuation is the result of transcription of a leader sequence that undergoes translation. Coupling of transcription and translation dictates whether transcription continues past the leader sequence and into the structural genes.

8. The CAP binding site is part of the *lac* promoter and is located at approximately -60. It binds the CAP–cAMP complex and opens DNA slightly to allow efficient RNA polymerase binding at the *lac* promoter.

10. A *Cap⁻* mutation would alter the CAP binding site sequence and render it unrecognizable by CAP–cAMP. The required positive regulation of transcription would not occur, and *lac* operon transcription would be minimal. The strain would be *lac⁻*.

12. Transcription occurs under both conditions because allolactose, the inducer, is present. Transcription is higher in the absence of glucose because CAP-cAMP levels, which stimulate transcription, are higher.

14. Antisense RNAs are single-stranded RNAs that are complementary to a portion of specific mRNA transcripts. Bound to their mRNA targets, antisense RNAs can either block translation or lead to the destruction of mRNA. Blocking translation prevents the production of proteins that might initiate unnecessary or harmful actions.

16a. Blocks all transcription

16b. Produces constitutive transcription

16c. Blocks all transcription (this is an I^S mutation)

16d. Produces constitutive transcription (this is an I^- mutation)

16e. Only minimal transcription will occur.

18. See table.

Genotype	β-Galactosidase		Permease		Phenotype
	No Lactose	**Lactose**	**No Lactose**	**Lactose**	
Example: $I^+ P^+ O^+ Z^+ Y^+$	+	−	+	−	lac^+
a. $I^S P^+ O^+ Z^+ Y^+ / I^- P^+ O^+ Z^+ Y^+$ −	−	−	−	−	lac^-
b. $I^- P^+ O^+ Z^- Y^+ / I^+ P^+ O^C Z^+ Y^-$ +	+	+	+	−	lac^+
c. $I^+ P^+ O^+ Z^- Y^+ / I^+ P^- O^+ Z^+ Y^-$ −	−	−	+	−	lac^-
d. $I^- P^+ O^C Z^+ Y^+ / I^+ P^- O^+ Z^+ Y^+$ +	+	+	+	+	lac^+
e. $I^+ P^+ O^C Z^+ Y^- / I^+ P^+ O^+ Z^+ Y^-$ +	+	−	−	−	lac^-
f. $I^+ P^+ O^+ Z^- Y^+ / I^S P^+ O^+ Z^+ Y^-$ −	−	−	−	−	lac^-
g. $I^S P^+ O^+ Z^- Y^+ / I^+ P^+ O^C Z^+ Y^-$ +	+	+	−	−	lac^-

20a. $I^- P^+ O^+ Z^- Y^+ / I^+ P^+ O^+ Z^+ Y^+$ will have inducible transcription of both genes. $I^+ P^+ O^C Z^- Y^+ / I^+ P^+ O^+ Z^+ Y^+$ will have constitutive transcription of *lacY* and inducible transcription of *lacZ*. $cap^+ I^+ P^- O^+ Z^+ Y^+ / I^+ P^+ O^+ Z^+ Y^+$ will have inducible transcription of both genes. $cap^- I^S P^+ O^+ Z^+ Y^+ / I^+ P^+ O^+ Z^+ Y^+$ will be noninducible.

20b. The first three partial diploids will be able to grow on a lactose medium, but the final partial diploid ($I^S P^+ O^+ Z^+ Y^+ / I^+ P^+ O^+ Z^+ Y^+$) will not.

22a. No; permease is not produced.

22b. Transcription of *lacZ* is inducible from the $cap^+ I^- P^+ O^+ Z^+ Y^-$ chromosome. Only minimal transcription occurs from the other chromosome, so permease is noninducible.

22c. The *lacI* gene has its own promoter and is not affected by *lac* operon regulation of gene mutations. The cap^- mutation minimizes transcription, but repressor protein produced from this chromosome is trans-active and binds O^+ on the other chromosome to induce *lacZ* expression.

24. Gene *Z* is the enzyme, gene *W* is the repressor, and *G* is the operator.

26a. This would prevent the lac repressor from binding to the operator, which would cause constitutive transcription of the *lac* operon.

26b. This would prevent the repressor from binding to O_{R1}, allow *cro* binding to O_{R3} and O_{R2}, prevent transcription of P_{RM}, allow transcription of P_R, promoting the lytic life cycle.

26c. This would prevent *cro* from binding to O_{R3}, allow repressor binding to O_{R2} and O_{R1}, prevent transcription of P_R, allow transcription of P_{RM}, promoting the lysogenic life cycle.

28a. The mutant is incapable of establishing lysogeny. Lytic gene transcription from the O_R sites cannot be repressed.

28b. The mutant is incapable of establishing lysogeny.

28c. The mutant will be unable to carry out lysis. No transcription activation occurs from O_L or O_R.

28d. The mutant will be unable to establish lysogeny. The mutant cannot undertake site-specific recombination to integrate the lysogen.

28e. The mutant will be unable to carry out lysis due to the *cro* mutation, and it will be unable to establish lysogeny due to the *cII* mutation.

28f. The mutant will be unable to carry out lysogeny. The expression of the late gene that takes place through the antiterminator activity of *N* at t_L, t_{R1}, and t_{R2} will not occur.

30a. The same band in both lanes

30b. No band in lane 1; band in lane 2

30c. No band in either lane

30d. The same band in both lanes

30e. No band in lane 1 and a band in lane 2

30f. No band in either lane

32a. The mutation would cause the levels of charged tRNA trp to be low regardless of the available levels of tryptophan in the medium and remove attenuation as a regulatory mechanism controlling trp operon transcription.

32b. The 3–4 stem loop will be formed less frequently in this mutant because ribosomes will pause at the trp codons in region 1, preventing formation of the 1–2 stem-loop. This would favor formation of the 2–3 stem loop, which prevents formation of the 3–4 stem loop.

Chapter 13

2a. UAS elements are found in the yeast genome, where they operate as enhancer-like regulatory sequences. Gal4 protein binds yeast UAS elements to activate transcription of galactose utilization genes.

2b. Insulator sequences shield genes from enhancer effects. The mechanism of action may be through the formation of specific DNA loops that protect particular genes from enhancers.

2c. Silencer sequences prevent transcription of particular genes. The mechanism of action may be through competitive protein binding at silencer sequences that overlap with enhancer sequences. The yeast Mig1 and Tup1 proteins bind a silencer sequence during glycolysis to prevent transcription of galactose utilization genes.

2d. The protein complexes that assemble at enhancers to facilitate transcription are known as enhanceosomes. The enhanceosome complex known as Mediator assembles at yeast enhancers. It contacts promoter-bound proteins to activate transcription.

2e. RNA interference describes the posttranscriptional regulation of mRNAs by regulatory RNA molecules. RNAi is a prominent feature of the regulation of gene expression in most eukaryotic genomes.

4. Acetylation occurs when acetyl groups are added to amino acids of the histone protein by acetylase enzymes. These acetylation events are most often associated with transcription activation, though there are many exceptions.

6. mRNAs are transcribed from DNA and carry the information to be translated into protein. rRNAs provide both scaffold and enzymatic activities to ribosomes. tRNAs binds an amino acid at their 3′ ends and recognize codons in mRNA via their anticodons, thus translating nucleic acid sequence information into protein sequence information. miRNAs and siRNAs act to regulate gene expression via RISC, either to slice or inhibit translation of mRNA targets, or to facilitate recruitment of chromatin modifying enzymes to chromosomal loci. Some lncRNAs act as scaffolds to bring chromatin regulatory proteins to chromosomal loci.

8. Several factors can be cited, including the following: (1) the presence of a nucleus in eukaryotic cells, (2) the chromatin structure of eukaryotic genomes, (3) multicellularity that is frequent in eukaryotes, and (4) differential gene expression among different types of eukaryotic cells.

10. Heterochromatin regions will decondense for DNA replication during the S phase of the cell cycle to allow replisome access.

12. Chromatin is classified into euchromatin and heterochromatin based on the chemical modifications on the histone proteins. Euchromatin is characterized by H3K9-acetylation and is transcriptionally active. Heterochromatin is transcriptionally inactive and may be either constitutive, in which case it is marked with H3K9-methylation, or facultative, in which case it is marked with H3K27 methylation. Facultative heterochromatin can be converted to euchromatin, and vice versa, by chromatin modification.

14. One potential role of lncRNAs in gene regulation is to act as scaffolds to recruit chromatin modifying enzymes to the chromatin. An example is Xist, which acts to recruit the polycomb complex to the X chromosome that is destined to be inactivated.

16. dsRNA leads to posttranscriptional silencing of genes that encode mRNAs with sequences corresponding to the dsRNA. One mechanism involves the destruction of the mRNA and the other involves inhibition of translation of the mRNA.

18a. Region B contains a promoter element that is required for transcription whereas F does not.

18b. Region D contains a negative, cis-acting regulatory element that functions in leaf but not stems.

18c. Mutant E contains a positive, cis-acting regulatory region required for transcription in leaves but not stems. This region could be a leaf-specific enhancer.

20a. Enhancer and silencer sequences are each detected in this analysis. The enhancer sequence is located in the deleted region that is common to mutant E and mutant F. The silencer sequence is located in the deletion region unique to mutant E.

20b. The deletion in mutant D deletes the *ME1* promoter sequence.

20c. It seems likely that regulation of *ME1* is developmentally controlled by the combined activity of an enhancer and a promoter that activate transcription and a silencer sequence that represses transcription at particular times during development.

Chapter 14

2. Difference suggests posttranscriptional regulation. One possibility is that the protein is stable in only one cell type and is rapidly degraded in other cell types. Another possibility is that the mRNA is translated in only one cell type.

4.

E. coli:	4.64×10^6 bp / 100 minutes $= 4.64 \times 10^4$ bp / minute
Arabidopsis:	130×10^6 bp / 600 cM $= 2.17 \times 10^5$ bp / cM
Saccharomyces:	12×10^6 bp / 4500 cM $= 2.67 \times 10^3$ bp / cM
C. elegans:	100×10^6 bp / 300 cM $= 3.33 \times 10^5$ bp / cM
Drosophila:	180×10^6 bp / 275 cM $= 6.55 \times 10^5$ bp / cM
Danio rerio:	2000×10^6 bp / 3000 cM $= 6.67 \times 10^5$ bp / cM
Mus:	3000×10^6 bp / 1400 cM $= 2.14 \times 10^6$ bp / cM
Homo female:	3000×10^6 bp / 4460 cM $= 6.73 \times 10^6$ bp / cM
Homo male:	3000×10^6 bp / 2590 cM $= 1.16 \times 10^6$ bp / cM
Homo average:	3000×10^6 bp / 4460 cM $= 8.51 \times 10^6$ bp / cM

There will always be a balance between increasing the size of the mapping population and thereby having a more accurate map position and identifying the physical DNA spanning flanking mapped markers. In organisms with a large number of base pairs per cM, it is often worthwhile to increase the number of individuals in a mapping population and thereby decrease the number of base pairs of DNA potentially encoding the locus of interest.

6. Although PCR or northern blotting approaches can give some perspective on expression patterns, observing them in situ provides more information. For this, either a transcriptional or translational fusion to a reporter gene (e.g., *lacZ* or *GFP*) would be best. The difficulty may be in initially identifying the sequences responsible for proper expression of the gene. These experiments are judged by the following standards: (1) How well does the observed expression pattern of the marker line match with all other data on expression patterns? and (2) Can a translational fusion gene complement a loss-of-function mutant phenotype?

8. The CRISPR-Cas system from Staphylococcus was modified by using its single endonuclease gene and creating a guide RNA gene that contains the crRNA fused to the tracer RNA. This created a simple, two-component system that can be used to target any DNA sequence by cloning a copy of that sequence into the position of the crRNA.

10. The advantage of chemical mutagens (and radiation) over transposon-based mutagens is that chemical mutagens can be used to mutate essentially every gene in the genome (saturation mutagenesis) while creating a relatively small number of mutant individuals, because every individual carries multiple mutations. Transposon-based mutagenesis is less efficient, however; it has the advantage of adding a "DNA tag" that allows each gene that is mutated to be rapidly identified and cloned.

12. To prove that the genomic clone contains the gene mutated in the bristle mutant, you could use the genomic clone to complement the mutation. This could be done by inserting the cloned gene into a Drosophila *P* element transformation vector and transforming the recombinant *P* element into fertilized eggs that are homozygous for the bristle mutation. Transformants identified as harboring the *P* element would then be examined to determine whether they had a wild-type or mutant bristle pattern. If transformants had a wild-type bristle pattern, then the cloned gene corresponds to the gene mutated in the bristle mutant.

14a. Use reverse genetics to create a loss-of-function allele by homologous recombination and gene replacement. This would remove the gene from the genome and create a null allele of the gene.

14b. Generate a transgenic yeast containing a translational fusion of the all the gene's regulatory sequences fused to a reporter gene, such as *GFP*. GFP fluorescence can then be used to indicate the location of the protein product of the gene being studied.

16. The mouse ortholog of the human dystrophin gene is located on the X chromosome. Use reverse genetics to create mice female mice containing a loss-of-function mutation in the mouse DMD gene and then mate these females with wild-type males. Half the male offspring of the mating should contain no functional DMD gene. Strategies for creating the loss-of-function mutation include using CRSPR-Cas or homologous recombination.

18. If the transposon supplies additional regulatory elements, insertion of the transposon adjacent to a gene may result in ectopic or overexpression of the adjacent gene, resulting in a dominant gain-of-function allele. Alternatively, if the transposon is inserted into the coding region of a gene, it will result in a loss-of-function allele.

20. Since meiosis is not required for viability, a genetic screen searching for mutants that fail to undergo meiosis properly would work. However, the ability to cross the mutant for complementation tests would be useful, and thus a screen for conditional mutants would be desirable. Since chemical mutagenesis induces the broadest spectrum of alleles, it would be a better choice of mutagen than insertion of deletion alleles, which are often null. Finally, the simplest genetic system in which meiosis occurs would be the best system to examine this question. *S. cereviseae*, where many genetic tools are available, would be a good choice.

22. Because you have no a priori information on the nature of the gene product, homology-based techniques are not applicable. Positional cloning would work and requires only a mutant phenotype to go from map position to gene. Since the genome of *Drosophila* has been sequenced, one could take a sequence-based approach as outlined in Figure 16.12. Transposon tagging would work by starting with an organism heterozygous for a mutation in one of the genes and mobilizing the *P* element. Since identifying the mutants is the most time-consuming, the sequence-based approach is the better choice.

24. The mutation can be mapped to a particular chromosome region using deletion mapping (see Figure 10.18). Genomic DNA clones containing genes in that region can then be used to transform the *Drosophila* mutant to determine which clone contains a gene that complements the mutation.

26a. Since *Arabidopsis* is a flowering plant, the female gametophyte (egg) is retained on the female parent, on the placenta. Female gametogenesis can be directly observed within the ovules. Mutations resulting in female gametophytic mutations (e.g., lethality) can be observed as a 1:1 ratio.

26b. Since the male gametophyte (pollen) is produced in excess and is not retained on the plant, to observe male gametophytic mutations, I would observe the developing pollen directly.

28a. Screen for mutants in which the pupae either eclose at a time other than dawn or eclose at random times during the day/night. Although this phenotype might be detrimental in nature, in the laboratory it is likely to be completely viable.

28b. Screen for mutations in which the expression of genes encoding photosynthetic machinery is no longer synchronized with the circadian rhythm. Again, although this phenotype in nature would be detrimental, in the laboratory it is likely to be viable, though a change in the color of the plants (e.g., lighter green) might be observed.

28c. Positional cloning, or since the genomes of these organisms have been sequenced, a sequence-based method (i.e., Figure 14.7).

Application Chapter C

2a. Benign tumors are composed of precancerous cells that are growing excessively but are well encapsulated and contained within their tissue. Malignant tumors are composed of cancer cells whose growth is extensive and highly disorganized. Cancer cells of malignant tumors have the potential to metastasize, escaping their tissue and spreading to other locations within the body.

2b. An example from the reading is the progression from benign adenoma to malignant colon cancer (see Figure C.6).

2c. The progression from benign to malignant tumors typically requires multiple genetic changes (mutations) that activate oncogenes and/or inactivate tumor suppressor genes. In the example of colon cancer, *APC, DCC,* and *p53* are examples of tumor suppressor genes and *KRAS* is an example of an oncogene.

4a. The chromosome mutation producing the Philadelphia chromosome is a reciprocal translocation that creates a gene fusion of the *BCR* gene on chromosome 22 and the *c-Abl* gene on chromosome 9. The normal *c-Abl* gene codes for a membrane-bound tyrosine kinase that signals cell cycle regulatory proteins and promotes the proliferation of white blood cells in response to proper extracellular signals. The *BCR-c-Abl* gene fusion codes for a fusion protein that has a constitutively active *c-Abl* tyrosine kinase, which sends a constant, unregulated signal stimulated continuous proliferation of white blood cells, leading to chronic myelogenous leukemia.

4b. The chromosome mutation that causes Burkitt's lymphoma is a reciprocal translocation involving chromosome 8 and chromosomes 2, 14, or 22. The translocation places the *c-Myc* gene on chromosome 8 near immunoglobulin genes, which are highly actively transcribed. This causes unregulated, high levels of *c-Myc* transcription. Because c-Myc is a transcription factor that activates transcription of genes that promote cell division, unregulated high-level *c-Myc* expression leads to unregulated cell division of B-lymphocytes.

6a. Radiation damages the DNA of all cells and initiates responses that halt cell division, initiate DNA repair, and cause cell death by apoptosis when repair cannot be completed in a timely manner. Cancer cells are among the most rapidly dividing cells in an individual and are, therefore, the most sensitive to DNA damage-induced cell death.

6b. Radiation can cause mutations in noncancer cells if those cells do not repair the damage and do not respond to signals for cell cycle arrest and apoptosis. Cells that continue to divide without repairing damage suffer additional mutations, which can lead to loss of tumor suppressor genes and activation of proto-oncogenes, which can lead to cancer.

6c. Radiation therapy should be effective for any cancer in which the cancer cells can respond to DNA damage by inducing cell death. One concern in radiation therapy is the dose needed to destroy any particular cancer; therefore, cancer cells that are sensitive to low doses of radiation provide the best circumstance for the use of radiation therapy, since low doses can be used and damage to surrounding normal tissue can be minimized.

8a. One cannot conclude with certainty that a woman with an *BRCA1* mutation will get breast cancer. It is true that 60% of women with certain *BRCA1* mutations are expected to develop breast cancer by age 70; however, 40% will not.

8b. In addition to the *BRCA1* mutation, which is inherited, mutations in other tumor suppressor genes or oncogenes and/or environmental factors must combine with the *BRCA1* mutation to cause breast cancer. It is thought that the absence of these additional factors explain the 40% chance that a woman with a *BRCA1* mutation will not get breast cancer by age 70.

10. The Cancer Genome Atlas will identify the most common genetic changes that occur in the somatic cells in different types of cancer. It is hoped that this knowledge will lead to more effective strategies for cancer detection and custom-designed treatments.

Chapter 15

2a. *Sau*3A, 1.17×10^7; *Bam*HI, 7.32×10^5; *Eco*RI, 7.32×10^5; *Not*I, 4.58×10^4

2b. *Sau*3A, 1.08×10^7; *Bam*HI, 4.32×10^5; *Eco*RI, 9.72×10^5; *Not*I, 7.68×10^3

4a. The genomic libraries

4b. The two genomic libraries should completely overlap. The cDNA libraries should be a subset of the genomic libraries. The two cDNA libraries should only partially overlap.

6. A 16-bp sequence is predicted to occur randomly once in 4.3×10^9 bp; thus, oligonucleotides should be of at least this length to have a reasonable probability of being unique in the genome.

8. The principles are identical for both species, but the techniques differ because homologous recombination occurs frequently in yeast and rarely in mice. Thus, positive–negative selection techniques are required in mice, whereas only positive selection is required in yeast.

10. Gene therapy often targets blood diseases because blood circulates throughout the body. Thus, replacement of mutant bone marrow cells with corrected ones allows the defect to be corrected throughout the body.

12. Both methods use "naturally" occurring biological entities. In plants, the Ti-plasmid is reengineered to have the gene of interest and then is reintroduced into *Agrobacterium*, which naturally transfers the T-DNA into the genome at random locations of plant cells. In *Drosophila*, the *P* element is reengineered to have the gene of interest and then injected into embryos, where it integrates into the genome at random locations.

14. Most recombinant DNA manipulations involving combining of DNA fragments of less than 10 kb, including changing specific base pairs in a known sequence, can be accomplished by synthesis. However, for instances where the exact sequence of the DNA in question is not known, standard recombinant DNA techniques will continue to be needed.

16. The sticky ends can be religated since the single strand overhangs can anneal, but neither enzyme can cut the resulting sequence following ligation.

22a. Loss-of-function alleles in *S. cerevisiae* can be produced by homologous recombination (see also Figure 17.5). Gain-of-function alleles, such as those that produce the gene product constitutively, can be constructed by making a gene fusion combining a promoter that drives transcription constitutively in *S. cerevisiae* with the coding region of the gene of interest (see also Figures 17.14 and 17.17).

22b. Since homologous recombination is not routine in tomato, loss-of-function alleles can be created by using RNAi-mediated mechanisms. In this case, a promoter that drives transcription constitutively can be transcriptionally fused with a sequence containing an inverted repeat, such that the mRNA produced can form a stem loop including double-stranded RNA (see also Figure 17.18). The chimeric gene can be introduced into tomato using *Agrobacterium* (see also Figures 17.6 and 17.7). Gain-of-function alleles would be produced in a similar manner as described for *S. cerevisiae*, except the regulatory sequences need to be suited to tomato and the transgenic organisms produced by *Argobacterium*-mediated transformation.

24. There are two possible approaches: (1) Mutagenize the bacterial strain and screen for mutants that can no longer metabolize crude oil. Then clone the corresponding gene(s) using a complementation assay, as outlined in Chapter 16. (2) Alternatively, clone the gene(s) by transferring large genomic clones from the strain of interest into a related *Pseudomonas* strain that cannot metabolize crude oil. This approach often works in bacteria with specialized traits since the gene conferring the trait is often found within a single operon.

26a. There are two possible approaches: (1) perform in situ hybridization using probes made from each of the two genes or (2) construct translational or transcriptional fusion genes with a reporter gene (*LacZ, GFP*) via homologous recombination methods. Translational fusions may retain their functionality as long as the marker gene fusion does not disrupt function of the protein of interest. If in a gene replacement, transcriptional fusions would result in a loss-of-function allele, but if in a recessive gene, transcription fusions would still provide information about gene expression in a phenotypically wild-type mouse.

26b. Use homologous recombination techniques to replace the coding region of the gene with a selectable marker. Alternatively, you can use an RNAi-based approach to create a loss-of-function phenotype. The former approach has the advantage of heritability.

26c. Create loss-of-function alleles via homologous recombination for each of the genes and examine the mutant phenotypes. Cross the two single mutants to create an F_1 population, interbreed the F_1s to produce an

F$_2$, and identify a double-mutant strain and examine its phenotype. If the double-mutant strain exhibits phenotypic defects beyond what is expected by the addition of the single-mutant phenotypes, then the two genes have redundant functions. Alternatively, you can use an RNAi-based approach to create a loss-of-function phenotype, but again, this approach is not heritable.

28. Because the original sequence (highlighted) was from reverse translation of the protein sequence, in nucleotide positions where there is degeneracy in potential sequences, these may differ from the actual sequence encoded in the genome.

30. The mutant sequence can be created using site-directed mutagenesis. These clones could be used to create wild-type and mutant protein to be studied in vitro. To study in vivo consequences, it would be best to introduce the mutant version of the gene into its endogenous chromosomal location. Unlike the creation of loss-of-function alleles, where a selectable marker replaces the endogenous gene, the creation of gain-of-function mutations is slightly more complicated. One solution is to create the point mutation in the genome via homologous recombination and then remove the selectable marker using a Cre–*lox*-based system. However, care must be taken not to leave a "footprint" of nonendogenous sequences in any coding or regulatory sequences.

Chapter 16

2a. Repetitive DNA can often be assembled in many different ways, making unambiguous assembly difficult. On a finer scale, repetitive DNA can also lead to polymerase slippage causing sequence errors.

2b. Dispersed, repetitive DNA that is longer than a single sequencing read and is found at many locations in the genome is particularly problematic.

2c. Paired-end sequencing is one approach to identify unique sequences flanking repetitive DNA.

4. cDNA sequences provide information on which genomic sequences are transcribed and processed into mature mRNAs. Different forms of full-length cDNAs from the same region of genomic DNA can indicate alternative splicing.

6. In eukaryotic genomes, one must account for the possible presence of introns; in prokaryotic genomes, open reading frames should be contiguous. Predictive algorithms must also take into account differences in promoter and enhancer elements/consensus sequences.

8. *Bioinformatic Method:* Use an algorithm to search for potential open-reading frames within the sequence. This method is only predictive and not very accurate, so experimental data are needed to confirm accuracy. *Comparative Method:* BLAST the sequence against the database of known sequences. If sequences are conserved, they are likely to be functional. This method also needs experimental verification. *Experimental Method:* Use the sequence as a probe against a cDNA library or other technique (e.g., microarray, rtPCR) to determine which sequences are transcribed. This is the best method, but it is also much more time- and labor-intensive than the others.

10. Human proteins are closer to fungal proteins than to plant proteins; plant proteins are equidistant from either human or fungal proteins.

12. The reference genome refers to the initial genome sequence of a species, which is usually based on one or a few individuals. As additional individuals from the same species are sequenced, their sequence can be compared with the reference genome to identify differences, which correspond to genetic variations.

14. This DNA sequence is the synthetic version (the nucleotide sequence inferred from reverse translation of the protein sequence) of the human insulin gene.

16a. All three genes are orthologs.

16b. *AY1* and *AY2* are paralogs; *AY1* and *BY* are orthologs; *BY* and *CY* are orthologs.

16c. *AZ1* and *AZ2* are paralogs; *BZ1* and *BZ2* are paralogs; *BZ2* and *BZ3* are paralogs; *BZ1* and *BZ3* are paralogs; *CZ1* and *CZ2* are paralogs; *AZ1* and *AZ2* are orthologous to *BZ1, BZ2,* and *BZ3*; *AZ1* and *AZ2* are

orthologous to *CZ1* and *CZ2*; *CZ1* is orthologous to *BZ1* and *BZ2*; *CZ2* is orthologous to *BZ3*.

18. Although large-scale chromosomal rearrangements appear to have been rare in primate evolution during mammalian evolution, small-scale rearrangements appear to be common and frequent.

20. Segmental duplications, resulting in large-scale gene duplication, can often lead to genetic redundancy, especially if the duplication is evolutionarily recent. Using reverse genetics (see Chapter 17), loss-of-function alleles can be created in the duplicate genes. Due to potential genetic redundancy, double mutants of the two paralogs might have to be constructed to observe an aberrant mutant phenotype.

22a. Any of these approaches are possible: (1) create a loss-of-function allele by gene replacement and examine for mutant phenotype, (2) create a gain-of-function allele by constitutive expression of the gene and examine for mutant phenotype, (3) create a reporter gene fusion allele by gene replacement to examine where and when in the cell the protein is expressed, (4) perform a synthetic enhancer screen in the loss-of-function background, (5) perform a two-hybrid screen to identify interacting proteins, (6) perform transcriptome analysis to examine the expression pattern of the gene.

22b. In a human genome, the possibilities are much more limited: only (5) and (6) from the answer to question 22a would work.

24. The first step is to organize the data to identify genes that behave similarly and those that behave differently. For example *a, c, d, e, f, g, i, j, k, n, q,* and *r* all increase in expression with both high salt and high temperature; *b, p,* and *s* all decrease in expression with both high salt and high temperature; *h* and *o* decrease in response to salt but increase in response to high temperature; *l* and *m* increase in response to salt but decrease in response to high temperature. This analysis provides information into possible roles of genes that may be involved in a general stress response versus genes that may have specific roles in response to salt or temperature stress.

26. The *PEG10* gene is likely derived from the insertion of a retrotransposon, and its protein-coding sequences have been co-opted to perform a role in placenta formation. Retrotransposons contain a gene encoding reverse transcriptase, a nucleic-acid-binding protein that could be co-opted to have a role in binding and regulating endogenous nucleic acid sequences. The presence of the gene in placental mammals only suggests that the insertion of the retrotransposon occurred in the common ancestor of therian mammals, after the divergence of the monotremes from the rest of the mammals.

Chapter 17

2. Their membrane system, chromosomal organization, replication, transcription, and translation (ribosome structure) are all similar to those in bacteria.

4. Sequencing of eukaryotic genomes has revealed evidence of transfers that are recent and transfers that are ancient. Transferred sequences that are highly similar must have been transferred recently.

6. See Table 17.1 for variations in the genetic code in mitochondria. A consequence of tRNA gene number reductions and the change in the code minimizes errors such that the two closely related codons, UGA and UGG, are both Trp.

8. There are three steps in this process: (1) Transfer of organelle DNA from organelle to nucleus and integration into the nuclear genome. (2) Acquisition of nuclear transcriptional regulatory elements such that the organellar gene is transcribed in the nucleus. Translational regulatory elements are similar (except where there are changes in the genetic code or RNA editing, both of which might inhibit production of a functional protein). (3) For the protein to be targeted back to the organelle, protein sequences facilitating efficient subcellular targeting need to be acquired from adjacent genomic sequences.

10. The most appropriate advice would be the following: for III-1, none of your progeny will be afflicted; for III-2, all of your progeny will be afflicted, and the extent may vary between individuals depending on levels of homo- and heteroplasy; for III-3, all of your progeny will be afflicted, though the extent may vary between individuals depending on levels of homo- and heteroplasy.

12. Maternal inheritance

14. *pet1* is a segregational (nuclear) mutation; *pet2* is a neutral mutation. The expected progeny is 2 wild type : 2 *petite.*

16. Since inheritance of this syndrome is maternal and not paternal, there is no need to worry, but if the mother exhibits symptoms, then there is a probability that their children would be affected. The extent to which their children will be affected depends on whether the mother is homoplasmic (all offspring would be affected) or heteroplasmic (possibility that some might not be affected).

18. Sibling II-2's children will be afflicted, but II-5's children will not be afflicted because MERRF is maternally, not paternally, inherited.

20. The presumptive Anastasia's mitochondrial DNA should be identical to that of her mother, so differences in the two sequences could eliminate the claim. However, if the two sequences are identical, the claim would not be proven, because mitochondrial haplotypes are not unique to one family.

22. The CMS genes are maternally inherited mitochondrial alleles, whereas the Rf loci are nuclear. The F_1 will be CMS1 $\frac{rf1}{rf1} \frac{Rf2}{rf2}$ and will be male sterile.

24. *Plasmodium falciparum* is in the phylum, Apicomplexa, which includes members with functional chloroplasts. If *P. falciparum*, contains functional chloroplast that are important for reproduction, then aminoglycoside antibiotics may be effective for treating malaria. If it does not, then these antibiotics will not be effective treating malaria.

Chapter 18

2. The neural crest cells differentiate autonomously with the identity of the species from which they are derived. However, they can recruit host cells to contribute to the beak, suggesting that the neural crest cells nonautonomously influence the developmental fate of neighboring host cells.

4a. In a syncytium, factors that determine pattern formation are not partitioned into separate cells, therefore other mechanisms are required to partition these factors into different domains of the embryo.

4b. Gradients of morphogens such as *bicoid* and *nanos* either must not exist or the gradients must be established in another manner, such as cell-to-cell communication.

6. Segments correspond to the clear morphological and anatomical divisions in the larva or adult organism. Parasegments are offset from the segments, spanning the posterior part of one segment and the anterior part of its neighbor, and correspond to domains of gene expression. Developmental biologists consider parasegments as the subdivisions that are produced during fly development because they correspond to the domains of gene expression that control pattern formation and identity in the organism.

8. Similarities: Both segmentation in *Drosophila* and floral organ whorls in *Arabidopsis* are serially repeated structures/segments with identities controlled by related sets of transcription factors that act combinatorially and exhibit cross-regulation. **Differences:** In *Drosophila* the genes are *Hox* genes and are encoded in complexes in the genome, whereas in *Arabidopsis* the genes are *MADS*-box genes that are dispersed throughout the genome.

10a. In a loss-of-function mutant, the phenotype is vulva-less.

10b. In a gain-of-function mutant, the phenotype is multi-vulval.

12a. This phenomenon can occur only when cells are totipotent. Once cells are only pluripotent, the identities of possible differentiation pathways are limited and may not be able to form a complete organism.

12b. The resulting individual will be a genetic mosaic, consisting of two distinct genotypes. This probably happens more than is acknowledged, but it is detected only when multiple parts of an individual are genotyped.

14. Extra copies of *bicoid* would increase the amount of *bicoid* mRNA that the mother puts into her eggs, thus increasing the amount of *bicoid* protein. This would result in a posterior shift in threshold levels of *bicoid*

required to activate downstream targets; hunchback expression would be increased; other gap genes and pair-rule genes are also likely to be affected, with a general shift of anterior gene expression patterns (and subsequent fates) to more posterior positions—shifting the other gap gene expression patterns to more posterior positions.

16a. Pair-rule genes might be expected to influence the expression of the segment polarity genes, which act at a later time in development.

16b. The *fushi tarazu* single mutant likely has a loss of the even-numbered parasegments (*fushi tarazu* is Japanese, meaning "too few segments"), and the engrailed single mutant likely has defects in the anterior part of each parasegment. Thus, one might predict that the double mutant would be a combination of these two single-mutant phenotypes.

18. This pattern could be established by lateral inhibition.

20a. Gain-of-function alleles in *let-23* and *let-60* would result in a vulva being produced in the *lin-3* loss-of-function background.

20b. Loss-of-function alleles of *let-60* would suppress the gain-of-function *let-23* multi-vulva phenotype and result in a vulva-less worm.

22a. The difference between the two sticklebacks would be due to differences in cis- or trans-acting regulatory sequence controlling expression of *Eda.*

22b. The phenotype of loss of *Eda* function in humans indicates that *Eda* controls multiple aspects of human development. *Eda* could do by directly controlling each tissue type independently, or by controlling a developmental precursor to all of the affected tissue.

24a. In an otherwise wild-type background, the phenotypic effects of *agamous* mutations are confined to the third and fourth whorls, but in an *apetala2* mutant background, phenotypic effects of *agamous* mutations are also seen in the first and second whorls. This implies that in an *apetala2* mutant background, *AGAMOUS* is ectopically expressed in the first and second whorls, and the converse is true for the phenotypic effects of *apetela2* mutations.

24b. Yes; cross-regulatory interactions occur among *Hox* genes in animals. Posteriorly expressed *Hox* genes often repress the expression of *Hox* genes normally expressed in respective anterior positions. This is a common, though not universal, feature in the regulation of *Hox* genes.

26. Based on the phylogeny of eukaryotes (see Figure 18.11), the last common ancestor of Basidiomycota and animals (or plants) was likely a single-celled organism. Thus, as in the comparison of multicellular development of plants and animals, Basidiomycota are likely to utilize a unique set of genes to direct their development. Although the genes might be expected to encode transcription factors and signaling molecules, they are not likely to be homologous to those directing development in plants and animals. Thus, a forward genetic screen to identify pattern formation mutants in mushrooms would likely be a more successful approach than any reverse genetic screens.

Chapter 19

2. Traits 1a through 1d are likely to be multifactorial. Dietary nutrition and temperature are two environmental conditions likely to influence each trait.

4. $V_E = 2.25$, $V_G = 5.40 - 2.25 = 3.15$.

6. The mean is 165.75, $s^2 = 1137.22/11 = 103.38$, and $s = 10.17$.

8. A random sample is a subset of a population selected at random (no bias for any particular attribute). It can be used to represent an entire population because it can be representative of the population: that is, it can contain the same representation of types of individuals in the population.

10a. $A_1A_1B_1B_1C_1C_1 = 36$ cm and $A_2A_2B_2B_2C_2C_2 = 18$ cm.

10b. 27 cm

10c. 24 cm

10d. Any genotype with five "1" alleles and one "2" allele yields $[(5)(6 \text{ cm})] + (3 \text{ cm}) = 33$ cm.

10e. There are $(3)^3 = 27$ possible genotypes.

10f. Seven different phenotypes are possible.

12a. $V_E = 3.5$ and $V_G = 7.4 - 3.5 = 3.9$.

12b. $H^2 = 3.9/7.4 = 0.527$.

14. $H^2 = 34.48/38.10 = 0.905$.

16a. For the cross involving 12-gram tomatoes, $S = -4$ g; for the cross involving 24-gram tomatoes, $S = 8$ g.

16b. For the cross involving 12-gram tomatoes, $R = (-4)(0.8) = -3.2$ g; for the cross involving 24-gram tomatoes, $R = (8)(0.8) = 6.4$ g.

18. Blood type is known (see Chapter 4) to be the result of three alleles of a single gene, and the MZ results confirm the exclusive genetic determination of blood type. Chicken pox is an infectious disease, and there is no reason to suspect gene-dependent differences in infection as the equal concordance values indicate. For the five other conditions, MZ concordance is considerably higher than DZ concordance, suggesting that genes have a pronounced effect on the appearance of the conditions.

22. QTL analysis screens a large number of SNP and other DNA sequence variants and plots the results on the phenotype of interest, running speed in this case. Any DNA markers associated with faster running speed could potentially indicate the nearby location of a gene (quantitative trait locus) influencing running speed.

24a. For protein content, $S = 22.7 - 20.2 = 2.5\%$; for butterfat content, $S = 7.4 - 6.5 = 0.9\%$.

24b. Response to selection will be greater for protein content $[(2.5)(0.60) = 1.5\%]$ than for butterfat content $[(0.9)(0.80) = 0.72\%]$.

26a. 100%. Blood type is controlled by genotype alone, and MZ twins are genetically identical.

26b. 50%. Blood types A ($I^A i$) and B ($I^B i$) are both expected, with a probability of 1/2. The chance that DZ twins will have the same blood group is 1/4 for blood type A plus 1/4 for blood type B, or 1/2. It is also possible that since DZ twins are the result of independent fertilization events, one twin could be blood type A and the other blood type B.

Chapter 20

2. Inbreeding is a genome-wide phenomenon that increases homozygosity and reduces heterozygosity. It does not change allele frequencies; rather, it nonrandomly distributes alleles into genotypes. Inbreeding can increase the probability that inbred organisms might be homozygous for a rare recessive allele.

4. Natural selection conferring the highest relative fitness on particular heterozygous organisms will eliminate the two alleles when they occur in homozygous genotypes. Equilibrium allele frequencies are established as a ratio of the selection coefficients operating against the alleles.

6. Among a very small number of population samples, each outcome contributes a large percentage to the total; in much larger samples, each individual outcome contributes a much smaller percentage to the total.

8. A genetic bottleneck substantially reduces the number of organisms in a population. Elimination and survival are random. Some alleles may be lost, and others may survive at much different frequencies than were present before the bottleneck. The overall result is less genetic diversity after the bottleneck. As populations increase in size after a bottleneck, they display a reduced level of genetic variability in comparison with diversity before the bottleneck.

10a. $\sqrt{0.28} = 0.53$.

10b. $1 - 0.53 = 0.47$.

10c. Using $p = 0.47$ for the dominant allele T and $q = 0.53$ for the recessive allele t, $TT = (0.47)^2 = 0.22$, $Tt = 2(0.47)(0.53) = 0.50$, and $tt = (0.53)^2 = 0.28$.

12. Mutation can generate new antibiotic-resistant alleles that confer improved survival on bacteria carrying the mutant alleles that are exposed to an antibiotic.

14. Evolutionary processes, including directional selection, require inherited variability for their operation. In the absence of inherited variation, there is just a single allele of a gene, and selection has no alternative alleles on which to exert selective pressure.

16. Inbreeding may be reduced by carefully managing matings to ensure that the level of relationship is minimized to the extent possible when matings take place.

18. The expected frequencies of rabbits are black ($C_1 C_1$) = $(0.70)^2 = 0.49$, tan ($C_1 C_2$) = $2(0.70)(0.30) = 0.42$, and white ($C_2 C_2$) = $(0.30)^2 = 0.09$.

20. In this problem, $s = 1 - 0.82 = 0.18$, and $t = 1 - 0.32 = 0.68$. The estimated equilibrium frequencies are $\beta^A = t/s + t = 0.68/0.86 = 0.791$ and $\beta^S = s/s + t = 0.18/0.86 = 0.209$.

22a. A genetic bottleneck is a substantial population reduction that eliminates population members at random.

22b. Since the loss of population members is random in a genetic bottleneck, the overall level of genetic diversity is reduced; certain alleles are eliminated and other alleles retained at frequencies that are higher or lower than before the bottleneck. In Ashkenazi populations, repeated bottlenecks followed by population growth generated a founder effect that brought alleles such as the recessive for Tay–Sachs disease to high frequency.

22c. In this population, the recessive allele frequency, $f(t)$, is 0.0365.

22d. The dominant allele frequency is $f(T) = 1 - 0.0365 = 0.9635$, and the carrier frequency is $2(0.9635)(0.0365) = 0.070$, or about 7 per 1000 people.

26a. Following one generation of natural selection, the relative genotype frequencies are $C_1 C_1 = 0.421, C_1 C_2 = 0.526$, and $C_2 C_2 = 0.032$. The approximate allele frequencies are $C_1 = 0.421 + (0.5)(0.526) = 0.684$, and $C_2 = 0.053 + (0.5)(0.526) = 0.316$.

26b. Following reproduction of the survivors of predation, the genotype frequencies are $C_1 C_1 = (0.684)^2 = 0.468$, $C_1 C_2 = 2(0.684)(0.316) = 0.432$, and $C_2 C_2 = (0.316)^2 = 0.010$.

26c. The equilibrium allele frequencies are predicted to be $C_1 = 0.2/0.6 + 0.2 = 0.25$, and $C_2 = 0.6/0.6 + 0.2 = 0.75$.

28. Assuming $f(I^A) = p, f(I^B) = q$, and $f(i) = r$, the frequency of the frequency of P is and the frequency of Q is $1 - (0.579 + 0.290) = 0.131$.

30a. For dimpling, the genotype frequencies are estimated to be $DD = (0.62)^2 = 0.3844, Dd = 2(0.62)(0.38) = 0.4712$, and $dd = (0.38)^2 = 0.1444$. For PTC tasting ability, the genotype frequencies are estimated to be $TT = (0.76)^2 = 0.5776, Tt = 2(0.76)(0.24) = 0.3648$, and $tt = (0.24)^2 = 0.0576$.

30b. The expected phenotypes are dimpled taster $(D-T-) = (0.8556)(0.9424) = 0.8063$; dimpled nontaster $(D-tt) = (0.8556)(0.0576) = 0.0493$; undimpled taster $(ddT-) = (0.1444)(0.9424) = 0.1361$; undimpled nontaster $(ddtt) = (0.1444)(0.0576) = 0.0083$.

32a. 0.032

32b. 0.062

32c. 0.0038

34a. Individuals V-1, V-2, and V-3 are inbred.

34b. Common ancestors are I-1 and I-2.

34c. $F = 4(1/2)^8 = 0.015625$.

38. The recessive allele producing achromatopsia was present in the original (pretyphoon) Pingelapese population, though the original allele frequency is unknown. The typhoon produced a genetic bottleneck that produced a frequency of approximately 1 copy in 40 alleles, or $Q = 0.025$ for the recessive allele. Subsequent repopulation of the island was affected by genetic drift and inbreeding that may have acted to increase the frequency of the allele (genetic drift) and to increase the likelihood of individuals who are homozygous IBD (inbreeding).

Application Chapter D

2. Analyses of human mitochondrial DNA sequence variation support the recent African origin (RAO) hypothesis, which states that modern humans are derived from an ancestral population that migrated out of Africa about 170,000 years ago.

4. Human specific variation in noncoding regulatory elements are hypothesized to contribute to derived traits in humans (traits present in humans but lacking in other great apes) by altering the regulation of gene expression. Examples discussed in this chapter include alteration of gene expression leading to a human-specific structure of the mandible, reduction in cell surface antigens used by pathogens, increased growth of certain brain regions, loss of facial hair, and penile spikes.

8. Natural selection increases the frequency of adaptive alleles in a population. Tightly linked alleles also increase in frequency by a process called "genetic hitchhiking," resulting in a haplotype that includes the selected and hitchhiking alleles that exists in linkage disequilibrium. Selection for the adaptive allele indirectly selects for the entire haplotype reducing the variation in all loci in that haplotype. Variation will be restored after enough time has passed for mutation and recombination to return the haplotype to linkage equilibrium.

10. One hypothesis for the presence of Denisovan alleles in the genomes of Australians and Malenesians is that the modern humans who migrated eastward out of Africa interbred with Denisovans.

12. The presence of the same 9-bp deletion in the mitochondrial DNA of all these populations implies that it originated in an ancestral population and is derived in the others. Since the frequency is lowest in the Taiwanese population, then members of the Taiwanese population are most likely the ancestors of the western Polynesian, eastern Polynesian, and New Zealand populations.

14. An early population of modern humans may have interbred with Neanderthals at a time after the split between Neanderthals and Denisovans. The resulting Neanderthals would have an admixture of human and Neanderthal DNA. Natural selection could have selected for retention of the human mitochondrial DNA but not the majority of the nuclear DNA, resulting in a Neanderthal population that shares more mitochondrial DNA homology with humans than with Denisovans.

Application Chapter E

2. The paternity index is a measure of the likelihood that a child inherited a nonmaternal allele from a particular male. It is calculated as the ratio of the probability of the child inheriting the allele from the male to the frequency of the allele in the population. The combined paternity index is the product of the paternity indices for multiple CODIS STR markers. If the combined paternity index is greater than 100, then there is greater than a 99% chance that the male in question is the child's father.

4. The statistical principle behind the genetic health risk assessment is that some DNA markers are associated with genetic conditions at a frequency greater than that predicted by chance alone. This indicates that inheritance of the DNA marker is associated with a higher likelihood of having the disease. This assessment is probabilistic and not predictive because some individuals who inherit the DNA marker do not also inherit the condition.

6a. Suspects A and C are excluded by the results.

6b. Suspect B is not excluded by the results.

8. The frequency of the genotype shown in the Figure E.1 for the three CODIS alleles is $2(0.017)(0.125) \times 2(0.131)(0.119) \times 2(0.134)(0.270) = 9 \times 10^{-6}$

10a The combined paternity index for F_1 for the four genes in the analysis is $(0.5/0.18) \times (0.5/0.23) \times (0.5/0.13) \times (0.5/0.14) = 83$.

10b. A CPI of 83 indicates a high likelihood that F_1 is the father.

12a. S1 and S2 can be ruled out by Marker C because neither carries the nonmaternal Marker C allele.

12b. The PI for Markers A is 0.5/0.12, the PI for Marker B is 0.5/0.17, and the PI for Marker C is 0.5/0.11. The CPI is $(0.5/0.12) \times (0.5/0.17) \times (0.5/0.11) = 56$.

Glossary

3′ polyadenylation (3′ poly-A tailing) During eukaryotic pre-mRNA processing, an enzyme-driven modification that removes the 3′ end of the pre-mRNA and adds numerous adenines.

3′ splice site In eukaryotic pre-mRNA processing, the location of cleavage at the 3′ end of an intron. Contains an AG dinucleotide in a consensus sequence.

3′ to 5′ exonuclease activity DNA- and RNA-digesting activity that progresses in the 3′ to 5′ direction to remove nucleotides. See also *DNA proofreading*.

3′ untranslated region (3′ UTR) The untranslated segment of mRNA between the stop codon and the 3′ end of the transcript.

5′ capping In eukaryotic pre-mRNA processing, the addition of 7-methylguanosine to the nucleotide at the 5′ end of pre-mRNA by a triphosphate bridge. Methylation of adjacent nucleotides may also occur.

5′ splice site In mRNA processing, the location of cleavage at the 5′ end of an intron. Contains a GU dinucleotide in a consensus sequence.

5′ to 3′ exonuclease activity DNA- or RNA-digesting activity that progresses in the 5′ to 3′ direction to remove nucleotides.

5′ to 3′ polymerase activity DNA synthesizing activity of DNA polymerases that progresses in the 5′ to 3′ direction to add new nucleotides to a growing DNA strand. Requires a template strand.

5′ untranslated region (5′ UTR) The untranslated segment of mRNA between the 5′ end of the transcript and the start codon.

6-4 photoproduct A DNA lesion and potential mutagenic event caused by exposure to ultraviolet (UV) irradiation.

−10 consensus sequence See *Pribnow box*.

10-nm fiber The "beads-on-a-string" form of chromatin, in which DNA is wrapped around nucleosomes.

30-nm fiber A structure of chromatin in which histone 1 (H1) partially condenses chromatin fibers into a coiled form. Also known as *solenoid* or *solenoid structure*.

30S initiation complex In bacterial translation, the complex formed by a small ribosomal subunit, mRNA, and the tRNA carrying fMet.

−35 consensus sequence A specific consensus sequence of the bacterial promoter at which RNA polymerase is bound.

70S initiation complex The fully assembled bacterial ribosome that is prepared to initiate translation.

300-nm fiber A structural state of chromatin in which chromatin fibers are looped and condensed.

α-helix (alpha helix) A form of secondary protein structure in which segments of proteins form helical structures that are held together by hydrogen bonds.

α-proteobacteria Lineage of bacteria that are the closest extant relatives of the lineage that gave rise to mitochondria.

β-pleated sheet (beta-pleated sheet) A form of secondary protein structure in which segments of proteins form n parallel arrays that are held together by hydrogen bonds.

θ (theta) value A variable indicating a recombination distance between genes. Used in lod score analysis.

A site See *aminoacyl site*.

acentric fragment (acentric chromosome) A chromosome fragment without a centromere.

acrocentric chromosome A eukaryotic chromosome in which the centromere is very near one end. Forms a chromosome with long and short arms of distinctly different lengths.

activator binding site DNA sequence to which an activator protein binds to regulate gene expression. Term refers to regulatory sites in bacteria; in eukaryotes, the equivalent sequence would be called an enhancer element.

activator protein A transcription factor that binds to regulatory sequences associated with a gene and upregulates that gene's expression.

adaptive mutation hypothesis A disproven theory of the source of gene mutations proposing that mutated copies of genes were available in the genome or could rapidly occur in the genome given specific changes in the physical environment of an organism.

addition rule See *sum rule*.

additive genes Genes contributing to a polygenic trait and producing their effect by their cumulative contributions that are approximately equal for each gene.

additive variance (V_A) For quantitative traits, the component of genetic variance contributed by genes having an additive effect on phenotypic variance.

adenine (A) One of four nitrogenous nucleotide bases in DNA and RNA; one of the two types of purine nucleotides in DNA and RNA.

adjacent-1 segregation A pattern of chromosome segregation that can occur following reciprocal balanced translocation. Leads to gametes carrying gene duplications and deletions.

admixed population A population whose members are a blend of formerly distinct populations.

agarose An inert material derived from agar that is mixed with buffer and used to form gels for gel electrophoresis.

allele An alternative form of a gene.

allele-counting method A method for determining allele frequency in a sample by tabulating the number of alleles of each type.

allelic phase The arrangements of alleles of linked genes on homologous copies of a chromosome pair.

allelic series A group of alleles of a gene that display a hierarchy of dominance relationship among them.

allolactose A modified form of lactose that binds to the lac repressor protein, inducing an allosteric change that reduces the DNA binding ability of the complex.

allopatric speciation The development of new species in geographic isolation.

allopolyploidy A polyploidy organism arising through the union of chromosome sets from different species.

allosteric domain Domain of a protein that allows the protein to change shape when it binds to a specific molecule; the protein in the new shape is altered in its ability to bind to a second molecule (e.g., DNA). Also known as *allostery*.

allosteric effector compound Molecule that binds to the allosteric protein domain and subsequently induces a change in the bound protein.

allostery Reversible interactions of a small molecule with a protein that lead to changes in the shape of the protein and to a change in the interaction of the protein with a third molecule.

alternate segregation A pattern of chromosome segregation that can occur following reciprocal balanced translocation that leads to the production of viable gametes.

alternative pre-mRNA splicing (alternative intron splicing, promoter, polyadenylation) In eukaryotic pre-mRNA processing, alternative processes by which different mRNAs can be produced from the same gene using different promoters or polyadenylation sites or by removal of different exon elements.

alternative sigma (σ) subunit Different forms of the sigma subunit of bacterial RNA polymerase that induce distinct conformational changes to the RNA polymerase core and to the recognition of distinct promoters.

Ames test A laboratory method commonly used to determine whether a compound or one of its breakdown products is mutagenic.

amino acid An aminocarboxylic acid that is a component of a polypeptide or protein.

aminoacyl site (A site) The site on a ribosome at which incoming charged tRNAs match their anticodon sequence with mRNA codons.

aminoacyl-tRNA synthetase (tRNA synthetase) A group of enzymes whose specific functions are to identify particular tRNAs and catalyze the attachment of the appropriate amino acid at the 3′ terminus.

amniocentesis A method used as part of prenatal genetic screening to collect amniotic fluid for chromosome, DNA, and biochemical analysis.

amorphic mutation See *null mutation*.

anaphase The phase of mitosis during which sister chromatids separate (*anaphase A*) and move to opposite poles (*anaphase B*).

aneuploid An uneven number of chromosomes. Usually the result of the gain or loss of a chromosome—that is, $2n + 1$ (trisomy) or $2n - 1$ (monosomy).

angiogenesis The growth of blood vessels to supply new tissue with a blood supply.

annotation (gene annotation, genome annotation) The process of attaching biological functions to DNA sequences. Genome annotation is the process of identifying the location of genes and other functional sequences within the genome sequence; gene annotation defines the biochemical, cellular, and biological function of each gene product the genome encodes.

***Antennapedia* complex** One of two homeotic gene clusters in *Drosophila* consisting of five genes (*labial, Deformed, Sex combs reduced, proboscipedia,* and *Antennapedia*) that act in combination to specify the cephalic and thoracic parasegments.

antibiotic resistance An inherited trait of a microbe that permits it to grow in the presence of a compound that kills or prevents the growth of antibiotic-sensitive microbes.

anticodon The nucleotide triplet sequence of transfer RNA that pairs with an mRNA codon sequence in translation.

antiparallel Opposite 5′ and 3′ orientations of two complementary nucleic acid strands.

antisense RNA An RNA molecule that is complementary to a portion of a specific mRNA.

antisequestor stem loop A stem loop structure forming in mRNA that exposes the Shine–Dalgarno sequence, leading to translation.

antitermination stem loop A stem loop that allows RNA polymerase to continue transcription through the leader region of bacterial attenuator controlled operons and into the structural genes of an operon (e.g., *the 2–3 stem loop* in trp operon regulation).

antiterminator A transcription-regulating DNA sequence that when bound by proteins is unable to terminate transcription.

apurinic (AP) site The location of a nucleotide that has lost its purine base.

apoptosis Programmed cell death; part of the normal process of eliminating aged or damaged cells.

Archaea One of the three domains of life; separate from Bacteria and Eukarya.

archaeal initiation factor (aIF) The transcription initiation proteins found in archaeal cells.

Argonaute Protein subunit of RISC (RNA-induced silencing complex) that binds small RNA molecules and provides either the catalytic "slicer" activity or the translational repressor activity.

artificial cross-fertilization A controlled cross between plants made by an investigator who transfers pollen from one plant to fertilize the other plant.

association The relationship between certain alleles and phenotypes that results in bearers of an allele being statistically more likely to express a particular phenotypic trait or characteristic.

aster The structure forming during cell division that contains microtubules emanating from centrosomes.

attachment site (att site) Identical or nearly identical sequences on the bacterial and bacteriophage chromosomes that are cut and used to integrate or to excise the bacteriophage chromosome from the bacterial chromosome.

attenuation A gene regulatory mechanism that fine-tunes transcription to match the momentary requirements of the cell, achieving a more or less steady state of compound availability.

attenuator region A regulatory region downstream of the promoter of repressible amino acid operons that exerts transcriptional control (in the form of *transcription termination*) based on the translation of a leader peptide, the efficiency of which is determined by the availability of specific amino acids.

autopolyploidy A pattern of polyploidy produced by the duplication of chromosomes from a single genome.

autosomal dominant inheritance A pattern of hereditary transmission in which the dominant allele of an autosomal gene results in the appearance of the dominant phenotype.

autosomal inheritance Hereditary transmission of genes carried on autosomes.

autosomal recessive inheritance A pattern of hereditary transmission in which the recessive allele of an autosomal gene results in the appearance of the recessive phenotype.

auxotroph (auxotrophic strain) A microbe with one or more mutations that prevents its growth on a minimal medium.

Bacteria One of the three domains of life; separate from Archaea and Eukarya.

bacterial artificial chromosome (BAC) Cloning vector used in bacteria that utilizes the F plasmid origin of replication; can accept DNA inserts up to 500 kb.

bacterial chromosome The main, usually singular, chromosome encoding the genome of a bacterium.

bacteriophage (phage) A virus whose host is a bacterium.

balanced polymorphism A genetic polymorphism maintained in a population because organisms with the heterozygous genotype have higher relative fitness than do organisms with either of the homozygous genotypes.

balancer chromosome A chromosome with inversions used to maintain specific allele combinations (e.g., recessive lethal alleles) in genetic stocks.

barcode Short DNA sequences that identify specific strains in knockout libraries.

Barr body The darkly staining inactive X chromosome visible in mammalian female nuclei. The result of random X inactivation.

basal transcription The very low level of transcription characteristic of a bacterial promoter that requires an inducer to initiate transcription.

base excision repair DNA repair that excises a damaged nucleotide base and then replaces the entire nucleotide.

base-pair substitution mutation A DNA sequence change resulting in the substitution of one base pair for another.

base stacking A phenomenon of DNA base-pair interaction that rotates the base pairs around a central axis of symmetry and imparts twisting to the double helix.

basic local alignment search tool (BLAST) A computer program designed to search for homologous sequences in databases.

Bayesian analysis An application of predictive statistical analysis that adjusts the predicted likelihood of an event based on past outcomes.

benign tumor Abnormal growth of tissue (a tumor) that is confined or encapsulated and does not invade surrounding tissues.

bidirectional DNA replication The standard method of DNA replication that synthesizes new DNA in both directions from a replication origin.

binary fission A process of cell division common in bacteria that splits the original cell into two cells following replication of the bacterial chromosome.

binomial probability A probability function using two coefficients, a and b, whose sum equals 1 and whose products predict the probability of events.

bioinformatics The use of computational approaches to decipher DNA-sequence information.

biological species concept The theory of species that says separate species are reproductively isolated and are unable to produce viable hybrids with members of other species.

biparental inheritance Condition in organellar inheritance where both parental gametes make contributions of cytoplasmic organelles to the zygote; contributions are often unequal because one gamete contributes more of the cytoplasm and the other gamete makes a smaller contribution.

bithorax complex One of two homeotic gene clusters in *Drosophila* consisting of three genes (*Ultrabithorax*, *abdominal-A*, and *abdominal-B*) that act in combination to specify the thoracic and abdominal parasegments.

blending theory of heredity An obsolete theory of heredity proposing that the traits of offspring are the average of parental traits.

blunt end 5′ or 3′ ends of double-stranded DNA lacking any single-stranded overhangs.

branch point adenine In intron splicing, an adenine nucleotide near the 3′ splice site of an intron that joins with a guanine located at the 5′ splice site by a 2′-to-5′ phosphodiester bond to form a lariat intron.

broad sense heritability (H^2) The proportion of total phenotypic variance that is contributed by total genetic variance.

bypass polymerase A group of DNA polymerases that are unstable and synthesize short regions of DNA under conditions in which the main DNA polymerase is unable to function, such as when faced with DNA lesions that block replication. See also *translesion DNA polymerase*.

CAAT box A common consensus sequence component of eukaryotic promoters.

CAP binding site A bacterial DNA regulatory sequence to which the CAP–cAMP complex binds to positively regulate gene expression. See also *CAP–cAMP complex*.

CAP–cAMP binding region A region of the bacterial *lac* operon promoter that binds the complex containing the catabolite activator protein (CAP) and cyclic AMP (cAMP) to positively regulate the transcription of operon genes.

CAP–cAMP complex Formed by joining catabolite activator protein to cAMP, this complex binds to the CAP binding site of the bacterial *lac* promoter to regulate gene expression.

carrier genetic testing Genetic testing intended to determine whether or not a person is heterozygous for a mutant allele.

Cas genes CRISPR-associated genes. Cas proteins act as the catalytic component (endonuclease) of the CRISPR–Cas complex, creating double-strand breaks in target DNA molecules. In *Staphylococcus*, a single protein, Cas9, is sufficient.

catabolite repression Situation where the presence of the preferred catabolite (e.g., glucose) represses the transcription of genes for an alternative catabolite (e.g., lactose).

cell cycle Consisting of interphase (*G₁ phase*, *S phase*, and *G₂ phase*) and *M phase* (mitosis or meiosis) in cells. The transition from one phase to the next is controlled by protein-based interactions.

cell cycle checkpoint Protein-mediated activities that monitor a cell's progression through the cell cycle, pausing the cell cycle to allow required

activity to take place and advancing the cell cycle when conditions in the cell are appropriate.

cellular blastoderm Stage of *Drosophila* embryogenesis in which the nuclei are located at the periphery of the embryo and are enclosed by cell membranes.

central dogma of biology The description of the functional relationship between DNA, RNA and proteins (DNA to RNA to protein).

centromere A specialized DNA sequence on eukaryotic chromosomes that is the site of kinetochore protein and microtubule binding.

centrosome A cytoplasmic region, containing a pair of centrioles in many eukaryotic species, from which the growth of microtubules forms the spindle apparatus during cell division.

Chargaff's rule The observation that the percentage of adenine equals that of thymine and that guanine percentage equals cytosine percentage in DNA.

charged tRNA A tRNA to which the correct amino acid has been attached.

chiasma (plural: chiasmata) Points of contact between homologous chromosomes that are coincident with crossover locations between the homologs.

chimeric gene A gene sequence composed of sequences from two or more sources.

chi-square test (χ^2 test) A statistical test to compare the observed results of an experiment with the results predicted by chance.

chloroplast An organelle, bounded by a double membrane, where photosynthetic reactions convert light energy and CO_2 into fixed organic carbon.

chorionic villus sampling (CVS) A method used as part of prenatal genetic testing that collects a sample of the chorionic villus for chromosomal, DNA, or biochemical analysis.

chromatin The complex of nucleic acids and proteins that compose eukaryotic chromosomes.

chromatin modifier Proteins that chemically modify histone proteins in the nucleosomes by adding or removing specific chemical groups, thereby modifying chromatin structure and regulating gene expression.

chromatin remodeler Proteins that reposition nucleosomes within chromatin in such a way as to open or close promoters and other regulatory sequences or that change the composition of nucleosomes, altering their biological activity (e.g., SWI/SNF, ISWI, SWR1).

chromatin remodeling Processes that modify the structure or composition of chromatin. Usually associated with alterations of nucleosome binding to DNA and affecting the regulation of gene transcription.

chromosome A structure composed of DNA and associated proteins that in total contain the genome of an organism.

chromosome arm [long arm (q arm), short arm (p arm)] The segments of eukaryotic

chromosomes between the centromere and the telomeres.

chromosome banding A group of laboratory methods that stain eukaryotic chromosomes to reveal distinctive patterns of light and dark bands. Chromosome banding by Giemsa staining produced standardized patterns for different chromosome of selected species. Also known as *Giemsa (G) banding*.

chromosome break point The location of a chromosome break.

chromosome fusion See *Robertsonian translocation*.

chromosome inversion (paracentric, pericentric) A structural alteration of a chromosome in which a segment breaks away from the chromosome and subsequently reattaches after 180° rotation. See also *inversion heterozygote*.

chromosome scaffold Composed of numerous nonhistone proteins, the superstructure of eukaryotic chromosomes.

chromosome territory The region within an interphase nucleus occupied by a particular chromosome during interphase.

chromosome theory of heredity The theory developed in the early 20th century that genes are carried on chromosomes and that the meiotic behavior of chromosomes is the physical basis of Mendel's laws.

chromosome translocation The relocation of a chromosome or chromosome segment to a non-homologous chromosome.

cis-acting Acting on the same chromosome (e.g., DNA sequences that control expression of genes encoded on the same piece of DNA).

cis-acting regulatory sequence Sequences to which proteins bind to regulate transcription of genes located on the same chromosome as the sequences.

cis-dominant The principle that the operator can influence only the transcription of adjacent downstream genes.

clade In phylogenetics, a group of organisms defined by characteristics that are unique to the group and distinguish the group from others.

cladistics The classification of organisms by characteristics that are unique to the group and distinguish it from other groups. Involves branching of new species from ancestral species. See also *clade*.

cloning vector A piece of DNA derived from a plasmid, virus, or other biological source that can be stably maintained in an organism and into which heterologous pieces of DNA can be inserted.

closed chromatin Chromatin in which regulatory DNA is covered by nucleosomes, thus restricting the access of regulatory proteins to the sequences rendering genes in closed chromatin transcriptionally silent.

closed promoter complex The initial stage of transcription that forms when RNA polymerase loosely binds the promoter.

coding region The region of a gene that encodes the gene product.

coding strand (nontemplate strand) The nontemplate strand of DNA that has the same 5′-to-3′ polarity as its transcript and the same sequence, except for T in DNA and U in RNA.

codominance The equal and detectable expression of both alleles in a heterozygous organism.

codon The nucleotide triplet of mRNA that encodes a single amino acid.

codon bias The preferential use of specific codons where there is redundancy in encoding a specific amino acid.

coefficient of coincidence (c) The ratio of the observed number of double recombinants to the number of double recombinants expected to occur by chance.

coefficient of inbreeding (F) The probability that two alleles carried in an individual are homozygous identical by descent (IBD).

cohesive compatible end Short, single-stranded overhangs at 5′ and 3′ ends produced after digestion with certain restriction ends. The cohesive ends are termed compatible if they can base-pair with complementary single-stranded ends of another DNA molecule. Compare with *cohesive end sequence (cos) sites*.

cohesive end sequence (cos) site The single-stranded ends of phage lambda that facilitate circularization or concatamerization of lambda phage genomes and that interact with coat proteins during packaging of phage particles. Compare with *cohesive compatible ends*.

colony A large number of bacteria forming a visible cluster on a growth plate that are derived by many cycles of binary fissioning from a single cell deposited at that location on the growth plate.

combined paternity index (CPI) An estimate of the joint probability of paternity based on the paternity index (PI) values derived from genetic analysis of alleles of multiple genes shared by a putative father and a child.

complementary base pairs The specific pattern of purine-pyrimidine pairing of nucleic acid strands. In DNA, G with C and A with T; RNA uses U instead of T.

complementary DNA (cDNA) library Collection of DNA clones, originally derived via reverse transcription of mRNA molecules into DNA (cDNA) and cloned into a vector.

complementary gene interaction (9:7 ratio) A characteristic ratio of phenotypes produced by the interaction of two complementary genes that control a trait.

complementation group A group of mutations that affect the same gene.

complete medium A microbial growth medium supplemented with a wide array of vitamins, nucleotides, amino acids, and other compounds that will support the growth of wild-type and mutant microbes.

complete penetrance The observation that the phenotype for a trait is always produced when the corresponding genotype(s) are present (in contrast, see *incomplete penetrance*).

composite transposon In bacteria, a transposable element containing multiple genes located between terminal insertion sequences.

concordance In twin studies, the observation that both twins exhibit the trait.

conditional probability A probability prediction that is dependent on another previous event having taken place.

conjugation The short-term union of two bacterial cells for the unidirectional transfer of DNA from the "donor" to the "recipient." The transferred material may be plasmid DNA or donor bacterial chromosome DNA.

conjugation pilus The hollow filament extending from the donor bacterium to the recipient bacterium through which DNA is transferred.

consanguineous mating See *inbreeding*.

consensus sequence A nucleotide sequence in a DNA segment derived by comparing sequences of similar segments from other genes or organisms. The most commonly occurring nucleotides at each position comprise the sequence.

conservation genetics The field of applied genetics that seeks to protect endangered species in native and captive populations.

conservative DNA replication A disproven model of DNA replication positing that one duplex produced by replication contained the two original strands and the other two daughter strands.

conserved noncoding sequence (CNS) Sequences that do not code for amino acids and are conserved across significant phylogenetic distances.

constitutive heterochromatin Chromosome regions containing chromatin that is always densely compacted. Usually containing highly repetitive DNA sequences.

constitutive mutants Mutants in which a gene is always expressed rather than being under regulatory control.

constitutive transcription State in which a gene is continuously transcribed.

consultand The person seeking information from a genetic counselor or medical genetics specialist.

contiguous sequence (contig) Overlapping DNA clones that together cover an uninterrupted continuous stretch of DNA sequence.

continuous variation In polygenic and multifactorial traits, the observation of phenotypic distribution over a continuous range.

controlled genetic cross Genetic crosses controlled by an investigator who usually knows the genotypes and/or phenotypes of the organisms being crossed.

convergent evolution Processes of independent evolution of similar structures in unrelated species. Also known as *homoplasmy*.

co-option A common theme in the evolutionary history of genes by which genes and genetic modules are reused in a new manner to direct the patterning or growth of novel organs.

coordinate gene Genes, often with maternal effects, that establish the major axes of the embryo, especially the anterior-posterior and dorsal-ventral axes; examples include *bicoid* and *nanos*.

copy number variant (CNV) A specific type of structural variant due to insertions or deletions (indels) greater than 1 kb in length.

core DNA The approximately 146 base pairs of eukaryotic DNA that wrap each nucleosome.

core element Consensus sequences in the active regions of promoters recognized by RNA polymerase I.

corepressor An accessory molecule required for a repressor protein to exert its function.

cosuppression The silencing, via a small RNA mediated mechanism, of an endogenous gene due to the presence of a homologous transgene or virus. Cosuppression can occur at the transcriptional or posttranscriptional level.

cotransduction The simultaneous transduction of two or more genes contained on a donor DNA fragment into a recipient cell, where it undergoes homologous recombination to be spliced into the transductant chromosome.

cotransduction frequency The frequency with which two genes are transduced.

cotransduction mapping A method of mapping donor bacterial genes based on their frequency of cotransduction.

cotransformation Simultaneous transformation of two or more genes carried on a donor DNA fragment into a recipient.

covered promoter Promoter in which nucleosomes are found adjacent to the transcription start site, preventing efficient transcription initiation. This feature is common at highly regulated genes.

CpG island Region in which the frequency of CpG dinucleotides is higher than the average for the genome; commonly found near the transcription start sites of animal genes. The cytosines are often methylated when the gene is inactive and demethylated when the gene is transcriptionally active.

CRISPR *Clustered Regularly Interspaced Short Palindromic Repeats*. Transcribed repetitive sequence that is processed into unique crRNAs acting in a bacterial or archael immune system.

CRISPR-Cas9 Complex of the Cas9 protein with tracrRNA and crRNA that acts to target invading nucleic acids in *Staphylococcus*. This system has been modified for use in gene editing.

crossing over The breakage and reunion of homologous chromosomes that results in reciprocal recombination.

crossover suppression The significant reduction, or complete absence, of progeny with recombinant chromosomes due to duplications and deletions of genetic material following crossing over within the inversion loop in organisms that are heterozygous for an inversion.

crRNA Unique small RNAs derived from CRISPR loci that combine through complementary base pairing with tracrRNAs in the CRISPR-Cas complex.

cryptic splice site A 5′ or 3′ splice site that is not normally used except when a mutation either inactivates an authentic splice site or creates a new splice site at the cryptic site location. See also *splicing mutation*.

cyanobacteria Lineage of photosynthetic bacteria that are the closest extant relatives of the lineage that gave rise to the plastids.

cytokinesis Part of telophase, the process of cytoplasmic division between daughter cells.

cytoplasmic inheritance Transmission of genes outside of the nucleus, e.g., in the mitochondrial or chloroplast genome.

cytosine (C) One of four nitrogenous nucleotide bases in DNA and RNA; one of the two types of pyrimidine nucleotides in DNA and RNA.

daughter cell The genetically identical cells produced by mitotic cell division.

daughter strand A newly synthesized strand of DNA that is complementary to a template strand.

deamination A DNA lesion resulting in the loss of an amino group (NH_2) from a nucleotide base.

dedifferentiation The loss of cell-type specific differentiation during the process of cancer development.

degrees of freedom (*df*) The number of independent variables in an experiment. In a chi-square test, most often the number of outcome class minus 1 ($n - 1$).

delayed age of onset The appearance of an abnormal phenotype that is not present at birth but appears later in life and is caused by an inherited mutation.

delayed early genes A group of genes in λ (lambda) bacteriophage that are expressed following expression of the early genes that initiate the lytic cycle.

deletion The loss of genetic material. See also *interstitial, microdeletion, partial deletion, partial deletion heterozygote*, and *terminal deletion*.

deletion mapping A method for mapping genes utilizing partial chromosome deletions with known locations to expose recessive mutants by pseudodominance.

deoxynucleotide monophosphate (dNMP) Monophosphate forms of deoxynucleotides.

deoxynucleotide triphosphate (dNTP) Triphosphate forms of deoxynucleotides.

deoxyribonucleic acid (DNA) The hereditary molecule of organisms. Composed of two complementary strands of nucleotides with purine bases adenine (A) and guanine (G) and pyrimidine bases thymine (T) and cytosine (C).

depurination A DNA lesion occurring when a deoxyribose molecule loses its purine nucleotide base. See *apurinic (AP) site*.

dicentric bridge In a dicentric chromosome, the portion between the two centromeres that are drawn to opposite poles of the cell during division.

dicentric chromosome A chromosome with two centromeres.

Dicer Ribonuclease that acts on double-stranded RNA responsible for the generation of small regulatory RNA molecules, such as microRNAs and small interfering RNAs; typically 21–30 nucleotides in length.

dideoxy DNA sequencing (dideoxynucleotide DNA sequencing) A method of DNA sequencing devised by Fred Sanger that uses a mixture of deoxynucleotide and dideoxynucleotide triphosphates to selectively block DNA replication, producing a ladder of partially synthesized DNA strands of different lengths. Also known as the *Sanger method*.

dideoxynucleotide triphosphate (ddNTP) Rare DNA nucleotides absent oxygen molecules at the 2′ and the 3′ carbons that are most commonly used in dideoxynucleotide DNA sequencing.

differential reproductive fitness See *relative fitness (w)*.

differentiation Process by which cells become restricted in their developmental potential and take on specialized morphologies and physiological activities.

dihybrid cross A cross between organisms that are heterozygous for two loci.

diploid number The characteristic number of chromosomes (*2n*) in somatic cell nuclei during the diploid phase of the eukaryotic life cycle. Equal to twice the haploid (*n*) number of chromosomes found in the nuclei of gametes of sexually reproducing diploid species.

direct-to-consumer genetic testing Genetic testing requested by an individual subscriber to whom the results and related information are then made directly available.

directional cloning Technique whereby a DNA insert is cloned with a specific directionality with respect to sequences of the cloning vector; usually accomplished by using two different restriction enzymes.

directional selection Natural or artificial selection that continuously changes the frequency of an allele in a direction toward fixation (frequency = 1.0) or toward elimination (frequency = 0.0).

discontinuous variation A phenotype distribution containing discrete or separable categories.

discordance In twin studies, the observation that the traits exhibited by the twins are different.

disjunction The normal process separation of homologous chromosomes or of sister chromatids during cell division.

dispersive DNA replication A disproven model of DNA replication positing that each strand of daughter duplexes is composed of segments of original DNA and segments of newly synthesized DNA.

displacement loop (D loop) During DNA damage repair and homologous recombination, the displacement of a single strand of DNA by strand invasion.

disruptive selection Natural or artificial selection of phenotypic extremes in a population, leading eventually to two strains with distinctive phenotypes.

DNA-binding domain The segment of a protein that interacts with DNA and usually binds to DNA containing one or more specific sequences.

DNA clone A fragment of DNA that is inserted into a vector, such as a plasmid, cosmid, or artificial chromosome.

DNA double helix (DNA duplex) The two complementary strands of DNA arranged in antiparallel orientation.

DNA fingerprinting Production by gel electrophoresis of a DNA band pattern for multiple genes for purposes of comparison and identification (usually a DNA band pattern specific to an individual).

DNA intercalating agents Mutagenic compounds of a size and shape that allow them to access to the space between nucleotide base pairs, thereby distorting the DNA duplex and potentially causing insertion or deletion mutations.

DNA library Collection of DNA clones in which the DNA is usually derived from a single source.

DNA ligase An enzyme active in DNA replication that joins together segments of a DNA strand by catalyzing formation of a phosphodiester bond.

DNA loop In gene regulation, a condition where the DNA sequences between regulatory elements form an extended loop that allows distant regulatory sequences with associated DNA-binding proteins to interact.

DNA microarray Collections of synthesized DNA fragments attached to a solid support and representing sequences present in a genome; can be used to assess transcription patterns, transcription factor binding sites, and recombination patterns, among other uses.

DNA nucleotides DNA building blocks composed of deoxyribose sugar, a nitrogenous base, and one or more phosphate groups. See also *adenine (A), thymine (T), cytosine (C),* and *guanine (G)*.

DNA pol A shorthand term for *DNA polymerase*.

DNA polymerase (pol I, pol II, pol III) The large multisubunit complex responsible for the synthesis of new strands of DNA during DNA replication or DNA repair.

DNA profiling DNA analysis intended to develop a genetic profile that can be attributed to an individual.

DNA proofreading The capacity of many types of DNA polymerase to utilize a $3'$ to $5'$ exonuclease activity to remove and replace mismatched or damaged nucleotides during replication. See also $3'$ to $5'$ *exonuclease activity.*

DNA replication The synthesis of new DNA strands by complementary base pairing of nucleotides in a daughter strand to those in a template strand.

DNA transposon One type of transposable genetic element encoding a transposase and capable of transposition.

DNase I hypersensitive site Any region of chromatin sensitive to cleavage by DNase I; often representing open chromatin that is transcriptionally active.

dominance variance In polygenic and multifactorial inheritance, the portion of genetic variance attributed to the dominance effects of contributing genes.

dominant allele An allele that is expressed in the phenotype if the genotype contains one or more copies of the allele.

dominant epistasis (12:3:1 ratio) A characteristic ratio of phenotypes produced by the interaction of two genes that control a trait in which a dominant allele of one gene masks or reduces the expression of alleles of a second gene.

dominant interaction (9:6:1 ratio) A characteristic ratio of phenotypes produced by the interaction of two genes that control a trait in which the presence of dominant alleles of both genes produces one phenotype, one dominant allele of either gene produces a second phenotype, and organisms with only recessive alleles for the interacting genes have a third phenotype.

dominant negative mutation A dominant mutation that behaves as a loss-of-function, often due to blocking the formation or normal function of a multimeric protein complex.

dominant phenotype The phenotype observed in a heterozygous organism that is identical to the phenotype observed in a homozygote. The phenotype produced when an organism is homozygous for the dominant allele or carries a single copy of the dominant allele in the heterozygous genotype. Compare with *recessive phenotype.*

dominant suppression (13:3 ratio) A characteristic ratio of phenotypes produced by the interaction of two genes that control a trait in which the dominant allele of one gene suppresses he expression of the dominant allele of the second gene.

donor cell (bacterial donor) The bacterial cell that is the source of DNA transferred to a recipient cell by either conjugation, transduction, or transformation.

dosage compensation mechanism A mechanism for equalizing the expression of X-linked genes in males and females of a species.

double Holliday junction (DHJ) An intermediate structure temporarily connecting chromatids of homologous chromosomes that forms during homologous recombination.

double recombinant (double crossover) The occurrence of two crossovers between homologous chromosomes in a particular region. May involve two, three, or all four chromatids.

double-strand break (DSB) Breakage of phosphodiester bonds on both strands of DNA; associated with DNA damage or with the initial steps of the process leading to homologous recombination.

double-strand break repair Following phosphodiester bond breakage on both strands of a DNA duplex, a mechanism of DNA damage repair. Related to the mechanism for homologous recombination.

downstream Referring to a gene or sequence location that is toward the $3'$ direction on the *coding strand.*

Drosha Ribonuclease that processes primicroRNA molecules into pre-microRNA molecules in animals.

duplicate gene action (15:1 ratio) A characteristic ratio of phenotypes produced by the interaction of two genes that duplicate each other's action due to genetic redundancy.

duplication The gain of genetic material by the inclusion of one or more additional copies of a chromosome segment. See also *microduplication, partial duplication,* and *partial duplication heterozygote.*

dysplasia Abnormal, but noncancerous, growth of tissue.

E site See *exit site.*

early operators The operator sequence in the genome of bacteriophage λ (lambda) that controls transcription of early genes. See also *delayed early genes* and *late genes.*

early promoters Regulatory sequences responsible for the activation of early genes or operons in bacteriophage. See also *delayed early genes* and *late genes.*

electrophoretic mobility A measurement of (1) the distance of migration or (2) the speed of migration of a nucleic acid or protein in gel electrophoresis.

elongation factor (EF) A group of proteins associated with ribosomes that contribute to the elongation of the polypeptide product.

embryonic stem cell In vertebrates, totipotent cells of early embryos that can give rise to any and all cell types of the organism.

endosymbiont An organism that lives within the body or cell of another organism.

endosymbiosis An (often) mutually beneficial relationship between organisms in which one organism, the endosymbiont, inhabits the body of the other.

endosymbiosis theory Hypothesis that the mitochondrion and chloroplast are evolutionarily derived from bacterial endosymbionts related to extant α-proteobacteria and cyanobacteria, respectively.

enhanceosome Protein complex that binds enhancer elements and directs DNA bending into loops that bring the protein complex into contact with RNA polymerase and transcription factors bound at the core promoter or with protein complexes bound to proximal promoter elements.

enhancer (enhancer sequence) A eukaryotic cis-acting DNA regulatory sequence to which trans-acting factors bind and stimulate transcription.

enhancer screen A genetic screen designed to identify mutations in genes that worsen the phenotypic effects of mutations in another gene.

enhancer trapping A transgenic construct inserted randomly into the genome that allows identification of enhancer elements controlling specific patterns of gene expression.

environmental variance (V_E) For quantitative traits, the proportion of the total phenotypic variance contributed by differences in the environment experienced by population members.

epigenetic Heritable patterns or changes in gene expression that are not associated with any change in DNA sequence.

epigenetic marks A collection of chemical marks and modifications, such as acteylation and methylation of histone proteins, that are functional in chromatin remodeling. Also known as *epigenetic modification.*

epigenetic modification Chemical modifications of DNA or associated histones, such as acetylation and methylation, that alter chromatin structure and influence gene transcription.

epistatic interaction A group of specific patterns of gene interaction in which an allele of one gene modifies or prevents the expression of alleles of another gene. Also known as *epistasis.*

ethidium bromide (EtBr) A compound used to stain DNA and RNA in electrophoresis gels.

euchromatin (euchromatic regions) Chromosome regions containing chromatin that is not densely compacted. Most expressed genes are located within euchromatic regions of chromosomes.

Eukarya One of the three domains of life; separate from Archaea and Bacteria.

eukaryotic expression vector A vector that contains all the necessary cis-regulatory sequences to enable gene expression in a eukaryotic cell.

eukaryotic initiation factor (eIF) A group of eukaryotic proteins that associate with ribosomal subunits and help initiate translation.

euploid A number of chromosomes that is an exact multiple of the haploid number.

E (var) mutation Mutations that enhance position effect variegation in *Drosophila.* Mutated genes produce proteins that are active in chromatin remodeling.

evo-devo The study of the evolution of development.

evolution (1) Any change in the genetic characteristics of a population, strain, or species over time. (2) The theory that all organisms are related by common ancestry and have diversified from common ancestors over time.

evolutionary genetics The study of evolution and evolutionary processes using genetic techniques and tools.

evolutionary genomics The comparison of genomes, both within and between species. It illuminates the genetic basis of similarities and differences between individuals or species.

exconjugant cell The cell that is the product of conjugation between a donor cell and a recipient cell.

exit site (E site) On the ribosome, the site through which an uncharged tRNA exits.

exon A nonintron segment of the coding sequence of a gene. Joined together following intron splicing, exons correspond to the mRNA sequence that is translated into a polypeptide.

expression array DNA microarray that carries unique sequences from every annotated gene of the genome and is used to monitor gene expression patterns.

expression vector Cloning vector possessing DNA sequences required for DNA fragments inserted into the vector to be transcribed and translated. Vectors with sequences facilitating expression in eukaryotes are called *eukaryotic expression vectors.*

F (fertility) plasmid The plasmid containing genes that confer the ability to act as a donor cell on a bacterium. May be either an extrachromosomal plasmid or may be incorporated into the donor bacterial chromosome. Also known as *F plasmid.*

F plasmid See *F (fertility) plasmid.*

F$^+$ cell (F$^+$ donor) A donor bacterium containing an extrachromosomal fertility plasmid.

F- (F- cells) A bacterial recipient cell; does not contain an F (fertility) plasmid.

F′ cell (F′ donor) A bacterial donor cell harboring an F (fertility) plasmid.

F′ factor An extrachromosomal fertility plasmid into which a portion of the donor bacterial chromosome has been incorporated.

F$_1$ generation (first filial generation) The first generation of offspring. In genetic experiments, usually the offspring produced by crossing pure-breeding parents.

F$_2$ generation (second filial generation) The second generation, produced by crossing F$_1$ organisms.

F$_3$ generation (third filial generation) The third generation, produced by crossing F$_2$ organisms.

facultative heterochromatin Heterochromatic chromosome regions whose level of compaction can vary. Often contains repetitive DNA, but may also contain some expressed genes.

familial cancer (hereditary cancer) Cancer cases developing in part through the inheritance of germ-line gene mutations that predispose individuals to cancer; an inherited susceptibility to cancer.

familial adenomatous polyposis (FAP) An inherited condition caused by a specific gene mutation that leads to the development of a large number of abnormal growths (polyps) in the colon; a condition that can be followed by the development of colon cancer.

fetal cell sorting A method used as part of pre-natal genetic testing that isolates fetal cells from maternal blood circulation for DNA, chromosomal, and biochemical testing.

first-degree relative (first-degree relationship; also second-degree, third-degree) A genetic relationship between individuals who share 50% of their genes in common, i.e., a parent-child relationship.

first filial generation See F_1 *generation.*

flanking direct sequence repeat (flanking direct repeat) Identical repetitive sequences flanking the sites of insertion of transposable genetic elements.

fluctuation test The term used to identify an experiment performed by Salvador Luria and Max Delbrück that identified the random nature of gene mutations.

fluorescent in situ hybridization (FISH) A laboratory method for identifying genes or DNA sequences using molecular probes labeled with a compound that can emit fluorescent light upon excitation.

forensic genetics (forensic genetic analysis) DNA-based analysis of biological material recovered from a crime scene or crime victim, or DNA analysis intended to identify individuals following a disaster or mass casualty event.

forked-line diagram A method for diagramming the probabilities of outcomes in a branching format.

forward genetic analysis The classical approach to genetic analysis whereby genes are first identified by mutant phenotypes caused by mutant alleles and the gene sequence is subsequently identified by recombinant DNA technologies. Also known as *forward genetics.*

forward genetics See *forward genetic analysis.*

forward mutation A mutation that alters a wild type and generates a mutant. Also known as *mutation.*

forward mutation rate (μ) The frequency of mutation from wild-type alleles to mutant alleles.

founder effect The random occurrence of allele and genotype frequency differences between a new population established by a small number of founders and the larger parental population.

frameshift mutation The insertion or deletion of DNA base pairs resulting in translation of mRNA in an incorrect reading frame.

frequency distribution A visual display or histogram of quantitative data.

fully penetrant Synonymous with the *term* complete penetrance. An allele that expresses itself in the phenotype every time it is present in the genotype.

functional domain A protein region with a specific function or interaction.

functional genomics Using genomic sequences and genome-wide patterns of transcripts and protein expression to understand gene function in an organism.

fusion gene A recombinant gene composed of DNA sequences from more than one source (e.g., the codon sequences derived from one gene and the sequences responsible for expression derived from a second gene).

fusion protein A recombinant protein encoded by DNA sequences from more than one source; made by combining the open reading frames of two unrelated genes.

G$_0$ phase The "G zero" phase of the cell cycle, an alternative to G$_1$ of the cell cycle entered by mature cells that generally do not divide again until they die. Compare with G$_1$ *phase* and G$_2$ *phase.*

G$_1$ phase The "Gap 1" phase of the cell cycle during which genes are actively transcribed and translated and cells carry out their normal functions. Compare with G$_0$ phase and G$_2$ *phase.*

G$_2$ phase The "Gap 2" phase of the cell cycle during which the cell prepares to divide. Compare with G$_0$ phase and G$_1$ *phase.*

GC-rich box A regulatory segment of DNA, usually of a promoter, that is rich in guanine and cytosine nucleotides.

gain-of-function mutation A mutation causing a gene to be overexpressed, to be expressed at the wrong time, or to encode a constitutively acting protein; usually inherited as a dominant mutation.

gamete The reproductive cells produced by male and female reproductive structures; sperm or pollen in male animals and plants and eggs in females.

gap gene In *Drosophila*, genes that control development in large contiguous regions along the anterior-posterior axis; examples include *hunchback, giant, Krüppel,* and *knirps.*

gel electrophoresis A laboratory method for separating proteins or nucleic acid molecules or fragments using electrical current in a gel matrix.

gene The physical unit of heredity, composed of a DNA sequence that is transcribed and encodes a polypeptide or another functional molecule.

gene dosage The number of copies of a gene.

gene drive Phenomenon in which the Mendelian pattern of segregation is altered in response to an increase in the frequency of inheritance of a particular allele (or locus) over the wild-type allele (or locus).

gene–environment interaction Interactions taking place between particular genes and specific environmental factors.

gene family A group of genes that is evolutionarily related via successive gene duplication events that are followed by diversification.

gene flow The movement of genes into, out of, or between populations as a consequence of the movement of organisms. See also *migration*.

gene interaction Referring to genes that interact with one another due to their participation in the production of a particular product or trait.

gene knockout Loss-of-function allele of a gene usually obtained via a reverse genetic approach.

gene pool The total of all alleles present in breeding members of a population at a given moment.

gene therapy The use of genes as therapeutic agents to cure or alleviate symptoms of a genetic disease.

general transcription factors (GTFs) Eukaryotic transcription-activating proteins that bind the promoter region to form part of the apparatus that initiates basal transcription.

generalized transducing phage In transduction, a bacteriophage that carries a random segment of the chromosome of a donor cell to the recipient cell.

generalized transduction The transduction of a random segment of a donor chromosome into a recipient cell by a transducing phage. See also *generalized transducing phage*.

genetic bottleneck A period or event characterized by a substantial random reduction in population size. Loss of genetic diversity and allele frequency changes usually occur.

genetic carrier screening See *carrier genetic testing*.

genetic chimera A tissue or organism composed of cells of two or more distinct genotypes.

genetic code The universal set of correspondences of mRNA codons to amino acids. Used in translation to synthesize polypeptides.

genetic complementation (1) The observation of a wild-type phenotype in an organism or cell containing two different mutations. (2) The cross of two pure-breeding mutants that yields progeny that are exclusively wild type.

genetic complementation analysis The experimental pairwise comparison of genetic mutants designed to determine whether mutants complement one another by producing wild types.

genetic dissection The use of mutations and recombinants in genetic analyses to identify and assemble the genetic components of a biological property or process.

genetic drift A process of evolution referring to random changes in allele frequencies that result from sampling errors. Occurs in all populations but is strongest in small populations.

genetic fine structure The method of high-resolution analysis of intragenic recombination to map genes at the nucleotide level.

genetic heterogeneity The observation of the same phenotype produced by mutation of any one of two or more different genes.

genetic hitchhiking The phenomenon in which specific alleles of genes that are closely linked to a gene undergoing positive natural selection have their frequencies increased by virtue of their presence on the same chromosomes as the favored allele.

genetic instability The tendency of a genome containing numerous gene or chromosome mutations to acquire more mutations.

genetic liability See *threshold of genetic liability*.

genetic linkage The result of genes being located so near one another on a chromosome that their alleles do not assort independently. Identified by detecting certain pairs of alleles (parentals) that are transmitted together significantly more often than expected by chance and of other pairs of alleles (nonparentals or recombinants) that are transmitted together significantly less often than expected.

genetic linkage mapping Process for creating maps of genes based on their linkage relationships to other genes.

genetic markers Alleles of either expressed genes or noncoding chromosomal regions identifying a specific region of a chromosome. Can be used to trace or identify another gene, the chromosome, or a cell, organ, or individual.

genetic mosaic An organism whose body consists of cells of at least two different genotypes.

genetic network Set of interacting genes identified from double mutants or other analyses indicating gene interaction.

genetic redundancy The situation where the functions of one gene are compensated for by the actions of another gene.

genetic screen A procedure whereby a population of organisms is mutagenized and their progeny are propagated and examined for mutant phenotypes. Also known as *mutagenesis*.

genetic variance (V_G) In polygenic and multifactorial inheritance, the proportion of total phenotypic variance contributed by genetic variation.

genome The entire complement of DNA sequences in a chromosome set of an organism.

genome editing A type of genetic engineering in which DNA is modified, inserted, or deleted in the genome of a living organism; most commonly done using the CRISPR–Cas system.

genome-wide association study (GWAS) Association analysis performed using genetic marker genes distributed throughout the genome. Designed to locate genes that may influence the variation of quantitative traits.

genomics The study of the structure, function, composition, and evolution of genomes.

genomic imprinting Epigenetic phenomena that create differential expression of alleles depending on whether they were maternally or paternally inherited.

genomic island Genome segments that differ in sequence makeup from the surrounding genome sequence. Often these are a consequence of lateral gene transfer.

genomic library A set of clones consisting of the DNA representing the genome of an organism.

genotype (1) The genetic composition of an organism or a cell (i.e., all the alleles of all the genes). (2) The alleles of a single gene or a specified set of genes in a cell or organism.

genotype proportion method A method for estimating allele frequencies in a population by manipulation of genotype frequencies.

genotypic ratio (1:2:1 ratio) (1) A ratio or set of relative proportions between organisms with different genotypes. (2) The ratio of 1/4 : 1/2 : 1/4 observed among the homozygous and heterozygous F_2 progeny of a monohybrid cross.

germinal gene therapy Gene therapy aimed at correcting the genetic defect in the germ cells, such that progeny would not inherit the genetic defect.

germ-line cell See *gamete*.

germ-line mutation A mutation present in sperm, pollen, or an egg.

Giemsa (G) banding See *chromosome banding*.

Goldberg–Hogness box See *TATA box*.

green fluorescent protein (GFP) A gene, derived from the jellyfish *Aequoria victoria*, that is the source of the natural bioluminescence of this species, fluorescing green (a 509-nm wavelength) when illuminated with UV light (a 395-nm wavelength). When used as a reporter gene, GFP allows a noninvasive means of visualizing gene and protein expression patterns in living organisms.

guanine (G) One of four nitrogenous nucleotide bases in DNA and RNA; one of the two types of purine nucleotides in DNA and RNA.

guide RNA (gRNA) In RNA editing, the nucleic acid that directs the addition or removal of nucleotides from mRNA. Also known as *guide strand*. In genome editing, the RNA molecule designed to operate in a CRISPR–Cas complex to target double-strand breaks in a specific DNA molecule or genomic locus.

guide strand See *guide RNA (gRNA)*.

Guthrie test The name given to the initial version of a biochemical test used to detect the hereditary condition phenylketonuria (PKU)

hairpin structure See *stem loop*.

haploid Possessing a single set of chromosomes (n); a cell or organism that possesses one-half the number of chromosomes found in diploid cells of the organism.

haploid number The number of chromosomes (n) typically found in nuclei during the haploid phase of the eukaryotic life cycle. One-half the diploid ($2n$) number.

haploinsufficient A wild-type allele that is unable to support wild-type function in a heterozygous genotype. Classified as a recessive wild-type allele. Compare with *haplosufficient*.

haplosufficient A wild-type allele that supports wild-type function in heterozygous organisms.

Classified as a dominant wild-type allele. Compare with *haploinsufficient*.

haplotype The specific array of alleles encoded by linked genes in a segment of a single chromosome.

Hardy–Weinberg equilibrium The population genetic principle that in a population practicing random mating and in the absence of natural selection, mutation, migration, or random genetic drift, allele frequencies are stable at frequencies $p + q = 1.0$ for two alleles and are distributed into genotypes at frequencies $p2$, $2pq$, and $q2$.

Hayflick limit The name given to the observation that normal human cells in cell culture usually experience a limited number of cycles of cell division before they die.

helicase In DNA replication, the enzyme responsible for breaking hydrogen bonds between complementary nucleotides of a DNA duplex. Unwinding of the strands occurs ahead of the advancing replication fork.

helix-turn-helix (HTH) motif A DNA-binding protein domain consisting of two alpha helices: one helix binds to a specific DNA sequence, and the second helix stabilizes the interaction.

hemizygous Referring to the genotype of males that carry a single copy of each X-linked gene.

hereditary retinoblastoma The form of retinal cancer that is bilateral and is caused by the inheritance of a mutation of a specific gene in either sperm or egg.

heritability See *broad sense heritability* and *narrow sense heritability*.

heterochromatin (heterochromatic region) A chromosome region containing densely compacted chromatin and few, if any, expressed genes. See also *constitutive heterochromatin* and *facultative heterochromatin*.

heteroduplex DNA A DNA duplex created during homologous recombination by combining complementary strands of DNA from nonsister chromatids. Also known as *heteroduplex region*.

heteroplasmic cell or organism A cell or organism that harbors a mixture of alleles of an organellar gene. Also known as *heteroplasmy*.

heteroplasmy See *heteroplasmic cell or organism*.

heterozygous genotype A diploid genotype characterized by the presence of two different alleles of a gene.

high-frequency recombination (Hfr) Pertaining to Hfr chromosomes or to Hfr donors in bacterial conjugation.

Hfr chromosome See *Hfr donor*.

Hfr donor A donor bacterial strain containing an F factor integrated into its chromosome. Also known as *Hfr chromosome*.

histone acetyltransferase (HAT) Chromatin-modifying enzyme that adds acetyl groups to specific positively charged amino acids (e.g., lysine) in the N-terminal tails of histones.

histone deacetylase (HDAC) Chromatin-modifying enzyme that removes acetyl groups to specific positively charged amino acids (e.g., lysine) in the N-terminal tails of histones.

histone demethylase (HDMT) Chromatin-modifying enzyme that removes methyl groups to specific positively charged amino acids (e.g., lysine) in the N-terminal tails of histones.

histone methyltransferase (HMT) Chromatin-modifying enzyme that adds methyl groups to specific positively charged amino acids (e.g., lysine) in the N-terminal tails of histones.

histone protein (H1, H2A, H2B, H3, H4) Five proteins encoded by a gene family that form octameric nucleosomes (H2A, H2B, H3, and H4) and adhere to DNA to condense chromatin (H1).

Holliday junction A DNA structure that forms during meiotic recombination in which single strands are crossed over between nonsister chromatids of homologous chromosomes.

Holliday model Proposed originally by Robin Holliday; a model intended to explain meiotic recombination at a molecular level.

holoenzyme A fully functional multisubunit protein complex in bacteria, for example, the RNA polymerase holoenzyme.

homeobox A conserved sequence of DNA of 180 nucleotides encoding a *homeodomain* composed of three α-helices in a family of transcription factors found throughout eukaryotes; in metazoans some genes with homeobox genes are homeotic genes.

homeodomain A 60-amino acid DNA-binding domain.

homeolog Paralogs whose origin lies in a polyploidization event. Homeologous chromosomes are chromosomes derived from chromosome (or whole genome) duplication events.

homeotic gene Gene that controls the developmental fate of a region of the body of an organism; examples include the *Hox genes* in metazoans and the *MADS-box* genes in flowering plants.

homeotic mutation Mutation in which an apparently normal organ or body part develops in an inappropriate location.

homologous chromosomes (homologous pair) Chromosomes that synapse (pair) during meiosis. Chromosomes with the same genes in the same order. Also known as *homologs*.

homologous genes Genes descended from a common ancestral gene. Also known as *homologs*.

homologous nucleotides Nucleotides descended from a common ancestral nucleotide.

homologous recombination Exchange of genetic information between homologous DNA molecules.

homologs Homologous chromosomes or genes that have the same genes and structure and pair with one another during meiosis.

homology Evolutionarily related, having descended from a common ancestor.

homoplasmic cell or organism A cell or organism in which all copies (alleles) of a cytoplasmic organelle gene are the same. Also known as *homoplasmy*.

homoplasmy The presence of one allelic version of DNA in the organellar genomes of a cell.

homozygous genotype A diploid genotype characterized by the presence of two identical alleles of a gene.

mutation hotspot A location within a gene or genome at which mutations occur much more often than average.

housekeeping gene Genes that have essential cellular or physiological functions.

Hox **gene** Members of the homeobox gene clusters found throughout metazoans; the genes often pattern the anterior-posterior axis and are homeotic genes.

hybrid dysgenesis In *Drosophila*, the failure of F_1 progeny of P-cytotype males crossed with M-cytotype females to develop due to the presence of *P* elements.

hybrid vigor The greater growth, survival, and fertility of hybrids produced by crossing highly inbred lines.

hybridization In an electrophoresis gel or in gel blotting, the binding of a single-stranded nucleic acid probe to a single-stranded target nucleic acid by complementary base pairing. In other contexts, the formation of a double-stranded nucleic acid molecule by the base pairing of two wholly or largely complementary single-stranded molecules.

hydrogen bond Weak electrostatic attraction formed by the sharing of a positively charged hydrogen atom by negatively charged oxygen and nitrogen atoms. Hydrogen bonds form between complementary nucleotides to hold nucleic acid strands together.

hypermorphic mutation A mutant whose phenotype is similar to, but greater than, the wild-type phenotype.

hypomorphic mutation See *leaky mutation*.

hyperplasia The overactive growth of abnormal, but noncancerous, tissue.

identical by descent (IBD) A homozygous genotype in an organism in which both copies of the allele in an individual can be traced back to a common ancestor.

illegitimate recombination Exchange of genetic information between non-homologous DNA molecules.

immediate early genes Genes expressing immediately upon infection of a host bacterial cell by bacteriophage λ (lambda). See also *delayed early genes* and *late genes*.

imprinting control region (ICR) Master regulatory cis-acting DNA sequences to which trans-acting factors bind to regulate genomic imprinting.

in vitro fertilization (IVF) The method of assisted reproduction in which sperm and egg are mixed together outside the body to generate fertilized eggs.

inbreeding Mating between relatives. Also known as *consanguineous mating.*

inbreeding depression A reduction in vigor, survival, or reproductive fitness of offspring due to inbreeding.

incomplete dominance The observation that the phenotype occurring in heterozygous organisms is intermediate between the phenotypes of homozygous organisms, but more similar to one homozygous phenotype than to the other. Also known as *partial dominance.*

incomplete penetrance The occurrence of individual organisms that have a particular genotype or allele but not the corresponding phenotype.

incorporated error An abnormality of DNA, usually a base-pair mismatch, that occurs through a replication error or through damage done to DNA.

induced mutation Mutations generated by exposure to physical, chemical, or biological mutagens.

inducer An accessory molecule that binds to a protein that leads to activation of gene expression. The inducer can bind to a repressor protein and prevent its function or bind to an activator protein and stimulate its function.

inducer–repressor complex A molecular complex consisting of a repressor protein and a bound inducer molecule.

inducible operon Operon that is not expressed under one set of environmental conditions, but whose transcription is activated under an alternative environmental condition (i.e., the *lac* operon).

induction Process by which one cell or tissue promotes a particular developmental fate in neighboring cells or tissues.

inductive signal A molecule that acts on cells autonomously to influence cell fate; in *C. elegans* vulval development, the lin-3 protein secreted from the anchor cells acts as an inductive signal to influence the fate of vulval precursor cells.

informational gene Class of genes that encode protein products that perform informational processes in the cell such as DNA replication, packaging of chromosomes, transcription, and translation.

ingroup A species within a clade used to compare with other members of the clade.

inhibition Process by which one cell or tissue prevents a particular developmental fate in neighboring cells or tissues.

inhibitor An accessory molecule that converts activator proteins to an inactive conformation by binding to an allosteric binding domain of the activator protein.

initial committed complex In eukaryotic transcription, a partially completed multiprotein complex that is preparing to bind RNA polymerase II.

initiation complex A protein complex formed prior to the initiation of transcription or translation that directs RNA polymerase or the ribosome to the locations at which they begin synthesis.

initiation factor (IF) A group of proteins, associated with ribosomes, that contribute to ribosome assembly and translation initiation.

initiator tRNA The first charged tRNA associated with the ribosome.

inosine (I) A modified nucleotide found occasionally in anticodons that can base-pair with uracil, cytosine, or adenine.

insertion sequence (IS) A bacterial DNA sequence that is the target of insertion of a transposable genetic element or is the site of integration of a plasmid such as an F plasmid.

insertional inactivation A process of mutation in which the insertion of DNA into a gene renders it nonfunctional.

in situ hybridization A laboratory method for hybridizing a molecular probe to a DNA sequence or a gene on an intact chromosome.

insulator sequence Cis-acting sequences that act to prevent cross-talk between regulatory elements of an adjacent gene and are located between enhancers and promoters of genes that are to be insulated from the effects of the enhancer.

interactive variance (V_I) In polygenic and multifactorial inheritance, the proportion of total phenotypic variance that is due to the interactions of genetic and environmental factors.

interactome The sum of all of the protein–protein interactions in an organism.

interchromosomal domain Open spaces between chromosome domains in the interphase nucleus.

interference (*I*) Measured on a zero to 1.0 scale, the measurement of the independence of crossovers. Expressed as 1.0 minus the *coefficient of coincidence (c).*

internal control region (ICR) Promoter consensus sequences of certain rRNA and tRNA genes that are downstream of the start of transcription (i.e., sequences that are internal to the transcriptional region of the gene).

interphase The multiphase period of the cell cycle between cell divisions. See also G_1 *phase, S phase,* and G_2 *phase.*

interrupted mating A technique used to map bacterial genes that stops conjugation at timed intervals to determine which genes have transferred from the donor cell to the recipient cell.

interspecific comparison Any comparison between different species. Compare with *intraspecific comparison.*

interstitial deletion The loss of a portion of a chromosome from within one arm.

intragenic reversion A reversion produced by a second site mutation within a single gene.

intraspecific comparison Any comparison between individuals of the same species. Compare with *interspecific comparison.*

intrinsic termination In bacterial transcription, the DNA sequence-dependent mechanism for *transcription termination.* Inverted repeat DNA sequences induce formation of 3′ mRNA stem loop (hairpin) structures that are followed by multiple uracils (transcribed from adenines).

introgression line (IL) Line of experimental organisms in which genome segments from two or more other lines are present due to repeated back crosses between hybrids and organisms of one parental line. Also called *near isogenic line (NIL).*

intron Intervening sequences between the exons of many eukaryotic genes. Present in DNA and pre-mRNA, but spliced out during pre-mRNA processing.

intron splicing The spliceosome complex-driven process that removes introns from eukaryotic pre-mRNA and ligates exons to form mature mRNA.

inversion heterozygote Organisms whose homologous chromosomes have different structural organization. Most commonly, one has normal structure whereas the homolog carries an inversion.

inversion loop At homologous chromosome synapsis in an *inversion heterozygote,* the structure that forms by the looping of one chromosome to align homologous regions.

inverted repeat (IR) sequence Identical or nearly identical DNA sequences located on the same molecule but with opposite orientations.

IS (insertion sequence) element Mobile DNA elements in bacteria that cause mutations by inactivating the expression of genes into which they insert.

island model In evolutionary genetics, a model of species evolution in which new species are reproductively isolated from an ancestral population.

isoaccepting tRNA The group of tRNAs that carry the same amino acid but recognize synonymous codons.

ISWI complex Imitation switch complex that functions primarily to control the placement of nucleosomes into an arrangement that causes a region to be transcriptionally silent.

karyokinesis Part of telophase, the process of nuclear division between daughter cells.

karyotype A digital or analog photograph of chromosomes arranged by conventional chromosome numbering.

kinetochore The site of attachment of multiple proteins that connects a spindle fiber microtubule to the centromeric region of a chromosome. Forms during *M phase* of cell division.

knockout library Collections of mutants in which most or all genes of a particular organism have been mutated by inactivating (or "knocking out") their expression.

Kozak sequence A specific consensus sequence of eukaryotic mRNA that contains the authentic start codon (AUG) sequence.

lac- phenotype Bacteria that are not able to grow on a medium containing lactose as the only sugar. Compare with *lac⁺ phenotype*.

lac⁺ phenotype Bacteria that are able to grow on a medium containing lactose as the only sugar. Compare with *lac⁻ phenotype*.

lacA gene A gene of the bacterial *lac* operon; encodes lac transacetylase. Compare with *lacY gene* and *lacZ gene*.

lactose (lac) operon An inducible operon consisting of genes (*lacA*, *lacY*, *lacZ*) encoding enzymes allowing the use of lactose as a carbon source. The operon is repressed by the lac repressor regulatory protein that binds to the lac operator sequence and is activated by the CAP–cAMP complex that binds to sequences of the CAP binding site.

lacY gene A gene of the bacterial *lac* operon; encodes lac permease, which facilitates import of lactose into the cell. Compare with *lacZ gene* and *lacA gene*.

lacZ gene A gene of the bacterial *lac* operon; encodes β-galactosidase, which breaks down lactose into glucose and galactose. Compare with *lacY gene* and *lacA gene*.

lagging strand In DNA replication, the discontinuously synthesized strand whose Okazaki fragments are ligated to complete new strand synthesis. Compare with *leading strand*.

large ribosomal subunit The larger of two subunits of the ribosome.

lariat intron structure During intron splicing, the structure formed by covalent bonding of the 5′ guanine of an intron to the branch point adenine of the intron.

late genes Bacteriophage genes expressed late in the lytic cycle. Encode protein products required for packaging of phage particles and lysis of the host cell. *Late promoters* and *late operators* are the regulatory sequences responsible for late gene activation.

late operators (late promoters) Regulatory sequences in lambda (λ) bacteriophage that regulate the transcription of genes late in the infection cycle.

lateral gene transfer (LGT) Transfer of genetic material between organisms belonging to the same or to different taxonomic groups.

lateral inhibition Process by which one cell or tissue prevents neighboring cells or tissues from acquiring a developmental fate similar its own.

law of independent assortment (Mendel's second law) The random distribution of alleles of unlinked genes into gametes.

law of segregation (Mendel's first law) The separation of alleles of a gene during gamete formation.

leader region Transcribed region upstream of the major enzyme encoding genes of repressible amino acid biosynthesis operons (e.g., *trpL*). Region encodes a small peptide whose rate of translation reflects the concentration of the amino acid (e.g., tryptophan) in the cells

and consequently regulates transcription of the operon.

leading strand In DNA replication, the continuously synthesized strand. Compare with *lagging strand*.

leaky mutation A mutant whose phenotype is similar to, but less than, the wild-type phenotype. Also known as *hypomorphic mutation*.

lethal allele See *lethal mutation*.

lethal mutation An allele that results in the premature death of the organisms that carry it. Lethality most often affects homozygous organisms. Also known as *lethal allele*.

linkage disequilibrium The nonrandom distribution into gametes of alleles of linked genes.

linkage equilibrium The random distribution into gametes of alleles of linked genes achieved by crossing over between the genes.

linkage group A group of genes displaying genetic linkage.

linker A short, chemically synthesized oligonucleotide that can be ligated to DNA molecules.

linker DNA DNA between nucleosomes in the 10-nm fiber structure of chromatin.

locus control region (LCR) Specialized enhancer element that regulates the transcription of multiple genes, often complexes of closely related genes.

lod score (log of the odds ratio) Based on analysis of transmission in pedigrees, the statistic used to calculate the likelihood of genetic linkage between genes.

long noncoding RNA (lncRNA) A transcribed RNA molecule that does not possess an extended open reading frame and that does not represent a tRNA, RRNA, or miRNA.

long terminal repeats (LTRs) Arrays of scores to hundreds of nucleotides that bracket the ends of retroviruses integrated into host chromosomes.

loss-of-function mutation A mutant that prevents the production of the wild-type protein or renders it inactive. Most commonly a recessive mutation.

lysis See *lytic cycle*.

lysogenic cycle The life cycle of a bacterium infected by a temperate bacteriophage that integrates into the host chromosome and replicates along with it.

lysogeny See *lysogenic cycle*.

lytic cycle The life cycle of a bacterium infected by a bacteriophage that replicates within the host cell and lyses the host to release progeny bacteriophage.

LUCA An acronym for the last universal common ancestor, meaning the last ancestor from which all living organisms are descended.

M phase The cell division phase of the cell cycle. Follows *interphase*.

MADS-box A conserved sequence of DNA of 168–180 nucleotides encoding a 56–60 amino acid DNA-binding domain in a family

of transcription factors found throughout eukaryotes; in flowering plants, some MADS-box genes are homeotic genes.

major gene A gene that has a substantial effect on phenotypic variation.

major groove The larger of two grooves formed in the DNA sugar-phosphate backbone by the helical twist of the double helix and exposing certain base pairs.

malignant tumor A cluster of cells that are cancerous.

mapping function Corrective calculations used to more accurately estimate recombination frequencies between linked genes. Mapping functions differ among certain species.

map unit (m.u.), centiMorgan (cM) A theoretical unit of distance between linked genes on a chromosome.

maternal effect gene Genes that act in the mother to impart gene products (RNA or protein) into the egg and subsequently the embryo. For maternal effect genes, the embryonic phenotype is determined by the genotype of the mother rather than that of the embryo.

maternal inheritance Transmission of genes via the maternal parent only; observed with mitochondrial or chloroplast genomes.

maternal serum screening (MSS) A method used in prenatal genetic testing that uses maternal blood as a source of three hormones whose significantly elevated or reduced levels are associated with specific chromosome abnormalities of a fetus; also known as the triple test.

matrix attachment region (MAR) Portions of the chromosome scaffold to which loops of chromatin are attached.

mature mRNA The fully processed product of eukaryotic transcription that moves to the cytoplasm for translation.

mean The average value of a group of values.

median In a sample distribution, the middle-most values. Also known as *median value*.

median value See *median*.

Mediator An enhanceosome complex that forms a bridge between activator proteins bound to enhancer elements and the basal transcriptional machinery bound to the promoter.

megabase (Mb) Equal to 1,000,000 nucleotide bases. Refers to DNA or to RNA molecules or fragments.

meiosis The process of cell division occurring in germ-line cells. Produces four haploid gametes or spores through two successive nuclear divisions in diploid species.

meiosis I First nuclear division characterized by homologous chromosomes separating. Compare with *meiosis II*.

meiosis II Second nuclear division characterized by sister chromatids separating. Compare with *meiosis I*.

Mendelian genetics Referring to genetic applications and analyses using the law of segregation and the law of independent assort-ment originally described through experiments and analysis by Gregor Mendel.

meristem Organized groups of pluripotent cells at the growing tips of plants that both generate organs and self-maintain to ensure that a pool of stem cells is always present.

messenger RNA (mRNA) A form of RNA tran-scribed from a gene and subsequently translated to produce a polypeptide or protein.

metabolomics The study of proteins, processes, and interactions involved in the metabolism of organisms.

metacentric chromosome A chromosome with a centrally located centromere that produces long and short arms of approximately the same length.

metagenome Sequence derived from whole-genome shotgun sequencing of DNA from entire natural communities consisting of a range of organisms.

metaphase The stage of *M phase* during which chromosomes align in the middle of the cell.

metaphase plate The cell midline along which chromosomes align during metaphase.

microdeletion A small chromosome deletion detectable only by using molecular methods of analysis.

microduplication A small chromosome duplica-tion detectable only by using molecular methods of analysis.

microRNA (miRNA) Small (21–24 nuts) regula-tory RNAs produced by Dicer and acting in a RISC complex to either repress translational or cleave target mRNA molecules. Compare with *RNA interference (RNAi)*.

microsynteny Conservation of the order of a small number of genes in related species.

migration A process of evolution referring to the movement of organisms and genes between populations. Also known as *gene flow*.

minimal medium A microbial growth medium containing a nitrogen source and a carbon source and with water and oxygen available; only prototrophic (wild-type) microbes typically grow on minimal medium.

minor groove The smaller of two grooves formed in the sugar-phosphate backbone by the helical twist of the double helix, exposing cer-tain base pairs.

mismatch repair The DNA repair process that repairs noncomplementary base pairs that occur through errant DNA replication or through nucleotide base modification. The process restores normal complementary base pairing.

missense mutation A DNA base-pair substitu-tion that leads to production of a polypeptide in which one amino acid substitutes for another.

mitochondria Eukaryotic cytoplasmic organ-elles, bounded by a double membrane, car-rying their own DNA (mtDNA), encoding polypeptides that interact with nuclear gene

polypeptides in oxidative phosphorylation to generate ATP. In many species, mitochondria also participate in other metabolic processes and biochemical reactions, including ion homeosta-sis and biosynthetic pathways.

mitosis The process of cell division in somatic cells that produces genetically identical daugh-ter cells through a single nuclear division.

mitosome Double-membrane-bound organelles that are evolutionarily derived from mitochon-dria but have lost all of the ancestral genome; proteins requiring an anaerobic environment to function are imported into them.

mode In a sample distribution, the most com-monly occurring value. Also known as *modal value*.

modern synthesis of evolution Referring to the broad-based effort beginning in the middle of the 20th century to unite Mendelian genetics with Darwin's theory of evolution by natural selection.

modifier gene A gene that modifies the effect of a major gene.

modifier screen A genetic screen designed to identify mutations in genes that modify, either enhance or suppress, the phenotypic effects of mutations in another gene.

molecular genetics The subfield of genetics that studies hereditary transmission, variation, mutation, and evolution through the analysis of nucleic acids and proteins.

molecular probe (probe) A single-stranded nucleic acid or antibody protein labeled with a detectable marker that attaches to a specific tar-get molecule, allowing target molecule detection in subsequent analysis. Single-stranded nucleic acid probes detect target nucleic acids, and anti-body probes bind specific target proteins.

monohybrid cross A genetic cross between organisms that are heterozygous for one gene.

monophyletic group A group of organisms with a single common ancestor.

monosomy The presence of a single chromo-some instead of a homologous pair, resulting in a chromosome number that is $2n - 1$.

morphogen Substance whose presence in dif-ferent concentrations directs different develop-mental fates.

morphospecies concept The method of iden-tifying species on the basis of their anatomy or appearance.

multifactorial inheritance The inheritance of traits whose phenotypic variation is the result of polygenic inheritance and environmental influ-ences. See also *multifactorial trait*.

multifactorial trait Traits whose phenotypic variation is the result of polygenic inheritance and environmental influences. See also *multifac-torial inheritance*.

multiple cloning site (MCS) A vector DNA sequence containing several unique restriction enzyme target sequences facilitating cloning of inserted DNA fragments.

multiple gene hypothesis The hypothesis that alleles of multiple genes contribute to the pro-duction of certain traits.

multiplication rule See *product rule*.

mutagen A chemical, physical, or biological agent capable of damaging DNA and creating a mutation.

mutagenesis A procedure whereby a population of organisms is mutagenized and their progeny are propagated and examined for mutant specific phenotypes. See also *genetic screen*.

mutation An inherited change in DNA.

mutation rate The rate at which mutations occur per gene per unit of time. Most often expressed per gene per generation.

mutation–selection balance An arithmetic expression used to determine the equilibrium frequencies of alleles in populations as a result of allele elimination by natural selection and new allele creation by mutation.

narrow sense heritability (h^2) The proportion of total phenotypic variance that is contributed by additive genetic variance.

natural selection The evolutionary process operating through differences in survival, fecun-dity, and relative fitness of organisms with dif-ferent genotypes and phenotypes.

near isogenic line (NIL) One of two or more experimental lineages of organisms that are nearly genetically uniform. See also *introgres-sion line*.

negative control (of transcription) Condition where binding of a repressor protein to a regula-tory DNA sequence prevents transcription of a gene or a cluster of genes.

negative interference Occurring when the *coefficient of coincidence (c)* is greater than 1.0, the observation of more double crossovers than expected between a pair of genes.

negative supercoiling Twisting of the DNA duplex in the direction opposite to the turns of the double helix.

neofunctionalization The process, following gene duplication, whereby a mutation in one of the duplicates provides a function not performed by the original gene.

neomorphic mutation A mutant expressing a new or novel function not seen in the wild type.

neoplasia A general term for a cancerous condi-tion or tumor.

next-generation sequencing (NGS) High throughput massively parallel DNA sequencing by synthesis.

newborn genetic screening A group of bio-chemical and DNA genetic tests mandated for all newborn infants in 50 of the United States and in many countries around the world.

N-formylmethionine (fMet; tRNAfMet) A modi-fied methionine amino acid usually used as the amino acid that initiates bacterial translation. Carried by a specialized tRNA.

nick translation An experimental method for incorporating new nucleotides into one strand of DNA beginning at a site where a phosphodiester bond on that strand has been broken.

node An evolutionary branch point in a phylogenetic tree.

noncomposite transposon Bacterial transposable genetic elements that lack insertion sequences.

nondisjunction The failure of homolog or sister chromatid separation during cell division. Results in nuclei with the wrong number of chromosomes.

nonhistone protein Numerous nuclear proteins that are not histones associated with chromosomes.

nonhomologous end joining (NHEJ) An error-prone mechanism of double-stranded DNA break repair in eukaryotic genomes in which damaged nucleotides are removed and blunt ends of strands are joined.

noninducible Condition in which transcription of bacterial genes or operons cannot be activated.

nonpenetrant An organism with a genotype corresponding to a mutant phenotype that instead displays the wild-type phenotype.

nonrecombinant vector Produced in a cloning experiment when the intended vector does not pick up a DNA insert.

nonreplicative transposition A transposable genetic element that transposes by excision from the original genome location, followed by insertion into a new location.

nonrevertible mutants Mutations caused by partial deletion of DNA nucleotides that cannot be reverted to wild type.

nonsense mutation A type of point mutation producing a stop codon in mRNA.

nonsister chromatid A chromatid belonging to a homologous chromosome. Nonsister chromatids of homologs are involved in crossing over.

nontemplate strand See *coding strand*.

non–Watson-and-Crick base pair Base-pair mismatches or base pairing involving modified nucleotides.

northern blotting A method for transferring mRNA from an electrophoresis gel to a permanent membrane or filter.

nuclear mitochondrial sequence (NUMTS) Mitochondrial DNA sequences found in the nucleus as a result of recent transfer from the mitochondrial genome to the nuclear genome.

nuclear plastid sequence (NUPTS) Plastid DNA sequences found in the nucleus as a result of recent transfer from the plastid genome to the nuclear genome.

nucleoid The region of bacterial and archaeal cells (or mitochondria or chloroplasts) where the main chromosome resides.

nucleolus (plural: nucleoli) Nuclear organelle containing rRNA-encoding genes.

nucleomorph In a secondary endosymbiosis, the nuclear genome of the secondary endosymbiont.

nucleosome An octameric protein complex composed of two polypeptides each of histones H2A, H2B, H3, and H4, around which DNA wraps in chromatin.

nucleosome core particle The octameric histone protein complex (two molecules each of H2A, H2B, H3, and H4) around which core DNA can wrap.

nucleosome-depleted region (NDR) A 100- to 150-bp region containing few nucleosomes, which lies immediately upstream of the start of transcription.

nucleotide base analog A compound with a size and shape that mimics a natural nucleotide base.

nucleotide excision repair A mechanism of DNA damage repair in which a segment of one strand containing damaged nucleotides is excised and replaced.

null mutation A mutant that produces no functional product. Most commonly a recessive allele. Also known as *amorphic mutation*.

Okazaki fragment A short segment of newly synthesized DNA that is part of a lagging strand and is ligated to other Okazaki fragments to complete lagging strand synthesis.

oncogene A mutated form of a proto-oncogene; frequently associated with cancer development.

one gene–one enzyme hypothesis Proposed by George Beadle and Edward Tatum in 1941, the hypothesis proposing that each gene encodes a specific protein product and controls a distinct function.

open chromatin Chromatin in which the association of DNA with nucleosomes is relaxed in regions containing regulatory sequences, allowing access by regulatory proteins and giving genes in open chromatin the potential to be transcriptionally active.

open reading frame (ORF) A reading frame that has the potential to be translated into a protein sequence.

open promoter Promoters that reside in open chromatin, resulting in constitutive transcription. See also *open promoter complex*.

open promoter complex At transcription initiation, the stage at which RNA polymerase is bound and a short region of DNA opens to allow transcription from the template strand. See also *open promoter*.

operational gene Class of genes that encode proteins involved in cellular metabolic processes (e.g., amino acid biosynthesis, biosynthesis of cofactors, fatty acid and phospholipid biosynthesis, intermediary metabolism, energy metabolism, nucleotide biosynthesis).

operator Regulatory DNA sequences to which repressor or activator proteins bind. Term used in bacterial systems.

operon A set of adjacent genes that are transcribed in a polycistronic mRNA and are thus coordinately regulated; an operon is generally considered to include associated regulatory sequences (e.g., promoter, operator, etc.). Primarily found in bacteria and archaea.

opposite sense resolution One possible process for resolving the DNA connections between homologous chromosomes (Holliday junctions) following crossing over as part of homologous recombination. See also *same sense resolution*.

organelle inheritance The transmission of genes on mitochondrial and chloroplast chromosomes.

organizer Groups of cells that possess the ability to influence the fates of cells in the surrounding tissues via nonautonomous signals.

origin of migration The starting point of nucleic acid or protein migration in gel electrophoresis.

origin of replication The specific sequence at which DNA replication begins.

origin of transfer (*oriT*) The site within the fertility (F) factor sequence where transfer to the recipient cell is initiated.

orthologous genes Genes in different species whose origin lies in a speciation event and that can be traced to a single gene in a common ancestor of the two species. Also known as *orthologs*.

orthologs See *orthologous genes*.

outgroup A species related to members of a *clade* but outside the clade; used to root the clade.

***P* element** A specific type of transposable genetic element prevalent in the *Drosophila* genome.

***P* site** See *peptidyl site*.

***P* value** See *probability value*.

paired-end sequencing Sequence generated from both ends of a DNA clone; provides evidence of physical linkage of the two paired sequences.

pair-rule gene In *Drosophila*, genes that delimit parasegments along the anterior-posterior axis; examples include *even-skipped* and *odd-skipped*.

pangenome The entire gene set of a species.

paracentric inversion A chromosome inversion in which the inverted segment does not include the region of the centromere.

paralogous genes Genes whose origin lies in a gene duplication event within an extant or ancestral species. Also known as *paralogs*.

paraphyletic group A group of organisms that includes some but not all the members descended from a common ancestor.

parasegment In *Drosophila*, the posterior part of one segment and the anterior part of its neighbor. The stripes of gene expression of pair-rule genes correspond to parasegments, straddling the boundaries between segments.

parental (nonrecombinant) chromosome Chromosomes in gametes produced when crossing over does not take place between linked genes. Alleles marking each gene are retained in their initial (parental) configurations.

parental generation (P generation) The parents of F_1 progeny. In controlled genetic crosses, the parents are pure-breeding.

parental strand The DNA strand acting as a template to direct the synthesis of a new ("daughter") strand of DNA.

partial chromosome deletion The loss of a segment of a chromosome.

partial deletion The loss of a segment of a chromosome. Results in partial monosomy for the affected chromosome segment.

partial deletion heterozygote An organism with one wild-type chromosome and a homolog that is missing a segment.

partial diploid An exconjugant bacterium that acquires a second copy of one or more genes by conjugation with an F′ donor cell.

partial dominance See *incomplete dominance.*

partial duplication The duplication of a segment of a chromosome.

partial duplication heterozygote An organism with one wild-type chromosome and a homologous chromosome with a duplicated segment.

particulate inheritance Mendel's theory that genetic information is transmitted from one generation to the next as discrete units or elements of heredity.

Pascal's triangle A diagram listing the coefficients of a given binomial expansion in which the binomial expression is expanded n number of times.

paternity index (PI) An arithmetic computation used as part of the estimate of the genetic likelihood of paternity for a putative father and a child. See also *combined paternity index (CPI).*

pathogenicity island Regions of laterally transferred DNA that contain genes with pathogenic function.

pedigree A family tree composed of standard symbols that depicts relationships in successive generations and often displays individual phenotypes.

penetrant Expression of the phenotype corresponding to a particular genotype.

peptide bond A type of covalent bond that joins amino acids in polypeptide chains. Formed between the amino end of one amino acid and the carboxyl end of the adjoining amino acid.

peptidyl site (P site) The site on the ribosome where amino acids are joined by a peptide bond.

pericentric inversion A chromosome inversion in which the inverted segment includes the region of the centromere.

permissive condition Environmental condition in which environmentally sensitive (e.g., temperature sensitive) mutants exhibit the wild-type phenotype or can survive.

pharmacogenetic screening A method of genetic screening used to identify individuals who carry specific alleles that make them more or less sensitive than average to specific drugs or medications.

phenotype (1) The observable physical characteristics or traits of an organism. (2) The physical manifestation of a specific genotype.

phenotypic ratio A ratio or set of relative proportions between organisms with different phenotypes—for example, the ratio of progeny produced by a monohybrid cross (3:1) or a dihybrid cross (9:3:3:1).

phenotypic variance (V_P) The total variance observed for a trait.

phosphodiester bond A type of covalent bond formed between two nucleotides in a nucleic acid strain. Formed between the 5′ phosphate group of one nucleotide and the 3′ OH of the adjacent nucleotide.

photoproduct A characteristic DNA lesion produced by exposure to ultraviolet light.

photoreactive repair A mechanism of DNA damage repair in bacteria that uses light in the visible part of the spectrum to provide the energy to remove the damage done by ultraviolet irradiation.

phylogenetic footprinting Technique whereby conserved sequences are identified by searching for similar sequences in species separated by large evolutionary distances.

phylogenetic shadowing Technique whereby conserved sequences are identified by first eliminating sequences that are not conserved in closely related species.

phylogenetic species concept The concept that a species is the smallest group with a definably unique genetic history.

phylogenetic tree A diagram of evolutionary relationships among organisms or genes based on morphological or molecular characteristics.

physical gap Sequence gap between scaffolds for which there is no clone to supply the sequence.

pioneer factor Any of a class of transcription factors that can directly bind condensed (heterochromatic) chromatin. Can be either an activator or a repressor.

plasmid One of multiple types of extrachromosomal circular DNA molecules that may be found in bacterial cells.

plastid Organelle, bounded by a double membrane, descended from the cyanobacterial endosymbiont; specialized types of plastids include chloroplasts and chromoplasts.

pleiotropy A single gene mutation that affects multiple and seemingly unconnected properties of an organism.

pluripotent State of a cell when it can give rise to many but not all cell types of an organism.

point mutation A DNA lesion at a defined location. Usually either a base pair substitution or the insertion or deletion of one or a small number of base pairs.

polar mutation Mutations affecting downstream genes in an operon by reducing production or altering translation of polycistronic mRNA.

poly-A tail The sequence of approximately 20 to 200 adenines that are enzymatically added to the 3′ end of most eukaryotic mRNAs as part of the posttranscriptional processing of precursor mRNA (pre-mRNA). This process is accompanied by cleavage of a 3′ segment of pre-mRNA.

polyacrylamide A synthetic compound mixed with buffer and used to form electrophoresis gels.

polyadenylation signal sequence A hexanucleotide sequence of mRNA, usually AAUAAA, that identifies the location of 3′ pre-mRNA cleavage and polyadenylation.

polycistronic mRNA In bacteria, an mRNA containing the transcripts of two or more genes.

polygenic inheritance (polygenic trait) A quantitative trait dependent on the contributions of multiple genes. Also known as *polygenic trait.*

polymerase chain reaction (PCR) A laboratory method for controlled replication of a specific target sequence of DNA in successive cycles. Using two short single-stranded primers that bind to sequences on opposite sides of the target sequence, exponential replication of the target sequence occurs.

polypeptide A chain of amino acids joined by peptide bonds. Formed at ribosomes during translation.

polyploidy The presence of more than two complete sets of chromosomes in a genome. See also *allopolyploidy* and *autopolyploidy.*

polyribosome In translation, the simultaneous translational activity of multiple ribosomes on a single mRNA.

population A group of organisms that mate with one another to establish the next generation.

population genetics The subfield of genetics that studies the genetic structure and evolution of populations.

positional information Process by which gene expression or other chemical cues establish geographical addresses along the axes of a developing embryo or organ primordium.

position effect variegation (PEV) The observation in *Drosophila* of a specific type of mutation producing variegation of eye color due to the abnormal positioning of the *w* (white) gene for eye color.

positive control (of transcription) Condition where binding of an activator protein to a regulatory DNA sequence stimulates transcription of a gene or a cluster of genes.

positive–negative selection The use of both negative and positive selectable markers to follow the fate of introduced DNA to select for homologous recombination events.

positive supercoiling Superhelical twisting of DNA.

posttranslational polypeptide processing In eukaryotes, modifications to polypeptides in the endoplasmic reticulum and Golgi apparatus after the completion of translation.

postzygotic mechanism Mechanisms operating after mating to reduce or prevent the possibility of producing hybrids between populations or species.

precursor mRNA (pre-mRNA) The initial transcript of a eukaryotic gene requiring mRNA processing prior to translation.

preimplantation genetic screening Isolation of a single cell from a newly fertilized embryo before implantation, done to test DNA for a specific hereditary disease or condition. May be used as part of assisted reproduction.

preinitiation complex (PIC) In eukaryotic transcription, a large multiprotein complex containing several general transcription factors and RNA polymerase II.

prenatal genetic testing Genetic testing conducted on a fetus in utero.

presymptomatic genetic testing Genetic testing of individuals who may have inherited a disease-causing gene mutation, to screen for a mutant allele before symptoms of the disease appear.

prezygotic mechanism Mechanisms operating before mating to reduce or prevent the possibility of producing hybrids between populations or species.

Pribnow box (− 10 consensus sequence) A specific consensus sequence component of the bacterial promoter with a location centered at approximately − 10 relative to the start of transcription.

primary structure In regard to a polypeptide, the order of amino acids composing the polypeptide.

primase (DnaG) The specialized RNA polymerase that synthesizes the RNA primer during DNA replication.

primer walking Technique for sequencing long DNA molecules where new sequencing primers are synthesized based on successive DNA sequence reads. Compare with *shotgun sequencing*.

prior probability A statistical prediction of an outcome before the event. In genetics, the prediction of the possible outcomes of a genetic cross based on Mendelian genetics.

probability value (*P* value) In the chi square test, the likelihood that a repeat experiment will produce a result as deviant or more deviant than expected in comparison with the experimental result being tested.

product rule The probability of an event requiring the sequential or simultaneous occurrence of two or more contributing events. The probabilities of contributing events are multiplied, and their product is the event in question. Also known as the *multiplication rule*.

proliferation Active cell reproduction and tissue growth.

prometaphase In *M phase* of the cell cycle, sometimes identified as a stage between prophase and metaphase.

promoter A regulatory sequence of DNA near the 5′ end of a gene that acts as the binding location of RNA polymerase and directs RNA polymerase to the start of transcription.

promoter mutation A mutation altering promoter sequence and function.

prophage The designation for bacteriophage that has integrated into the host bacterial chromosome.

prophase The stage of *M phase* during which chromosome condensation occurs.

protein A string of amino acids encoded during translation of mRNA and linked together by peptide bonds. See also *polypeptide*.

proteome Set of the proteins in a cell, tissue, or organism.

proteomics The study of all the proteins, collectively known as the proteome, within a cell, tissue, or organism.

proto-oncogene A broad category of normal genes producing protein whose generalized functions promote cell proliferation. It is often mutated in carcinogenesis.

prototroph (prototrophic strain) The wild-type strain of a microorganism. Also, any organism that can synthesize its nutrients from inorganic material.

pseudoautosomal region (PAR) Homologous regions on the X and Y chromosomes that synapse and cross over.

pseudodominance The phenotypic expression of a recessive allele on one chromosome due to deletion of a portion of the homologous chromosome containing the dominant allele.

pseudogene Sequences recognizable as mutated gene sequences often derived from gene duplication or retrotransposition events.

Punnett square Named in honor of early 20th-century geneticist Reginald Punnett, a checkerboard-like diagram that predicts the genotypes and genotype frequencies of progeny from a genetic cross.

pure-breeding strains A group of genetically identical homozygous organisms that, when self-fertilized or intercrossed, only produce offspring that have a phenotype identical to the parents. Also known as *true-breeding strains*.

QTL mapping A method for locating quantitative trait loci in a genome.

quantitative genetics The subfield of genetics that studies quantitative traits.

quantitative trait A trait exhibiting polygenic inheritance and displaying continuous phenotypic variation.

quantitative trait locus (QTL) A gene contributing to the phenotypic variation of a quantitative trait.

quaternary structure The state of protein function requiring the joining of two or more

polypeptides to form a functional protein (e.g., hemoglobin protein).

R-group The functional groups that give each amino acid their distinctive characteristics.

R (resistance) plasmid A type of bacterial plasmid conferring resistance to one or more antibiotic compounds.

random mutation hypothesis The correct theory that gene mutations occur at random. See also *fluctuation test*.

random X inactivation (Lyon hypothesis) Proposed by Mary Lyon in the mid-20th century, the process of randomly inactivating one copy of the X chromosome in each mammalian female nucleus early in zygotic development.

reading frame The partitioning of sequential sets of mRNA trinucleotide segments (codons) that are used in translation to determine amino acid order of a polypeptide.

realizator gene In *Drosophila*, the *Hox* target genes whose expression contributes to the characteristic morphology of each segment.

RecBCD pathway A complex of three bacterial proteins that cut DNA and facilitate homologous recombination; a foundation of eukaryotic homologous recombination.recessive allele An allele that can only be expressed in a phenotype if two copies of the allele make up the genotype.

recessive epistasis (9:3:4 ratio) A characteristic ratio of phenotypes produced by the interaction of two genes that control a trait in which alleles of one gene mask or reduce the expression of alleles of a second gene.

recessive phenotype The phenotype observed in an organism that is homozygous for the recessive allele. Compare with *dominant phenotype*.

recipient cell (F⁻ cell) A bacterial cell that does not contain fertility factor DNA sequence and can conjugate with a donor bacterium.

reciprocal cross Paired crosses involving distinct parental phenotypes in which the sexes are switched (i.e., if one cross is ♂ phenotype A × ♀ phenotype B, the reciprocal cross is ♂ phenotype B × ♀ phenotype A).

reciprocal translocation (balanced, unbalanced) Exchange of chromosome segments between non-homologous chromosomes. If all genes are present, the translocation is "balanced," but if genes are missing, the translocation is "unbalanced."

recombinant (nonparental) chromosome Chromosomes in gametes produced by crossing over between linked genes. Alleles marking each gene are rearranged on chromatids by crossing over.

recombinant clone A combination of DNA molecules from different sources (e.g., vector and insert DNA) that are joined together using *recombinant DNA technology*.

recombinant DNA molecule A DNA molecule formed in the laboratory using molecular genetic techniques, such as molecular cloning.

recombinant DNA technology The set of laboratory techniques developed for amplifying, maintaining, and manipulating specific DNA sequences in vitro as well as in vivo.

recombination coldspot A chromosome region with a recombination rate that is lower than average for the number of nucleotide base pairs present.

recombination hotspot A chromosome region with a recombination rate that is higher than average for the number of nucleotide base pairs present.

recombination frequency (r) The rate of occurrence of recombination between a pair of linked genes. Expressed as the number of recombinants divided by the total number of meioses.

recombination nodule Protein aggregations along the synaptonemal complex that are thought to play a role in crossing over.

Recommended Uniform Screening Panel (RUSP) The list of approximately three dozen hereditary conditions that are recommended for newborn genetic testing in the 50 United States and many countries around the world. See also *newborn genetic screening.*

reference genome sequence The DNA sequence of the individual or individuals used to construct the initial complete genome sequence.

regulated transcription Condition in which gene expression is controlled at the transcriptional level in response to changing environmental conditions.

regulatory mutation A mutation altering a regulated attribute of gene expression.

relative fitness (w) In evolutionary genetics, the measurement of the reproductive fitnesses of organisms in a population relative to one another. The organism class with greatest fitness has a relative fitness of $w = 1.0$.

relaxosome The bacterial structure that participates in the transfer of donor DNA during conjugation.

release factor (RF) Molecules that bind mRNA stop codons and contribute to translation termination.

replica plating The microbial method for transferring all the growing colonies from an original growth plate to one or more new growth plates.

replicate cross Repeated crosses involving parents with the same genotypes and phenotypes.

replicated error DNA damage, usually a base-pair mismatch, that is made part of a DNA strand after a cycle of DNA replication. See also *incorporated error.*

replication bubble A region of active bidirectional DNA replication containing replication forks on each end, an origin of replication in the middle, and leading and lagging strands in each half of the bubble.

replication fork In DNA replication, the site of the replisome structure, and the site of synthesis of leading strand and lagging strand DNA.

replicative segregation Random segregation of organelles during cell division.

replicative transposition Transposition carried out by replicating a copy of a transposable element and inserting the copy in a new genome location.

replisome The large molecular machine located at the replication fork that coordinates multiple reaction steps during DNA replication.

reporter gene A gene whose expression is easy to assay phenotypically. Fusion of reporter genes with heterologous sequences allows both transcriptional and translational expression patterns to be visualized.

repressible operon Operon that is expressed under one set of environmental conditions, but whose transcription is repressed under an alternative environmental condition (i.e., the *trp* operon).

repressor protein A transcription factor that binds to regulatory sequences associated with a gene and represses that gene's expression.

reproductive isolation The absence of inter-breeding between populations or species; often involves geographic, physical, or behavioral mechanisms or conditions.

response to selection (R) The amount of change in the phenotype of a trait between parental and offspring generations as a result of selection on the parents.

restriction endonuclease (restriction enzyme) One of a large number of DNA-digesting enzymes, usually of bacterial origin, that cut DNA at specific recognition sites called restriction sequences. Each enzyme has its own specific base-pair sequence, known as a *restriction sequence,* for double-stranded cleavage of DNA.

restriction fragment A fragment of DNA produced by treating DNA with a restriction endonuclease.

restriction fragment length polymorphism (RFLP) A fragment of DNA generated by treatment with a restriction endonuclease.

restriction map A map showing the numbers and relative positions of target sites for restriction enzymes of a DNA molecule.

restriction–modification system System of a restriction enzyme with a specific recognition sequence and a modifying enzyme that adds methyl groups to bases of the recognition sequence. The system protects the bacteria's own DNA from being digested by endogenous restriction enzymes but allows restriction of invading exogenous DNA.

restrictive condition Environmental condition in which environmentally sensitive (e.g., temperature sensitive) mutants exhibit the mutant phenotype.

retrotransposon A transposable element that uses reverse transcriptase to transpose through an RNA intermediate.

reverse genetics Genetic analysis that begins with a gene sequence, which is used to identify or introduce mutant alleles and subsequently to identify and evaluate the resulting mutant

phenotype. It is the complementary approach to forward genetics.

reverse transcriptase Enzyme, derived from retroviruses or retrotransposons, that catalyzes the synthesis of a DNA strand (cDNA) from an RNA template.

reverse transcription The process of DNA synthesis from an RNA template by the enzyme reverse transcriptase.

reversion mutation (reverse mutation) A mutation that alters a mutant to wild-type sequence and function. Also known as reversion.

reversion rate The rate at which reversion (reverse) mutations occur in an organism.

revertible mutant A point mutation caused by base-pair substitution or deletion of one or a few base pairs that can be reverted to wild type.

rho-dependent termination (rho protein) The process of bacterial *transcription termination* involving rho protein.

rho utilization site (rut site) The site of attachment of rho protein that aids in rho-protein-driven bacterial *transcription termination.*

ribonucleic acid (RNA) A family of polynucleotides that are transcribed from DNA. RNAs are composed of nucleotides containing the sugar ribose, one or more phosphate atoms, and one of four nitrogenous bases (A, G, C, and U).

ribonucleotide Composed of ribose, one or more phosphate groups, and one of four nitrogenous bases, the nucleotides that make up RNA. See also *adenine (A), uracil (U), guanine (G), and cytosine (C).*

ribose The 5-carbon sugar molecule in ribonucleotides.

ribosomal RNA (rRNA) A group of RNA molecules that compose part of the structure of ribosomes.

ribosome Ribonucleoprotein particles, composed of rRNAs and numerous proteins, at which translation takes place.

riboswitch A group of genetic regulatory processes in bacteria that are mediated by mRNA sequences.

RNA editing The process of posttranscriptional addition or removal of nucleotide of certain mRNAs.

RNA interference (RNAi) A regulatory gene-silencing mechanism based on double-stranded RNA, which can target complementary sequences for inactivation. The machinery can be harnessed to silence gene expression in a reverse genetic approach.

RNA pol A shorthand term for *RNA polymerase.*

RNA polymerase The enzyme that catalyzes the synthesis of RNA. See also *RNA pol, RNA pol I, RNA pol II,* and *RNA pol III.*

RNA polymerase I (RNA pol I) In eukaryotic transcription, the enzyme that transcribes certain rRNA genes.

RNA polymerase II (RNA pol II) In eukaryotic transcription, the enzyme that transcribes protein-coding genes to produce mRNA.

RNA polymerase III (RNA pol III) In eukaryotic transcription, the enzyme that transcribes tRNA genes.

RNA polymerase core The five-polypeptide component of bacterial RNA polymerase that actively carries out transcription.

RNA primer In DNA replication, the short, single-stranded RNA segment synthesized by primase. The 3′ end of the RNA primer is used by DNA polymerase to begin synthesis of DNA.

RNA-induced silencing complex (RISC) Complex containing Argonaute protein that binds small RNA molecules and targets complementary RNA molecules for degradation or translational repression.

RNA-induced transcription-silencing (RITS) complex RISC-like complex that mediates small RNA-induced transcriptional gene silencing.

Robertsonian translocation The fusion of two non-homologous chromosomes, often with the deletion of a small amount of nonessential genetic material. Also known as *chromosome fusion*.

rolling circle replication A unidirectional mode of DNA replication used to replicate circular plasmid molecules in which the replicating circular molecule appears to reel off its nontemplate DNA strand, using the other as the template for replication.

S phase (synthesis phase) The middle phase of interphase, during which DNA replication takes place.

same sense resolution One of the possible patterns for resolving a Holliday junction to separate homologous chromosomes before meiotic anaphase.

Sanger method See *dideoxy DNA sequencing*.

saturation mutagenesis Mutagenesis aimed at identifying multiple mutant alleles for all loci in the genome of an experimental organism.

scaffold A set of contigs that are physically linked.

scaffold protein A protein contributing to the structure of a chromosome.

scanning In eukaryotic translation, the process used by the small ribosomal subunit to locate the authentic start codon.

secondary endosymbiosis (tertiary endosymbiosis) Endosymbiotic event where one eukaryotic, usually photosynthetic, is an endosymbiont within another eukaryote resulting in an organism with genomes derived from at least two nuclear genomes and multiple organellar genomes.

secondary structure A form of protein folding in which hydrogen bonds between amino acids of a polypeptide stabilize α-helical twists or β-sheets.

second filial generation (F_2 generation) The offspring produced by mating F_1 organisms to one another.

second-site reversion A specific type of reversion taking place at a location separate from the site altered to generate the original mutation.

segment polarity genes In *Drosophila*, genes that delimit the anterior and posterior regions of individual parasegments along the anterior-posterior axis; examples include *wingless*, *engrailed*, *hedgehog*, and *gooseberry*.

selected marker screen An experimental method used to detect microorganisms with a specific genotype.

selection coefficient (s, t) The value of the reduction in reproductive fitness for an organism (i.e., $w = 1.0 - s$).

selection differential (S) The difference between the population mean value for a phenotype and the phenotype value of population members selected as parents for the next generation.

selective growth medium The growth medium used in a selective marker screen.

selective sweep The reduction or elimination of polymorphism spanning a locus under selection.

self-fertilization Reproduction by organisms that contain both male and female reproductive structures; the natural reproductive mechanism on many plants, including pea plants.

semiconservative DNA replication The established method of DNA replication in which each strand of a parental duplex acts as a template for daughter strand synthesis and each daughter duplex is composed of one parental strand and a complementary daughter strand.

sequence gap Gap between two contigs for which a clone is available for further sequencing that could close the gap.

sex chromosome Homologous chromosomes that differ between the sexes. Designated X and Y in species in which females are XX and males XY. Designated Z and W in species in which females are ZW and males are ZZ.

sex determination The genetically controlled processes that determine the sex of offspring.

sex-influenced trait A gene, usually autosomal, whose expression differs between males and females of a species. Also known as *sex-influenced expression*.

sex-limited trait A gene or trait expressed exclusively in one sex. Also known as sex-limited gene.

sex-linked inheritance The inheritance of genes on the sex chromosomes.

shared derived characteristics Characteristics or traits of organisms that evolve from more ancestral characteristics or traits found in ancestral organisms.

shelterin A protein complex helping to protect chromosome telomeric regions from damage during DNA replication.

Shine–Dalgarno sequence In bacterial translation, the 5′ UTR mRNA consensus sequence that pairs with nucleotides near the 3′ end of 16S rRNA in the small ribosomal subunit to orient the start codon on the ribosome.

short tandem repeat (STR) Clusters of variable numbers of repetitive DNA sequences of less than 10 base pairs each that are variable among individuals; can be used as genetic markers.

shotgun sequencing Method for sequencing large molecules of DNA that relies on redundant sequencing of fragmented target DNA in the hope that all regions will be sequenced at least a few times. Contrast with *primer walking*.

shuttle vector A vector that can replicate in two species and thus can be used to shuttle DNA sequences between them.

sickle cell disease (SCD) A human autosomal recessive disorder resulting from homozygosity; a specific mutant allele (β^S) of the β-globin gene that is part of hemoglobin protein.

sigma (σ) subunit Accessory protein that changes the promoter-recognition specificity of the bacterial RNA polymerase core.

signal hypothesis The accepted hypothesis proposing that the polypeptide signal sequence identify posttranslational processing and transport.

signal sequence A string of amino acids at the N terminal and of certain eukaryotic polypeptides containing information directing posttranslational processing and the extracellular destination of the polypeptide.

silencer (silencer sequence) A eukaryotic cis-acting DNA regulatory sequence to which trans-acting factors bind to repress transcription.

single nucleotide polymorphism (SNP) A single base-pair difference in a specific genome location detected by comparing individual DNA sequences.

single-stranded binding protein (SSB) In DNA replication, a protein that adheres to each template strand following unwinding by helicase to prevent strand reannealing before the arrival of the replication fork.

sister chromatids The identical DNA duplexes that are produced by DNA replication and are temporarily joined to one another during the early stages of cell division.

sister chromatid cohesion The protein-based temporary attachment of sister chromatids facilitated by cohesin protein that resists the pulling forces of spindle fibers in metaphase.

site-specific recombination An exchange between two DNA molecules that requires specific sequences in common and that is catalyzed by an enzyme specific to that recombination (e.g., integration of phage lambda into the *E. coli* genome).

sliding clamp In bacterial DNA replication, the multisubunit protein complex that joins with DNA polymerase to hold polymerase on the template and helps drive polymerase along the template.

small interfering RNA (siRNA) Single-stranded 21- to 24-nucleotide RNA molecules derived from either endogenous or exogenous double-stranded RNA molecules that are incorporated in RISC to mediate RNAi. Endogenously produced siRNAs are most often from nongenic regions (e.g., repetitive RNA or products of an RNA-dependent RNA polymerase). Exogenously produced siRNAs are often derived from invading nucleic acids (e.g., transposons and viruses).

small nuclear RNA (snRNA) Regulatory RNAs operating in the nucleus.

small ribosomal subunit The smaller of two subunits of the ribosome.

solenoid structure See *30-nm fiber.*

somatic gene therapy Gene therapy aimed at correcting a genetic defect in the somatic cells.

somatic mutation A mutation occurring in a somatic (structural) cell of an organism. See also *germ-line mutation.*

Southern blotting A laboratory method devised by Edwin Southern for transferring DNA from an electrophoresis gel to a permanent membrane or filter.

specialized transduction (specialized transducing phage) Transduction from a donor cell to a recipient cell of a few select genes located near the site of bacteriophage integration.

spindle fiber microtubule (kinetochore, nonkinetochore, and astral microtubule) Composed of tubulin proteins, the fibers emanating from centrosomes that attach to kinetochore regions (kinetochore), overlap to control cell shape (polar), or attach to the cell membrane to stabilize centrosomes (astral).

spliceosome The multiprotein complex that carries out intron splicing.

splicing mutation A mutation altering the normal splicing pattern of a pre-mRNA.

spontaneous mutation Mutations occurring due to spontaneous events or changes involving nucleotides or nucleotide bases.

sporadic cancer A term describing 90% or more of all cases of cancer, that develop as the result of the accumulation of multiple somatic mutations; these cancers occur without the inheritance of a specific mutation that increases an individual's susceptibility to cancer.

sporadic retinoblastoma Cases of retinal cancer that occur as a result of homozygous somatic mutation of a specific gene in the same cell of a retina.

square root method A method for estimating allele frequencies based on manipulation of the frequency of a homozygous genotype.

stabilizing selection A pattern of natural or artificial selection that reduces population variation by removing organisms with extreme phenotypes.

standard deviation (s) A statistical value that measures the scatter of outcome values around the mean or average outcome value. Expressed as the square root of the sum of squared deviations of each value from the mean value.

start codon Most commonly AUG, encoding methionine, the first codon translated in polypeptide synthesis.

start of transcription The DNA location at which transcription begins.

stem loop structure Short double-stranded segments of RNA topped by a single-stranded loop containing unpaired nucleotides. Also known as a *hairpin structure.*

sticky end Short single-stranded overhangs created by the cleavage of DNA by specific restriction endonucleases, which can potentially base-pair with complementary single-stranded sequences.

stop codon One of three codons that bind a release factor instead of base-pairing with tRNA to initiate a series of events that stops translation.

strand invasion During synthesis-dependent strand annealing and meiotic recombination, the entry of the 3′ end of a displaced DNA into the intact sister chromatid.

strand polarity (5′ and 3′) The orientation of a nucleic acid strand indicating its 5′ phosphate and 3′ hydroxyl ends.

strand slippage During DNA replication, a mutational event leading to increased or decreased numbers of repeating nucleotides in newly synthesized DNA and caused by slippage of DNA polymerase on the template strand or slippage of the newly synthesized strand on DNA polymerase.

structural genomics The sequencing of whole genomes and the cataloging, or annotation of sequences within a given genome.

Su(var) mutations Mutations that suppress position effect variegation in *Drosophila.* Mutated genes produce proteins that are active in chromatin remodeling.

subcloning Process by which DNA clones are further subdivided to clone still smaller fragments for analyses.

subfunctionalization The process, following gene duplication, whereby mutations in each of the two copies can result in the two genes having complementary activities such that their combined activity is the same as the activity of the gene before duplication.

submetacentric chromosome A chromosome with a centromere located near the midpoint that produces long and short arms of different lengths.

sugar-phosphate backbone The alternating sugar (deoxyribose or ribose) and phosphate molecule pattern of nucleic acid strands formed by the formation of phosphodiester bonds linking nucleotides in the strand.

sum rule The probability of an event that can result from two or more equivalent outcomes. The probabilities of the contributing events are added, and their sum is the probability of the event in question. Also known as the *addition rule.*

supercoiled DNA The superhelical twisting of covalently closed circular DNA. See also *positive supercoiling* and *negative supercoiling.*

supplemented minimal medium A microbial growth medium that begins as a minimal medium and has selected additional compounds added to support the growth of specific auxotrophs (mutants).

suppressor mutation A mutation whose effect is to reverse the effect of another mutation. Acts to restore wild-type, or near wild-type, function.

suppressor screen A modifier genetic screen designed to identify mutations in genes that suppress the phenotypic effects of mutations in another gene.

SWI/SNF (switch/sucrose nonfermentable) complex A yeast chromatin-remodeling complex that modulates nucleosome positioning in an ATP-dependent manner.

SWR1 complex (switch remodeling 1) A chromatin-remodeling complex responsible for replacing the common histone 2A protein of nucleosomes with a variant form known as H2AZ.

sympatric speciation An evolutionary process in which new species form in overlapping regions. Reproductive isolation mechanisms accompanying speciation are usually behavioral or mechanical.

synapsis The close approach and contact between homologous chromosomes during early prophase I in meiosis.

synaptomorphy A characteristic present in an ancestral species and shared, perhaps in a modified form, by its evolutionary descendants.

synaptonemal complex A specialized three-layer protein complex, consisting of a central element and two lateral elements, that forms between homologous chromosomes at synapsis.

syncytial blastoderm Stage of *Drosophila* embryogenesis in which the nuclei are located at the periphery of the embryo but are not separated by cell membranes.

syncytium A multinucleated cell in which the nuclei are not separated by cell membranes.

synonymous codon The groups of codons that specify the same amino acid.

synonymous mutation A base substitution mutation that changes one codon to a synonymous codon and does not alter the amino acid sequence of a polypeptide.

syntenic genes Genes located on the same chromosome.

synteny The conserved order of genes together on a chromosome in species that share a common ancestor.

synthesis-dependent strand annealing (SDSA) An error-free mechanism for repair of DNA double-strand breaks occurring after the completion of DNA replication and utilizing strand invasion to provide wild-type sequences for repair.

synthetic lethality The situation where a particular double mutant results in lethality but the two respective single mutants are viable.

systems biology Prediction of biological functions of genes based on correlations between different data sets.

T loop A structure formed during DNA replication of a telomeric repeat sequence.

T (transfer) strand The DNA strand of the T-DNA cleaved to initiate the transfer of plasmid DNA during rolling circle replication.

targeted induced local lesions in genomes (TILLING) A reverse genetic approach in which a population of organisms of an inbred strain is randomly mutagenized throughout the genome and this population is then screened to find mutations in a gene of interest for which the sequence is known.

TATA-binding protein (TBP) A general transcription factor protein that binds the TATA box and assists in binding other transcription factors and RNA polymerase II to promoters.

TATA box The thymine- and adenine-rich consensus sequence region found in most eukaryotic promoters. Also known as *Goldberg-Hogness box*.

TBP-associated factor (TAF) Specific general transcription factors that associate with TATA-binding protein.

telocentric chromosome A chromosome with a centromere located at one end, producing a long arm only.

telomerase The ribonucleoprotein complex whose RNA component provides a template used to synthesize repeating DNA segments that form chromosome telomeres.

telomerase RNA The RNA portion of the telomerase enzyme that provides a template for synthesis of the repeating sequence of the telomere.

telomere Repeating DNA sequences, synthesized by *telomerase*, at the ends of linear chromosomes in eukaryotes; contain dozens to hundreds of copies of specific short DNA sequence repeats that buffer the coding sequence of the chromosome from loss during successive cycles of DNA replication.

telophase The last stage of *M phase*, in which the nuclear contents are divided (*karyokinesis*) and the daughter cells are divided (*cytokinesis*).

temperate phage A bacteriophage, such as λ phage, that can integrate into the bacterial host chromosome and produce either the lytic or lysogenic life cycle.

temperature-sensitive allele A mutation evident only at or above a certain temperature due to an abnormality of the protein product that affects its stability.

template strand The DNA strand serving as a template for synthesis of a complementary nucleic acid strand.

terminal deletion The loss of a chromosome segment that includes the telomeric region.

terminal inverted repeat Identical sequences found at both ends of a transposable genetic element. The sequences are inverted relative to one another.

termination region The region of a gene containing the transcription-terminating sequence or region.

termination sequence DNA sequences that serve to stop transcription. Also known as *transcription termination*.

termination stem loop (3–4 stem loop) Stem loop of an mRNA transcript that signals RNA polymerase to terminate transcription in the leader region of bacterial attenuator-controlled operons (e.g., *trp* operon).

tertiary structure The state of protein folding stabilized by hydrogen bonds and covalent bonds that form the functional structure of a protein. A protein may have more than one tertiary structure.

test cross The cross of an organism with the dominant phenotype that may be heterozygous with an organism that is homozygous for a recessive allele. Also known as test-cross analysis.

theta value (θ value) See θ *(theta) value*.

third-base wobble The flexibility of purine-pyrimidine base pairing between the third base of a codon and the corresponding nucleotide of the anticodon.

third filial generation (F₃ generation) The offspring produced by mating F_2 organisms to one another.

third-generation sequencing (TGS) Advanced DNA sequencing methods that were the immediate predecessors of next-generation sequencing (NGS).

three-point test-cross analysis A test cross designed to identify genetic linkage between three genes and to provide data for determination of recombination frequency between linked genes.

threshold of genetic liability In polygenic and multifactorial inheritance, a trait with different phenotypes (e.g., affected and unaffected) that are determined by whether individual organisms are above or below a particular critical value on the phenotypic scale. Also known as *threshold trait*.

threshold trait See *threshold of genetic liability*.

thymine (T) One of four nitrogenous nucleotide bases in DNA; one of the two types of pyrimidine nucleotides in DNA.

thymine dimer The specific type of lesion formed on DNA due to exposure to ultraviolet irradiation.

time-of-entry mapping A method of donor gene mapping by conjugation that uses interrupted mating to determine the order and relative timing of gene transfer.

Ti plasmid A large (200 kb) circular plasmid of *Agrobacterium tumefaciens* that harbors genes for transfer of DNA into plants cells and genes that cause uncontrolled division of plant cells; hence, the tumor-inducing (Ti) plasmid. It has been engineered for the construction of transgenic plants.

DNA topoisomerase Enzyme that relaxes DNA supercoiling by controlled strand nicking and rejoining.

totipotency State of a cell when it can give rise to any and all cell types of an organism.

tracrRNA Small RNA that act to couple crRNAs with a Cas protein in the CRISPR–Cas complex.

trans-acting Acting between two molecules (e.g., DNA sequences that control expression of genes interacting with a diffusible protein product).

trans-acting regulatory protein Proteins that act in trans by binding to cis-acting regulatory sequences and consequently regulating nearby genes, either by activating or repressing transcription. Often referred to as *transcription factors (TFs)*.

transcription The cellular process that synthesizes RNA strands from a DNA template strand.

transcription factors (TFs) Proteins that bind promoters and are functional in transcription.

transcriptome Set of transcripts present in a cell, tissue, or organism.

transcriptomics The study of all the transcripts, collectively known as the transcriptome, within a cell, tissue, or organism.

transductant The bacterium that is the product of transduction.

transduction In bacterial systems, the process of transfer of DNA from a donor bacterial cell to a recipient cell using a bacteriophage as a vector. More generally can refer to the process by which foreign DNA is introduced into another cell via a viral vector.

transfer DNA (T-DNA) The portion of the Ti plasmid that is transferred from the bacterium into the nucleus of a plant cell.

transfer RNA (tRNA) A family of small RNA molecules that each bind a specific amino acid and convey it to the ribosome, where the anticodon sequence undertakes complementary base pairing with an mRNA codon during translation.

transformant The bacterium that is the product of transformation.

transformation (1) The bacterial process of gene transfer in which donated DNA fragments originating in a dead donor cell, or plasmid DNA, are taken up across the cell wall and membrane of a recipient cell and recombined into the transformant genome. (2) More generally refers to the process by which exogenous DNA is directly taken up by a cell resulting in a genetic alteration of the cell. (3) The conversion of animal cells to an abnormal unregulated state by an oncogenic virus or by transforming DNA.

transgene A gene that has been modified in vitro by recombinant DNA technology and introduced into the genome via transformation.

transgenic organism An organism harboring a transgene.

transition mutation A type of DNA base-pair substitution in which one purine replaces the other or one pyrimidine replaces the other.

translation The process taking place at ribosomes to synthesize polypeptides. Complementary base pairing between mRNA codons and tRNA anticodons determines the order of amino acids composing the polypeptide.

translation repressor protein In bacteria, proteins that regulate translation by binding mRNA in the vicinity of the Shine–Dalgarno sequence and thereby prevent ribosome binding.

translesion DNA synthesis Utilizing a bypass polymerase, a mechanism for replicating DNA in the presence of damage that blocks replication by the common polymerase.

translocation heterozygote An organism with chromosome translocation in which chromosome pairs consist of one normal chromosome and a homolog carrying a translocation.

transmission genetics The subfield of genetics concerned with assessment and analysis of gene transfer from parents to offspring. Synonymous with *Mendelian genetics.*

transposable genetic element A class of DNA sequences that can move from one chromosome location to another, either by excision and reinsertion or by replication and reinsertion of the replicated copy.

transposase The enzyme produced by transposons that cuts DNA to allow the excision and insertion of the transposon.

transposition The process by which mobile genetic elements move from one portion of a genome to another. See also *transposable genetic element.*

transversion mutation A type of DNA base substitution mutation in which a purine substitutes for a pyrimidine, or vice versa.

tree of life The phylogenetic tree depicting the evolutionary relationships between organisms.

trihybrid cross A genetic cross between organisms that are heterozygous for three genes.

trinucleotide repeat expansion disorder A hereditary disorder caused by a mutant gene containing an increased number of repeats of a DNA trinucleotide sequence.

trisomy The presence in a genome of three copies of a chromosome rather than a homologous pair of chromosomes and resulting in a number of chromosomes that is $2n - 1$.

trisomy rescue In a trisomic genome, the random loss of one extra chromosome to reduce the chromosome number to the diploid.

true-breeding strains See *pure-breeding strains.*

true reversion A type of reversion that exactly reverses the original mutation.

tumor A cancerous growth or tissue.

tumor suppressor gene A broad category of normal genes whose generalized functions slow, pause, or stop cell proliferation. It is often mutated in carcinogenesis.

two-hit hypothesis The genetic theory of cancer development proposing that both copies of a gene must be mutated to permit the development of certain cancers. See also *sporadic retinoblastoma.*

two-hybrid system A method for discovering whether two proteins interact using the GAL4 protein of yeast, which is separated into a DNA-binding domain and a transcriptional activation domain. The two GAL4 domains are fused with the two proteins of interest respectively, and the resultant fusion proteins are assayed for their ability to activate transcription, which indicates interaction of the two proteins of interest.

two-point test-cross analysis A test cross designed to identify genetic linkage between two genes and to provide data for determination of recombination frequency between linked genes.

ultrasound A clinical method used to visualize a fetus in utero.

ultraviolet (UV) repair A multiprotein DNA damage repair system that corrects lesions caused by exposure to ultraviolet irradiation.

unbalanced translocation A chromosome translocation resulting in the gain or loss of genetic material.

uncharged tRNA A tRNA not carrying an amino acid.

unequal crossover Resulting from the improper synaptic pairing of homologous chromosomes and crossing over between the mispaired chromosomes. A source of duplication and deletion of genetic material.

uniparental disomy In a genome, the presence of a pair of homologous chromosomes that originate from a single parent.

uniparental inheritance Condition in organellar inheritance whereby just one parental gamete—often the maternal gamete—contributes all of the cytoplasmic organelles.

unpaired loop At synapsis involving partial deletion or partial duplication of one chromosome of a homologous pair, the "extra" genetic material that does not have a homolog on the paired chromosome.

unselected marker screen An experimental technique used to screen microbial genotypes. Commonly used following selected marker screening.

upstream Referring to a gene or sequence location that is toward the 5′ direction of a *coding strand.*

upstream activator sequence (UAS) An enhancer-like sequence in yeast, located just upstream of the genes they regulate.

upstream control element An upstream consensus sequence found in certain eukaryotic gene promoters.

uracil (U) One of four nitrogenous nucleotide bases in RNA; one of the two types of pyrimidine nucleotides in RNA.

variable expressivity Variation in the degree, magnitude, or intensity of expression of a phenotype.

variable number tandem repeat (VNTR) Clusters of varying numbers of repetitive DNA sequences of more than 10 base pairs each that are variable among individuals; can be used as genetic markers.

variance A statistical measurement of the variation of sample values around the mean value.

vector A DNA fragment with attributes that will allow its amplification (origin of replication) in a biological system and serves as a carrier for foreign DNA inserted into it. Vectors usually also possess genes (e.g., encoding resistance to an antibiotic) that allow selection of hosts carrying the vector.

western blotting A method for transferring protein from an electrophoresis gel to a permanent membrane or filter.

whole-genome shotgun (WGS) sequencing An approach to genome sequencing whereby DNA representing the entire genome is fragmented into smaller pieces and a large number of fragments are chosen at random and sequenced with the aim that all genomic regions will be sequenced multiple times. Compare with *clone-by-clone sequencing.*

wild type The most common form of an allele or of a phenotype in a population.

X/autosome ratio (X/A ratio) The ratio of X chromosomes to a pair of autosomes. Used in *Drosophila* as the mechanism of sex determination.

X-linked dominant A pattern of inheritance consistent with the transmission of a dominant allele of a gene on the X chromosome. Compare with *X-linked recessive.*

X-linked inheritance The pattern of inheritance characteristic of genes located on the X chromosome.

X-linked recessive A pattern of inheritance consistent with the transmission of a recessive allele of a gene on the X chromosome. Compare with *X-linked dominant.*

Y-linked inheritance The exclusively male-to-male transmission of genes on the Y chromosome.

Z_{max} The most likely recombination distance (theta [θ] value) between genes as determined by lod score analysis.

zone of polarizing activity (ZPA) The posterior side of the limb bud that acts as an organizer, secreting Sonic hedgehog (Shh) protein that acts to pattern the developing limb.

Z/W system The sex chromosome inheritance system in species in which the male is homogametic (ZZ) and the female is heterogametic (ZW).

zygotic gene Genes that are active only in the zygote or embryo. For zygotic genes, the genotype of the embryo determines the phenotype.

Credits

Photo Credits

Cover Gunilla Elam/Science Source

Chapter 1 p. 1, CO-1, Michel & Gabrielle Therin-Weise/Alamy; p. 3, 1.1a, Scala/Art Resource, NY; p. 3, 1.1b, Andrew McRobb/Dorling Kindersley, Ltd.; p. 7, 1.3, Science History Images/Photo Researchers/Alamy; p. 7, 1.4, Omikron/Science Source; p. 8, 1.5, Science & Society Picture Library/Getty Images; p. 17, 1.13, Pearson Education, Inc.; p. 17, 1.14a, John L. Bowman/University of California at Davis; p. 17, 1.14b, Centers for Disease Control and Prevention; p. 19, 1.15, David Wacey; p. 25, 1.19, Photo by Frederick York, taken at London Zoo in 1870

Chapter 2 p. 30, CO-2, Villanova University; p. 41, EI 2.1, Denise Kappa/Shutterstock

Chapter 3 p. 67, CO-3, Science History Images/Photo Researchers/Alamy; p. 70, 3.2a–c, Jennifer Waters/Science Source; p. 71, 3.2d-f, Jennifer Waters/Science Source; p. 73, 3.5a, Don W. Fawcett/Science Source; p. 73, 3.5b, Dartmouth Electron Microscope Facility; p. 85, 3.17, Georg Halder; p. 91, 3.22a, top left, Catalin Petolea/Shutterstock; p. 91, 3.22a, top right, Margo Harrison/Shutterstock; p. 91, 3.22a, bottom left, Richard Peterson/Shutterstock; p. 91, 3.22a, bottom right, Margo Harrison/Shutterstock; p. 91, 3.22b, top left, Richard Peterson/Shutterstock; p. 91, 3.22b, top right, Potapov Alexander/Shutterstock; p. 91, 3.22b, bottom left, Catalin Petolea/Shutterstock; p. 91, 3.22b, bottom right, Margo Harrison/Shutterstock; p. 93, 3.23b, Garo/Phanie/Alamy; p. 97, 3.27, Susan Richey-Schmitz/123RF.com

Chapter 4 p. 105, CO-4, Claire Norman/Shutterstock; p. 111, 4.3, Dr. Karen E. Petersen, University of Washington; p. 116, 4.7, Courtesy of Ueli Grossniklaus, Institute of Plant Biology, University of Zurich; p. 117, 4.8a, INSADCO Photography/Alamy; p. 117, 4.8b, Stanton K. Short/The Jackson Laboratory; p. 120, 4.13, Biophoto Associates/Science Source/Getty Images; p. 129, 4.20a, c, d and f, Eric Isselee/Shutterstock; p. 129, 4.20b, Rosa Jay/Shutterstock; p. 129, 4.20e, Jagodka/Shutterstock

Chapter 5 p. 145, CO-5, From the book: *Meiosis*, by B. John, published by Cambridge University Press, 1990, p. 33, Fig. 2.3a part 1

Chapter 6 p. 185, CO-6, Eye of Science/Science Source; p. 191, 6.3, Huntington Potter/University of South Florida College of Medicine; p. 206, 6.15 top, Eye of Science/Science Source; p. 206, 6.15 bottom, Dr. Michel Wurtz/Biozentrum, University of Basel/Science Source; p. 211, 6.20, Lester V. Bergman/Corbis Documentary/Getty Images

Application A p. 223, CO-A, Garo/Phanie/Alamy

Chapter 7 p. 235, CO-7, Science History Images/Alamy; p. 237, 7.1, Centers for Disease Control and Prevention (CDC); p. 247, 7.10, Dr. Gopal Murti/Science Source; p. 250, 7.13a, Blumenthal et. al, Cold Spring Harbor Laboratory Symposia on Quantitative Biology, 1974, Figure 1, p. 207. Reprinted by permission of Cold Spring Harbor Laboratory Press; p. 265, 7.29b, Southern Illinois University/Science Source

Chapter 8 p. 275, CO-8, Science History Images/Alamy; p. 298, 8.21, Phillip A. Sharp

Chapter 9 p. 319, RT 9.1a–b, Ribosomal proteins. XII. Number of proteins in small and large ribosomal subunits of Escherichia coli as determined by two-dimensional gel electrophoresis. E. Kaltschmidt and H. G. Wittmann, *Proc Natl Acad Sci U S A.* 1970 Nov;67(3):1276–82, Fig. 1 and Fig. 2; p. 328, 9.11a, Professor Oscar Miller/Science Source

Application B p. 346, CO-B, Marmaduke St. John/Alamy; p. 349, B.1a–b, From the Huntington Disease Collaborative Research Group (1993); p. 351, B.4, Editorial Image, LLC/Alamy

Chapter 10 p. 361, CO-10, SPL/Science Source; p. 363, 10.1, Andreas Bolzer et al./PLoS Biol; p. 363, 10.2, Hesed M. Padilla-Nash, Antonio Fargiano and Thomas Reid, "Cancer Genomics," Genetics Branch, Center for Research, National Cancer Institute, National Institutes of Health, Bethesda, MD 20892; p. 364, 10.4a, James King-Holmes/Science Source; p. 364, 10.4b, L. Willatt/Science Source; p. 373, 10.10 left, Dionisvera/123RF.com; p. 373, 10.10 right, Stawomir Zelasko/123RF.com; p. 373, 10.11a, Vanessa Morgan, PSU-Center for Lakes and Reservoirs; p. 373, 10.11b, Miguel Sanz Alcántara; p. 373, 10.11c, FloralImages/Alamy; p. 374, 10.12a, Dr. Adina Breiman Ph.D; p. 374, 10.12b, Western Regional Research Center, Agricultural Research Service, U.S. Department of Agriculture; p. 374, 10.12c, James King-Holmes/Science Source; p. 374, 10.12d, W. John Raupp; p. 374, 10.12e, Bon Appetit/Alamy; p. 374, 10.12f, Arco Images GmbH/Alamy; p. 374, 10.12g, Bon Appetit/Alamy; p. 374, 10.12h, Redhen/Shutterstock; p. 374, 10.12i, ImageBroker/Alamy; p. 374, 10.12j, Redhen/Shutterstock; p. 387, 10.24b, Victoria Foe; p. 387, 10.24c, Dr. Barbara A. Hamkalo; p. 389, 10.26a, Power and Syred/Science Source; p. 389, 10.26b, Courtesy of Ulrich K. Laemmli

Chapter 11 p. 399, CO-11, Frank Augstein/AP Images

Chapter 12 p. 439, CO-12, Bettmann/Getty Images

Chapter 13 p. 476, CO-13.1, Jorgensen, Richard A./American Society of Plant Biologists; p. 476, CO-13.2, Napoli, C., C. Lemieux, and Jorgensen, Richard A./American Society of Plant Biologists; p. 476, CO-13.3, Jorgensen, Richard A./American Society of Plant Biologists; p. 478, 13.2 left, David Scharf/Science Source; p. 478, 13.2 right, Nigel Pavitt/John Warburton-Lee Photography/Alamy

Chapter 14 p. 507, CO-14, Courtesy of the Archives/California Institute of Technology; p. 529, 14.15a, Paul Sternberg; p. 529, 14.15b, John L. Bowman/University of California at Davis; p. 529, 14.15c, National Science Foundation; p. 529, 14.15d, Courtesy of John Wilson/Baylor College of Medicine; p. 529, 14.15e, Livet, Weissman, Sanes, and Lichtman/Harvard University; p. 530, 14.16, Stephen J. Small, A. Blair, and M. Levine. *EMBO J.* 1992 Nov; 11(11): 4047–57; p. 532, 14.18 top left, Eye of Science/Science Source; p. 532, 14.18 top right, Eye of Science/Science Source; p. 532, 14.18 bottom left, David Scharf/Science Source; p. 532, 14.18 bottom right, Eye of Science/Science Source; p. 534, 14.19a–d, John L. Bowman/University of California at Davis

Application C p. 538, CO-C, Paul A. W. Edwards

Chapter 15 p. 552, CO-15, Reproduced with permission from the *Annual Review of Plant Physiology and Plant Molecular Biology*, Vol. 49 © 1998 by Annual Reviews www.annualreviews.org; p. 556, GA 15.1, John L. Bowman/University of California at Davis; p. 557, 15.2, John L. Bowman/University of California at Davis; p. 560, 15.6b, John L. Bowman/University of California at Davis; p. 570, 15.13c, John L. Bowman/University of California at Davis; p. 574, 15.15c, Golden Rice Institute; p. 576, 15.17, Robert H. Devlin, Ph. D; p. 584, 15.22, Photo Courtesy of The Roslin Institute, The University of Edinburgh Roslin, Scotland, UK

Chapter 16 p. 593, CO-16, John L. Bowman/University of California at Davis; p. 616, 16.17b left, Tbx2 terminates shh/fgf signaling in the developing mouse limb bud by direct repression of gremlin1. H. F. Farin et al. *PLoS Genet.* 2013; 9(4):e1003467. doi: 10.1371/journal.pgen.1003467. Epub 2013 Apr 25. Fig. 1F. CC by 4.0; p. 616, 16.17b right, Robert Hill; p. 620, 16.21b, David J. Lockhart and Elizabeth A. Winzeler; p. 622, 16.22, Republished with permission of AAAS from S. Chu et al. "The transcriptional program of sporulation in budding yeast" *Science* 282(5389), October 23, 1998, pp. 699–705; permission conveyed through Copyright Clearance Center, Inc.

Chapter 17 p. 632, CO-17, Dartmouth Electron Microscope Facility; p. 645, 17.10, Dr. David Furness/Keele University/Science Source; p. 646, 17.11b, Don W. Fawcett/Science Source; p. 649, 17.14, Dr. Jeremy Burgess/Science Source; p. 650, 17.15a, Dr. Richard D. Kolodnar/Dana-Farber Cancer Institute

Chapter 18 p. 663, CO-18, FLPA/Alamy; p. 664, 18.1a, Courtesy of the Archives, California Institute of Technology; p. 664, 18.1b, Eye of Science/Science Source; p. 665, 18.02, © 2002 Steven J. Baskauf, http://bioimages.vanderbilt.edu/baskauf/17080; p. 666, 18.3b, Reproduced with permission of *Annual Review of Cell and Developmental*, Volume 20 © 2004 by Annual Reviews www.annualreviews.org.; p. 666, 18.3c, James B. Skeath; p. 668, 18.5a, Daniel St. Johnston and Wolfgang Driever; p. 668, 18.5b, John Reinitz; p. 668, 18.5c–d, James B. Jaynes; p. 670, 18.6b, Daniel St. Johnston and Wolfgang Driever; p. 672, 18.8, Mattias Mannervik; p. 672, 18.9c, Stephan J. Small; p. 674, 18.10b, William McGinnis; p. 679, 18.14a, Paul W. Sternberg; p. 680, 18.15a top, Dr. Erik M. Jorgensen, PhD; p. 680, 18.15a bottom left and right, Paul W. Sternberg; p. 684, 18.18c, Tatiana Popova/Shutterstock; p. 686, 18.19, John L. Bowman/University of California at Davis; p. 687, 18.20, John L. Bowman/University of California at Davis; p. 690, 18.22c left, Binns, W., James, L. F., Shupe, J. L., "Toxicosis of veratrum californicum in ewes and its relationship to a congenital deformity in lambs" *Annals of the New York Academy of Sciences*, December 15, 2006. Copyright © 2006 John Wiley and Sons. Used with permission.; p. 690, 18.22c center and right, Robert Hill

CREDITS

C-1

Chapter 19 p. 696, CO-19, Peter Morenus

Chapter 20 p. 725, CO-20, Andy Lidstone/
Alamy

Application D p. 758, CO-D, Pascal Goetghe-
luck/Science Source

Application E p. 778, CO-E, David Parker/
Science Source

Text and Illustration Credits

Chapter 1 p. 9, J. D. Watson and F. H. C. Crick,
1953, "Molecular structure of nucleic acids: A structure
for deoxyribose nucleic acid," *Nature* 171: 737–38;
p. 3, William Bateson (1861–1926); **p. 19,** Richard
Dawkins, *River out of Eden: A Darwinian View of Life*,
NY: Basic Books; **p. 21, 1.16,** Neil A. Campbell et al.,
Biology, 7th Ed., ©2008. Reprinted and Electronically
reproduced by permission of Pearson Education, Inc.,
New York, NY

Chapter 2 p. 37, Based on Gregor Johann
Mendel's first law, law of segregation; **p. 58,
Table 2.9,** Based on OMIM statistics as of September
2016 (http://www.omim.org/statistics/entry)

Chapter 3 p. 98, 3.28, Karin Jegalian and Bruce
T. Lah, "Why the y is so weird." *Scientific American*,
February 2001, pages 56–61, illustrator, Alfred Kama-
jian, directly regarding permission. Website: http://
www.kamajian.com

Chapter 4 p. 123, 4.16, Adapted from Monroe W.
Strickberger, *Genetics*, 3e, p. 543. Macmillan, 1969.
Used with permission of Pearson Education.

Chapter 5 p. 155, Thomas Hunt Morgan, 1911;
p. 155, A. H. Sturtevant (1965), *A History of Genetics*,
Harper & Row; **p. 165, 5.11,** J. L. Weber et al. 1993.
"Evidence for human meiotic recombination interference obtained through construction of a short tandem
repeat polymorphism linkage map of chromosome 19,"
American Journal of Human Genetics 53:1079–95;
p. 171, Experimental Insight 5.1, Data from J. Hall
et al. (1994)

Chapter 6 p. 200, 6.11, Based on E. L. Wollman,
F. Jacob, and W. Hayes, "Conjugation and genetic
recombination in escherichia coli K-12," *Cold Spring
Harbor Symposia on Quantitative Biology*, 21, 1956,
p. 141; **p. 202, 6.12,** Microbiology and molecular biology reviews: MMBR by American Society for Microbiology. Reproduced with permission of American
Society for Microbiology; **p. 215, 6.23,** Adapted from
Seymour Benzer, "On the topography of the genetic
fine structure," *Proceedings of the National Academy
of Sciences*, Vol. 47, No. 3 (1961), p. 406, Fig. 3.
Used with permission; **p. 215, 6.24,** Adapted from
Seymour Benzer, "On the topography of the genetic
fine structure," *Proceedings of the National Academy
of Sciences*, Vol. 47, No. 3 (1961), p. 410, Fig. 6. Used
with permission

Chapter 7 p. 236, Edmund Wilson, 1895; **p. 237,
7.2,** Based on F. Griffith, 1928, "The significance of
pneumococcal types," *J. Hyg.* 27: 113–59; **p. 238,
7.3,** Based on O. T. Avery, C. M. Macleod, and M.
McCarty, 1944, "Studies on the chemical nature of the
substance inducing transformation of pneumococcal
types: Induction of transformation by a desoxyribonucleic acid fraction isolated from pneumococcus
type III," *J. Exp. Med.* 79: 137–58; **p. 239, 7.4,** Based
on A. D. Hershey, and M. Chase, 1952, "Independent
function of viral protein and nucleic acid in growth of
bacteriophage," *J. Genet. Phys.* 36: 39–56; **p. 245, 7.8,**

Based on M. Meselson, and F. W. Stahl, 1958, "The
replication of DNA in Escherichia coli," *Proc. Natl.
Acad. Sci.* USA 44: 671–82; **p. 245,** J. D. Watson
and F. H. C. Crick, "A structure for deoxyribose
nucleic acid," April 25, 1953, *Nature*, 171, 737–38;
p. 246, 7.9, Based on M. Meselson, and F. W. Stahl,
1958, "The replication of DNA in Escherichia coli,"
Proc. Natl. Acad. Sci. USA 44: 671–82; **p. 249, 7.12,**
Reprinted from *Journal of Molecular Biology*, Vol. 32,
J. A. Huberman and A. D. Riggs, "On the mechanism
of DNA replication in mammalian chromosomes,"
pp. 327–41. Copyright 1968, with permission from
Elsevier; **p. 251, 7.14,** Scott Freeman, Kim Quillin,
Lizabeth Allison, *Biological Science*, 5th ed., ©2014.
Reprinted and electronically reproduced by permission
of Pearson Education, Inc., Upper Saddle River, New
Jersey

Chapter 8 p. 291, 8.12, *Science* by Moses King,
reproduced with permission of American Association
for the Advancement of Science; **p. 297, 8.19,** James
D. Watson et al., *Molecular Biology of the Gene*, 6th
ed., ©2008. Reprinted and Electronically reproduced
by permission of Pearson Education, Inc. Upper Saddle
River, New Jersey; **p. 301, 8.24,** Reprinted from *Cell*,
Vol. 103, D. L. Black, "Protein diversity from alternative splicing," pp. 367–370. Copyright 2000, with permission from Elsevier; **p. 302, 8.25,** From "Three novel
brain tropomyosin isoforms are expressed from the
rat cx-tropomyosin gene through the use of alternative
promoters and alternative RNA processing," *Molecular
and Cellular Biology*, J. P. Lees-Miller, L. O. Goodwin,
and D. M. Helfman, 10, 04, 1990. Republished with
permission of American Society of Microbiology

Chapter 9 p. 315, 9.1, Adapted from Scott
Freeman et al., *Biological Science* 5th ed., Pearson
Education; **p. 316, Table 9.2,** Data from Scott Freeman
et al., *Biological Science* 5th ed., Pearson Education;
p. 323, Table 9.8, Data from H. G. Khorana et al.
(1967), "Polynucleotide synthesis and the genetic
code," *Cold Spring Harbor Symp.* 31: 39–49

Chapter 10 p. 365, 10.5, Figure adapted from
J. J. Yunis and O. Prakash, "The origin of man: A
chromosomal pictorial legacy," *Science*, 215:1527.
Reprinted with permission from AAAS. http://www.
sciencemag.org/content/215/4539/1525.abstract?
sid=17df9c3a-287e-4f30-b241-c7b1c88b1126; **p. 370,
Table 10.3,** Data adapted from E. B. Hook and A.
Lindsjo, "Down syndrome in live births by single year
maternal age interval in a Swedish study: Comparison
with results from a New York State study," *Am. J. Hum.
Genet.* 30 (1978): 19–27

Chapter 11 p. 415, 11.16, H. H. Watson, J. D.
Winsten, J. A., eds., *Origins of Human Cancer*, 1977,
1431–50, Cold Spring Harbor Laboratory Press, Cold
Spring Harbor, N.Y. Used with permission

Chapter 12 p. 442, 12.3a, Based on James D.
Watson et al., *Molecular Biology of the Gene*, 7th
ed., 2013. Printed and electronically reproduced by
permission of Pearson Education Inc., Upper Saddle
River, New Jersey; **p. 442, 12.3b,** Based on Michael T.
Madigan et al., *Biology of Microorganisms*, 13th ed.,
2012. Printed and electronically reproduced by permission of Pearson Education, Inc., Upper Saddle River,
New Jersey

Chapter 13 p. 487, 13.15, Based on *Nature*,
Vol 461 no.7261, Bradley R. Cairns "The logic of
chromatin architecture and remodelling at promoters,"
copyright 2009; **p. 489, 13.16,** Based on James D.
Watson et al., *Molecular Biology of the Gene*, 6th ed.,
2008. Printed and electronically reproduced by permission of Pearson Education Inc., Upper Saddle River,

New Jersey; **p. 489, 13.17,** Reprinted by permission
from Macmillan Publishers Ltd.: *Nature*, Vol 461
no.7261, Bradley R. Cairns, "The logic of chromatin
architecture and remodelling at promoters," copyright
2009; **p. 493, 13.22,** Reprinted by permission from
Macmillan Publishers Ltd.: *Nature*, 461, p. 189,
Nicholas J. Fuda, M. Behfar Ardehali, and John T. Lis,
"Defining Mechanisms that regulate RNA polymerase
II transcription in vivo," copyright 2009.; **p. 497, 13.25,**
Based on James D. Watson et al., *Molecular Biology of
the Gene*, 6th edition, 2008. Printed and electronically
reproduced by permission of Pearson Education Inc.,
Upper Saddle River, New Jersey

Chapter 14 p. 514, 14.5, Reprinted by permission from Macmillan Publishers Ltd.: *Nature Reviews
Genetics*, 8, 437–49 © 2007

Application C p. 541, C.1, U.S. Centers for
Disease Control (2013)

Chapter 16 p. 603, 16.8a, Adapted by permission from Macmillan Publishers Ltd.: *Nature* Vol.
408 no. 6814, "The Arabidopsis Genome Initiative,
"Analysis of the genome sequence of the flowering
plant Arabidopsis thaliana," copyright 2000. www.
nature.com.; **p. 603, 16.8b,** Data from "The Genome
Sequence of *Drosophila melanogaster*," Mark D.
Adams, et al., *Science* 287, 2185 (2000), DOI:
10.1126/science.287.5461.2185.; **p. 616, 16.17,**
Adapted/Reprinted from *Current Biology* 9, J. Sharp
et al. "Identification of Sonic hedgehog as a candidate
gene responsible for the polydactylous mouse mutant
Sasquatch," 97–100, copyright 1999, with permission
from Elsevier.; **p. 617, 16.18,** Adapted from Macmillan
Publishers Ltd.: *Nature Reviews Genetics*, 5. Dario
Boffelli, Marcelo A. Nobrega, and Edward M. Rubin
"Comparative genomics at the vertebrate extremes,"
copyright 2004. www.nature.com/nrg/index.html.;
p. 618, 16.20, Adapted by permission from Macmillan
Publishers Ltd.: *Nature* Vol. 408 no. 6814. The Arabidopsis Genome initiative, "Analysis of the genome
sequence of the flowering plant Arabidopsis thaliana,"
copyright 2000. www.nature.com.; **p. 623, 16.23b,**
Adapted by permission from Macmillan Publishers
Ltd.: *Nature* Vol. 403 no. 6770. P. Uetz, L. Giot et al.,
"A comprehensive analysis of protein-protein interactions in saccharomyces cerevisiae," copyright 2000.
www.nature.com.; **p. 624, 16.24,** Adapted by permission from Macmillan Publishers Ltd.: *Nature Reviews
Genetics* Vol 8, no. 6, Charles Boone, Howard Bussey,
and Brenda J. Andrews, "Exploring genetic interactions
and networks with yeast," copyright 2007. www.nature.
com.; **p. 626, 16.26,** Adapted from Amy Hin Yan Tong
et al., "Systematic genetic analysis with ordered arrays
of yeast deletion mutants" *Science* 294, 2364–68,
Fig.3. Reprinted with permission from AAAS and
the author

Chapter 17 p. 640, 17.6, Reprinted from *Bio-
chimica et Biophysica Acta*, 1366, S. DiMauro et al.,
"Mitochondria in neuromuscular disorders," p. 206.
Copyright 1998, with permission from Elsevier, http://
www.sciencedirect.com/science/journal/00052736;
p. 641, 17.7, Based on *Mitochondrial DNA Mutations
in Human Disease*, vol. 6, no. 5, 2005; **p. 647, 17.12a
left,** Reprinted by permission from Macmillan Publishers Ltd.: *Nature Reviews Genetics*, vol. 6, no. 5,
Robert W. Taylor and Doug M. Turnbull, "Mitochondrial DNA mutations in human disease," copyright
2005. http://www.nature.com/nrg/index.html; **p. 647,
17.12a right,** From http://tolweb.org/Jakobida/97407
Copyright © 2000 OGMP (The Organelle Genome
Megasequencing Program), 26/Feb/00: http://megasun.
bch.umontreal.ca/ogmp/. Reproduced by permission;
p. 647, 17.12b, Adapted from *Trends in Genetics*, 19,

G. Burger and M. W. Gray, "Mitochondrial genomes: anything goes," 709–16. Copyright 2003, with permission from Elsevier, http://www.sciencedirect.com/science/journal/01689525; **p. 648, 17.13,** Adapted from *Molecular Cell*, 24, Bonawitz et al., "Initiation and beyond: Multiple functions of the human mitochondrial transcription machinery," p. 814. Copyright 2006, with permission from Elsevier, http://www.sciencedirect.com/science/journal/10972765; **p. 650, 17.15b,** Reprinted from *Trends in Genetics*, 3, K. Umesono and H. Ozeki, "Chloroplast gene organization in plants," p. 281. Copyright 1987, with permission from Elsevier, http://www.sciencedirect.com/science/journal/01689525; **p. 653, 17.17,** Laura A. Katz (2012), "Origin and diversification of eukaryotes." *Annu. Rev. Microbiol.* 66:411–27. Figure 3 on p. 421; doi 10.1146/anurev-micro-090110-102808. Reproduced by permission; **p. 655, 17.19,** Reprinted from *Trends in Genetics*, 19, D. Leister, "Chloroplast research in the genomic age," 47–56. Copyright 2003, with permission from Elsevier, http://www.sciencedirect.com/science/journal/01689525; **p. 658, 17.21,** Based on *Nature Genetics*, 4. R. Toni Prezant et al., "Mitochondrial ribosomal RNA mutation associated with both antibiotic–induced and non-syndromic deafness," copyright 1993. http://www.nature.com/ng/index.html

Chapter 18 **p. 668, 18.5,** Reprinted by permission from Macmillan Publishers Ltd.: *Nature*, 287, Christiane Nusslein-Volhard and Eric Wieschaus, "Mutations affecting segment number and polarity in Drosophila," copyright 1980. Adapted from *Developmental Biology*, 6th ed., Fig. 9.27, p.286. Sunderland: Sinauer Associates, 2000. Used with permission. http://www.nature.com/nature/index.html; **p. 678, 18.13,** Adapted from Macmillan Publishers Ltd.: *Nature*, vol. 399, no. 6738, Renaud de Rosa, Jennifer K. Grenier, Tatiana Andreeva, Charles E. Cook, Andre Adoutte, et al., "Hox gener in brachiopods and priapulids and protostome evolution," copyright 1999. http://www.nature.com/nature/index.html; **p. 683,** François Jacob, "Evolution and tinkering," *Science*, New Series, vol. 196, no. 4295. (Jun. 10, 1977), pp. 1161–66

Chapter 19 **p. 702, 19.4,** Adapted from "Biometrical Genetics" ed. K. Mather, Fig. 2, p. 6. Dover Publications (1949). Used with permission of the publisher; **p. 706, 19.8,** Data is from William Castle (1916) *Genetics and Eugenics*, Harvard University Press; **p. 712, Table 19.3,** Data from R. Plomin et.al, 1994, "The genetic basis of complex human behaviours," *Science* 264: 1733–39.; **p. 716, 19.14,** Adapted from Eyal Fridman et al., "Zooming in on a quantitative trait for tomato yield using interspecific introgressions," *Science* vol. 305, no 5691, p. 1787, Fig 2. Reprinted with permission from AAAS and the author; **p. 718, 19.15,** Data from Paul R. Burton, David G. Clayton, Lon R. Cordon, Nick Craddock, and Panos Deloukas et al., "Genomewide association study of 14000 cases of seven common diseases and 3000 shared controls," *Nature* 447, 2007

Chapter 20 **p. 726,** G. H. Hardy, 1908, "Mendelian proportions in a mixed population," *Science*, N. S., Vol. XXVIII: 49–50, (letter to the editor); **p. 734, 20.5,** Adapted from Scott Freeman and Jon C. Herron, *Evolutionary Analysis*, 4th ed., copyright 2007. Printed and electronically reproduced by permission of Pearson Education Inc., Upper Saddle River, New Jersey; **p. 744,** Charles Darwin, "On the Origin of Species by Means of Natural Selection," 1859; **p. 745, 20.11,** Based on Neil A. Campbell, Jane B. Reece, *Biology*, 8th ed., 2008. Printed and electronically reproduced by permission of Pearson Education Inc., Upper Saddle River, New Jersey; **p. 747, 20.13,** Adapted from Freeman Scott, Jon C. Herron, *Evolutionary Analysis*, 4th ed., copyright 2007. Printed and electronically reproduced by permission of Pearson Education Inc., Upper Saddle River, New Jersey

Application D **p. 762, D.2,** Linda Vigilant, Mark Stoneking, Henry Harpending, Kristen Hawkes, and Allan C. Wilson (1991), "African populations and the evolution of human mitochondrial DNA," *Science*, Vol. 253, 27 September 1991, pp. 1503–7; Fig. 3 on p. 1505. © 1991, reproduced by permission of AAAS and the author; **p. 764, D.3,** Linda Vigilant, Mark Stoneking, Henry Harpending, Kristen Hawkes, and Allan C. Wilson (1991), "African populations and the evolution of human mitochondrial DNA," *Science*, Vol. 253, 27 September 1991, pp. 1503–7, Fig. 3 on p. 1505. Permission conveyed through Copyright Clearance Center, Inc.; **p. 765, D.4,** Jun Z. Li, et al., "Worldwide human relationships inferred from genome-wide patterns of variation," Science, Vol. 319, 22 February 2008, p.1100, www.sciencemag.org; **p. 767, D.8,** Jobbing et al., *Human Evolutionary Genetics*, 2nd ed., 2014, Garland Science

Application E **p. 782, E.1,** Adapted from William S. Klug, *Essentials of Genetics*, 8th ed., ST 2–5, p. 506, 2013

Index

Note: A *b* following a page number indicates a box, an *f* indicates a figure, and a *t* indicates a table. Page numbers in **bold** indicate pages on which key terms are discussed.

1-2 stem loop, 456–457, 457*f*
2-3 stem loop, **456,** 456–459, 457*f*
3-4 stem loop, **456,** 456–459, 457*f*
3′-5′ exonuclease activity, **256**
3′ polyadenylation, **294**
3′ splice site, **298**
3′ untranslated region (3′ UTR), 281, 281*f*, **316**
5′ capping, **294**
5′ splice site, **298**
5′ untranslated region (5′ UTR), 281, 281*f*, **316**
5′-to-3′ exonuclease activity, **255**
5′-to-3′ polymerase activity, **255**
6-4 photoproduct, **413**
-10 consensus sequence, **281,** 281*f*
30-nm fiber, 387*f*, **388**
30S initiation complex, **322**
-35 consensus sequence, **281,** 281*f*
70S initiation complex, **322**
300-nm fiber, **389**

A

A-form DNA, 241, 243, 243*t*
AATD (alpha-1 antitrypsin deficiency), 358
ABO alleles
    dominance relationships, 110–113, 111*f*
    molecular basis of, 111–113
ABO blood group antigens, production of, 112*f*
Ac elements, 429, 429*f*
Acentric chromosome, **375**
Acetylation, histone, 489, 491, 492*f*
Acrocentric chromosome, **364**
Activator binding sites, **441**
Activator proteins, **441,** 442*f*
    eukaryotic, 478–480
Acute lymphoblastic leukemia (ALL), 550
Adaptive evolution, 20
Adaptive mutation hypothesis, **400,** 401*f*
Addition rule, 47
Additive genes, 698–699
    continuous phenotypic variation from multiple, 699, 701, 701*f*, 701*t*
    defined, **698**
Additive variance (V_A), **708**
Adenine (A), **7,** 240–241
    branch point, **298**
Adenosine triphosphate (ATP), 4, 644–645
Adjacent-1 segregation, **383,** 385*f*
Adjacent-2 segregation, 384, 385*f*
Admixed population, **738**
Affordable Care Act (ACA), 232
Aflatoxin B₁, mutagenicity of, 415, 415*f*
AFP (alpha fetoprotein), 356, 356*t*
AGAMOUS gene, 533*b*, 534*f*
Agarose, **15**
Agarose gel electrophoresis, 555, 555*f*, 556*b*, 557, 557*f*
Agouti gene, 117–118, 117*f*–118*f*, 505*b*
Agriculture, transgenic plants in, 573
Agrobacterium tumefaciens, 570–571, 570*f*
    lateral gene transfer, 216, 615
    Ti plasmid, 216
Albinism, 399*f*, 698
Alcohol dehydrogenase (Adh) gene, 734–735, 735*f*
Alkaptonuria, 2–3, 5, 124

Alkylating agents, 411–412, 412*f*
ALL (acute lymphoblastic leukemia), 550
Allele(s), **4,** 20
    ancestral *versus* derived, 766, 766*f*
    determining the number of mutant, 513–514
    dominance relationships and, 106–118
    dominant, **36**
    gain-of-function, 524, 527
    gene drive, 585*b*, 586*f*, 587*b*
    haploinsufficient, **107**
    haplosufficient, **107**
    independent assortment, 42
    lethal, 116–118, 116*f*–118*f*
    loss-of-function, 524
    Mendel's conceptual understanding of, 36
    notational systems for relationships, 109–110
    private, 761
    recessive, **36**
    segregation of, 35*f*, 36–37
    temperature-sensitive, **114,** 116
    that is both dominant and recessive, 118, 118*f*
Allele-counting method, **730**
Allele frequency
    determining autosomal in populations, 729–731
    directional natural selection, 733–735, 734*t*
    equilibrium and equalization, 739
    founder effect, 740
    genetic drift of, 739, 739*f*
    intensity of natural selection and, 734*f*
    quantifying the effects of mutation on, 737
Allele segregation, in quantitative trait production, 701–702
Allelic phase, **168,** 168–169, 169*f*
Allelic series, **113,** 113–116, 114*f*–115*f*
Allis, C. Davis, 489
Allohexaploid, 371
Allolactose, **443,** 444*f*
Allopatric speciation, **746,** 746–747, 747*f*
Allopolyploids, **371,** 373, 373*f*
Allosteric domain, **441**
Allosteric effector compound, **441,** 442*f*
Allostery, **441**
Alpha-1 antitrypsin deficiency (AATD), 358
Alpha fetoprotein (AFP), 356, 356*t*
α-helix (alpha-helix), **317**
α-proteobacteria, 652, 656
Alternative polyadenlylation, **301**
Alternative pre-mRNA splicing, **301,** 301–302, 302*f*, 307*b*–308*b*, 308*f*
Alternative promoters, **301**
Alternative segregation, **383,** 384, 385*f*
Alternative sigma (σ) subunit, **280,** 284, 284*t*, 459–461, **460,** 461*f*
Alu elements, 427, 431
Alzheimer disease, late-onset, 788–789
Ames, Bruce, 413
Ames test, **413,** 413–415, 414*f*–415*f*, 416*b*
Amino acid sequences, phylogenetic tree construction using, 22
Amino acids, **12**
    peptide bond formation, 315, 315*f*
    structure, 315, 316*t*
Aminoacyl site (A site), **318**
Aminoacyl-tRNA synthetases, **333,** 333*f*
Aminoglycosides, 340*b*, 658*b*–659*b*
Amish, Old Order, 740
Amniocentesis, 227, **354,** 354–355, 355*f*

Amorphic mutation, **107,** 108*f*
Anabolic pathways, 123, 124*f*, 189*b*
Anagenesis, **745**
Anaphase, 67*f*, **69,** 71*f*, 73, 74*f*
    anaphase A, 73
    anaphase B, 73
    anaphase I, 76, 78, 79*f*, 81*f*
    anaphase II, 79, 80*f*
Ancestral gene and protein reconstruction, 749–750
Ancient DNA, 24*b*–26*b*, 766–770
Andrews, Anthony, 136*b*
Androgen insensitivity syndrome (AIS), 90*b*
Anencephaly, 228
Aneuploidy, **366**
    in humans, 368–370, 369*t*, 370*t*
Angelman syndrome, 371, 503*b*
Angiogenesis, **542**
Animal cells, cytokinesis in, 73–74, 73*f*
Animal development, *Drosophila* development as paradigm for, 666–679
Animals
    cloning, 584–585, 584*f*
    dosage compensation in, 96, 96*t*
    lethal alleles, 116–118, 117*f*–118*f*
    reproduction in, 75–76
    transgenic, 574–578, 576*f*, 577*f*
Annotation, 214, **602,** 602–606
    bioinformatics, 602–603, 604*b*
    functional gene annotation, 603, 603*f*, 605
    gene families, 605
    interspecific genome comparisons, 605–606
    structural
        computational approaches to, 602–603
        experimental approaches to, 602, 603*f*
    variation in gene organization among species, 605–606, 606*f*
Antennapedia complex, 664, 664*f*, 673, **673,** 673–674, 674*f*
Antibiotic inhibitors of protein synthesis, 340*b*, 340*t*
Antibiotic resistance, evolution of, 217*b*
Antibiotic resistance genes, **191**
Anticodon, 13, 15*f*, 330–331, 330*f*–331*f*, 331*t*
Antifungal compounds, translation blockage by, 340*b*
Antimalarial drug, produced in *E. coli*, 569*b*
Antiparallel strands, DNA, **8,** 241
Antisequestor stem loop, **463,** 463*f*
Antitermination stem loop, **456,** 456–459, 457*f*
Antiterminator, **465**
APC gene, 547–548
Apurinic (AP) site, **409**
Arabidopsis thaliana, development in, 686*f*–687*f*, 687–689
Arber, Werner, 554*b*
Archaea, 2–3
    conjugation in, 203
    origins of replication, 249
    plasmids, 203
    polypeptide elongation in, 324, 324*t*, 327
    promoters, 292–293, 294*f*
    reproduction of, 74–75
    ribosomes, 318–319, 318*f*
    transcription, 292–293
Archaea (domain), **5–6,** 5*f*
Archaeal initiation factor (aIF), **323**
Archaeal translation initiation, 322–324, 324*t*
Argentina, identification of the disappeared in, 786
Argininemia (ARG), 223–224, 351

Argonaute, **500,** 501–502, 501*f*
Armstead, Ian, 56, 404*b*
Artemisinin, 569*b*
Artificial chromosomes, 561
Artificial cross-fertilization, **32,** 33*f*
Artificial selection, narrow sense heritability and, 712–713, 712*t*, 713*f*
ASD (autism spectrum disorders), 711–712, 718*b*–719*b*
Asexual reproduction, 74–75
Aspartame, 350–351, 351*f*
Association, of marker with a disease, 357–358, 358*t*
Aster, **72**
Astrachan, Lazarus, 277
Astral microtubules, **72,** 72*f*
ATM, 420
att site, **211**
Attenuation, **455**
    of the *trp* operon, 456–459, 457*f*, 460*b*
Attenuator region, **455,** 457*f*
Aubry, Sylvain, 56, 404*b*
Australia, human migration and, 771–772
Autism spectrum disorders (ASD), 711–712, 718*b*–719*b*
Autonomously replicating sequences, 250, 252*f*
Autopolyploids, **371,** 373
Autosomal aneuploidy, 369*t*
Autosomal genetic diversity, 763
Autosomal genetic linkage, detecting through test-cross analysis, 150–153, 152*f*
Autosomal inheritance, **52**
    dominant, **52,** 52–53, 53*f*, 53*t*
    Mendel's hereditary principles and, 51–54
    recessive, **53,** 54*f*, 54*t*
        argininemia, 224
Autotetraploid, 371
Auxotrophic strains, **125, 187**
Auxotrophs, **125, 187,** 189*b*–190*b*, 193–194, 193*f*
Avery, Oswald, 4, 238

B

B-form DNA, 241, 243, 243*t*
Bacillus thuringiensis, 573
BACs (bacterial artificial chromosomes), **561**
Bacteria
    chromosome, 3, **188,** 189, 191*f*
    conjugation, 185*f*, 191, **191,** 192*f*–197*f*, 193–198, 196*t*, 198*t*, 199*b*, 200–203, 200*f*–203*f*, 204*b*–205*b*
    culture and growth analysis, 186–188, 187*f*–188*f*
    DNA replication in, 251*f*
    expression of heterologous genes in, 566–570, 567*f*
    features useful to geneticists, 186
    gene expression regulation, 439–470, 441*t*
        antiterminators and repressors in, 464–469
        attenuation, 455–459, 457*f*, 459*f*, 460*b*
        inducible operon system, 443–454
        repressible operon system, 454–459
        riboswitches, 462–464, 463*f*–464*f*
        stress response and, 459–461, 461*f*, 469*b*–470*b*
        transcriptional control, 439*t*, 440–461, 461*t*, 462–463, 463*f*
        translational regulation, 461–462, 463–464, 463*f*
    gene transfer processes, 191, 192*f*, 193
    genetic analysis and mapping in, 185–222
    plasmids in cells of, **189,** 191, 191*f*
    polypeptide elongation in, 324, 325*f*
    polyribosomes in, 328*f*
    reproduction of, 74–75
    ribosomes, 318, 318*f*
    transduction, **191,** 192*f*, 193, 205–211, 208*f*–210*f*, 212*t*
    transformation, **191,** 192*f*, 203, 205, 206*f*
    whole-genome shotgun sequencing of the *Haemophilus influenzae* genome, 597–598, 598*f*
Bacteria (domain), 5–6, 5*f*
Bacteria genome
    alteration by lateral gene transfer, 214–217
    characteristics of, 188–189
    transposable elements in, 426–427
Bacterial artificial chromosomes (BACs), **561**
Bacterial RecBCD pathway, 422
Bacterial transcription
    elongation, 284
    initiation, 281, 282*f*, 284
    process, 279–286, 282*f*
    promoters, 280–281, 281*f*, 283
    RNA polymerase, 280, 280*f*
    termination mechanisms, 284–285, 285*f*, 286*f*
Bacterial translation initiation, 320–322, 321*f*
Bacteriophage(s), **239**
    generalized transducing, **208,** 209
    life cycles, 205–208, 207*f*
    site-specific recombination systems, 578, 578*f*
    specialized transduction, **211**
    structure, 205, 206*f*
    temperate, **207**
    transduction, **191,** 192*f*, 193, 205–211, 208*f*–210*f*, 212*t*
Bacteriophage chromosome mapping by fine-structure analysis, 211, 213–214, 213*f*–215*f*
Bacteriophage λ, 464–469, 466*f*–469*f*
    early gene transcription, 465–466
    genome, 465, 466*f*
    lysogenic cycle, 467*f*, 468, 469
    lytic cycle, 466, 467*f*, 468
    regulation of entry into lytic or lysogenic cycle, 467*f*
    restriction mapping of, 555*f*
Bacteriophage T2, 239
Balanced polymorphism, **735**
Balancer chromosomes, **511,** 511–512, 512*f*
Band shift assay, 288*b*
Barcodes, **624**
Barr, Murray, 96
Barr body, **96,** 496
Basal transcription, **445**
Base excision repair (BER), **417,** 417*f*, 417*t*
Base-pair substitution mutations, **401,** 401–402, 402*f*
Base stacking, **241**
Basic biological research, 554*b*
Bateson, William, 3, 132, 149–150
Baur, Erwin, 632–635
Bayes, Thomas, 229
Bayesian analysis, **229,** 230–231, 231*t*
BCR gene, 544
Beachy, Philip, 691
Beadle, George, 124–125, 125*b*, 314, 775
Belling, John, 366
Benign tumors, **541**
Benzer, Seymour, 211, 213–214, 377, 511
Berg, Paul, 554*b*
β-globin complex, locus control region of, 481
β-globin gene, 22, 23*f*
    mutations, 401–402, 401*f*
    promoter, 290, 291*f*
β-interferon gene, 482, 482*f*
β-pleated sheet (beta-pleated sheet), **317**
Beyer, Peter, 573
Bhattacharyya, Madan, 56
Bicoid gene, 670, 670*f*, 671*f*
Bidirectional DNA replication, **247,** 247–248, 248*f*, 249*f*
Binary fission, **186**
Binomial expansion formula, 48
Binomial probability, **48,** 48–49, 49*f*
    application to progeny phenotypes, 48–49, 49*f*
Bioinformatics, **602,** 602–603, 604*b*
Biological species concept (BSC), **743,** 743–744
Biparental inheritance, 633, 641–642, 644, 644*f*
Bison, genetic analysis of, 639*b*
Bithorax complex, **673,** 674–675, 674*f*, 677*b*
Bithorax genes, 664, 664*f*
Blackburn, Elizabeth, 259
Blakeslee, Albert Francis, 366
BLAST (Basic Local Alignment Search Tool), 608, 610*b*
Blastoderm
    cellular, 667
    syncytial, 667
Blending theory of heredity, **32,** 36
Blobel, Günter, 334
Blood proteins, testing for genetic carriers, 353
Bloom syndrome, 269*b*–270*b*
Blots, 17
Blue *versus* white screening, 560, 560*f*
Blunt ends, **554**
Bonacum, James, 747
Boveri, Theodor, 2–3, 80, 83, 236
Branch point adenine, **298**
BRCA1 (breast cancer 1) gene, 171, 171*b*, 233, 419, 548, 548*t*
BRCA2 (breast cancer 2) gene, 233, 548, 548*t*
Breast cancer, 233, 548–549, 548*t*
Brenner, Sydney, 277–278, 615, 679, 682
Bridges, Calvin, 87, 87*f*, 89, 145, 366
Broad sense heritability (H^2), **709,** 710, 711*t*
Brock, Louise, 262
Brock, Thomas, 262
Brown, Robert, 2
Bt toxins, 573
Burkitt's lymphoma, 544–545, 544*f*

C

C-gene system for mammalian coat color, 113–116, 114*f*–115*f*
    molecular basis of, 114, 116
c-MYC gene, 545
C-to-U RNA editing, 650, 651*f*
CAAT box, **287**
Caenorhabditis elegans, development in, 679–683, 679*f*–682*f*
CAG repeat, 348–349, 349*f*, 350*f*
CAH (congenital adrenal hyperplasia), 90*b*
Calcitonin/calcitonin gene-related peptide (CT/CGRP) gene, 301
Calico coat pattern, 96, 97*f*
Cancer, 538–550. *See also specific cancers*
    epigenetics, 549–550
    familial or hereditary, **543**
    genetic basis of, 543–549
    genome sequencing, 549
    hallmarks of cancer cells and malignant tumors, 541–543
    incidence, 539, 540*t*
    predisposition, 548, 548*t*
    progression of abnormalities, 540–541, 541*f*
    as somatic genetic disease, 540
    targeted therapy, 550
Cancer Genome Atlas (TCGA), 549
CAP binding site, **444,** 445*f*
CAP-cAMP binding region, **445,** 445*f*, 446*f*
CAP-cAMP complex, **446,** 446*f*
Capecchi, Mario, 576
Capillary gel electrophoresis, 781–782
Capping 5′ pre-mRNA, 294–295, 295*f*
CARD15 gene, 174, 174*f*
Carrier genetic screening, **348,** 353–354
Carriers
    genetic testing to identify, 226–227, **348,** 353–354
    obligate, 230–231

Carter, Jimmy, 538–539
Cas endonuclease, 519
Case study
    ancient DNA, 24b–26b
    antibiotics and translation interference, 340b
    complementation groups in a human cancer-
            prone disorder, 136b–137b, 137f
    cyclopia and polydactyly, 690b–691b, 690f
    degenerative evolution of the mammalian
            Y chromosome, 97b–98b, 98f
    DNA helicase gene mutations and human
            progeroid syndrome, 269b–270b, 269t
    environmental epigenetics, 502b–503b
    gene drive alleles can rapidly spread through
            populations, 585b–587b, 586f
    genetics of autism spectrum disorders, 718b–719b
    genomic analysis of insect guts, 627b
    human chromosome evolution, 392b–393b, 392f
    Mendel's peas are shaped by transposition,
            431b–432b
    OMIM, gene mutations, and human hereditary
            disease, 57–59
    ototoxic deafness, 658b–659b, 658f
    reverse genetics and genetic redundancy in
            flower development, 532b, 534f
    sexy splicing, 37b–308b, 308f
    sickle cell disease evolution and natural selection
            in humans, 750b–751b, 751f
    Vibrio cholerae, 469b–470b
Castle, William, 726
Catabolic pathways, 123–124, 124f, 189b
Catabolite repression, **446**
Cavalli-Sforza, Luigi Luca, 196
Cavener, Douglas, 734
cDNA library. See Complementary DNA (cDNA)
            libraries
Cech, Thomas, 302, 304
Celiac disease, 789
Cell cycle, **68**, 68–69, 69f
    in germ-line cells, 76
Cell cycle checkpoints, **74**, 75f
Cell death
    during development, 682–683
    resistance to, 542
Cell differentiation, 665
Cell division. See also Meiosis; Mitosis
    chromosome heredity and, 67–104
    completion of, 73–74
    in somatic cells, 68–74
Cell fate, cellular interactions specifying, 679–683,
            679f–682f
Cell plate, 73f
Cell theory, 2–3
Cellular blastoderm, **667**
Centers for Disease Control, 539
CentiMorgan (cM), **156**
Central dogma of biology, **11**, 12f, 235, 276
Centromere, **70**, 71
Centrosomes, **72**, 72f
CFTR (cystic fibrosis transmembrane conductance
            regulator), 58, 175b–176b
CGH (congenital generalized hypertrichosis), 92–93,
            92t, 94f
Chalfie, Martin, 530
Chargaff, Erwin, 7
Charged tRNAs, **320**
Chase, Martha, 239–240, 239f
Chemical mutagens, 410–412, 411f–412f, 411t
Chi-square analysis, 49–51
    of genetic linkage data, 156
    of Mendel's data, 50–51, 52t
Chi-square statistic, 147
Chi-square table, 51t
Chi-square (χ^2) test, **50**
    of Hardy-Weinberg predictions, 731–732

Chiasmata (chiasma), **77**, 78f
Chiba, Yasutane, 634
Chilton, Mary-Dell, 570
Chimeric gene, **532**
Chimpanzee genomes, human genome compared,
            765–766
ChIP (chromatin immunoprecipitation), 488
ChIP-seq, 619, 620f
Chlamydomonas, 632f
Chlamydomonas reinhardii, mating type and chloro-
            plast segregation in, 640–641, 642f
Chloroplast(s), **4, 632**
    endosymbiosis theory, 651–657, 653f–655f
    evolution of, 4
    genome structure and gene content, 648–649,
            650f
    maternal inheritance of, 632–634, 634f
    nuclear plastid sequences (NUPTS), **654**, 655
    RNA editing, 650–651, 651f
    segregation in Chlamydomonas, 640–641, 642f
    as sites of photosynthesis, 648–651
    structure and function, 648, 649f
Cholera, 469b–470b
Chorionic villus sampling (CVS), 227–228, **355**, 355f
Chromatids
    nonsister, 76, **77**
    sister, **69**, 71, 72–73, 74, 76, 79
Chromatin, 287, **291**, 292, 362, 476–477
    chemical modifications of, 488–493
    closed, **487**
    compaction, 386
    euchromatin, **292, 365**, 366
    eukaryotic chromosome organization and,
            385–391
    heterochromatin, **292, 366**
    higher-order organization, 389
    nucleosome-based model of, 388
    open, **487**
    position effect variegation (PEV), 485–486,
            485f, 496
    stabilization of cellular memory by architecture
            of, 678–679
    writers, erasers, and readers, 489, 491f
Chromatin-based regulation of RNA Pol II transcrip-
            tion, 291–292
Chromatin immunoprecipitation (ChIP), 488, 619
Chromatin modifiers, 486, **488**, 489
Chromatin remodeling, 484–498, **487**
    chemical modification, 488–493
    DNase I hypersensitivity sites, 487–488, 487f
    epigenetic heritability and, 494–496
    histone modification, 489, 491–492, 491f–492f
    mechanisms of, 487
    open and closed promoters, 486–487, 487f
    overview of, 486
Chromatin remodels, 486, **498**
Chromosomal heredity
    cell division and, 67–104
    disease and, 225–226
Chromosome(s), 2, **3**
    acentric, **375**
    acrocentric, **364**
    artificial, 561
    bacterial, **188**, 189, 191f
    balancer, **511**, 511–512, 512f
    CIB, 382b–383b
    condensation, 76–78, 386, 387f, 477
    dicentric, **381**
    DNA in, 236
    DNA replication at the ends of linear, 257–259,
            260f
    eukaryotic organization of, 385–391
    evolution of human, 392b–393b, 392f
    gene order on, 159–160
    genetic linkage and mapping, 145–184

homologous, 3
    meaning and usage of term, 71
    metacentric, **363**
    movement and distribution, 72–73
    nondisjunction, 87, 87f, 366, 367f
    nonrecombinant, **146**
    parental, **146**, 157–160
    recombinant, **146**
    sex determination and, 87, 89–91, 89f, 91f
    shape, 364f
    submetacentric, **363**
    telocentric, **364**
Chromosome arms, **363**
Chromosome banding, **364**, 364–365, 365f
Chromosome break point, **375**
Chromosome breakage
    inversion and translocation of chromosomes,
            378–384
    mutation by loss, gain, and rearrangement of
            chromosomes, 375–378
Chromosome deletion, partial, 375
Chromosome fusion, **383**
Chromosome inversion, **378**, 380–381, 380f, 383
Chromosome number, 362
    aberrations of, 225–226
    aneuploidy, 366, 368–370, 369t, 370t
    nondisjunction and, 366
    polyploidy, 371–375
    in selected animal species, 362t
Chromosome scaffold, **389**, 389f
Chromosome segregation
    adjacent-1, **383**, 385f
    adjacent-2, 384, 385f
    alternative, **383**, 384, 385f
Chromosome structure, higher order chromatin organi-
            zation and, 389, 389f
Chromosome territory, **362**, 362–363, 363f
Chromosome theory of heredity, **68**, 145–146
    testing of, 86–87
Chromosome translocations, 361f, **378**, 383–384,
            384f–385f
Chromosome trisomy, 225
Chromosome visualization, 363–364, 363f–364f
Chronic myelogenous leukemia (CML), 544, 544f, 550
Chronic obstructive pulmonary disease (COPD), 358
CIB chromosome, 382b–383b
Cis-acting mutations, **448**
Cis-acting regulatory sequences, 478–484, **479**
Cis-dominant, **450**
Clades, **21**, 22, 22f
Cladistic approach to phylogenetic tree construction, **21**
Cladogenesis, **746**
Cleavage furrow, 73, 73f
Clegg, Michael, 734
Clinton, Bill, 599
Clone-by-clone sequencing, **596**
Cloning, 516
    directional, **558**, 558–559, 558f
    genes by complementation, 516–517, 517f
    molecular, 557–561, 558f–561f
    of plants and animals, 583–585
    subcloning, 555
Cloning vector, **516**
Closed chromatin, **487**
Closed promoter complex, **281**
CML (chronic myelogenous leukemia), 544, 544f,
            550, 619
CNS (conserved noncoding sequences), **615**, 615–616,
            616f, 766, 767f
Co-option
    defined, **683**
    evolution through, 683–685
Co-suppression, 476f
Coat colors in Labrador retrievers, 105f, 131b, 133
Coding region, **279**

Coding strand, **12**, 12*f*, 13*f*, 15*f*, **279**
CODIS (Combined DNA Index System), 780–784, 781*t*, 782*f*–783*f*, 784*t*
Codominance, **110**
Codominant inheritance of a VNTR, 167, 167*f*
Codon bias, **566**, 566*t*
Codons
    genetic code, 13
    synonymous, **329**, 329–330
    third-base wobble, 305
Coefficient of coincidence, **161**
Coefficient of inbreeding, **742**, 742–743, 742*f*, 744*b*
Coffin-Lowry syndrome, 426
Cohesin, 73, 73*f*, 77, 81*f*
Cohesive compatible ends, **557**
Cohesive (*cos*) ends, **465**
Collins, Francis, 176*b*, 599
Colony, bacterial, **186**
Color blindness, 92, 92*t*, 93*f*
Colorectal cancer, 547
Combinatorial homeotic activity, 686–689
Combined DNA Index System (CODIS), 780–784, 781*t*, 782*f*–783*f*, 784*t*
Combined Paternity Index (CPI), **785**
Community-based carrier testing, 226–227
Comparative genomics. *See* Evolutionary genomics
Complementary base pairing, 330, 330*f*
Complementary base pairs, **7**, 8–9, 9*f*, 241, 242*f*, 243–244
Complementary DNA (cDNA) libraries, **516**, 517, **562**, 563–564, 563*f*–564*f*
Complementary gene interaction (9:7 ratio), 129*f*, 130*b*, **132**
Complementation
    cloning genes by, 516–517, 517*f*
    genetic, 132
    genetic complementation analysis, 213, 213*f*
Complementation analysis, 133–136, **135**, 135*f*, 136*b*–137*b*
    lac operon, 447–448
Complementation group, **135**, 135–136, 136*b*–137*b*, 137*f*
Complementation tests, 513
Complete medium, **187**
Complete penetrance, **119**
Composite transposons, **427**, 427*f*
Compound heterozygosity, 353
Concordance, **711**
Condensation, chromosome, 477
Conditional alleles, 512–513, 513*f*
Conditional probability, **47**, **229**, 230–231
Congenital adrenal hyperplasia (CAH), 90*b*
Congenital generalized hypertrichosis (CGH), 92–93, 92*t*, 94*f*
Conjugation, archaea, 203
Conjugation, bacterial, 185*f*, **191**, 192*f*
    consolidation of Hfr maps, 200–201, 202*f*
    definition, 191
    F factor transfer, 194–196, 195*f*
    with F' strains producing partial diploids, 201–203, 203*f*
    Hfr gene transfer, 196–198, 196*f*–197*f*, 198*t*
    identification of, 193–194, 193*f*
    interrupted mating, **198**, 199*b*
    outcomes of, 196*t*
    time-of-entry mating, **198**, 200*f*
Conjugation pilus, **194**, **195**
Consanguineous mating, **741**
Consensus sequences, **249**
Conservation genetics, **743**
Conservative DNA replication, **245**
Conserved coding sequences, 615
Conserved noncoding sequences (CNS), **615**, 615–616, 616*f*, 766, 767*f*
Constitutive heterochromatin, **484**, 491*f*, 501–502

Constitutive mutants, **448**, 450
Constitutive repressor protein mutations, 450
Constitutive transcription, **440**
Consultands, 227
Contiguous sequence (contig), **595**
Continuous (phenotypic) variation, **697**
    from multiple additive genes, 699, 701, 701*f*
Contractile ring, 73, 74*f*
Controlled crosses, **33**, 34*f*
Convergent evolution, **773**
Coordinate genes, **668**, 668*f*, 669–670, 671*f*, 672*f*
Copia elements, 431
Copy number
    of genes, 225
    plasmid, 191
Copy-number variants (CNVs), **600**, 601*f*, 719*b*
    in humans, 761
Core DNA, **388**
Core element, promoter, 292
Core promoter region, 481
Corepressor, **441**, 441*f*
Corn, genetics of bicolor, 41*b*
Corolla length in tobacco, 701–702, 702*f*
Correns, Carl, 3, 632–634
Cosuppression, **499**
Cotransduction, **209**
Cotransduction frequency, **209**
Cotransduction mapping, **209**, 209–211, 210*f*, 210*t*, 212*t*
Cotransformation, **205**
Covered promoters, **487**, 487*f*
CpG dinucleotides, **498**
CpG islands, **498**
CPI (Combined Paternity Index), **785**
Cre-*lox* recombination system, 578–579, 578*f*
Creighton, Harriet, 153, 155
Cremer, Christoph, 362
Cremer, Thomas, 362
Cri-du-chat syndrome, 225
Crick, Francis, 4, 6–7, 8*f*, 9, 11, 12*f*, 240, 241, 245, 331
CRISPR-*cas* system, **519**, 519–522, 520*f*–521*f*
    applications of, 521–522
    structure and mechanisms in microbes, 520*f*
CRISPR-Cas9-mediated genome editing, 576, 581–583, 582*f*, 585*b*, 586*f*, 587*b*
Cro protein, 465–466, 468
Crohn's disease, 717–718, 718*f*
Cross-fertilization, artificial, **32**, 33*f*
Cross-pollination, 33
Crosses
    controlled, **33**, 34*f*
    dihybrid, **40**
    monohybrid, 34–40
    reciprocal, **34**
    replicate, **34**
    test, **34**
    trihybrid, **45**
Crossing over, 76, **77**, 78–79, 146–147
    biological factors affecting, 164–165, 165*f*
    identifying parental, single-crossover, and double-crossover gametes in three-point mapping, 157–158, 157*f*
    interference, 160–161
    in inversion loop, 380–381, 380*f*–381*f*, 383
    Morgan's hypothesis, 152*f*
    sex affect on rate, 164, 165*f*
Crossover
    double, 523, 523*f*
    gene duplication by unequal, 610, 611*f*
    single, 523, 523*f*
    unequal, 376–377, 376*f*
Crossover suppression, **381**
crRNAs, **520**, 520*f*, 521*f*
Cryo-electron microscopy (cryo-EM), 320
Cryptic splice sites, **404**, 405*f*

Cuenot, Lucien, 116, 118
CVS (chorionic villus sampling), 227–228, **355**, 355*f*
Cyanobacteria, **653**
Cyclopia, 690*b*–691*b*, 690*f*
Cystic fibrosis, 232
    genetic testing for, 353–354
    mapping the gene for, 175*b*–176*b*, 176*t*
Cystic fibrosis transmembrane conductance regulator (CFTR), 58, 175*b*–176*b*
Cytokinesis, **70**, 71*f*, 73–74, 74*f*, 78, 79, 79*f*, 80*f*
Cytological evidence of recombination, 153, 153*f*, 155
Cytoplasmic inheritance, **4**
Cytoplasmic male sterility in flowering plants, 651*b*–652*b*
Cytosine (C), **7**, 240–241

D

Dalgarno, Lynn, 322
Damage repair, DNA. *See* DNA damage repair
Darwin, Charles, 2, 19–22, 30, 725*f*, 744–745, 775
Darwin's finches, evolution of, 748
Daughter cells, **68**
Daughter strand, **9**, 11*f*
Davis, Bernard, 193–194, 193*f*
Dawkins, Richard, 189
Dawson, Martin, 238
De novo derivation of genes, 611, 611*f*
de Vries, Hugo, 3, 46
Deacetylation, histone, 491, 492*f*
Deafness, ototoxic, 658*b*–659*b*
Deaminating agents, 411, 412*f*
Deamination, **409**, 409–410, 410*f*
Dedifferentiated cells, **540**
Degrees of freedom (*df*), **50**, 707
Delayed age of onset, **118**, 119*f*
Delayed early genes, phage λ, **465**
Delbrück, Max, 400, 401*f*
Deletion, of nucleotide repeats, 405–406
Deletion, partial chromosome
    detecting, 377
    interstitial, **375**, 375–376, 376*f*
    mapping, 377–378, 378*f*
    microdeletion, **377**
    terminal, **375**, 375*f*
    unequal crossover and, 376–377, 376*f*
Deletion mapping, 213, **214**, 215*f*, **377**, 377–378, 378*f*
Denaturation, step in PCR, 261, 261*f*
Denisovans, 18, 25*b*–26*b*, 768*f*, 769–770, 769*f*
Deoxynucleotide monophosphates (dNMPs), 240*f*, **241**
Deoxynucleotide triphosphates (dNTPs), **241**
Deoxyribonucleic acid. *See* DNA
Deoxyribose, 240
Depurination, **409**, 409*f*
Development
    as building of a multicellular organism, 664–666, 664*f*–666*f*
    cell death during, 682–683
    Drosophila, 666–679
    in plants, 685–689, 686*f*–688*f*
Developmental genes, facultative heterochromatin and, 494, 495*f*
Developmental genetics, 663–691
Developmental pathways, 124
Diagnostic test, 356
Diakinesis, 76–77, 79*f*, 81*f*
Dicentric bridge, **381**
Dicentric chromosome, **381**
Dicer, **499**, 500–502, 500*f*–501*f*
Dichotomous traits, 31, 32*f*
Dideoxynucleotide (dideoxy) DNA sequencing, 260–261, **263**, 265–266, 265*f*, 267
Dideoxynucleotide triphosphate (ddNTP), **263**, 265
Differential reproductive fitness, **733**
Differentiated cells, **665**
Differentiation mechanisms, 665–666, 666*f*

Digestive microbiome, 601*b*
Digits
    development of, 683, 684*f*
    polydactyly, 690*b*–691*b*, 690*f*
Dihybrid-cross analysis of two genes, 40–43, 40*f*–42*f*
Dihybrid crosses, **40**
Dihydrotestosterone, 90*b*
Dinosaurs, 22
Diploid, **4**, 75
Diploid number, **68**, 362
Diploid species, 362
Diplotene, 76–77, 78*f*, 81*f*
Direct repeats, 425, 425*f*
Direct-to-consumer genetic testing, **348**, 357–359, 358*t*
Directional cloning, **558**, 558–559, 558*f*
Directional natural selection (directional selection), **713**, 734*t*
Discontinuous variation, **697**
Discordance, **711**
Disease-causing genes, 58–59
    linked to genetic markers, 167–168
Disjunction, **73**
Disomy, uniparental, 371
Dispersed repetitive DNA, 606
Dispersive DNA replication, **245**
Displacement (D) loop, **421**, 423*f*
Disruptive selection, **713**
DNA (deoxyribonucleic acid), **6**. *See also* Mitochondrial DNA (mtDNA)
    alignment of DNA, mRNA, and polypeptide, 316*f*
    altering and synthesizing molecules, advances in, 564–565
    ancient, 24*b*–26*b*, 766–770
    in central dogma of biology, 11, 12*f*
    in chromosomes, 236
    core, 387*f*, **388**
    as hereditary molecule, 2, 4, 6, 19, 236–240
    heteroduplex, **422**, 424
    linker, 387*f*, **388**
    stains, 16–17, 17*f*
    transfer DNA (T-DNA), 570–571, 570*f*, 572*f*
    as transformation factor, 238, 238*f*
DNA analysis for genealogy, genetic ancestry, and genetic health risk assessment, 786–789
DNA-binding domain, **441**
DNA-binding proteins, regulatory, 441–443, 442*f*
DNA clones, **557**
DNA damage, radiation-induced, 412–413, 413*f*
DNA damage repair, 415–420
    base excision repair, **417**, 417*f*, 417*t*
    direct, 415, 417–419, 417*f*–418*f*, 417*t*
    double-strand breaks, 420–421, 421*f*
    mismatch repair, 417*t*, **418**, 418–419, 419*f*
    nucleotide excision repair, **417**, 417–418, 417*t*, 418*f*
    photoreactive repair, 415, **417**, 417*t*
    signaling systems for, 419–420
    ultraviolet (UV) repair, **417**
DNA double helix, **6**
    A-form, B-form, Z-form, 241, 243, 243*f*, 243*t*
    complementary and antiparallel strands in, 240–244
DNA duplex, **6**, 240, 241, 243–244
DNA fingerprinting, **779**
DNA footprint protection, 288*b*–289*b*
DNA gel electrophoresis, 15–17, 17*f*
DNA helicase, gene mutations and, 269*b*–270*b*, 269*t*
DNA Identification Act, 780
DNA intercalating agents, **412**, 413*f*
DNA isolation, 10*b*–11*b*
DNA library, **562**
    cDNA, constructing, 563–564, 563*f*–564*f*
    expression library, 564

genomic, constructing, 562–563, 562*f*
    uses of, 564
DNA ligase, **255**
DNA loop, **454**
DNA methyltransferase, 543, 550
DNA microarrays, **619**
DNA nucleotides, **7**, 7–8, 8*t*, 9*f*, 240–241, 240*f*
DNA polymerase
    processivity of, 255
    proofreading abilities, 256–257, 257*f*
    properties of, 256*t*
    translesion, **420**
DNA polymerase I (DNA pol I), **254**, 255–256, 256*t*
DNA polymerase II (DNA pol III), **254**, 255–256, 256*t*
DNA profiling, **779**
DNA proofreading, **256**, 256–257, 257*f*
DNA replication, **6**, 9
    in bacteria, 251*f*
    bacteriophage, 205–206
    bidirectional, **247**, 247–248, 248*f*, 249*f*
    conservative, **245**
    continuous strand, 253–254
    discontinuous strand, 253–254
    dispersive, **245**
    at ends of linear chromosomes, 257–259, 260*f*
    initiation of, 253, 253*f*
    Meselson-Stahl experiment on, 245–247, 246*f*
    models of, 245, 245*f*
    molecular genetic analytic methods using processes of, 260–268
    nucleosome disassembly, synthesis, and reassembly during, 389–390
    nucleosome inheritance after, 390*f*
    Okazaki fragment ligation, 254–255, 255*f*
    origins of replication, **247**, 247–249, 248*f*
        DNA sequences at, 249–250, 252, 252*f*, 252*t*
        multiple in eukaryotes, 248–249, 250*f*
    precisely duplicating genetic material, 249–260
    RNA primer removal, 254–255, 255*f*
    in S phase of mitosis, 69, 80, 248–249
    semiconservative, **245**
    shared attributes in all organisms, 244–245
    spontaneous errors, 405–408, 408*f*–409*f*, 408*t*
    strand elongation, 242*f*
DNA sequence polymorphisms. *See* Genetic markers
DNA sequences
    manipulation in vivo, 578–579
    phylogenetic tree construction using, 22, 23*f*
    at replication origins, 249–250, 252, 252*f*, 252*t*
DNA sequencing, 18. *See also* Whole-genome shotgun (WGS) sequencing
    ancient DNA, 25*b*–26*b*
    clone-by-clone, 596
    dideoxynucleotide, 260–261, **263**, 264*f*, 265–266, 265*f*, 267
    genome sequencing, 18
    of Huntington disease gene, 349–350, 349*f*
    next-generation, **266**, 268*f*
    paired-end, 596–599, 597*f*–599*f*
    third-generation sequencing, **266**
DNA strand elongation, 242*f*
DNA structure, 6–9, 9*f*
    A-form, B-form, Z-form, 241, 243, 243*f*, 243*t*
    complementary and antiparallel strands in, 240–244
    discovery of, 6–7, 7*f*
    nucleotides, 7–8, 8*t*, 240–241, 240*f*
    supercoiling, **257**, 258*f*
    table-top model, 7, 8*f*
DNA synthesis
    of leading and lagging strands at the replication fork, 255–256
    translesion, 420

DNA topoisomerases, **257**, 258*f*
DNA transposons, **425**, 425–427, 425*f*
DnaA, DnaB, DnaC proteins, 253, 253*f*
DNase I, 388
DNase I footprint protection analysis, 453*b*
DNase I hypersensitive sites, **487**, 487–488, 490*b*
Dobzhansky, Theodosius, 21, 725
Doebley, John, 775
Dolly, 584–585, 584*f*
Domains of life, 5–6, 5*f*
Domestication of plants and animals, 775
Dominance
    Agouti (A^Y) allele, 117–118, 117*f*
    codominance, **110**
    incomplete (partial), **110**, 110*f*
    molecular basis of, 106–107
    pseudodominance, **377**, 379*b*
Dominance relationships
    of ABO alleles, 110–113, 111*f*
    allele interactions producing, 106–118
    in allelic series, 113–116, 114*f*–115*f*
Dominance variance (V_D), **708**
Dominant allele, **36**
Dominant epistasis (12:3:1 ratio), 129*f*, 131*b*, **133**
Dominant gene interaction (9:6:1 ratio), 129*f*, 130*b*, **132**, 132–133
Dominant mutation
    identification of, 510–511, 511*f*, 513
    negative, 108*f*, **109**
Dominant phenotype, **35**
Dominant suppression (13:3 ratio), 129*f*, 131*b*, **133**
Donor, **191**
Doppler, Christian, 31–32
Dosage compensation, **96**
Double crossovers, 151–161, 157*t*, **159**, 523, 523*f*
Double Holliday junctions (DHJs), **424**, 424*f*
Double recombinants, **159**
Double-strand break repair, **420**, 420–421, 421*f*
Double-strand breaks (DSBs), **420**
Double-stranded RNA, gene silencing by, 499–501, 500*f*–501*f*
Down syndrome, 225, 228–229, 356, 370, 370*t*, 372*b*
Down syndrome critical region (DSCR), 370
Downstream, **280**
Drosha enzyme complex, **499**
Drosophila CIB chromosome method, 382*b*–383*b*
Drosophila melanogaster
    complete genetic linkage in males, 147
    Copia elements, 431
    crossover frequency in females, 164
    development, 666–679
        Hox genes, 673–678, 674*f*–676*f*, 677*b*, 678*f*
        overview, 666–667, 667*f*
        stabilization of cellular memory by chromatin, 678–679
        toolkit, 667–669
    diversification of *Drosophila* species on the Hawaiian Islands, 746–747, 747*f*
    DNA replication origins in, 248, 250*f*
    genetic complementation analysis of eye color, 135–136, 136*f*
    genetic linkage and, 150–153, 151*f*–152*f*
    genetic linkage mapping, 155–156, 155*t*, 156*f*
    juvenile hormone, 122
    Morgan's work with, 83, 85–86
    P element, 429–430, 430*f*, 574–575, 575*f*
    Polycomb group and Trithorax group genes, 492, 494, 495*f*
    position effect variegation (PEV), 390–391, 391*f*, 485–486, 485*f*, 496
    sex determination, 87, 89, 275*f*, 307*b*–308*b*, 308*f*
    whole-genome shotgun sequencing of the genome, 598–599, 599*f*
    X-linked inheritance, 85–86, 85*f*–86*f*, 88

Ds elements, 429, 429*f*
DSBs (double-strand breaks), **420**
Dubochet, Jacques, 320
Duchenne muscular dystrophy (DMD), 583, 583*f*
Duplicate gene action (15:1 ratio), 129*f*, 130*b*, **132**
Duplication
    detecting, 377
    microduplications, 377, 377*f*
    partial, 376
    whole-genome, 618, 618*f*
Dysplasia, **541**, 541*f*
dystrophin (DYS) gene, **400**

E

E(var) mutations, **485**, 485*f*
Early operators, phage λ, **465**
Early promoters, phage λ, **465**
East, Edward, 701–702
*Eco*RI, 553–554, 557
Edward syndrome, 228
Eiberg, Hans, 175*b*
Electrophoresis
    agarose gel, 555, 555*f*, 556*b*, 557, 557*f*
    capillary gel, 781–782
Electrophoretic analysis, in forensic genetic analysis,
        781–782, 782*f*
Electrophoretic mobility, **15**, 15–17
Elephant seal, 741
Ellis-van Creveld syndrome, 740
Elongation
    in bacterial transcription, 284
    translation, 324, 324*t*, 325*f*, 327
Elongation factor (EF), **324**, 324*t*, 327
Embryonic axes, 665, 665*f*
Embryonic stem (ES) cells, **665**
    somatic gene therapy using, 579
    transformation of, 578
Emerson, Rollins, 158
EMS (ethyl methyanesulfonate), 510, 511
Endosymbiont, **652**
Endosymbiosis, **651**
    secondary and tertiary, 656–657
Endosymbiosis theory, **651**, 651–657, 653*f*–655*f*
Energy metabolism, reprogramming of, 542
Enhanceosome, **480**
Enhancer screen, **514**
Enhancer sequences (enhancers), **291**, 292*f*, **479**,
        480–484, 480*f*, 482*f*, 484*f*
Enhancer trapping, **531**, 531*f*
Environment
    gene-environment interactions, **121**, 121–122,
        658*b*–659*b*, 658*f*, 702, 704, 704*f*
    phenotypic variation, effects on, 702, 704, 704*f*
Environmental epigenetics, 502*b*–503*b*
Environmental variance, 704, 707, **708**
Ephrussi, Boris, 642
Epigenetic irregularities in cancer, 549–550
Epigenetic modification, important features of, 486
Epigenetics, **292**, **495**
    environmental, 502*b*–503*b*
    epigenetic heritability, 494–496
    genomic imprinting, 497–498
    nucleotide methylation, 498
Epistasis, **129**
    dominant, 129*f*, 131*b*, **133**
    recessive, 129*f*, 131*b*, **133**
Epistatic (gene) interactions, **129**, 129–133, 130*b*–131*b*
    complementary (9:7 ratio), 129*f*, 130*b*, **132**
    dominant (9:6:1 ratio), 129*f*, 130*b*, **132**
    dominant epistasis (12:3:1 ratio), 129*f*, 131*b*, **133**
    dominant suppression (13:3 ratio), 129*f*, 131*b*,
        133
    duplicate (15:1 ratio), 129*f*, 130*b*, **132**
    no interaction (9:3:3:1 ratio), 129, 129*f*, 132
    recessive epistasis (9:3:4 ratio), 129*f*, 131*b*, 133

Epistatic ratios, in the F₂ generation of dihybrid
        crosses, 130*b*–131*b*
Equus, evolution of the genus, 745, 745*f*
Erasers, chromatin, 489, 491*f*
Escherichia coli
    expression vector, 565–566, 565*f*
    genome characteristics, 188
    lac operon, 443–454
    lambda phage infection of, 464–469
    mismatch repair in, 418–419, 419*f*
    origin of replication, 249, 252*f*, 252*t*, 253, 253*f*
    pathogenicity islands, 217
    plant-derived antimalarial drugs produced in,
        569*b*
    production of human insulin, 566–568, 567*f*
    ribosomes, 318, 318*f*
    SOS system, 420
Estriol (uE3), 356, 356*t*
Ethical, Legal, and Social Implications, 232
Ethical issues
    genetic counseling and, 232–233
    in genetic medicine, 231–232
Ethidium bromide (EtBr), **16**, 16–17, 17*f*
Ethyl methyanesulfonate (EMS), 510, 511
Euchromatic regions, 365
Euchromatin, **292**, 365
Eukarya (domain), **5**–6, 5*f*
Eukaryotes
    cell cycle, 69, 69*f*
    gene expression, regulation of, 476–503
    mitochondria as sites of ATP production,
        644–645
    multiple replication origins in, 248–249, 250*f*
    polymerase II transcription of mRNA in eukary-
        otes, 287
    polypeptide elongation in, 324, 324*t*, 327
    reproduction in, 75–76
    ribosomes, 318, 318*f*
Eukaryotic chromosomes, organization into chromatin,
        385–391
Eukaryotic expression vectors, **566**
Eukaryotic genomes, transposable elements in, 427
Eukaryotic initiation factor (eIF), **322**
Eukaryotic transcription, 286–294
Eukaryotic translation initiation, 322, 323*f*
Euploid, **366**
Europe, human migration and, 770–771
Evans, Martin, 576
even-skipped (eve) gene, 530*f*, 531, 671–673, 672*f*
Evo-devo, **683**
Evolution, **19**
    adaptive, 20
    of antibiotic resistance, 217*b*
    of chloroplasts, 4
    comparative transcription, 293–294
    convergent, **773**
    Darwin's theory, 2, 19–20
    endosymbiosis theory, 651–657, 653*f*–655*f*
    enhancer-sequence conservation, 482, 482*f*
    of *Equus* genus, 745, 745*f*
    of eukaryotes, 656, 657*f*
    genetic basis of, 19–23
    human, 25*b*–26*b*, 25*f*, 758–776
    human chromosome, 392*b*–393*b*, 392*f*
    lateral gene transfer and genome evolution,
        215–216
    linkage disequilibrium and evolutionary analysis,
        174–175
    mammalian Y chromosome, 97*b*–98*b*, 98*f*
    modern synthesis, **21**, 725–726
    molecular evolution changes genes and genomes
        through time, 748–750
    molecular genetics in Darwin's finches, 748

    morphological, 21*f*
    multicellular, in plants, 685–689
    mutation and, 399
    by natural selection, 2, 19–20
    nonadaptive, 20
    of novelty, 750
    plant, 685–689
    polypeptide elongation, 324
    by polyploidy, 374–375, 374*f*
    processes, 20–21
    processes of speciation, 744–746
    recombination and, 146
    reproductive isolation and speciation, 746–747,
        746*t*, 747*f*
    of RNAi, 502
    Robertsonian translocation, 384
    sickle cell disease and, 750*b*–751*b*, 751*f*
    through co-option, 683
    vertebrate steroid receptor, 749–750
Evolutionary genetics, **6**
Evolutionary genomics, 607–618
    defined, **594**
    interspecific genome comparisons, **607**, 608–618
        gene content, 608, 609*f*, 610–615
        gene order, 616–618, 617*f*
        genome annotation, 605–616
    intraspecific genome comparisons, 607
    tree of life, 608, 609*f*
Evolutionary relationships, tracing, 21–23, 21*f*–23*f*,
        24*b*
Exconjugant cell, **194**
Exit site (E site), **318**
Exon shuffling, 605, 610, 611*f*
Exons, **13**, 13*f*, 18
Exporter structure, **194**
Expression array, **619**
Expression library, 564
Expression of heterologous genes in bacterial and fun-
        gal hosts, 565–570
Expression vectors, 565–566, **565**, 565*f*
eyeless gene, 532–533, 532*f*

F

F⁺ (F⁺ cells), **194**
F⁻ (F⁻ cells), **194**
F′ cells, **201**
F′ (F prime) donor, **201**
F′ factor, **201**
F factor/plasmid (fertility factor), **191**
    structure, 194, 194*f*
    transfer of, 194–196, 195*f*
F₂ self-fertilization, hypothesis testing by, 38, 38*f*,
        40, 40*t*
Factor VIII, 93
Facultative heterochromatin, **485**, 491*f*, 492, 494, 495*f*
Familial adenomatous polyposis (FAP), **547**, 547–548,
        547*f*
Famine effects, inheritance of, 503*b*
Federal Bureau of Investigation (FBI), 780
Fertilization, 67–68
    artificial cross, **32**, 33*f*
    self, **32**, 32*f*, 75
        genotype frequency and, 741, 741*t*
        reproduction in, 75–76
Fetal cell sorting, **356**
Finch speciation, Galapagos, 748
Fine-structure analysis, mapping bacteriophage
        chromosomes by, 211, 213–214,
        213*f*–215*f*
Fire, Andrew, 499
First-cousin mating, 742–743, 742*f*
First-degree relationships, **787**
First-degree relatives, **705**
First filial generation (F₁ generation), **34**, 34*f*
FISH (fluorescent in situ hybridization), **364**, 364*f*

Fisher, Ronald, 20–21, 706
Flanking direct repeats, **425**, 425*f*
Fleming, Alexander, 217*b*
Fleming, Walter, 2–3
Floral-organ identity, 686–689, 687*f*–688*f*
Florey, Howard, 217*b*
Fluctuation test, **400**, 401*f*
Fluorescent in situ hybridization (FISH), **364**, 364*f*
Folstein, Susan, 718*b*
Forensic genetic analysis, **779**
    CODIS and, 780–784, 781*t*, 782*f*–783*f*, 784*t*
    electrophoretic analysis, 781–782, 782*f*
    identification of 9-11 attack remains, 785
    identification of disappeared in Argentina, 786
    individual identification, 785–786
    paternity testing, 784–785, 784*t*
Forensic genetics, **779**
Forked-line diagram, **41**, 41*f*, 45, 45*f*
Forward genetic analysis, **508**
Forward genetic screens, 509–516, 515*b*
    analysis of mutagenesis, 513–514
    general design of, 509
    genes of interest revealed by, 533*b*, 534*f*
    modifier screens, 514–516, 514*f*
    specific strategies of, 509–513, 511*f*
        balancer chromosome use, 511–512, 512*f*
        conditional alleles in haploid organisms, screening for, 512–513, 513*f*
        dominant and recessive mutation identifications, 510–511, 511*f*
        mutagen choice, 510, 510*t*
        organism choice, 510
Forward genetics, **508**
    general strategy of, 508, 508*f*
Forward mutation, **405**
Forward mutation rate, **736–737**
Founder effect, **740**
Fraenkel-Conrat, Heinz, 336
Fragile X syndrome, 406, 718*b*
Frameshift mutation, **336**, 401*t*, **402**, 403*f*
Franklin, Rosalind, 4, 6–7, 7*f*, 235*f*, 240, 241, 242
Frequency distribution, **706**, 706*f*
Fridman, Eyal, 717
Fruit fly. *See Drosophila melanogaster*
Fully penetrant, **120**
Functional gene annotation, 603, 603*f*, 605
Functional genomics, 618–626
    defined, **594**
    genetic networks, 625–626, 626*f*
    interactome, 623
    proteomics, 621
    reverse genetics, 623–624
    transcriptiomics, 619–621, 620*f*
    yeast mutants to categorize genes, using, 624–625
Fusion
    transcriptional, 528, 528*f*
    translational, 528, 528*f*
Fusion genes, **568**
Fusion protein, **568**

G
G (Giemsa) banding, **365**
G_0 (G zero) state, **69**
G_1 checkpoint, 75*f*
G_1 (or Gap 1) phase of interphase, **69**, 69*f*, 74, 74*f*, 75*f*, 76
G_2 checkpoint, 75*f*
G_2 (or Gap 2) phase of interphase, **69**, 69*f*, 76
Gaertner, Carl Friedrich, 46*b*
Gain-of-function allele, 524, 527
Gain-of-function mutation, **107**, 108*f*, 109, 532–533, 532*f*, 677*b*
Galactose utilization in *S. cerevisiae*, 482–483, 483*f*
Galápagos Islands finches, 21–22, 21*f*

Gametes, **4**, **68**, 74–76, 79
    frequency determined from genetic maps, 161–162
    identifying parental, single-crossover, and double-crossover gametes in three-point mapping, 157–158, 157*f*
Gap genes, **668**, 668*f*, 669, 670–671, 671*f*, 672*f*
Garrod, Archibald, 2–3, 124, 314, 509
Gaucher disease, 353
GC-rich box, **287**
Gel electrophoresis, **15**, 15–18, 16*f*, 17*f*
    agarose, 555, 555*f*, 556*b*, 557, 557*f*
    separation of PCR products, 262
    two-dimensional, 319, 319*b*
Gene(s), **3**
    additive, **698**, 698–699, 700*f*, 701, 701*f*, 701*t*
    births and deaths of, 608, 610–611, 611*f*
    coordinate, **668**, 668*f*, 669–670, 671*f*, 672*f*
    copy number of, 225
    functional annotation, 603, 603*f*, 605*f*
    gap, **668**, 668*f*, 670–671, 671*f*, 672*f*
    homeotic, **668**, 669, 673–678, 674*f*–676*f*, 678*f*
    homologous, 612
    housekeeping, **668**, 668*f*
    informational, **656**
    major, **698**
    maternal effect, **669**
    modifier, **698**
    number revealed by mutagenesis, 513
    operational, **656**
    orthologous, 612
    pair-rule, **668**, 668*f*, 671–673
    paralogous, 612
    pleiotropic, 122, 123*f*
    reporter, 621
    segment polarity, **668**, 668*f*
    structure and associated nomenclature, 279–280, 280*f*
    syntenic, 146–148
    transgenes, **516**
    zygotic, **669**
Gene-counting method, 729–730
Gene dosage, 366–368, **367**
Gene drives, 585*b*, 586*f*, 587*b*
Gene duplication, 612–613
    by duplication of genomic DNA, 608, 611*f*
    fates of duplicate genes, 612*f*
    by unequal crossover, 610, 611*f*
Gene-environment interactions, **121**, 121–122, 702, 704, 704*f*
    mitochondrial, 658*b*–659*b*, 658*f*
Gene expression, 276
    in bacteria and bacteriophage, regulation of, 439–470, 441*t*
        antiterminators and repressors in, 464–469
        attenuation, 455–459, 457*f*, 459*f*, 460*b*
        inducible operon system, 443–454
        repressible operon system, 454–459
        riboswitches, 462–464, 463*f*–464*f*
        stress response and, 459–461, 461*f*, 469*b*–470*b*
        transcriptional control, 439*t*, 440–461, 461*t*, 462–463, 463*f*
        translational regulation, 461–462, 463–464, 463*f*
    bacterial and eukaryotic compared, 478–479, 478*t*
    in eukaryotes, regulation of, 476–503
        chromatin remodeling, 484–498
        cis-acting regulatory sequences, 478–484
        overview, 477–478, 477*f*
        RNA-mediated mechanisms, 498–502
    monitoring with reporter genes, 528–531, 529*f*–530*f*
Gene expression machine, 298–299, 300*f*
Gene families, **605**

Gene fission, 611, 611*f*
Gene flow, **737**
    effects of, 738
    examples in humans, 738
Gene fusion, 611, 611*f*
Gene hypothesis, 83
Gene identification, genome sequencing to determine, 517–519, 518*f*
Gene interactions, 105–144, **122**
    allele interactions and dominance relationships, 106–118
    complementation analysis, 133–137
    epistatic, **129**, 129*f*, 130*b*–131*b*, 132–133
    Mendelian ratio modification and, 122–133
    notation systems for, 109–110
    in pathways, 122–124, 124*f*
    variable phenotypes and, 118–122
Gene knockouts, **524**
Gene mutations. *See* Mutation(s)
Gene order, 159–160, 616–618
Gene pools, mutation diversification of, 736–737
Gene silencing by double-stranded RNA, 499–501, 500*f*–501*f*
Gene structure, 13*f*
Gene therapy, 579–583
    curing sickle cell disease in mice, 581–582, 582*f*
    defined, **579**
    Duchenne muscular dystrophy, 583, 583*f*
    germinal, **579**
    hemophilia B, 583
    proof of principle, 581–582
    somatic, **579**, 579–583
Genealogical relationships, assessing, 786–787
Genealogical tree of modern humans, 762*f*
General transcription factors (GTFs), **290**, 479
Generalized transducing phages, **208**, 209
Generalized transduction, **208**, 208*f*, 209
Genetic analysis of quantitative traits, 696–719
Genetic ancestry, assessing, 787–788
Genetic bottleneck, **740**, 740–741, 740*f*
Genetic code, **13**, 329–338, 330*f*
    deciphering, 337–338, 337*f*
        experiments in, 334–338
    lack of gaps in, 336–337
    lack of overlap in, 335–336, 336*f*
    mitochondrial, 647–648, 648*t*
    modifications, 331*t*
    redundancy, 329, 331
    third-base wobble, 330–331, 331*f*, 331*t*
    triplet, 336
    universal (almost), 331
Genetic complementation, 132
Genetic complementation analysis, 133–136, **135**, 135*f*, 136*b*–137*b*, 213, 213*f*
Genetic counseling, 227–233
    assessing and communicating risks and options, 228–231
    assessment of future risk, 229
    ethical issues, 232–233
    example cases, 228–231, 229*f*–231*f*, 231*t*
    immediate decision making, 228–229
    indicators and goals of, 227–228, 228*t*
Genetic crosses, controlled, **33**, 34*f*
Genetic disease. *See* Hereditary disease
Genetic dissection, **127**, 127*f*
Genetic diversity
    generation by recombination, 146
    in humans, 759–763, 762*f*, 764*f*, 765*f*
Genetic drift, **20**, **739**
    founder effect, 740
    genetic bottlenecks, 740–741, 740*f*
Genetic fine structure, **211**
Genetic heterogeneity, **135**
Genetic hitchhiking, **772**

Genetic Information Nondiscrimination Act (GINA), 232
Genetic liability, 704–706
    defined, **704**
    threshold of, **705**
Genetic linkage, **146**
    autosomal, test-cross analysis to detect, 150–153, 152*f*
    chi-square analysis of data, 156
    complete, 147, 149*f*
    consequences of, 147–148, 148*f*
    detection, 147–149, 148*f*, 150–153
    discovery of, 149–150, 150*t*
    incomplete, 147–148, 149*f*
    linkage group, **166**
Genetic linkage mapping/maps, **147**
    allelic phase, 168–169, 169*f*
    basis of, 155–156, 156*f*
    constructing a three-point recombination map, 158–161, 158*t*
    correction of genetic map distances, 162, 162*f*, 164
    first, 155–156, 156*f*
    gamete frequencies determined from, 161–162
    gene order determined from, 159–160
    genetic markers, **166**, 166–168, 167*f*–168*f*
    identifying parental, single-crossover, and double-crossover gametes, 157–158, 157*f*
    lod score analysis, 169–171, 170*f*, 170*t*, 171*b*, 172*b*
    three-point test-cross analysis, **156**, 156–164
Genetic map distances, correction of, 162, 162*f*, 164
Genetic markers, **166**, 166–168, 167*f*–168*f*
    for *BRCA1* gene, 171*b*
    disease-causing genes linked to, 167–171
    mapping with, 166–167
Genetic material
    identification of, 4
    location of, 3–4
Genetic medicine. *See* Medical genetics
Genetic mosaic, **574**
Genetic networks, **625**, 625–626, 626*f*
Genetic potential, 697–698
Genetic predisposition, testing for, 233
Genetic redundancy, **515**, 515–516
    in flower development, 533*b*, 534*f*
Genetic screening/testing, 346–359
    biochemical analysis, 226
    blood proteins and, 353
    carrier, 226–227, **348**, 353–354
    chromosome analysis, 226
    direct-to-consumer, **348**, 357–359, 358*t*
    ethical issues, 232–233
    genetic carrier, **348**, 353–354
    genetic predisposition, testing for, 233
    Huntington disease, 346–349, 347, 349*f*, 350*f*
    maternal serum screening, 356
    molecular analysis, 226
    newborn, 227, 232, **348**, 349–353, 352*t*
    opportunities and choices, 359
    preimplantation, **348**, 356–357
    prenatal, 227, 232, **348**, 354–357, 354*t*
    presymptomatic, 227, **348**
    Recommended Uniform Screening Panel (RUSP), 351–353, 352*t*
Genetic screens, **508**
    enhancer, 514
    forward, 509–516
    modifier, 514–516, 514*f*
    suppressor, 514
Genetic variance (V_G)
    defined, **707**
    partitioning, 708
Genetic variation, detection of, 15–19
Genetics
    ancient applications of, 3, 3*f*

branches of, 6
of cancer, 538–550
conservation, 743
development of modern, 2
forensic, 778–789
four phases of modern, 3–5
human evolutionary, 758–776
Naudinian, 46*b*
overview of, 1–2
Genome(s), **5**
    cancer cell, 543, 549–550
    chloroplast, 648–649, 650*f*
    Denisovan, 769–770
    great apes, 763, 765–766, 765*f*–766*f*
    human, 599
    instability and mutation, 543
    interspecific comparisons of, **607**, 608–618
    lambda phage, 467, 468*f*
    lateral gene transfer alteration of, 214–217
    lateral gene transfer identification in, 216–217
    metagenome, **600**
    mitochondrial, 645–646, 646*f*, 647*f*
    Neandertal, 768–769, 788
    nucleotide-base composition of various, 8*t*
    pangenome, **600**
    reference, 599–600
    resequencing, 600
    variation in genome organization among species, 605–606, 606*f*
Genome annotation of human chromosome 21, 607*f*
Genome editing, 519–522, 521*f*
Genome evolution, lateral gene transfer and, 215–216
Genome replication in organelles, 635–636, 636*f*
Genome sequences
    human genetic diversity, revealed by, 759–760
    insights from, 606
Genome sequencing, 18
    ancient DNA, 25*b*–26*b*
    cancer cell, 549
    to determine gene identification, 517–519, 518*f*
Genome-wide association studies (GWAS), 172–174, 174*f*, **717**, 788
    quantitative trait loci identification, 717–718, 718*f*
Genomic imprinting, **497**, 497–498, 497*f*
Genomic islands, 217
Genomic libraries, **516**, **562**, 562–563, 562*f*
Genomics, 18, 593–627
    annotation, **602**, 602–606, 603*f*, 605*f*–607*f*
    evolutionary, **594**, 607–618
    examples of sequenced genomes, 595*t*
    functional, **594**, 618–626
    gene identification, 517–519, 518*f*
    insect guts, analysis of, 627*b*
    metagenomics, 600–602, 601*b*–602*b*
    structural, **594**, 594–602
Genomics era, 4–5
Genotype, **4**
    dominant, **35**
    recessive, **35**
Genotype frequencies
    consequences of self-fertilization for, 741*t*
    inbreeding alteration of, 741
Genotype proportion method, **730**
Genotypic ratio, **36**
Genotyping using microbial growth, 189*b*–190*b*
Germ-line cells, **68**, 76
Germ-line mutations, **401**, 543
Germ plasm theory, 2
Germinal gene therapy, **579**
GFP (green fluorescent protein), **529**, 529–530, 529*f*
Giardia, 656
Gilbert, Walter, 263
GINA (Genetic Information Nondiscrimination Act), 232
Glaeser, Robert, 320

Gleevec, 550
Globin gene family, 613*f*
Goldberg-Hogness box, **287**
Golden Rice, 573–574, 574*f*
Goss, John, 46*b*
Grapes, cloning of, 583–584
Great apes, genomes of, 763, 765–766, 765*f*–766*f*
Green fluorescent protein (GFP), **529**, 529–530, 529*f*
Greider, Carol, 259
Griffith, Frederick, 236–238, 237*f*
Growth, bacterial, 186–188, 187*f*
GTFs (general transcription factors), **290**
Guanine (G), **7**, 240–241
Guide strand, **499**, 500
guideRNA (gRNA), **307**, 307*f*, **520**, 521–522, 521*f*, 585*b*, 587*b*
Gurdon, John B., 581
Guthrie test, **350**
GWAS. *See* Genome-wide association studies

H

Haemophilus influenzae, genome sequencing of, 597–598, 598*f*
Hairpin, **285**
Haldane, J. B. S., 20–21, 164
Hanahan, Douglas, 542
Haploid, **3**, 74–76, 361
Haploid number, **68**
Haploid organisms, screening for conditional alleles in, 512–513, 513*f*
Haploinsufficient, **107**
Haplosufficient, **107**
Haplotypes, **167**, 167–168, 168*f*
    evolutionary analysis involving, 175
    genetic ancestry and, 787
Hardy, Godfrey, 726–727
Hardy-Weinberg (H-W) equilibrium, **726**, 727–729, 730*f*
    application of the, 727–728, 728*f*
    assumptions and predictions, 727–729, 727*t*
    for autosomal genes, 728*f*, 729*t*
    chi-square analysis, 731–732
    history of, 726–727
    for more than two alleles, 731, 731*t*
    for two autosomal alleles, 728*f*, 729*t*
Hayes, William, 194, 198
Hayflick, Leonard, 259
Hayflick limit, **259**
HCG (human chorionic gonadotropin), 356, 356*t*
Health risk assessment, genetic, 788–789
Heat shock genes, alternative sigma (σ) factor for, 460–461, 461*f*
Heijmans, Bastiaan, 503*b*
Helicase, **253**
Helix Bridge, 1*f*
Helix-turn-helix (HTH) motif, **442**, 442–443, 442*f*
Hellens, Roger, 404*b*
Hemizygous, **86**
Hemoglobin, 16
    sickle cell disease and, 750*b*–751*b*, 751*f*
Hemophilia A, 92–93, 94*f*, 95*b*, 426
Hemophilia B, 583
Hereditary disease. *See also specific diseases*
    chromosomal conditions, 225–226
    environmental modification to prevent, 121–122
    genetic counseling, 227–233
    genetic testing and diagnosis, 226–227
    Mendelian conditions, 225
    types of, 225–226
Hereditary retinoblastoma, **545**
Hereditary transmission, 2–3
Heredity
    blending theory of, **32**, 36
    chromosome theory of, **68**, 86–87, 145–146

Heritability
artificial selection and, 712–713, 712t, 713f
broad sense, **709**, 710, 711t
defined, **709**
epigenetic, 494–496
erroneous understanding of, 709–710
measuring genetic component of phenotypic variation, 708–713
narrow sense, **709**, 712–713, 712t, 713f
twin studies, 710–712, 711t, 712t
Hershey, Alfred, 239–240, 239f
Heterochromatic region, **366**
Heterochromatin, **292, 366**
constitutive, **484**, 491f, 501–502
facultative, **485**, 491f, 492, 494, 495f
Heterochromatin protein-1 (HP-1), 485–486, 486f
Heteroduplex DNA, **422**, 424
Heteroduplex region, **422,** 423f
Heteroplasmic cell/organism, **634**, 635f, 636, 637f
Heteroplasmy, **634,** 634–635, 635f, 637f
Heterotetramer, 317
Heterozygote, natural selection favoring, 735, 735t
Heterozygous genotype, **35**
Hexon, 298, 298f
Hfr chromosome, **196**, 196f
F factor excision from, 201, 203f
Hfr gene transfer, 196–198, 197f, 198t
Hfr maps, consolidation of, 200–201, 202f
HGMD (Human Gene Mutation Database), 761
High altitude, adaptations to, 774–775
High-frequency recombination (Hfr) bacteria, **196**
High-throughput sequencing, 619
HindII, 554b
Histone acetyltransferases (HATs), **489,** 492f
Histone code, 489
Histone deacetylases (HDACs), **489,** 492f
Histone demethylases (HDMTs), **491**
Histone methyltransferases (HMTs), 485–486, 486f, **491**
Histone proteins, 295, **386,** 386t, 387f, 388–390
modification of, 489, 491–492, 491f–492f, 502b
Hoelzel, A. Rus, 741
Holliday, Robin, 422
Holliday junction, **422,** 423f, 424, 424f
Holliday model, **422**
Holoenzyme, **280,** 280f
Holoprosencephaly, 690b–691b
Homeobox, **673**
Homeodomain, **673**
Homeologs, **618**
Homeotic genes, **668,** 669
in floral-organ identity, 686–689, 687f–688f
Homeotic mutations, **664**
Homo erectus, 770
Homo floresiensis, 770
Homologous chromosomes, 145f
crossing over, 76–77
separation, 78, 81f
Homologous genes, **612,** 613f
identification of, 532b
Homologous nucleotides, **608**
Homologous pairs, 3, 52
Homologous recombination, **146, 422,** 423f, 424, 424f, **523**
double-stranded break model of, 422, 423f, 424
genome editing, 519, 521, 521f, 576
in reverse genetics, 522–524, 523f
Homologs, **3, 612,** 613f
Homology, **21**, 22, 23f, 612
Homoplasmic cell/organism, **634,** 635–636, 635f, 637f
Homoplasmy, **21, 634,** 634–635, 635f, 637f
Homotetramer, 317
Homozygous genotype, **35**
Honeybees, 502b
Hooke, Robert, 2

Horowitz, Norman, 127
Horvitz, Robert, 679, 682
Hotspots, of recombination, 165–166, 165f
Housekeeping genes, 668
Hox genes, 494, **673,** 677b
downstream targets of, 675–676
evolution and, 683, 684f, 685
specification of parasegments by, 673–675
throughout metazoans, 676–678, 678f
Huberman, Joel, 247–248
Human chorionic gonadotropin (HCG), 356, 356t
Human evolution, 758–776
adaptation to new environments, genetic evidence for, 772–775, 773f
African origin of modern humans, 761–763
autosomal genetic diversity, 763, 764f, 765f
cladogram showing genetic distances, 764f
CNV variation, 761
conserved noncoding sequences, 766, 767f
Denisovans, 768f, 769–770, 769f
fossil hominins, 766–768, 767f
future, 776
genealogical tree of modern humans, 761–763
genes that make us human, 770
genetic diversity revelated by genome sequences, 759–760
great ape genomes compared, 763, 765–766, 765f–766f
high altitude, adaptations to, 774–775
lactose tolerance, 772–775, 773f
migration of humans around the globe, 770–772
migration of modern humans out of Africa, 769f
models of human migration, 759, 760f
Neandertals, 758, 758f, 768–769, 768f, 769f
skin pigmentation, 774
SNP variation, 760–761
Y chromosome phylogeny, 762–763
Human evolutionary genetics, 758–776
Human Gene Mutation Database (HGMD), 761
Human genetic disease, mitochondrial mutations and, 638, 640, 640f
Human genome, 57–59
origins of replication, 248
Human Genome Diversity Project, 760
Human genome mapping, 166
Human Genome Project, 5, 18, 232, 593, 599, 759
Human hereditary disease, 57–59, 58t
Human migrations around the globe, 770–772
Australia, 771–772
Europe, 770–771
Human mitochondrial transcription, 648f
Human progeroid syndrome, 269b
hunchback gene, 671, 671f, 672, 672f
huntingtin gene, 347–349
Huntington disease, 118, 119f, 227, 233, 346–349, 349f, 350f
Hybrid dysgenesis, **429,** 429–430, 430f
Hybrid vigor, **374,** 651b
Hybridization, **17**
Hydrogen bonds, **8**
Hydroxylating agents, 412, 412f
Hypermorphic mutations, 108f, **109**
Hyperplasia, **541,** 541f
Hypomethylation, 550
Hypomorphic mutation, 108f, **109**
Hypothesis testing
by F_2 self-fertilization, 38
by test-cross analysis, 37, 37f
Hypoxia-inducible factor (HIF) pathway, 774

I

IARC (International Agency for Research on Cancer), 539
ICR (internal control region), **292**
Identity by descent (IBD), **742,** 742–743, 786

IGF2 gene, 497–498, 497f, 503b
Illegitimate recombination, **523,** 574, 576
Illumina sequencing, 266, 268f
Immediate early genes, phage λ, **465**
Immortality, cellular, 542
Immune system avoidance by cancer, 543
Imprinting control region (ICR), **497,** 497–498, 497f
In vitro fertilization (IVF), **356,** 356–357
Inborn error of metabolism, 3
Inbreeding, **741,** 741–743
Inbreeding depression, **743**
Incomplete dominance, **110,** 110f
Incomplete penetrance, 119, **120,** 120f
Incorporated error, **406,** 407, 409f
Independent assortment, 41–46, 42f
genetic linkage *versus,* 148f
law of, **42**
of syntenic genes, 146–147
testing by test-cross analysis, 43, 43f, 45
testing by trihybrid-cross analysis, 45–46, 45f
Individual identification, forensic genetic analysis and, 785–786
Induced mutations, **410,** 410–415
Induced pluripotent stem cells (iPS cells), 581–582, 582f
Inducer, **441**
Inducer compound, 443
Inducer-repressor complex, **445**
Inducible operon, **443**
Induction, lysogeny, **468, 665,** 666, 666f
Inductive signal, **680**
Inflammation, tumor-promoting, 543
Informational genes, **656**
Ingroup, **22**
Inheritance. *See also* Organellar inheritance
biparental, **633**
haplotype, 168, 168f
nucleosome, 390f
particulate, **36**
uniparental, **633**
Inhibition, **665,** 666, 666f
lateral, **682,** 682f
Inhibitor compound, **441,** 442f
Initial committed complex, **290**
Initiation
in bacterial transcription, 281, 281f, 284
translation, 320
Initiation complex, **322**
Initiation factors, 320, **321,** 321–322, 321f
archael, 323, 324t
bacterial, 321–322, 321f, 324t
eukaryotic, 322, 323f, 324t
Initiation of transcription, 440
Initiator tRNA, **320,** 321f
Inosine, **331**
Insects. *See also Drosophila melanogaster*
genomic analysis of guts, 627b
Insertion
mutants in reverse genetics, 524–525, 524f
of nucleotide repeats, 405–406
Insertion sequence (IS), **194, 426,** 427, 428b
Insertional inactivation, **426**
Insulator sequences, **484,** 484f
Insulin, producing human in *E. coli,* 566–568, 567f
Insulin growth factor 2 *(IGF2),* 497–498, 497f, 503b
Interactive variance (V_I), **708**
Interactome, **623**
Interchromosomal domain, **363**
Interference, 160–161, **161**
negative, **161**
Internal control region (ICR), **292**
International Agency for Research on Cancer (IARC), 539
Interphase
chromosome territories, 362–363, 363f
of the germ-line cell cycle, 76

Interrupted mating, **198**, 199*b*
Interspecific comparisons of genomes, **607**, 608–618
   gene content, 608, 610–615
   gene order, 616–618, 617*f*
   genome annotation, 615–616
Interstitial deletion, **375**, 375–376, 376*f*
Intragenic recombination, 213–214, 214*f*
Intragenic reversion, **405**, 406*f*
Intraspecific comparisons of genomes, **607**
Intrinsic termination, **285**, 285*f*
Introgression, of Neandertal DNA into the modern
     human genome, 768
Introgression lines, **717**, 717–718, 717*f*
Intron splicing, **294**
Introns, **13**, 13*f*, 18, 296–297, 297*f*, 297*t*
   self-spicing, 302, 304, 304*f*
   splicing and, 297–298, 299*f*
   types of, 297*t*
Inversion heterozygotes, **378**, 380–381, 381*f*, 383
Inversion loop, **380**, 380*f*, 381
Inverted repeats, **285**, 285*f*, 425, 425*f*
iPS cells (induced pluripotent stem cells), **581**–582, 582*f*
IS10 insertion sequence, **462**, 462*f*
Island model of migration, **738**, 738*f*
Isoaccepting tRNA, **330**, 330*f*
ISWI (imitation switch) complex, **488**, 489*f*
IVF (in vitro fertilization), **356**, 356–357

J

Jacob, François, 198, 277–278, 439*f*, 440, 447–448
Jansen, Hans, 2
Jansen, Zacharias, 2
Jeffreys, Alec, 779
Jenuwein, Thomas, 489
Joint probability, **229**, 230–231
Jorgensen, Richard, 499
Juvenile hormone, of *Drosophila*, 122

K

Karyokinesis, **70**, 78
Karyotype, 355, **363**, 363*f*
Kelp, development of body plan in, 689*b*
Keytruda, 538–539
Khorana, Har Gobind, 338
Kidwell, Margaret, 429
Kinetochore, **71**, 72–73, 72*f*–73*f*, 78, 81*f*
Kinetochore microtubules, **72**, 72*f*, 73, 77–78, 81*f*
King, Mary-Claire, 171*b*, 786
Knight, Thomas Andrew, 46*b*
Knock-in, 526
Knockout library, **522**, 624, 624*f*
Knockouts, 524
Knudson, Alfred, 545
Kornberg, Roger, 388
Kosambi, Damodar, 164
Kowalczykowski, Stephen, 256
Kozak, Marilyn, 322
Kozak sequence, **322**, 323*f*, 326*b*–327*b*
Krüppel gene, 671, 672, 672*f*

L

lac⁻ phenotype, **443**
lac operator (*lacO*), **444**, 445*f*, 447*t*
lac (lactose) operon, 439*f*, 440, **443**, 445*f*
   eukaryotic regulation compared, 478, 480
   function, 444–445, 446*f*
   "leaky" regulation, 478
   molecular analysis, 451, 454
   mutational analysis, 447–450
      regulatory mutations, 447*t*, 448–451, 449*f*
      structural gene mutations, 447–448, 447*t*
   regulatory proteins binding to regulatory
       sequences, 453*b*
   structure, 444, 445*f*
   transcription conditions, 451*t*

lac operon promoter (*lacP*), 444, 445*f*, 447*t*
lac⁺ phenotype, **443**
Lac repressor, 478
lacA, **444**, 445*f*
lacI, 444, 445*f*, 447*t*
Lactase, 772–774, 773*f*
Lactose metabolism, 443, 444*f*
Lactose tolerance, 772–774, 773*f*
lacY, **444**, 445*f*, 447*t*
lacZ, **444**, 445*f*, 447*t*, 528, 559–560, 568
Lagging strand, **254**, 254*f*
Lahn, Bruce, 97*b*–98*b*
Lambda (λ) phage. *See* Bacteriophage λ
Lanktree, Matthew, 697
Large ribosomal subunit, **318**
Lariat intron structure, **298**
Last universal common ancestor (LUCA), **5**, 5*f*
Late age of onset, 227
Late genes, phage λ, **465**
Late operators, phage λ, **466**
Late promoters, phage λ, **466**
Lateral gene transfer (LGT), **215**, 611, 611*f*, 613, 615
   genomes altered by, 214–217
   identifying in genomes, 216–217
   processes, 191, 192*f*, 193
Lateral inhibition, **682**, 682*f*
Law of independent assortment, **42**, 80–81, 83*f*, 105, 146
Law of segregation, **37**, 80, 82*f*, 105
LCR (locus control region), **481**, 481–482, 481*f*, 482*f*
Leader regions, **333**, 455
Leading strand, **254**, 254*f*
Leaky mutation, **107**, 108*f*, 109
Leber hereditary optic neuropathy, 638, 640*f*
Leder, Philip, 338
Lederberg, Joshua, 193–194, 193*f*, 196
Leeuwenhoek, Anton van, 2
Lenormand, Thomas, 164
Leptotene, 76, 78*f*
Lester, Diane, 56, 404*b*
Lethal alleles, 116–118, 116*f*–118*f*
Lewis, Edward B., 664, 666
Lewis, Mitchell, 454
Li-Fraumeni syndrome, 546, 546*f*
Liability alleles, **705**
Life-forms, early, 19, 19*f*
Life on Earth, origin of, 19
Limb evolution, 683, 684*f*, 685
LINE (long interspersed nuclear elements), 430–431
Linkage, genetic. *See* Genetic linkage
Linkage disequilibrium, **173**, 173–175, 772
Linkage equilibrium, **173**
Linkage groups, **166**
Linker DNA, **388**
Linkers, **559**
Locus control region (LCR), **481**, 481–482, 481*f*, 482*f*
Lod score analysis, **169**, 169–171, 170*f*, 170*t*, 171*b*,
    172*b*
   BRCA1 gene, 171*b*
   cystic fibrosis gene, 175*b*–176*b*, 176*t*
Long arm, **363**, 364*f*
Long noncoding RNAs (lncRNAs), **496**
Long terminal repeats (LTRs), **430**
Loss-of-function alleles, 524
Loss-of-function mutations, **107**, 108*f*, 109, 511, 513,
    532–533, 532*f*, 677*b*
LUCA (last universal common ancestor), **5**, 5*f*
Luciferase, 529
Luria, Salvador, 400, 401*f*
Lwoff, André, 439*f*, 440, 447
Lyon, Mary, 96
Lyon hypothesis, **96**
Lysis, **205**
Lysogenic cycle, 207*f*, **208**
Lysogeny, **207**, 208
   in phage λ, 467*f*, 468, 469

Lytic cycle, 207*f*, **208**
   in phage λ, 466, 467*f*, 468

M

M phase
   of eukaryotic cell cycle, 69, 69*f*, 74
   of meiosis, 76
   substages of, 69–71, 70*f*–71*f*
MacLeod, Colin, 4, 238, 238*f*
MADS box genes, **688**, 688–689
Maize, 775–776, 775*f*, 776*f*
   discovery of Ds and Ac elements in, 427–429,
    429*f*
Major genes, **698**
Major groove, DNA, **241**
Malaria, 750*b*–751*b*, 751*f*
Male sterility in plants, 651*b*–652*b*
Maleszka, Ryszard, 502*b*
Malignant tumors, **541**
Mammals
   coat color determination, 113–116, 114*f*–115*f*
   degenerative evolution of the mammalian Y
    chromosome, 97*b*–98*b*, 98*f*
   dosage compensation and, 96, 96*t*
   mitochondrial inheritance in, 637–640, 638*f*
   random X inactivation, 96–97, 97*f*
   ribosomes, 318
   sex determination in, 89, 89*f*
Map unit (m.u.), **156**
Mapping. *See also* Genetic linkage mapping/maps
   allelic phase, 168–169, 169*f*
   consolidation of Hfr maps, 200–201, 202*f*
   cotransduction, **209**, 209–211, 210*f*, 210*t*, 212*t*
   cystic fibrosis gene, 175*b*–176*b*, 176*t*
   gene for breast and ovarian cancer susceptibil-
    ity, 171*b*
   with genetic markers, 166–168, 167*f*–168*f*
   genome-wide association studies, 172–174, 174*f*
   lod score analysis, 169–171, 170*f*, 170*t*, 171*b*,
    172*b*
   by transformation, 205
Mapping deletion, 213, **214**, 215*f*
Mapping function, **164**
Mapping time-of-entry, **198**, 200*f*
Marchantia polymorpha, chloroplast genome of, 649,
    650*f*
Martin, Cathie, 426
Martin, David, 56, 404*b*
Maternal effect genes, **669**
Maternal inheritance, **633**
   of chloroplasts, 632–634, 634*f*
   of mitochondria, 637
Maternal serum screening, **356**, 356*t*
Mating type and chloroplast segregation in *Chlamydo-
    monas*, 640–641, 642*f*
Matrix attachment regions, **389**
Matthei, Johann Heinrich, 337
Mature mRNA, **294**
Mavaddat, Nasim, 498
Maxam, Allan, 263
Mayr, Ernst, 21, 743
McCarty, Maclyn, 4, 238, 238*f*
McClintock, Barbara, 153, 155, 427–429
McKusick, Victor, 58
Median, **707**
Median value, **707**
Mediator, **483**
Medical genetics
   ethical issues, 231–232
   genetic counseling, 227–233
   overview of, 224
Megabases (Mb), **18**
Meiosis, **4**, **68**, 74–82
   chromosome aberration errors, 226
   Mendelian ratios generated by, 80–81

mitosis compared to, 76, 76t
molecular model of homologous recombination in, 423f
nuclear content of cell through phases of, 79, 82f
overview of, 76, 77f
stages of, 78f–79f
X-chromosome nondisjunction in, 87, 87f
Meiosis I, **76**, 76–79, 77f–79f, 81f
Meiosis I nondisjunction, 367f
Meiosis II, 79, 80f
Meiosis II nondisjunction, 367f
Melanin, 698, 774
Mello, Craig, 499
Mendel, Gregor, 2–3, 30–31, 30f
autosomal inheritance and hereditary principles of, 51–57
basic principles of genetic transmission discovered by, 31–34
chi-square analysis of data of, 50–51, 52t
experimental innovations of, 33–34
modern experimental approach of, 31–33
molecular genetics of traits examined by, 54, 56–57, 57t
mutations and, 402, 404b
peas shaped by transposition, 431b–432b
rediscovery of his work, 46
Mendelian disease conditions, 225
Mendelian genetics, **6**
Mendelian Index in Man (MIM), 58
Mendelian inheritance, extensions of, 106
Mendelian ratios
gene interactions modifying, 122–133
mechanistic basis of, 80–81, 82f–83f
Mendelism, 3, 30
in the produce aisle, 41b
Mendel's first law, **37**
Mendel's second law, **42**
Meristems
defined, **685**
development at, 685–686, 686f
MERRF (myoclonic epilepsy with ragged red fibers), 640
Meselson, Matthew, 245–247, 246f, 278
Meselson-Stahl experiment, 245–247, 246f
Messenger RNA (mRNA), 4, **6**, 11–13, 276, 278, **279**. See also Precursor messenger RNA (pre-mRNA); Transcription; Translation
alignment of DNA, mRNA, and polypeptide, 316f
codons, 13, 15f
editing of chloroplast, 650–651, 651f
experimental discovery of, 277–278
genetic code and, 329–338
polycistronic, **329**, 329f
polymerase II transcription of mRNA in eukaryotes, 287
stability, riboswitch control of, 464, 464f
synthetic, 337–338, 337f–338f, 337t
translation, 13, 15f
Metabolomics, **18**
Metacentric chromosome, **363**
Metagenome, **600**
Metagenomics, 600–602, 601b–602b
Metaphase, **69**, 71f, 74f, 75f
Metaphase checkpoint, 75f
Metaphase chromosome, chromosome scaffold of, 389, 389f
Metaphase I, 76–78, 79f, 81f
Metaphase II, 79, 80f
Metaphase plate, **73**
Metastasis, **541**, 542
Metazoans, *Hox* genes in, 676–678, 678f
Methionine biosynthesis, genetic dissection of, 127, 127f

Methylation
epigenetics and, 502b–503b
histone, 502b
of nucleotides, 498
Meyers, Matthias, 25b
Mice
curing sickle cell disease in mice, 581–582, 582f
gene therapy studies in, 581–583, 582f, 583f
transgenic, 576–578, 577f, 580b
Microbial growth
genotyping using, 189b–190b
visualizing, 189b
Microbiome
digestive, 601b
skin, 601b–602b
Microdeletions, **377**, 377f
Microduplications, **377**, 377f
microRNA (miRNA), 12, 12f, **279**, 279t, **499**, 500f–501f, 550
Microsynteny, **617**
Microtubules
astral, **72**, 72f
in dividing cells, 72–73, 72f
kinetochore, **72**, 72f, 73, 77–78, 81f
nonkinetochore, **72**, 72f
Miescher, Friedrich, 236
MIF (Müllerian-inhibitory factor), 89, 90b
Mlf1, 484
Migration, **20**
MIM (Mendelian Index in Man), 58
Minimal medium, **187**
Minor groove, DNA, **241**
Mismatch repair, **418**, 418–419, 419f
Missense mutation, 401t, **402**, 402f, 404b
Mitochondria, **4**, **645**, 645f
endosymbiosis theory, 651–657, 653f–655f
as energy factories of eukaryotic cells, 644–648
evolution of, 4
nuclear mitochondrial sequences (NUMTS), **654**, 655
Mitochondrial DNA (mtDNA), 24b–25b
bison, 639b
forensic genetic analysis use of, 785–786
human evolutionary genetics and, 761–762
mother-child identity of, 637–638
mutations in, 761
sequences and species evolution, 638
Mitochondrial Eve, 762
Mitochondrial genetic codes, 647–648, 648t
Mitochondrial genome
gene content of humans, 647f
structure and gene content, 645–646, 646f, 647f
Mitochondrial inheritance in mammals, 637–640, 638f
Mitochondrial transcription and translation, 646–648, 648t
Mitosis, **4**, 68
meiosis compared to, 76, 76t
nuclear contents of a cell through the phases of mitosis, 74, 74f
overview of, 75f
in somatic cell division, 68–74
Mitosomes, **656**
MN blood group, 113b, 732b
Modal value, **707**
Mode, **707**
Model organisms, 18
Modern synthesis of evolution, **21**, 725–726
Modifier genes, **698**
Modifier screen, **514**, 514–516, 514f
Molecular analysis of the *lac* operon, 451
Molecular biology
of transcription and RNA processing, 275–308
of translation, 314–340
Molecular cloning, 557–561, 558f–561f
Molecular genetics, **6**
of Mendel's traits, 54, 56–57, 57t

Molecular genetics of evolution in Darwin's finches, 748
Molecular probes, **17**, 17–18
Monod, Jacques, 439f, 440, 447–448
Monohybrid cross(es), 34–40, **36**
Monohybrid traits, 36t
Monophyletic groups, **21**, 22
Monosomic, **366**
Monosomies, 369, 370
Morgan, Lilian, 146
Morgan, Thomas Hunt, 83, 85–86, 107, 145, 507, 664
crossing-over hypothesis, 152f
genetic linkage and, 150–153, 151f–152f, 155
Morphogens, **665**
Morphological evolution, 21f
Morphospecies concept, **744**
Morton, Newton, 169
Mosaicism, 96, 370, 371f
Motor proteins, 72
mRNA. *See* Messenger RNA
mtDNA. *See* Mitochondrial DNA (mtDNA)
Muller, Hermann, 382b–383b, 390–391, 412, 509
Müllerian ducts, 89, 89f, 90b
Müllerian-inhibitory factor (MIF), 89, 90b
Mullis, Kary, 261
Multicellular evolution, plants and, 685–689
Multifactorial conditions, 226
Multifactorial traits, **697**
Multimers, 317
Multiple cloning site (MCS), **559**, 559–560, 560f
Multiple-gene hypothesis, **698**
Multiplication rule, 47
Multiregional (MRE) hypothesis, 759, 760f, 762
Mus musculus, transgenic, 576–578, 577f, 580b
Mutagenesis, **508**
analysis of mutants obtained by, 513–514
common mutagens used for, 510t
forward genetic screens, 508–516
genomics approach to gene identification following, 517–519, 518f
insertional, 524f
saturation, **510**
strategies, 511f
Mutagens, **410**
alkylating agents, 411–412, 412f
chemical, 410–412, 411f–412f, 411t, 510, 510t
deaminating agents, 411, 412f
DNA intercalating agents, 412, 413f
for forward genetic screens, 510, 510t
hydroxylating agents, 412, 412f
insertional, 510t
nucleotide base analog, 410–411, 411f, 411t
radiation, 412–413, 413f, 510t
Mutants
constitutive, **448**, 450
forward genetic screen identification of, 509–516
gain-of-function, 532–533, 532f
insertion, 524–525, 524f
loss-of-function, 532–533, 532f
noninducible, **450**
nonrevertible, **214**
promoter, 450
revertible, **214**, 215f
Mutation(s), **20**, 399
adaptive mutation hypothesis, **400**, 401f
altering human sex development, 90b
attenuation, 461, 461f
base-pair substitution, **401**, 401–402, 401f
cancer and, 542, 543–546
in cell cycle control, 74
cis-acting, **448**
complementation analysis, 133–136, 135f, 136b–137b
complementation of, 213, 213f
diversification of gene pools by, 736–737

dominant negative, 108*f*, **109**
driver, 549
E(var), **485**, 485*f*
forward, **405**
frameshift, **336**, 401*t*, **402**, 403*f*
frequency of, 58–59
functional effects of, 107–109, 108*f*
gain-of-function, **107**, 108*f*, 109, 677*b*
germ-line, **401**
hypermorphic, 108*f*, **109**
identifying dominant and recessive, 510–511, 511*f*, 512*f*, 513
identifying type of, 407*b*
induced, **410**, 410–415
    Ames test for, 413–415, 414*f*–415*f*, 416*b*
    chemical mutagens, 410–412, 411*f*–413*f*, 411*t*
    radiation, 412–413, 413*f*
insertion, 404*b*
leaky (hypomorphic), **107**, 108*f*, **109**
loss-of-function, **107**, 108*f*, 109, 511, 513, 677*b*
Mendel's, 402, 404, 404*b*
missense, 401*t*, **402**, 402*f*, 404*b*
mitochondrial, 638, 640, 640*f*, 641*f*, 761
mutagenic effect of transposition, 426
neomorphic, 108*f*, **109**
noll (amorphic), **107**, 108*f*
nonsense, 401*t*, **402**, 402*f*
in OMIM, 58, 58*t*
operator, 448–450, 449*f*, 454*f*
passenger, 549
PEV, 485–486, 485*f*
point, **401**, 401*t*
polar, **448**
polyadenylation, 404–405
promoter, 401*t*, **403**, 403*f*
quantification of effects of mutation on, 737
random mutation hypothesis, **400**, 401*f*
regulatory, 401*t*, 402–405, **403**, 403*f*
reverse, **405**, 414
reversion, **336**
silent, 402
somatic, **401**
splicing, 403–404, 403*f*, **404**, 404*b*
spontaneous, **405**, 405–410
    DNA replication errors, 405–408, 408*f*–409*f*, 408*t*
    nucleotide base changes, 409–410, 409*f*–410*f*
strand slippage, 405–406, 408*f*
Su(var), **485**, 485*f*
suppressor, **405**
synonymous, 401*t*, **402**, 402*f*
transition, **401**, 402
transversion, 401–402
X-ray induced, 382*b*–383*b*
Mutation hotspots, **400**
Mutation rate, **400**
Mutation-selection balance, **737**
Mutational analysis of the *lac* operon, 446–450
Myers, Richard, 290

N

N-formylmethionine (fMet), **322**
Naegeli, Karl, 31
Narrow sense heritability (*h²*)
    artificial selection and, 712–713, 712*t*, 713*f*
    defined, **709**
Nathans, Daniel, 554*b*
National DNA Index System (NDIS), 780
Natural selection, 19–20, **20**, 399
    bacterial promoters and, 281
    directional, 733–735, 735*f*
    favoring heterozygotes, 735, 735*t*
    lactase persistence and, 773

operating through differential reproductive fitness within a population, 732–735
    sickle cell disease and, 750*b*–751*b*, 751*f*
Naudin, Charles, 46, 46*b*
Neandertals, 18, 25*b*–26*b*, 758, 758*f*, 768–769, 768*f*, 769*f*, 788
Near isogenic lines (NILs), **717**
Negative control of transcription, **441**, 441*f*
Negative interference, **161**
Negative regulation of transcription, 480
Neofunctionalization, **612**, 612*f*, 613
Neomorphic mutations, 108*f*, **109**
Neoplasia, **541**
Neural tube defects, 228
Neurospora crassa, 124–125, 125*b*–126*b*, 127
Newborn genetic screening, **348**, 349–353, 352*t*
Newborn testing, 227, 232
Next-generation sequencing (NGS), 18, **266**, 268*f*
Nick translation, **417**
Nilsson-Ehle, Hermann, 698
Nirenberg, Marshall, 337
Nitrous acid, 411
Nodes, **608**
Noll, Markus, 388
Non-Hodgkins lymphoma, 550
Non-Watson-and-Crick base pairs, **406**
Nonadaptive evolution, 20
Noncomposite transposon, **427**, 427*f*
Nondisjunction, **87**, 87*f*, **366**, 367*f*
Nonhistone proteins, **386**
Nonhomologous end joining (NHEJ), 420, **421**, 421*f*
    genome editing, 519–520, 521*f*
Noninducible mutants, **450**
Nonkinetochore microtubules, **72**, 72*f*
Nonparental phenotypes, 42
Nonpenetrant, **120**
Nonrecombinant chromosomes, 146
Nonrecombinant vector, **558**
Nonreplicative transposition, **425**
Nonrevertible mutants, **214**, 215*f*
Nonsense mutation, 401*t*, **402**, 402*f*
Nonsister chromatids, 76, **77**
Nontemplate strand, **279**
Northern blotting, 17
Notational systems for genes and allele relationships, 109–110
Notch gene, 377–378, 378*f*
Novelty, evolution of, 750
Nuclear genome, organellar gene transfer into, 654–655, 654*f*–655*f*
Nuclear mitochondrial sequences (NUMTS), **654**, 655
Nuclear plastid sequences (NUPTS), **654**, 655
Nuclei, chromosomes in, 362–363
Nuclein, 2, 236
Nucleoid, **4**, 635
Nucleoli (singular, nucleolus), **292**
Nucleomorph, **657**
Nucleosome, 387*f*, **388**
    disassembly, synthesis, and reassembly during replication, 389–390
    displacement of, 489, 489*f*
    inheritance after DNA replication, 390*f*
Nucleosome-based model of chromatin, 388
Nucleosome core particle, **386**, 388
Nucleosome-depleted region, **486**
Nucleosome structure, 388, 388*f*
Nucleotide base analog, **410**, 410–411, 411*f*, 411*t*
Nucleotide excision repair (NER), 136*b*–137*b*, **417**, 417–418, 417*t*, 418*f*
Nucleotide repeats, 405–406, 408*f*
Nucleotides, 240–241, 240*f*. *See also* DNA nucleotides
    deamination, **409**, 409–410, 410*f*
    depurination, **409**, 409*f*
    homologous, 608
    methylation of, 498

mispaired, 406–408, 409*f*
RNA, 12, 276–277, 277*f*
spontaneous base changes, 409–410, 409*f*–410*f*
used in DNA sequencing reactions, 263, 264*f*
Null mutation, **107**, 108*f*
Nüsslein-Volhard, Christiane, 509, 666–668

O

Obligate carrier, 230–231
Okazaki, Reiji, 254
Okazaki fragments, **254**, 254*f*
    ligation, 254–255, 255*f*
Olfactory receptor genes, 765
On the Origin of Species by Means of Natural Selection (Darwin), 744
Oncogenes, **542**
One gene-one enzyme hypothesis, 124–125, **125**, 125*b*–126*b*, 315
Online Mendelian Index in Man (OMIM), 58, 58*t*, 225
Open chromatin, **487**
Open promoter complex, **281**
Open promoters, **486**, 486–487, 487*f*
Open reading frames (ORFs), **602**, 602–603
Operational genes, **656**
Operator mutations, 448–450, 449*f*, 454*f*
Operators, **441**, 441*f*
Operons, **443**. *See also lac* (lactose) operon; *trp* (tryptophan) operon
    with attenuator control of transcription, 459, 459*f*
    inducible, **443**
    repressible, **454**
Opposite sense resolution, **424**, 424*f*
Organellar inheritance
    defined, **633**
    discovery of, 633–634
    modes of, 636–644
    summary of, 644
Organellar proteins, encoding of, 655–656
Organelle genomes
    replication in, 635–636, 636*f*
    replicative segregation of, 635–636
Organelles, continual DNA transfer from, 654–655, 654*f*–655*f*
Organizer region, **665**
OriC, 249, 252*f*, 253, 253*f*
Origin of replication, 9, **15**, **247**, 247–248, 248*f*
    DNA sequences, 249–250, 252, 252*f*
    multiple in eukaryotes, 248–249, 250*f*
    plasmid, 559
Origin of Species by Means of Natural Selection (Darwin), 20
Origin of transfer (*oriT*), **194**
Origin recognition boxes (ORBs), 250–251
Origin replication complex (ORC), 253
Orthologous genes, **612**, 613*f*
Orthologs, **612**, 613*f*
Osteogenesis imperfecta, 109
Otto, Sarah, 164
Outgroup, **22**
Ovarian cancer, 233, 548–559, 548*t*

P

P arm, **363**, 364*f*
P element, **429**, 429–430, 430*f*, 574–575, 575*f*
P1 bacteriophage, 208–209, 208*f*
p53, 420
Pääbo, Svante, 25*b*, 767
Pachytene, 76–77, 78*f*
Page, David, 97*b*–98*b*
Pair-rule genes, **668**, 668*f*, 669, 671–673
Paired-end sequencing, **596**, 596–599, 597*f*–599*f*
Palade, George, 278
Pancreatic cancer, 549

Pangenome, **600**
Paracentric inversion, **378**, 380*f*, 391
Paralogous genes, **612**, 613*f*
Paralogs, **612**, 613*f*
Parasegments, **669**
Parental chromosomes, 146, 157–160
Parental generation (P generation), **34**, 34*f*
Parental phenotypes, 42, 147
Parental strand, **9**, 11*f*
Partial deletion, **376**
Partial deletion heterozygotes, **375**
Partial diploids, **202**, 203, 203*f*
    lac operon and, 447–448, 449*t*
Partial dominance, **110**, 110*f*
Partial duplication, **376**
Partial duplication heterozygote, **376**
Particulate inheritance, **36**
Pascal's triangle, **49**, 49*f*
Paternity Index (PI), **785**
Paternity testing, 784–785, 784*t*
Paterson, Andrew, 715
Pathogenicity islands, **217**
Pathways, gene action in, 122–124, 124*f*
Pattern formation, 665–666
    maternal effects on, 669
Pauling, Linus, 16, 17*f*
PAZ site, 499
PCR. *See* Polymerase chain reaction
PCR thermal cycler, 261
PD-1 protein, 539
Pea plant (*Pisum sativum*)
    artificial cross-fertilization of, 32, 33*f*
    incomplete dominance in, 110, 110*f*
    life cycle of, 32, 32*f*
    Mendel's research on, 31–38, 32*f*–35*f*, 36*t*,
        37*f*–38*f*, 38*t*, 40–43, 40*t*, 41*f*–43*f*,
        45–46, 45*f*
    mutations, 402, 404, 404*b*
    seed shape, transposition and, 431*b*–432*b*
    self-fertilization, 75
Pearson, Karl, 726
Pedigrees, **52**, 52*f*
Penetrance
    complete, **119**
    incomplete, 119, **120**, 120*f*
    variable penetrance of mitochondrial mutations,
        640, 641*f*
Penetrant, **120**
Peptide bond, **13**, 15*f*, **315**, 315*f*
Peptidyl site (P site), **318**
Pericentric inversion, **378**, 380*f*
Permissive condition, **512**
Petite phenotypes in *Saccharomyces cerevisiae*, 642,
    644, 644*f*
PEV. *See* Position effect variegation
Phages, **239**. *See also* Bacteriophage(s)
Pharmacogenetic screening, **354**
Phenotype(s), **4**
    application of binomial probability to progeny,
        48–49, 49*f*
    dominant, **35**
    genes producing variable, 118–122, 119*f*–121*f*,
        123*f*
    nonparental, 42
    parental, 42
    recessive, **35**
Phenotypic ratio, **36**
    in epistatic gene interactions, 129, 129*f*,
        130*b*–131*b*, 132–133
Phenotypic variance (V_P)
    defined, **707**
    partitioning, 707–708
    sources of, 708*f*
Phenotypic variation
    effects of environmental factors on, 702, 704, 704*f*

heritability measuring the genetic component of,
    708–713
    statistical description of, 706–707, 706*f*
Phenylketonuria (PKU), 121–122, 349–351, 351*f*
    Guthrie test, **350**
    living with, 350–351, 351*f*
PHO5 gene, 493–494, 493*f*
Phosphodiester bonds, 7, 9*f*, 277, 278*f*
Photolyase, 417
Photoproducts, **413**, 413*f*
Photoreactive repair, 415, **417**, 417*t*
Photosynthesis, chloroplasts as sites of, 648–651
Phylogenetic footprinting, 533, **615**, 616*f*
Phylogenetic shadowing, **615**, 617*f*
Phylogenetic species concept, **744**
Phylogenetic tree, **21**, 21–22, 21*f*–23*f*, 24*b*
    constructing using morphology and anatomy,
        22, 22*f*
    constructing using proteins or nucleic acids, 22,
        23*f*, 24*b*
Phylogenomics. *See* Evolutionary genomics
Physical gaps, **597**
Pigmentation, skin, 774
Pioneer factors, **480**, 480*f*, 492, 493*f*
PKU. *See* Phenylketonuria
Plant cells, cytokinesis in, 73–74, 73*f*
Plants
    cloning, 583–584
    development, 685–689, 686*f*–688*f*
    domestication of, 775–776
    lethal alleles, 116
    male sterility in, 651*b*–652*b*
    multicellular evolution in, 685–689
    reproduction in, 75
    transformation of genomes by *Agrobacterium*,
        570–571, 570*f*, 572*f*
    transgenic, 571, 572*f*, 573–574, 574*f*
Plaque formation, 211, 211*f*, 213
Plasmids
    in archaea, 203
    in bacterial cells, **189**, 191, 191*f*
    as cloning vectors, 559–560, 560*f*
    expression vectors, 565–566, 565*f*
    resistance (R), **191**
    Ti, 216, 570–571, 570*f*, 572*f*
    yeast, 570
Plasmodium, 585*b*
    apicoplast of, 657
    mitochondrial genome of, 646
Plastid, **648**
Pleiotropy, **122**, 123*f*
Pluripotent cells, **665**
PMS gene, 376–377
Pneumococcus, 237, 237*f*
Point mutations, **401**, 401*t*
Polar mutations, **448**
Poly-A tail, **294**
Polyacrylamide, **15**
Polyadenylate polymerase (PAP), 295
Polyadenylation
    of 3′ pre-mRNA, 295, 296*f*
    alternative, **301**
    mutations, 404–405
Polyadenylation signal sequence, **295**
Polycistronic mRNAs, **329**, 329*f*
    lac operon, **444**, 444–445
Polycomb group (PcG), 492, 494, 495*f*
Polydactyly, 120, 120*f*, 690*b*, 690*f*, 691, 691*b*
Polygenic inheritance, **697**
    of wheat kernel color controlled by two additive
        genes, 699, 699*f*
Polygenic traits, **696**
Polymerase chain reaction (PCR), 260, **261**
    in forensic genetic analysis, 780
    Huntington disease gene, 349, 350*f*

process, 261–262, 261*f*
    separation of PCR products, 262, 263*f*
Polypeptide(s), **13**, 15*f*, **315**
    alignment of DNA, mRNA, and polypeptide, 316*f*
    as amino acid chains that are assembled at
        ribosomes), 315–320
    elongation, 324, 324*t*, 325*f*, 327
    structure, 315–317, 317*t*
Polyploid species, 362
Polyploidy, **4**, **371**, 371–375
    allopolyploidy, **371**, 373, 373*f*
    autopolyploidy, **371**
    consequences of, 373–374
    evolution and, 374–375, 374*f*
    fruit size and, 373–374, 373*f*
Polyribosomes, **328**, 328*f*
Population-based carrier testing, 226–227
Population genetics, 20, 725–750, **726**
    Hardy-Weinberg equilibrium, 726–732, 728*f*,
        729*t*, 730*f*, 731*t*
Position effect variegation (PEV), **390**, 390–391, 391*f*
    mutations, 485–486, 485*f*, 496
Positional information, **665**, 666, 666*f*
Positive control of transcription, **441**, 441*f*
Positive-negative selection, **577**, 580*b*
Positive regulation of transcription, 478
Posttranscriptional processing, 294–307
Posttranslational polypeptide processing, **333**, 333–
    334, 334*f*
Postzygotic mechanisms of reproductive isolation,
    746, 746*t*
Potrykus, Ingo, 573
Prader-Willi syndrome, 371, 503*b*
Pre-mRNA splicing, 297–298
Precursor messenger RNA (pre-mRNA), 276, **294**
    alternative splicing, 301–302, 302*f*, 307*b*–308*b*,
        308*f*
    capping 5′, 294–295, 295*f*
    coupled transcription and processing, 298–299,
        300*f*
    polyadenylation of 3′, 295, 296*f*
Predictions, prospective and retrospective in human
    genetics, 53–54, 54*f*
Preimplantation genetic screening, **348**, 356–357
Preinitiation complex, **290**, **322**, 323*f*
Prenatal testing, 227, **348**, 354–357
Presymptomatic genetic testing, 227, **348**
Prezygotic mechanisms of reproductive isolation, **746**,
    746*t*
Pribnow box sequence, 281
Primary microRNA (primiRNA), 499, 501*f*
Primary structure, polypeptide, 316*f*, 317*t*
Primase, **253**
Primer annealing, step in PCR, 261, 261*f*
Primer extension, step in PCR, 261, 261*f*
Primer walking, **594**, 596*f*
Prior probability, **47**, **229**, 231
Probability
    Bayesian analysis, **229**, 230–231, 231*t*
    conditional, **229**, 230–231
    joint, **229**, 230–231
    prior, **47**, **229**, 231
Probability theory
    binomial probability, **48**, 48–49, 49*f*
    conditional probability, **47**
    predicts Mendelian ratios, 47–49
    product rule, **47**
    sum rule, **47**
Probability value (*P* value), **50**
Product rule, **47**
Proliferation of cancer cells, 540, 542
Prometaphase, **69**, 70*f*
Promoters, **12**, 12–13, 13*f*, **279**
    alternative, **301**
    archaeal, 292–293, 294*f*

bacterial, 280–281, 281*f*, 283
closed, **487**, 487*f*
eukaryotic
β-globin gene, 290, 292*f*
consensus sequences, 287*f*
detecting consensus elements, 290
RNA polymerase I, 292, 293*f*
RNA polymerase III, 292, 293*f*
techniques for finding, 288*b*–289*b*
mutations, 401*t*, **403**, 403*f*, 450
open, **486**, 486–487, 487*f*
Proofreading, DNA, **256**, 256–257, 257*f*
Prophage, **208**, 465
Prophase, **69**, 70*f*, 74*f*
Prophase I, 76–77, 78*f*–79*f*, 146
Prophase II, 79, 80*f*
Protein, reporter, 528
Protein folding, 333
Protein motifs, 605, 605*f*
Protein-protein interaction networks, 621, 623, 623*f*
Protein synthesis inhibition by antibiotic compounds, 340*b*, 340*t*
Proteins, **13**
in central dogma of biology, 11, 12*f*
control of translesion DNA synthesis and repair of double-strand breaks, 420–421
gel electrophoresis, 15–17, 17*f*
Proteome, **18, 621**
Proteomics, **18, 621**
Proto-oncogenes, **541**, 542
Prototroph, **125, 187**, 189*b*, 193–194, 193*f*
Prototrophic strains, **125, 187**
Proximal elements, 479
Prune-killer (K-pn) mutation, 514, 514*f*
Pseudoautosomal regions (PARs), **78**, 82*f*
Pseudodominance, **377**, 379*b*
Pseudogenes, **611**
Pseudohermaphroditism, 90*b*
Pulse-chase experiments, 277
Punnett, Reginald, 132, 149–150, 726
Punnett square, **36**, 36–37, 37*f*
Pure-breeding strains, **34**, 34*f*
Purines, 240–241, 240*f*, 276, 277*f*
Pyrimidines, 240–241, 240*f*, 276, 277*f*

Q
Q arm, **363**, 364*f*
QTL mapping, **713**
QTL mapping strategies, 714–715, 714*f*–715*f*, 715*t*
Quagga, 24*b*–25*b*
Quantitative genetics, **697**
Quantitative trait analysis, statistical nature of, 706–708
Quantitative trait loci (QTLs), **713**
genome-wide association studies, 717–718, 718*f*
identification of QTL genes, 716–717, 716*f*
Quantitative trait locus, **713**
Quantitative traits
allele segregation in production of, 701–702
defined, **697**
displaying continuous phenotype variation, 697–706
Quaternary structure, protein, **317**, 317*t*
Quinn, chip, 509
Quorum sensing, 439

R
R-group, **315**, 316*t*
R-loop, 298, 298*f*
R (resistance) plasmid, **191**
Radiation-induced DNA damage, 412–413, 413*f*
Raly gene, 118, 118*f*
Ramakrishnan, Venki, 320
Random mutation hypothesis, **400**, 401*f*
Random X inactivation, 370, 496–497, 497*f*

Random X inactivation hypothesis, **96**
Readers, chromatin, 489, 491*f*
Reading frame, **336**
Realizator genes, **675**
RecBCD pathway, **422**
Recent African origin (RAO) hypothesis, 759, 760*f*, 762
Recessive allele, **36**
Recessive epistasis (9:3:4 ratio), 129*f*, 131*b*, **133**
Recessive lethal allele, directional selection against, 734, 734*t*
Recessive mutations, identification of, 511, 511*f*, 512*f*, 513
Recessive phenotype, **35**
Recessiveness, molecular basis of, 106–107
Recipient, **191**
Reciprocal balanced translocation, **383**, 383–384, 384*f*–385*f*
Reciprocal crosses, **34**
Reciprocal translocation
balanced, **383**, 383–384, 384*f*–385*f*
in Burkitt's lymphoma, 544–545, 544*f*
in chronic myelogenous leukemia, 544, 544*f*
Reclinomonas americana, mitochondrial genome of, 646, 647*f*
Recombinant chromosomes, 146
Recombinant DNA molecule
amplifying, 560–561, 561*f*
creating, 557–559, 558*f*, 559*f*
defined, **557**
Recombinant DNA technology, 508, 516–519, 552–587
altering and synthesizing DNA molecules, advances in, 564–565
applications of, 552–587
cloning genes by complementation, 516–517, 517*f*
defined, **553**
DNA libraries, 562–564, 562*f*–564*f*
gene therapy, 579–583
molecular cloning in, 557–561, 558*f*–561*f*
restriction enzymes in, 553–557, 554*b*, 555*f*, 556*b*, 557*f*
transgenic organisms, creating, 565–579
Recombination, 145*f*. *See also* Crossing over
bacterial transformation, produced by, 203, 205
biological factors affecting, 164–165, 165*f*
crossing over and, 77
cytological evidence of, 153–154, 153*f*
evolution and, 146
genetic diversity generated by, 146
genetic linkage mapping, 155–156, 155*t*, 156*f*
homologous, **422**, 423*f*, 424, 424*f*, 519, 521, 521*f*, 522–524, **523**, 523*f*
illegitimate, **523**, 574, 576
intragenic, 213–214, 214*f*
in inversion heterozygotes, 381, 383
site-specific, 578–579, 578*f*
three-point recombination map, constructing, 158–161, 158*t*
Recombination coldspots, **165**, 165–166, 165*f*
Recombination frequency, **147**, 148–149, 149*f*
biological factors affecting, 164–165, 165*f*
genetic linkage mapping based on, 155–156, 156*f*
map units and, 156
physical distance between genes, relationship to, 162, 162*f*, 164
Recombination hotspots, **165**, 165–166, 165*f*
Recombination nodules, **77**, 81*f*
Recommended Uniform Screening Panel, 351–353, 352*t*
RECQ helicases, 269*b*–270*b*, 269*t*
Reduction division, 77*f*, 78
Reference genome sequence, **600**
Reference genomes, 599–600

Regulated transcription, **440**
Regulatory mutation, 401*t*, 402–405, **403**, 403*f*
lac operon, 447*t*, 448–451, 449*f*
Regulatory sequences
evolutionary loss or gain of, 766
molecular evolution in, 22
Reich, David, 26*b*
Relative fitness, **733**, 736*b*
Relaxosome, **194**
Release factor, **327**, 328*f*, 328*t*
Repair systems. *See* DNA damage repair
Repetitive DNA, 596–597, 597*f*, 606
dispersed, 606
Replica plating, **188**, 188*f*, 189*b*–190*b*
Replicate crosses, **34**
Replicated error, **407**, 407–408
Replication. *See also* DNA replication
bacteriophages, 205–206
of organellar genome, 635–636, 636*f*
plasmid, 191
rolling circle, **195**, 195*f*
Replication bubble, **247**, 247*f*, 250*f*, **254**, 254*f*
Replication forks, **247**, 247*f*, 248*f*, 250*f*
Replicative segregation, 635–**636**, 636, 637*f*
Replicative transposition, **425**
Replisome, **254**, 256
Reporter genes, **527**, 621
Repressible operons, **454**
Repressor protein(s), **441**, 442*f*
constitutive mutations of, 450
eukaryotic, 478–480
Lac, 444, 446*f*, 450–451, 451*f*, 454, 454*f*
phage λ, 468, 469
translation, 462
Reproduction
in animals, 75–76
asexual, 74–75
binary fission, 186
meiotic production of cells for, 74–82
in plants, 75
sexual, 74–75
in single-celled eukaryotes, 75
Reproductive isolation, **746**
mechanisms of, 746, 746*t*
speciation and, 746–747, 746*t*, 747*f*
Resequencing, 599–600
Response to selection, **712**
Restriction endonucleases. *See* Restriction enzymes
Restriction enzymes, **167**, 553–557, 554*b*, 555*f*, 556*b*, 557*f*
Restriction fragment length polymorphism (RFLP), **167**
Restriction fragments, **167**
Restriction map, 554*b*, **555**, 555*f*, 556*b*
Restriction-modification systems, **553**
Restrictive condition, **512**
Retinoblastoma, 545, 545*f*
hereditary, 545
sporadic, **545**
Retrotransposons, **425**, 430–431, 431*f*
Retroviruses, 12, 12*f*
Reverse genetic analysis, 508
Reverse genetics, **508**, 519–526
general strategy of, 508, 508*f*
genetic redundancy in flower development, 533*b*, 534*f*
genome editing, 519–522, 520*f*–521*f*
genomic approaches to, 623–624
homologous gene functions revealed by, 533*b*, 534*f*
homologous recombination, 522–524, 523*f*
insertion mutants, 524–525, 524*f*
in model genetic organisms, 522*t*
overview of, 519
RNA interference, 525, 525*f*
by TILLING, 525–526, 526*f*
Reverse mutation, **405**, 406*f*

Reverse mutation rate, **737**
Reverse transcriptase, 425, 430–431, **563**
Reverse transcription, **12,** 12*f,* 610–611, 611*f*
Reversion, **405,** 406*f*
Reversion mutation, **336,** 414
Reversion rate, **737**
Reversions, **214**
Revertible mutants, **214,** 215*f*
RFLP (restriction fragment length polymorphism), **167**
Rho-dependent termination, **285,** 286*f*
Rho protein, **285,** 286*f*
Ribonucleic acid. *See* RNA
Ribonucleotides, **276,** 276–277, 277*f*
Ribose, **277**
Ribosomal proteins, 319, 319*b*
Ribosomal RNA (rRNA), 5, **11,** 11–12, 276, 278, **279,** 279*t*
Ribosomal RNA processing, 304, 305*f*
Ribosomes, **6,** 314*f*
    endoplasmic reticulum-bound, 334, 335*f*
    polypeptides assembled at, 315–320
    structure, 317–319, 318*f,* 320*f*
    three-dimensional view of, 319–320, 320*f*
    in translation, 13, 15*f*
Riboswitch, **462**
    control of mRNA stability, 464
    regulation of transcription, 462–463, 463*f*
    regulation of translation, 463–464, 464*f*
Rice, golden, 573–574, 574*f*
Richmond, Timothy, 388
Riggs, Arthur, 247–248
RISC (RNA-induced silencing complex), **499,** 500, 500*f*–501*f*
RITS (RNA-induced transcriptional silencing) complex, 501*f,* **502**
RNA, **6.** *See also* Transfer RNA (tRNA)
    antisense, **462,** 462*f*
    categories of, 278–279, 279*t*
    in central dogma of biology, 11, 12*f*
    gel electrophoresis, 15–17, 17*f*
    guideRNA (gRNA), **307,** 307*f,* **520,** 521–522, 521*f,* 585*b,* 587*b*
    long noncoding RNAs (lncRNAs), **496**
    microRNA (miRNA), 12, 12*f,* **279,** 279*t,* **499,** 501*f*–501*f,* 550
    ribosomal RNA (rRNA), 5, **11,** 11–12, 276, 278, **279,** 279*t*
    small interfering RNA (siRNA), **279,** 279*t,* **499,** 500*f,* 502
    small nuclear RNA (snRNA), **279,** 279*t*
    stains, 16–17, 17*f*
    structure, 276–277, 277*f*
    telomerase, **279,** 279*t*
    tracrRNA, **520,** 520*f*
RNA editing, **307,** 307*f*
    chloroplast mRNA, 650–651, 651*f*
RNA-induced silencing complex (RISC), **499,** 500, 500*f*–501*f*
RNA-induced transcriptional silencing (RITS) complex, 501*f,* **502**
RNA interference (RNAi), **499,** 499–502, 500*f*–501*f*
    evolution and applications of, 502
    in gene activity, 525
    reverse genetics using, 525, 525*f*
RNA-mediated mechanisms of gene expression control, 498–502
    constitutive heterochromatin maintenance, 501–502
    evolution and applications of RNAi, 502
    gene silencing by double-stranded RNA, 499–501, 500*f*–501*f*
RNA polymerase, 12–13, **277**
    bacterial, 280, 280*f*
    eukaryote, 286–287
RNA polymerase core, **280,** 280*f*

RNA polymerase I (RNA Pol I), **287**
RNA polymerase I promoters, 292, 293*f*
RNA polymerase II (RNA Pol II), **287,** 481
    promoter recognition, 289–290
RNA polymerase III (RNA Pol III), **287**
RNA polymerase III promoters, 292, 293*f*
RNA primer, **253**
RNA primer removal, 254–255, 255*f*
RNA processing
    posttranscriptional, 294–307
    ribosomal RNA, 304, 305*f*
    transfer RNA, 304–307, 305*f*
RNA synthesis, 277, 278*f*
RNA transcripts, carrying the messages of genes, 276–279
RNAi. *See* RNA interference
RNase, 296, 301
Roberts, Richard, 298
Robertsonian translocation, **383,** 384, 384*f*
Rolling circle replication, **195,** 195*f*
Rothmund-Thompson syndrome, 270*b*
Rowley, Janet, 544
rpoH gene, 461, 461*f*
rRNA. *See* Ribosomal RNA (rRNA)
Rs or rsid number, **358**
Rubin, Gerald, 574–575
Russell-Silver syndrome, 498
Rut site, **285,** 286*f*
Rutter, Michael, 718*b*

S

S-phase checkpoint, 75*f*
S phase (synthesis phase) of interphase, **69,** 69*f,* 74, 74*f,* 75*f,* 76, 248–249, 252
Saccharomyces cerevisiae. See also Yeast
    biparental inheritance in, 641–642, 644, 644*f*
    genome comparisons, 608, 609*f*
    mutants to categorize genes, 624–625
    transcriptome analysis, 621, 622*f*
    use in forward genetic screens, 510
Salmon, transgenic, 575, 576*f*
Salmonella typhimurium, in Ames test, 413–415, 414*f*–415*f,* 416*b*
Same sense resolution, **424,** 424*f*
Sanger, Frederick, 261, 263
Sanger sequencing, 263
Saturation mutagenesis, **510**
Scaffold, **596**
Scaffold proteins, **389**
Scanning, **322**
Schizosaccharomyces pombe, 501–502
Schleiden, Matthias, 2
Schwann, Theodor, 2
Scientific method, steps in, 33
Screening test, 356
SDSA (synthesis-dependent strand annealing), **421,** 421*f*
Second-degree relationships, **787**
Second filial generation (F$_2$ generation), **34,** 34*f*
Second-site reversion, **405,** 406*f*
Secondary endosymbiotic events, **656,** 657
Secondary structure, polypeptide, **317,** 317*t*
Segment polarity genes, **668,** 668*f,* 669
Segregation
    of alleles, 35*f,* 36–37
    of the homologous chromosomes, 76
    law of, 37
Selander, Robert, 741
Selected marker screen, **209**
Selection
    artificial, 712–713, 712*t,* 713*f*
    directional, **713,** 733–735, 734*t,* 735*f*
    disruptive, **713**
    mutation-selection balance, 737
    response to, 712
    stabilizing, **713**

Selection coefficient, **733**
Selection differential, **712,** 713
Selective growth medium, **197**
Selective sweep, **772,** 773*f*
Self-fertilization, **32,** 32*f,* 75
    genotype frequency and, 741, 741*t*
    reproduction in, 75–76
Self-splicing introns, 302, 304, 304*f*
Self-splicing processes, 297
Semiconservative DNA replication, **9,** 11*f,* **245**
Separase, 73, 73*f*
Sequence gaps, **597**
Sequencing
    high-throughput, 619
    transcriptome analysis by, 619
Serial founder effect, 763
Sex, recombination frequency and, 164–165, 165*f*
Sex chromosome(s), 4, **52, 68**
    pseudoautosomal regions (PARs), 78, 82*f*
    sex determination and, 87, 89, 91
Sex chromosome aneuploidy, 369*t*
Sex chromosome monosomy, 225
Sex chromosome trisomies, 225
Sex determination, **87**
    diversity of, 89, 91, 91*f*
    in *Drosophila,* 87, 89, 307*b*–308*b,* 308*f*
    in fruit flies, 275*f*
    mammalian, 89, 89*f*
    molecular basis of, 275*f*
Sex-influenced traits, **119,** 119–120, 119*f*
Sex-limited traits, **119**
Sex-linked genes, and expression equalization by dosage compensation, 96–97
Sex-linked inheritance, **85**
Sex-linked transmission, human, 91–93, 92*t,* 93*f*–94*f,* 95*b*
Sexual reproduction, meiotic production of cells for, 74–82
Shared derived characteristics, **21**
Sharp, Phillip, 298
Shelterin, **259**
Shimomura, Osamu, 532
Shine, John, 322
Shine-Dalgarno sequence, **322,** 322*f,* 323, 329, 448, 462–464, 646
Short arm, **363,** 364*f*
Short tandem repeats (STRs), 778*f,* 780–784, 781*t,* 782*f*–783*f,* 784*t*
Shotgun sequencing, **594.** *See also* Whole-genome shotgun sequencing
Shuttle vector, **570**
Sickle cell disease (SCD), 16, **750***b,* 750*b*–751*b,* 751*f*
    carrier testing, 353
    evolutionary analysis, 175
    genetic therapy for mice with, 581–582, 582*f*
    pleiotropy in, 122, 123*f*
Sigma subunit (σ), **280,** 280*f,* 284, 284*t*
Signal hypothesis, **334,** 335*f*
Signal sequence, 298, **334**
Signal transduction pathways, 124
Signaling systems, DNA damage, 419–420
Silencer sequences (silencers), **291, 479,** 480, 480*f*
Silent mutation, 401*t,* **402,** 402*f*
SINE (short interspersed nuclear elements), 430–431
Singh, Nadia, 166
Single-celled eukaryotes, reproduction in, 75
Single crossover, 523, 523*f*
Single-crossover event, 157–158, 157*f*
Single nucleotide polymorphism (SNP), **167,** 167*f,* 786–788
    association with a disease, 357–358
    differentiating the human and chimpanzee genomes, 766
    quantitative trait loci and, 713–714
    variation in humans, 760–761

Single-stranded binding protein, 253
Sister chromatid cohesion, 73, 73*f*
Sister chromatids, 69, 71, 72–73, 74, 76, 79
    separation in anaphase, 73
Site-specific recombination, 578, 578–579, 578*f*
Skin microbiome, 601*b*–602*b*
Skin pigmentation, 698, 774
Sliding clamp, 255, 256, 256*f*
Small interfering RNA (siRNA), 279, 279*t*, 499, 500*f*,
    502
Small nuclear ribonucleoproteins (snRNPs), 298
Small nuclear RNA (snRNA), 279, 279*t*
Small ribosomal subunit, 318
Smith, Hamilton, 554*b*
Smithies, Oliver, 576
SNP. *See* Single nucleotide polymorphism
Solenoid structure, 387*f*, 389
Somatic cells, division of, 68–74
Somatic gene therapy, 579, 579–583
Somatic mutations, 401
Sonic hedgehog (SHH), 480–481, 480*f*, 690*b*–691*b*,
    690*f*
SOS system, 420
Southern, Edwin, 17
Southern blotting, 17
Specialized transducing phage, 211
Specialized transduction, 211
Speciation
    allopatric, 746–747, 747*f*
    Galapagos finches, 748
    processes of, 744–746
    reproductive isolation and, 746–747,
        746*t*, 747*f*
    sympatric, 747
Spina bifida, 228
Spindle fiber microtubules, 72
Spliceosome, 297, 298, 299*f*
Splicing
    alternative, 301–302, 301*f*
    cryptic, 404, 405*f*
    pre-mRNA, 297–298
Splicing mutations, 403–404, 403*f*, 404, 404*b*
Splicing signal sequences, 298
Sporadic cancer cases, 543
Sporadic retinoblastoma, 545
Spradling, Allan, 574–575
Square root method, 730, 730–731
SRY (sex-determining region of Y), 89, 89*f*, 90*b*,
    98*b*, 98*f*
Stabilizing selection, 713
Stahl, Franklin, 245–247, 246*f*
Stains, 16–17, 16*f*
Standard deviation, 707
Start codon, 13, 15*f*
Start of transcription, 13, 13*f*
Statistically significant, 50
Steitz, Thomas, 320
Stem-loop structure, 285, 285*f*
Stern, Curt, 153, 155
Stevens, Nettie, 85
Sticky ends, 554, 554*b*
Stop codon, 13, 15*f*
Strand invasion, 421, 423*f*
Strand polarity, 8
Strand slippage, 405, 405–406, 408*f*
Streisinger, George, 405
Stress response genes, regulation of, 459–461, 461*f*,
    469*b*–470*b*
STRs. *See* Short tandem repeats
Structural annotation
    computational approaches to, 602–603
    experimental approaches to, 602, 603*f*
Structural genomics, 594–501
    defined, 594
    human genome and, 599

metagenomics, 600–602
reference genomes and resequencing, 599–600
whole-genome shotgun sequencing, 595, 596–
    599, 598*f*–599*f*
Sturtevant, Alfred, 145–146, 155, 164, 514, 664
Su(var) mutations, 485, 485*f*
Subcloning, 555
Subfunctionalization, 612, 612*f*, 613
Submetacentric chromosome, 363
Sugar-phosphate backbone, 241, 242*f*
Sulston, John, 679, 682
Sum rule, 47
Supercoiling, 257, 258*f*
Supplemented minimal medium, 187
Suppressor mutations, 405
Suppressor screen, 514
Sutton, Walter, 2–3, 80, 83, 236
SV40 genome map, 554*b*
SWI/SNF complex, 488, 489*f*
SWR1 complex, 488, 489*f*
Sympatric speciation, 747
Synapsis, 76, 77
Synaptomorphies, 21
Synaptonemal complex, 76, 77, 81*f*
Syncytial blastoderm, 667
Syncytium, 667
Synonymous codons, 329, 329–330
Synonymous mutation, 401*t*, 402, 402*f*
Syntenic genes, 146, 146–148
Synteny, 617, 617*f*
Synthesis-dependent strand annealing (SDSA), 421,
    421*f*
Synthetic enhancement, 514, 514*f*, 515
Synthetic lethality, 514, 514*f*, 515, 625, 626*f*
Systems biology, 18, 18–19, 626
Szostak, Jack, 259

T

T cells, 539, 550
T-DNA, 524–525, 524*f*, 533*b*, 534*f*
T loop, 259
T (transfer) strand, 194
Taq polymerase, 261–262
Targeted induced local lesions in genomes (TILLING),
    526, 526*f*
TATA-binding protein (TBP), 290
TATA box, 287
Tatum, Edward, 124–125, 125*b*, 193–194, 193*f*, 196,
    314
Tay-Sachs disease, 227, 353
TBP-associated factor (TAF), 290
TDF (testis-determining factor), 89
Telocentric chromosome, 364
Telomerase, 258, 259, 260*f*
Telomerase RNA, 279, 279*t*
Telomeres, 258, 259, 260*f*
Telophase, 69, 71*f*, 73, 74*f*, 75*f*
Telophase I, 76, 78, 79*f*
Telophase II, 79, 80*f*
Temperate bacteriophages, 207
Temperature-sensitive allele, 114, 116
Template strand, 12, 12*f*, 13*f*, 15*f*, 242*f*, 279
Tenebrio molitor, 85
Teosinte, 775–776, 775*f*, 776*f*
Terminal deletion, chromosome, 375, 375*f*
Terminal inverted repeats, 425, 425*f*
Termination
    of transcription, in bacteria, 284–285, 285*f*, 286*f*
    translation, 327, 328*f*
Termination region, 280
Termination sequence, 13, 13*f*
Termination stem loop, 456, 456–459, 457*f*
TERT (telomerase reverse transcriptase) gene, 259
Tertiary endosymbiotic events, 656, 657
Tertiary structure, polypeptide, 317, 317*t*

Test-cross(es), 34
    autosomal genetic linkage detection through,
        150–153, 152*f*
    two-point test-cross analysis, 150
Test-cross analysis
    hypothesis testing by, 37, 37*f*, 387*t*
    testing independent assortment, 43, 43*f*, 45
    testing segregation, 37, 37*f*, 387*t*
Testosterone, 90*b*
Tetrahymena, 259, 302
TGS (third-generation sequencing), 266
Thalassemia, 482
Thermus aquaticus, 262
θ value (theta value), 169, 170–171, 170*f*, 170*t*, 171*b*,
    172*b*
Thiamin pyrophosphate (TPP), 462–464, 463*f*
Third-base wobble, 305, 330, 331, 331*f*, 331*t*
Third-degree relationships, 787
Third filial generation (F₃ generation), 34, 34*f*
Third-generation sequencing (TGS), 266
Thornton, Joseph, 749–750
Three-point recombination map, 158–161, 158*t*
Three-point test-cross analysis, 156, 156–164
Threshold traits, 704, 704–706, 704*f*–705*f*
Thymine (T), 7, 240–241
Thymine dimer, 413, 413*f*
Ti plasmid, 216, 570, 570–571, 570*f*, 572*f*
Time-of-entry mapping, 198, 200*f*
Tishkoff, Sarah, 772
TLF (*TBP*-like factor), 290
Tn10, 427, 427*f*
Tobacco, corolla length in, 701–702, 702*f*
Tomato, QTL mapping in, 715, 715*f*
Torpedo model of transcription termination, 296, 297*f*
Tortoiseshell coat-color patterning, 96
Totipotent cells, 571, 665
Toxins, *Vibrio cholerae*, 469*b*–470*b*
TP53 protein/gene, 546–547, 549
tracrRNA, 520, 520*f*
Trans-acting, 450
Trans-acting regulatory proteins, 479
Transcription, 3–4, 6. *See also* Bacterial transcription
    alternative patterns, 301–302
    archaeal, 292–293
    bacteriophage λ, 465–466
    basal, 445
    of chloroplast genes, 649
    chromatin structure and, 390–391
    constitutive, 440
    couple with pre-mRNA processing, 298–299,
        300*f*
    coupled with translation, 328, 328*f*
    eukaryotic
        chromatin remodeling regulating, 484–498
        cis-acting regulatory sequences, 478–484,
            479*f*
        overview of regulatory interactions,
            479–480
        yeast model, 479*f*, 482–484, 483*f*–484*f*,
            493–494, 493*f*
    evolutionary implications of comparative tran-
        scription, 293–294
    gene structure and, 12–13, 13*f*
    mitochondrial, 646, 648*f*
    molecular biology of, 275–308
    negative control of, 441, 441*f*, 442*f*, 478
    of open and covered promoters, 486–487, 487*f*
    overview of, 12–13, 12*f*, 15*f*
    positive control of, 441, 441*f*, 442*f*, 478
    regulated, 440
    regulation in bacteria and bacteriophage
        attenuation, 456–459, 457*f*, 459*f*, 460*b*
        bacteriophage λ, 465–468, 467*f*–468*f*
        DNA-binding proteins and, 441–443, 442*f*
        lac operon, 443–454

negative control, 441, 441*f*
positive control, 441, 442*f*, 469*b*–470*b*
riboswitch, 462–463, 463*f*
stress response genes, 459–461, 461*f*, 469*b*–470*b*
trp operon, 454–459
Transcription factors, 287, **289**, 289–290, 290*f*, 478
Transcription termination, torpedo model of, 296, 297*f*
Transcriptional fusion, 528, 528*f*
Transcriptome, **18, 619**
Transcriptomics, **18, 619**, 620*f*, 621
Transductant, **205**, 209
Transduction, 205
  cotransduction, **209**, 209, 209–211
  definition, 191, 193
  generalized, **208**
  specialized, 211
Transfer DNA (T-DNA), **570**, 570–571, 570*f*, 572*f*
Transfer RNA (tRNA), **11**, 11–12, 13, 15*f*, 276, 278, **279**, 279*t*
  charged, **320**
  charging tRNA molecules, 333, 333*f*
  chloroplast, 649
  initiator, **320**, 321*f*
  isoaccepting, **330**, 330*f*
  structure, 306*f*
  uncharged, **320**
Transfer RNA (tRNA) genes, mitochondrial, 646–648
Transfer RNA processing, 304–307, 305*f*
Transformant, **205**
Transformation
  bacterial, **191**, 192*f*, 203, 205, 206*f*
  definition, 191
  for introducing recombinant DNA molecules, 560, 561*f*
  mapping by, 205
  P element-mediated transformation in *Drosophila*, 575*f*
  of plant genomes by *Agrobacterium*, 570–571, 570*f*, 572*f*
  steps in, 205
Transformation factor
  DNA as, 238, 238*f*
  Griffith's experiments, 236–238, 237*f*
Transgenes, **516**, 527–533, **565**
  chimeric genes, 532–533
  enhancer trapping and, 531, 531*f*
  reporter genes, 528–531, 529*f*–530*f*
Transgenic animals, 574–578, 576*f*, 577*f*
Transgenic organism, **516**, 550–551
  creating, 565–579
  defined, **565**
  expression of heterologous genes in bacterial and fungal hosts, 565–570
  manipulation of DNA sequences in vivo, 578–579
Transgenic plants, 571, 572*f*, 573–574, 574*f*
Transition mutations, **401**, 402
Translation, 3–4, **6**
  antibiotic interference with, 340*b*, 340*t*
  chloroplast, 649–650
  coupled with transcription, 328, 328*f*
  genetic code and, 329–338
  mitochondrial, 646–648
  molecular biology of, 314–340
  nick, **417**
  overview of, 13, 15*f*, 316*f*
  phases, 320–327, 321
    elongation, 324, 324*t*, 325*f*, 327
    initiation, 320–324
    termination, 327, 328*f*
  of polycistronic mRNA, 329, 329*f*
  riboswitch regulation of, 463–464, 464*f*
  speed and efficiency of, 327–329
Translation complex, 327–328

Translation repressor proteins, **462**
Translational regulation in bacteria, 461–462, 463–464, 463*f*
Translesion DNA polymerase, **420**
Translesion DNA synthesis, **420**
Translocation, chromosome, 153, **378**, 383–384, 384*f*–385*f*
  reciprocal balanced, **383**, 383–384, 384*f*–385*f*
  Robertsonian, **383**, 384, 384*f*
  unbalanced, **383**, 384*f*
Translocation heterozygotes, **383**
Transmission genetics, **6, 30,** 30–66
Transposable elements
  in bacterial genomes, 426–427
  characteristics and classification of, 425
  in eukaryotic genomes, 427
  RNAi evolution and, 502
Transposable genetic elements, 18, **425**, 425–431. *See also* Transposons
  discovery of Ds and Ac elements, 427–429
  insertion sequences, 426–427, 428*b*
Transposase, **425**
Transposition, **425**
  Mendel's peas and, 431*b*–432*b*
  mutagenic effect of, 426
  nonreplicative, **425**
  replicative, **425**
Transposons
  composite, **427**, 427*f*
  derivation of exons from, 611, 611*f*
  DNA, **425**, 425–427, 425*f*, 429–431
  general structure, 425, 425*f*
  insertion of, 425, 426*f*
  noncomposite, **427**
  P elements, 429–430, 430*f*, 574–575, 575*f*
  retrotransposons, **425**, 430–431, 431*f*
Transversion mutations, **401–402**
Tree of life, **608**, 609*f*, 656
Trihybrid cross, **45**
Trihybrid-cross analysis, 45–46, 45*f*
Trinucleotide repeat expansion disorders, **406**, 408*t*
Trinucleotide repeat expansions, 348–349
Trisomic, **366**, 369*f*
Trisomy, 356, 369
Trisomy 18, 228
Trisomy 21, 225–226, 227, 228, 356, 369–370, 369*t*, 370*t*, 372*b*
Trisomy rescue, 371
Trithorax group (TrxG) genes, 492, 494, 495*f*
tRNA. *See* Transfer RNA (tRNA)
tRNA synthetases, **333**, 333*f*
trp (tryptophan) operon, 210–211, 210*f*, 210*t*, 454–459
  attenuation of, 456–459, 457*f*, 460*b*
  feedback inhibition of, 455–456, 456*f*
  structure, 455, 455*f*
True-breeding strains, **34**
True reversion, **405**, 406*f*
Tryptophan. *See trp* (tryptophan) operon
Tschermak, Erich von, 3
Tsien, Roger Y., 530
Tsui, Lap-Chee, 175*b*–176*b*
Tumor suppressor genes, **542**
Tumors
  benign, **541**
  defined, **541**
  malignant, **541**
Turner syndrome, 369*t*, 370
Twin studies, heritability and, 710–712, 711*t*, 712*t*
Twitch (film), 347–348
Two-dimensional gel electrophoresis, 319*b*
Two-hit hypothesis, **545**
Two-hybrid system, **621**, 623, 623*f*
Two-point test-cross analysis, **150**
Ty retrotransposons of yeast, 431
Tyrosinase, 114, 116

U
UAS (upstream activator sequence), **483**, 483*f*–484*f*, 484
Ultrabithorax gene, 494, 674–676, 674*f*, 675*f*, 676*f*
Ultrasound, prenatal, 356
Ultraviolet (UV) irradiation
  DNA damage from, 412–413, 413*f*
  repair of DNA damage from, 415, 417
Ultraviolet (UV) repair, **417**
Unbalanced translocation, **383**, 384*f*
Uncharged tRNAs, **320**
Unequal crossover, **376**, 376–377, 376*f*
Unger, Franz, 31
Uniparental disomy, 371
Uniparental inheritance, 633
Unpaired loop, **377**, 377*f*
Unselected marker screen, **209**
Upstream, 279
Upstream activator sequence (UAS), **483**, 483*f*–484*f*, 484
Upstream control element, **292**
Uracil (U), **12, 276**
UTRs
  3′ untranslated region (3′ UTR), 281, 281*f*, **316**
  5′ untranslated region (5′ UTR), 281, 281*f*, **316**

V
Van Goethe, Johann Wolfgang, 664
Variable expressivity, **120**, 120–121, 121*f*
Variable number tandem repeats (VNTRs), **167**, 167*f*, 262, 263*f*, 780
Variance, **707**
  additive, **708**
  dominance, **708**
  environmental, 704, 707, **708**
  genetic, **707**, 708
  interactive, **708**
  phenotypic, **707**, 707–708, 708*f*
Variation
  continuous, **697**
  discontinuous, **697**
Vector, **557**
  eukaryotic expression, 566
  expression, 565–566, 565*f*
  nonrecombinant, **558**
  plasmids as cloning, 559–560, 560*f*
  shuttle, **570**
Venter, J. Craig, 599, 759
Vertebrate steroid receptor evolution, 749–750
Vertebrates, transgenic, 575–578, 576*f*, 577*f*
Vibrio cholerae toxins, 469*b*–470*b*
Virchow, Rudolph, 2
Virus. *See also* Bacteriophage(s)
  retroviruses, 12, 12*f*
VNTRs. *See* Variable number tandem repeats
Volkin, Elliot, 277
Volvox, 663*f*
von Ettinghausen, Andreas, 31
von Tschermak, Erich, 46
Vulval precursor cells (VPCs), 679–682, 679*f*–681*f*

W
Waardenburg syndrome, 120–121, 121*f*
Wacey, David, 19
WAGR syndrome, 375–376
WAGRO syndrome, 375–376
Wallace, Alfred, 19
Warnecke, Falk, 627*b*
Watson, James, 4, 6–7, 8*f*, 9, 240, 241, 245
Weinberg, Robert, 542
Weinberg, Wilhelm, 726–727
Weismann, August, 2
Wells, Robert, 243
Werner syndrome, 270*b*

Western blotting, **17**
Wheat, evolution of modern, 374–375, 374*f*
Whole-genome duplication, 618, 618*f*
Whole-genome shotgun (WGS) sequencing
    of a bacterial genome, 597–598, 598*f*
    defined, **595**
    of a eukaryotic genome, 598–599, 599*f*
    repetitive DNA problem, 596–597, 597*f*
Wieschaus, Eric, 511, 666–668
Wild type, **83,** 107
Wilkens, Horst, 710
Wilkins, Maurice, 4, 6–7
Williams-Beuren syndrome, 376–377, 376*f*
Wilson, Allan, 24*b*–25*b*, 762
Wilson, Edmund Beecher, 2, 236
Woese, Carl, 5
Wolbachia, 216
Wolffian ducts, 89, 89*f,* 90*b*
Wollman, Ellie, 198
Wright, Sewall, 20–21
Writers, chromatin, 489, 491*f*

X

X/A ratio, **89**
X/autosome ratio, **89**
X chromosome(s), 67
    absence of Neandertal DNA from human, 768
    inactivation, 96–97, 97*f,* 370
    nondisjunction, 87, 87*f*
    pseudoautosomal regions (PARs), 78, 82*f*
    X-ray induced mutations, 382*b*–383*b*

X chromosome monosomy, 369*t,* 370
X-gal, 528
X inactivation, 96–97, 97*f,* 370
X-inactivation center (XIC), 496, 497*f*
X-inactivation-specific transcript *(XIST),* 97, 496–497, 497*f*
X-linked genes
    genetic linkage mapping, 155–156, 155*t,* 156*f*
    genetic linkage of, 150, 151*f*
X-linked inheritance, **85,** 85–86, 85*f*–86*f,* 88
    dominant, **91,** 92*t,* 93, 94*f*
    recessive, **91,** 91–93, 92*t,* 93*f*–94*f,* 95*b*
X-ray diffraction, 6–7, 7*f,* 235*f*
X-Y shared genes, 98
Xeroderma pigmentosum, 136*b*–137*b,* 137*f,* 418

Y

Y chromosome(s), 67
    degenerative evolution of the mammalian, 97*b*–98*b,* 98*f*
    forensic genetic analysis use of, 785
    phylogeny, 762–763
    pseudoautosomal regions (PARs), 78, 82*f*
Y chromosome short tandem repeats (Y-STR), 762–763
Y-linked inheritance, **92,** 93
Y-STR (Y chromosome short tandem repeats), 762–763
Yamanaka, Shinya, 581
Yamanaka factors, 581
Yamnaya, 771, 772, 774

Yanofsky, Charles, 210–211, 210*f,* 210*t*
Yeast, 75. *See also Saccharomyces cerevisiae*
    autonomously replicating sequences, 250, 252*f*
    biparental inheritance in, 641–642, 644, 644*f*
    cloning genes by complementation, 516–517, 517*f*
    conditional lethal allele in, 512–513, 513*f*
    constitutive heterochromatin maintenance, 501–502
    homologous recombination in, 523–524
    inducible transcriptional regulation in *S. cerevisiae,* 493–494, 493*f*
    mutants to categorize genes, 624–625
    recombination hotspots in, 165–166, 165*f*
    synthetic genome, 564
    transcriptional regulation in, 479*f,* 482–484, 483*f*–484*f*
    transcriptome analysis, 621, 622*f*
    Ty elements of, 431
Yeast plasmids, 570
Yonath, Ada, 320
Yule, George Udny, 726

Z

Z-form DNA, 243, 243*t*
Z/W system, **91,** 91*f*
Zebra, 24*b*–25*b*
Z_{max}, **170,** 170*t,* 171, 171*b,* 172*b*
Zone of polarizing activity (ZPA), **683**
Zygotene, 76, 78*f*
Zygotic genes, **669**

Model Organisms

Life Cycle	E. coli	A. thaliana (mouse ear cress)	S. cerevisiae (baker's yeast)	C. elegans (nematode)
m, meiosis; f, fertilization				
Generation time	20–40 minutes	10 weeks	2–3 hours	3 days

Genome	E. coli	A. thaliana (mouse ear cress)	S. cerevisiae (baker's yeast)	C. elegans (nematode)
Size	4.64 Mb	136 Mb	12.2 Mb	103 Mb
Chromosomes	1 circular chromosome + plasmids	5 chromosomes ($2n = 10$)	16 chromosomes ($2n = 32$)	5 autosomes + X chromosome ($2n = 10 + XX$ or $X0$)
Number of protein-coding genes (estimate)	4262	27,352	6728	20,452
Genetic distance	100 minutes	600 cM	4500 cM	300 cM

Nomenclature	E. coli	A. thaliana (mouse ear cress)	S. cerevisiae (baker's yeast)	C. elegans (nematode)
Wild-type allele	lacZ+	PHB	CDC28	dpy-10
Mutant allele	lacZ	phb	cdc28	dpy-10(allele#)
Allele designation style	Superscript	Hyphenated number	Hyphenated number	Parenthetical
Specific mutant allele	$lacZ^3$	phb-6	cdc28-3	dpy-10(e128)
Dominant mutant allele		phb-1d		
Protein product	LacZ	PHB	CDC28p	DPY-10
Gene name style	Genes are usually named based on their presumed wild-type function. They are three letters, sometimes followed by a fourth letter for genes with similar functions.	Genes are usually named based on the mutant phenotype. They are three letters, sometimes followed by a number for genes with similar mutant phenotypes.	Genes are usually named based on their presumed wild-type function. They are three letters, sometimes followed by numbers for genes with similar mutant phenotypes.	Genes are usually named based on the mutant phenotype. They are three letters, sometimes followed by a hyphen and number for genes with similar mutant phenotypes.

Website	E. coli	A. thaliana (mouse ear cress)	S. cerevisiae (baker's yeast)	C. elegans (nematode)
	www.ecolicommunity.org	www.arabidopsis.org	www.yeastgenome.org	www.wormbase.org